MACNAB'S

BACKACHE

Third Edition

MACNAB'S

BACKACHE

Third Edition

John McCulloch, M.D., F.R.C.S.C.
Professor of Orthopaedics
Northeastern Ohio Universities
College of Medicine
Rootstown, Ohio

Ensor Transfeldt, M.D., B.Ch., F.R.C.S.C.
Associate Professor, Department of Orthopaedic Surgery
University of Minnesota
Twin Cities Scoliosis Spine Center
Minneapolis, Minnesota

SANS TACHE

Williams & Wilkins
A WAVERLY COMPANY

BALTIMORE • PHILADELPHIA • LONDON • PARIS • BANGKOK
HONG KONG • MUNICH • SYDNEY • TOKYO • WROCLAW

Editor: Darlene Barela Cooke
Managing Editor: Frances M. Klass
Production Coordinator: Danielle Santucci
Copy Editor: Arlene Sheir-Allen
Designer: Nancy Hagan Abbott
Cover Designer: Nancy Hagan Abbott
Typesetter: Graphic Sciences Corporation
Printer: RR Donnelley & Sons Company
Digitized Illustrations: Trinity Graphics
Binder: RR Donnelley & Sons Company

351 West Camden Street
Baltimore, Maryland 21201-2436 USA

Rose Tree Corporate Center
1400 North Providence Road
Building II, Suite 5025
Media, Pennsylvania 19063-2043 USA

Accurate indications, adverse reactions and dosage schedules for drugs are provided in this book, but it is possible that they may change. The reader is urged to review the package information data of the manufacturers of the medications mentioned.

Printed in the United States of America

First Edition, 1977

Library of Congress Cataloging-in-Publication Data

98 99
2 3 4 5 6 7 8 9 10

To Gillian and Ian

Dedication

This textbook is dedicated to the memory of:

The late Ian Macnab, M.B., ChB., F.R.C.S.
Former Chief, Division of Orthopaedic Surgery
The Wellesly Hospital
Former Emeritus Professor of Surgery
University of Toronto
Toronto, Ontario, Canada

Preface to the Third Edition

It is now 20 years since Dr. Macnab sat down in his study to write the first edition of *Backache.* And he did it in one weekend! Originally published as a soft cover primer by the Workmen's Compensation Board of Ontario, this text was so good that Williams & Wilkins published it in hardcover in 1977.

Dr. Macnab was one of a handful of spine specialists in North America at the time. He was a brilliant researcher and teacher; but his greatest quality was his command of the written and spoken word. With one sentence (or even a word) he could bring a resident or fellow up short (orthopedic rounds in Toronto at that time showed no mercy for the unprepared resident!). He sometimes needed to bring his staff members back to reality, but we watched him do that with a few sentences and a gentleness that allowed for a soft landing. We had no trouble accepting that the first edition of *Backache* was written in a weekend, because we had watched the master at work over many years.

What we had trouble with, in trying to triplicate Ian's effort, was to produce the third edition of *Backache* in less than a year! Two matters urged us on. First, *Backache* has enjoyed a reasonable amount of success as a primer on back pain. Second, after we, as residents and fellows, watched and experienced Dr. Macnab and worked with him as members of the University of Toronto Medical School Staff, we lived in even more awe of his prowess as a thinker, researcher, and writer on issues of spinal pain. All the while, as members of the "Macnab Club," we each became a special friend of Ian and his lovely wife Rita. Now that he is gone, we wish to see his ideas continue to be popularized through his students. This has led to the publication of the third edition of *Backache,* which is now renamed *Macnab's Backache.*

Will this text be as useful as the first edition? We will let time tell. We had fun rewriting Ian's work with the original intention that we did not want a reference type text, but an easy reading dogmatic statement of our views, as shaped by Ian. Incidentally, to make it easier reading, for orthopods especially, we put in lots of pictures!

John McCulloch
Ensor Transfeldt

Preface to the Second Edition

"The more things change, the more they stay the same."

— Anonymous

Back disability is still all too prevalent. In fact, the treatment of back pain has become an industry unto itself, generating $14 billion a year in medical costs in the United States just in the workmen's compensation population, let alone private practice. As more practitioners, medical and otherwise, enter the field, costs continue to escalate. "Experts" abound with the "magic cure," while the costs to industry to insure its workers go out of sight, and the social costs of long-term disability multiply manyfold.

One is hard pressed to explain why the incidence of laminectomy on the West Coast of the United States is twice that on the East Coast, and why the incidence of laminectomy in North America is so much higher than in European countries. Are "West Coasters" possessed of weaker backs than their East Coast compatriots; are American lumbar spines inferior to European low backs? There are, perhaps, twice as many orthopedic surgeons on the West Coast of the United States compared with the East Coast. Do spine surgeons increase back disability? The corollary question has to be asked: Do you think back disability would go away if we stopped treating the malady? Obviously, this is not acceptable to the patient, employer, physicians, physical therapists, chiropractors, and the lawyers. So what is the answer?

As the field of lumbar disc disease unfolded, many early pioneers, including Dr. Macnab, stressed the importance of clinical medicine. Newman, Wiltse, Verbiest, and others helped us understand "the vital necessity to know as much about the patient who has the backache as about the backache the patient has."

To this end, Dr. Macnab instilled the promise of clinical medicine in Dr. McCulloch. The teacher taught, and the pupil learned, the essence of a thorough history and physical examination. Both skills were learned under the restraints of oil-based myelography as the "gold standard" of investigation. How things have changed; but this time, they will not stay the same!

We have available to us today incredibly sophisticated investigative techniques. When you compare what magnetic resonance imaging and computed tomography offer to the clinician with what oil-based myelography offered, we have entered a new era of spine surgery for degenerative spinal conditions. It is only after a perfect marriage of clinical acumen with investigative modalities, documenting not only the nature of the pathology but its exact location, that surgery will be indicated. This represents the major section of rewriting in this second edition: understanding the importance of MRI and CT in improving clinical medicine.

The original purpose of this book was to describe, in a clear and concise fashion, the various conditions afflicting the lumbar spine, in a form readable by all professionals: young orthopedists and neurosurgeons, family practitioners, therapists, and others desiring an understanding of the basic principles of lumbar disorders. It is hoped that this new edition lives up to that original intention.

The burden and thrill of authorship would not be possible without the help of so many others. Our thanks (and apologies) go out to Faye Poole, who typed, and retyped, and retyped; and Darlene Jones and Mary Kingstone, invaluable secretaries to two workaholics. To complete this second edition, the junior author relied heavily on many Akron colleagues. Thanks go to: Tina Powell for her splendid photographs; Tina Cauller and Maggie Meenan for their artwork; and Drs. Mark Leeson (tumors), Dan Bethem (fracture), Tony Passalaqua and Joe Crawford (bone scans), and Michael Modic (MRI) for so many of the new illustrations. Akron colleagues in radiology (Drs. Pepe, Taylor, Bury, McCloskey, and Kurman) were always more than willing to provide radiographic examples of pertinent cases. The junior author would like to single out for special thanks the research assistant for Crystal Clinic, Mr. Frank Hurst, whose help in numerous research and authorship projects has been invaluable. Every time JM thinks he can wear out Frank's abilities to produce, Frank delivers: it is a great pleasure to work with and against, his indefatigability.

Many of our colleagues offered constructive criticism to both editions; it does not take alot of criticism for a bad idea to go away, and it is in the milieu of critique that new ideas flourish and grow. To hide from criticism is to expose inherent weakness in one's ideas.

The real instigator for this second edition was Mr. Timothy Grayson of Williams & Wilkins, who has recently taken over the responsibility for orthopedic texts. He skillfully bridged the gap between mentor and pupil, rewrite after rewrite, to bring this second edition to fruition.

Ian Macnab
John McCulloch

Preface to the First Edition

"In seeking absolute truth we aim at the unattainable and must be content with finding broken portions."

— Sir William Osler

Low back pain is a remarkably common disability. Hirsch stated that 65% of the Swedish population was affected by low back pain at some time during their working lives. Rowe stated that, at Eastman Kodak, back pain was second only to upper respiratory tract infections as the reason for absence from work. In 1967, the US National Safety Council reported that 4,000,000 workers were disabled by back pain each year and, in Ontario, Canada, 20,000 claims for disability resulting from backache are received annually by the Workmen's Compensation Board. However, despite its frequency, backache is not a dramatic disease that arouses the scientific curiosity and interest of medical practitioners. Physicians are understandably disenchanted by the frequently obscure etiology of this irksome syndrome and the commonly disappointing response to treatment.

In an attempt to dispel some of the clouds of confusion that obscure the problem, this book has been designed to present a working classification of the common causes of low back pain and to act as a guide to the examination and management of a few commonly seen syndromes.

Some readers may have no intention of entering into the field of spinal surgery. Surgeons in training always find that a surgical textbook is a poor substitute for experience in the operating room. Because of the rapid changes in the minutiae of surgical technique, a textbook is "dated" as soon as it is written, and a description of surgical techniques is of little value to the practicing surgeon who must depend on articles published in medical journals to modify the surgical procedures employed. However, one has to accept the fact that, on occasion, a patient suffering form discogenic backache comes to the end of the road as far as conservative treatment is concerned. The back becomes a malevolent dictator determining what the patient can do at work and play. The physician directing treatment must then decide whether surgical intervention is indicated. In order that he/she can give intelligent and informed advice to patients, he/she must have some knowledge of the operative procedures, including the preoperative investigation that must be undertaken, factors involved in the postoperative investigations that must be undertaken, and factors involved in postoperative care. The surgeon in training also needs to know the indications for considering operative intervention and, in addition, must have some knowledge of the general principles of operative technique. The practicing surgeon will understandably skip over the descriptions of operative technique but may find value in a detailed description of the preoperative investigation of obscure lesions.

For these reasons, chapters have been devoted to the preoperative evaluation and operative technique of laminectomy and fusion, and space has been devoted to discussion of that bête noire of orthopedic surgeons and neurosurgeons alike, the failure of spinal surgery.

Because this book is designed to discuss only the principles of diagnosis and treatment, it has been illustrated by simple line drawings. No attempt has been undertaken to make this text into an authoritative atlas of clinical syndromes, radiological changes, or operative techniques.

Although diagnosis and treatment are presented with unmitigated dogmatism, it must be remembered that, with the frequent absence of scientific facts, any treatise on the management of back pain must, perforce, be regarded as a philosophy and, moreover, a philosophy that must be modified to fit the needs of the physician's community.

It is almost impossible to acknowledge all of the people who have played a role in the preparation of this book and to thank them adequately. To Mr. Philip Newman, I owe special thanks for initiating my interest in the problem of low back pain while I was still a Registrar at the Royal National Orthopaedic Hospital in London, England. The late R.I. Harris made it possible for me to investigate the pathological and mechanical changes associated with disc degeneration, and his contagious enthusiasm encouraged me to study the clinical aspects of the problem in greater depth.

It was with considerable reluctance that I later accepted the offer made by Dr. A. W.M. White to study a group of patients under the care of the Workmen's Compensation Board of Ontario, Canada, who continued to be disabled by back pain despite all forms of treatment, including only too often, several surgical assaults. I shall be eternally grateful for Bill White's persistent insistence that I should take on this unenviable task, because it was from this study that I learned of the vital necessity to know as much about the patient who has the backache as about the backache the patient has. Dr. Allan Walters led the world on his observation on pain syndromes, and it was from him that I learned of the varying and variable relationship of the disability complained of to the pain experienced.

For the preparation of the manuscript, I would like to pay my special thanks to: Margot McKay for illustrations; Kathleen Lipnicki for photographic prints; and Jennifer Widger for typing, retyping, and retyping the script without complaint.

Finally, I would like to express my gratitude to Sara Finnegan of Williams & Wilkins, who patiently and gently guided me through the task of transforming my handwritten notes and sketches into a form more suitable for publication.

I sincerely hope that our combined efforts have produced a text that the reader can use as a basis on which he/she can build a personal philosophy of the management of this commonplace syndrome.

Ian Macnab

Acknowledgments

No project this size can be completed without the help of many. The "backbone" of it all was Nancy Vickroy, BS, PA-C, a young physician assistant who edited and transcribed our thoughts and words, while carrying a heavy clinical load in our spine practice.

A number of orthopedic colleagues in Akron were a tremendous source of material, including Drs. Scott Weiner and Mark Leeson for tumors, and Drs. Rick Brower and Dan Bethem for general spine cases. Rhematological colleagues Drs. Raynor and Bacha provided material, as did Dr. Tom File, an infectious disease specialist (and next door neighbor of JM, who had little chance of resisting requests!). There is extensive radiological input from Drs. Bill Taylor and Ed Bury, who helped rewrite the Investigation" chapter. Dr. Tony Passalaqua helped rewrite the nuclear medicine section and provided many of the scans. Probably the most stressed radiology colleague was Madeline Vincent, the radiographic technologist for Summit Orthopaedic Group, who tore her hair out and my scalp off every time I saw to it that a good teaching radiograph would disappear into my mile-high teaching file.

The bulk of the book's pages are covered with pictures, rather than print, which were provided by artist Maggie Littlefield and photographer Tina Schoch.

As always, many at Williams and Wilkins played a key role. Timothy Grayson was again in on the ground floor, stimulating us to take on the third edition. Will Passano took over from Tim and quickly turned things over to Darlene Cooke. Darlene was so pleasant to deal with, but she did not tell me about Fran Klass, whose job it was to see that the manuscript arrived to the editorial department in a timely fashion. On a number of occasions, we thought that Fran was trained by the Marines, but she informed us that she is simply in the process of raising two teenage sons and did not see us any differently.

Although the bulk of the writing and production for the third edition came out of Akron, the junior author (ET) has put his stamp on the work. To him, the senior author (Macnab Fellow 1969–1970) passes the responsibility for any future editions.

John McCulloch
Ensor Transfeldt

Contents

1

Musculoskeletal and Neuroanatomy of the Lumbar Spine

"You will have to learn many tedious things which you will forget the moment you have passed your final examination, but in anatomy it is better to have learned and lost than never to have learned at all."

— W. Somerset Maugham

INTRODUCTION

It is a convention observed by most authors of medical texts to start the book with a chapter devoted to the anatomy of the subject covered. In many instances, this is a form of brownian movement having very little purposive significance. Having skipped through many such essays with ill-concealed impatience, it was with considerable trepidation that we continued to follow this well-established precedent. The only purpose of this long introductory chapter is to remind the reader of anatomical terminology and to correlate the gross anatomical features of the lumbar vertebrae with pathological changes of clinical significance. You probably will not read the whole chapter, and in fact, you may see how long this chapter is and might be tempted to put the book down forever. But remember, the key to understanding disease and completing exacting surgical techniques is an intimate knowledge of anatomy. You will find this chapter to be in three sections: (1) Functional Musculoskeletal Anatomy, (2) Neuroanatomy, and (3) Surgical Anatomy.

(1) FUNCTIONAL MUSCULOSKELETAL ANATOMY

There are five lumbar vertebrae and the sacrum making up the lumbar spine. We can consider each vertebra as having three functional components: the vertebral bodies, designed to bear weight; the neural arches, designed to protect the neural elements; and the bony processes (spinous and transverse), designed as outriggers to increase the efficiency of muscle action.

The vertebral bodies are connected together by the intervertebral discs, and the neural arches are joined by the facet (zygapophyseal) joints (Fig. 1.1). The discal surface of an adult vertebral body demonstrates on its periphery a ring of cortical bone. This ring, the epiphysial ring, acts as a growth zone in the young and in the adult as an anchoring ring for the attachment of the fibers of the annulus. The hyaline cartilage plate lies within the confines of this ring (Fig. 1.2). The size of the vertebral body increases from L1 to L5, which is indicative of the increasing loads that each lower lumbar vertebral level has to absorb.

The neural arch (Fig 1.1) is composed of two pedicles and two laminae. The pedicles are anchored to the cephalad half of the vertebral body and form a protective cover for the cauda equina contents of the lumbar spinal canal. The ligamentum flavum fills in the interlaminar space at each level (Fig. 1.1).

The outriggers for muscle attachment are the transverse processes and spinous process.

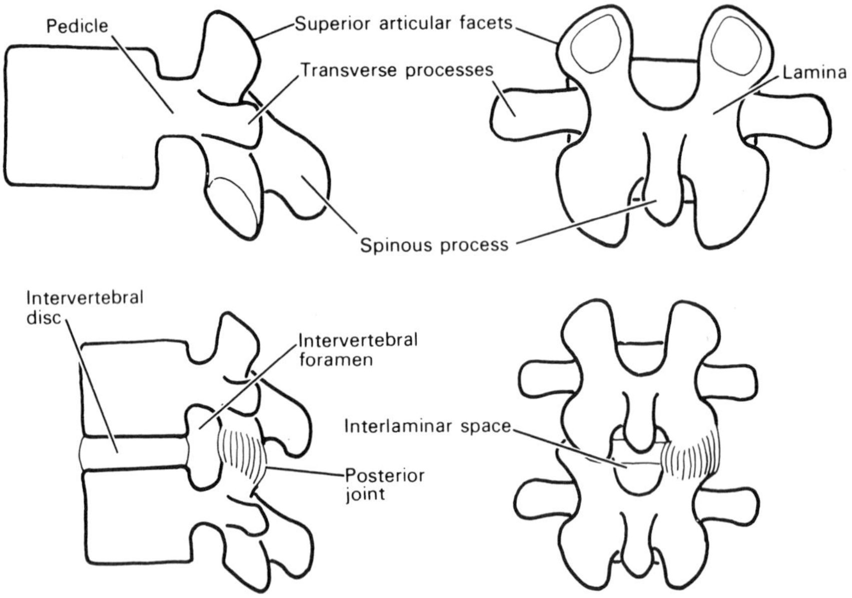

Figure 1.1 *The components of a lumbar vertebra: the body, the pedicle, the superior and inferior facets, the transverse and spinous processes, and the intervertebral foramen and its relationship to the intervertebral disc and the posterior joint.*

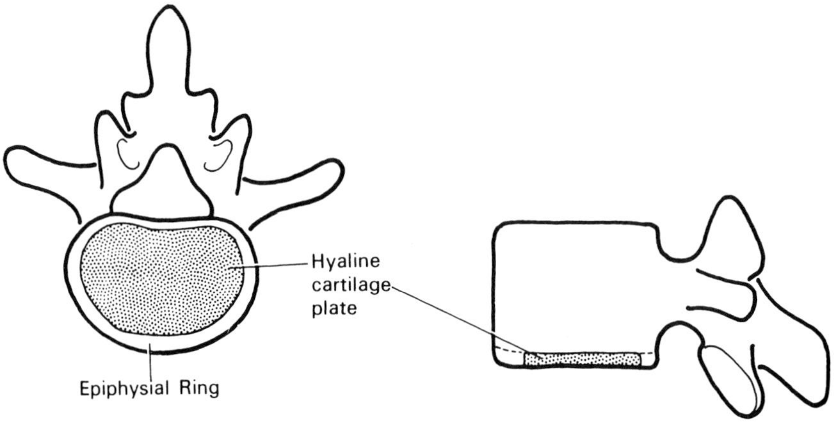

Figure 1.2 *The epiphysial ring is wider anteriorly and surrounds the hyaline cartilaginous plate.*

The Intervertebral Disc

The intervertebral discs (Fig. 1.3) are complicated structures, both anatomically and physiologically. Anatomically, they are constructed in a manner similar to that of a car tire, with a fibrous outer casing, the annulus, containing a gelatinous inner tube, the nucleus pulposus. The fibers of the annulus can be divided into three main groups: the outermost fibers attaching between the vertebral bodies and the undersurface of the epiphysial ring; the middle fibers passing from the epiphysial ring on one vertebral body to the epiphysial ring of the vertebral body below; and the innermost fibers passing from one cartilage endplate to the other. The anterior fibers are strengthened by the powerful anterior longitudinal ligament. The posterior longitudinal ligament affords only weak reinforcement, especially at L4–5 and L5–S1, where it is a midline, narrow, unimportant structure attached to the annulus. The anterior and middle fibers of the annulus are most numerous anteriorly and laterally but are deficient posteriorly, where most of the fibers are attached to the cartilage plate (Fig. 1.3). With the onset of degenerative changes in the disc, abnormal movements occur between adjacent vertebral bodies. These abnormal movements apply a considerable traction strain on the outermost fibers of the annulus, resulting in the development of a spur of bone, the so-called traction spur.(10) Because the outermost fibers attach to the vertebral body beneath the epiphysial ring, this spur

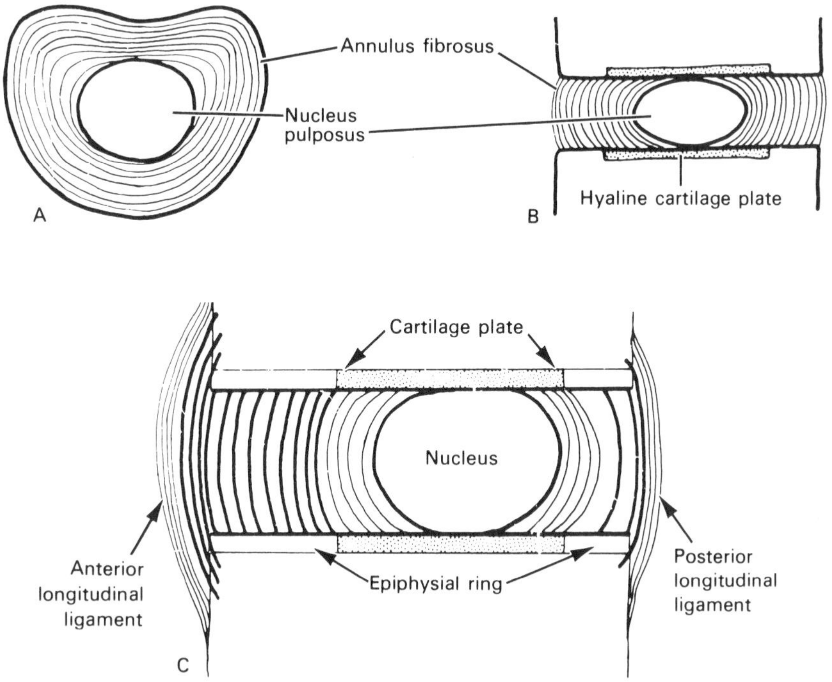

Figure 1.3 *The annulus fibrosus is composed of concentric fibrous rings that surround the nucleus pulposus* **(A)**. *The nucleus pulposus abuts against the hyaline cartilage plate* **(B)**. *The outermost annulus fibers are most numerous anteriorly and are attached to the vertebral body immediately deep to the epiphysial ring.* **(C)** *The epiphysial fibers run from one epiphysial ring to the other. The cartilaginous fibers run from one cartilage plate to the other cartilage plate. These comprise 90% of the annulus fibers posteriorly. The anterior fibers of the annulus are strongly reinforced by the powerful anterior longitudinal ligament, but the posterior longitudinal ligament only gives weak reinforcement to the posterior fibers of the annulus.*

develops about 1 mm away from the discal border of the vertebral body and projects horizontally. This differs in its radiological morphology from the common claw-type osteophyte, which develops at the edge of the vertebral body and curves over the outer fibers of the intervertebral disc (Fig. 1.4). The clinical significance of a traction spur lies in the fact that it indicates the presence of an unstable vertebral segment.

The first stage of a disc rupture would appear to be detachment of a segment of the hyaline cartilage plate. The integrity of the confining ring of the annulus is then disrupted. Nuclear material can escape between the vertebral body and the displaced portion of the cartilage plate. On occasion, as a result of a compression force, a whole segment of the annulus may be displaced posteriorly, carrying with it the nucleus pulposus and displaced portion of the hyaline plate (Fig. 1.5). This pathology is more common in younger patients (Fig. 1.5B).

The fibers of the annulus are firmly attached to the vertebral bodies and are arranged in lamellae, with the fibers of one layer running at an angle to those of the deeper layer (Fig. 1.6). This anatomical arrangement permits the annulus to limit vertebral movements. This important function is reinforced by the investing vertebral ligaments.

Because the nucleus pulposus is gelatinous, the load of axial compression is distributed not only in a vertical direction but also radially throughout the nucleus as well.(8, 11) This radial distribution of the vertical load (tangential loading of the disc) is absorbed by the fibers of the annulus and can be compared with the hoops around a barrel (Fig. 1.7).

Weight is transmitted to the nucleus through the hyaline cartilage plate. The hyaline cartilage is ideally suited to this function because it is avascular. If weight were transmitted through a vascularized structure, such as bone, the local pressure would shut off blood supply, and progressive areas of bone would die. This phenomenon is seen when

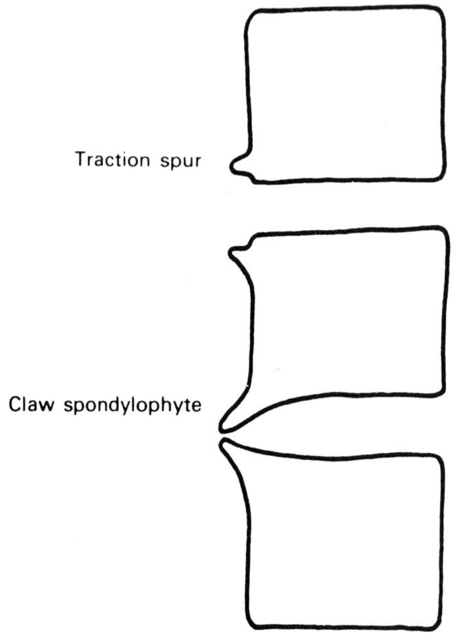

Figure 1.4 *The traction spur projects horizontally from the vertebral body about 1 mm away from the discal border. It is indicative of segmental instability. The common claw spondylophyte, on the other hand, extends from the rim of the vertebral body and curves as it grows around the bulging intervertebral disc. It is associated with disc degeneration. It* does not *represent the radiological manifestation of osteoarthritis.*

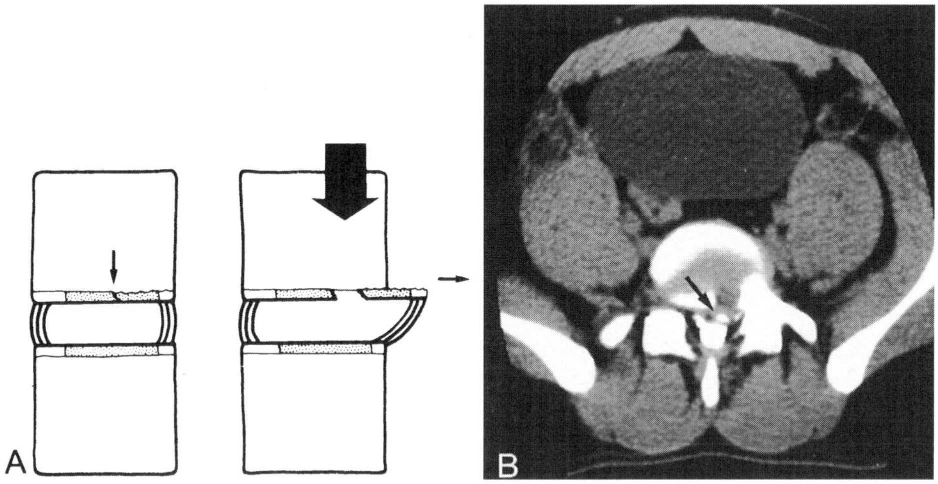

Figure 1.5 **A.** *The first morphological change to occur in a disc rupture is a separation of a segment of the cartilage plate from the adjacent vertebral body. Fissures run through the annulus on each side of the detached portion of the cartilage. When a vertical compression force is then applied, the detached portion of the cartilage plate is displaced posteriorly, and the nucleus exudes through the torn fibers of the annulus.* **B.** *CT of young patient with end-plate fracture arrow and herniated nucleus pulposus.*

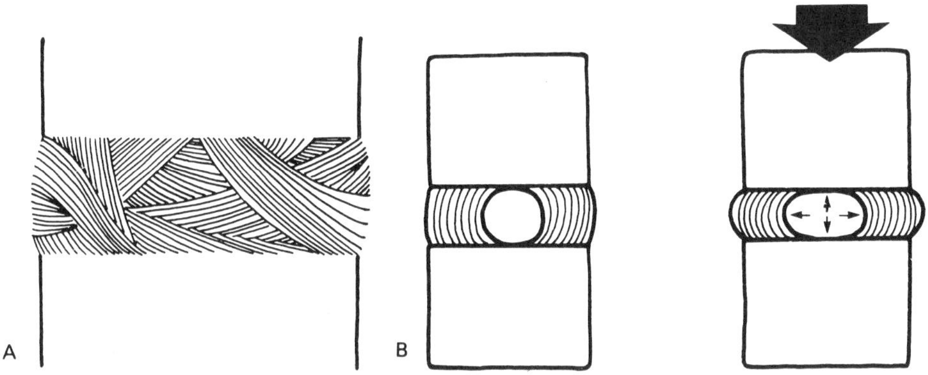

Figure 1.6 **A.** *The annulus is a laminated structure with the fibrous lamellae running obliquely. This disposition of the fibers permits resistance of torsional strains.* **B.** *The nucleus pulposus is constrained by the fibers of the annulus. When a vertical load is applied to the vertebral column, the force is dissipated radially by the gelatinous nucleus pulposus. Distortion and disruption of the nucleus pulposus are resisted by the annulus.*

the cartilage plate presents congenital defects and the nucleus is in direct contact with the spongiosa of bone. The pressure occludes the blood supply; a small zone of bone dies; and the nucleus progressively intrudes into the vertebral body. This phenomenon was first described by Schmorl and Junghanns,(13) and the resulting lesion bears the name Schmorl's node (Fig. 1.8).

The annulus acts like a coiled spring, pulling the vertebral bodies together against the elastic resistance of the nucleus pulposus, with the result that when a spine is sectioned sagittally, the unopposed pull of the annulus makes the nucleus bulge. This has been referred to as "turgor" of the nucleus, but in actual fact, it is the manifestation of a springlike action, the compressing action of the annulus fibrosus. This makes for a very

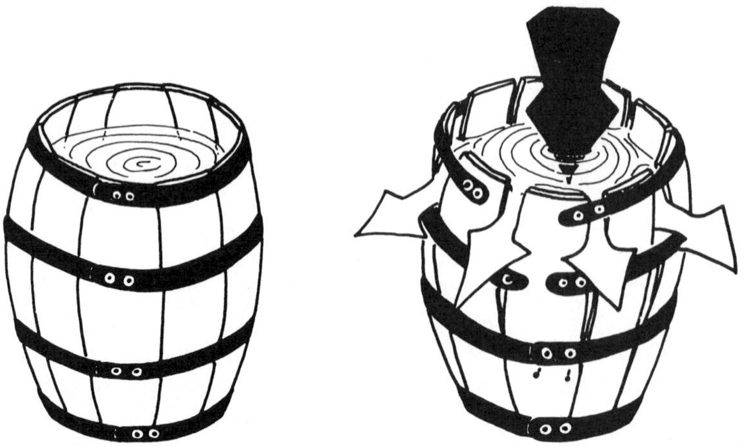

Figure 1.7 *Hoop stress. This diagram shows how the load of water in a barrel is resisted by the hoops around the barrel. When too great a load is applied, the hoops will break. The annulus functions in a manner similar to that of the hoops around a water barrel.*

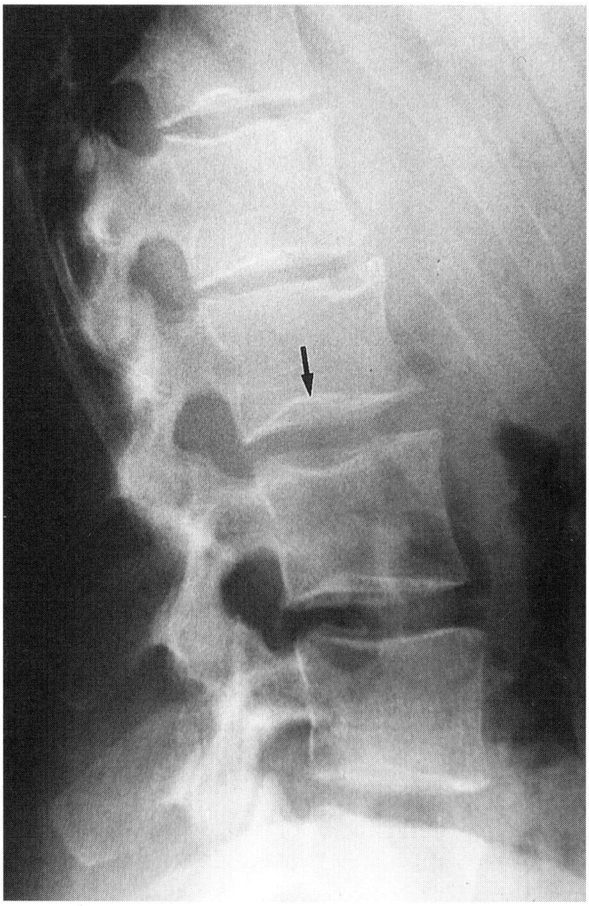

Figure 1.8 *A Schmorl's node* (L2–3) (arrow), *likely of no clinical significance. Have you ever seen a herniated nucleus pulposus at the same disc space as a Schmorl's node?*

good coupling unit, provided that all of the structures remain intact. The nucleus pulposus acts like a ball bearing, and in flexion and extension the vertebral bodies roll over this incompressible gel while the posterior joints guide and steady the movements (Fig. 1.9).

The intervertebral discs of a person up to the age of 8 have a blood supply, but thereafter they are dependent for their nutrition on diffusion of tissue fluids. This fluid transfer is through two routes: (a) The bi-directional flow from vertebral body to disc and from disc to vertebral body, and (b) the diffusion through the annulus from blood vessels on its surface. This ability to transfer fluid from the disc to the adjacent vertebral bodies minimizes the rise in intradiscal pressure on sudden compression loading. This fluid transfer acts like a safety valve and protects the disc. Clinical experience supported by experimental observations has shown that the fibers of the annulus are less commonly ruptured by direct compression loading (Fig. 1.10). Sudden severe loading of the spine, however, may produce a rise in fluid pressure within the vertebral body great enough to produce a "bursting" fracture.

Although this has been a very cursory review of the structure and function of the intervertebral disc, one can see that the components of a disc act as an integrated whole, subserving many functions, in addition to being a roller bearing between adjacent vertebral bodies.

The Facet Joints

The zygapophyseal joints are synovial joints that permit simple gliding movements. Although the lax capsule of the zygapophyseal joints is reinforced to some extent by the ligamentum flavum anteriorly and the supraspinous ligament posteriorly (Fig. 1.11), the major structures restraining movement in these joints are the outermost fibers of the annulus. When these annular fibers exhibit degenerative changes, excessive joint play is permitted. This is the reason why degenerative changes within the discs render the related posterior joints vulnerable to strain. The intimate relationship between the disc and its two facet joints has led to Kirkaldy-Willis (6) labeling the unit "the three joint complex" (Fig. 1.11).

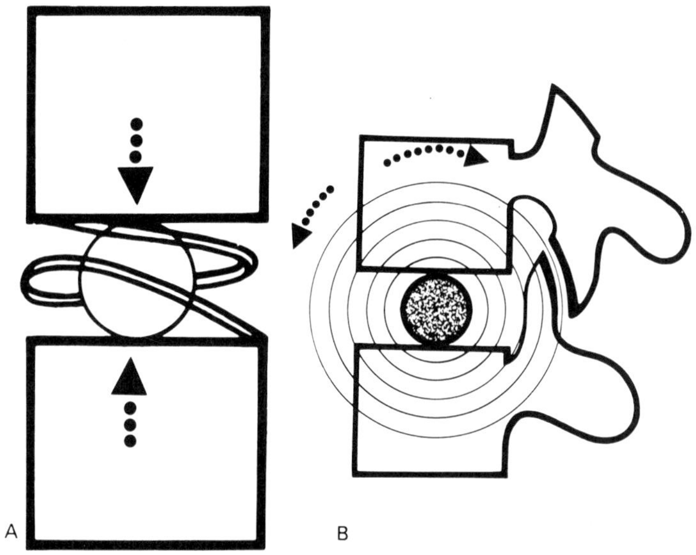

Figure 1.9 **A.** *The annulus acts like a coiled spring, pulling the vertebral bodies together against the elastic resistance of the nucleus pulposus.* **B.** *The nucleus pulposus acts as a ball bearing with the vertebral bodies rolling over this incompressible gel in flexion and extension while the posterior joints guide and steady the movement.*

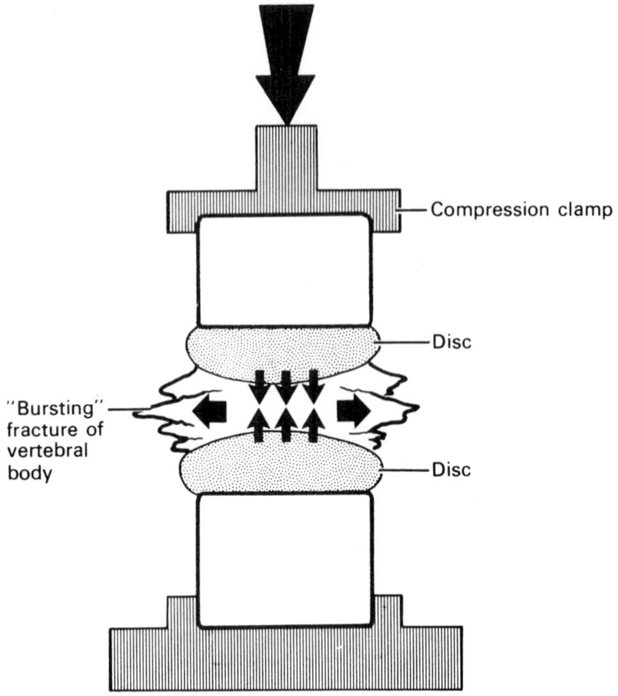

Figure 1.10 *Diagram shows the experimental testing of vertical loading of the spine. When a very high compressive force is applied, the discs will remain intact, but the vertebral body shatters.*

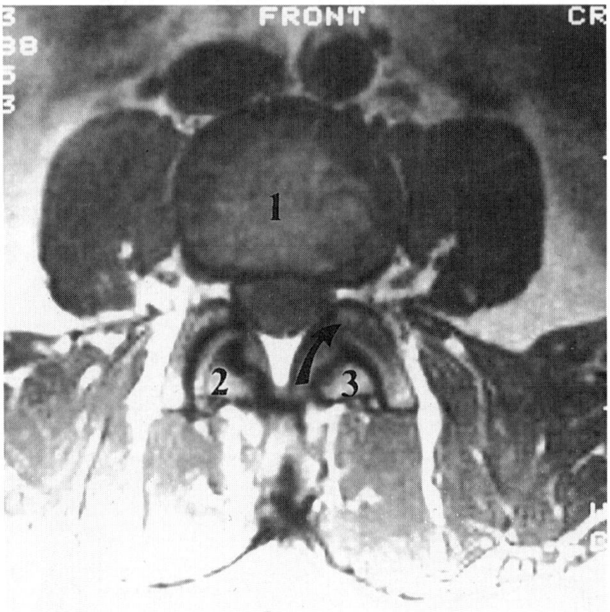

Figure 1.11 *The ligamentum flavum inserts into the capsule on the superior facet (arrow). The three joint complex is composed of the disc space (1) and two facet joints (2 and 3).*

The Muscles and Ligaments of the Lumbar Spine

The Muscles

It is somewhat futile to learn the names of the muscles of the low back. Each time we learn their names, we promptly forget them! But every now and then a consultant will ask you to name them, and for completeness, here they are. The muscles of the lumbar spine are divided into extensor, flexors, rotators, and lateral flexors:

Extensors (Fig. 1.12) The extensors of the lumbar spine when viewed posteriorly are covered by the fascial origin of the latissimus dorsi. Deep to this fascia are three layers of muscles:

1. The superficial group is the erector spinae (sacrospinalis) that fans out over the lumbar spine as three bands (Fig. 1.12).
2. The intermediate group is semispinalis, multifidus, and the rotators.
3. A deep group of short muscles running from one segment to the next (intersegmental) (Fig. 1.12).

These muscles are all supplied by the posterior primary ramus (Fig. 1.13).

Flexors The next large group of muscles are the flexors of the lumbar spine (Fig. 1.14) and include the:

1. Extrinsics: the abdominal wall muscles (rectus abdominis, the external and internal obliques, and the transversus).
2. Intrinsic: iliopsoas.

Rotators and lateral flexors The rotator muscles are various combinations of the extensors and flexors. Lateral flexion is accomplished by contraction of unilateral flexors and extensors.

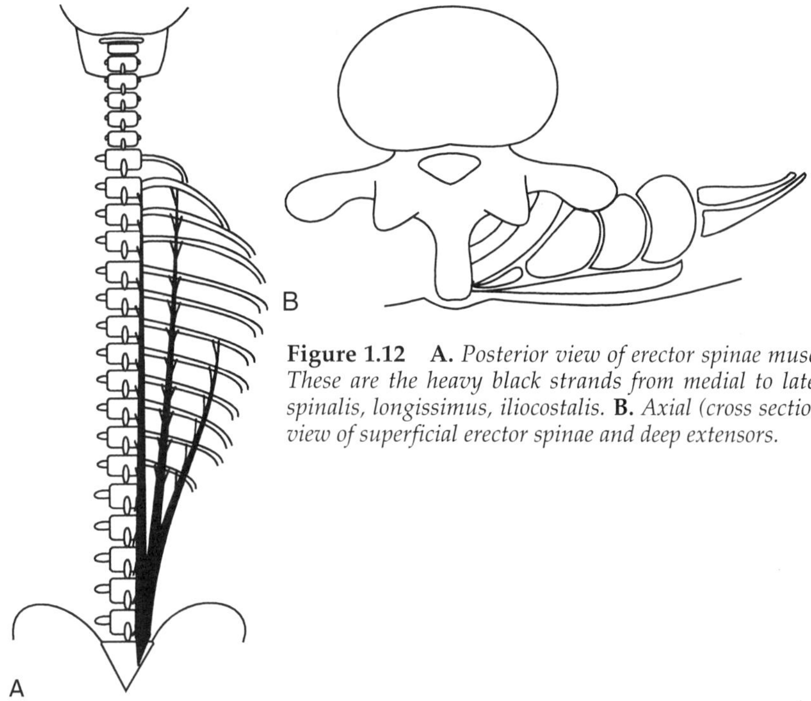

Figure 1.12 **A.** *Posterior view of erector spinae muscles. These are the heavy black strands from medial to lateral: spinalis, longissimus, iliocostalis.* **B.** *Axial (cross sectional) view of superficial erector spinae and deep extensors.*

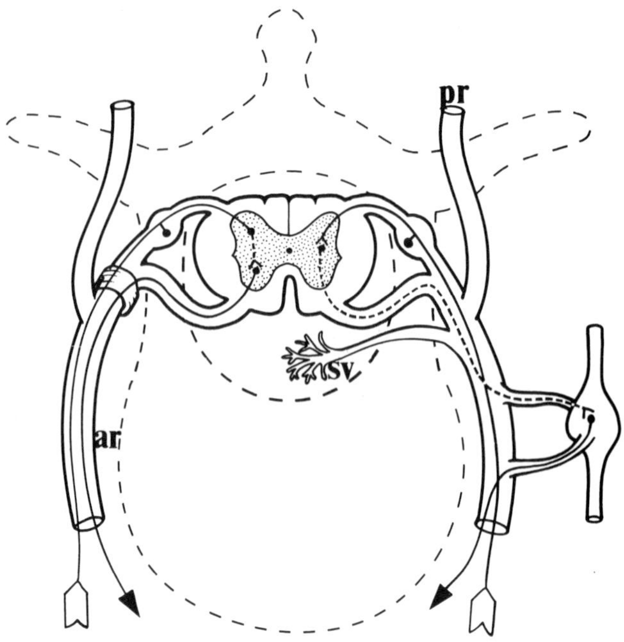

Figure 1.13 *The posterior primary ramus (pr) and anterior primary ramus (ar). The sinuvertebral nerve is labeled sv.*

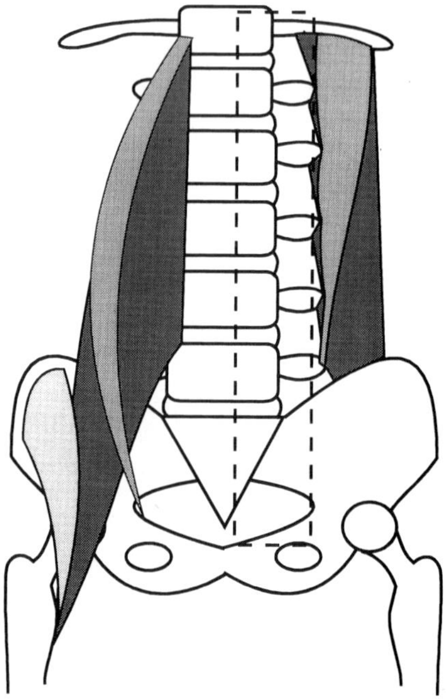

Figure 1.14 *The extrinsic flexors (rectus abdominis is most anterior and represented by dotted rectangle) and intrinsic flexors (shaded), including iliopsoas on left and quadratus on right.*

The Ligaments

Although the ligaments of the lumbar spine are no more important than the muscles, their names and functions are required knowledge.

Anterior longitudinal ligament Obviously, this ligament runs the length of the anterior aspect of the spine (Fig. 1.15). It is intimately attached to the anterior annular fibers of each disc and is a fairly strong ligament useful in fracture reduction (see Chapter 4, Spondylogenic Back Pain: Osseous Lesions).

Posterior longitudinal ligament This is the posterior mate to the anterior longitudinal ligament (Fig. 1.16). It is a significant ligament in all areas of the spine except the lower lumber region. Although frequently mentioned in the discussion of lumbar disc disease, the ligament itself is rather flimsy and inconsequential in the lower lumbar spine where lumbar disc problems are most common.

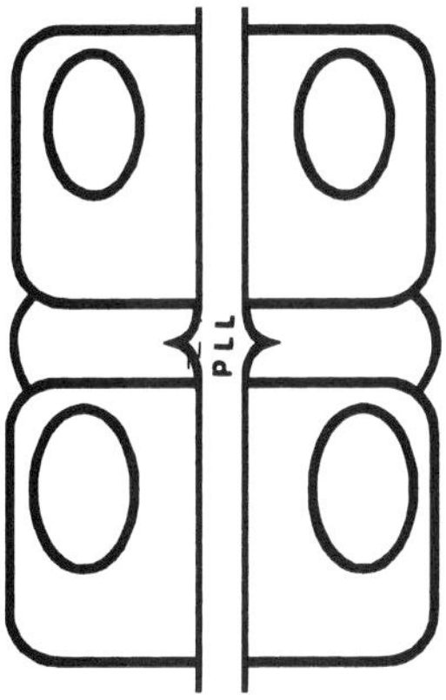

Figure 1.15 *The anterior longitudinal ligament (arrow) on proton density MRI.*

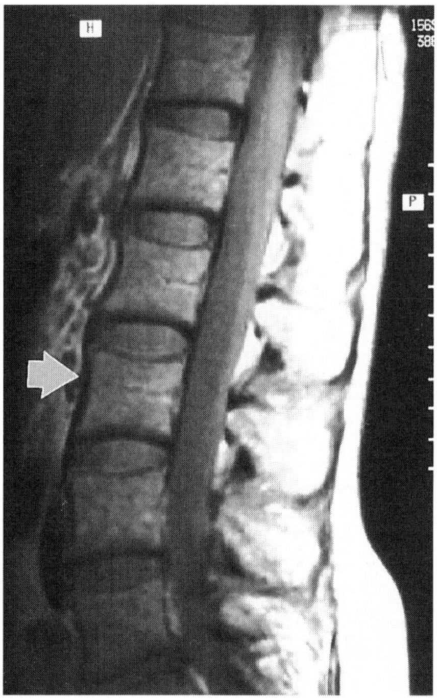

Figure 1.16 *The posterior longitudinal ligament (PLL), which at L4–5 and L5–S1 is very thin and narrow.*

Interspinous/supraspinous ligament complex Although most authors draw these two ligaments backwards and as separate structures (Fig. 1.17), it does not take a rocket scientist to figure out that if you want to flex the lumbar spine, the ligaments have to be structured as depicted in Figure 1.18.

Ligamentum flavum (the yellow ligament) This ligament is so named because of the yellowish color that is given to it by the high content of the elastin fibers. The ligamentum flavum bridges the interlaminar interval, attaching to the interspinous ligament medially and the facet capsule laterally (Fig. 1.11). Normally, it maintains a taught configuration, stretching for flexion and contracting its elastin fibers in neutral or extension. In this way, it always covers but never infringes on the epidural space (Fig. 1.19). With aging, the ligamentum flavum loses its elastin fibers, and the collagen hypertrophies, which results in buckling of the ligamentum flavum and encroachment on the thecal sac (Fig. 1.20).

The Bony Lumbar Vertebral Column

Normally, there are five vertebrae in the lumbar spine. But approximately 10% of the adult patients seen with symptomatic degenerative conditions of the low back have a congenital lumbosacral anomaly.(4) These anomalies are mainly failures of segmentation, which may be symmetrical or asymmetrical. Our involvement with percutaneous spinal surgical procedures led to early recognition of the many traps these congenital lumbosacral anomalies present to the surgeon. There are two potential technical pitfalls for the surgeon operating on a patient with these anomalies. First, when using an image intensifier for a procedure such as discolysis, the surgeon has available a very limited image intensifier field (Fig. 1.21). If the surgeon is unaware of

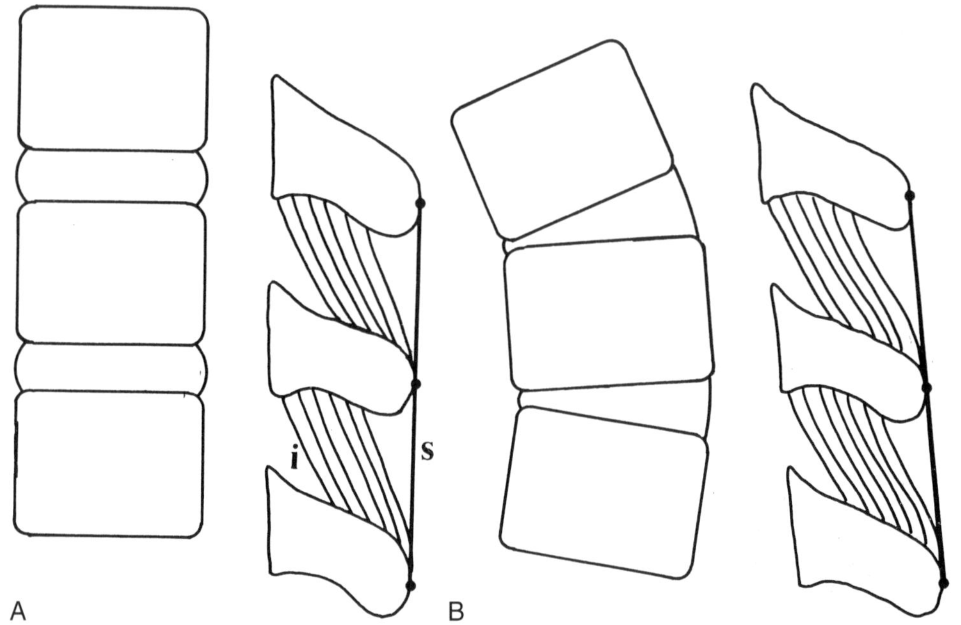

Figure 1.17 **A.** *The usual way for the supraspinous ligament (S) and interspinous ligaments (i) to be drawn.* **B.** *Now, try to flex your spine—no give!*

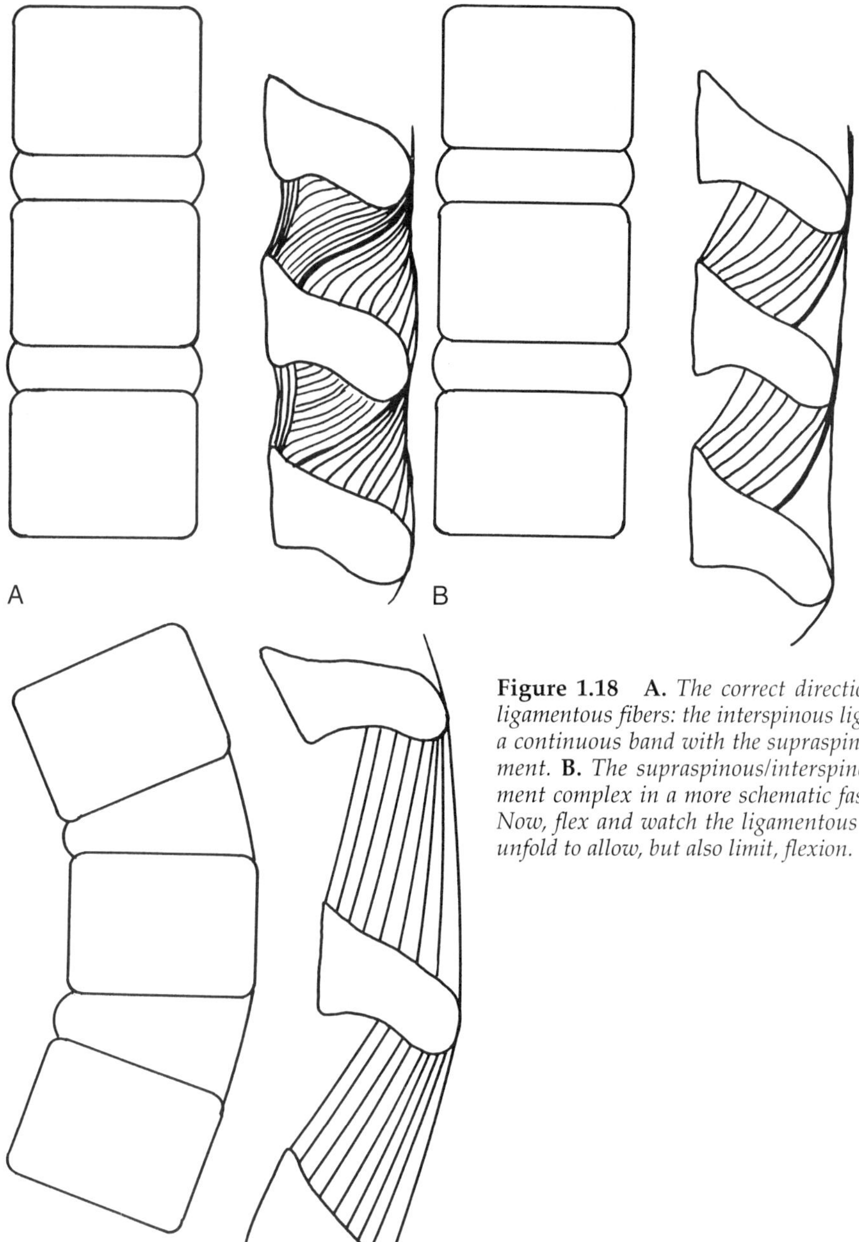

Figure 1.18 **A.** *The correct direction of the ligamentous fibers: the interspinous ligament is a continuous band with the supraspinous ligament.* **B.** *The supraspinous/interspinous ligament complex in a more schematic fashion.* **C.** *Now, flex and watch the ligamentous complex unfold to allow, but also limit, flexion.*

congenital lumbosacral anomalies, it is easy to inject chymopapain into the wrong disc space. Second, when operating through the midline microsurgical approach, the limited exposure available to the surgeon (Fig. 1.22) makes it very easy to enter the wrong level surgically. Thus, congenital lumbosacral anomalies, to the unwary, can lead to the injection of chymopapain into the wrong disc space or to a microsurgical exposure of the wrong disc space level.

Figure 1.19 *A normal ligamentum flavum is taut (arrow), ready to be flexed, and does not encroach on the common dural sac.*

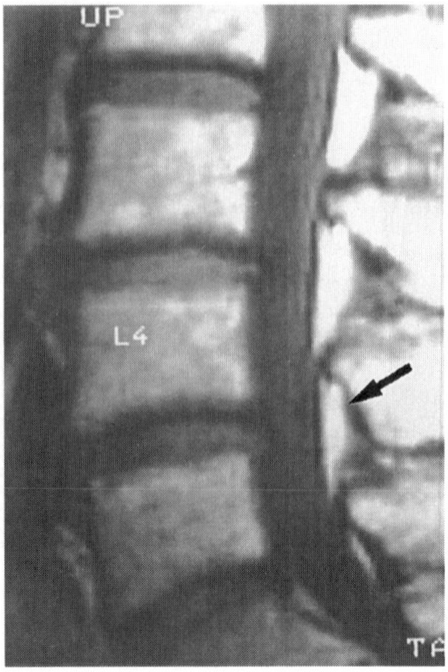

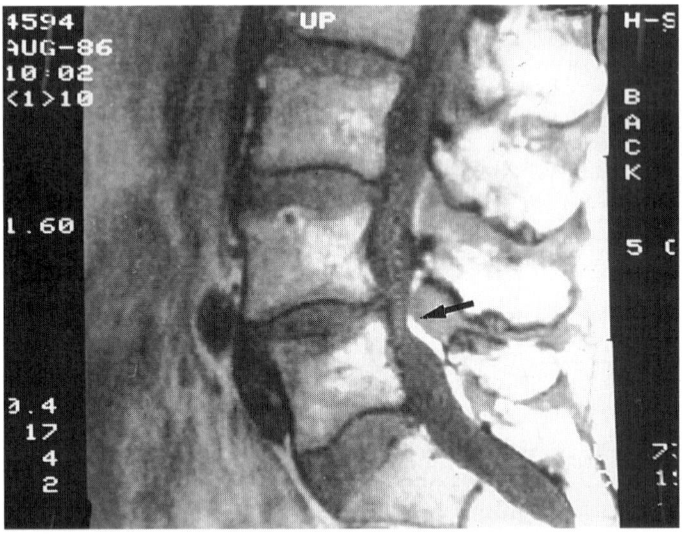

Figure 1.20 *Spinal canal stenosis at a slip (degenerative spondylolisthesis) level. Note the infolding of the ligamentum flavum (arrow).*

Definitions

It is best to designate a disc-space level as an interspace between two vertebral bodies; that is, the disc space between the fifth lumbar vertebral body and the first sacral vertebral body is the L5–S1 disc space. Further, it is best to designate a nerve root according to the pedicle beneath which it passes. Thus, the fifth lumbar nerve root passes beneath the fifth lumbar pedicle. Proximal to this, it passes across the L4–5 disc space, where it can be encroached upon by an L4–5 disc herniation. Distal to the pedicle, the fifth lumbar nerve root lies just lateral to the L5–S1 disc space, and a lateral disc herniation at L5–S1 can encroach on the fifth lumbar nerve root at this level (Fig. 1.23).

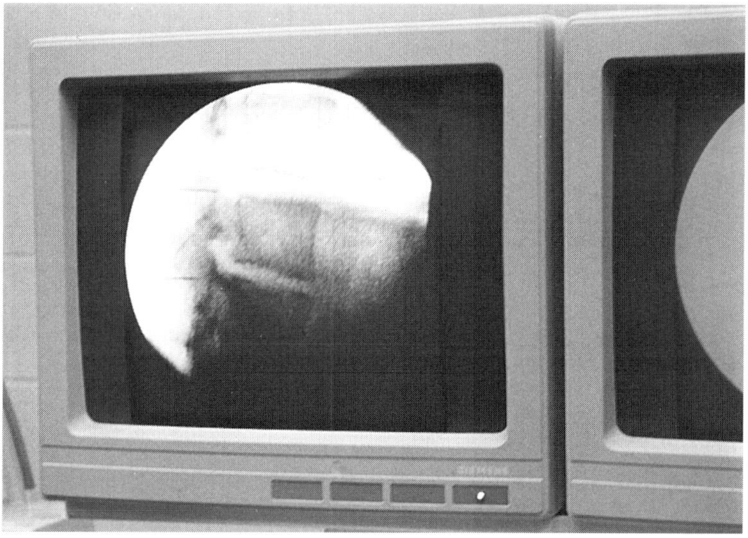

Figure 1.21 *The limited image intensifier field. The needles are opposite which levels? (If you guessed L4–5 and L5–S1, you are wrong! On shifting the image intensifier a few inches caudally, it became evident that L3–4 and L4–5 had been marked.)*

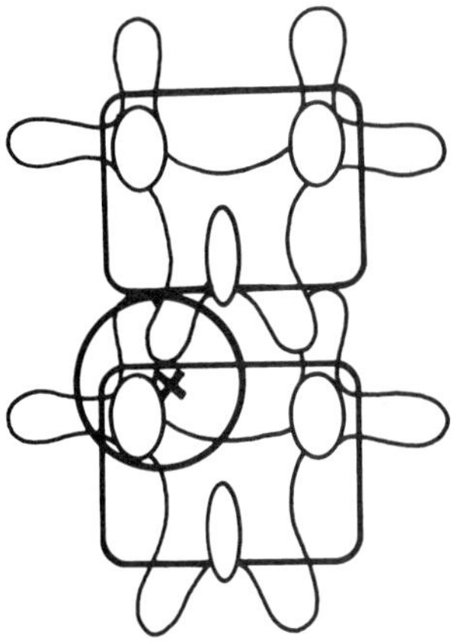

Figure 1.22 *The relative size of the microsurgical field is shown against a schematic of an anatomic segment.*

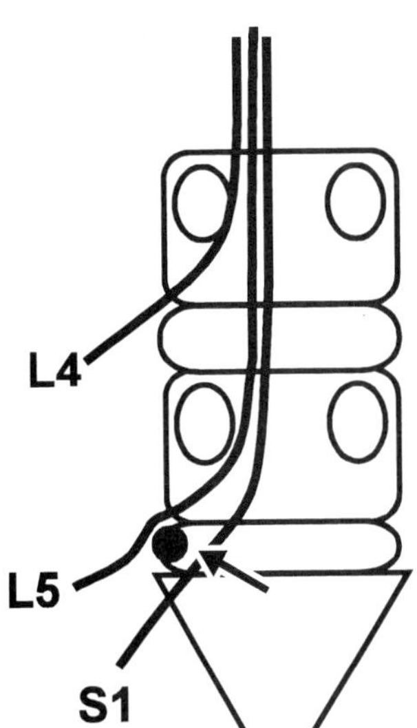

Figure 1.23 *A foraminal disc at L5–S1 will compress the L5 nerve root (arrow).*

It is not uncommon to see radiologic designations of congenital lumbosacral anomalies such as L4–S1 and L6–S1. In addition, the terms sacralization and lumbarization are very common in reporting radiographs with lumbosacral anomalies (15, 16). The frequent disagreement between radiologists and clinicians as to designation of levels is due to the fact that radiologists always have an AP and a lateral radiograph to view, and invariably count down from the last rib to number the lumbar vertebrae. On the other hand, spinal surgeons, who often count vertebrae in the operating room, have only a spot lateral radiograph and count from the sacrum up. If the patient has a normal lumbar spine, the radiologist and the surgeon will meet at the same L4–5 level (Fig. 1.24). If the patient has six lumbar vertebrae, the radiologist and the surgeon will be at different levels (Fig. 1.24), and a wrong level exposure may result.

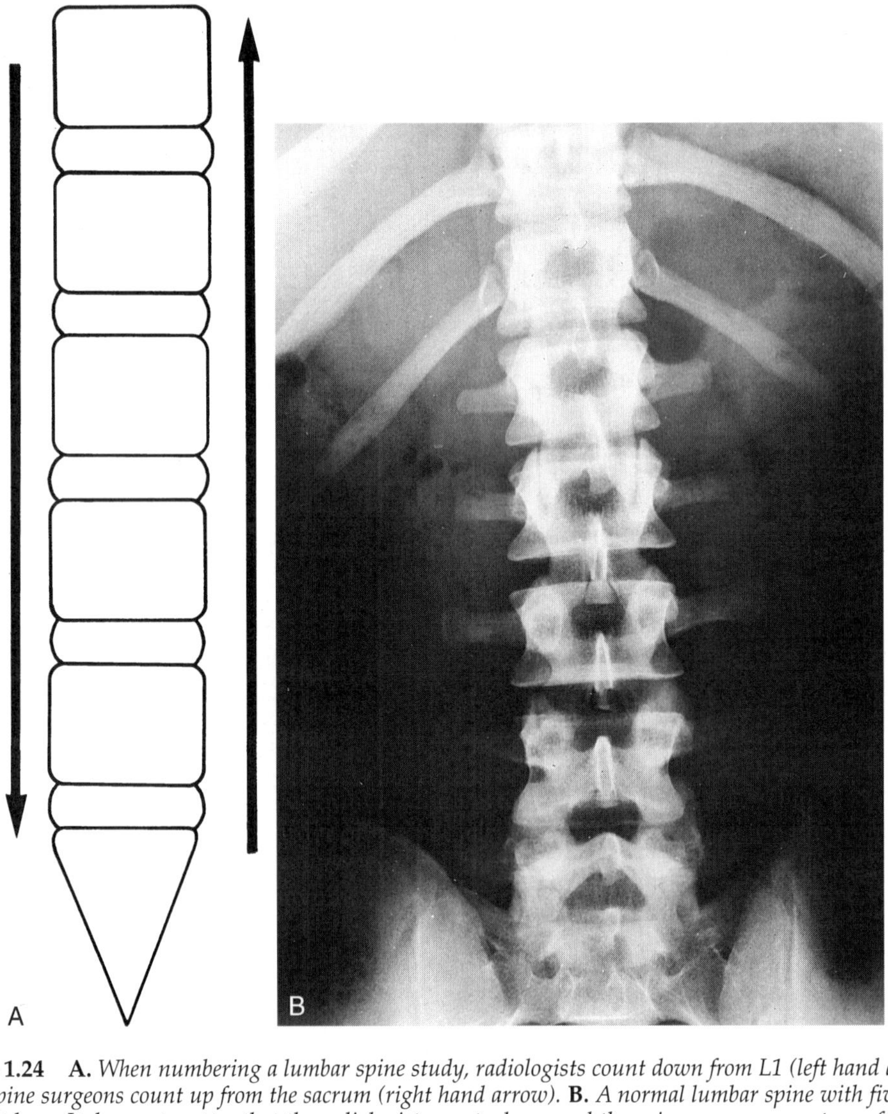

Figure 1.24 **A.** *When numbering a lumbar spine study, radiologists count down from L1 (left hand arrow), while spine surgeons count up from the sacrum (right hand arrow).* **B.** *A normal lumbar spine with five lumbar vertebrae. It does not matter that the radiologist counts down and the spine surgeon counts up from the sacrum: they will both be talking about the same disc when they use the terminology L4–5.*

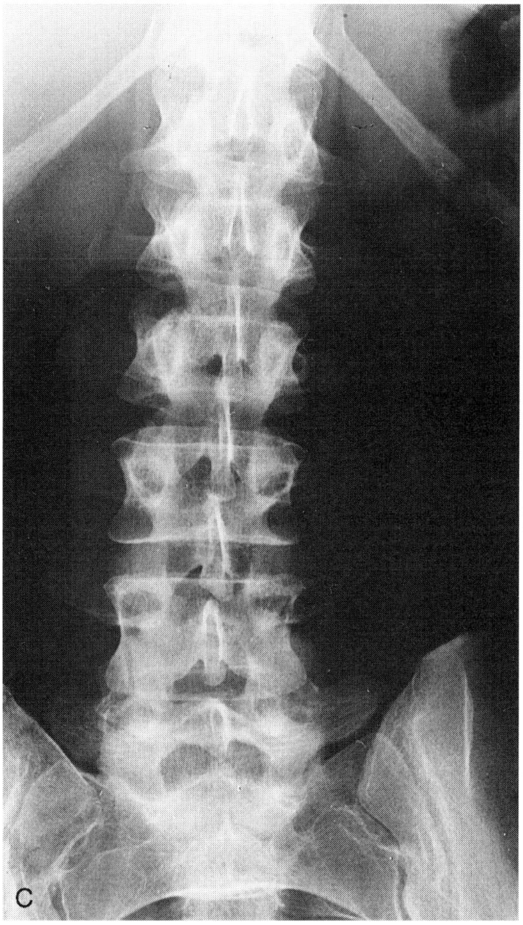

Figure 1.24 (continued) C. *Now, count down to L4–5 (like a radiologist) and then count up (like a spine surgeon). Are you each talking about the same disc space?*

It is proposed that we use the terms formed levels and mobile levels to designate levels in congenital lumbosacral anomalies. A formed level is described as any level of the lumbar spine that has an interlaminar space and a disc space. The extent of interlaminar space formation usually parallels disc-space formation (Fig. 1.25). In a normally formed lumbar level, there is a transverse process that is free of any attachments to the pelvis or sacrum, and there are two facet joints.

A normally formed level such as the level between L5 and S1 should be a fully mobile level; failure of complete segmentation may result in the transverse process being fixed to the pelvis or to the sacrum. This takes away mobility from that level, but still leaves an interlaminar space and a disc space with various degrees of formation of transverse processes and facet joints. In this situation, the last mobile level is the level above the fixed level and is designated the last mobile level (Fig. 1.26).

Thus, the last formed level is any level that has an interlaminar space (and usually a disc space, however rudimentary), with or without facet joints, and transverse processes that may or may not be attached to the pelvis. The last mobile level is the last formed level that is free of all bony attachments to the pelvis and is a fully mobile level. In a normal lumbar spine, the L5–S1 level is both the last formed level and the last mobile level (Fig. 1.24).

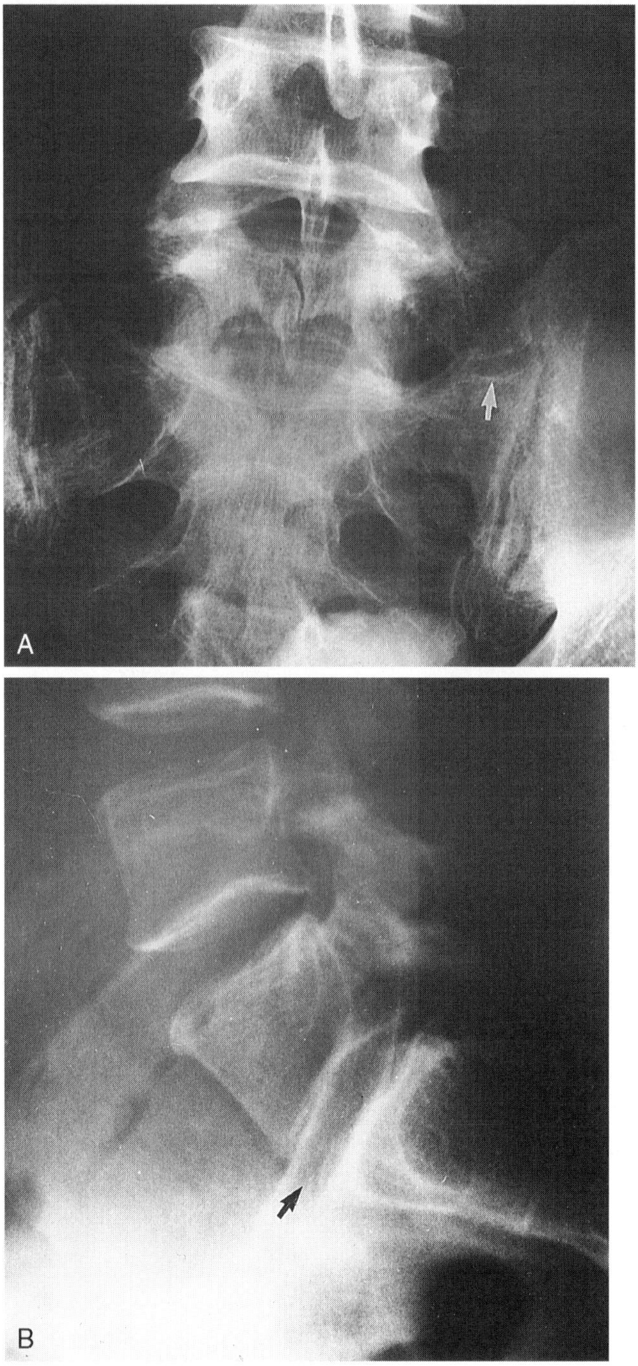

Figure 1.25 **A.** *A fixed last formed level (arrow), with a wide interlaminar space.* **B.** *Note a well formed disc space on lateral radiograph (arrow).*

Discussion

The first anomaly that is of concern has already been mentioned; that is, the presence of six lumbar vertebrae with a pathologic condition reported by the radiologist at the L4–5 level. Figure 1.27 demonstrates this problem.

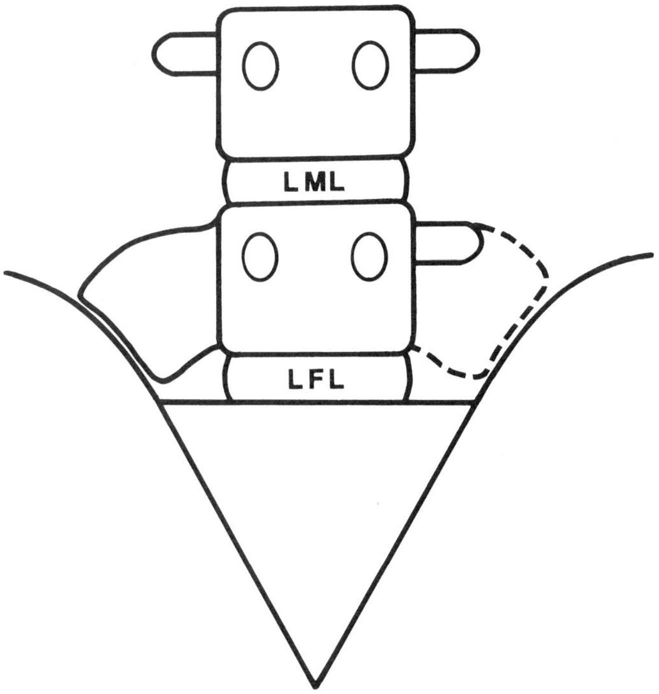

Figure 1.26 *The fixed level (on the left of the spine and shown dotted in on the right) takes mobility away from the last formed level (LFL). The level above becomes the last mobile level (LML).*

The second problem is the partially fixed last formed level, with five vertebrae above that are free of rib attachments. A radiologist may report a pathologic condition at the L5–S1 level. Figure 1.28 demonstrates this problem. If one is doing an image intensifier procedure with the patient in the lateral position, it is very easy, with the limited image intensifier field, to try to enter the last disc space level (last formed level). In fact, one should be entering the second-to-last formed level, which is the last mobile level, the level that the radiologist may have designated as L5–S1.

The third congenital anomaly of concern is demonstrated in Figure 1.29. Here, the patient had five lumbar vertebrae, with the last formed level being fixed and, to a certain extent, rudimentary. The pathologic condition was reported to be at the L4–5 level, and it would have been very easy to enter the third last formed, second last mobile level to perform discolysis.

Figure 1.30 demonstrates the newest problem that has arisen with congenital lumbosacral anomalies. Here, the patient had plain radiographs done in one radiography unit and a CT scan done in a separate radiography unit. Different numbering was used at the two units, which led to confusion as to designation of the level of the pathologic condition.

In congenital lumbosacral anomalies (with the various degrees of fixation between the last formed level and the pelvis), the last formed disc space is always narrow.(5) A rudimentary level is narrowed in a parallel fashion, but does not have any of the reaction of degenerative disc disease such as sclerosis, osteophyte formation, wedging of the disc space, retrospondylolisthesis, or air in the disc space (Fig. 1.25B).

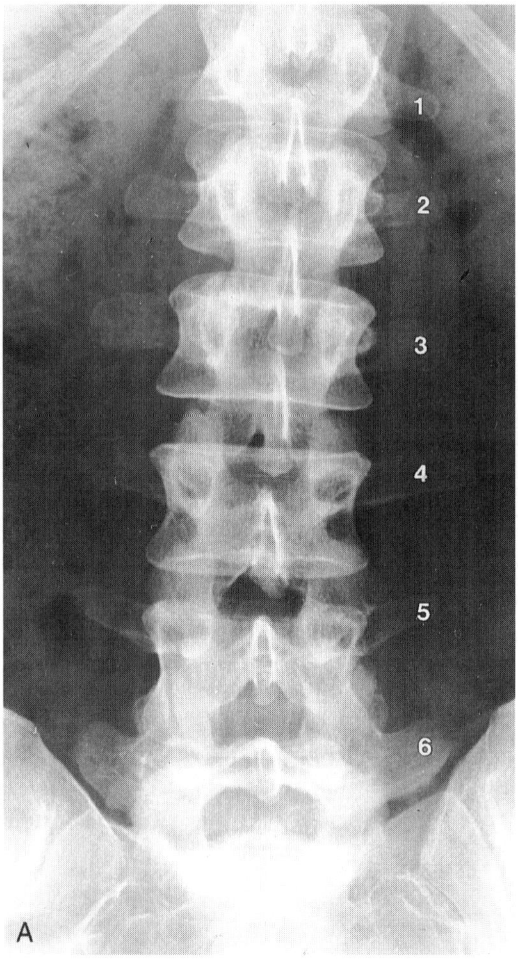

Figure 1.27 **A.** *Six lumbar vertebrae numbered from the top down. Now, number them from the bottom up, designating the LFL/LML L5–S1 as in most normal spines. You will be at a different L4–5 space, which is marked with a needle on an image intensifier screen in Figure 1.27 B.*

Conclusion

With the advent of less invasive spinal surgery such as discolysis and microdiscectomy, the surgeon must be very aware of congenital lumbosacral anomalies that might lead to injection or exposure of the wrong disc-space level. The high percentage of these anomalies puts 10% of patients at risk. In the past, rib counts and identification of the interiliac crest line and the longest and broadest transverse processes have been used to help localize levels. These clinical and radiologic parameters have been adequate, but we think that it is time to introduce the terminology last mobile level and last formed level.

The Canals of the Lumbar Spine

Think of the canals of the spine as you would of the canals of Venice. There is one main canal and many tributary canals. The main canal is called the spinal canal through which traverses the cauda equina, bathed in spinal fluid and contained by the common dural sac (Fig. 1.31). At each vertebral level, L1 to L5 nerve roots have to exit the lumbar spine and do so through the tributary canals or foramina.

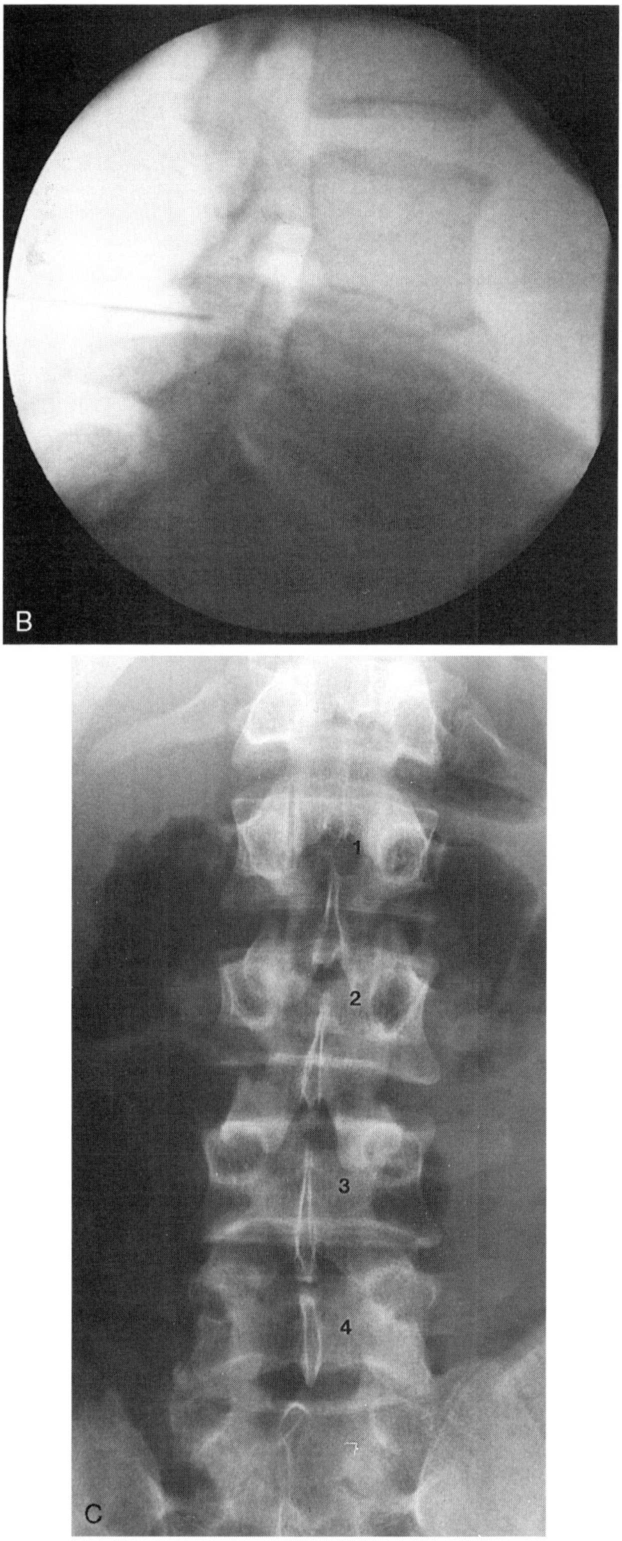

Figure 1.27 (continued) **B.** *This is one way wrong level exposures occur.* **C.** *Here is a little more confusion: four lumbar vertebrae with a well fixed last formed level. Is L3–4 really L4–5?*

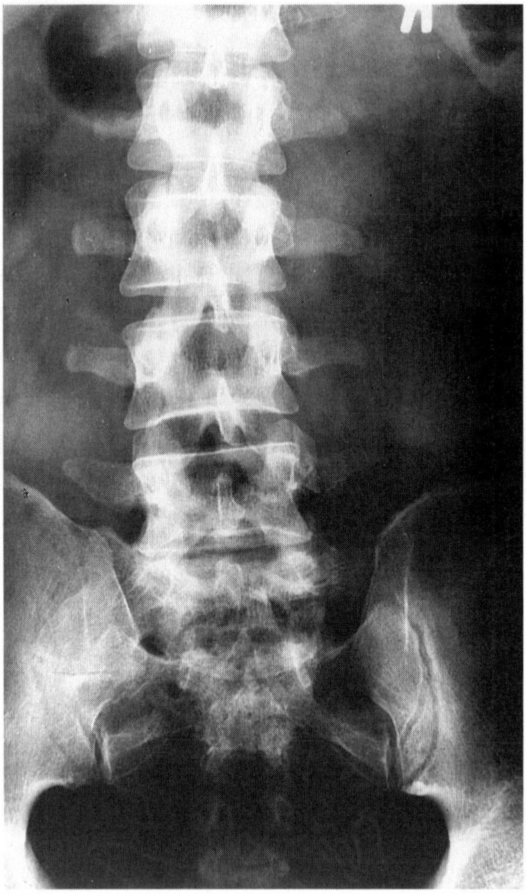

Figure 1.28 *A fixed last formed level (fixed on the left side by "bat-wing" transverse processes), with five lumbar vertebrae above.*

The (Common) Spinal Canal

Boundaries of the Spinal Canal

The spinal canal is bounded in front by the vertebral bodies and discs (Fig. 1.32). Each side is formed by the medial border of the pedicles, between which are the foramina. The posterior boundary is completely covered by the laminae/facet joint complexes, which are linked by the ligamentum flavum.

Dimensions of the Spinal Canal

Normally, the spinal canal offers lots of room for the common dural sac, adequate at L1 and more than adequate at L5 (Fig. 1.33). The canal is wider in a transverse dimension than in its anterior-posterior depth (Table 1.1).

The spinal canal can be narrower at birth (congenital canal stenosis) or become narrowed by degenerative changes. Both conditions are discussed in Chapter 17, Disc Degeneration with Root Irritation: Spinal Canal Stenosis.

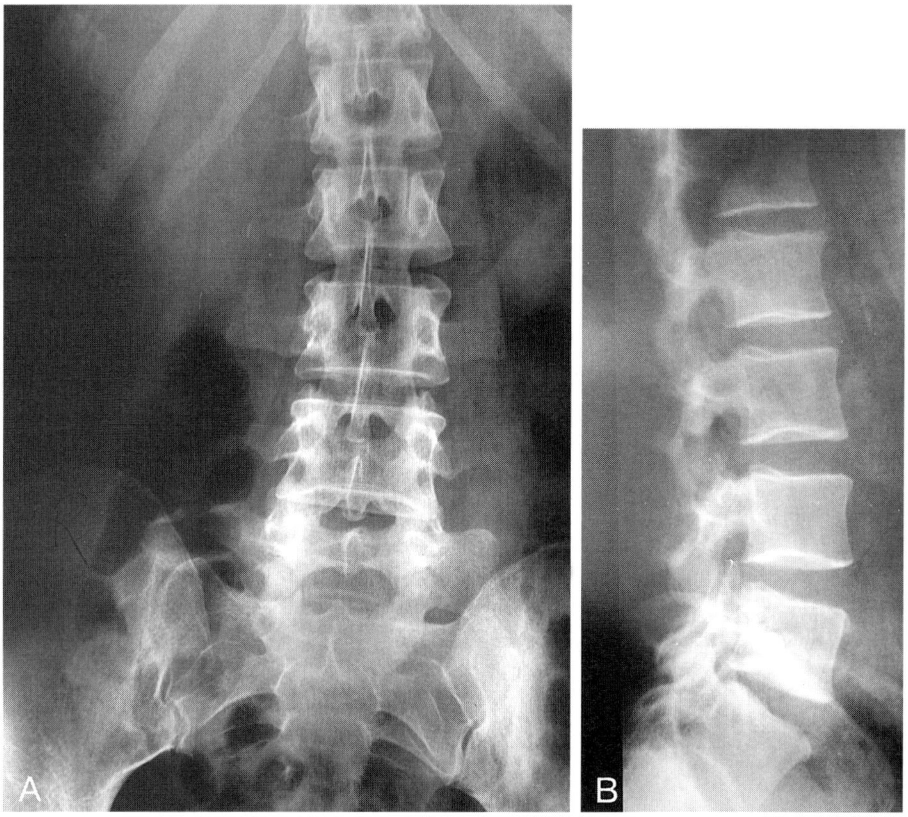

Figure 1.29 **A.** *Five lumbar vertebrae with the last level fixed to the pelvis and nonmobile. Some radiologists might try to label the last mobile level (L5–S1), which would present serious problems to the surgeon looking at Figure 1.29* **B.**

Shape of the Lumbar Spinal Canal

The upper levels of the lumbar spinal canal are fairly consistent in their shape and are shown in (Fig. 1.33). It is the L4 and L5 (S1) regions that may vary in shape (Fig. 1.34), a characteristic that can be significantly altered by degenerative changes.

The Foramen

Beneath each pedicle (actually, between two adjacent pedicles) exits the nerve root, two per level (one on each side, right and left) (Fig. 1.35). The exit is known as the foramen (opening or hole); it allows each nerve root a passage into the retroperitoneal space, where they unite to form the lumbosacral plexus. There is no agreement as to what constitutes the foramen, so we recommend that the word be changed to lateral zone of the spinal canal (Fig. 1.36). Its boundaries will be discussed later in this chapter in the section on surgical anatomy.

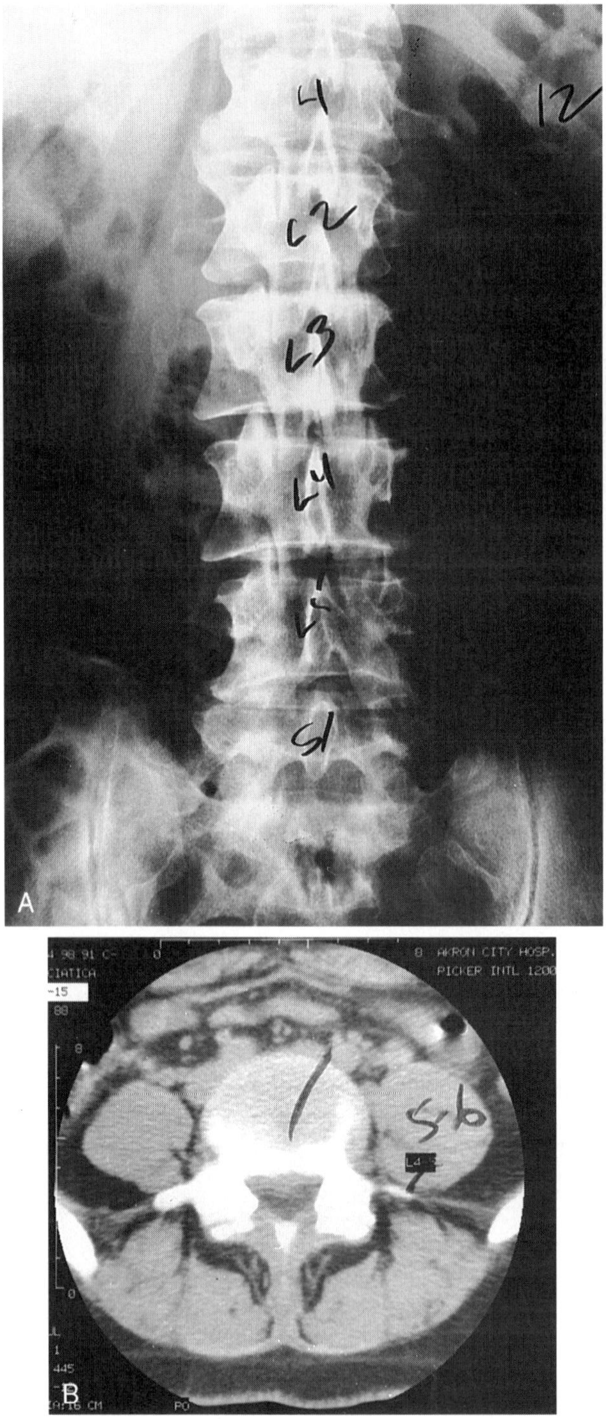

Figure 1.30 **A.** *AP radiograph numbered by a radiologist (he/she was kind enough to write the numbers very large so there would be no misunderstanding as to his/her position!).* **B.** *At another unit, patient underwent a CT scan, which showed a disc herniation at a level labeled L4–5 by the technologist but changed to L5–L6 by the radiologist (Does anybody know who's on 1st?)*

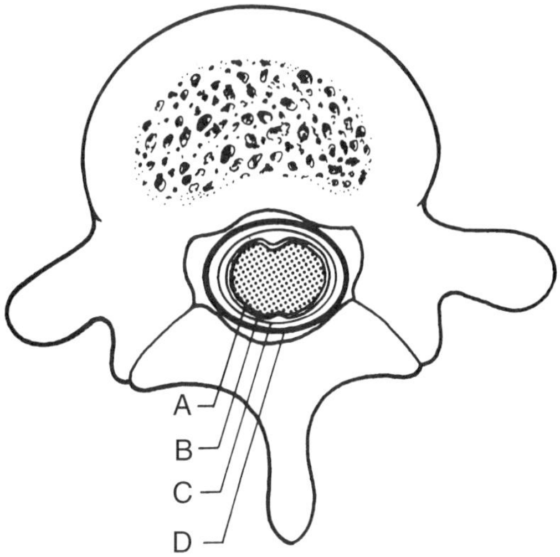

Figure 1.31 *Cross-section of the spinal canal:* **(A)** *cauda equina,* **(B)** *pia mater lining the spinal nerves,* **(C)** *arachnoid membrane,* **(D)** *common dural sac.*

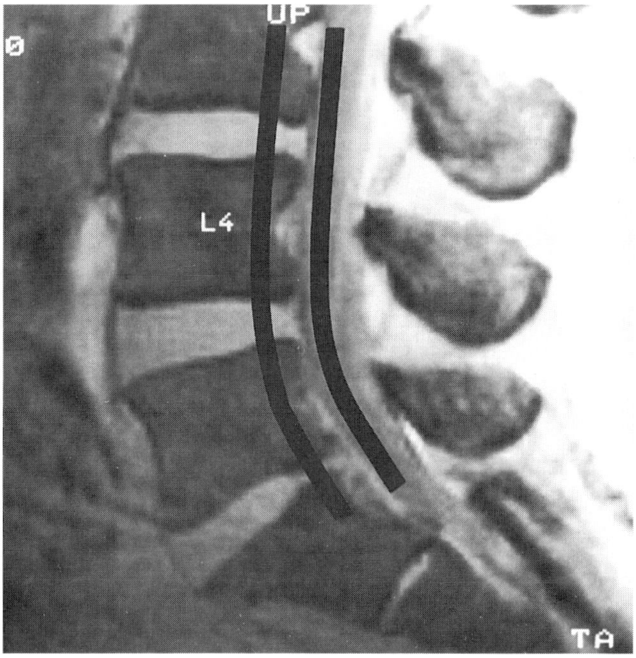

Figure 1.32 *Degenerative spine surgeons spend their entire efforts sorting out problems in the interval between the disc/vertebral column anteriorly and the common dural sac posteriorly.*

The Blood Supply to the Lumbar Spinal Canal

Arterial

Each lumbar segment is supplied by a paired set of lumbar arteries arising from the aorta (Fig. 1.37). The exception is L5, which receives its paired arterial supply from the internal iliacs (the iliolumbar arteries). As the lumbar arteries pass posteriorly from the aorta, they do so deep to the sympathetic trunk, hugging the midpoint of the vertebral body and psoas and providing a rich network of blood supply to each vertebral segment.

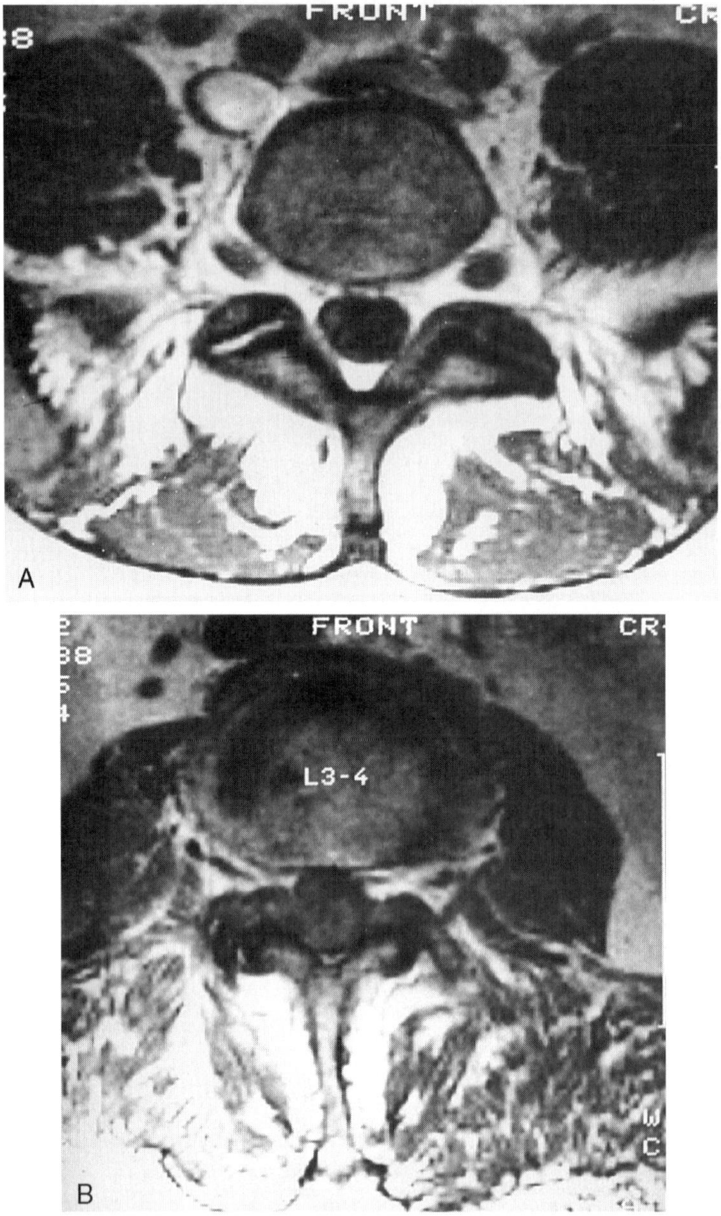

Figure 1.33 **A.** *There is much more room in the spinal canal (and less in the way of nerve roots at L5–S1) than at L3–4* **(B).**

Table 1.1. Approximate Dimensions of the Lumbar Spinal Canal

	AP	TRANSVERSE
L1	15 mm	20 mm
L3	15 mm	22 mm
L5	18 mm	28 mm

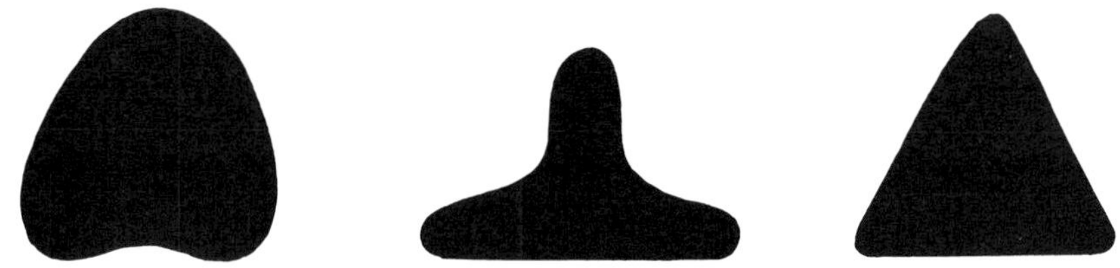

Figure 1.34 *The three canal shapes seen at L5–S1: left, oval; middle, trefoil; right, triangular.*

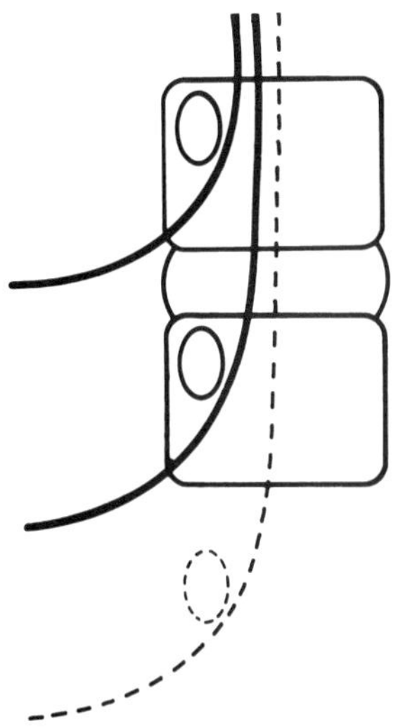

Figure 1.35 *Nerve roots exiting beneath pedicle; only the roots on the left are shown.*

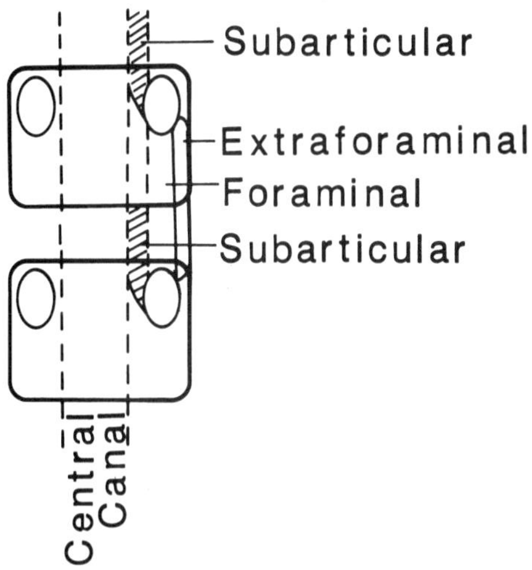

Figure 1.36 *The lateral zone is subdivided into three regions.*

At the level of the vertebral foramen, three terminal branches to the lumbar segmental artery arise (Fig. 1.37):

1. Anterior branch to the anterior abdominal wall following the anterior aspect of the transverse process and then lying on the quadratus lumborum.

2. An intermediate branch (spinal artery) that penetrates the foramen and supplies the walls and contents of the spinal canal.
3. A posterior branch (muscular artery) that passes posteriorly at the lateral edge of the pars (Fig. 1.38). Just proximal to this location at the pars, articular branches are given off. The location of this posterior branch adjacent to the lateral border of the pars is constant. If the surgical exposure requires exposure of the lateral border of the pars, this vessel will have to be cauterized.(10) From this location lateral to the pars, the muscular artery continues its posterior direction to supply to posterior paraspinal muscles.

Venous

Batson's Plexus

The valveless venous system inside the spinal canal and around the vertebral body constitutes Batson's plexus. Its importance in the spread of infection and cancer was

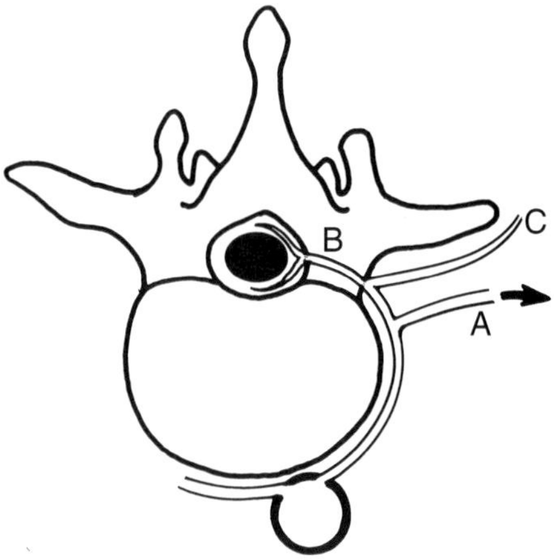

Figure 1.37 *Representation of one side of paired lumbar arteries:* **(A)** *anterior branch,* **(B)** *intermediate branch,* **(C)** *posterior branch.*

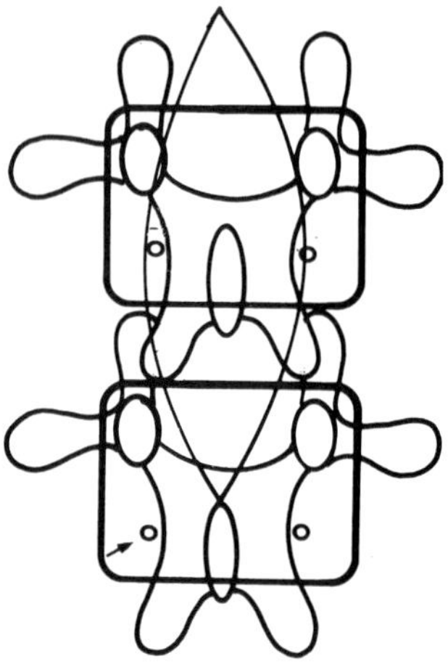

Figure 1.38 *Macnab's artery: it's always there, just lateral to pars (arrow).*

first described by Batson in 1940.(2) He described the plexus as a pathway for tumor cells and bacteria that bypass the great venous system (inferior vena cava, superior vena cava, and pulmonary circulation) to lodge in the vertebral bodies. This results in metastatic malignancy (most commonly breast and prostate) or osteomyelitis. For the purpose of this discussion, venous blood can flow through Batson's plexus to pool in the spinal surgical field.

There are three components to Batson's plexus (Fig. 1.39):

1. The internal venous system;
2. The external venous system; and
3. Rich connecting or anastomotic veins.

Components of Batson's plexus

1. Internal venous system.

   Within the spinal canal lie the following:

   a. Anterior internal vertebral veins (AIVV) on the posterior surface of the vertebrae. The basivertebral vein drains into this part of the system.
   b. Posterior internal vertebral veins (PIVV) in the anterior surface of the lamina (posterior part of the canal).
      i. Anastomotic veins connect the two systems within the spinal canal.
      ii. The internal venous systems represents a continuous venous pathway from the sacrococcygeal region to the base of the skull.
2. The external venous system.

   Longitudinally traveling veins lie:

   a. Anterior to the vertebral bodies,
   b. On the outer aspect of the lamina (posterior external vertebral plexus), and
   c. On the outer aspect of the transverse process.
3. Connectors.

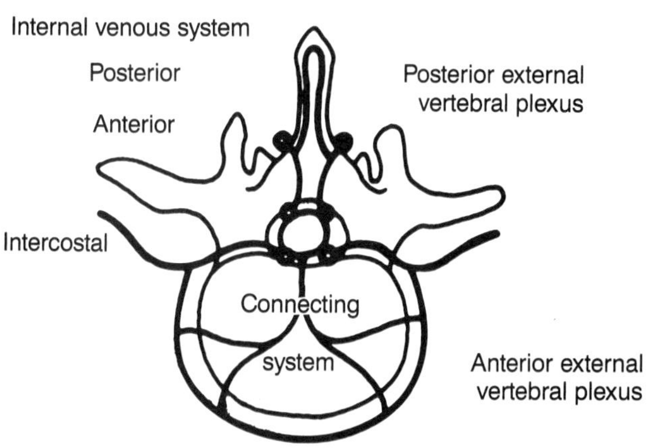

Figure 1.39 *Batson's plexus.*

There is a rich anastomotic system of veins connecting the internal to the external vertebral system and connecting both parts of the vertebral venous system to the vena cava circulation. It consists of the following:

a. basivertebral branches that pass laterally and forward to penetrate vertebral bodies;
b. radicular branches of veins that lie with spinal roots (intervertebral veins);
c. posterior anastomotic channels that penetrate ligamentum flavum; and
d. anastomotic links between the AIVV and PIVV within the spinal canal.

This rich venous plexus surrounding the spinal structures is an alternate route to the inferior vena cava system. By raising the intra-abdominal pressure or obstructing the inferior vena cava in some other fashion, blood flow will go through Batson's plexus into the spinal canal, vertebral bodies, discs, or posterior elements. It is for this reason that proper patient positioning (Fig. 1.40) is an important step in preparing for lumbar microsurgery.

NEUROANATOMY

Conus Medullaris

The spinal cord ends at approximately L1 at the conus medullaris (Fig. 1.41). The conus itself is approximately 1 vertebral body in length, and tends to end a little lower in men than in women. Connecting the tip of the conus to the coccyx is the filum terminale, a thin nonneural filament.

The conus contains the cell bodies and dendrites (axons) exiting to the peripheral nerves of the sacral plexus between L5 and S3. Pure lesions of the conus medullaris are rare but can occur in burst fractures of the thoracolumbar junction. The neurological lesion is characteristically midline and symmetric, that is, bladder and bowel sphincter disturbances with saddle anesthesia and occasionally distal lower extremity weakness (L5 and lower roots, obviously). The resulting autonomous neurogenic bladder is characterized by loss of voluntary initiation of micturition and increased residual urine (Table 1.2).

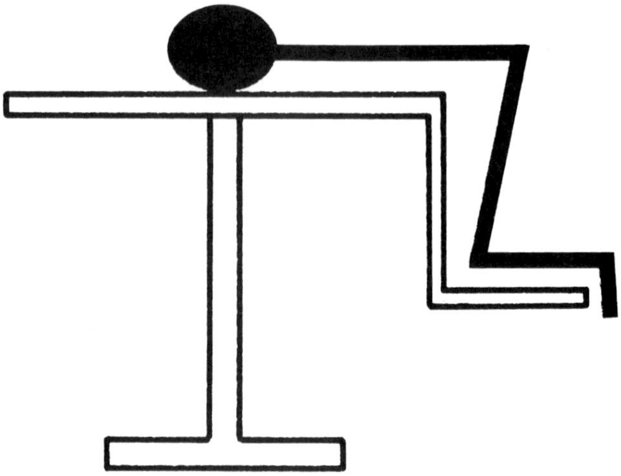

Figure 1.40 *Proper patient position in the kneeling position on the operating table so that there is no pressure on the belly to obstruct the inferior vena cava.*

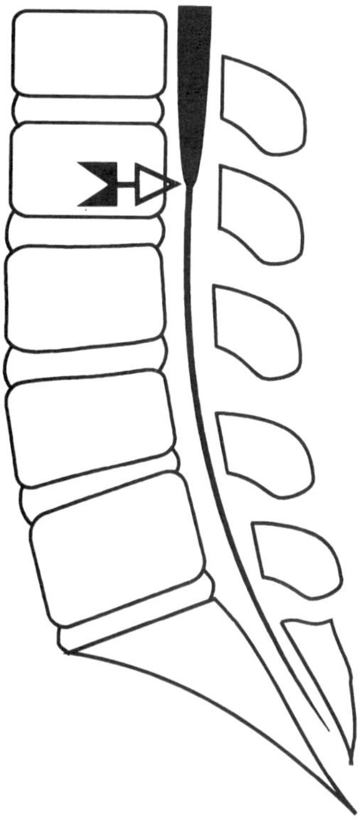

Figure 1.41 *The spinal cord ends (arrow) and the cauda equina is well formed at the L1–L2 region.*

Table 1.2. Neurogenic Bladder Dysfunction[a]

OLD TERMINOLOGY	NESBIT/LAPIDES TERMINOLOGY	CLINICAL CONCEPT
1) Upper motor neuron (UMN)[b] (Spastic) (Lesion above T11 cord)	Uninhibited neurogenic Reflex neurogenic	Failure to store
2) Lower Motor Neuron (LMN) (Flaccid) (Lesion of conus or cauda equina)	Sensory neurogenic Motor neurogenic Autonomous	Failure to empty
3) Mixed UMN LMN (Lesion T12-L1 cord)	Any of above, mixed to start, Evolving from one to the other	Failure to store or empty

[a]Modified from O'Donnell WF Urological management in the patient with acute spinal cord injury. Crit Care Clin;1987; 3:599-617.

[b]Note: It is relatively poor anatomical terminology to use *upper motor* and *lower motor* to apply to lesions of the autonomic nervous system. It is probably better to say *suprascaral* for upper motor and sacral for lower motor lesions.

The Cauda Equina

The cauda equina (horse's tail) is the collection of peripheral nerves in the common dural sheath within the lumbar spinal canal. The cauda equina begins its takeoff at the bony vertebral level T10, where the L1 nerve root exits the spinal cord (Fig. 1.41). The L2 and L3 nerve roots leave the spinal cord opposite the T11 vertebral body. As these roots start to descend in the spinal canal, they envelop the conus, which explains why a pure conus lesion is so rare. When a pure conus lesion does occur, it is said to be "root sparing" or "root escape," that is, the conus lesion involves L5 to S5 segments but spares the L1 to L3 roots that envelope the conus. The reason this can occur is that the peripheral nerve roots L1 to L3 are ensheathed in tough fibrous nerve sheaths that have a higher threshold of injury than the conus.

Slowly progressing (nontraumatic) lesions of the cauda equina more readily result in an asymmetric neurological presentation. Partial or complete lesions of the cauda equina are lower motor neuron lesions which produce degrees of flaccid paralysis (LMNL), with a sensory loss below the level of the lesion. The more significant the mass effect, the more significant the neurological presentation of multiple, bilateral root encroachment. This results classically in perineal paraesthesia; urinary retention, with or without overflow incontinence; and lower extremity pain, weakness, sensory loss, and reflex depression.

NEUROANATOMY OF BLADDER CONTROL

The previous discussions of conus and cauda lesions included loss of bladder control mechanism. What are those mechanisms?

Bladder Neurophysiology

Despite hundreds of articles available on the subject of lower urinary tract control, it is impossible to find a consensus on how lesions in the lumbar spine affect bladder functions.(7, 12, 17) There is a lack of agreement among the various authors because of one or more of the following reasons:

1. Variations in the degree of the neurological lesion.
   a. Lesions may be complete or incomplete.
   b. Lesions may be pure motor/pure sensory or mixed. These variations are not different than the variations that occur when a herniated nucleus pulposus compresses a nerve root.
2. Unilateral neurological lesions occur in a bilaterally innervated system.
3. Variations in an individual's neurological control of bladder function.
4. Complications, such as bladder infections or outflow obstruction (prostatic hypertrophy), that confuse the neurological lesion.
5. Over time, overdistention of the bladder will lead to loss of inherent neuronal activity in the bladder wall.

Derangement in micturition due to a neurological lesion has been designated "neurogenic bladder." It is better to be called neurogenic micturition abnormalities to remove focus on the bladder, which is only a part of the micturition system. On the other hand, the bladder is the center of activity for micturition, storing, and when appropriate, expelling urine. Table 1.2 presents a classification of neurogenic bladder dysfunction.

Neurogenic bladder symptoms can be divided into two groups.

1. Retention.
2. Incontinence.
   a. Failure of storage (nonneurogenic stress incontinence);
   b. Failure of emptying (leading to overflow incontinence); and
   c. Failure of control (uninhibited or reflex voiding).

Symptoms secondary to infection (dysuria, urgency, frequency) are not included.

Physiology of Micturition

Let's step back for a moment and consider bladder innervation. There are basically four neurological systems involved in bladder control (Table 1.3).

1. Higher centers,
2. Parasympathetic system: autonomic nervous system,
3. Sympathetic system: autonomic nervous system, and
4. Somatic voluntary nervous system.

Let us focus on the autonomic system (Fig. 1.42).

Autonomic Nervous System

The autonomic nervous system is the visceral or vegetative nervous system that stimulates and controls structures not under conscious (somatic) control. The (autonomic nervous) system stimulates and modulates three types of tissue:

1. Heart muscle,
2. Glands, and
3. All smooth muscle, for example, detrusor (bladder wall and internal sphincter).

Table 1.3. The Four Neurological Systems Involved in Bladder Control

SYSTEM	NERVE	INNERVATION	ACTION
1) Higher centers	Spinal tracts	Modifier of systems below	Inhibit and facilitate systems below
2) Parasympathetic	Pelvic nerves (S2,3,4)	Smooth muscle: Bladder wall (detrusor) Internal sphincter	Promotes micturition (emptying), causes contraction of detrusor, relaxes internal sphincter
3) Sympathetic	From lower thoracic upper lumbar via hypogastric plexus	Smooth muscle: Bladder wall (α & β) Internal sphincter (α)	Promotes storage, relaxes detrusor, contracts internal sphincter
4) Somatic	Pudendal	Striated (voluntary) muscle: external sphincter	Promotes micturition, relaxes sphincter by decreasing nerve stimulus to sphincter

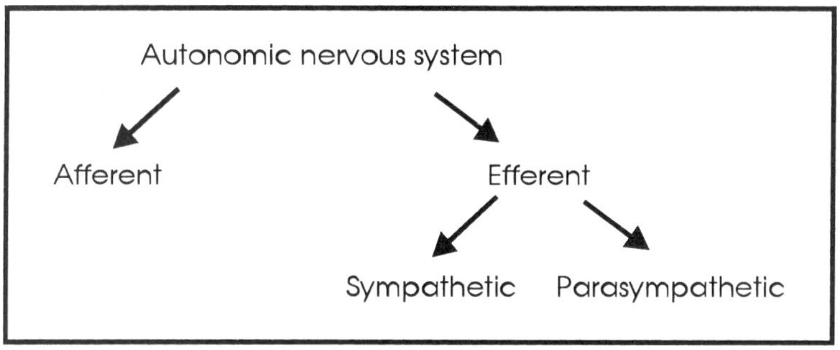

Figure 1.42 *The autonomic nervous system.*

The autonomic nervous system is structured like the somatic nervous system (Fig. 1.42) in that it has both an afferent and efferent system. The afferent system is often not described when considering the autonomic nervous system. It includes those visceroreceptive fibers that travel from smooth muscle, glands, and heart muscles to transmit messages to the central nervous system. In bladder physiology, the afferent fibers are in the parasympathetic system (sensory in function) and synapse in the sacral cord (conus) with the pudendal motor nuclei (somatic voluntary system). This system forms the bladder reflex arc, somewhat akin to the ankle reflex arc. Now here we go mixing you up by telling you we will talk about the autonomic nervous system and proceeding to talk about the somatic voluntary system!

So let us talk about the classical efferent side of the autonomic system. There are two components to the efferent side:

1. Sympathetic, and
2. Parasympathetic (it has both afferent and efferent functions).

By and large, the separate sympathetic and parasympathetic systems innervate structures together and work in an antagonistic fashion. Together, they balance vegetative activity. This balance can be upset by:

1. Stimulating one of the efferents, and
2. Blocking the other efferent.

Sympathetic Nervous System

The sympathetic nervous system dominates in stress—fight or flight. It is a two-neuron system, with the cell body of the first neuron located in the lateral gray horn of the spinal cord, T1 to L3 (Fig. 1.43). The sympathetic efferent system is known as the thoracolumbar outflow.

The fibers of this first-level neuron leave the cord by way of the ventral roots, from which they leave as a communicating ramus. The nerve fibers in this ramus enter the sympathetic trunk. On entering the sympathetic trunk, these first-order neurons follow one of three courses (Fig. 1.44).

1. The neurons synapse in the sympathetic ganglion, to become second-order neurons that travel to the end-organ.
2. The first-order neuron travels up and down the sympathetic trunk before synapsing to become a second-order neuron.
3. The first-order neuron travels directly through the sympathetic trunk to arrive at another ganglion before synapsing with the second-order neuron. These particular nerves leave the sympathetic chain as splanchnics. They enter the superior and inferior mesenteric ganglia as preganglionic fibers. The postganglionic (second-order) fibers spread out over the blood vessels and other smooth muscles of the organs: urinary bladder, genital organs, and the descending and sigmoid colon.

Because the first-order neuron is myelinated, the ramus leaving the ventral root is a communicating white preganglionic ramus. The second-order neuron that returns the nerve root is a nonmyelinated fiber and thus, is a communicating gray postganglionic ramus.

This system is known as the adrenergic nervous system.

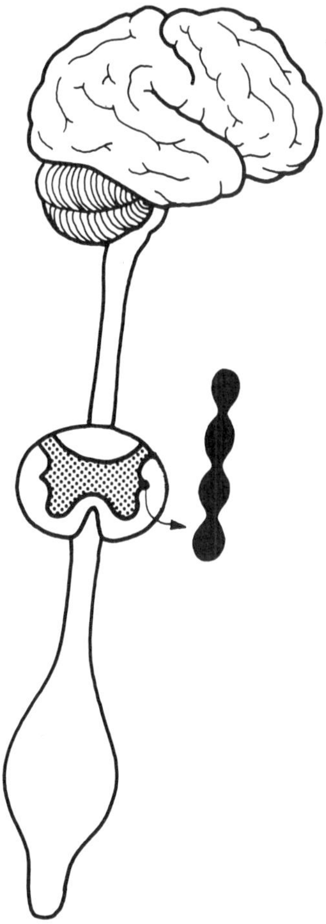

Figure 1.43 *The origin of the preganglionic sympathetic fibers is from the thoracolumbar spinal cord levels. The fibers enter the chain of sympathetic ganglia.*

We have done something else to confuse you. We have taken the usual tack of describing the sympathetic side of the efferent autonomic nervous system, when in fact it is much less important and less understood in bladder control when compared with the parasympathetic system. Do not despair; it gets clearer in a moment.

Parasympathetic Nervous System

The parasympathetic nervous system dominates in relaxed situations; that is, it slows the heart and increases bladder and bowel activity. It is also a two-neuron system with preganglionic and postganglionic components.

The cell body of the first neuron is in the cranial or sacral sections of the central nervous system (Fig. 1.45). This is why the parasympathetic nervous system is sometimes known as the craniosacral outflow. The cranial nerves that are parasympathetic in nature are the third, seventh, ninth, and tenth. The sacral preganglionic fibers have their cell body in the lateral area of the gray matter from S2 to S4. The preganglionic fibers leave by way of the ventral roots and then split off to form the pelvic splanchnic nerve (nervi erigentes) (Fig 1.46). The pelvic splanchnic nerve synapses in the walls of the descending colon, ureter, bladder, and genital organs.

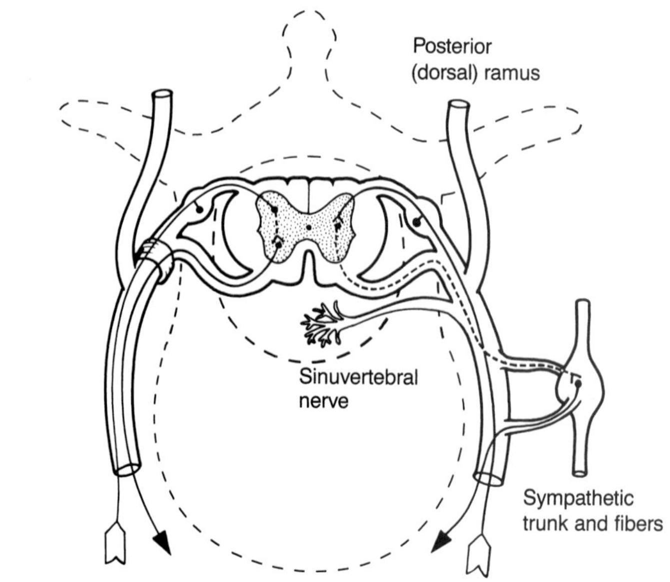

Figure 1.44 *The proximal portion of the peripheral nerve fiber tracts. The sympathetic nervous system: first- and second-order (first- and second-level) neurons. The second-order lumbar neuron will innervate the blood vessels and sweat glands of the lower extremity. The sinuvertebral nerve will also carry second-order neurons to the blood vessels of the spinal canal.*

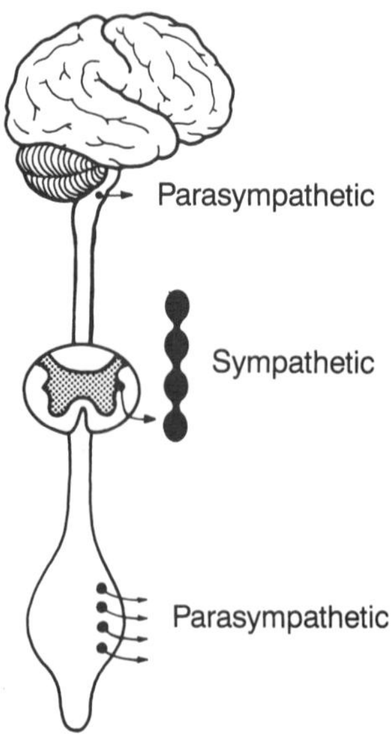

Figure 1.45 *The preganglionic parasympathetic fibers originate in the cranial and sacral regions of the brain stem and spinal cord.*

The Somatic (Voluntary) Nervous System

This is shown in Figure 1.47.

We have described four neurological systems involved in bladder control (the higher centers, two autonomic [parasympathetic and sympathetic], and the somatic). Now let us describe the four loops or reflex arcs they form.(12)

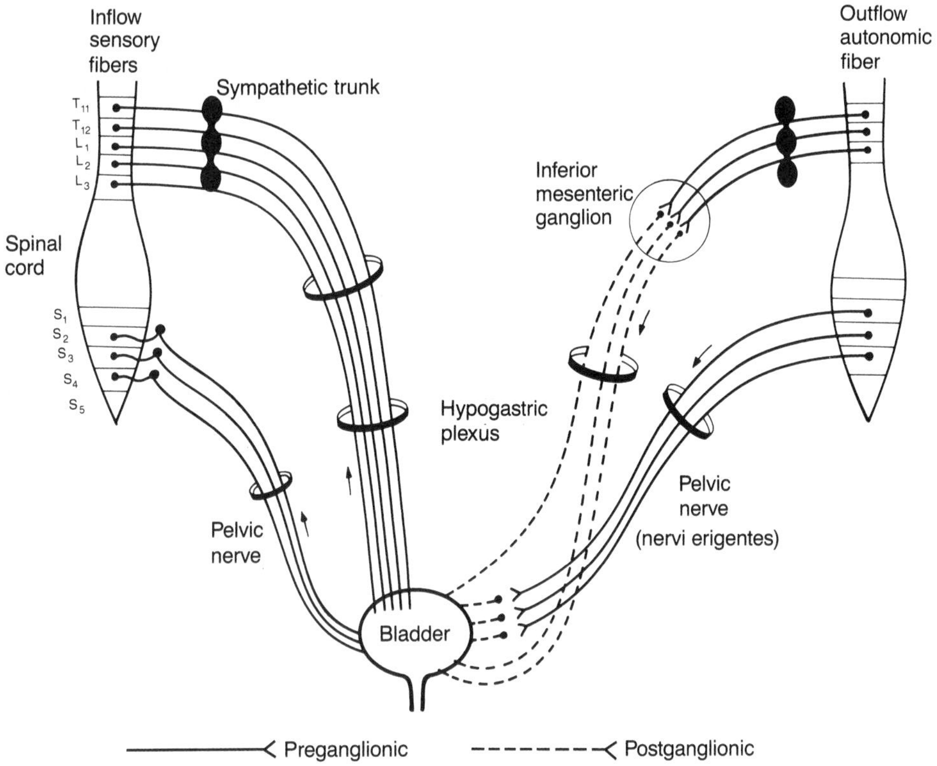

Figure 1.46 *Autonomic efferent (right) and afferent (left) fibers, including the nervi erigentes.*

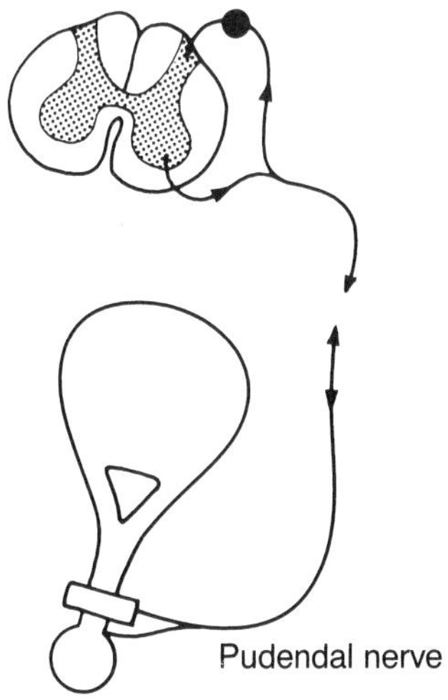

Figure 1.47 *The somatic (voluntary) control of bladder function. The pudendal nerve arises from the 2nd, 3rd, and 4th sacral segments. It supplies sensory fibers to the perineum and motor control to the anal sphincter and the external bladder sphincter.*

Loop 1 Figure 1.48 presents the pathways from frontal lobes to the brain stem and is concerned with volitional micturition.

Loop 2 Figure 1.48 represents the motor and sensory fiber innervation to the detrusor muscle. These travel peripherally in the pelvic nerve and in the retrospinal tracts in the spinal cord.

Figure 1.48 *Loop 1: The higher-center loop, above the brain stem. Loop 2: The spinal cord and peripheral autonomic motor and sensory pathways.*

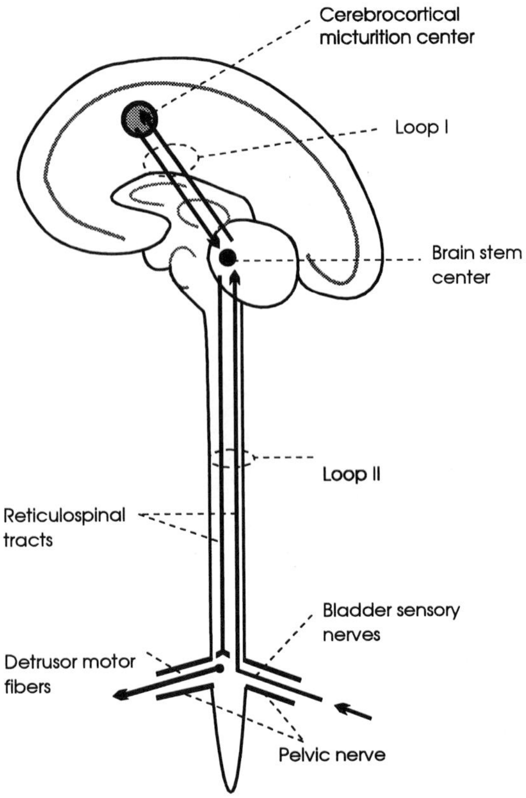

Loop 3 Figure 1.49 is made up of sensory fibers from the detrusor muscle, which, in the sacral spinal cord, synapses on the pudendal motor nucleus. This results in inhibition of the motor nerve impulses and relaxation of the periurethral striated musculature.

Loop 4 Figure 1.50 is made up of supraspinal and segmented innervation of the periurethral striated musculature in the bulbocavernosus reflex.

Loops 1 and 2 are responsible for initiating the micturition reflex, and Loops 3 and 4 are responsible for sustaining voiding.

Physiology of micturition can be seen as three separate phenomena:

1. Bladder filling,
2. Bladder emptying, and
3. Bladder control.

Bladder Filling

This portion of micturition occurs as a result of two phenomena:

1. Contraction of the external sphincter (somatic motor leads to increased activity in Loop 3), and
2. Relaxation of the bladder wall (autonomic motor leads to decreased parasympathetic activity in Loop 2).

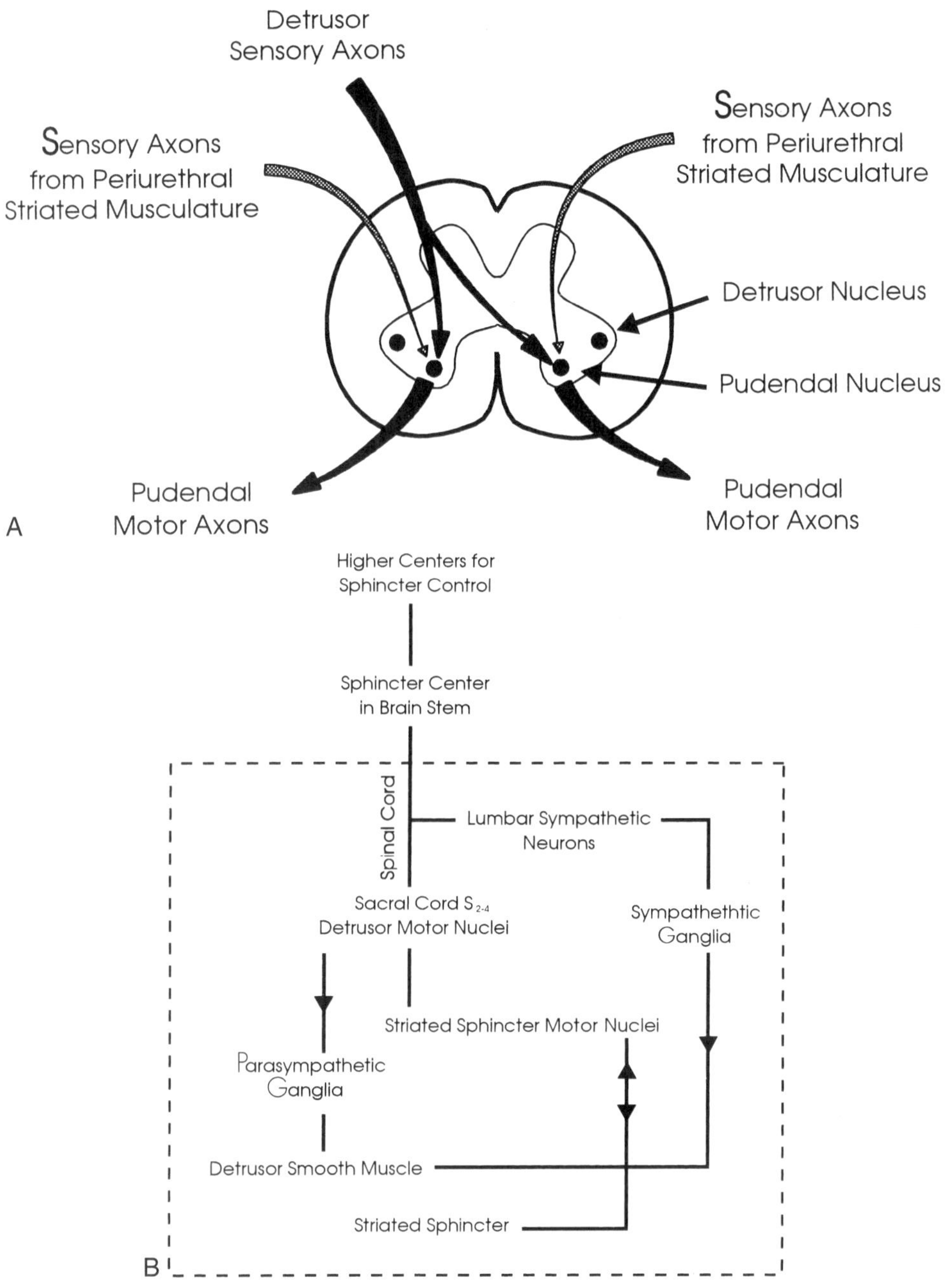

Figure 1.49 **A.** *Loop 3: Probably the most difficult loop to understand; its interrelationship is diagramed in Figure* **B.**

Role of the Sympathetic Nervous System The role of the sympathetic nervous system in bladder filling is controversial. It appears to provide active sensory supply to the trigone. As a result of increased bladder volume, there is stimulation of the sympathetic fibers that lead to internal sphincter contraction in the bladder neck and proximal urethra, thereby allowing further urine storage.

Figure 1.50 *Loop 4: The voluntary system (Fig. 1.47), with higher center modulation.*

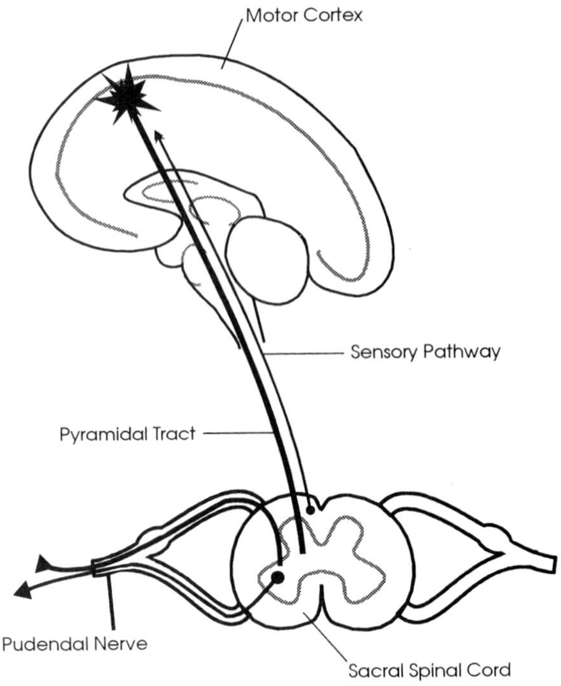

Bladder filling is also known as the sympathetic state or parasympathetic inhibition stage. Bladder filling occurs because of three factors:

1. Accommodation of increased volumes of urine at low bladder pressure,
2. Closed bladder outlet at rest and during increased intra-abdominal pressure, and
3. Absence of involuntary (uninhibited) bladder contraction.

Bladder Emptying

Bladder emptying is considered the parasympathetic phase of micturition. It depends on the following factors (Loops 2 and 3):

1. Coordinated bladder smooth muscle contraction.
2. Lowering of resistance at the level of:
   a. Smooth muscle of the bladder neck and proximal sphincter (smooth muscle sphincter);
   b. Striated musculature surrounding proximal urethra (striated muscle sphincter); and
3. No anatomic obstruction from conditions such as an enlarged prostrate or infection.

The bladder that is filled and then prepares for emptying introduces the subject of bladder control. The increased intravesical pressure leads to the sensation of distention, which results in the initiation of voluntary-induced bladder contraction (Loop 1).

Bladder Control

There are two types of bladder control:

1. Afferent (autonomic and somatic impulses to signify fullness); and
2. Efferent.

It is best to consider efferent bladder function from the central nervous system distally:

1. Ascending and descending spinal cord pathways from the micturition center in the brain stem offer facilitatory and inhibitory influences on bladder control. It is at this level where conscious control of micturition is effected (Loop 1).
2. The second factor is multifactorial:
   a. The highly coordinated parasympathetically induced contraction of the bladder wall, and
   b. The depression of sympathetic inhibitory reflexes. In addition, there is
   c. Inhibition of somatic neural discharge to the striated pelvic floor musculature, and
   d. Shaping, or funneling, of the bladder outlet (Loop 2).

Mechanical factors such as intra-abdominal pressure and outflow obstruction ultimately affect the continuity of urine excretion.

Abdominal pressure

Abdominal pressure can have a direct effect on urinary control (Fig. 1.51). The abdominal musculature is innervated from a level cephalad to L1. Thus, stimulation of the nerves that control the abdominal wall can lead to an increase in intra-abdominal pressure which, in turn, increases the pressure in the pelvic floor and increases the pressure to close down the proximal urethra. This, in turn, offers obstruction to the outflow of urine.

Paralysis of the pelvic floor through a cauda equina lesion can lead to weakening of the pelvic floor mechanism and a resulting leaking of urine under stress.

Types of Bladder Lesions Encountered in Spine Conditions (Table 1.2)

Reflex Neurogenic Bladder (Complete Upper Motor Neuron Lesion)

Lesion The etiology of this bladder problem is interruption of the ascending and descending spinal cord tracts above the spinal cord segment of T11. This leaves the bladder reflex intact but interferes with higher function control.

Cause The cause of this lesion is traumatic paraplegia (after spinal shock has passed); transverse myelitis; multiple sclerosis; extradural abscesses; syringomyelia; and tumors of the spinal cord.

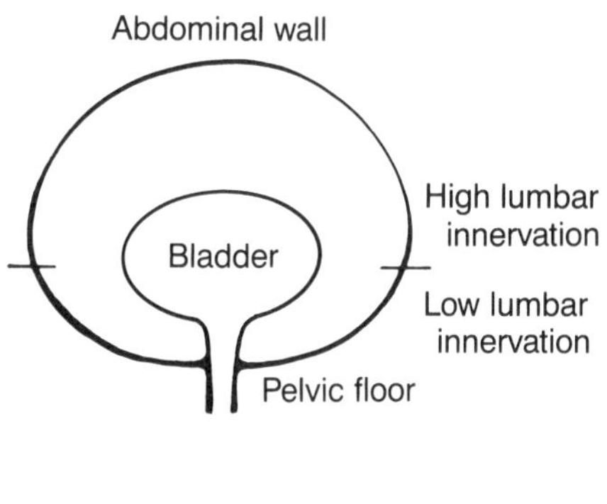

Figure 1.51 *The effect of abdominal pressure on bladder control; see text for discussion.*

The result The actual lesion interrupts bladder sensation and allows for uninhibited contractions to occur. The patient is unable to initiate micturition voluntarily, but there are involuntary spurts of voiding. This incontinence usually occurs without the sensation of urgency.

Spinal shock Spinal shock is the state that intervenes between the onset of a total spinal cord section and the re-establishment of reflex function (eg, the reappearance of the bulbocavernosus reflex or the anal wink). It is manifested by urinary retention resulting from (1) flaccid paralysis, and (2) suppression of deep tendon reflexes. After spinal shock passes (2–14+ days), there is detrusor hyperreflexia with the reflex bladder as previously described.

Uninhibited Neurogenic Bladder (Incomplete Upper Motor Lesion)

Lesion There is a loss in inhibiting impulses from the supraspinal centers that occurs as a result of interruption in the descending pathways of the spinal cord.

Cause The etiology of such lesions resides in cerebrovascular accidents (CVAs), brain tumors, and disseminated cord lesions such as multiple sclerosis. On occasion, cervical spondylosis will cause an uninhibited neurogenic bladder.

The result The patient can initiate micturition voluntarily but cannot store enough urine to do so normally. The patient establishes the voiding pattern of an infant. As the bladder fills, the patient suddenly becomes aware of a desire to void at a volume less than normal bladder capacity. Thus, the clinical presentation is one of increased urinary frequency and incontinence.

The Autonomous Neurogenic Bladder (Complete Lower Motor Neuron Lesion)

Lesion This lesion occurs as a result of the loss of all nerve connections between the bladder and the sacral reflex center in the conus. Most often, it is a lesion of the cauda equina.

Causes The causes include such conditions as massive midline lumbar disc herniation, myelomeningocele, radical pelvic surgery, trauma, infection, and tumor affecting the cauda equina.

The result As a result of this, bladder sensation is lost, and the ability of the bladder to contract is absent, leading to urinary retention and overflow or dribbling incontinence.

Incomplete Lower Motor Neuron Lesion (Sensory Paralytic Bladder)

Lesion This lesion is either an interruption of the sensory limb of the sacral reflex arc or an interruption of the long ascending spinal cord tracts.

Causes Causes include such conditions as a herniated nucleus pulposus, spinal stenosis, diabetes mellitus, and central nervous system syphilis.

The result The patient is unaware that the bladder is filling, and he/she does not receive any stimuli to void when the bladder is full, leading to chronic overdistention of the bladder and chronic overflow incontinence.

Incomplete Lower Motor Neuron Lesion (Motor Paralytic Bladder)

Lesion This lesion involves the motor or parasympathetic outflow from the second, third, and fourth sacral spinal cord segments.

Cause Causes include a disc herniation and cauda equina lesion, such as spinal stenosis. It may also occur in a peripheral neuropathy.

The result Bladder sensation is still intact, but the patient cannot initiate the voiding action, resulting in acute, painful, urinary retention. Subsequently, bladder atony intervenes.

Chemistry of Autonomic Nervous System Control

The nature of the chemical transmission in the autonomic nervous system is outlined in Table 1.4. The neurotransmitters for excitation of the autonomic nervous system are either norepinephrine (sympathetic) or acetylcholine (parasympathetic). The acetylcholine- receptor sites are also divided into:

1. Muscarinic: activated by muscarine and blocked by atropine. (Bethanechol [Urecholine] [Merck & Co., Inc., West Point, Penna.] stimulates at this level. It is the cholinergic drug with the most selective action on the bladder.) Bethanechol is used orally or subcutaneously in a dose of 10–25 mg to stimulate bladder action. It should not be used in patients in whom a general parasympathetic stimulation could be a problem. This includes patients with coronary artery disease (because of the hypotensive effect of bethanechol) and those with peptic ulcer disease (because of the increased gastric stimulation). Note that atropine will block the effect of bethanechol.
2. Nicotinic: activated by nicotine and blocked by curare.

Table 1.4. Chemical and Drug Aspects of Autonomic Nervous Systems

- Parasympathetic effect (postganglionic cholinergic)
  - Stimulation (slow heart, $\uparrow$ peristalsis, $\uparrow$ bladder activity)
    - Acetylcholine
    - Pilocarpine
  - Indirect stimulation by blocking cholinesterase
    - neostigmine
  - Inhibitors of parasympathetic effect ($\uparrow$ heart rate, pupillary dilation, $\downarrow$ Bronchial secretions, vasodilation and $\uparrow$ bladder activity)
    - Atropine
    - Scopolamine
- Sympathetic effect (postganglionic adrenergic)
  - Stimulation ($\uparrow$ heart rate, $\uparrow$ blood pressure, $\downarrow$ bladder contraction)
    - adrenaline
  - Inhibitors (α-blockers)
  - Inhibitors (β=blockers)

Norepinephrine-receptor sites are adrenergic and are further divided into α and β segments.

The α effect includes vasoconstriction and contraction of smooth musculature of the lower urinary tract. This effect is achieved with norepinephrine and epinephrine and is inhibited by Dibenzyline (phenoxybenzamine) (Smith Kline Beecham Consumer Brands, LP, Pittsburgh, Penna.).

The β effects are cardiac stimulation, vasodilation, and smooth muscle relaxation. The β effects in the adrenergic system are stimulated by isoproterenol and antagonized by propranolol (Inderal) (Wyeth - Ayerst Laboratories, Philadelphia, Penna.).

It is thought that there are α-adrenergic receptor sites in the bladder neck, the presence of which results in bladder neck contraction and can be blocked with an α-adrenergic blocking agent such as Dibenzyline.

The Cerebrospinal Fluid (CSF)

The cauda equina and the spinal cord float in a CSF bath (Fig. 1.31) that is contained by the common dural sac (in actuality, the arachnoid). If you have had the surgical thrill of viewing the cauda equina through the intact dura, you will have noticed that the rootlets pulsate and move within the CSF, like minnows at the edge of a pond.

Lumbar spinal surgeons spend much of their operating time looking at pulsating dura. Have you ever asked any of the following questions?

1. What makes the dura pulsate?
2. What makes the dura stop pulsating?
3. Is there any prognostic significance in the fact that the dura pulsates (or does not pulsate) after a decompressive laminectomy for spinal stenosis?

Pulsating dura is always present after a microdiscectomy for a simple disc herniation and is usually present after a microdecompression for lateral zone stenosis. After a midline decompression for spinal stenosis, a pulsating dura may or may not be present. Is that prognostically significant? The question is not answerable from any reading we have done. Although the issue seems off topic for the book, it is an interesting neurophysiological phenomenon, and perhaps including it in this book will provoke discussion and more observation.

Cerebrospinal Fluid Formation

Cerebrospinal fluid is secreted from the epithelial cells of the choroid plexus at a rate of 500 mL/d. It enters the four ventricles, and from there it flows to surround the brain, spinal cord, and cauda equina, filling and distending the subarachnoid space (Fig. 1.52). The rate of cerebrospinal fluid production is constant; any increase in CSF volume or pressure is due to causes other than increased production.

Cerebrospinal Fluid Absorption

Cerebrospinal fluid is constantly circulating in a pulsatile fashion (1) around the spinal cord and cauda equina. From the sacral dural sac, CSF flows proximally in the posterior aspect of the dural sac to become absorbed through arachnoid granulations or villi in the

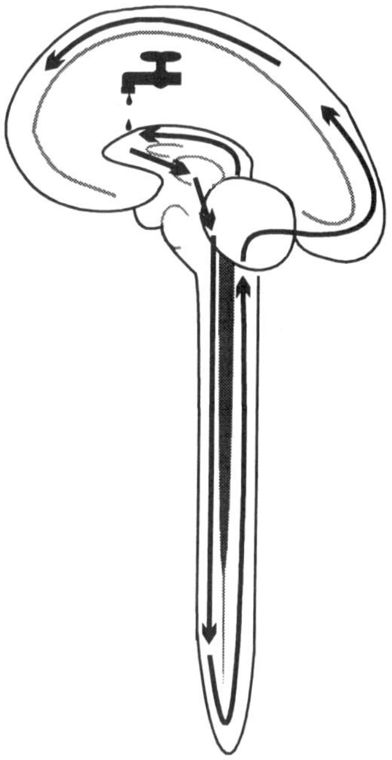

Figure 1.52 *CSF is produced by the choroid plexus (top) and travels through the ventricles, down the ventral aspect of the spinal canal, bathing the cord and cauda equina (arrows). The flow pattern reverses itself at the end of the common dural sac (sacrum), with the CSF returning posteriorly to the surface of the brain, where it is absorbed by the arachnoid granulations.*

venous sinuses over the surface of the brain. These are most numerous in the superior sagittal sinus, and therefore most absorption occurs in this sinus.

Absorption depends on a pressure gradient between the venous system and the cerebrospinal fluid:

1. High cerebrospinal fluid pressure leads to increased absorption.
2. A low cerebrospinal fluid pressure results in decreased absorption.

Causes of Pulsation in Cerebrospinal Fluid

There are two pulsatile waves in the cerebrospinal fluid:

1. Arterial A waves, and
2. Pulmonary P waves.

Arterial Pulsations

Pulsations transmitted from the arterial vessels in the circle of Willis and the cerebral cortex present the main source of cerebrospinal fluid pulsations (1). The resulting A wave is most prominent in the cervical canal and decreases toward the lumbar portion of the subarachnoid space where the cauda equina is located. The waves have the same pulsatile characteristics as the arterial pulse and are easily identified under the microscope.

Pulmonary Pulsations

A secondary source of a pulsatile wave in the cerebrospinal fluid is the pulmonary system. During inspiration there is an increase in the intrathoracic pressure that is transmitted through the valveless venous system, including Batson's plexus. This results in a momentary increase in cerebrospinal fluid pressure, which causes a wave of cerebrospinal fluid pulsation corresponding to respiration. This P wave is superimposed on the arterial pulsations. It is a little harder to discern than the arterial pulsations but is present in the normal subarachnoid space.

Change in Cerebrospinal Fluid Pulsations

It is generally hoped that when a spinal stenosis decompression is finished, the dura, which was nonpulsatile at the beginning of the decompression, will show renewed vigor with bounding pulsations. This fails to happen often, yet so many of these patients go on to get good results that there must be other causes of decreased dural pulsations. A variation in this consideration is the phenomenon of no dural pulsations at the end of a spinal stenosis decompression, yet obvious cerebrospinal fluid flow and arterial flow within the subarachnoid space as evidenced by the "swimming minnows" (nerve roots). This observation can be made through the nonpulsatile thinned dura that occurs in spinal stenosis.

Causes of Decreased or Absent Dural Pulsations

1. Decreased volume of cerebrospinal fluid.
   a. Cerebrospinal fluid leakage resulting from a tear during surgery or during a prior myelogram.
2. Obstruction to cerebrospinal fluid flow.
   a. Cervical,
   b. Lumbar, or
   c. Both a and b: the presence of cervical obstruction will abolish all lumbar pulsations regardless of the extent of lumbar decompression.
3. Alteration in cerebrospinal fluid dynamics.
   a. Deceased arterial pulsations (eg, hypotension),
   b. Low respiratory volume, or
   c. Positioning of patient on operating room table.
      i. Neck extension, which may further lower cervical cerebrospinal fluid pulsations; or
      ii. abdominal pressure, which prevents transmission of respiratory wave.
4. Drugs. It is possible that some of the sedative/analgesic agents used during anesthesia may decrease or abolish pulsations.
5. Dural insult. The constant dural contact with surgical instrumentation has reduced dural pulsations (in the authors' experience).

The Future

Magnetic resonance imaging (MRI) may represent a new tool for investigating cerebrospinal fluid pulsations in spinal stenosis. Articles are now appearing in the radiological literature (14) describing the increase in signal intensity (increased whiteness on T2 weighted images) in disease processes or anatomical derangements that decrease the normal amplitude of cerebrospinal fluid pulsations. In time, studies of patients with spinal stenosis, before and after decompression, will appear and help us determine the significance of dural pulsations, present or absent, at the end of a spinal stenosis decompression.

MICROSURGICAL ANATOMY OF THE LUMBAR SPINE

Introduction

This section is written largely for the spine surgical resident. We think it is fun to read, but if you do not have a surgical beat in your heart, we suggest that you "skip" to the next chapter!

Two trends are apparent in spine surgery today: (1) instrumentation, especially pedicle fixation, has opened new treatment avenues for deformity, fractures, tumors, and infections; (2) minimally invasive surgical techniques are being used to handle more and more degenerative spine problems. It would appear that the middle ground in spine surgery is fast shrinking!

If a procedure can be successfully completed through a limited surgical approach—saving normal bone and soft tissues—the spine and the patient are better off for it. These least-invasive surgical techniques have been made possible by the newer imaging modalities of MRI and computed tomography (CT), which can pinpoint the nature and location of pathology. Once localized, however, the use of percutaneous or microsurgical procedures to deal with degenerative spine lesions raises the potential for complications, such as wrong level exploration and missed pathology. The surgeon quickly learns that the problems and opportunities in least-invasive spine surgery are best mastered through an intimate understanding of spinal anatomy. To develop this understanding, the surgeon should accept the following concepts:

Concept 1: The Skeletal Anatomy of the Lumbar Spine

The anatomical unit of the lumbar spine is a vertebral body and disc below (Fig. 1.53). Just as the brain needs a skull for protection, the spinal cord and cauda equina need skeletal coverings. To provide this protection, each vertebral segment has attached posterior elements. For a moment, ignore the disc space and concentrate on an imaginary line joining the inferior pedicle borders (Fig. 1.54). There are six named posterior elements, three lying above that line (all paired) and three lying below that line (two of three paired) (Fig. 1.55). Lying right on that dividing line is the pars interarticularis.

Concept 2: Nerve Root Anatomy

The neurological structures in the lower lumbar spinal canal include the dural sheath containing the cauda equina and bilaterally exiting nerve roots for each anatomical segment. The exiting nerve root is numbered according to the pedicle beneath which it passes (Fig. 1.56), unlike the cervical spine, where a nerve root is numbered according to the pedicle above which it passes. Lumbar nerve roots are intimately related to the pedicle beneath which they pass; when looking for a nerve root in the spinal canal, a good rule to obey is to locate its adjacent pedicle. Not only does each anatomical segment have paired exiting roots, there are also the more medial traversing nerve roots (Fig. 1.57).

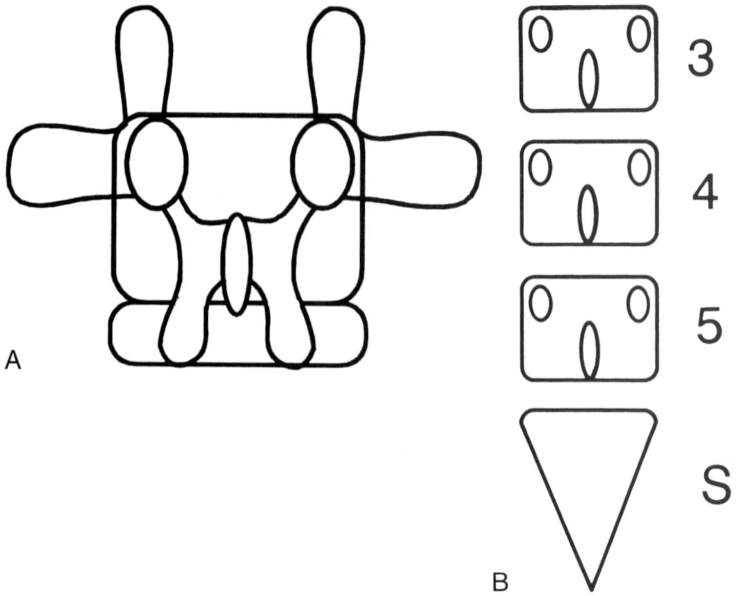

Figure 1.53 **A.** *The anatomic spine unit is the vertebral body with its disc below and the attached posterior elements.* **B.** *An assembled lower lumbar spine with bodies, pedicles, and spinous processes.*

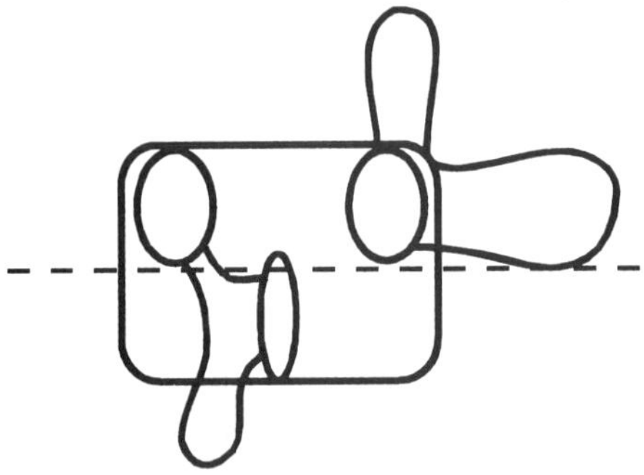

Figure 1.54 *This is the anatomic unit missing some posterior elements and the disc. Note the infrapedicular line (broken line).*

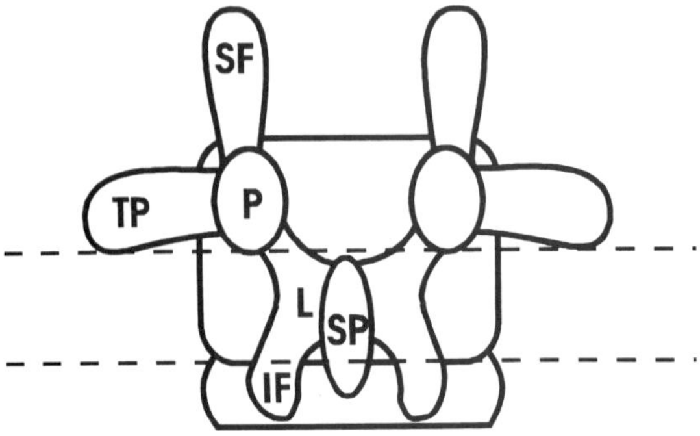

Figure 1.55 *We are now back to Figure 1.53, with the posterior elements missing on the right. The three posterior elements above the infrapedicular line are the transverse process (TP), superior facet (SF), and obviously the pedicles (P); the three posterior elements below this line are the lamina (L), spinous process (SP), and inferior facet (IF).*

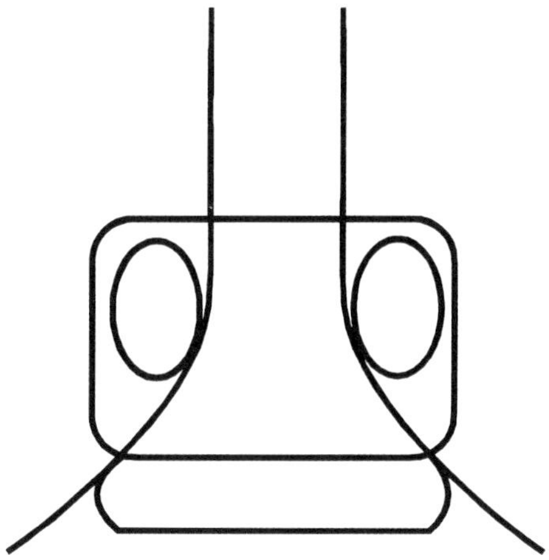

Figure 1.56 *The paired exiting roots at each level. Nerve roots are numbered according to the pedicle beneath which they pass. If this is the 4th lumbar anatomic segment, these are the 4th lumbar nerve roots.*

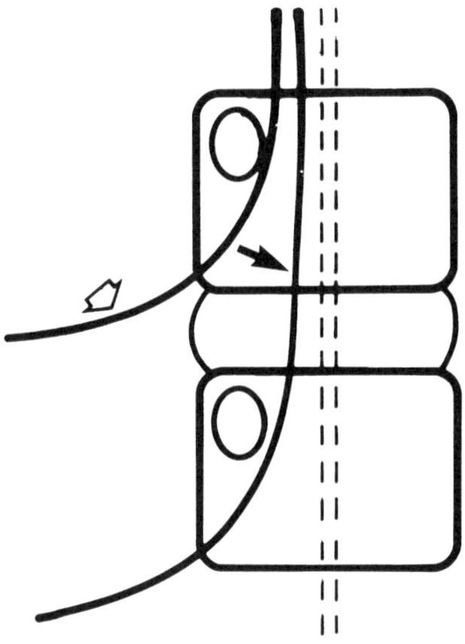

Figure 1.57 *Exiting and traversing nerve roots. The cephalad root is the exiting root (open arrow); the root beside it is the traversing root (arrow) of the upper anatomical segment. In turn, the traversing root becomes the exiting nerve root of the segment below, and the dotted roots are traversing roots of the lower segment.*

Concept 3: Imaging Localization of Pathology

The eyes of today's microsurgeon are the sensitive imaging modalities of MRI and CT. To help localize lesions within the spinal canal, a "three storied anatomical house" for each spinal segment is proposed (Fig. 1.58). This concept helps the surgeon reformat in his/her mind the exact location of pathology in the interface between the disc/vertebral column and the neurological column (Fig. 1.59).

Using the inferior border of the pedicles as an artificial division line, each anatomical segment can be divided into three "stories," as in a house. (The choice of the concept "stories in a house" will become evident in the next few pages.) Now, let us reconsider the posterior elements (take another look at Fig. 1.55). Of these six elements, two only are located in a single story: the pedicle and transverse process are located exclusively in the third story. The superior facet is not only in the third story but overlies the disc space (first

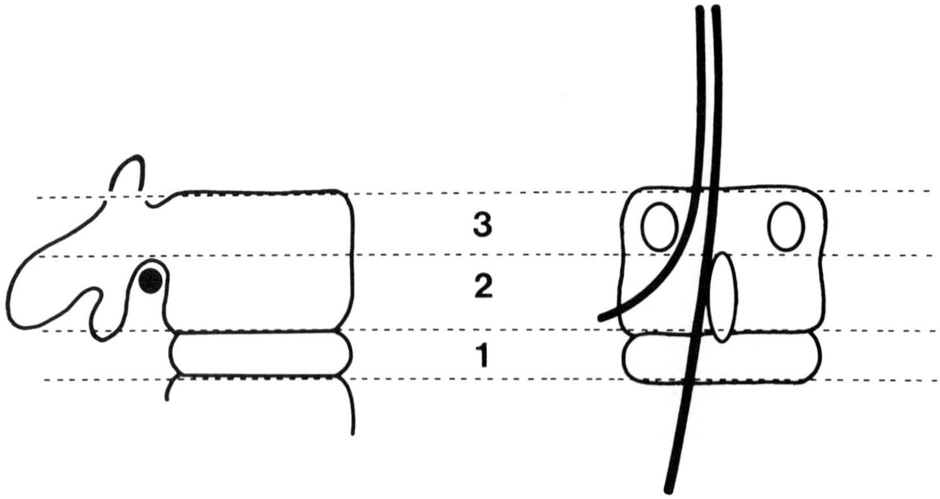

Figure 1.58 *The anatomical "house": first story, the disc; second story, the foramen; third story, the pedicle level. Note that the first and second stories are "nonpedicle" levels.*

story) of the segment above. Similarly, the inferior facet straddles the territory of the first and second stories; the cephalad border of the lamina encroaches on the third story of the same anatomical level as does the caudal border overhang the first story of that anatomical segment (Figs. 1.55, 1.56).

The next exercise is to "read the stories," an exercise that allows the surgeon to reformat and exactly localize pathology within the interface between the disc/vertebral column and the neurological column. Figures 1.60 and 1.61 show examples of "reading the stories."

Concept 4: Windows of Opportunity into the Spinal Canal

Linking the anatomical segments and studying the posterior elements, it is possible to construct three "windows of opportunity" into the spinal canal (Fig. 1.62). You are already familiar with the routine interlaminar window. This unilateral interlaminar window can be used to enter the opposite side of the spinal canal (window 2 in Fig. 1.62). The third window of opportunity into the spinal canal is the intertransverse window. The use of these three windows of opportunity into the spinal house is facilitated by the magnification and illumination inherent in the microscope.

The Interlaminar Window

The so-called "standard laminectomy," has used the interlaminar window. The salient anatomical features of this window are:

The Dimensions of the Window Note on the radiograph that with descending levels in the lumbar spine the dimensions of the interlaminar window become broader and higher (Fig. 1.63). This makes entry into the canal for an L5–S1 discectomy a relatively easy procedure, compared to, say, an L2–3 discectomy.

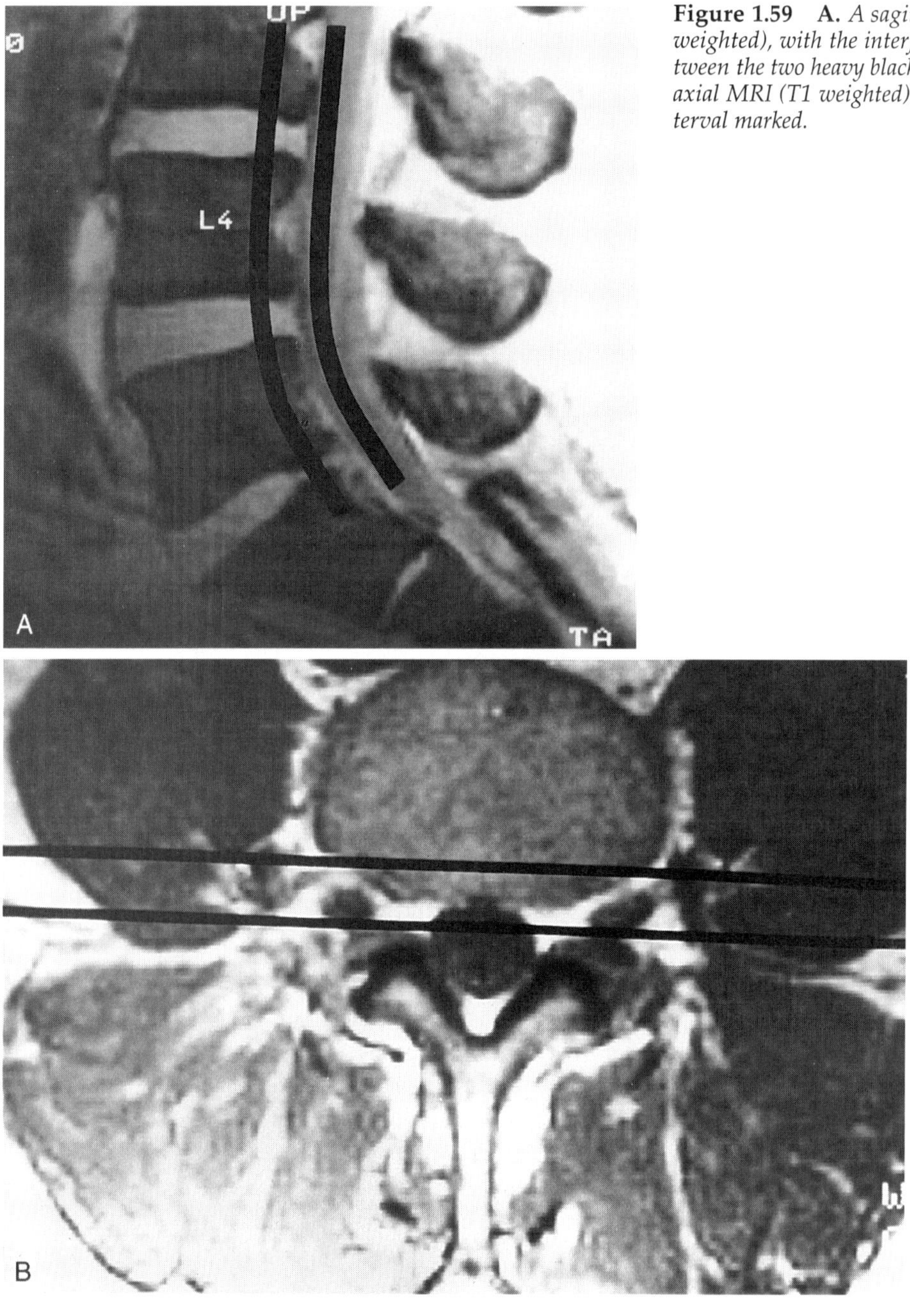

Figure 1.59 **A.** *A sagittal MRI (T1 weighted), with the interface lying between the two heavy black lines.* **B.** *An axial MRI (T1 weighted), with the interval marked.*

Laminar Overhang Also note that with ascending levels there is more of the inferior edge of the lamina that overhangs the disc space (Fig. 1.64). This is a fact that is lessened by surgical frames that flex the lumbar spine, and increased by surgical frames that allow positioning of the patient in a neutral or lordotic position (Fig. 1.65). It is also an important fact when trying to retrieve a disc herniation from the second story of L1, L2, L3, and L4 in that a considerable portion of the cephalad lamina has to be removed for a direct view of this pathology.

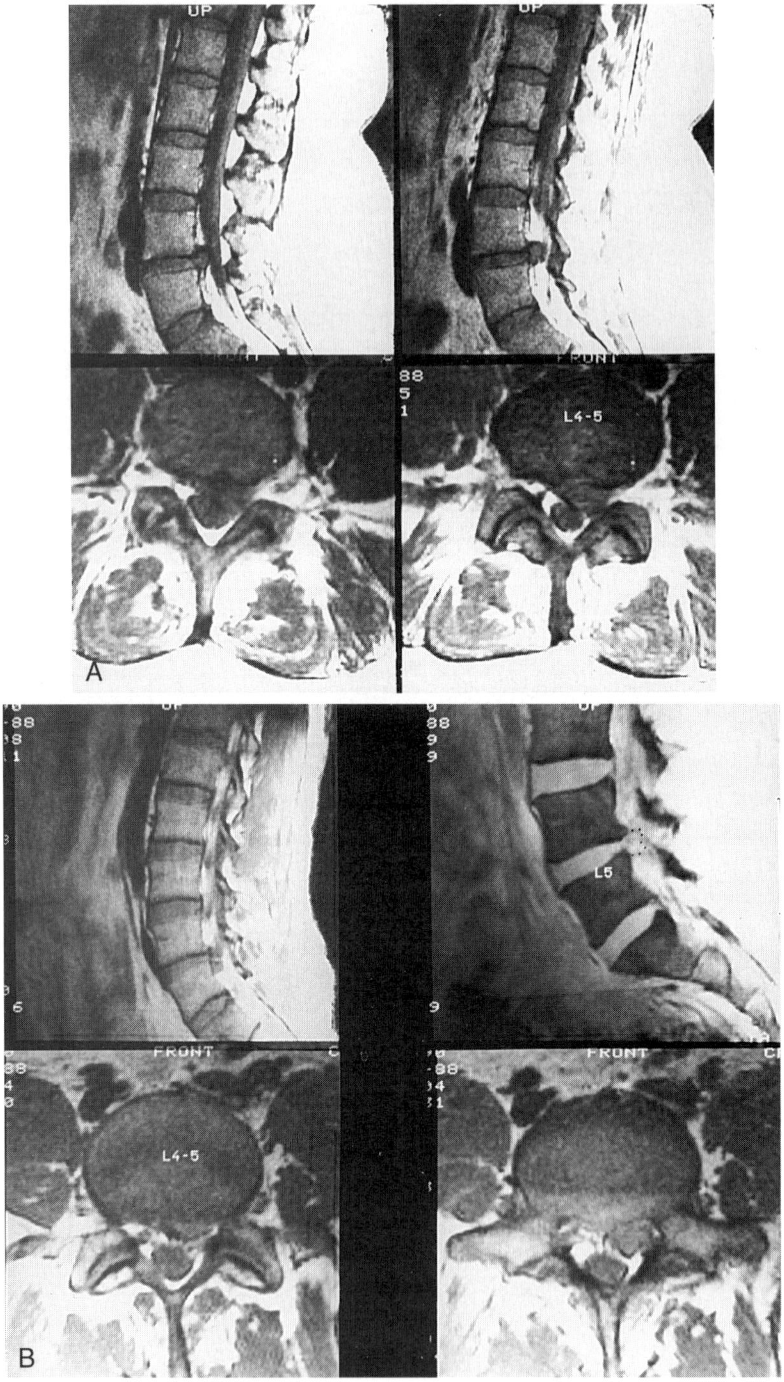

Figure 1.60 *Reading the stories:* **A.** *A disc herniation in the 1st story of L4–5.* **B.** *A disc herniation (L4–L5 [left]) starting to migrate down into the 3rd story of the anatomic segment below (the L5 anatomic segment).*

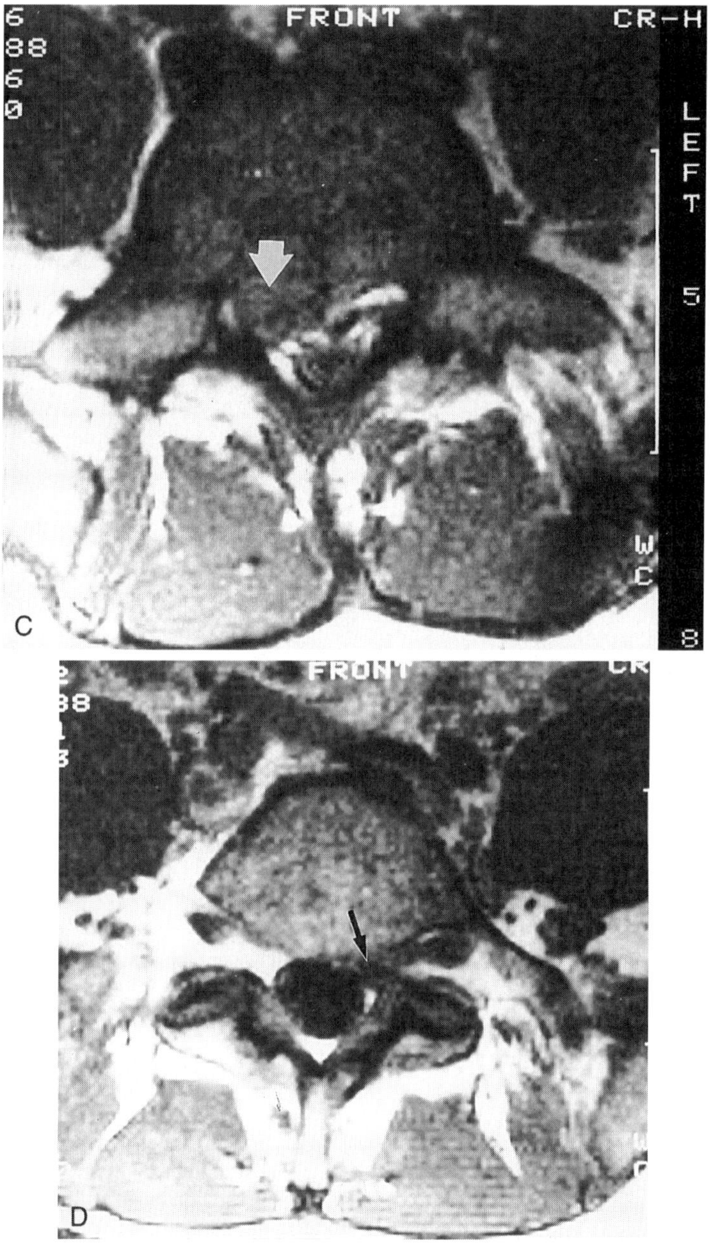

Figure 1.60 (continued) **C.** *A disc herniation that is in the 3rd story of S1 (arrow).* **D.** *A disc herniation up into the 2nd story of L5 (arrow).*

Laminar Overhang and Wrong Level Exposures Laminar overhang and the anteriorly sloping lamina create the setting for wrong level exposures (Fig. 1.66). Add to this a patient with degenerative disc disease; a narrowed interlaminar distance; a short, obese, loose jointed body on the Andrew's frame (OSI, Union City, Calif.), which cannot reduce lordosis (Fig. 1.65), and it is a reasonable expectation that a limited surgical incision will result in wrong level exposure (Fig. 1.67)! Get ready!

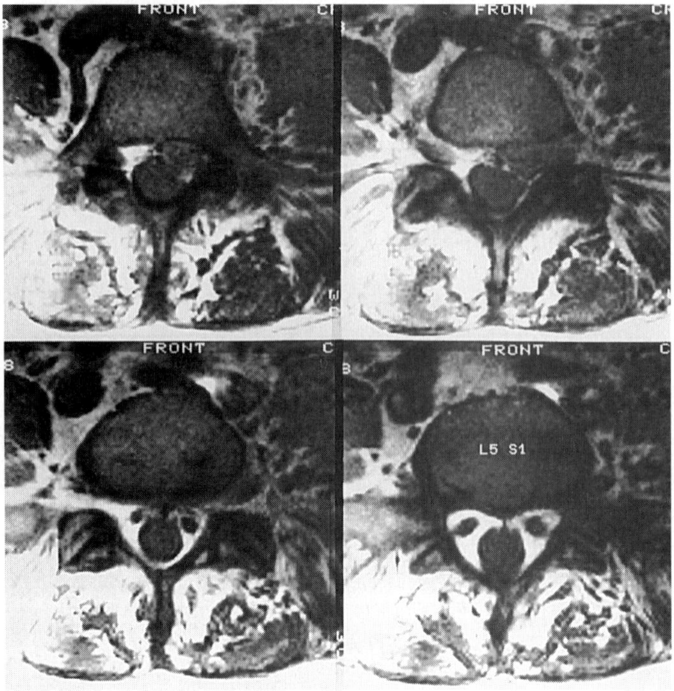

Figure 1.61 *From where did this large disc fragment arise to occupy the 3rd and 2nd stories of the 5th anatomic segment? The sagittal MRI showed that it migrated down from L4–5.*

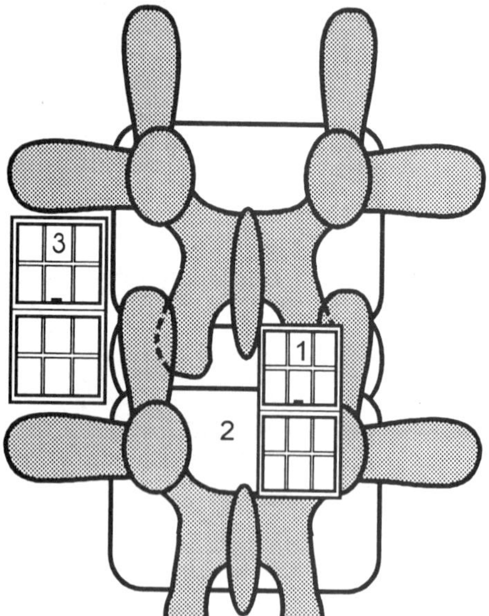

Figure 1.62 *The two windows of opportunity into the spinal house:* **(1)** *The interlaminar window on the right, and* **(3)** *the intertransverse window on the left.*

Contents of the Lumbar Spinal Canal The more proximal lumbar spinal canal levels have three salient anatomical features.

1. The more proximal levels in the lumbar spinal canal contain more neurological tissue (L1 has conus, and all the lumbar and sacral roots compared with L5, which has no cord, and only the L5 to S5 sacral roots.)

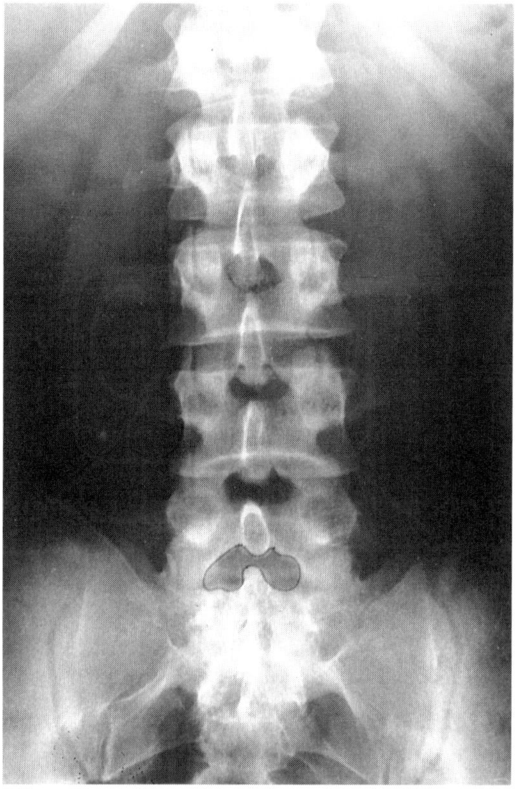

Figure 1.63 *The dimensions of the interlaminar window are outlined at L5–S1. Compare that with the interlaminar window at L2–3. Which window seems easier to enter? (If you guessed L2–3, go directly to internal medicine!)*

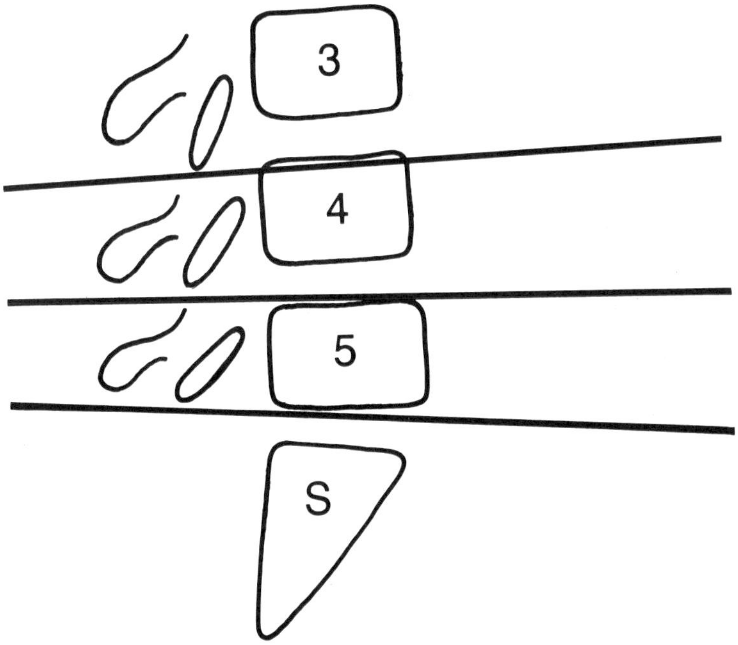

Figure 1.64 *Laminar overhang. As you ascend in lumbar spine levels, there is more overlapping of the inferior edge of the lamina with the disc space. Refer back to Figure 1.63 to see this on radiograph.*

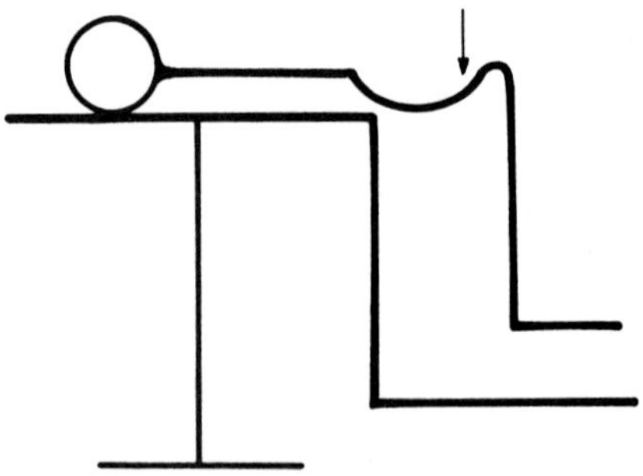

Figure 1.65 *The kneeling frames for spine surgery have one major drawback—they will not reverse lumbar lordosis in some patients, which aggravates laminar overhang from Figure 1.64.*

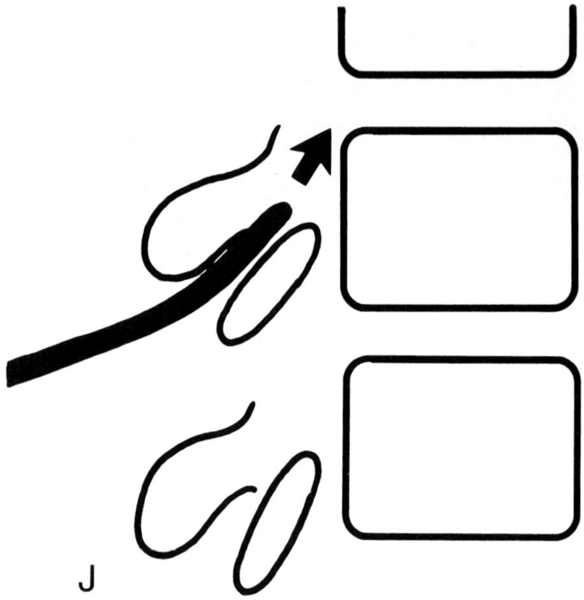

Figure 1.66 *Laminar overhang and sliding up one lamina to end up at the wrong disc space.*

2. The canal space available for neurological tissue at L1 is much reduced compared with L5 (Fig. 1.33A).
3. The proximal lumbar roots take a more horizontal course in exiting through the foramen (Fig. 1.68). This makes the L1 root less mobile than the S1 root (Fig. 1.69).

Summary

An exposure of an L2–3 disc is a much more difficult technical exercise than an L5–S1 disc because of laminar overhang, a smaller canal with greater neurological contents, and the more horizontally exiting roots. If the disc herniation is up in the second story of a proximal lumbar anatomical segment (Fig. 1.70), you have a real microsurgical challenge.

The Axillary Disc Rupture The axilla of the L5 traversing nerve root and the S1 traversing root are related to the disc space in Figure 1.71. This is an important relationship to appreciate because an axillary disc, which is more prone to occur at L5–S1 (Fig. 1.72), can displace a nerve root far into the subarticular region and out of direct view, where it can be damaged by the unwary surgeon.

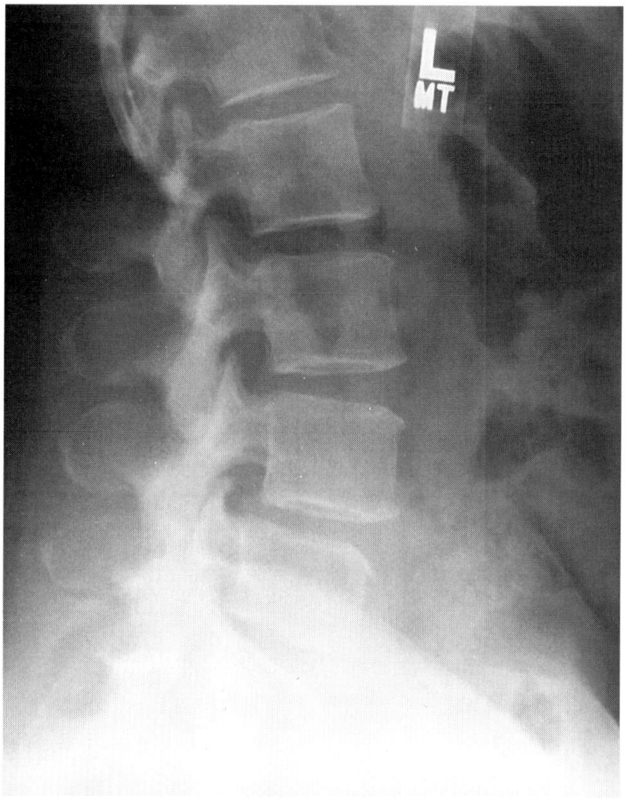

Figure 1.67 *A lateral radiograph of a patient with degenerative spondylolisthesis at L4–5, degenerative disc disease at L5–S1, and facet joint degeneration above L4–5. On the Andrews frame (OSI, Union City, Calif.), the spondylolisthesis will be increased, and laminar overhang will be significantly aggravated.*

The Migrating Disc Rupture Disc herniations usually occur in the posterolateral quadrant of the disc space, but they can migrate as extruded and sequestered fragments (Fig. 1.73). MRI scans in Figure 1.60 show migrated discal fragments, and Figure 1.74 shows how the posterior element anatomy is used to arrive at the exact location of the migrated fragment.

Locating the Interlaminar Window: "The Safety Net" After dissecting soft tissue off the interspinous/interlaminar windows and positioning the frame retractor, look for the "safety net" at the inferior tip of the inferior facet (Fig. 1.75). This area is labeled the "safety net" because it is marked by the facet fat pad (a "whiter" fat than normal); deep to the safety net lies the joint surface of the superior facet. Plunging a sharp instrument into the safety net is harmless because the cartilaginous surface of the superior facet protects the nerve root (Fig. 1.75).

Once the safety net has been identified, it is then easy to move along the cephalad or caudal laminar borders (Fig. 1.76).

Entering the Spinal Canal through the Interlaminar Window There are basically three ways to cross the ligamentum flavum to enter the spinal canal:

1. Transligamentous (Fig. 1.77).
2. Through the cephalad lamina (Fig. 1.78).
3. Through the caudal lamina (Fig. 1.80).
   a. Transligamentous (Fig. 1.77)

Figure 1.68 *Note that the proximal lumbar roots come off at a more horizontal direction compared with the S1 root, which has a much more vertical course through the spinal canal.*

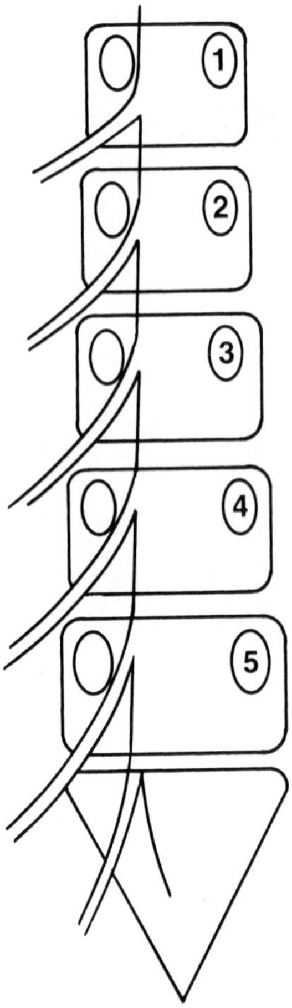

Figure 1.69 *Retraction of the L4 root is limited compared with the 1-cm retraction for the S1 root. The S1 root can easily be retracted to the midline, but this is not so for the roots above L4.*

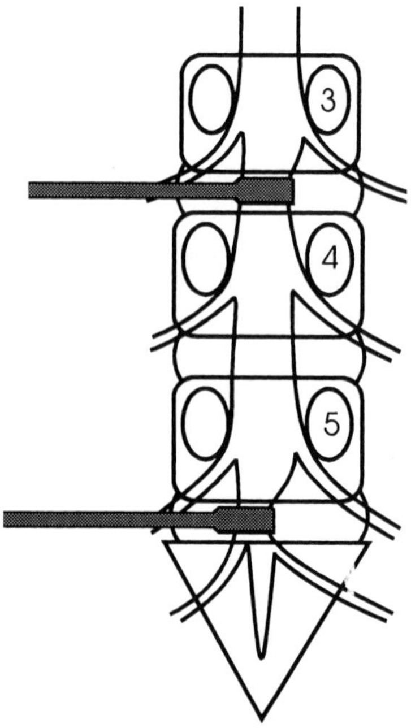

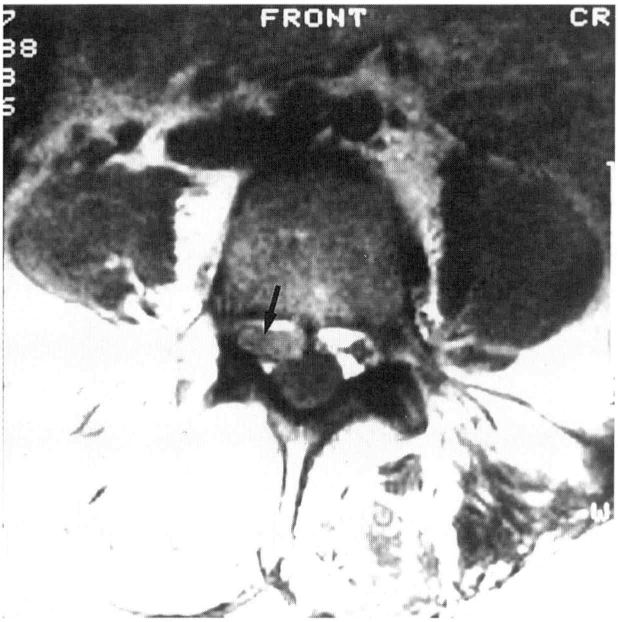

Figure 1.70 *Axial (T1) MRI showing a free fragment of disc (arrow) behind the vertebral body of L2.*

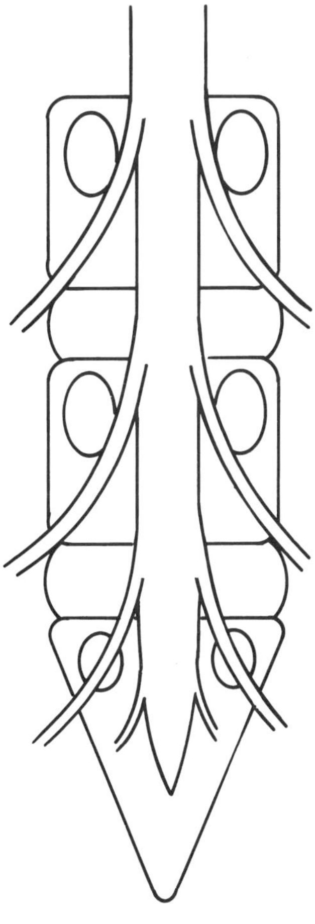

Figure 1.71 *The relationship of the axilla of the nerve root to the disc space: note that at L5–S1 the axilla is at the bottom end of the disc space, but at L4–5 the axilla is below the inferior edge of the disc space.*

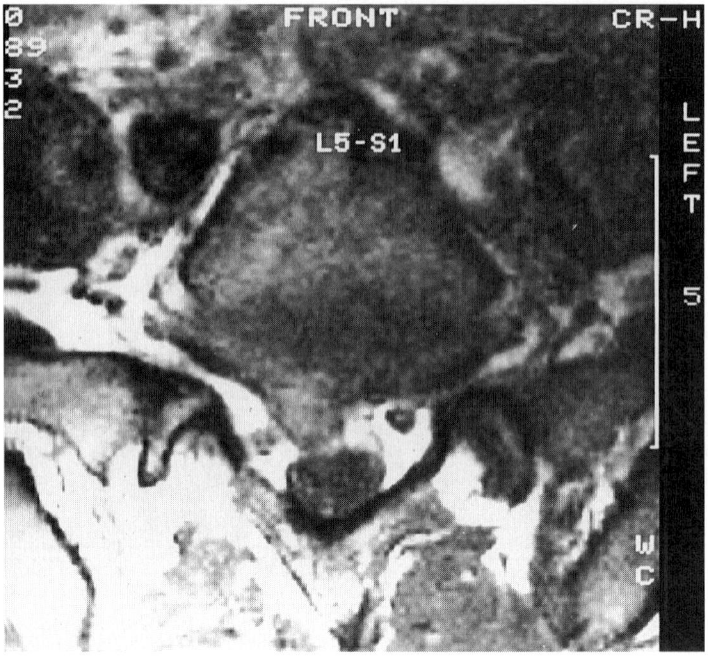

Figure 1.72 *A disc herniation at the top end of the 1st story of L5 (L5–S1 herniated nucleus pulposus [HNP]) lies medial to the nerve root. This is an easily recognized axillary disc herniation. Look back at Figure 1.60, C and see a more difficult to recognize axillary HNP.*

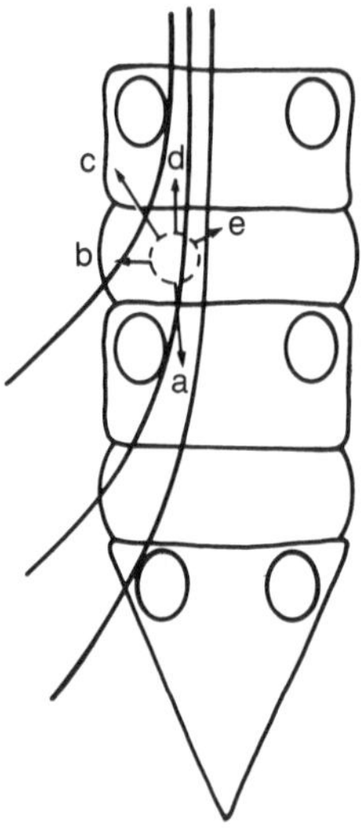

Figure 1.73 *Disc herniations usually occur in the posterolateral corner of the disc space. But many disc herniations migrate:*
a. Into the 3rd story of the anatomic segment below (see Figure 1.60, C).
b. Lateral.
c. Foraminal.
d. Into the 2nd story (see Figure 1.60, D).
e. Midline.

1. Transligamentous (Fig. 1.77).

Only if a normal interlaminar space is present is the transligamentous opening a viable option. If degenerative changes have narrowed the disc space and / or resulted in facet hypertrophy or shingling of the lamina, the interlaminar window will be so narrowed that this approach should not even be tried. When directly crossing the ligamentum flavum, one word of caution; the L5–S1 ligamentum flavum has a tremendous variation in thickness from patient to patient. It can be very thin, especially in the presence of any congenital lumbosacral anomaly, such as spina bifida at L5–S1; one bold stroke used to cross the midportion of such a ligament may land you in a sea of cerebrospinal fluid because of a dural laceration.

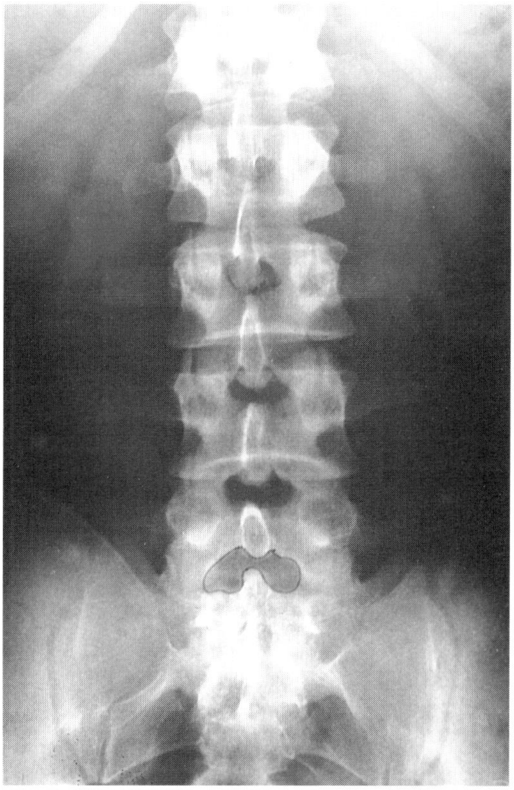

Figure 1.74 *The inferior border of L5 and the wide interlaminar space make a disc excision at L5–S1 easy. A disc herniation at L3–4 that migrates down into the third story of L4 is also an easy surgical exercise. A disc herniation at L2–3 that migrates up into the second story of L2 (Figure 1.70) requires excision of a reasonable amount of lamina.*

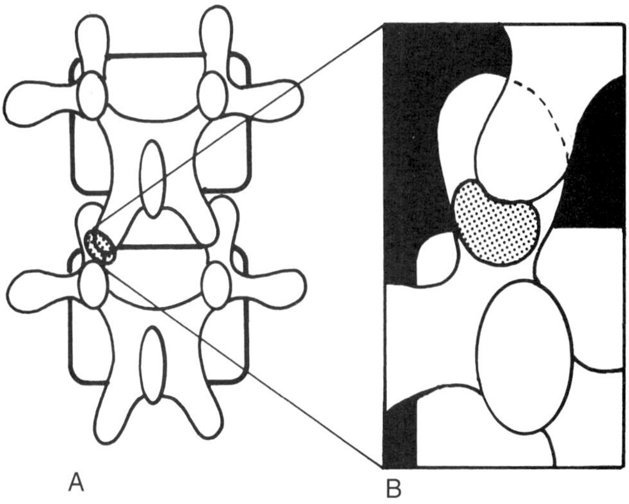

Figure 1.75 **A.** *The "safety net" to be located outside the spinal canal.* **B.** *Plunging a sharp instrument down into the safety net is stopped by the cartilaginous surface of the superior facet.*

2. Through the cephalad lamina (Fig. 1.78).

Because of the frequency of a narrowed interlaminar space in laminectomy, many surgeons prefer to remove a portion of the proximal (or cephalad) lamina before crossing ligamentum flavum. Often, it is recommended that the ligamentum flavum be

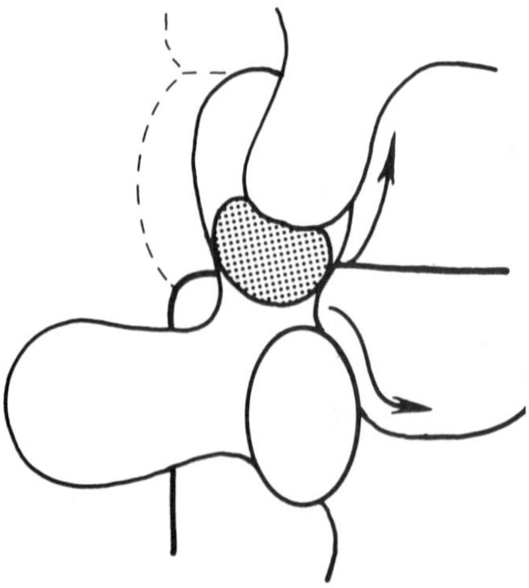

Figure 1.76 *From the safety net, move either cephalad along the inferior laminar border above or caudad to the superior edge of the lamina below.*

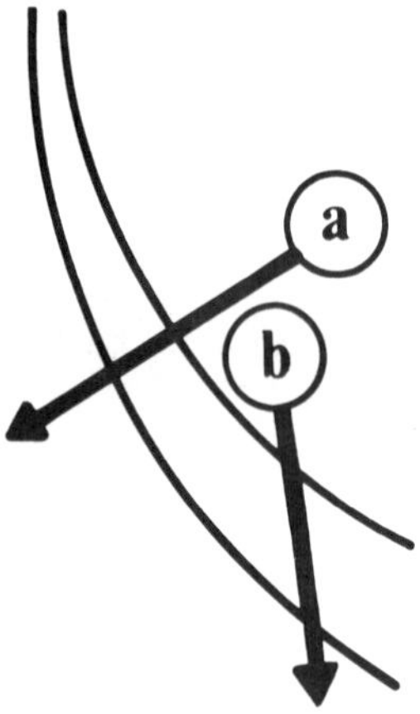

Figure 1.77 *Crossing the ligamentum flavum. Cut a is the direct route into the spinal canal; cut b is the incorrect route through the ligament.*

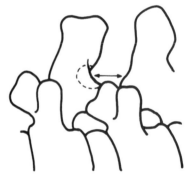

Figure 1.78 *Entry by taking off the edge of the cephalad lamina (dotted line). The line with the double-headed arrow is the transligamentous route in Figure 1.77.*

detached with an elevator before the proximal laminectomy is attempted. Rather, remember that the lamina is thicker laterally and thinner medially (Fig. 1.79). Use this knowledge with the Kerrison rongeur medially on the lamina, and dissect sublaminarly as you are removing the edge of the lamina.

3. Through the caudad lamina (Fig. 1.80).

Probably the easiest way to enter the spinal canal is through the superior edge of the caudad lamina. This is easy because of two anatomical factors:

i. The ligamentum flavum attaches to the posterosuperior edge of the caudad lamina and is easy to remove (Fig. 1.81).
ii. The shape of the dural sheath and adjacent nerve root leaves a small, safe area of entry along the midportion of the lamina (Fig. 1.82).

Spinal Stenosis and Window 2

The salient anatomical features of spinal stenosis and the unilateral interlaminar window for bilateral canal surgery (Fig. 1.62) are as follows:

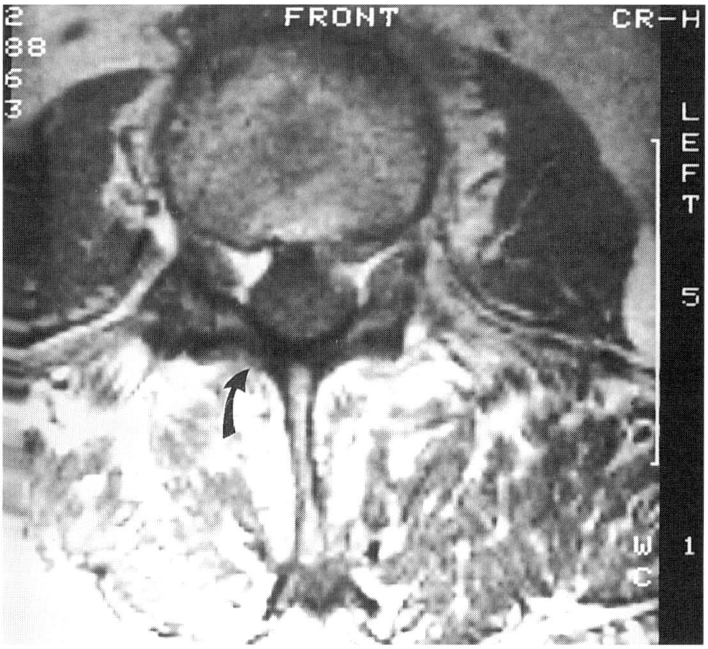

Figure 1.79 *The lamina medially (arrow) is thinner than the lamina laterally; that is, it is easier to get a Kerrison rongeur around the medial edge of the lamina.*

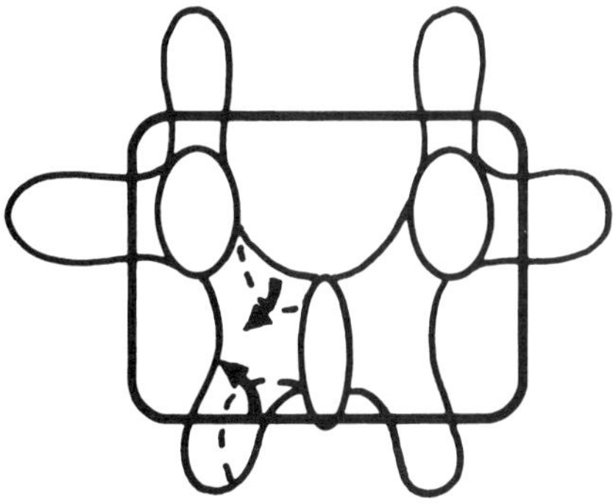

Figure 1.80 *Both entry points for one anatomical segment are shown. If this is the 5th anatomic segment, the upper arrow represents entry through the caudad lamina in an L4–5 exposure; the lower arrow represents entry to the spinal canal through the cephalad lamina in an L5–S1 exposure.*

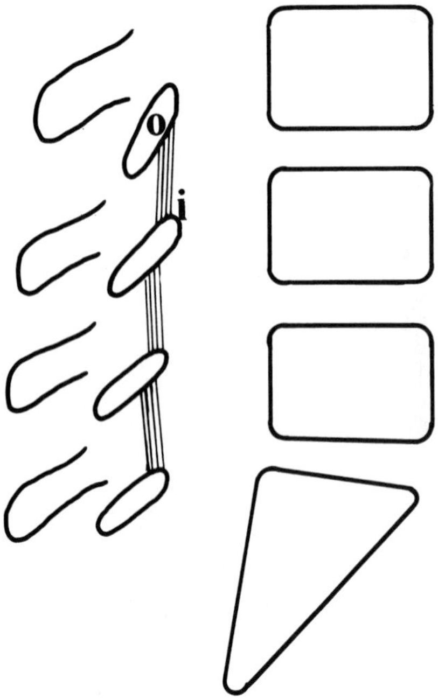

Figure 1.81 *The ligamentum flavum origin (o) is from the anterior surface of the lamina above, and its insertion (i) is into the posterior edge of the lamina below.*

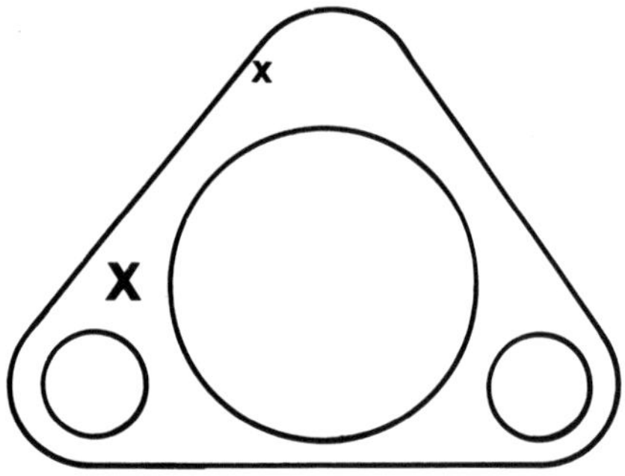

Figure 1.82 *The safe entry points along the edge of the lamina are the large X, or as described in Figure 1.79 and designated by the small x.*

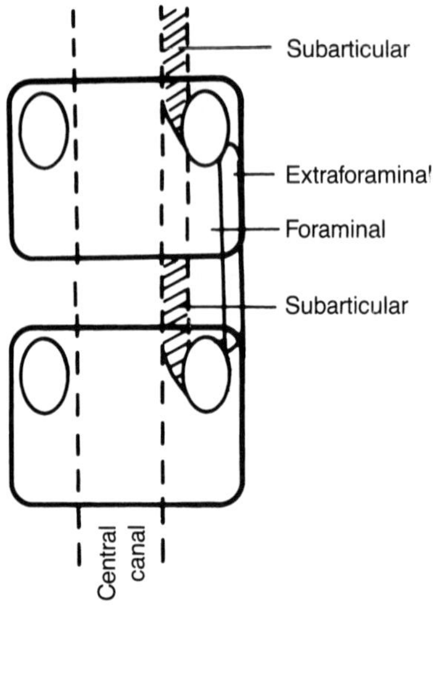

Figure 1.83 *The central canal (between the dotted lines) and the lateral zone divided into three regions.*

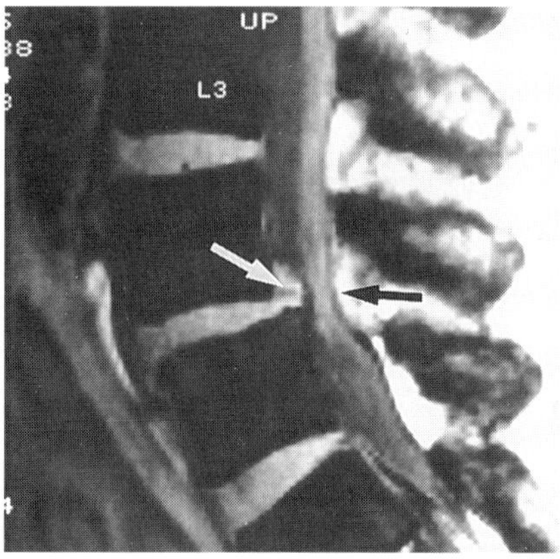

Figure 1.84 *Spinal canal stenosis at a degenerative spondylolisthesis level showing annular bulging (white arrow) from in front of the common dural sheath, and ligamentum flavum infolding (black arrow) from behind. (This is a spin echo sequence MRI, known as proton density.)*

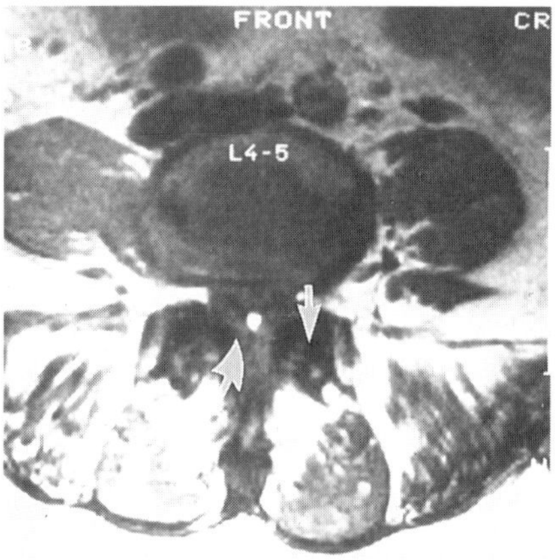

Figure 1.85 *Spinal canal stenosis on a T1 axial MRI. The straight arrow is on top of the hypertrophied facet, and the curved arrow is pointing to the thick ligamentum flavum.*

The Central and Lateral Zones (Fig. 1.86) Spinal stenosis can be divided into central canal stenosis (Fig. 1.83) or lateral zone stenosis (Fig. 1.83). Central canal stenosis is a true circumferential encroachment on cauda equina territory with annular bulging anteriorly (with or without a spondylolisthesis) (Fig. 1.84); facet joint hypertrophy laterally (Fig. 1.85); and ligamentum flavum infolding posteriorly (Fig. 1.84). Note that the predominant location of the lesion in acquired spinal canal stenosis is largely in the first story of the anatomical segment, with some extension of the lesion into contiguous portions of the second story of the same segment and the third story of the adjacent caudad segment (Fig. 1.86).

The Attachments of the Ligamentum Flavum Using the knowledge of attachment of the ligamentum flavum (Fig. 1.81), it is possible to decompress the lesion in spinal canal stenosis with a limited microsurgical exposure (Fig. 1.87). The cephalad lamina is removed proximally until the origin of the ligamentum flavum fibers is seen. This is evident as a thinning of the ligamentum proximally as well as the sighting of "blue" dura. Next, remove the medial edge of the facet joint (Fig. 1.88). Finally, complete the interlaminar decompression by removing the superior edge of the caudad lamina, which removes the insertion of the ligamentum flavum (Fig. 1.89).

Figure 1.86 *Remember the three story concept of the anatomical segment and look at Figure 1.84. You will appreciate that the stenosed portion of the spinal canal lies largely in the 1st story of an anatomic segment, with extension up into the 2nd story above and down into the 3rd story below.*

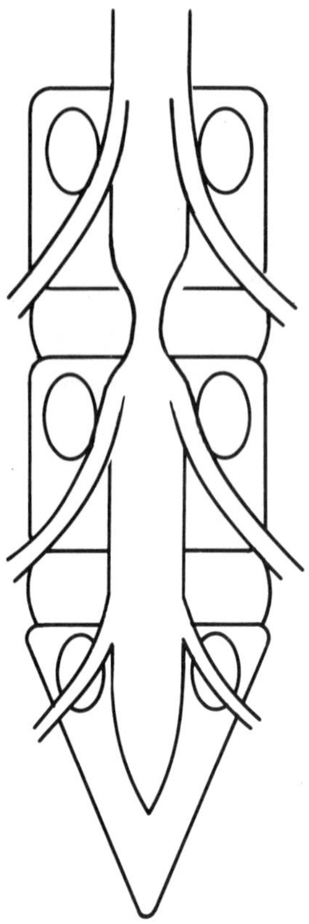

Figure 1.87 *Remove the lower half of the cephalad lamina, which takes you above the origin (Figure 1.81) of the ligamentum flavum.*

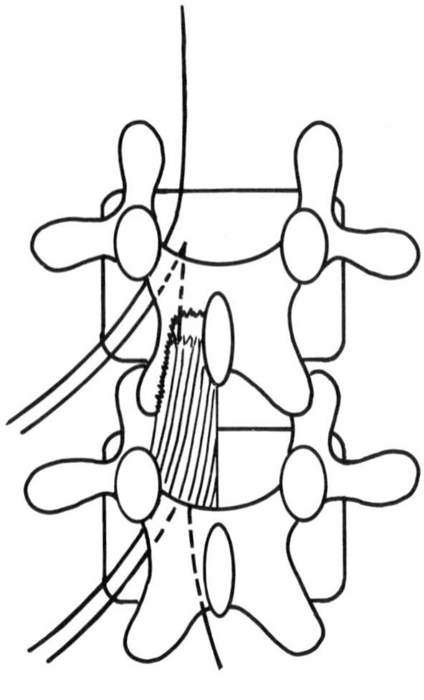

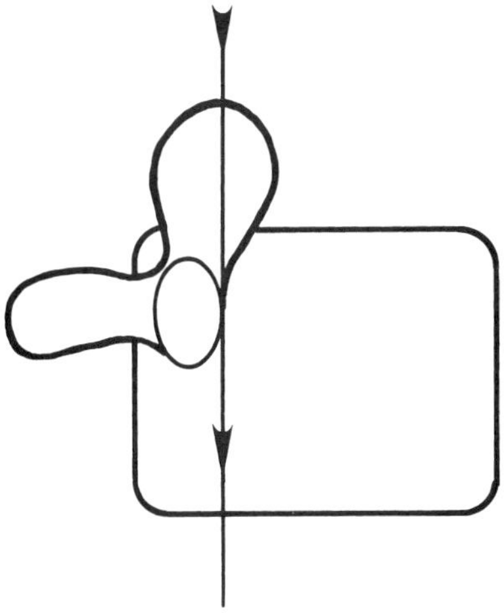

Figure 1.88 *The next step in a spinal canal stenosis decompression is to take off the medial edge of the facet joint (arrow), flush with the medial border of the pedicle.*

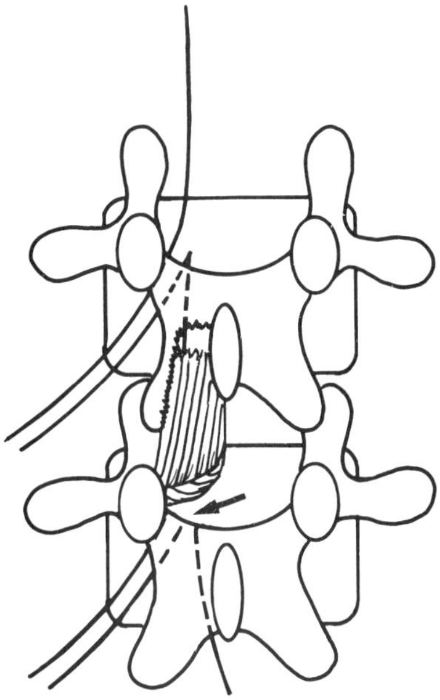

Figure 1.89 *The last step is removing the superior edge of the lamina below to detach the insertion of the ligamentum flavum (arrow).*

The Two Leaves of the Ligamentum Flavum Another useful anatomical fact during this decompression is the cleft that usually separates the right and left leaves of the ligamentum flavum (Fig. 1.90). Using this natural division, it is easy to remove the medial portion of the ligamentum flavum, moving cephalad to caudad.

The View of the Contralateral Canal from the Ipsilateral Interlaminar Window By retracting (and saving) the interspinous ligament and rotating the patient away from the ipsilateral side, it is possible to use the magnification and illumination of the microscope to see the contralateral side of the spinal canal. With careful preparation, it is possible to do a bilateral decompression of spinal stenosis through a unilateral interlaminar window (Fig. 1.91).

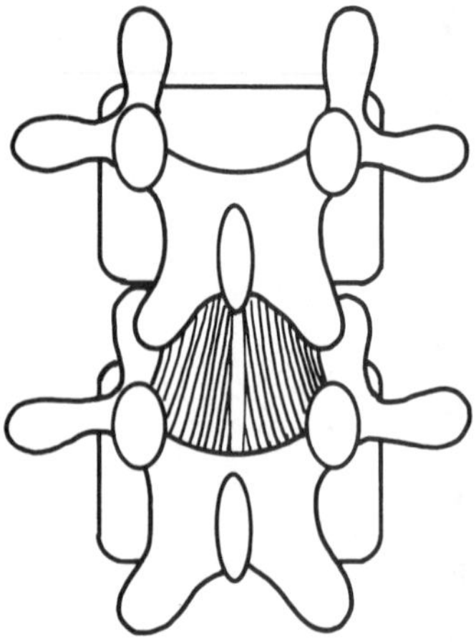

Figure 1.90 *The ligamentum flavum is contiguous with the interspinous ligament, but a cleft separates the two halves of the ligamentum flavum when viewed from the midline.*

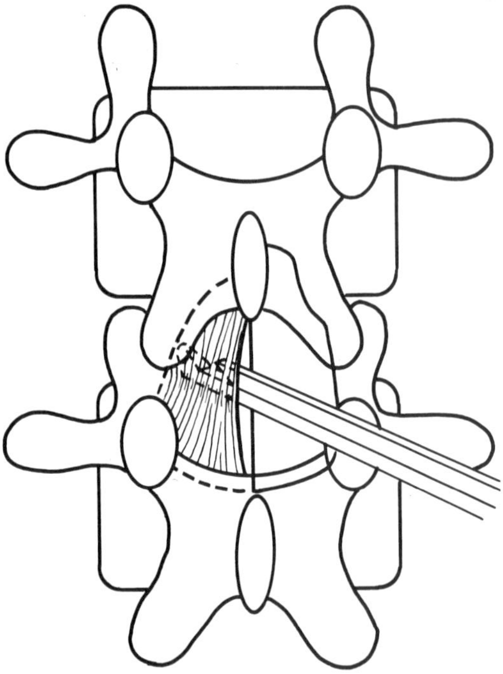

Figure 1.91 *The interlaminar window (Fig. 1.62) can be used to gain entry to the opposite side of the spinal canal.*

Window 3: The Intertransverse Window

For years, spine surgeons have been using the interlaminar window for entry to the spinal canal. With the discovery of the foraminal disc (Fig. 1.92) by CT and MRI, it seemed only natural to try and retrieve that disc rupture through the "tried and true" interlaminar window. Unfortunately, these disc ruptures lie in Macnab's hidden zone (Fig. 1.93), and retrieval is difficult through the interlaminar window. All too often in the orthopedic community, the disc fragment was missed, in order to save the facet joint and maintain stability, while in the neurosurgical community, the facet was sacrificed to properly see the nerve root and the pathology. To avoid this dilemma, the intertransverse window is proposed as a route to retrieve foraminal pathology.

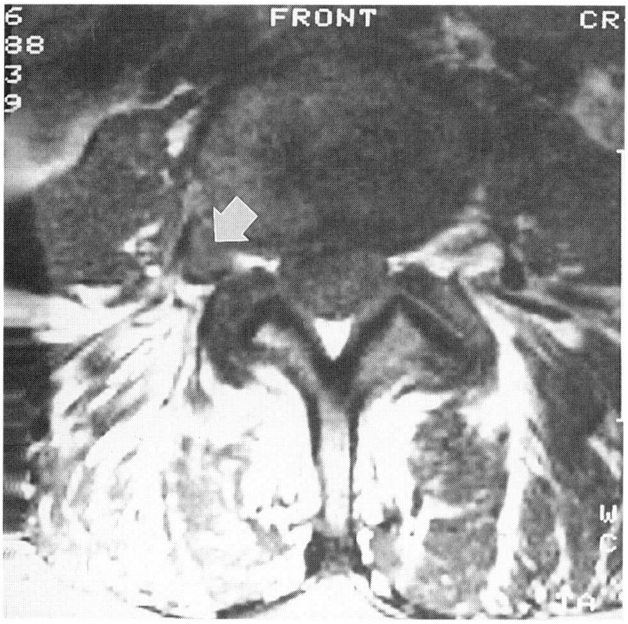

Figure 1.92 *A lumbar foraminal disc (arrow) at L4–5.*

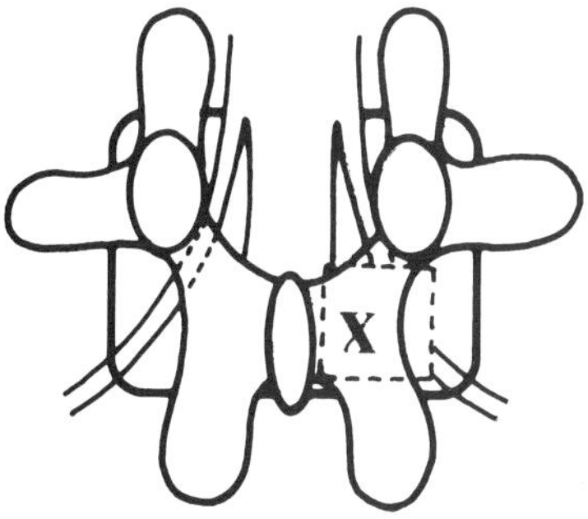

Figure 1.93 *Macnab's hidden zone (X).*

The Intertransverse Window to the Foramen The salient anatomical features are as follows:

1. Foramen.

The boundaries of the foramen are shown in Figure 1.94.

2. Roof of the foramen.

At the L1, L2, L3, or L4 anatomic segments, note that the lateral border of the pars is on the same sagittal plane as the medial border of the pedicle (Fig. 1.95). The only exception to this rule is at the L5 anatomic segment, where the sagittal plane for the lateral border of the pars is at midpedicle (Fig. 1.95). If you accept that the foramen is bordered by adjacent pedicles (Fig. 1.94), then the foramen has no bony roof. Rather, the roof of the foramen is the intertransverse ligament. To enter the L1, L2, L3, or L4 foramen from within the spinal canal, it is necessary to cross the pars (sacrificing the inferior facet) to gain a direct view of pathology (Fig. 1.96). Using this anatomical concept, it becomes evident that to retrieve a

Figure 1.94 *The boundaries of the foramen are easy to remember (pedicle to pedicle and pedicle to pedicle); that is, from the inferior border of one pedicle to the superior border of the pedicle below, and between the medial borders and lateral borders of the same two pedicles.*

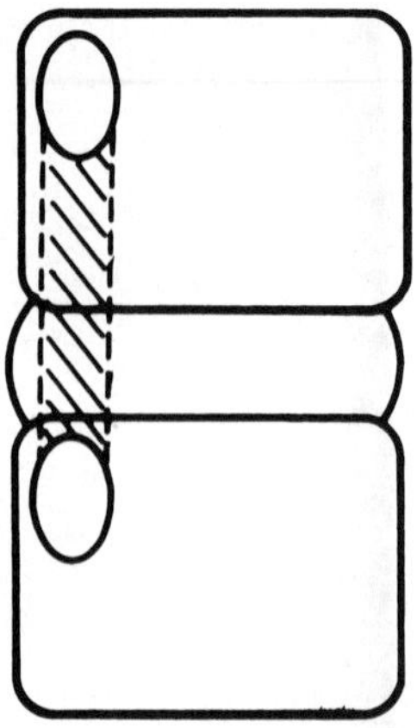

Figure 1.95 *The top segment represents L1, L2, L3, L4, showing the medial border of the pedicle and the lateral border of the pars interarticularis on the same sagittal plane. Not so at L5, which is shown in the bottom anatomic segment.*

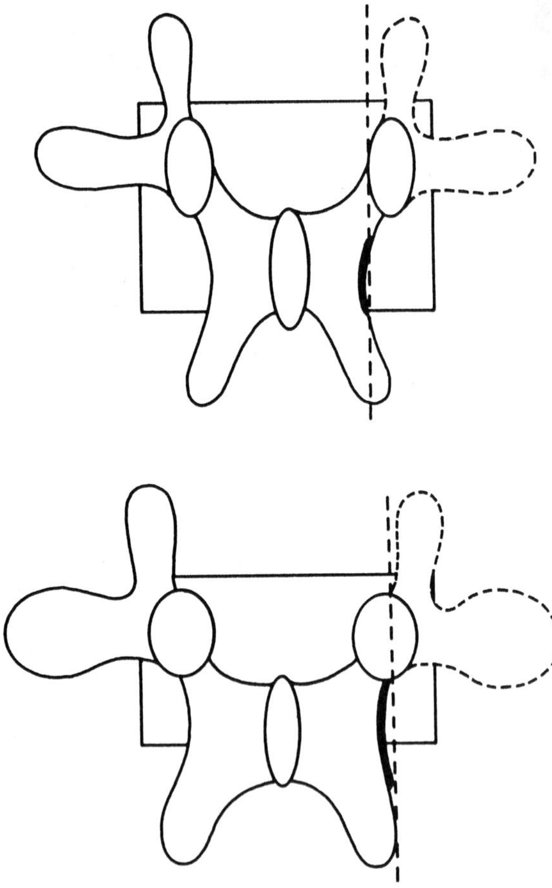

foraminal disc fragment, it is much easier to take the paraspinal approach, crossing the soft tissue intertransverse ligament roof of the foramen (Fig. 1.97).

The Lateral Border of the Pedicle The little-mentioned accessory process at the proximal inferior border of the transverse process marks the lateral edge of the pedicle (Fig. 1.99).

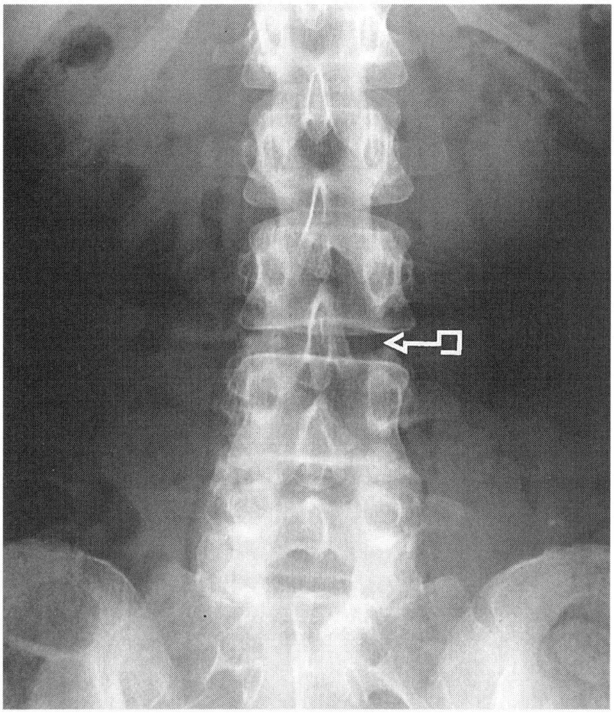

Figure 1.96 *Loss of the inferior facet occurred (arrow) when trying to reach a foraminal disc from within the canal.*

The Disc Lateral to the Pars Looking at Figure 1.96, it becomes evident that a reasonable portion of the disc space lies lateral to the pars. This is more obvious in the proximal lumbar segments, but even at L4 a reasonable portion of the disc space lies lateral to the pars. It is necessary to remove a small portion of the tip of the superior facet to gain entry to the disc space (Fig. 1.98).

The Paraspinal Surgical Approach The paraspinal surgical approach to a foraminal disc is discussed in more detail in Chapter 16.

Surgical Anatomy Necessary to Understand Lumbar Fracture Patterns

Most fractures of the lumbar spine occur around the thoracolumbar junction, and the anatomy described will be used to classify fractures of this region (Chapter 4).

Denis (3), after studying 400 CT scans of thoracolumbar and lumbar spine fractures, developed a three-column anatomical basis for classifying injuries. The basic premise of the three-column classification is that spinal stability is dependent on the status of the middle spinal column and not on the posterior ligamentous complex. In the three-column theory, the thoracolumbar and lumbar spine can be viewed as consisting of the anterior, middle, and posterior columns (Fig. 1.99). Table 1.5 outlines the various components of each column.

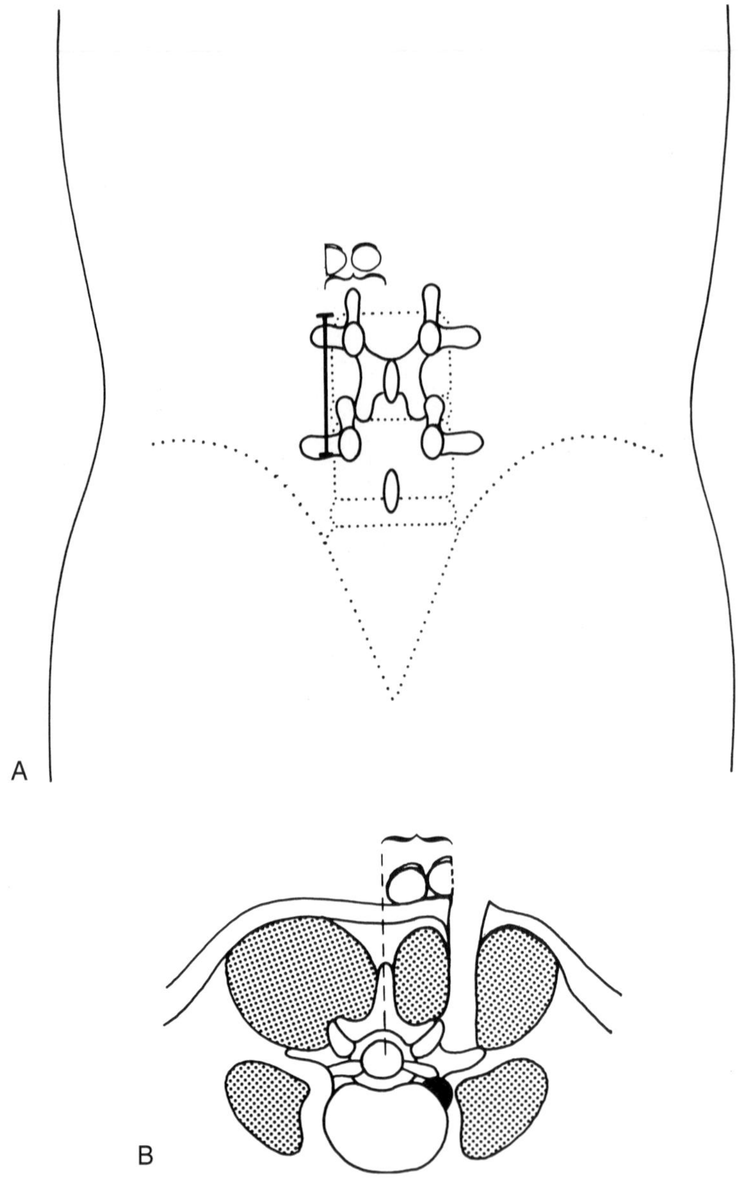

Figure 1.97 **A.** *The more direct way to the foramen is a direct paraspinal approach (off the midline) as shown in Figure 1.97* **B** *(an axial view).*

CONCLUSION

Now that we have the spine formed—vertebrae upon vertebrae with a disc between, and tiny compartments with stories in a house and columns in a row—of what use is it? The biggest problem with such classifications is the occurrence of situations that cannot be classified. This is especially true of the numerous varieties of fractures that affect the thoracolumbar spine. But in order to mature one's understanding of disease mechanisms

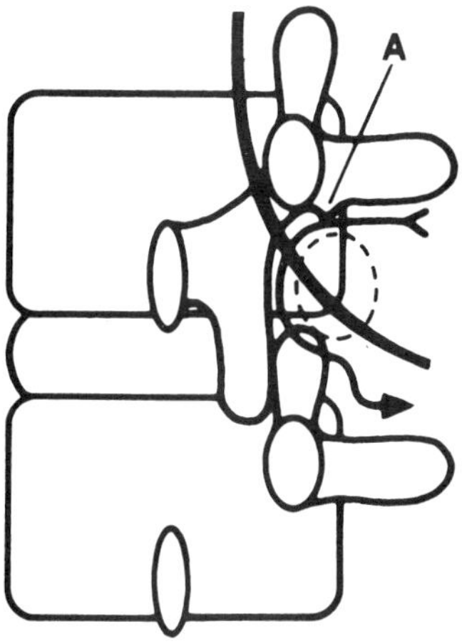

Figure 1.98 *The accessory process (A) marks the lateral border of the pedicle. The wandering arrow shows how to take down the intertransverse ligament to get to the foraminal disc, a technique discussed in detail in Chapter 16.*

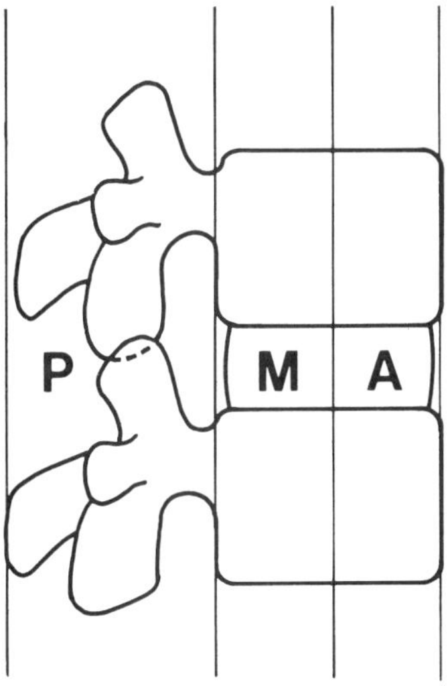

Figure 1.99 *The final piecing, or sectioning, of the spinal column to help understand fracture patterns and stability in spine trauma. A, Anterior column; M, middle column; P, posterior column.*

Table 1.5. Anatomical Basis for Classification of Fractures

Column	Components
Anterior	Anterior longitudinal ligament Anterior half of vertebral body Anterior portion of annulus fibrosus
Middle	Posterior longitudinal ligament Posterior half of the vertebral body Posterior portion of annulus fibrosus
Posterior	Neural arch with facet joints Ligamentum flavum Supraspinous/interspinous ligament complex

in the lumbar spine, it is essential to have some anatomical basis. It is a fitting conclusion to this chapter to make the iconoclastic observation that the first question the physician must ask himself, when he has recognized an anatomical abnormality on radiograph, is: "I wonder what the cause of this patient's backache is?"

REFERENCES

1. Adolph RJ, Fukusumi H, Fowler NO. Origin of cerebrospinal fluid pulsations. Am J Physiol 1967;212(4):840–846.
2. Batson OV. The function of the vertebral veins and their role in the spread of metastases. Ann Surg 1940;112:138–142.
3. Denis F. The three column spine and its significance in the classification of acute thoracolumbar spinal injuries. Spine 1983;8:817–831.
4. Gibson ES, Martin RH, Terry CW. Incidence of low back pain and pre-employment x-ray screening. J Occup Med 1980;22:515–519.
5. Hasner E, Jacobsen HH, Schalimtzek M, Snorrason E. Lumbosacral transitional vertebrae. A clinical and roentgenological study of 400 cases of low back pain. Acta Radiology 1953;39:325–335.
6. Kirkaldy-Willis WH, Wedge JH, Yong-Hing K, Reilly J. Pathology and pathogenesis of lumbar spondylosis and stenosis. Spine 1978;3:319–328.
7. Lapides J, Diokno AC. Urine transport, storage and micturition. In: Lapides J, ed. Fundamentals of Urology. Philadelphia: WB Saunders, 1976; pp 190–241.
8. Lucas DB, Bresler B. Stability of the ligamentous spine. Biomechanics Lab, University of California, Berkeley, Report No. 40, 1961.
9. Macnab I. The traction spur. J Bone Joint Surg 1971;53A:663–670.
10. Macnab I, Dall D. The blood supply of the lumbar spine and its application to the technique of spinal fusion. J Bone Joint Surg 1971;53B:628–638.
11. Nachemson AL, Elfstrom G. Intravital dynamic pressure measurements in the lumbar discs. A study of common movements, maneuvers and exercises. Scand J Rehab Med 1970; 2(suppl 1): 1–40.
12. O'Donnell WF. Urological management in the patient with acute spinal cord injury. Crit Care Clin 1987;3:599–617.
13. Schmorl G, Junghanns H. The Human Spine in Health and Disease. Besemann EF, translator. New York: Grune & Stratton; 1971.
14. Sherman JL, Citrin CM, Gangarosa RE, Bowen BJ. The MR appearance of CSF pulsations in the spinal canal. AJNR 1986;7:879–884.
15. Southworth JD, Borsack SR. Anomalies of the lumbosacral vertebrae in five hundred and fifty individuals without symptoms referral to the low back. AJR 1950;64:624–634.
16. Timi PG, Wieser C, Zinn WM. The transitional vertebrae of the lumbosacral spine: its radiological classification, incidence, prevalence and clinical significance. Rheum Rehab 1977;16: 80–187.
17. Wein AJ. Classification of neurogenic voiding dysfunction. J Urol 1981;125:605–689.

2

Biomechanics

[Mechanical surgeons] have been the bane of the science; intruding themselves into the ranks of the profession, with no other qualification but boldness in undertaking, ignorance of their responsibility, and indifference to the lives of their patients; proceeding according to the special dictates of some author, as mechanical as themselves, they cut and tear with fearless indifference, utterly incapable of exercising any judgment of their own in cases of emergency; and sometimes, without possessing even the slightest knowledge of the anatomy of the parts concerned. The preposterous and impious attempts of such pretenders, can seldom fail to prove destructive to the patient, and disgraceful to the science. It is by such this noble science has been degraded in the minds of many, to the rank of an art.

— Ephraim McDowell (1771–1830)
The Eclectic Repertory and Analytical Review, Medical and Philosophical 9:546, 1819.

INTRODUCTION

The spine is a flexible, multisegmental column bridging the interval between the base of the skull and the pelvis. Its requirements include maintaining an upright posture, yet allowing for flexibility, while at the same time providing a protective conduit for neurological structures. The fact that it provides all of these functions in most of us, with little upset, is an astonishing fact.

For most of us the "microtrauma" of repetitive movements will take its toll in degeneration; for an unfortunate few, major trauma, such as a motor vehicle accident, will devastate the vertebral and neurological structures of the spine and cause paraplegia. A study of these accumulated microtraumas and sudden major forces is known as biomechanics.

LUMBAR DISC DEGENERATION

Nutritional changes in proteins and the resulting alteration in the histochemical makeup of the discs and facet joints cannot alone explain how discs degenerate and nuclear material herniates through a rent in the annulus. It is the addition of mechanical forces that adds a further dimension to understanding degeneration in the lumbosacral region. On the other hand, numerous young persons absorb tremendous loads in the lumbar spine during sporting activities. The fact that we do not see degenerative disc disease to any great extent in the younger population suggests that most of the biomechanical effects on the spine are the result of accumulated, rather than momentary, trauma. If, at autopsy, one takes a normal disc and makes a longitudinal incision in the posterior part of the annulus through to the nucleus and then loads the specimen, no disc herniation occurs. This is further evidence (3) for the resilience of the young disc.

The final determinant in disc degeneration (Table 2.1), and perhaps the most important, is the individual's genetic code. It is a recurrent theme in medical practice that some patients age faster than others. Although there is a common middle ground of aging, there are many young patients who are seen with degenerative disc disease that cannot be explained by nutritional and biomechanical forces alone. At the other end of the spectrum is the well preserved older patient, who on radiograph has little in the way of degenerative spine changes. They commonly carry with them the house officer's statement "looking much younger than their stated age." Obviously, these individuals have a genetic code that has determined a slower aging process.

THE MOTION SEGMENT

In the Chapter 1, you were introduced to the anatomic segment. Now, meet the motion segment, or the functional spinal unit (FSU) (Fig 2.1).

Movement Forces

Movement forces applied to the axial skeleton are absorbed and dissipated through the special hydrostatic nature of the disc. The fluid nature of the nuclear gel allows for absorption of forces, and the intimate contact between nucleus and annulus allows for dissipation of these loads into the elastic coil structure of the annulus. Further support for this force transmission is found in the various ligaments and muscles attached to processes, body, and posterior arch of the vertebral segment.

Abnormal nuclear movement or disc failure can occur in one of three ways:

Table 2.1. Determinants of Disc Degeneration

Age and the accumulation of microtraumas
Age and disc nutritional changes
Genetic code

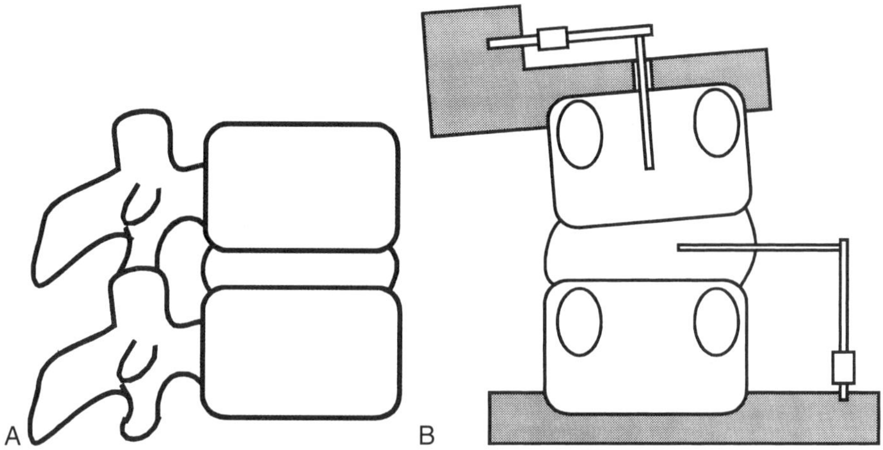

Figure 2.1 **A.** *The motion segment or functional spinal unit (FSU) is the disc space and two adjacent vertebral bodies.* **B.** *The motion segment is set up in a testing gauge: the lower vertebral body is fixed, whereas the upper vertebrae is stressed. Forces are measured in the disc space by a probe.*

1. Nuclear material may herniate throughout the endplate (a Schmorl's node).
2. Nuclear-annular integrity can be altered from within, resulting in a progressive disruption of annular integrity from within, progressing toward the outer boundary of the annulus.
3. Annular integrity can be altered from without when forces applied to the motion segment exceed the normal resistance of the annulus, cleaving the outer fibers. With further injury, this rent extends inward and eventually communicates with the nucleus, thereby creating a path for nuclear migration.

Forces

There are numerous forces that can be applied, alone or in combination, to a spinal motion segment. Complex mathematical equations (4) are used to describe the resulting distortion of the disc architecture. For the purpose of this monograph, a simple concept of only three forces, acting singly, will be considered.

Compression

The main support for compressive loads is the anterior and middle columns (Fig 2.2). Discs can be subjected to very high compressive loads. These forces increase the pressure within the nucleus (5) and result in a minor loss (5%) of nuclear water, with a decrease in volume of the nucleus. Further absorption of the force occurs through bulging of the annulus. In normal discs, this increased annular fiber tension results in increased angulation in the collagen lamellar pattern. With increasing compression in a normal disc, the nuclear pressure and annular tension changes will sustain until the endplate fails (1500–2000 lb): so-called "endplate fracture." As previously mentioned, this herniation of nuclear material through the endplate, combined with the subsequent healing of bone, has the characteristic appearance (on radiograph) of a Schmorl's node (Fig. 2.3).

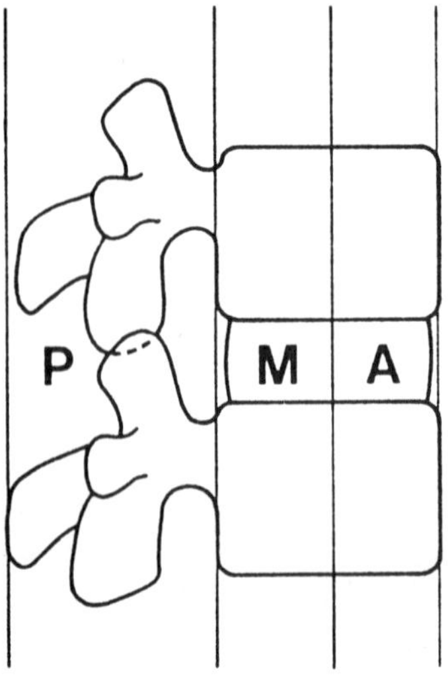

Figure 2.2 *Do you remember this figure from Chapter 1? It shows the three columns of Denis, of which the anterior and middle are the main support for compressive loads.*

With alteration of the nucleus-annulus junction through aging, repeated compressive loads may initiate annular fissures from within the disc. Eventually, nuclear material may protrude partway through the annulus but may still be enclosed by the annulus. This nuclear material creates a localized bulge in the annulus, which subsequently may compromise an adjacent nerve root (Fig. 2.4, A). On discography, this disc will be contained (Fig. 2.4, B) (see Chapter 10).

Torsion

Experimental evidence would suggest that torsion, along with bending, is the most damaging force applied to a disc.(1) The application of torsion (twisting or rotation on the long axis) produces tensile and shear stresses in the annulus. These forces are greatest on the outermost fibers of the annulus and decrease as one moves toward the center of the disc, where very little force is applied to the nucleus. In addition, the facet joints may be damaged by absorbing some of these torsional strains. At times, the facet joints are damaged by torsion to the point where the vertebral segment is permanently rotated. Farfan (3) believes that this rotation can compress the root because the medial migration of the pedicle may kink the existing nerve root; in such an instance, the resulting myelographic defect may mimic a disc herniation.

A forced rotational injury will damage the annulus but not the endplates. This is because the force is greatest on the outer annular fibers, and it is here that the first radial fissures start. With repeated torsional strains, the radial fissure will work its way inward, ultimately connecting with the nuclear cavity and forming a pathway through which nuclear material can extrude.

The posterolateral portions of the annulus are thinner and weaker than the rest of the annulus, and it is here that a torsion stress has its maximal effect. Further alteration in the localization of these stress risers comes through the shape of the posterior vertebral border, to which the annulus is attached. The rounder the shape (L5–S1), the more lateral will be the stress riser and resulting annular damage (Fig. 2.5).

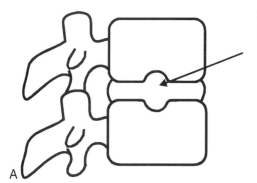

Figure 2.3 **A.** *A schematic of Schmorl's node (arrow), which are shown at multiple levels in* **B.**

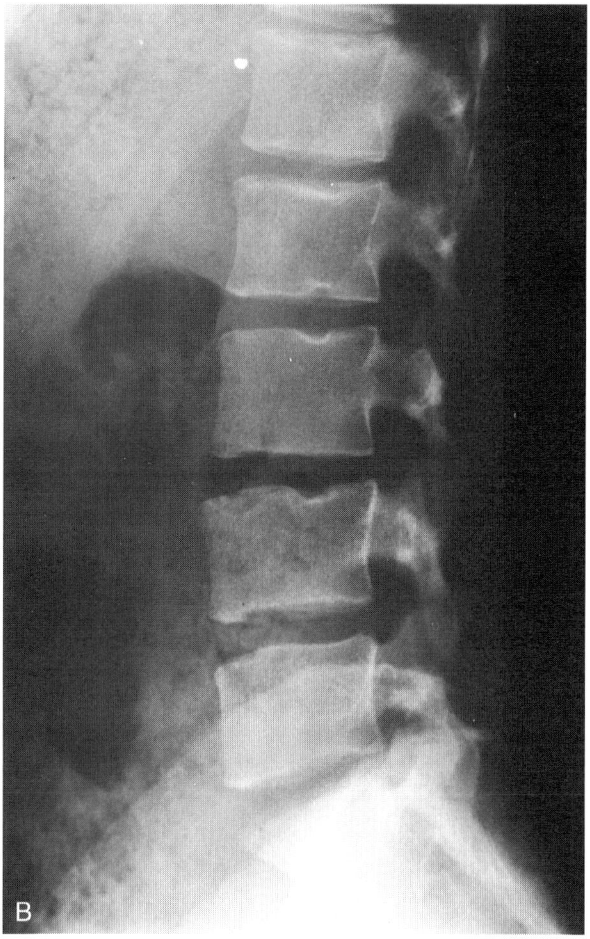

Approximately 95% of nuclear protrusions will occur at L4–5 and L5–S1. Younger patients tend to have an increased incidence of disc herniation at the L5–S1 level because stress increases at the junction of mobility (L5) and fixation (S1 and pelvis). With slow aging and degeneration, an inherent stability will develop in the L5–S1 disc through loss of turgor and elasticity, with subsequent fibrosis of the disc. This transfers more stress to the level above, which explains the higher incidence of nuclear protrusion at the L4–5 level that occurs with increasing age.

Figure 2.4 **A.** *A contained disc herniation that compresses and irritates a nerve root.* **B.** *A contained degenerative disc on discography at L4–5. This is almost a degenerative spondylolisthesis level. The discs above and below are normal on discography.*

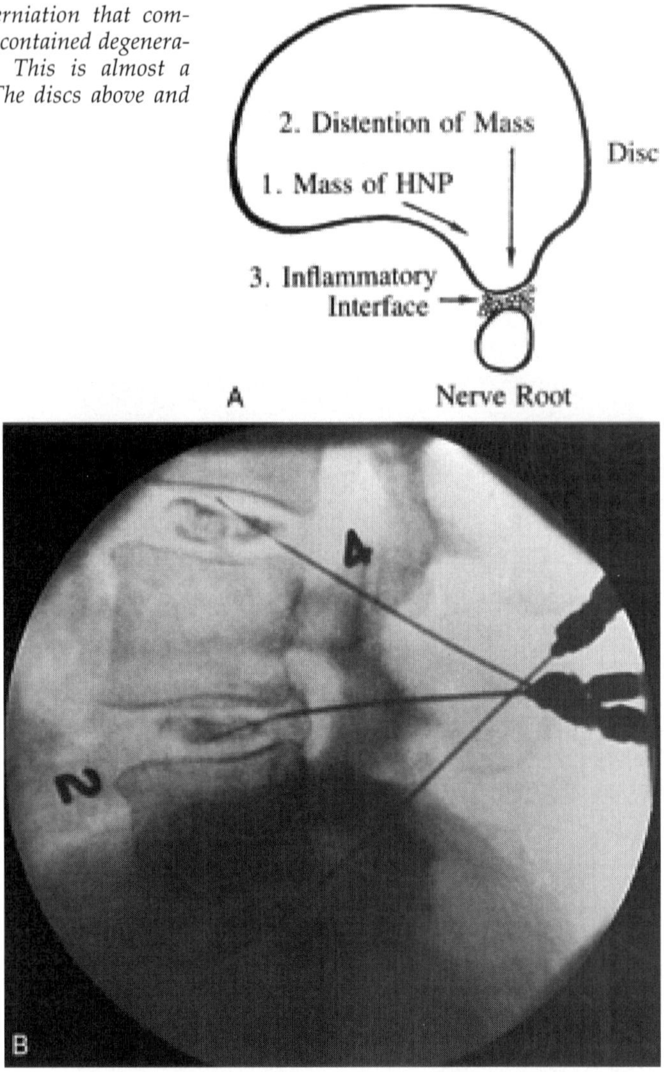

Further protection of the L5–S1 disc segment from torsion stress occurs when L5 has a long transverse process (and thus a short iliotransverse process ligament). This built-in stability of L5 to S1 offers protection from rotational forces and transfers the stress riser to the L4–5 disc (Fig. 2.6).

Bending (Forward Flexion, Backward Extension, Lateral Flexion)

Bending has occurred when the upper surface of a disc tilts with respect to its lower surface. As with torsion stresses, there is very little increase in nuclear pressure and thus, no endplate failure occurs. However, forward bending will cause increased tension (stretch) on posterior annular fibers and may cause failure of the annulus in this area. Compression and torsion distribute forces evenly around the cross-section of a disc, whereas forward bending

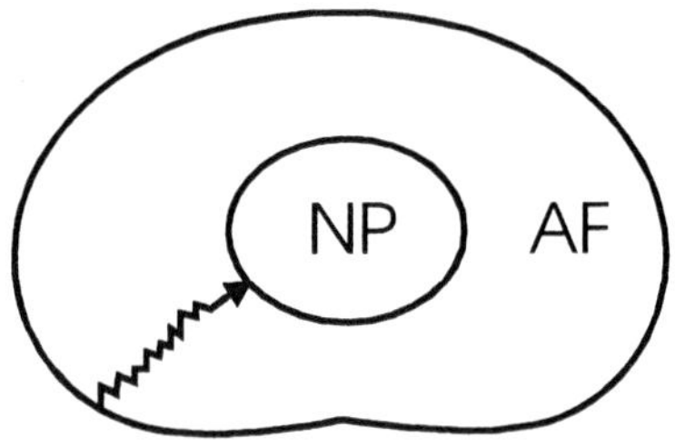

Figure 2.5 *Axial view of a disc space showing a radial fissure that starts at the periphery of the annulus fibrosis (AF) and works its way toward the nucleus (NP) with repeated stresses.*

localizes forces to the posterior collagenous fibers. This bending can have a very disruptive effect on the posterior annulus by cleaving the annulus or separating the annular fibers from the vertebral body or endplate. As with torsion injury, these annular disruptions can extend into nuclear territory and create a pathway for nuclear herniation.

LOAD BEARING

In lateral and posterior shear, axial compression, and flexion, the disc appears to be the major load-bearing element. In anterior shear and axial torque, the facets play a major role in dissipating the forces. The ability to absorb and dissipate these forces is significantly reduced by lumbar disc degeneration.

The Facet Joints

The facet joints are not major load bearers except in the lower lumbar spine, where they can accept up to 20% of a compressive load. This role is highest in extension movements. Rather, the normal facet joints guide the motion of the FSU. Viewing the orientation of the facet joints in the lumbar spine supports the concept that the facet joints facilitate movements in the sagittal plane (flexion/extension) and limit movements in rotation (torsion) and bending.

BIOMECHANICS OF LIGAMENTS

The ligaments of the lumbar spine act like rubber bands. They have an elastic physical property that allows the ligament to stretch and resist tensile forces. Under compression, the ligaments buckle and serve little function. In resisting tensile forces, ligaments allow just enough movement without injury to vital structures. Passively, they maintain tension in a segment so that muscles do not have to work as hard.

LIGAMENT LOAD BEARING

The strongest ligaments in the spine are the anterior longitudinal ligament and the facet joint capsules. The interspinous-supraspinous ligament complex is of intermediate strength, and weakest of all is the posterior longitudinal ligament. The ligamentum flavum contains significant amounts of elastin fiber, which indicates that its function is one of stretching rather than restraining.

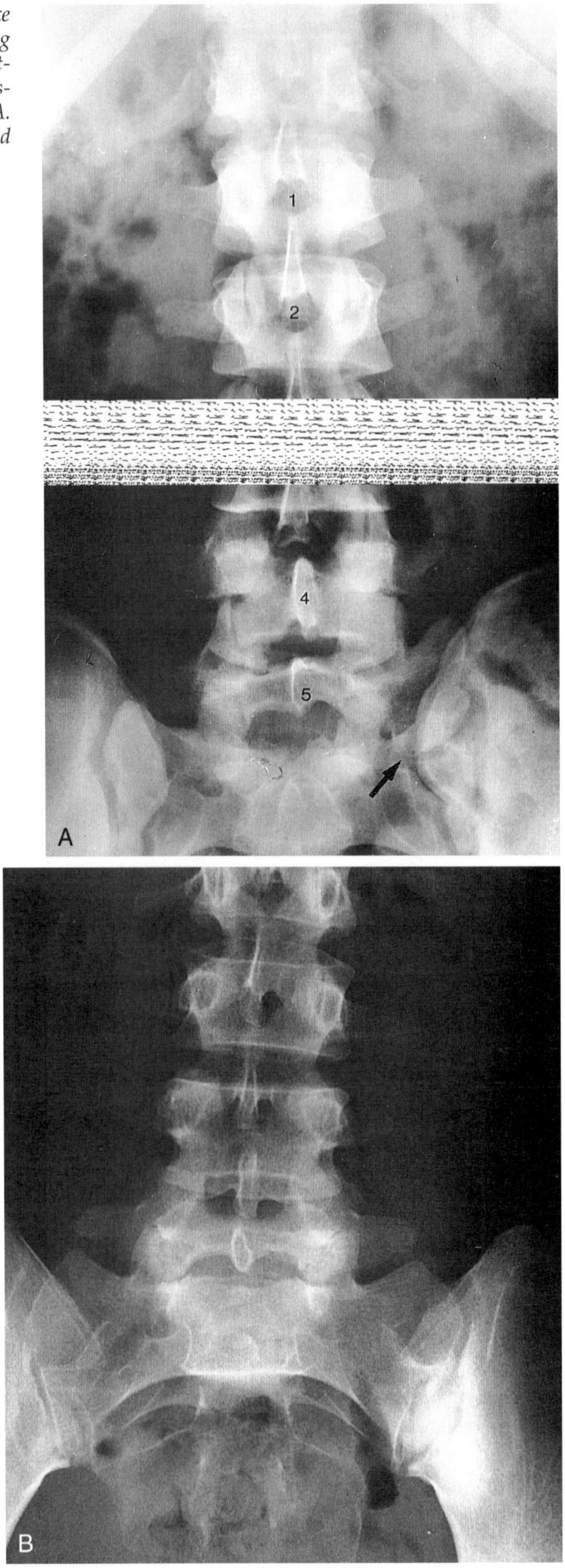

Figure 2.6 **A.** *There are many ways to make the L5–S1 level more stable, such as a long transverse process. This example is even better: L5 is fixed to the pelvis with a large transverse process (arrow).* **B.** *Just the reverse of A. the L5 segment sits high out of the pelvis and is more unstable than normal.*

ROLE OF THE ABDOMINAL CAVITY

There is some controversy as to what role the abdominal cavity plays in sharing the load on the lumbar spine. Farfan (3) has theorized that an increase in intra-abdominal pressure serves to protect the lumbar spine, but Schultz et al (6) have concluded just the opposite. For now let us accept the fact that the abdominal cavity and its surrounding muscles stabilize the spine for activities such as lifting.

INTRADISCAL PRESSURE

Regardless of both the loads on the spine and the support of the muscles and ligaments, the final determining factor in biomechanical injury to the spine is the intradiscal pressure. Nachemson (5) and co-workers are leaders in this field. They designed a special transducer that measured pressures within the L3–4 disc space under various conditions of load (Fig. 2.7).

These authors examined normal discs only and showed that in various postures and loading positions, there are different forces across the disc space. If these forces exceed what the disc space can absorb, then injury to the motion segment occurs, and pathological changes occur in the three-joint complex.

ERGONOMICS

Standing in our natural posture, and provided that body segments are normal and aligned with respect to the center of gravity, minor muscular activities are required to balance the spine. However, changes in the posture, such as flexion, require contraction of muscles to support the spine. This results in (1) an increased pressure in the disc, and (2) dissipation of forces. If a load is added, then further muscle forces are required to counterbalance the load. These concepts, as proposed by Nachemson,(5) GBJ Anderson et al,(2) and CK Anderson et al (1) have raised the field of ergonomics to important levels

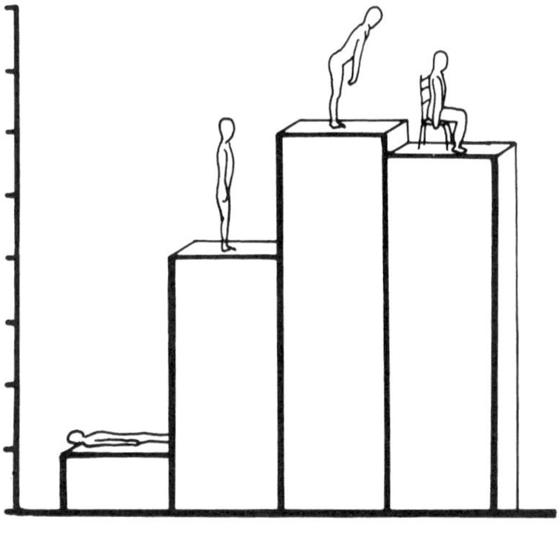

Figure 2.7 *Dr. Nachemson's very famous study that measured pressures in the L3–4 disc in varying positions. The lowest pressure occurs when laying down, the highest pressure when bending forward.*

in industry. Numerous studies, both those completed and ongoing, which look at the various forces on the lumbar spine and how they might be modified, will ultimately decrease the injury rate for workers. What is commonly taught now in industry is that externally applied loads, such as repetitively lifting an object away from the body (Fig. 2.8), will subject the lumbar spine to very damaging forces. To minimize those forces (during lifting or carrying), the distance between the object lifted and the trunk should be as short as possible (Fig. 2.8).

SUMMARY

It is obvious that disc degeneration and nuclear migration through the annulus represent a combined effect of (1) aging, with molecular alteration of the nucleus pulposus and annulus fibrosus, and (2) repeated mechanical stresses to the motion segment. The speed of the process is set up by the individual's genetic code. No one cause of disc degeneration and herniation can be pinpointed. This explains the many different clinical combinations of symptoms and signs confronting the clinician who tries to assess a patient with a low back pain syndrome.

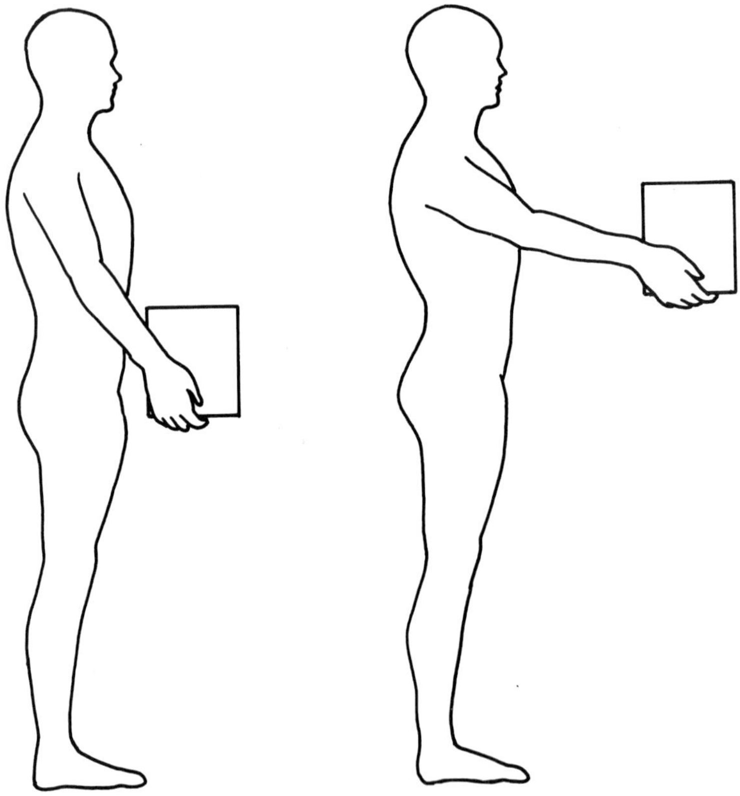

Figure 2.8 *The force on the lumbar discs is greatly increased by holding a load away from the body (right) during a lift, compared with the figure on the left.*

REFERENCES

1. Anderson CK, Chaffin DB, Herrin GD, et al. A biomechanical model of the lumbosacral joint during lifting activities. J Biomech 1985;18:571-584.
2. Anderson GBJ, Ortengren R, Herberts P. Quantitative electromyographic studies of back muscle activity related to posture and loading. Orthop Clin North Am 1977;8:85-96.
3. Farfan HF. A reorientation in the surgical approach to capital degenerative lumbar intervertebral joint disease. Orthop Clin North Am 1977;8:9-21.
4. Hickey DS, Hakins DWL. Relation between the structure of the annulus fibrosis and the function and failure of the intervertebral disc. Spine 1980;5:106-116.
5. Nachemson A. The load of lumbar discs in different positions of the body. Clin Orthop 1966;45:107-122.
6. Schultz AB, Haderspeck-Grib K, Sinkora G, et al. Quantitative studies of the lexion-relation phenomenon in the back muscles. J Orthop Res 1985;3:189-197.

3

Classification of Low Back Pain

"Seek facts and classify them and you will be the workmen of science."

— Nicholas Maurice Arthus

INTRODUCTION

Low back pain, like abdominal pain, is a symptom, not a disease. The pathological basis for the pain may be something within the spine, or a lesion outside of the spine. The causes are many but may be broadly classified as spondylogenic or neurogenic (causes within the spine) and viscerogenic, vascular, or psychogenic (causes outside of the spine).

SPONDYLOGENIC BACK PAIN

Spondylogenic back pain may be defined as pain derived from the spinal column and its associated structures. The pain is aggravated by general and specific activities and is relieved, to some extent, by rest.

The pain may be derived from lesions involving the bony components of the spinal column, changes in the sacroiliac joints, or, most commonly, changes occurring in the soft tissues (discs, ligaments, and muscles).

Because these lesions constitute the most common source of low back pain seen in clinical practice, the pathological changes and the pathogenesis of symptoms are discussed in detail in the chapters that follow.

NEUROGENIC PAIN

Tension, irritation, or compression of a lumbar nerve root or roots will usually cause referral of pain symptoms down one or both legs. Although this interference with root function constitutes the most common cause of neurogenic pain, it is prudent to remember there are other causes. Lesions of the central nervous system such as thalamic tumors may present or develop a causalgic type of leg pain, and arachnoid irritation from any cause as well as tumors of the spinal dura may produce back pain. The pathological lesions most likely to give rise to confusion in diagnosis are neurofibroma, neurilemmoma, ependymoma, and other cysts and tumors involving the nerve roots. These lesions usually occur in the upper lumbar spine outside of the field of view of computed tomography scanning and missed on sagittal magnetic resonance image scanning if not looked for. The history may be indistinguishable from nerve root pressure due to a disc herniation. Frequently, however, patients report a history of having to get out of bed at night to walk around in order to obtain relief of their symptoms.

The difficulties that may arise in diagnosis are best exemplified by a patient who presented with severe sciatic pain associated with paresthesia involving the lateral border of the foot and the lateral two toes. His symptoms were aggravated by provocative activity and relieved to some extent by recumbency. Examination revealed an impairment of first sacral root conduction, as evidenced by weakness of the plantar flexors of the ankle, a markedly diminished ankle jerk, and diminution of appreciation of pinprick over the lateral border of the foot. The patient's history and clinical findings resembled the classic picture of a herniated lumbosacral disc with first sacral root compression. Myelographic examination was performed and demonstrated a gross defect opposite the body of L2. At surgery, a lipoma involving the first sacral root was found at the point where the root emerged from the conus (Fig. 3.1).

This case emphasizes not only the fact that nerve root tumors can mimic disc herniation, but also the importance of looking at the conus region as an essential preoperative investigation in the surgical management of patients apparently suffering from discogenic root compression.

VISCEROGENIC BACK PAIN

Viscerogenic back pain may be derived from disorders of the kidneys or the pelvic viscera, lesions of the lesser sac, and retroperitoneal tumors (Fig. 3.2). Backache is rarely the sole symptom of visceral disease. Careful questioning will usually elicit description of other symptoms. The history of viscerogenic back pain can be differentiated from back

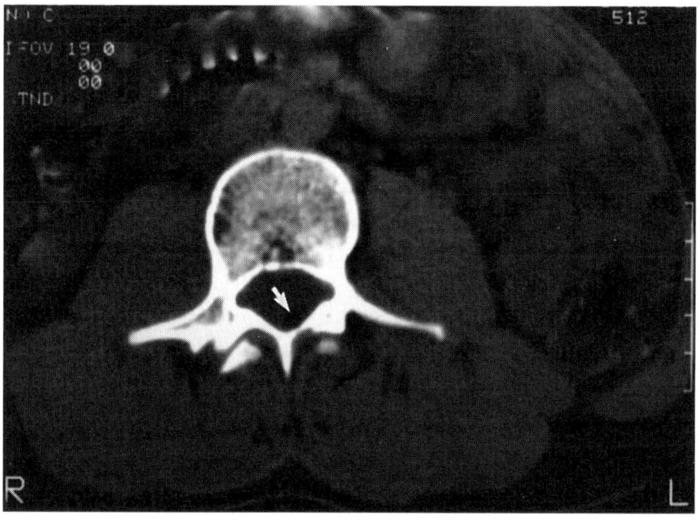

Figure 3.1 *Conus lipoma, as depicted on CT scan (arrow). The patient presented with sciatica and first lumbar nerve root symptoms. Notice posteriorly on the left in the cauda equina, a lesion with the density of fat. This was a lipoma extending up to the conus.*

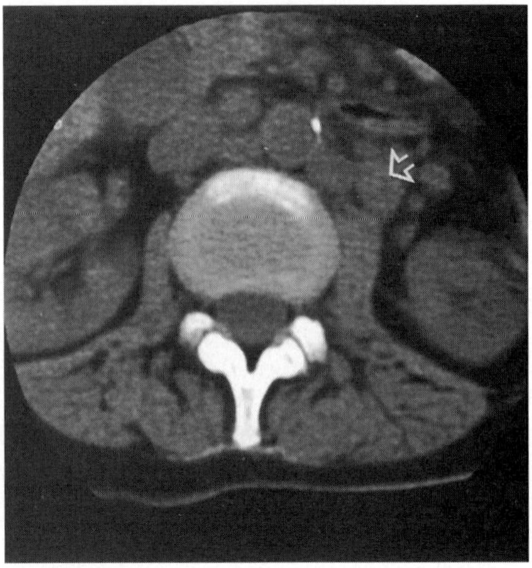

Figure 3.2 *Axial CT of a patient who presented with back pain. Note the extensive retroperitoneal nodes (arrow). The patient had Hodgkin's disease.*

pain derived from a disorder of the spinal column by one important feature. The pain is not aggravated by activity, nor is it relieved by rest. Indeed, with severe pain, the patient whose symptoms are visceral in origin will writhe around to get relief, whereas the patient suffering from the tortures of a septic discitis will lie perfectly still.

VASCULAR BACK PAIN

Abdominal aortic aneurysms or peripheral vascular disease may give rise to backache or symptoms resembling sciatica. Abdominal aneurysms may present as a boring type of deep-seated lumbar pain unrelated to activity (Fig. 3.3). Insufficiency of the superior gluteal artery may give rise to buttock pain of a claudicant character, which is aggravated by walking and relieved by standing still. The pain may radiate down the leg in a sciatic distribution. However, the pain is not precipitated or aggravated by other activities that put a specific stress on the spine (eg, bending, stooping, lifting, and so forth).

Intermittent claudication—intermittent pain in the calf—associated with peripheral vascular disease may on occasion mimic sciatic pain produced by root irritation, but the history of specific aggravation by walking and relief by standing still will make the clinician look for signs of peripheral vascular insufficiency.

The symptoms associated with peripheral vascular disease (PVD) may be mimicked by spinal stenosis. A patient suffering from PVD frequently complains of pain and weakness in the legs, which is initiated and aggravated by the act of walking a short distance. One distinguishing feature, however, is that in spinal stenosis the pain is not relieved by standing still. For a more detailed discussion of neurogenic claudication, the reader is referred to Chapter 17.

PSYCHOGENIC BACK PAIN

Pure psychogenic back pain is rarely seen in clinical (civilian) practice. Clouding and confusion of the clinical picture by emotional overtones are very commonly seen. Al-

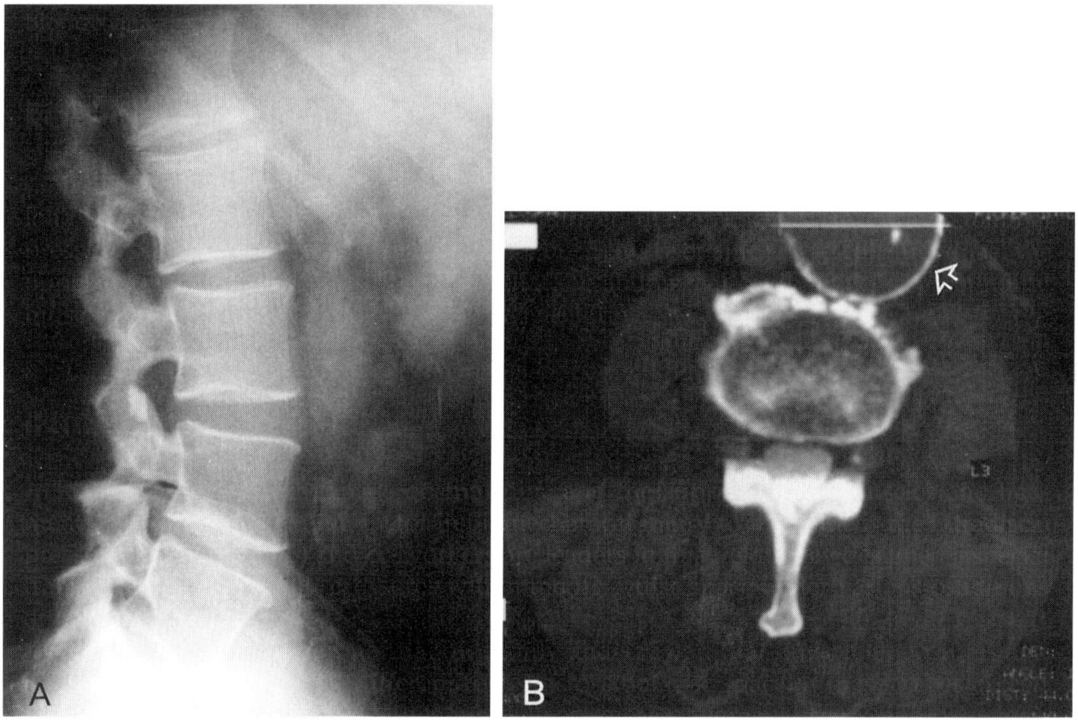

Figure 3.3 **A.** *Plain lateral lumbosacral radiograph showing calcified aortic aneurysm.* **B.** *CT scan (axial) showing degenerative changes. Note the aortic aneurysm (arrow), a condition that may cause back pain.*

though the physician must learn to recognize the presence of an emotional breakdown, he/she must never forget that emotional illnesses do not protect a patient against organic diseases. In such patients, although the task may be difficult, the physician must be prepared to accept the possibility of an underlying significant pathological process and investigate its probability thoroughly. Because this is such an important aspect of proper decision making in lumbar spine surgery, Chapter 12 will cover the topic in extensive detail.

4

Spondylogenic Back Pain: Osseous Lesions

"The spine is a series of bones running down your back. You sit on one end of it and your head sits on the other."

— Anonymous

INTRODUCTION

Patients with severe pathological processes involving the vertebrae (and the intervertebral joints), such as infections, neoplasms, and metabolic disorders, frequently present with pain in the back. Although there may be minor aggravation by activity, the significant distinguishing feature of these conditions is the fact that the pain is not relieved by rest. Major trauma resulting in fracture and fracture dislocations, although not the thrust of this book, will be covered briefly because it can result in back pain as a tiresome sequel. The diagnosis of all of these conditions is largely dependent on radiographic findings, and treatment is along well-established lines, with the exception of major trauma with vertebral fracture. New computed tomography (CT) scanning and magnetic resonance imaging (MRI) techniques are giving us a better understanding of these various conditions and allowing, in some cases, for a more aggressive surgical treatment option.

Although these lesions constitute a very small percentage of the backaches seen in clinical practice, some aspects of each group will be discussed very briefly.

The chapter has been divided into:

1. Trauma.
2. Infection.
3. Tumors (Neoplasms).
4. Metabolic bone disease.

TRAUMA

Introduction

The title of this book is Macnab's Backache. Why do we include a chapter on spine fractures? They do not cause backache; they cause severe immediate back pain. In fact, the severity of the pain is a good teaching point: if a patient with minor backache walks into the emergency room immediately after an accident, he/she probably does not have a fracture. However, if the patient arrives on a gurney in severe pain and unable to move, then that patient has a fracture and/or dislocation of the spine regardless of what the radiographs say. We have included this portion of the chapter to give you a basic working knowledge of thoracolumbar spine fractures to help in the primary care setting. The actual management of spinal fractures has become so advanced and technical that it has become a subspecialty of the subspecialty of spine, with whole textbooks written and whole cupboards full of new instrumentation with which to fix these injuries. But remember, those high-powered subspecialists all started with a basic fund of knowledge that we hope we can establish in a few pages. We are also stretching a little bit, because most fractures in this area occur at the thoracolumbar junction (upper lumbar region) rather than in the lower lumbar region, where degenerative disc disease is so common.

Trauma to the Neurological Contents of the Spine

The lumbar vertebral column has a number of functions, the most important of which is protection of the cord and cauda equina. If the vertebral column is injured, it becomes your duty as the primary caregiver to protect the neurological structures from any or further neurological damage. To do so, consider the following principles:

1. The first duty of a house officer, when a spine fracture is suspected, is to assure immobilization of the spine so that no further neurological damage occurs. Immobilization will be covered in the subsequent section on skeletal structures.
2. The first determination in cord or cauda equina injury is to establish the extent and level of the neurological and skeletal injury.

Neurological Structures That Can Be Injured

Lower thoracic and lumbar spine injuries can damage the lower end of the spinal cord, the conus medullaris, the cauda equina, or the individual roots, as isolated or combined lesions. Do you remember where the conus lies? (Look back at the section on neuroanatomy in Chapter 1 if this information slipped by!)

Injury to nerve tissue can be partial or complete and caused by either a stretching or compressive force. A complete lesion of the cord or the cauda equina causes complete paralysis of the lower extremities (paraplegia); a partial (incomplete) lesion leaves varying degrees of motor and sensory function known as paraparesis.

There are four clinical neurological concepts that you should be aware of. Remember, these concepts apply predominantly to cord injuries; there is very little spinal cord in the lumbar spine, with the spinal cord ending at approximately L1 to L2.

Concept 1

Spinal Shock Following a severe injury to the cord, the portion of the cord caudal to the lesion shuts down: it is in a state of shock, and no activity, including reflex activity, occurs. That means no (cord) reflex activity occurs; the bulbocavernosus and anal wink reflexes, for example, are absent (Fig. 4.1). The final prognosis in neurological injury cannot be determined until spinal shock has passed, something that occurs usually before 24 hours.

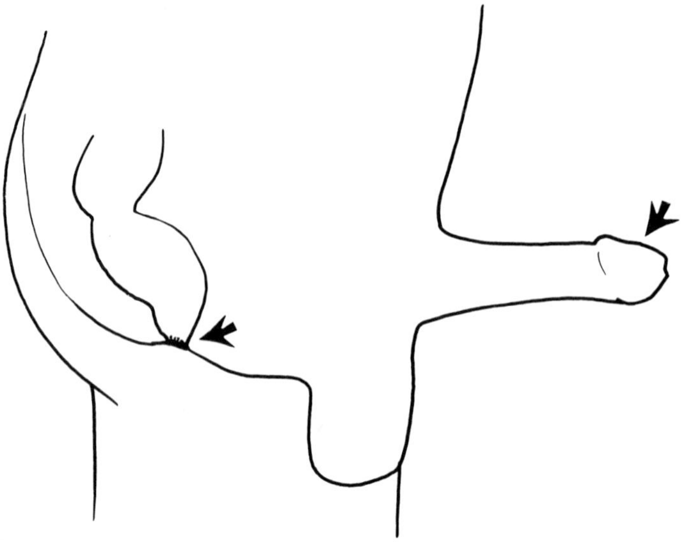

Figure 4.1 *The bulbocavernosus reflex is elicited by pinching the glans penis (right arrow) and either observing an anal wink (left arrow) or feeling contraction of the bulbocavernosus muscle. The peripheral nerve supply for this reflex is the pudendal nerve (S3–4).*

In the acute stage of a complete cord lesion with spinal shock, there is total flaccid paralysis with full loss of reflexes and sensation below the vertebral level of injury. The only difference between presentation of this state and a complete cauda equina lesion is the level of the neurological lesion, that is, a cord lesion will have paralysis of motor power and loss of sensation up to a cord level, whereas the cauda equina lesion will not extend above L1 on sensory or motor examination.

This shocklike state may or may not occur. If present, its duration is variable, lasting from a few hours to a few days. Its end is marked by the return of the bulbocavernosus and anal wink reflexes, at which time a detailed neurological examination can be completed.(1) If, after return of these cord reflexes, there is no discernible motor or sensory function below the level of the lesion, the patient is determined to have complete paralysis from which no functional recovery will occur. On the other hand, if a patient coming out of spinal shock shows some motor or sensory function, this patient has an incomplete cord lesion, which has a much more favorable prognosis.

Concept 2

Sacral sparing is a subtle set of neurological findings that include perianal sensation, some rectal tone, and great toe flexor movement. When present, it indicates some structural continuity of long tracts and a better prognosis regarding neurological recovery.

Concept 3

The most common means of describing the extent of neurological injury is the Frankel classification, (5) which describes the neurological status below the level of the fracture:

- Frankel Grade A: No neurological function (total paralysis) below level of neurological lesion and no sacral sparing.

- Frankel Grade B: Preservation of sensory function below level of neurological injury.
- Frankel Grade C: Motor function below level of neurological injury, but not useful for ambulation.
- Frankel Grade D: Motor function—able to work against gravity (muscle grade > 3).
- Frankel Grade E: Normal neurological function (sensory and motor).

Concept 4

The incomplete Frankel grades (5) of B, C, and D can be further subdivided according to the area of the cord that sustains the most injury (Fig. 4.2):

1. Brown-Séquard syndrome. In this partial neurological injury, one half of the spinal cord is damaged. This results in distal motor and posterior column loss on the same side, and sensory loss on the opposite side. It rarely occurs in its pure form but is a useful descriptive term when there is an asymmetric paresis of the lower extremities, with analgesia or hypalgesia on the least paretic side. Excellent recovery usually follows this lesion.
2. Central cord syndrome. This injury damages the central gray matter and the central long tracts of the white matter. Knowing the location of those tracts makes it easy to understand how the upper extremities, especially the hands, are more affected than the lower extremities. This is the most common type of spinal cord injury and is prone to occur in the older patient with spondylotic bars who falls and suffers a hyperextension injury to the neck. A reasonable degree of recovery (except for the hands) is possible after this injury.
3. Anterior cord syndrome. This lesion affects the anterior two thirds of the cord and is the most devastating of the incomplete lesions. Fortunately, it is less common than the Brown-Séquard and central cord syndromes, and leaves the patient with only posterior cord function (position and vibration sense). There is no significant motor or sensory function distally, and very few patients recover useful function.
4. Root injury. The nerve root exiting at the level of the vertebral injury may suffer from lower motor neuron lesion (LMNL) and may recover. For example, a vertebral lesion at C5 to C6 should allow for recovery of the C6 nerve root.

Concept 3 applies mostly to cervical cord injuries, but it is a useful concept to be aware of when evaluating any spinal cord injury.

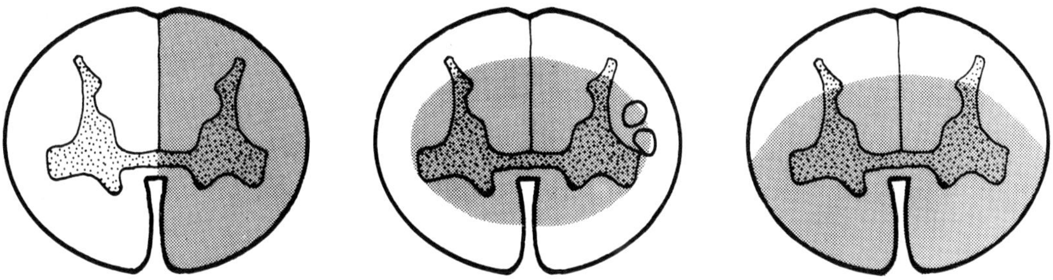

Figure 4.2 *The shaded areas represent the damaged area of the spinal cord: left—Brown-Séquard; middle—central cord; right—anterior cord syndrome.*

Trauma to the Skeletal Structures

Vertebral injuries in this area usually occur in the thoracolumbar region (T10–L1). Fractures or fracture dislocation in the mid or lower lumbar spine are rare and are usually of the "burst" variety.

There are two common fracture patterns that occur in the thoracolumbar region: (1) the burst fracture; (2) the fracture dislocation. Unfortunately, the majority of these patients present with complete neurological lesions to the cord, conus, or cauda equina. The fracture dislocation almost always is associated with a complete neurological lesion. The simple anterior wedge compression fracture (without neurological injury) will be covered later in this chapter.

As with neurological lesions, there are some basic concepts to appreciate in vertebral column fractures.

Concept 1

Forces That Can Be Applied to the Spine Figure 4.3 depicts the forces that can disrupt the thoracolumbar and lumbar spine: compression, tension or distraction, shear, rotation, and bending/flexion. These forces rarely occur in isolation, with most injuries representing the effect of combined forces. This combination of forces is known as coupling, often with one force dominating (such as compression), but another force (such as bending) determining the final fracture pattern. This detracts from the usefulness of classifications. To add to our woes in trying to understand these injuries is the fact that injury not

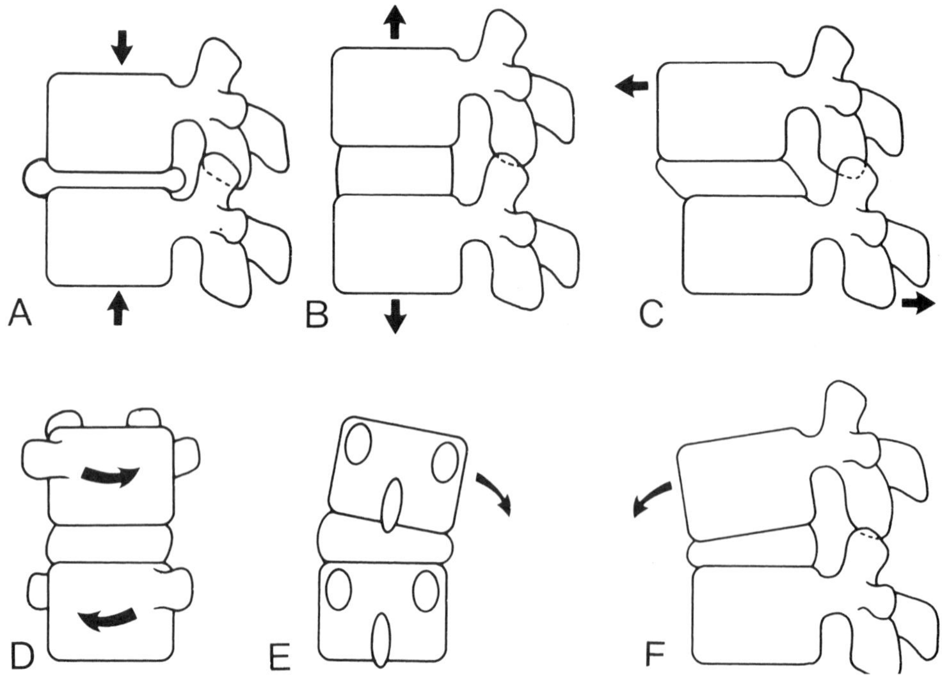

Figure 4.3 *The forces that may disrupt the thoracolumbar and lumbar spine.* **A.** *Compression.* **B.** *Tension or distraction.* **C.** *Shear.* **D.** *Rotation.* **E.** *Lateral bending.* **F.** *Flexion.*

only occurs to the skeleton, but it also affects the neurological tissues and the musculoligamentous support structures. The anatomical level and extent of the neurological injury can be determined by clinical examination, but the pathology affecting the neurological tissue is not known. We are even further in the dark with regard to ligamentous damage that cannot be seen on any imaging modality, including MRI. So, although there is a classification of forces and an anatomical basis for interpreting bony changes on radiograph (Fig. 4.4), there are many holes left in this attempt to adopt a universal language for lumbar fracture care.

Concept 2

Denis, (4) after studying 400 CT scans of thoracolumbar and lumbar spine fractures, developed a three-column anatomical basis for classifying injuries according to the forces applied to the spine (eg, compression). In the three-column theory, the thoracolumbar and lumbar spine can be viewed as consisting of the anterior, middle, and posterior columns (Fig. 4.4). Table 4.1 outlines the various components of each column.

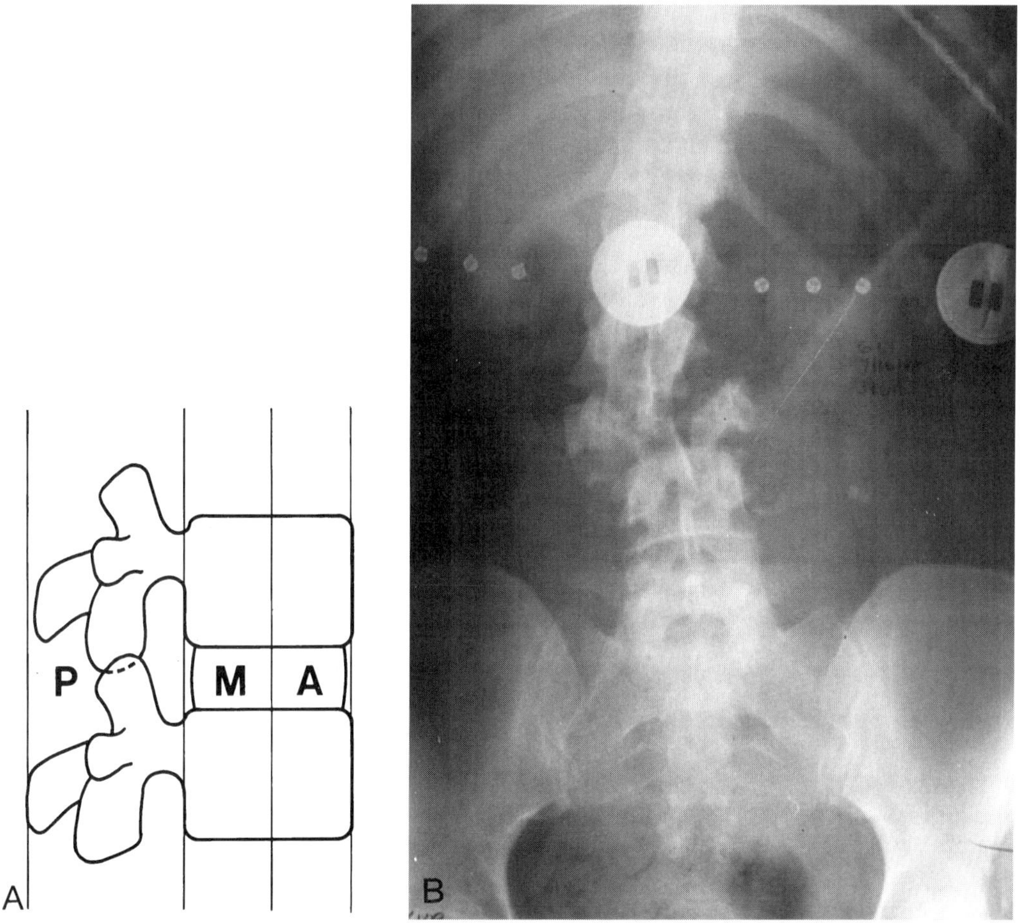

Figure 4.4 **A.** *Denis' three-column classification essential to understanding fracture patterns and spinal stability. See fig. 1.29.* **B.** *A spine fracture that is unclassifiable.*

Table 4.1. Anatomical Basis for Classification of Fractures

Column	Components
Anterior	Anterior longitudinal ligament Anterior half of vertebral body Anterior portion of annulus fibrosus
Middle	Posterior longitudinal ligament Posterior half of the vertebral body Posterior portion of annulus fibrosus
Posterior	Neural arch with facet joints Ligamentum flavum Supraspinous/interspinous ligament complex

Stability Versus Instability Spinal stability is defined as a state in which physiological loads can be absorbed by the spine without abnormal motion and/or damage to neurological structures occurring. Spinal instability is a state in which normal loads result in abnormal motion or deformity, with the potential for damage to neurological structures. The basic premise of the three-column theory of Denis(4) is that spinal stability is most dependent on the status of the middle spinal column and not the posterior ligamentous complex. In general, an unstable spinal fracture is defined as any fracture that has disrupted the middle spinal column, such that bone has burst into the spinal canal, with or without compromise of neurological structures, and/or any fracture that produces more than 15 degrees of kyphosis. By analyzing the three columns one can figure out the forces that caused the injury and the forces needed to stabilize an unstable fracture. A burst (compression) fracture should not be stabilized with instrumentation that compresses and a distraction injury should not be stabilized with instrumentation that distracts.

Damage to neurological structures automatically classifies a spinal fracture as unstable. This damage can occur at the level of the spinal cord, the conus medullaris, or the cauda equina, or to an isolated nerve root.

Concept 3

It is important to understand that the level of vertebral injury does not determine the level of neurological injury, that is, a fracture of L1 does not produce an L1 neurological level injury. The wide variation in the neurological picture in thoracolumbar injuries is due to the variation in the exact vertebral levels of the end of the cord, the end of the conus, and the beginning of the cauda equina. Do you remember the concept of root sparing? Figure 4.5 explains these differences.

Common Fracture Patterns

The two most common fracture patterns in the thoracolumbar column are the compression (burst) fracture and the flexion/bending/rotation fracture or fracture/dislocation.

The Burst Fracture

Figure 4.6 demonstrates the compression burst fracture. In the stable burst fracture, both the anterior and middle columns are involved, and the posterior column is intact. In the unstable burst fracture (14), the posterior column has also been damaged.(15) The ribs in the lower tho-

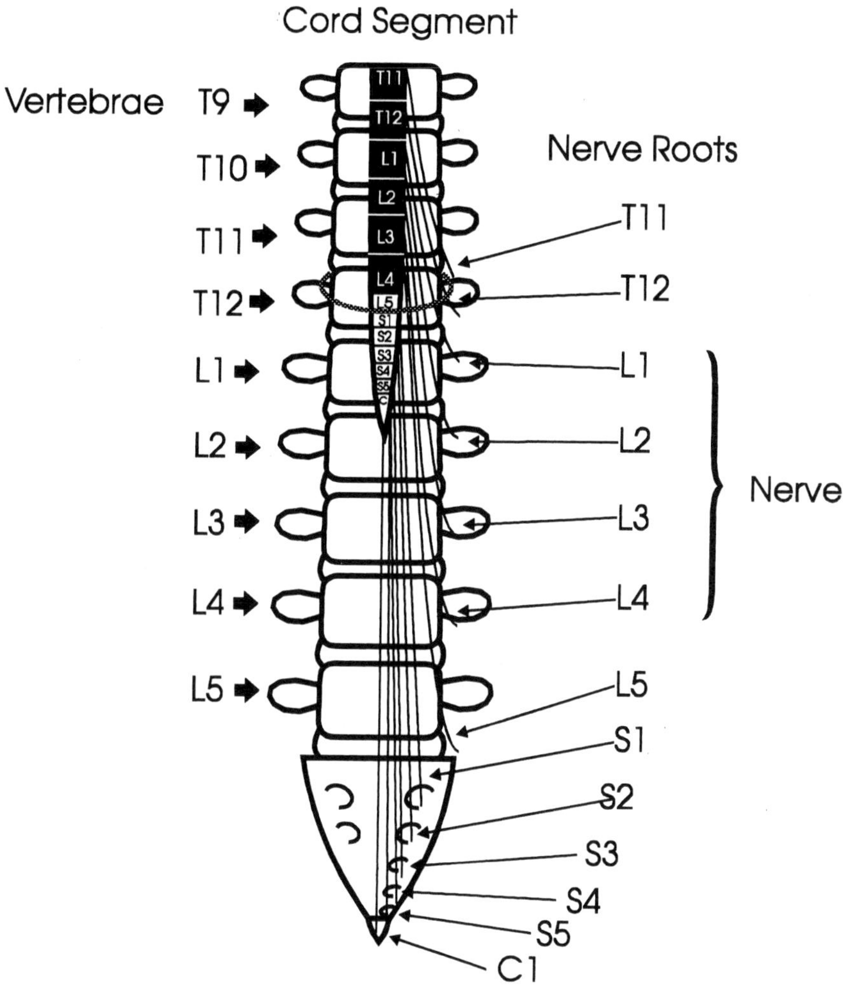

Figure 4.5 *Vertebral column injury at T12 (note the dotted ring at T12) will damage the spinal cord segments from L4 down, but the spinal roots above L4 may be spared damage because their nerve root sheaths are more resistant to injury: the concept of root escape or root sparing.*

racic region protect the area from this pure compression load so that most of these injuries are to the L1 or L2 vertebral bodies. "Burst" is a good description of what happens to the fracture fragments, with the most serious damage done by the superior corner of the middle column (posterior vertebral body) being displaced into the spinal canal (Fig. 4.6). The size of the fragment and the degree of displacement determine the extent of the neurological damage.

Fracture/Dislocations

This type of fracture occurs as a result of numerous forces, the two most common being flexion and rotation. These injuries are the result of severe forces and are often associated with multiple (other) injuries such as abdominal injuries and long bone fractures. In this fracture pattern, all three columns of Denis have failed, and the fracture is very unstable and requires surgical stabilization. Unfortunately, a very high percentage of these fractures have complete neurological lesions (Fig. 4.7).

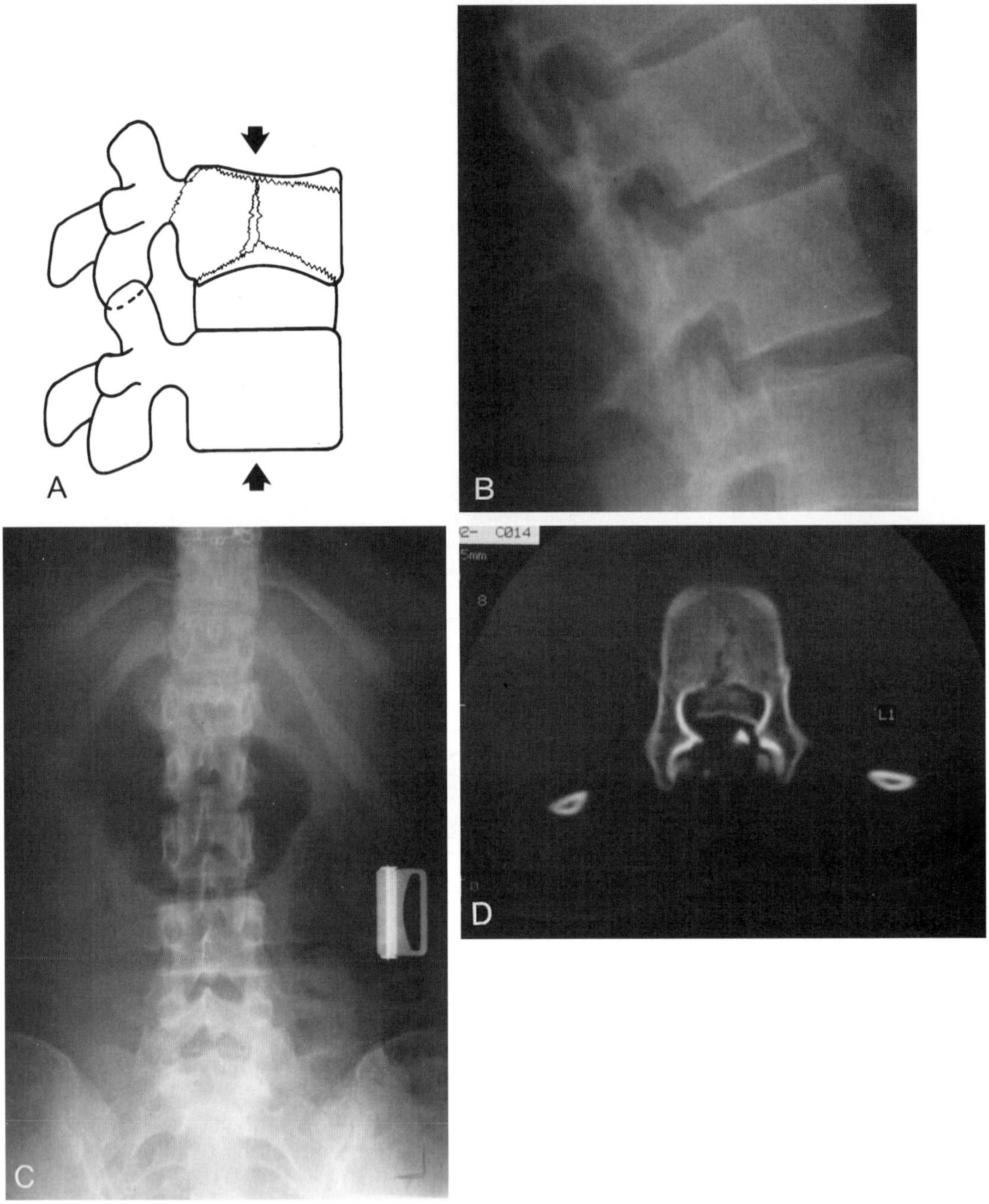

Figure 4.6 *The two most common major lumbar fractures.* **A.** *Schematic of burst fractures.* **B.** *Burst fracture of L1 (arrow).* **C.** *AP showing widening of pedicles in burst fracture.* **D.** *CT showing burst of posterior wall into spinal canal.*

Other Fracture Patterns

Less common injuries in the thoracolumbar region are the so-called "seat belt" injuries or flexion/distraction injuries. Often, there is coupling of the forces in this mechanism of injury that produces the fracture pattern shown in Figure 4.8.

The next most common area of injury is in the thoracic area above T10. These may be

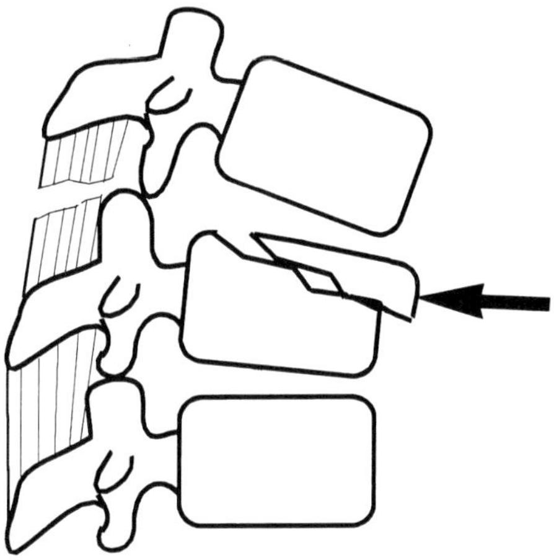

Figure 4.7 *A schematic of a fracture/dislocation with the proximal vertebral body forward on the middle vertebrae. Note the slice of the superior edge of the vertebral body (arrow).*

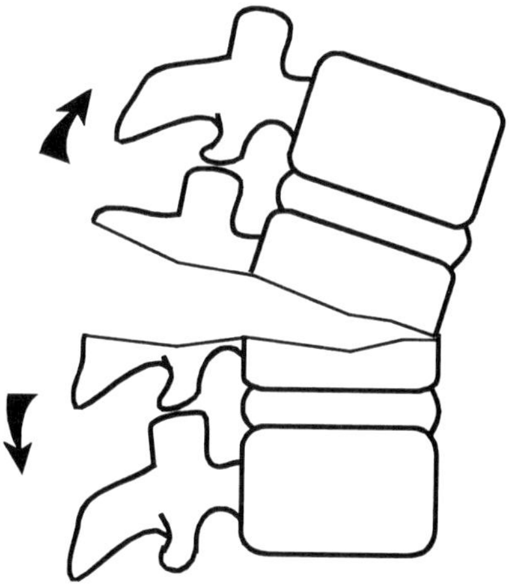

Figure 4.8 *A schematic of the seat belt or flexion/distraction thoracolumbar injury.*

compression injuries or the more devastating fracture mechanism of flexion, rotation, and shear. There is a very high incidence of associated life-threatening injuries to the cardiovascular and/or pulmonary systems. These injuries are also handled largely through a posterior approach, with various methods of reduction and fixation being used.

Investigation

These multiply injured patients have many specialists involved in their care who will all make the appropriate decisions to intervene for their specific system failure. How do you investigate the skeletal and neurological injuries to the spine? First, do no harm in transporting a patient with an unstable unsplinted spine.

Every patient requires, at minimum, an anteroposterior and a lateral radiograph of the injured area, plus radiographs of as many segments above and below the injury as possible. If one spine fracture is discovered, the entire spine has to be radiographed because up to one third of the patients will have another spine fracture. Special attention has to be paid to the junctional areas: craniocervical, cervicothoracic, thoracolumbar, and lumbosacral. Once the skeletal injury has been localized, CT scan is an appropriate next step.

If time and the patient's general condition permit, it is often very helpful to obtain an MRI of the area, which will give you information about soft tissue involvement (including the neurological structures), and also gives you sagittal cuts to supplement the axial CT scan cuts. Myelography now plays a limited role in the assessment of these patients.

Treatment

General Principles of Treatment

The goals of treatment are:

1. Treat the whole patient: approximately 50% of these patients will have other life-threatening injuries to their head, chest, or belly.
2. Treat the spine-injured patient to produce a reduced, stable, pain-free spine with minimal deformity and to allow for maximum neurological recovery.

Through interdisciplinary efforts, the patient's brain, pulmonary status, vascular tree, bowel (ileus), and bladder (paralysis) must be addressed. The early use (within 8 hours) of high doses of steroids has also been proposed for spinal cord injuries. Hypotension must be prevented at all costs to prevent further ischemic injury to neurological tissues.

The Absolute Indications for Surgery

Neurological Indications Partial neurological injuries, in the end, are best treated surgically, with the timing of surgery dependent on the other injuries. Most spine surgeons will intervene as early as possible (within 24 hours) if allowed. Incomplete neurological injuries that show increasing deficits are a surgical emergency (this is a rare situation).

Complete neurological injuries (determined after spinal shock has passed) have little chance of neurological recovery, and the treatment principles center around skeletal considerations and can be made electively.

Skeletal Indications

Burst Fractures Instability that merits a surgical decision is present if there is:

- Fifteen degrees or greater kyphosis (sagittal plane malalignment) (Fig. 4.9).
- Loss of more than 50% of anterior vertebral body height (implying posterior column damage) (Fig. 4.9).
- More than 25% of the spinal canal compromised by the retropulsed fragment with a partial neurological lesion (Fig. 4.9).

Unless, in these partial neurological lesions, there is gross canal compromise from the retropulsed fragment, most experts would agree that the initial surgical approach to this injury is better as a posterior rather than an anterior route. Because of a concern for late collapse, some surgeons add an anterior approach to bone graft the fracture.

The best results, especially with regard to reduction of the burst fragment by ligamentotaxis (using the intact posterior longitudinal ligament and annulus, in tension, to reduce the retropulsed fragment), occur when the posterior surgery is done within 48 hours of the injury.

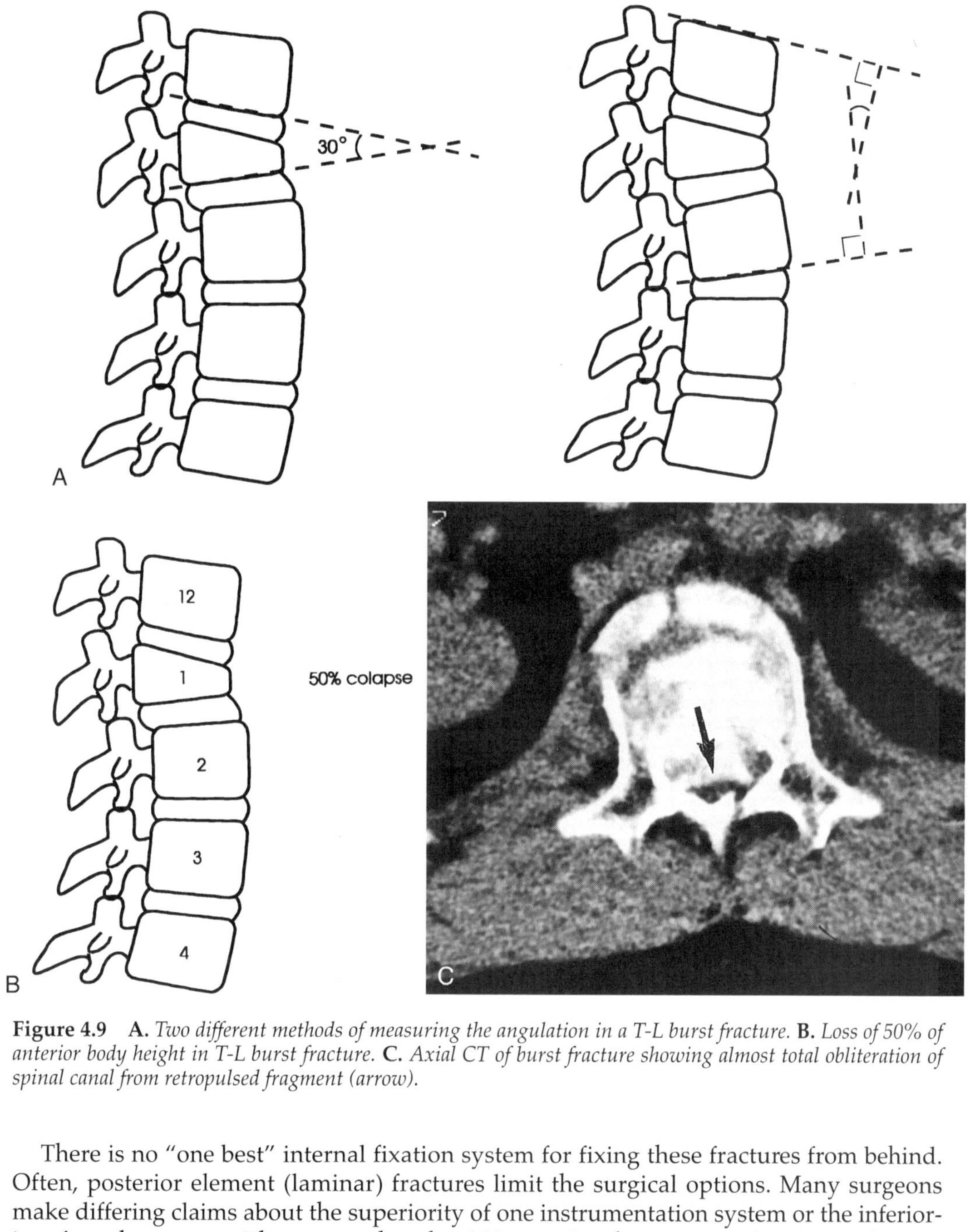

Figure 4.9 **A.** *Two different methods of measuring the angulation in a T-L burst fracture.* **B.** *Loss of 50% of anterior body height in T-L burst fracture.* **C.** *Axial CT of burst fracture showing almost total obliteration of spinal canal from retropulsed fragment (arrow).*

There is no "one best" internal fixation system for fixing these fractures from behind. Often, posterior element (laminar) fractures limit the surgical options. Many surgeons make differing claims about the superiority of one instrumentation system or the inferiority of another system. The system that should be used is the one most familiar to the surgeon and the institution and may include rods with various combinations of hooks, wires, or sleeves, or pedicle fixation with various rods, wires, and plates. Figure 4.10 shows two common examples of fixation for this injury. It is important that every system maintains lumbar lordosis.

The levels to be fixed and fused depend on the level of the burst fracture. Using as an example an L1 burst, the internal fixation would extend from T11 to the lamina of L2,

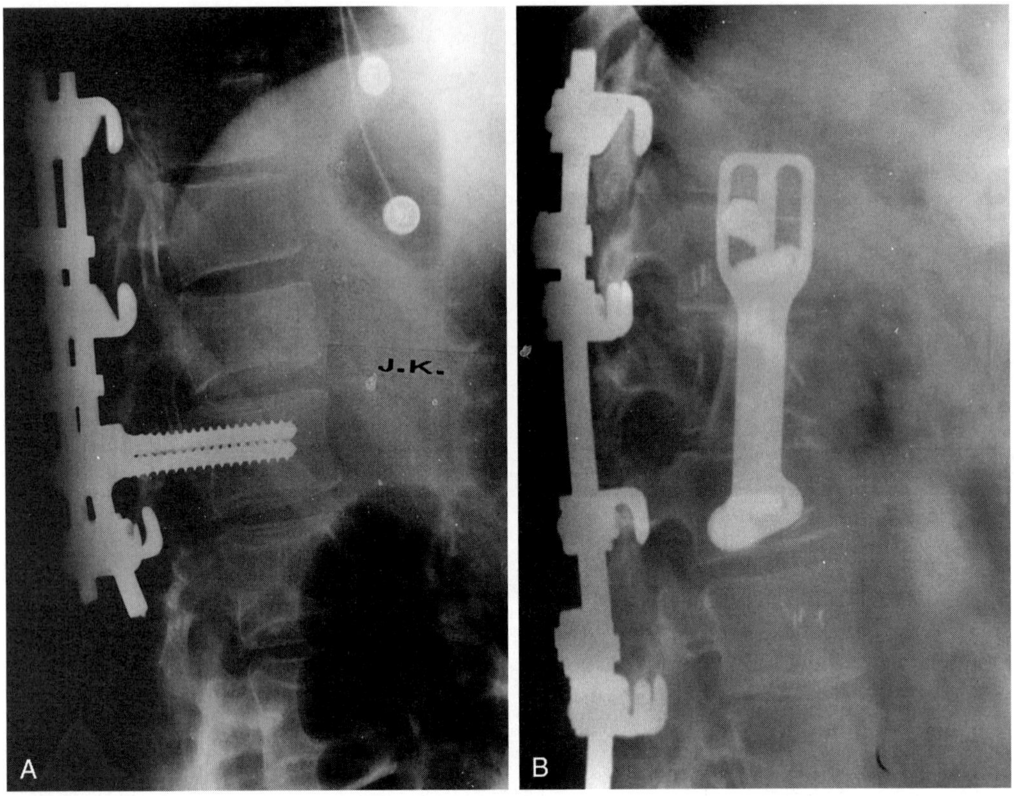

Figure 4.10 *Fixation of a burst fracture.* **A.** *Posterior instrumentation for L1 burst (the level above the screws).* **B.** *Posterior and anterior fixation (the fracture is behind the midportion of the plate).*

leaving the L2–3 interspace mobile. The associated fusion would extend from the transverse process and facet joints of T11 to L2.

Postoperatively, maintain the patient in an external support (Fig. 4.11) until the fracture heals (radiographic assessment including flexion/extension films).

There are two types of burst fractures that still have alot of support for management with conservative care (nonoperative management). (10)(18)

1. The burst fracture with no neurological involvement, good skeletal alignment (as determined by a standing radiograph in a thoracolumbar spinal orthosis [TLSO]), and less than 50% canal compromise.
2. The burst fracture with a permanent, complete neurological injury and acceptable skeletal alignment, regardless of the degree of canal compromise.

If you wish to alter skeletal alignment, do it early. Letting these fractures go beyond a week after injury reduces the chance of realignment (9); all fractures beyond a month of injury will require an anterior procedure to correct alignment.

Laminectomy has little role to play in the management of thoracolumbar burst fractures except to cause long-term instability and deformity. Burst fractures in the lower lumbar spine (L4/L5) have different fracture patterns, with more posterior element fractures, that may require laminectomy to free up impailed neurological tissue.

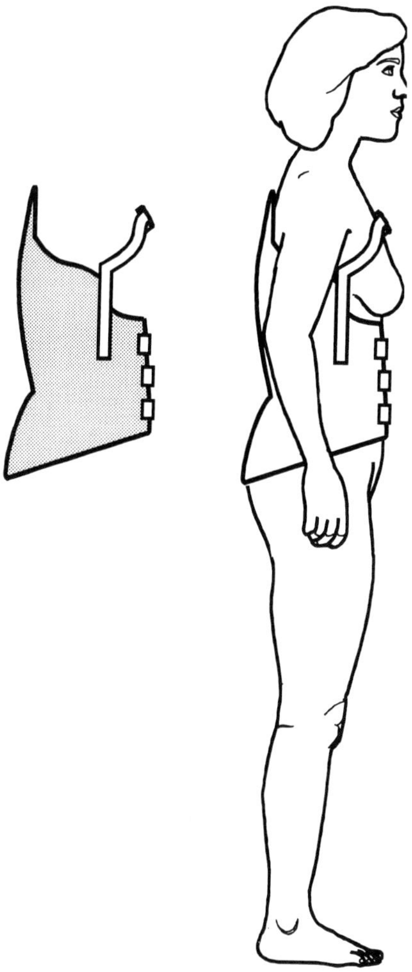

Figure 4.11 *A variety of the TLSO (thoracolumbosacral orthosis) lateral view (left) and on a patient (right).*

Flexion/Rotation Injuries These injuries are all very unstable skeletally and require surgical stabilization regardless of the neurological status. The mechanism of injury dictates a posterior surgical approach. This type of injury is so unstable that it is prudent to include at least two levels above and two levels below the fracture in the posterior instrumentation and fusion (Fig. 4.10).

Minor Traumatic Events Affecting the Lumbar Spine

The Osteoporotic Compression Fracture

The most common spine fracture you will see in the emergency department is the compression fracture in osteoporotic bone. Your patient will usually (but not always) be a woman and will describe the sudden onset of midback pain brought on by a simple maneuver such as a cough or lifting of a bag of groceries. In approximately 20% of the patients, the compression fracture will be asymptomatic and unrecognized until a radiograph is done for some other purpose.

Most patients will experience the sudden onset of pain so severe they will appear in the emergency department. Even though the fracture may be affecting a single vertebral level, the pain will be described as a diffuse discomfort; for example, a fracture of T9 will radiate widely, even to the lower lumbar region.

Careful palpation or percussion of the spinous processes will usually reveal the level of fracture. Rarely will there be evidence of radicular or cord involvement in simple compression fractures.

Plain radiographs will reveal one of three fracture patterns (Fig. 4.12). The anterior wedge is the fracture pattern most commonly seen in the thoracic vertebrae, with the biconcave endplate fracture being more common in the lumbar region.

Most patients with benign compression fractures can be treated outside of the hospital. Occasionally the pain is so severe that admission becomes a necessity. The rare complications of ileus, urinary retention, and neurological complications will require hospital admission. In this older population, excessive narcotic use (eg, oxycodone and hydrocodone), will cause more problems than solutions. Often strong analgesia is needed in the first couple of days, but this should be quickly reduced as the patient is ambulated in corset support (Fig. 4.13). Bracing is especially important in ambulating these patients, but the design has to be simple to accommodate frailty and the often accompanying arthritic hands. Obviously, severe osteoporosis or osteoporosis in the younger patient (less than 65 years of age) requires redress.

Healing is best followed by the patient's symptoms, although serial radiographs will show any progressive collapse. It will take 6 to 12 weeks before patients are comfortable enough to shed their brace and increase their activities. It takes a lot of reassurance on the part of the supervising physician to keep these patients pointed in the right direction. Once a comfort level is achieved, the institution of an extension exercise program and low impact aerobics is important.

Repeated compression fractures will lead to an increasing kyphotic deformity of the chest, with the ribs eventually settling on the pelvis. This causes discomfort and is associated with poor posture, a protuberant abdomen, and a very unhappy patient. There is little the physician can offer in this situation; thus, prevention is an important goal.

Osteoporotic Compression Fracture vs Tumor

The constant dilemma in the emergency room is to decide whether the thoracic fracture you are looking at is occurring in osteoporotic bone or bone weakened by a tumor.

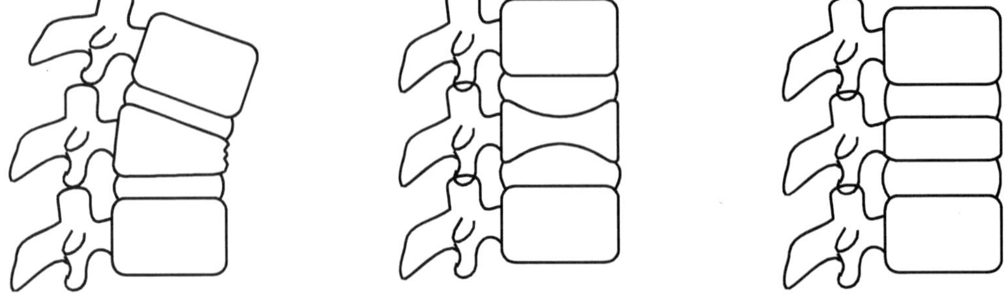

Figure 4.12 *The three varieties of compression fracture: left—wedge; middle—"codfish"; right—uniform compression, anterior and posterior.*

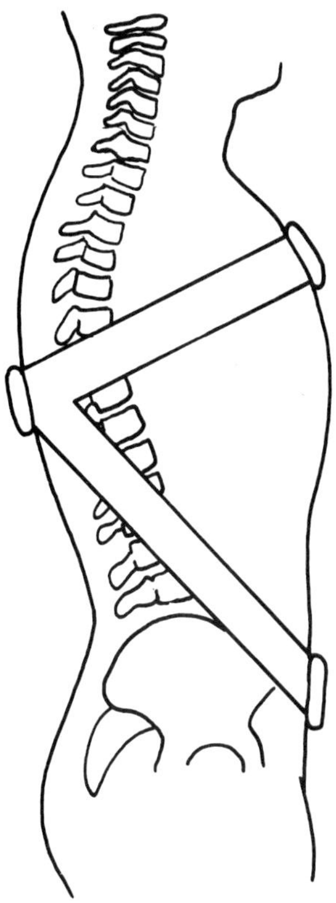

Figure 4.13 *Brace support: Three points of support—one posterior below fracture, one on sternum, and one on the symphysis pubis.*

The following points suggest that you are dealing with a secondary malignant lesion (or primary myeloma):

1. The patient presents with severe pain, and any attempt to roll or sit up becomes a moment of agony.
2. Radicular pain and or cord symptoms and signs are present.
3. Plain radiographs reveal:
   a. Destruction of cortex.
   b. Loss of pedicle (Fig. 4.14).
   c. A compression fracture above T7 or below L2.
4. The patient has a history of a past malignancy.
5. An MRI (Fig. 4.14) reveals:
   a. The marrow cavity is completely obliterated, with no fatty marrow left.
   b. The cortical margins are gray and mottled, rather than black and distinct.
   c. There is a soft tissue mass outside of the vertebral body such as cord effacement (Fig. 4.15).
   d. There are skip lesions (Fig. 4.16).
   e. Gadolinium injection on MRI is not a reliable way to sort out malignancy from benignity.
6. A bone scan is often helpful in distinguishing malignant from benign lesions (Fig. 4.17).

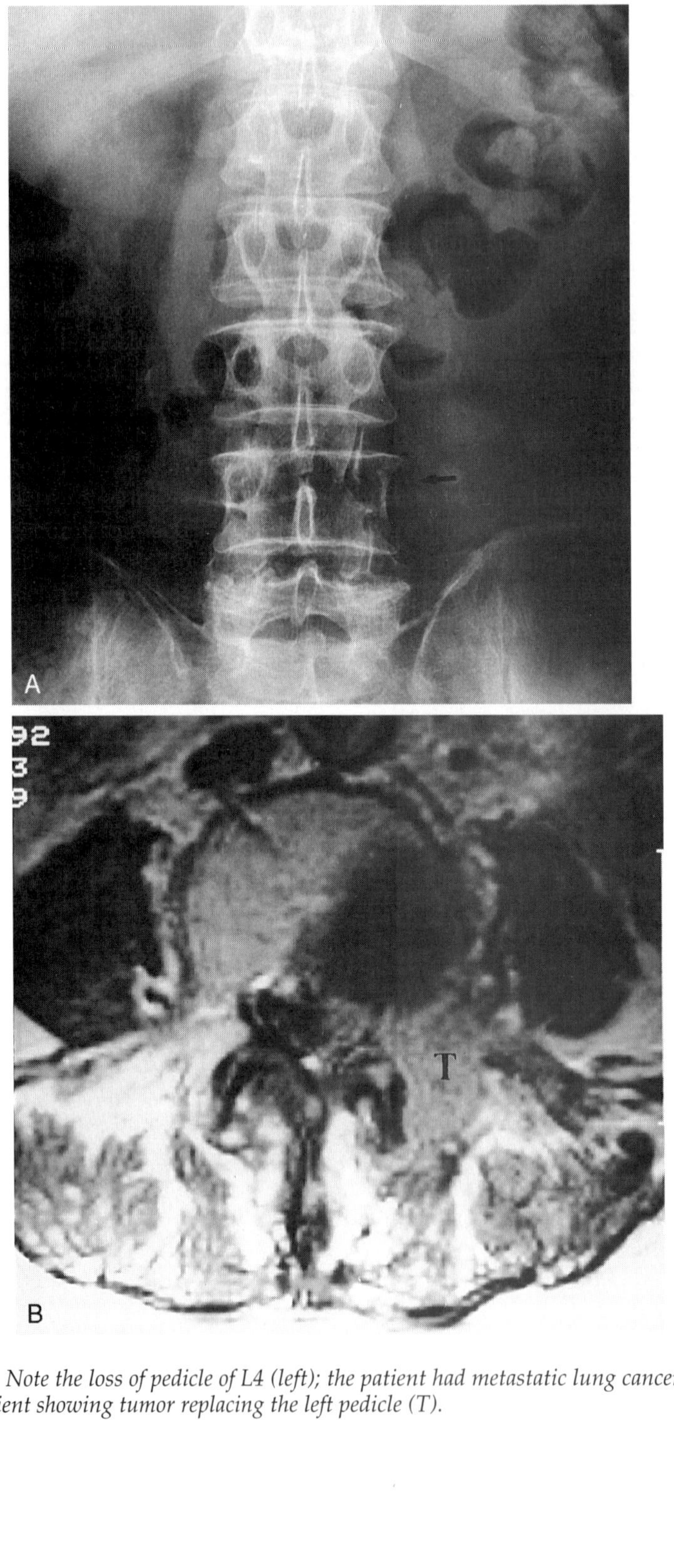

Figure 4.14 **A.** *Note the loss of pedicle of L4 (left); the patient had metastatic lung cancer.* **B.** *An axial (T1) MRI in same patient showing tumor replacing the left pedicle (T).*

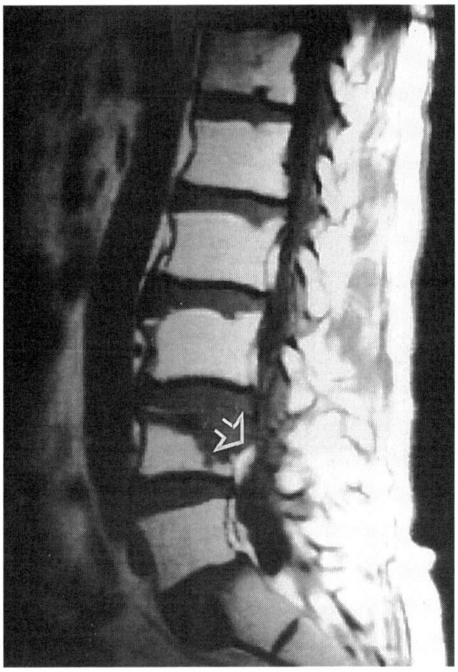

Figure 4.15 *The soft tissue mass of tumor on MRI (sagittal T1) is pressing on the cauda equina (arrow).*

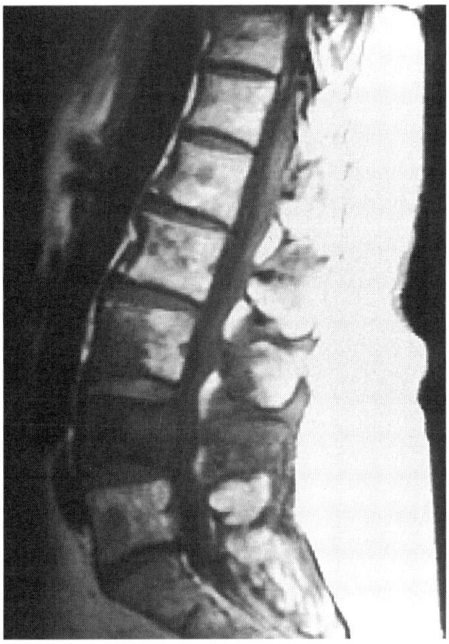

Figure 4.16 *Metastatic skip lesions on MRI (T1 sagittal): the main tumor mass (black or low signal intensity) is in L4. Note the additional "skip" lesions in L5, L3, L2, and L1, with preservation (skipping) of the disc spaces.*

If, after all of the considerations just mentioned, you have still not pinned down the diagnosis, a CT-guided biopsy will be required.

The management of osteoporosis will be discussed later in the chapter, in the section on metabolic bone disease.

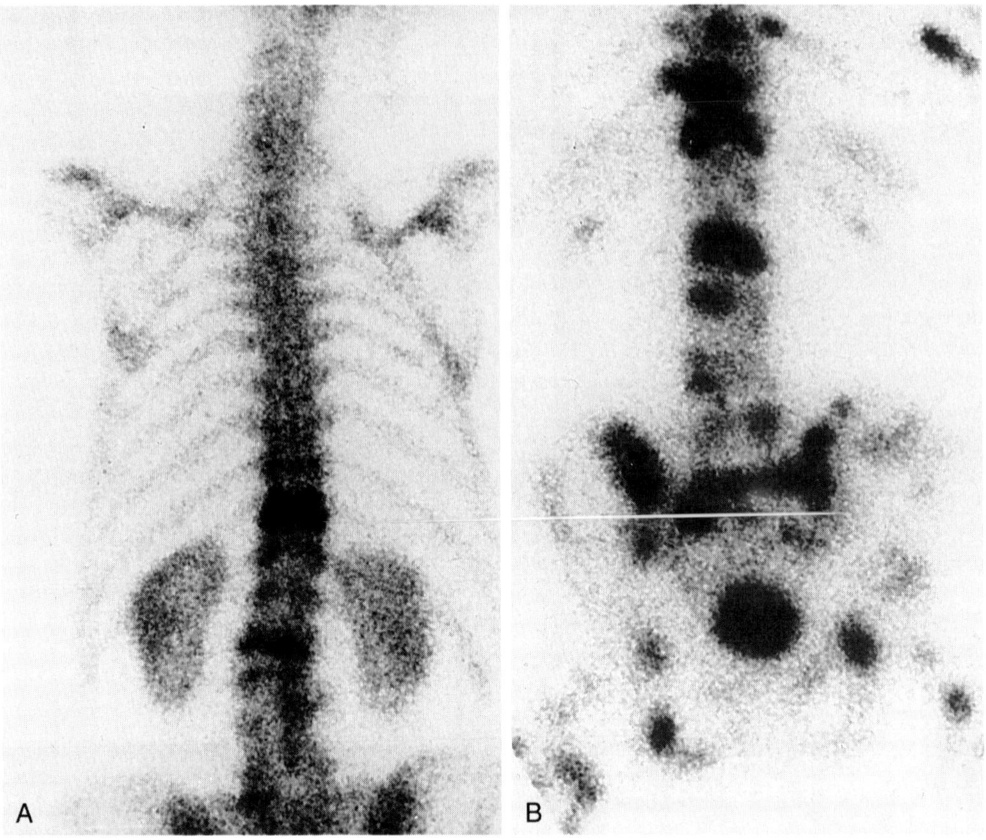

Figure 4.17 *Bone scans in a fracture* **(A)** *and tumor* **(B).** *There is no difference in the intensity of the hot spot, but there are multiple "hot spots" in B indicative of metastatic tumor.*

INFECTION

Spinal infections, despite their relative rarity, must be remembered as a potential source of back pain. For convenience of discussion, infections involving the vertebral column may be considered under the following clinicopathological syndromes:

1. Vertebral osteomyelitis.
   a. Pyogenic.
   b. Granulomatous (tubercle bacillus).
   c. Miscellaneous.
2. Epidural abscess.
3. Intervertebral disc "infection."
4. Intervertebral disc "inflammation."

Pyogenic Vertebral Osteomyelitis

Although pyogenic spinal lesions may result from discography, discectomy, and open wounds, most vertebral osteomyelitis results from hematogenous spread through an arterial or venous route. Probably the most common source of infection is from a pelvic inflammatory lesion (eg, bladder infection), with spread occurring through Batson's plexus (Fig. 4.18) after a surgical procedure such as cystoscopy.

The clinical features of vertebral osteomyelitis have altered from the preantibiotic era. Vertebral osteomyelitis used to be a disease of adolescents and was very acute in onset. The source of the infection was rarely known. Staphylococcus sp was by far the most common organism involved, and the disease had a dreadful mortality of approximately 60%.

Vertebral osteomyelitis is presently a disease of adults. The onset may still be acute, but more often than not the onset is insidious, and the course is chronic. This leads to more misdiagnoses than you can imagine; in fact, the first time you meet a patient with vertebral osteomyelitis, you will likely miss the diagnosis!

The source of infection can be localized in approximately 50% of patients and usually can be linked to infection or instrumentation of the genitourinary system. It is interesting to note that a significant portion of these patients are elderly, debilitated, or diabetic. Although Staphylococcus sp is still the most common infecting organism, Escherichia coli and other gram-negative organisms are increasing in frequency. The drug subculture has added a new dimension, with its own group of gram-negative organisms (*Pseudomonas* sp).

The lumbar spine is more commonly affected than the thoracic or cervical spine. Because the vertebral body has a richer vascular network than the posterior elements, the majority of infections involve the body. Commonly, two adjacent vertebrae and the intervening disc space are involved (Fig. 4.19). Varying degrees of vertebral body destruction and collapse occur. With the spread of the infection, an abscess may develop and extend either anteriorly or posteriorly.

Neurological damage may result from the development of an angulatory kyphosis, an epidural abscess, or a sequestrated disc or bone fragments. Occasionally, the spinal cord may be destroyed by obliteration of its vascular supply.

Clinical Presentation

Backache is the most common presenting symptom: indeed, early in its course, the disease may be indistinguishable symptomatically from a mechanical backache. The insidious onset and the lack of radiographic changes account for the usual delay of 8 to 10 weeks in diagnosis. With progression of the disease, the back pain increases in intensity, becoming constant, and is particularly noticeable in bed at night. More often than not, the back pain has reached severe proportions before the diagnosis is made. On occasion, pain will be referred to the abdomen, leading to a search for intra-abdominal disease.

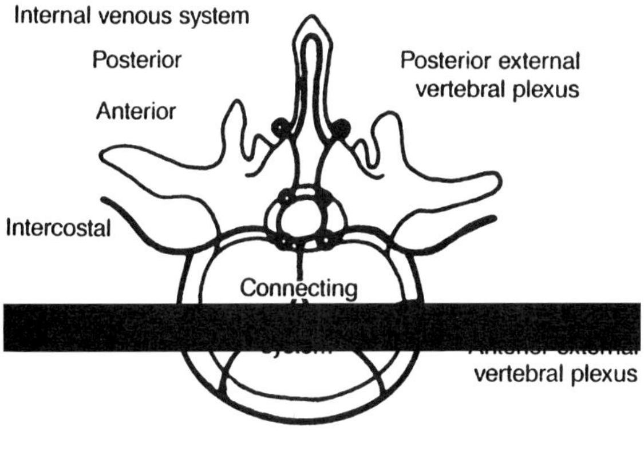

Figure 4.18 *Batson's plexus is a network of veins that connects the abdominal and thoracic cavities (via the vena cava) to the vertebral body and epidural space. The components of the plexus around the spinal column are shown and include the external vertebral veins, the internal (epidural) veins, and the connecting veins.*

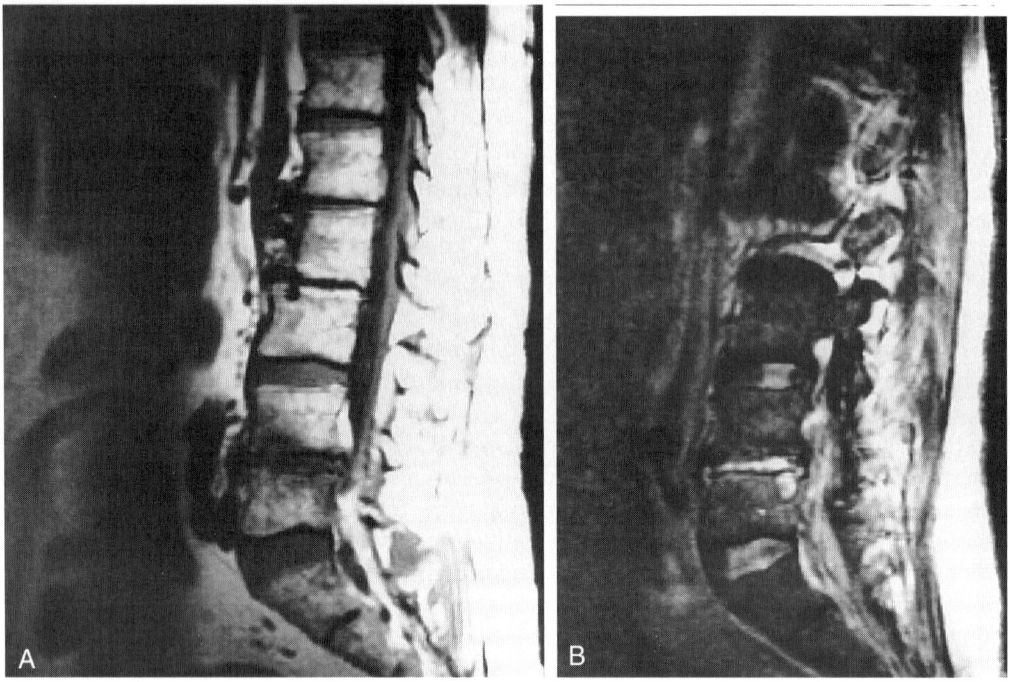

Figure 4.19 *MRI of osteomyelitis:* **A.** *Sagittal (T1) showing decreased signal intensity on either side of L4–5 disc space.* **B.** *Sagittal (T2) showing increased signal intensity in same area: this is the typical MRI picture of the edema of inflammation.*

The patient may appear sick and will have a variable temperature elevation. The findings at examination vary with the stage and severity of the disease. All spinal movements and jarring intensify the pain. Paravertebral muscle and hamstring spasms are sometimes severe. The patient may stand with a marked list of the spine to one side. Gross spinal rigidity is a characteristic feature. The spinous processes are usually tender on pressure. The back pain is intensified by percussion of the involved area. Straight leg raising (SLR) is restricted because of hamstring spasm. If the infection has spread to involve the meninges, SLR may be markedly reduced from the meningismus. On the rare occasion, neurological findings of root compression will be detected, but every so often a delay in diagnosis will be followed by epidural abscess formation, and either direct compression or a vascular lesion will damage the lower cord or cauda equina. If paralysis is the outcome, there is little chance for recovery from this tragic sequence of events.

Laboratory

In half of the patients, the white blood count (WBC) will be within normal limits, and even when elevated, the WBC rarely rises above 15,000/cu mm. The erythrocyte sedimentation rate (ESR), however, is consistently elevated and is the most useful test for monitoring disease activity and the efficacy of treatment. On occasion, a very debilitated patient will show no signs of fever, no elevated WBC, or increased ESR. Blood cultures may be positive in up to 50% of patients, particularly in those who present with a markedly febrile clinical course.

Radiology

Radiological evidence of the spinal disease lags 4 weeks or more behind the clinical manifestations. The earliest changes are localized rarefaction of the vertebral endplates (Fig. 4.20), followed rapidly by involvement of the adjacent vertebrae and narrowing of the disc spaces. With the increasing recognition of disc degeneration as a source of spondylogenic pain, there is an inherent danger of misinterpretation of the radiological changes. The early specific radiological features that distinguish the disc narrowing that is the result of infection from the disc narrowing that is associated with degenerative changes are very subtle and include fuzziness of the cortical endplate and a "divot" out of the anterior-superior or anterior-inferior portion of the vertebral body (Fig. 4.20). This raises another distinguishing feature of infection vs tumor: early radiological changes reflective of infection affect the endplate region and are anterior, whereas tumors affect the medullary/marrow space and tend to be posterior in the vertebral body.

The radiologist frequently is not provided with enough clinical information, and there is no reason why the minimal radiological changes should make him suspicious of

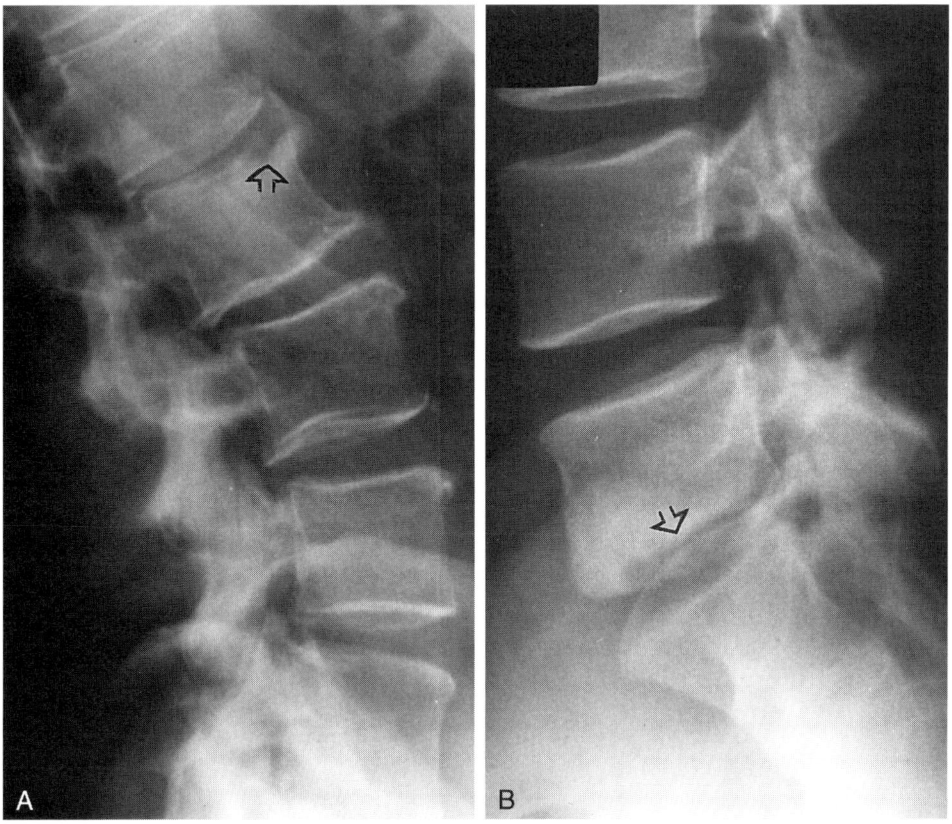

Figure 4.20 *Plain radiograph of the stages of discitis/osteomyelitis.* **A.** *Early: a small "divot" out of the anterior aspect of L2 (arrow).* **B.** *Midphase: irregularities of vertebral endplate of L5 (arrow) and disc space narrowing L5-S1.*

an infective lesion. So the diagnosis is suggested by the clinical findings: a sick patient with severe pain, a rigid back, fever, and a raised WBC and sedimentation rate. Early plain radiological changes are minimal but may give an indication of the site of the lesion. At this stage, the diagnosis is best made by an MRI (Fig. 4.19). (16) But even with these sophisticated tests, the diagnosis can be missed because of nonspecific changes.

Later in the course of infective disease, the plain radiographs reveal destructive erosion of the contiguous vertebral bodies, starting first and usually most extensive anteriorly (Fig. 4.21). Subsequently, there is sclerosis and the development of reactive bone. Evidence of soft tissue reaction is revealed on radiograph by distortion of the psoas shadow or by a localized paravertebral mass.

There may be some difficulty in distinguishing the radiological changes of an infective lesion from those produced by a neoplasm, but as a general rule it may be said that with infection the disc space is the first structure to be destroyed, whereas with secondary deposits in the vertebral body the disc space is spared (Fig. 4.22).

So many of these infections occur in the debilitated patient (elderly, rheumatoid, diabetic, or immunocompromised) that a special word needs to be said. The patients are sickly to start with and often are in chronic pain, so the addition of a disc space infection adds little to the clinical appearance. The onset and progress of infection in this group is very insidious and hidden. The fever and laboratory changes are not obvious. The radiographic changes can easily be ascribed to the patients' known disease process rather than osteomyelitis. It takes an especially vigilant clinician to recognize vertebral infections in this patient population.

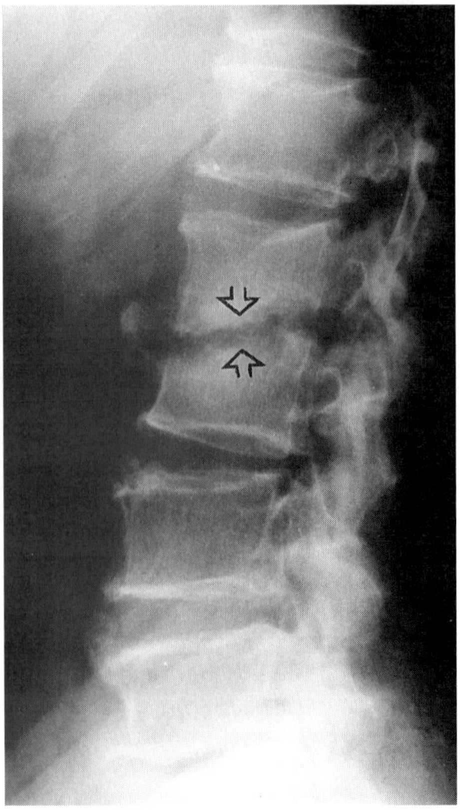

Figure 4.21 *The late stage: total destruction of disc space and adjacent vertebral bodies (arrows).*

Diagnosis

It is essential to search for the causative organism. The triad of cultures—blood, infection site, and potential source—are to be completed before institution of antimicrobial therapy. The blood culture and source culture (eg, urine or sputum) are readily obtained. A culture of the infection site requires a percutaneous biopsy (Fig. 4.23) and is mandatory because of the occasional case of blood cultures revealing organisms different from the actual organism cultured from the infected site.

Treatment is absolutely dependent on the isolation of the organism and on the stage of the disease. No longer is it safe to presume that the infection is staphylococcal. Because of the increasing incidence of gram-negative infections and infections by more than one organism, the offending organism must be identified by blood culture and/or a vertebral biopsy and culture, in order that its sensitivity may be determined. If needle biopsy fails to obtain enough material to permit isolation of the organism, then an open biopsy is necessary.

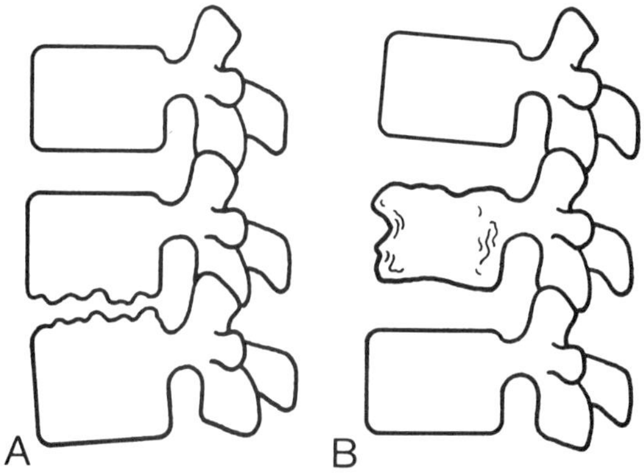

Figure 4.22 **A.** *Pyogenic infections attack and narrow the disc space early.* **B.** *Tuberculosis and neoplasms spare the disc space.*

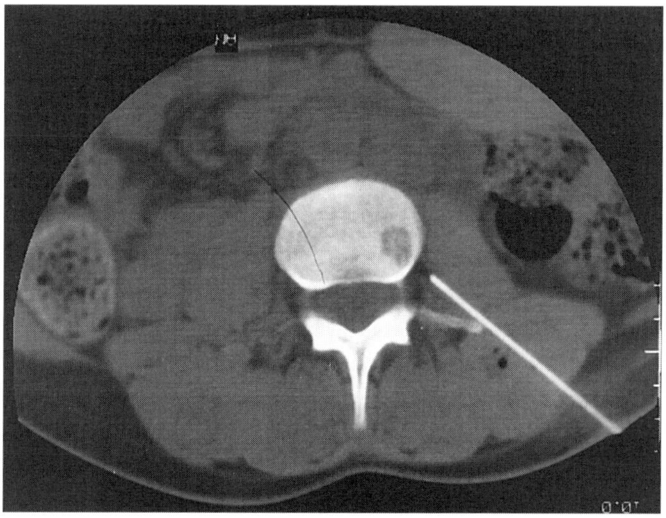

Figure 4.23 *A CT guided biopsy of a lytic lesion in L4.*

Treatment

Intravenous antibiotics and bed rest to start are followed by bracing, oral antibiotics, and activity limitation. Treatment should be continued until the sedimentation rate has returned to normal. The brace should be worn for an arbitrary period of 3 months, and antibiotic coverage should be continued during this period of time, providing the clinical course allows; serial sedimentation rates that return toward normal should be included in this regimen. Routine radiological assessment should be carried out at 6-week intervals. Fusion occurs in 50% of pyogenic disc space infections in approximately 1 year, and the majority of the remainder show bony obliteration of the disc space in 2 years. Routine radiological reassessment is of importance to evaluate effectiveness of antibiotic treatment as measured by no ongoing bone destruction.

The endpoint in medical treatment has been reached when the patient's pain and fever have resolved, there is radiographic evidence of fusion, and the ESR is back to normal for that patient. Remember, in alot of elderly debilitated patients there is no such occurrence as "normal" sedimentation rate. When you have met these four criteria, administration of antibiotics can be stopped, the brace can be shed, and rehabilitation for lost function can start.

Surgery

The indications for surgical intervention are:

1. Failure of medical management: despite rest and massive intravenous antibiotics, the patient's fever and pain persist.
2. A large abscess forms. Small abscesses, providing they are not in the epidural space, may be successfully treated with medical management. Never let the sun set on a large paraspinal or any sized epidural abscess.
3. Progressive neurological deficit. If the patient arrives on your service paraplegic, you must intervene on an emergency basis, but there is little likelihood of salvage. If on your watch (a neurological examination every 2 to 4 hours), you detect an increasing deficit despite medical treatment, take the patient to the operating room without delay.
4. Biomechanical instability is a likely outcome (eg, anticipated or actual kyphosis of > 15 degrees).
5. Failure to obtain an adequate biopsy specimen sufficient to make a definitive diagnosis.

Type of Surgery

The basic rule in spine infection (and almost any other spinal problem) is to go directly to the problem. Because these infections are in the vertebral body and disc space, the surgical approach is anteriorly. The only exception to this rule is an epidural abscess, which should be approached posteriorly (laminectomy).

The surgical goals anteriorly are adequate debridement, decompression of any material in the spinal canal, and stabilization of the interspace with rib strut grafts or tricortical iliac crest grafts. A satisfactory fusion rate with this approach, along with antibiotics and rest, is a very high likelihood.

The lumbar paraspinal approach or the thoracic costotransversectomy approach (Fig. 4.24) is acceptable to debride a paraspinal abscess and obtain a biopsy specimen but offers too many limitations for definitive treatment. This approach is limited to lesions in the posterolateral corner of the vertebral body. The laminectomy approach, except for epidural abscess evacuation, is mentioned only to be condemned.

Epidural Abscess

Introduction

It is highly unlikely that you will ever see a lumbar epidural abscess. If you happen upon it when it appears in the emergency department, you will probably miss it, something that happens most of the time. It does not sound very promising, does it?

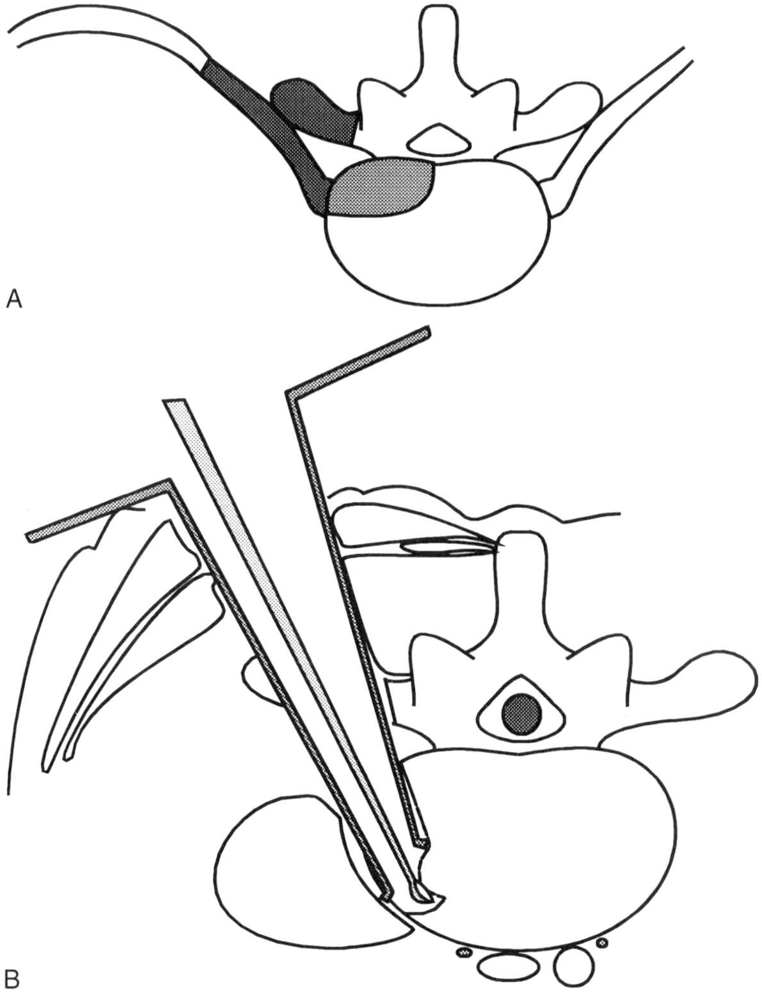

Figure 4.24 *Costotransversectomy approach.* **A.** *With the patient in the prone position on the operating table, the darkly shaded areas of the rib and transverse process are removed.* **B.** *Access is gained to the back of the vertebral body on the same side.*

Demography

Epidural abscess is predominantly an adult disease, affecting the thoracic and lumbar spinal canal more than the cervical region. As a spontaneous hematogenous event in a normal adult, it is highly unlikely. Most often it occurs after spine surgery, and more frequently it appears in debilitated (diabetic or alcoholic) or immunocompromised patients. If you work in an area with high drug abuse, you will see epidural abscess more frequently.

Bacteriology

The majority of patients will have cultures that reveal Staphylococcus aureus; drug abusers have a higher incidence of gram-negative infections such as Pseudomonas, but the majority of patients will have cultures that grow S. aureus.

Pathogenesis and Clinical Presentation

The mass of infective cells in the epidural space may be either granulation tissue or pus. Both occupy space needed for neurological structures. Initially, the patient will have local pain (especially nonmechanical nighttime pain). As the mass expands, radicular pain will appear, followed by weakness and, in the end, paralysis. How fast this clinical progression occurs is variable, but the pain to paralysis stage may take but a few hours, making the diagnosis and treatment of epidural abscess an emergency.

At the stage of radicular pain and early in the stage of neurological changes, the patient is usually unable to move in bed because of the severity of pain. The meningismus will be evident by a profound reduction in SLR due to back pain.

In the thoracic and lumbar spine, there is a posterior epidural space filled with fat. Because of this anatomy, it is easy to understand why epidural abscesses tend to occur posteriorly in the thoracic and lumbar regions. If abscesses occur after anterior spine surgery or discography, then obviously most epidural collections will be anterior. They may be confined to one segment, but more often the pus or granulation tissue collection spreads over multiple segments.

Diagnosis

The quickest path to diagnosis is a high index of suspicion in any adult, especially those debilitated by drugs, disease, or decay, and in whom there is presentation of nighttime back pain and stiffness with fever. Sometimes, because of immunosuppression, the fever, ESR, and WBC will show minimal change.

Any suspected infectious disease needs immediate identification of the underlying organism through direct abscess culture, blood culture, or culture of a remote but more accessible source, such as an infected skin lesion, kidney, or lung.

Unless there is associated discitis/osteomyelitis, plain radiographs are likely to be negative. Until the advent of MRI, myelography with CT scanning was needed for diagnosis. MRI is now the investigative modality of choice, which avoids all the dangers of subarachnoid puncture in a patient with a spinal infection (Table 4.2) (Fig. 4.25).

Table 4.2. MRI Epidural Abscess (Granulation Tissue) Appearance

MRI Sequence	Compared with Spinal Cord	Compared with CSF
T1-weighted spin echo	Most often isointense[b]; sometimes hypointense	Hyperintense
T2-weighted spin echo	Almost always hyperintense	Hyperintense
Gradient echo T2[a]	Same as T2 SE	Same as T2 SE
Gadolinium enhancement	Hyperintense periphery (granulation tissue) Hypointense core (abscess)	Not routinely done

[a]T2 is a fast imaging technique that appears somewhat like a T2 spin echo but requires much less time in the machine.
[b]Isointense: same signal intensity.
Hyperintense: higher (whiter) signal intensity.
Hyporintense: lower (grayer) signal intensity.

Treatment

An epidural abscess is an urgent medical situation. If you are fortunate enough to catch it early, before weakness has occurred, conservative care with the appropriate antibiotic is a choice. Most cases of epidural abscesses require surgical drainage because:

1. The disease is diagnosed late, and radicular pain and weakness are present.
2. The time interval between weakness and paralysis can be measured in hours. Some surgeons think this is because of venous or arterial thrombosis in the vascular tree of the spinal cord and/or cauda equina.
3. The lesion is not only a space-occupying lesion in neurological territory, it is an abscess with a necrotic center that may not be reached by antibiotics.
4. The presence of paralysis for more than 36 hours usually results in either no functional recovery or death.

Surgery should proceed under appropriate antibiotic coverage. Obviously, the goal of surgery is to evacuate the pus. As with any other spinal condition, the approach is dictated by the location of the pathology. If the pus is posterior, go posteriorly (laminectomy); if it is anterior, and confined to one segment in the conus or cord region, go anteriorly. If the pus is anterior in the cauda equina region (L2 and caudally), it is best to use a laminectomy approach. Pus spread over many segments will require a multisegmental decompression and/or catheter lavage of the site.

There is always the possibility that anterior destruction of the vertebral elements will lead to a deformity that will have to be corrected at a later date.

Tuberculous Vertebral Osteomyelitis

Tuberculous infections of the lumbar spine usually have a clinical course that distinguishes them from pyogenic infections (Table 4.3). Skeletal tuberculosis is almost always secondary to a focus elsewhere, particularly the pulmonary and urinary tracts. The most frequent site of vertebral involvement is the lower thoracic and upper lumbar region. The vertebral body, as in pyogenic osteomyelitis, is the site of localization. The intervertebral

Figure 4.25 *MRI of epidural abscess after gadolinium injection.* **A.** *Sagittal;* **B.** *Axial (arrow).*

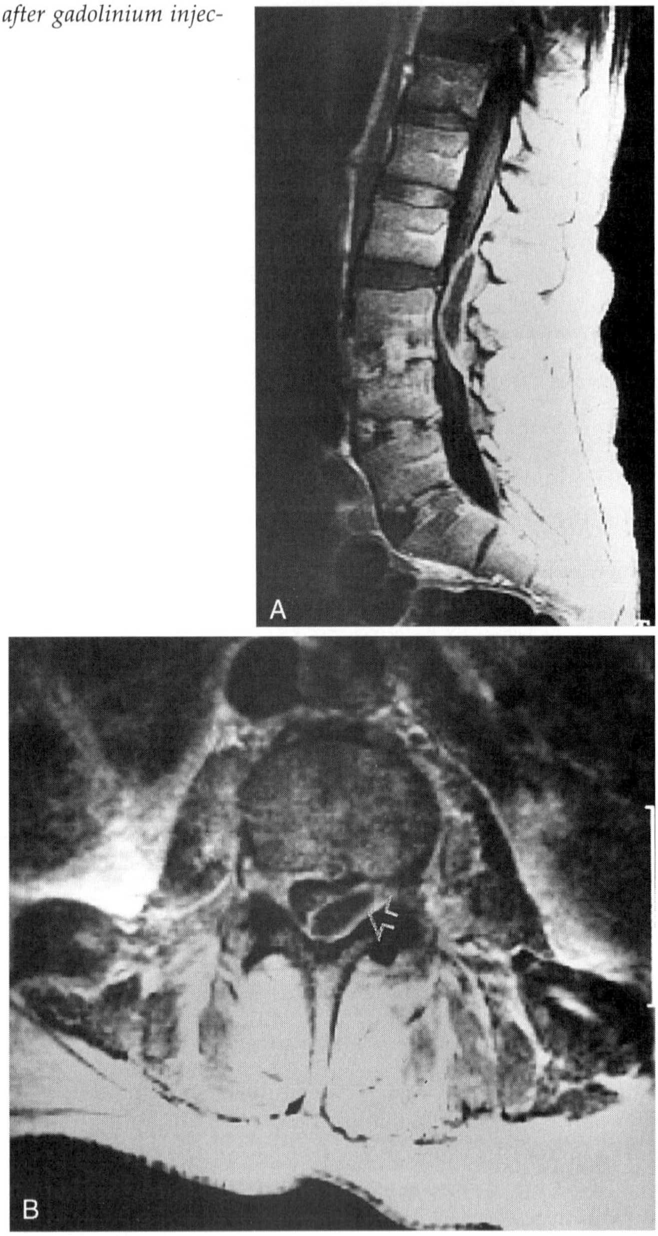

disc is relatively resistant to tuberculous destruction and the infection simply migrates under the anterior longitudinal ligament to the adjacent vertebral body.

The disease is very insidious, and the time that elapses from the onset of symptoms to hospital admission is often well more than 6 months. This is further complicated by the fact that, in North America, tuberculosis is now a much rarer condition and is frequently overlooked in differential diagnosis. However, over the past decade, there has been an increase in the incidence of pulmonary tuberculosis, and it is reasonable to assume there will be a subsequent increase in tuberculous osteomyelitis.

Table 4.3. Comparison of Pyogenic Vertebral Osteomyelitis (PVO) and Tuberculous Spondylitis (TS)[a]

Comparison Factors	PVO	TS
Onset	Some insidious; some acute	Always insidious
Average interval to diagnosis	3 mo +	8 mo +
Apparent antecedent infection or surgery	50%	100%
Back pain	Can be severe	Rarely severe
Neurological involvement	Unusual	Usual
Paralysis	More common	Less common
Levels	Single segment; lumbar most common	Multiple segments possible Equally lower thoracic and lumbar
ESR	Very high (over 100 not unusual)	Rarely over 50
Radiograph	Disc space narrowing occurs early	Disc space preserved
Requirement for surgery	Not usual	More common
Residual deformity	Unusual	Common

[a]The only surefire way to distinguish between these two diseases is histological and culture examination of a direct biopsy.

In the younger child, irritability and refusal to sit or walk are presenting features. Older children and adults present with simple backache. The symptoms do not have the dramatic disability characteristic of the later stages of a pyogenic vertebral osteomyelitis.

A careful history will reveal the association of constitutional symptoms of intermittent fever, sweats, anorexia, weight loss, and easy fatigability. At examination, marked splinting of the spine can usually be demonstrated. Although the gross tenderness associated with pyogenic osteomyelitis is rarely apparent, localized bony deformity associated with vertebral collapse, presenting as gibbus, is common.

Because of the insidious nature of the disease and the consequent delay in seeking advice, the patient may present with evidence of neurological impairment even when seen for the first time.

Laboratory and Radiograph

As in pyogenic lesions, the sedimentation rate is elevated. The white count is variable, however, and may even be depressed. The plain radiographic features that distinguish the lesion from pyogenic osteomyelitis are: (1) There may be multiple vertebral bodies affected. (2) There may be scalloping of the anterior surface of the vertebral bodies by the tuberculous abscess (Fig. 4.26). (3) The disc space is usually spared until late in the disease, when it may rupture into the tuberculous cavities within the vertebral bodies or paraspinal abscesses. In fact, the vertebral body destruction in tuberculosis is not unlike that caused by neoplasm, except that tuberculous lesions tend to be anterior in the vertebral body, and neoplasms, especially secondaries, are more posterior in the vertebral body and invade the posterior elements.

Figure 4.26 *When an abscess forms on the anterior surface of the vertebral column, the x-ray shows scalloping of the vertebral bodies. Because a similar type of scalloping is seen with abdominal aneurysms, this radiological lesion is sometimes referred to as "aneurysmal erosion." From Macnab I: Backache. Williams & Wilkins, Baltimore (1977) p. 27.*

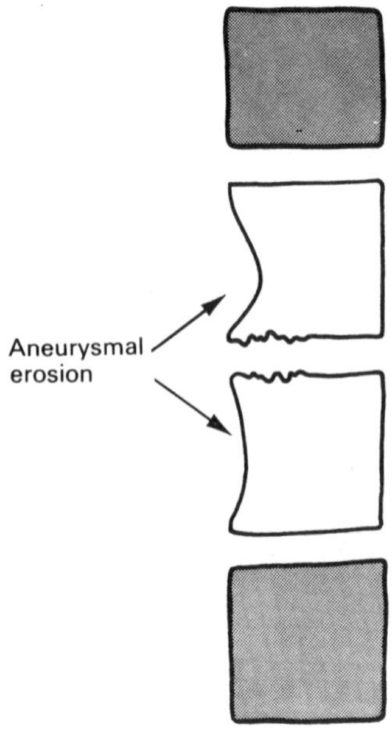

As noted earlier, tuberculous infections of the lumbar spine are rarely primary. They are commonly secondary to foci either in the lungs or the genitourinary tract. Radiographs of the chest and bacteriological examination of the urine must always be carried out in routine clinical assessment. The Mantoux test, when positive, can be regarded as suggestive but never diagnostic. As with pyogenic vertebral osteomyelitis, vertebral biopsy is essential for diagnosis.

Treatment

It is possible to treat the patient with antituberculous drugs and immobilization. However, anterior debridement of the lesion with immediate grafting is probably the treatment of choice, especially if there is neurological involvement. Surgical ablation of the tuberculous lesion significantly shortens the course of the disease process, and the incidence of deformity and residual neurological complications is markedly reduced. It must be emphasized once again that, unlike pyogenic osteomyelitis, tuberculous lesions of the vertebral column are commonly associated with neurological lesions. In such instances, the prognosis after decompression is carried out early is excellent. In contrast, in neglected cases, paraplegia caused by penetration of the dura and involvement of the cord by tuberculous granulation tissue produces irreversible changes.

Miscellaneous Infections of the Spine

Uncommon Pyogenic Lesions

The spine may be involved by actinomycosis, typhoid, or brucellosis. Unlike other pyogenic infections, the vertebral body frequently shows a reactive sclerosis appearing like a white block on radiograph.

Fungal

Fungi can establish growth within body tissue: mycotic osteomyelitis. The most common fungal infections seen are coccidioidomycosis and blastomycosis. The skeleton, however, is rarely involved except as part of a disseminated disease. From a clinical standpoint, it must be remembered that each one of these mycotic infections can mimic tuberculosis radiologically, again emphasizing the need for vertebral biopsy as an essential part of establishing the diagnosis and initiating appropriate treatment. Vertebral osteomyelitis may also rarely occur due to Candida sp as a complication of candidemia, which is increasing as a nosocomial occurrence.

Parasitic

Hydatid disease has been known as a clinical entity from ancient times. When bone involvement is present, the spine is also involved in approximately one fifth of patients. Diagnosis is difficult. Radiographs reveal lytic lesions in the vertebral body. Neurological involvement occurs early and relentlessly progresses to an irreversible paraplegia. To date, it would appear that treatment fails to obtain any significant response.

Syphilis

The incidence of syphilitic bone and joint involvement decreased from 36% in 1900 to less than 0.5% in 1936, and this decline has been maintained. Charcot's arthropathy is the most common manifestation of syphilitic involvement of the vertebral column and is seen most frequently at the thoracolumbar junction. Although the lesion may be symptomless and detected solely by incidental radiographs, pain may arise when destructive and hypertrophic changes are marked. Similar changes may be seen with diabetes, although this is rare. Complete collapse of the vertebral column may occur with transection of the cord or cauda equina.

Intervertebral Disc Space Infection

Disc space infections in adults most commonly occur following disc puncture, either at open surgery or closed percutaneous procedures, such as chemonucleolysis, discography, or percutaneous discectomy. The clinical picture is fairly characteristic. There is an initial relief of the preoperative sciatic pain after the procedure. Approximately 1 to 8 weeks later, severe backache occurs, with marked cramps of pain. The pain is described as being "excruciating" and is out of proportion to the objective findings.

There are very few constitutional symptoms, except in those patients who run a febrile course. If the sedimentation rate is elevated, it is useful in following the subsequent treatment program.

Radiographs do not show abnormality for approximately 4 or 6 weeks when, for the first time, narrowing of the disc space is revealed. This narrowing occurs much earlier than the anticipated narrowing subsequent to the physical act of discectomy and, of course, is much more marked. Later, irregularity and loss of definition of the vertebral endplates are noted, with subsequent vertebral destruction. More than half of the patients progress to disc space obliteration and interbody fusion. As with vertebral osteomyelitis, early diagnosis is facilitated by bone scanning (Fig. 4.27) and imaging with either CT or MR.

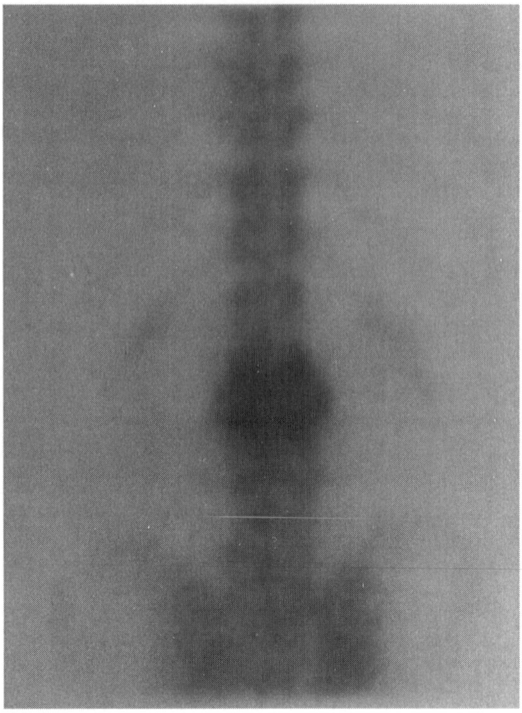

Figure 4.27 *A bone scan of an L2–3 discitis after surgery. Note how the increased tracer uptake is in adjacent portions of the L2 and L3 vertebral bodies.*

Aspiration by needle biopsy is essential to establish a bacteriological diagnosis in order that the lesion may be treated with appropriate antibiotics. The treatment, in essence, is the same as the treatment of pyogenic vertebral osteomyelitis.

The best approach to a potential postoperative disc space infection is prevention. Our approach is as follows:

1. Shaving of the back should be done in the operating room just before prepping and draping.
2. Our prepping solution is an alcohol wash followed by an iodine preparation.
3. If the procedure is a routine discectomy, intravenous antibiotics are given 20 minutes preoperatively. If there is an increased risk for infection, antibiotics are continued postoperatively.
4. Use of the microscope during surgery requires special diligence to assure that proper draping of the microscope is completed and that the uncovered eyepieces do not serve as a source of contamination.
5. At the end of the discectomy, the disc space is profusely irrigated with antibiotic solution.
6. The entire procedure (exposure and closure) is designed to leave behind no dead space.

Disc Space Infection in Children

Because the disc is a relatively avascular structure, primary hematogenous discitis is a rare entity. As with adults, discitis in children probably starts with the deposit of an infective embolus in the end arteries of the vertebral body circulation. These are located close to the endplate and are more prominent anteriorly. Thus, the initial focus of infection in children and adults is close to the endplate and anteriorly in the vertebral body. However, younger children differ from adults in that there is a rich vascular connection between the vertebral body and the disc. This disappears at approximately age 8 when the child's disc assumes the adult characteristic of an avascular space. Before the age of 8, this rich anastomosis between the vessels in the vertebral body and the disc space allows for a very early spread of infection to the child's disc. Thus, a purer form of "discitis" without significant osteomyelitis can occur in young children.

Aside from this anatomical difference in blood supply, there is little difference in the presentation, diagnosis, and treatment of discitis in the child. The disease is of more rapid progression in a child who often cannot adequately describe the symptoms. The parents may state that the child has become "sickly," refusing to eat and specifically refusing to walk. This should raise the suspicion of the examining physician to include discitis in the differential diagnosis. From there, laboratory test results, plain radiographs, bone scan, and CT or MR imaging are used to make the diagnosis.

Treatment depends on the organism, the extent of infection, and the presence of any complications such as abscess formation or compromise of neurological structures.

Note that this clinical syndrome is one of a sick and septicemic child with systemic symptoms, fever, elevated sedimentation rate and WBC count, and likely either a positive blood culture or a positive disc space biopsy. However, inflammatory lesions of the vertebrae and discs in children produce a wide spectrum of syndromes, from this obviously septic child to the child with back pain, no fever, some elevation of the sedimentation rate, and little change in the WBC count. This latter syndrome usually has disc space narrowing on plain radiograph, but a positive blood culture or a positive biopsy for infection is never obtained. This condition is known as intervertebral disc inflammation.

Intervertebral Disc Inflammation

This is a benign condition occurring only in children. Confusion regarding the etiology has resulted in a multitude of synonyms: acute infectious lesions of the intervertebral discs, spondyloarthritis in children, benign acute osteitis of the spine, nonspecific spondylitis, and discitis.

This confusion indicates that as yet the etiology is unknown. Objective data from the literature and personal experience lend support to an infectious etiology; however, until substantiated, the term inflammation is preferred to infection.

In contrast to vertebral osteomyelitis, intervertebral disc inflammation most commonly is first seen between the ages of 2 and 6. Infants refuse to walk, and older children complain of hip or back pain. There are few localizing signs early in the course of the disease. Later, typical findings of restricted spinal mobility, paravertebral and hamstring muscle spasm, and pain on percussion over the lumbar spine are present. The children are afebrile at examination.

The single most consistent laboratory finding is the elevated sedimentation rate, which may be considerably more than 50 mm/h. Blood cultures are not positive; indeed, if a positive blood culture is obtained, the condition should no longer be considered an inflammation but should be regarded as vertebral osteomyelitis or discitis and treated as such.

There is a 2- or 4-week delay before radiographic changes are present. The lumbar vertebrae are most commonly involved, especially the fourth lumbar vertebra. The earliest sign is narrowing of a disc space, which may be seen to progress for an additional 1 or 2 months. This change may be associated with irregular erosion of the vertebral endplates and, on occasion, the disc may balloon into the vertebral body. However, wedging and vertebral collapse do not occur. Tomography has occasionally demonstrated cavitation in the vertebral body that, interestingly enough, will persist after apparent healing. A bone scan may localize the level of pathology before radiographic changes are apparent.

In the natural history of the disease, the disc height is usually restored, and the endplates regain their definition.

The essence of treatment is immobilization. Without any knowledge of the presence and nature of any organisms, the empirical administration of antibiotics is illogical and of debatable value. Systemic signs, fever, leukocytosis, or failure to improve with bed rest are indications for biopsy to differentiate the syndrome of disc space inflammation from vertebral osteomyelitis, and, in the latter instance, to institute appropriate antibiotic therapy.

Whether discitis is inflammatory or infective at the time of presentation is often a difficult decision. Fraser et al(6) suggest that both conditions are initiated by bacterial contamination of the disc, but because of the particular nature of the disc cavity (relatively avascular), the bacteria initiate the damage and then are removed by the body's natural defense, never to be found on blood culture or biopsy. However, the damage done to the disc space progresses to its end state, which may be minimal damage and reconstitution or total obliteration of the space and a spontaneous fusion.

One might conclude from this discussion on vertebral body osteomyelitis and discitis in adults or children that we are looking at one disease entity (vertebral column infection), with many varieties of presentation.

TUMORS (NEOPLASMS)

The diagnosis of neoplasms of the vertebral column is largely dependent on radiographic examinations. This text is not intended as an atlas of lesions of the vertebral column, and no attempt is made here to describe the specific radiological and histological characteristics of the tumors that occur. An attempt is made to outline the principles of diagnosis and treatment. Benign neoplasms and primary malignancies in the vertebral column are rare. Secondary deposits are common. More generalizations include the following:

1. Almost all primary tumors of the spine can be seen on plain radiographs.
2. The older the patient, the more likely the primary tumor is malignant.
3. Except for giant cell tumor, eosinophilic granuloma, and hemangioma, most benign tumors are in the posterior elements.
4. Most primary malignant tumors will be found in the vertebral body.
5. The incidence of neurological compromise is high (75%) in malignant tumors and common (40–50%) in benign tumors. Neurological lesions occur through direct tumor extension, pathological fractures, and/or skeletal deformity.
6. The prognosis for malignant tumors, despite treatment, is not very good.

Benign Tumors

Benign tumors (8) predominantly affect the generation less than 30 years of age. Backache at the site of the lesion, is the dominant symptom, and this may be associated with a painful scoliosis. Idiopathic scoliosis is rarely painful. When a patient presenting with a scoliosis complains of severe backache, remember the possibility of a benign tumor and examine its likelihood with detailed radiological assessment.

Benign lesions usually occur in the posterior elements or accessory processes and present two specific difficulties in evaluation and treatment. First, there is the difficulty in demonstrating the lesion on regular radiograph. When clinical suspicion is high, but radiological findings are equivocal, a technetium bone scan is useful. If the scan can localize the tumor and confirm a lesion, CT or MR imaging may be employed to further define its exact site and characteristics. When the scan is negative, plain radiographs and the scan should be repeated after a 3-month interval if the clinical problem persists. Eventually, plain radiographs will show all benign lesions.

Second, benign lesions may be inaccessible for surgical removal. Fortunately, incomplete removal may be all that is necessary (except for giant cell tumor).

The following is a summary of the clinical features of the more commonly seen benign lesions:

Osteoid Osteoma

The classic clinical presentation is a gradual progressive backache, which is nonmechanical in nature and relieved by aspirin. The majority of the patients are men (2:1) and between 15 and 25 years of age. It can be said that backache in adolescents or young adults associated with marked paravertebral muscle spasm and the sudden onset of scoliosis warrants consideration of an osteoid osteoma. On radiograph, the small-sized lesion is most frequently seen to involve the posterior elements and is typically an area of dense sclerosis surrounding a central nidus (Fig. 4.28). On occasion, symptoms occur before it is possible to demonstrate the lesion on radiograph, at which time a single photon emissiopn computed tomography scan or computerized tomography is necessary to establish the diagnosis. The rarity of the lesion and its elusive radiographic diagnosis often lead to erroneous diagnoses, such as psychogenic pain.

The pain from an osteoid osteoma may resolve spontaneously with symptomatic treatment. If this does not happen, treatment is a local excision of the tumor.

Pathology will show a nidus of immature osteoblasts, osteoid, and some blood with a surrounding margin of dense mature, lamellar bone.

Osteoblastoma

In contrast to all other primary neoplasms of bone, osteoblastoma manifests a most distinct predilection for the spine. Forty percent of all osteoblastomata are found in the spine, almost invariably in the posterior elements of the lumbar spine and sacrum. The tumor is seen most commonly in boys / men, and 80% of the patients are less than 30 years of age.

Insidious, low-grade back pain is always the presenting symptom, with some scoliosis being demonstrated in more than half of the patients. Because of the expansile nature of the tumor, many of the patients will present at examination some evidence of a neurological irritation or compression. The tumor is larger than an osteoid osteoma and is often seen on plain radiograph (Fig. 4.29); if not, CT will make the diagnosis.

Treatment is by surgical excision, and even incomplete removal is compatible with complete symptomatic relief. The histology is often identical to osteoid osteoma, but at

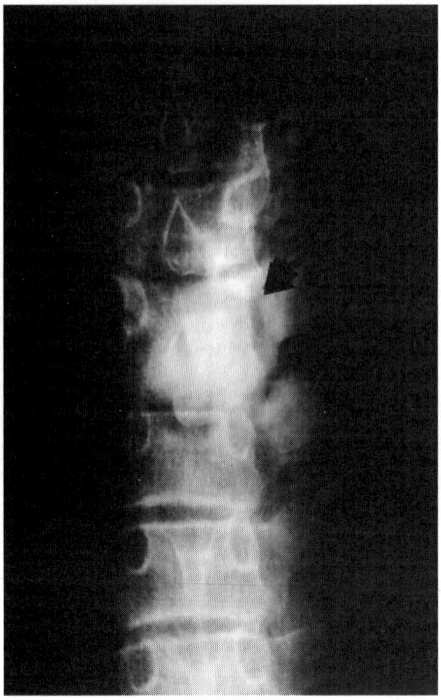

Figure 4.28 *Osteoid osteoma (arrow) in a thoracic vertebral body.*

times the cells are atypical enough to confuse the lesion with osteogenic sarcoma, thus requiring an experienced pathologist for interpretation of the slide.

Osteochondroma (Exostosis)

Although osteochondroma is much more common in extremity long bones, it does occur in the vertebral column, especially in patients with multiple exostoses. The age and sex distribution is similar to osteoid osteoma. Unlike osteoid osteoma, these lesions are often asymptomatic and an incidental discovery on spine films (Fig. 4.30).

Osteochondroma likely represents an abnormality in cartilage growth and is located close to the secondary centers of ossification (spinous process, pedicle, and neural arch). This lesion is typically a cortical stalk with a cartilaginous cap; the cartilage, obviously, is not apparent on plain radiograph (Fig. 4.31).

Because most of these lesions are asymptomatic, they merit observation alone. If they cause a local pressure phenomenon, then excision is required. Infrequently, and more prevalent in multiple exostoses, malignant transformation that requires surgical excision can occur in the cartilage portion.

Medullary Bone Island

These radiologically demonstrated discrete osteosclerotic foci seen on radiographs (Fig. 4.32) are composed of normal compact bone. They have no clinical significance, but care must be taken not to confuse them with osteoblastic metastases.

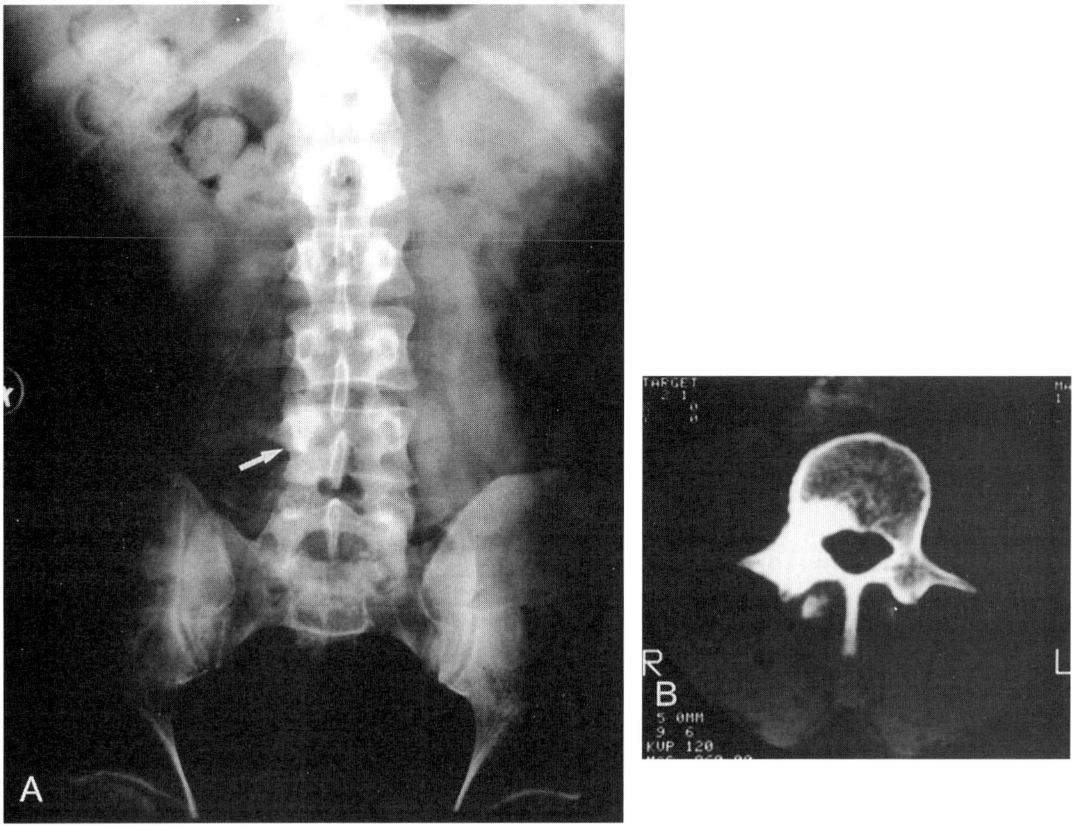

Figure 4.29 *Osteoblastoma.* **A.** *Plain AP x-ray showing a sclerotic pedicle, L4, right (arrow).* **B.** *Axial CT showing lesion in pedicle.*

Aneurysmal Bone Cyst

This tumor generally is first seen as a solitary expansile lesion involving the vertebra.(8) Although the tumor is seen in all age groups, 90% of the patients are less than 20 years of age. The clinical presentation is one of back pain with or without neurological symptoms that develops as a result of the expansile nature of the tumor.

Radiographs reveal a destructive expansile lesion, usually in the posterior elements (Fig. 4.33). Cortical bone is destroyed, but the periosteum is able to maintain a reactive rim of bone surrounding the lesion. It is the only benign lesion that may extend across a disc space to involve an adjacent vertebral element.

Treatment is by excision, with spinal fusion often unnecessary because posterior element excision may be limited. The operative procedure can be associated with a significant blood loss for which the surgical team should be prepared.

Histology reveals vascular lakes surrounded by reactive fibrous tissue with numerous giant cells and hemosiderin pigmentation.

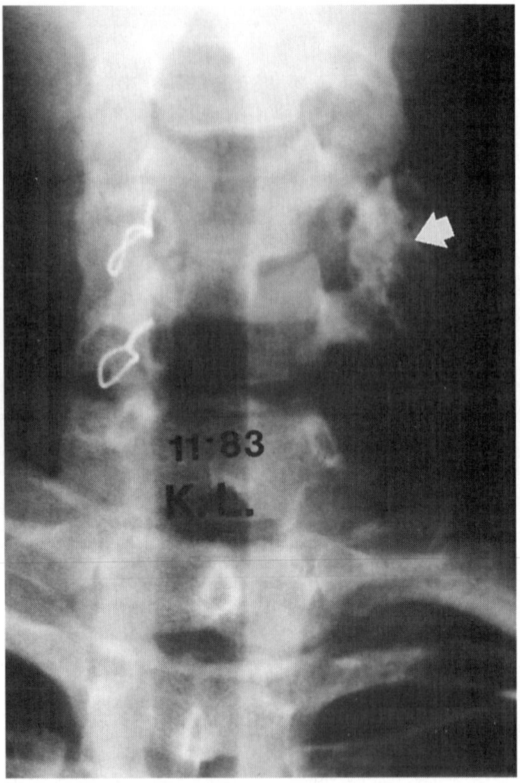

Figure 4.30 *Osteochondroma (arrow) in a cervical spine. Previous surgery on the opposite side was done to remove another osteochondroma.*

Hemangioma

Characteristically, on radiograph, the affected vertebra demonstrates linear striations that give rise to a corduroy cloth or honeycomb appearance (Fig. 4.34). This radiological finding can be demonstrated in nearly 12% of all vertebral columns, with the incidence increasing with age.(8) The incidence in the backache population is no greater, which emphasizes the fact that the mere demonstration of a hemangioma of a vertebral body on radiograph does not indicate that the source of the patient's backache has been found.

Treatment is simply observation. In a few patients with constant disabling pain, local radiotherapy may sometimes relieve the symptoms, but the risk of malignant degeneration is making this treatment less desirable. On the rare occasion that neurological compromise necessitates surgical intervention, embolization, followed by surgical excision, may be done. Surgery, and its attendant bleeding, carries with it a high morbidity, and even mortality, and should not be undertaken lightly.

Giant Cell Tumor

Although giant cell tumor is a relatively common benign tumor of long bones (most common on either side of the knee joint), it is relatively rare in the spine. When it does occur in the spine, it is most common in the sacrum and more prevalent in the female patient, tending to occur in an individual a little older than one with osteoid osteoma or osteoblastoma.

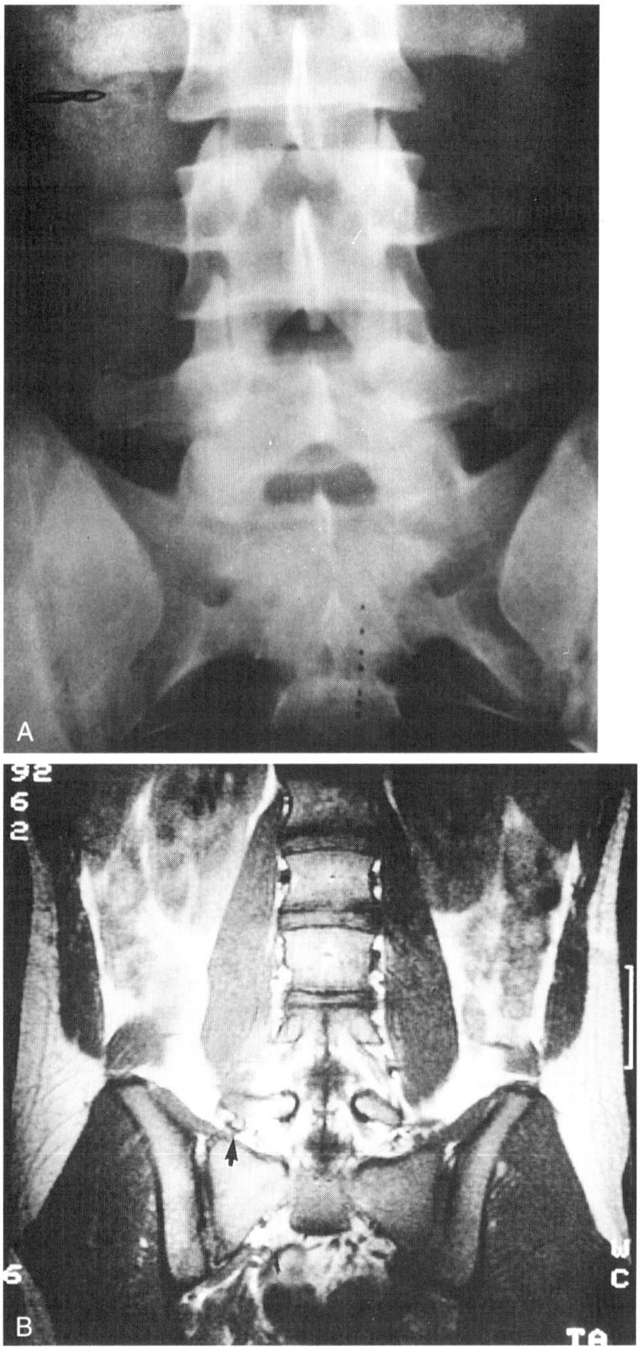

Figure 4.31 **A.** *Now that you have seen an osteochondroma in the neck, can you see one in this lumbar spine radiograph? (It is attached to the inferior border of the L5 transverse process.) If you find this hard to believe, here* **(B)** *it is on MRI (arrow).*

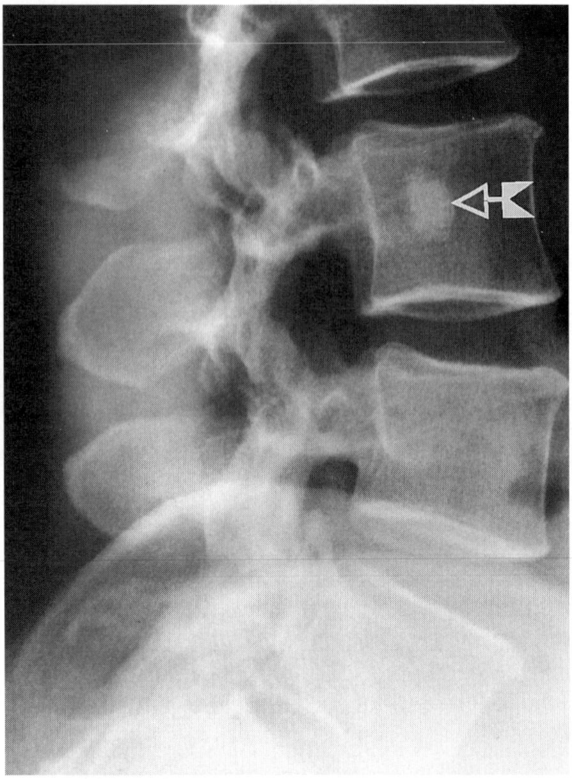

Figure 4.32 *A medullary bone island in the body of L3 (arrow).*

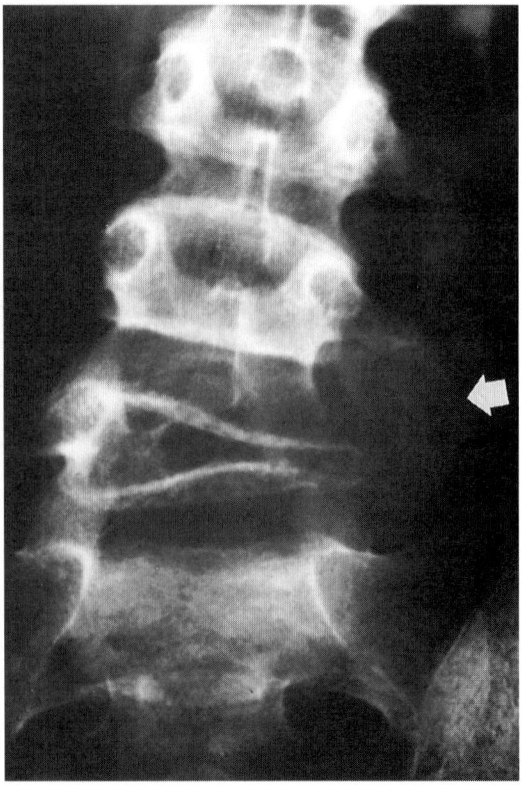

Figure 4.33 *Aneurysmal bone cyst (ABC) in the body of L5. The arrow points to the expanding margin of the lesion.*

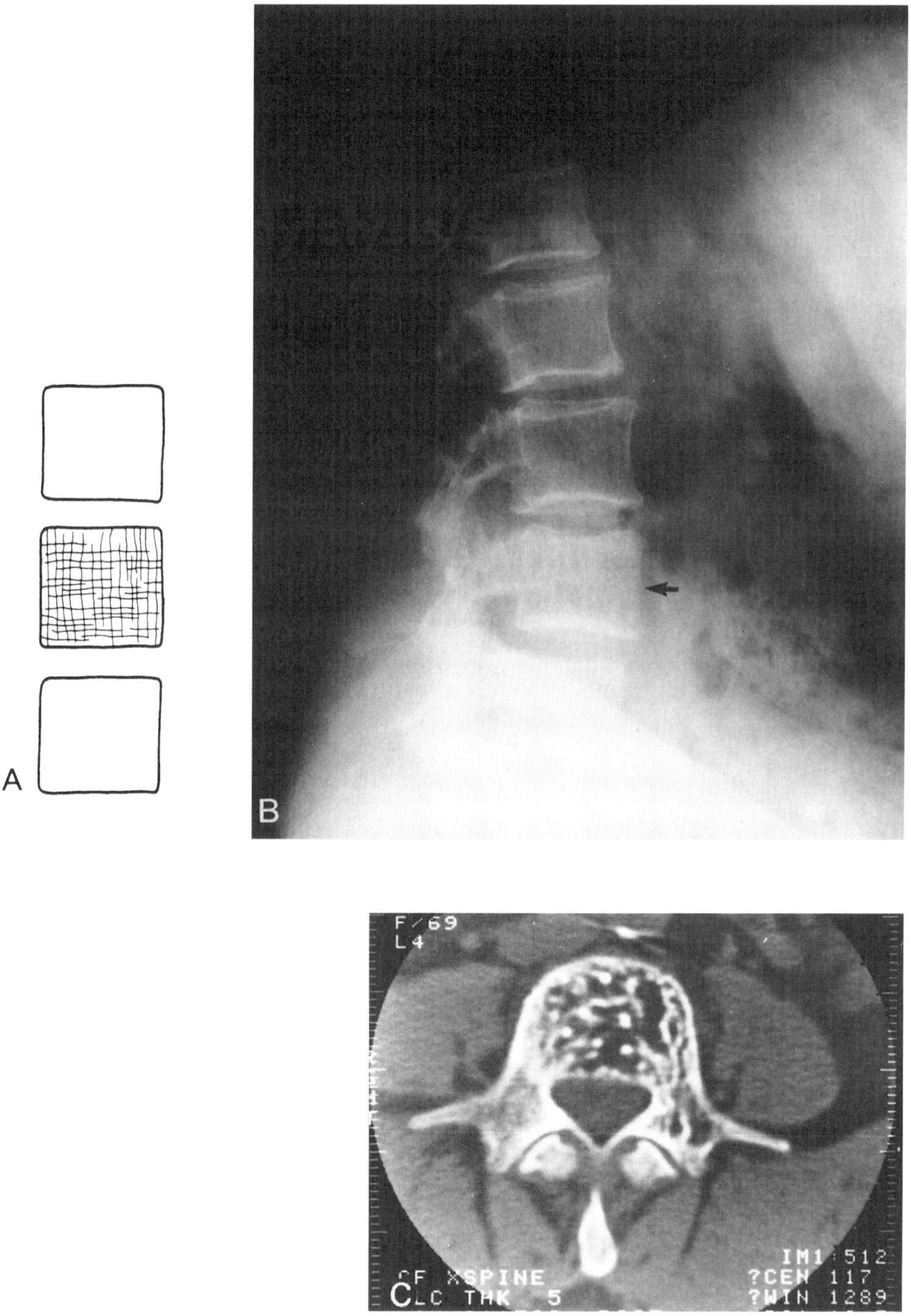

Figure 4.34 **A.** *Diagram to show the characteristic x-ray appearance of the so-called hemangioma of the vertebral body. The vertical and horizontal trabeculae are accentuated giving a corduroy cloth or honey-combed appearance.* **B.** *Hemangioma on plain x-ray (L4) (arrow).* **C.** *CT of hemangioma. From Macnab I: Backache. Williams & Wilkins, Baltimore, (1977), p. 31.*

The clinical presentation is no different from other benign lesions discussed and includes pain with occasional neurological compromise.

Although the lesion is not commonly malignant, it is certainly more malevolent than benign. From the moment the lytic, expansile lesion with little cortical reaction is seen on MRI (Fig. 4.35), the chase is on—with laboratory tests and pathology examination—to separate it from malignant lesions All laboratory test results will be normal, and pathological examination will reveal multiple giant cells. These cells can be confused with aneurysmal bone cysts, and brown tumor of hyperparathyroidism.

Treatment requires aggressive total excision of the tumor. Unfortunately, some of the lesions in the sacrum cannot be totally excised because of size and location. Radiotherapy used for these patients has the possibility of increasing the chances of malignant transformation. Of all the benign tumors of the spine, giant cell is the most difficult to treat, and if it is not treated aggressively (13), it will quickly change its behavior to a more aggressive and, eventually, maliganant lesion.

Eosinophilic Granuloma

This condition is a proliferative disorder of histiocytes. Vertebral involvement occurs early as a lytic lesion and subsequently as a variable degree of compression of a vertebral body, without any evidence of an adjacent soft tissue mass. In the extreme form, the vertebra is flattened to a thin disc, the so-called vertebra plana (Fig. 4.36). This spontaneous collapse of the vertebral body in children was first described by Calvé (2). It was thought to be a manifestation of osteochondritis juvenilis and is still referred to as "Calvé's disease." The disease is part of the complex of histiocytosis X disorders, which includes the

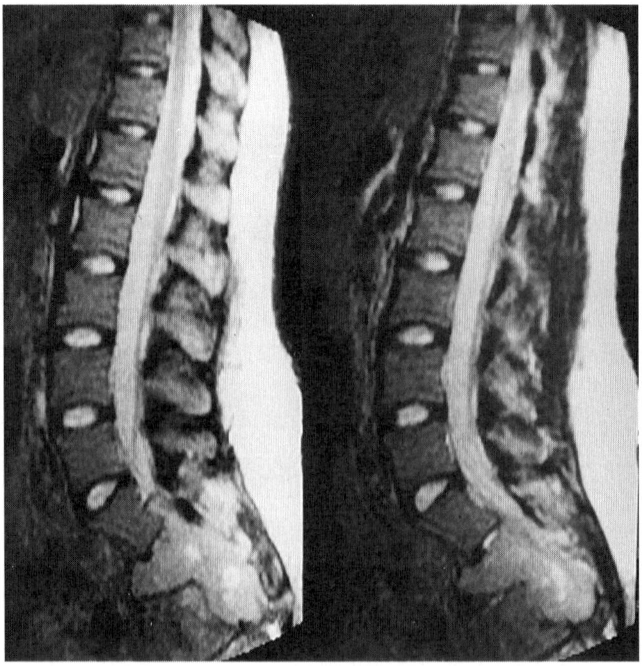

Figure 4.35 *A giant cell tumor is replacing most of the sacrum on MRI (a T2 weighted sagittal: two contiguous sagittal slices).*

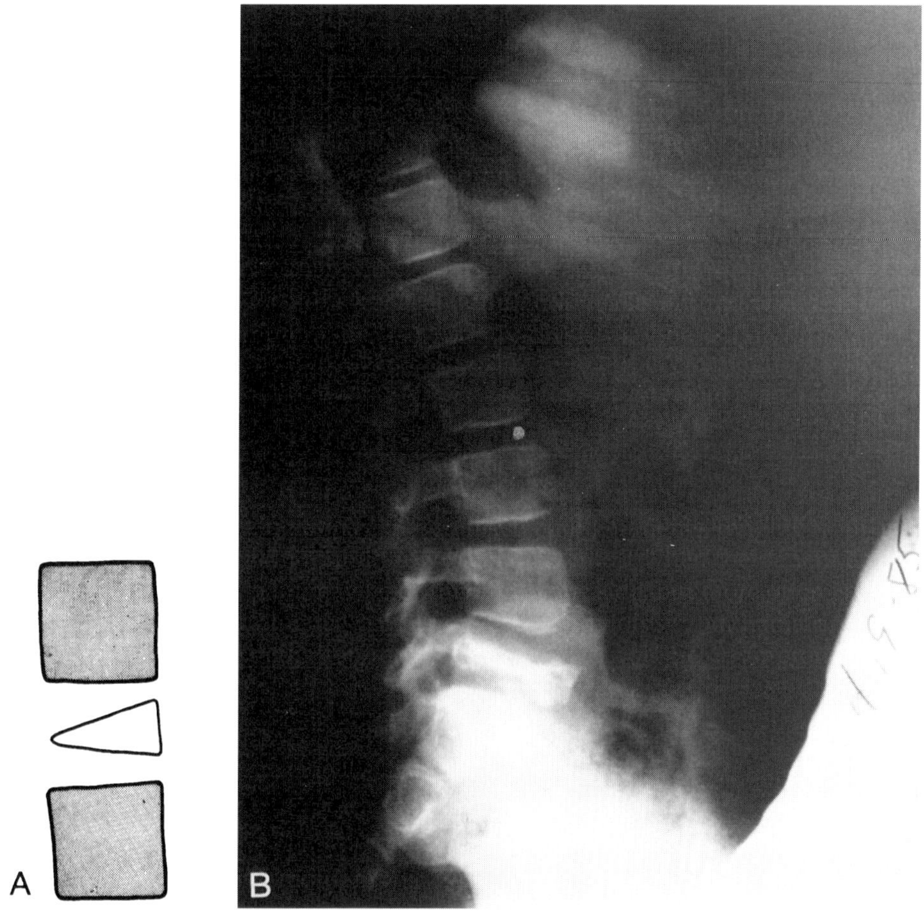

Figure 4.36 **A.** *Wedging of the vertebral body associated with Calvé's disease. From Macnab I: Backache. Williams & Wilkins, Baltimore (1977), p.* **B.** *Eosinophilic granuloma, vertebra plana, L5.*

more sinister forms of multiple histiocytic deposits in Hand-Schüller-Christian and Letterer-Siwe diseases. As long as the disease remains monostotic, it is the benign form of eosinophilic granuloma. If a biopsy is performed, the eosinophils may be mistaken for neutrophils, and the diagnosis of osteomyelitis is made; likewise, the phagocytic histiocytes may be erroneously confused with Hodgkin's disease.

The prognosis for the solitary lesion is excellent, and no treatment is necessary. A word of caution: Any secondary deposit may cause wedging of a vertebral body, and this possibility must be considered carefully before making the diagnosis of Calvé's disease.

Malignant Tumors

Malignant lesions, primary or secondary, are largely afflictions of persons more than 40 years of age; the incidence of malignant lesions increases with age. The tumors almost invariably involve the body, if primary, and the junction of the body and posterior elements, if secondary.

Backache is the presenting symptom, although neurological manifestations may arise not only because the lesion is expansile, but also from vertebral collapse and direct extradural extension. Early in the natural history of the disease, the lesion may not be demonstrated on radiograph. It must be remembered that 30% of the cortex of a bone must be destroyed before a lesion is radiologically evident. When routine radiographs fail to demonstrate any abnormality, a bone scan can be of value in defining the presence of the lesion and the extent of spinal involvement. CT and MR imaging are more sensitive in detecting these lesions before plain radiographic changes occur.

The concept of "disease extent" is critical in the treatment of spinal malignancies. Solitary metastatic lesions have a better prognosis for survival and warrant an active search for the primary lesion, with aggressive surgical or radiotherapeutic measures being applied to the secondary lesions.

The laboratory findings, such as alterations in the blood levels of calcium, phosphorus, alkaline and acid phosphatases, and globulins, may suggest malignant disease and can, on occasion, identify entities such as myeloma. Final confirmation of the nature of the lesion may require percutaneous or open biopsy.

Primary Malignant Tumors

Although primary malignant lesions are rare, the following may be seen.

Chordoma This is a slowly developing, locally invasive and destructive tumor originating from remnants of notochordal tissue, with a distinct predilection for the midline position at either end of the spinal column.

This lesion is uncommon before the age of 30 and is found more often in men. It is interesting that, although the tumor is locally aggressive with a 10% incidence of metastases, the symptoms are frequently of long duration; the average length of back pain before diagnosis is commonly more than 1 year. Pain in the lower back, sacrum, and coccyx are early and persistent symptoms. Characteristically, as with all tumors of the spinal column, the pain is not relieved by recumbency. As the tumor encroaches on the sacral foramina, neuropathies and bowel and bladder symptoms appear. Neurological involvement is usually later in the natural history of the tumor. A rectal examination is very helpful in diagnosing this tumor.

Radiographs reveal a large lytic lesion of the sacrum, with a large soft tissue mass almost indistinguishable from the radiographic appearance of a giant cell tumor (Fig. 4.37). However, a chordoma is slightly more common in men, whereas giant cell tumors occur with greater frequency in women. A chordoma is not seen until well beyond the third decade of life, whereas giant cell tumors are more frequently encountered before the age of 30. A giant cell tumor progresses usually more rapidly than a chordoma, and unlike a chordoma may be situated away from the midline.

Therapeutically, both lesions present problems. Total excision is the goal of any surgery, because the rate of recurrence is very high.

Sacral tumors in the upper sacral segments can be removed by a combined abdominal and sacral approach. This excision will leave satisfactory anal and bladder sphincter function. Those tumors in the lower sacral segments can be removed posteriorly.

Myeloma This is the most common primary malignant tumor of the spine. It is a malignant tumor of plasma cells that produce immunoglobulins and antibodies. The disseminated form of myeloma is uncommon before the age of 50 and is more often seen in men.

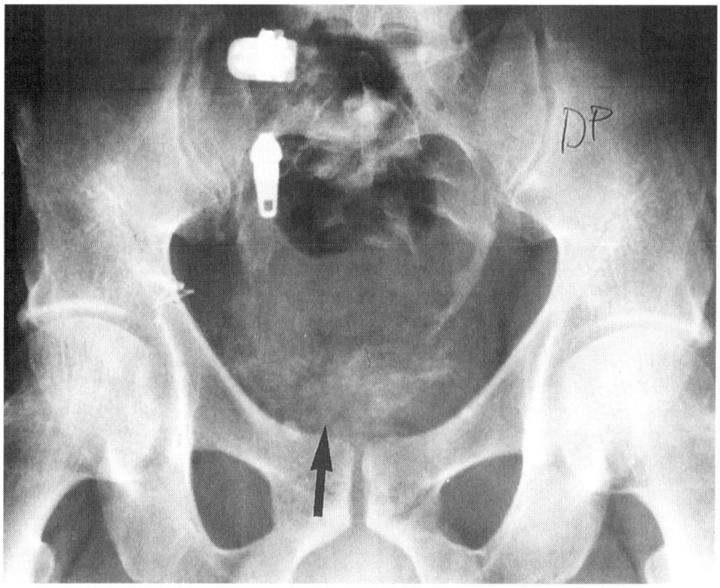

Figure 4.37 *A chordoma on plain radiograph completely replaces the lower half of the sacrum (arrow).*

Clinically, backache, weakness, weight loss, and other constitutional symptoms occur in nearly every patient with the generalized disease. The onset of pain may be sudden and is usually produced by the occurrence of a pathological fracture.

The sedimentation rate is consistently elevated and is usually greater than 50 mm/h. Almost all of these patients are very anemic. Laboratory investigations may also reveal nonspecific, minor hypercalcemia; hyperuricemia; and an elevation in the alkaline phosphatase level. Characteristically, the disease is associated with abnormal protein levels, which are best demonstrated by serum protein electrophoresis (Fig. 4.38). Bence Jones proteinuria may be demonstrated in approximately 50% of the cases. Generally, when the globulins are normal, the albumin is normal. The albumin decreases when the globulins are elevated, which reflects damage to the renal tubules.

On radiograph, the solitary lesions are purely lytic (Fig. 4.39) and do not show any attempt at regeneration of bone, a fact that renders bone scans negative in a high percentage of cases. The disseminated form frequently shows nothing more than a diffuse osteopenia with or without vertebral body crush. Bone marrow and lesion biopsy are the basis of investigation and will reveal many plasma cells.

Treatment of solitary plasmacytoma lesions is predicated on preservation of spinal stability and cord function. In the absence of gross spinal instability, management with radiotherapy and chemotherapy is probably the best mode of treatment. Spinal instability may require excision of the lesion and bypass bone grafting.

Cord impairment makes decompression mandatory. Depending on the number of segments affected and the type of encroachment on the cord, decompression may have to be performed either anteriorly or posteriorly. Because the neurological encroachment is coming from an anterior direction, the anterior approach to decompression, if feasible, is the preferred approach. This may seem to be excessive surgery for a malignant lesion, but it should be remembered that solitary lesions have a 5-year survival rate of approximately 60%.

Figure 4.38 *Top, a normal serum protein electrophoresis (SPEP); bottom, SPEP in multiple myeloma showing a spike in the gamma region.*

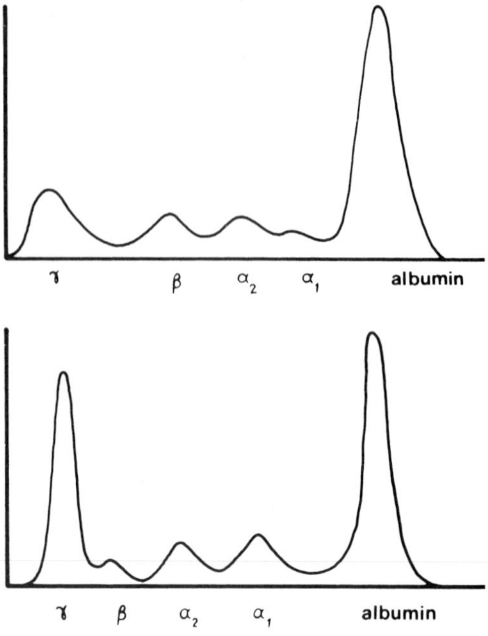

Figure 4.39 *MRI of multiple sites of myeloma involvement of the lumbar spine (T1).*

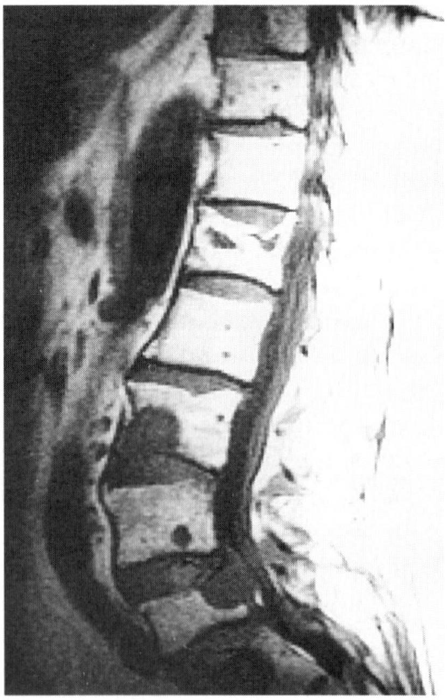

Other malignant tumors include chondrosarcoma, osteosarcoma, Ewing's sarcoma, fibrosarcoma, and lymphoma. They are not unlike any other malignant tumor, and patients present with pain and sometimes neurological involvement. Treatment depends on cell type and location; most patients with malignant tumors have a poor prognosis.

Metastatic Tumors The spine is the most common site of metastatic spread in the skeleton, and the lumbar vertebrae are the most frequently involved. The radiographs of the spine may be normal inasmuch as 30% cortical mass of a bone must be destroyed before a lesion is radiologically apparent. In autopsy specimens, only 15% of grossly affected vertebrae demonstrate recognizable lesions when the excised specimen is radiographed.

Most lesions in the vertebrae are osteolytic. Markedly osteolytic metastases are seen with hypernephroma and thyroid and large bowel carcinoma. Breast, prostate, and lung tumors may produce osteoblastic (increased bone density) metastases. Remember, both renal cell carcinoma and multiple myeloma might be silent when a bone scan is performed, which necessitates a skeletal survey.

Back pain due to spinal metastases may be the presenting finding in approximately 25% of patients suffering from malignant lesions. Any patient more than 50 years of age who presents with a history of low back pain of sudden onset without provocative trauma, unrelieved by bed rest, and associated with sudden cramps of pain, and a significantly elevated sedimentation rate, should be suspected of suffering from a secondary deposit in the spine unless proved otherwise. The concern is even greater if the patient has a previous history of a malignant lesion.

The radiographs may be normal, or the changes may indeed be minimal. A careful examination of the anteroposterior view of the spine may show the absence of one pedicle, the "winking owl sign" (Fig. 4.40).

When destructive lesions of the vertebral bodies are demonstrated, it is important to distinguish between neoplasms and infections. As a general rule, it may be said that the disc space is involved when infections occur and spared when neoplasms occur (Fig. 4.22). Occasionally, despite a clinical picture that is highly suggestive of secondary deposits in the spine, the only abnormality at radiographic examination is a diffuse osteoporosis of the vertebral column with or without a minor vertebral body crush. In such a patient, a disciplined use of laboratory findings followed, where indicated, by a bone scan and trephine biopsy is necessary to establish the diagnosis and define treatment.

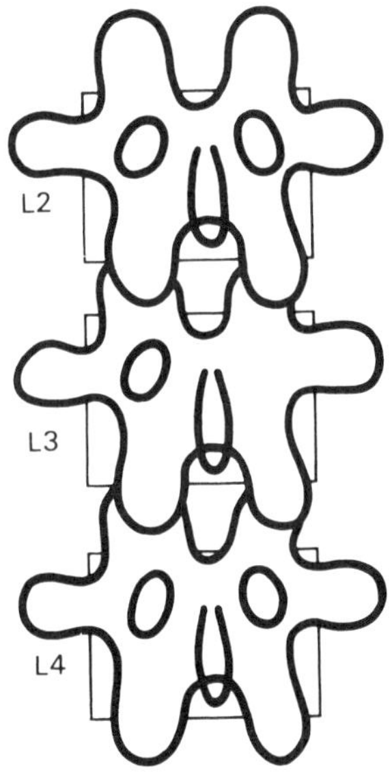

Figure 4.40 *Absence of one pedicle (the third lumbar vertrebra depicted in this diagram) is often the first and only sign of a secondary deposit in the lumbar spine. The x-ray appearance is sometimes referred to as the "winking owl sign." From Macnab I: Backache. Williams & Wilkins, Baltimore (1977), p. 36.*

In those patients in whom radiographs show a destructive vertebral lesion irrefutably due to a secondary malignant deposit and in whom there is no evidence of the site of the primary lesion, it is routine to perform a biopsy. But remember that the cell morphology in the secondary deposit is frequently so altered as to make it almost impossible to diagnose more specifically than "adenocarcinoma" or "epithelial tumor." However, the surgeon has to accept the fact that on occasion a specific diagnosis can be made, such as an unsuspected myeloma or a lymphoma. Under such circumstances, more specific modes of therapy can be instituted, depending on whether the lesion is hormone dependent or chemically controllable. The disease in such patients may run a slow course, and in certain instances, the surgeon might be justified in carrying out a biological stabilization with a bone graft.

On the other hand, when the prognosis is extremely grave in a patient whose general health is deteriorating, the debilitating pain can be humanely controlled by "grouting" the spine with methyl methacrylate (bone cement). The pain relief obtained by such means can, on occasion, be very gratifying, and the procedure, therefore, is justifiable despite the unremitting, relentless, and often rapid progress of the lesion.

More than one quarter of patients with spinal metastases present with neurological dysfunction. For tumors that frequently run a long clinical course, this is a disastrous complication. The prognosis is related to the following factors: (1) The level of neurological dysfunction: More than 80% of tumors producing neurological defects occur at the thoracic cord level. The more proximal the level of cord involvement, the poorer the prognosis. (2) Duration of neurological dysfunction: As a rule, the longer the signs are present, the worse the prognosis. (3) The onset of neurological signs: The more rapid the onset, the less favorable the prognosis. (4) Sphincter involvement: Sphincter involvement is indicative of an extremely poor prognosis.

It can be generally said that two thirds of patients who undergo operation for partial neurological defects can maintain their preoperative status. One third of those who are unable to walk before the operation can once again, for a period of time, get up and around. This improved prognosis has come about by the use of the anterior approach to remove the affected vertebrae (vertebrectomy) (Fig. 4.41). The less reliable laminectomy,

Figure 4.41 *The vertebra has been removed, and a bone graft is substituted and held into place by pedicle screws and plates.*

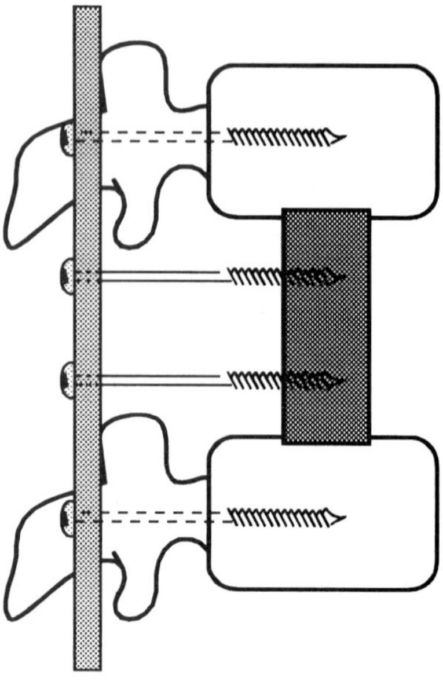

or posterior decompression, for masses that encroach on neurological tissue anteriorly, has largely been abandoned.

The timing of the decompression is of importance, and it appears that if a decompression is indicated, it must be carried out as an emergency procedure if any measure of recovery is to be expected. The surgical decompression must be performed with the meticulous technique employed in the decompression of acute traumatic lesions. Careless handling of the cord can convert a partial lesion into a complete lesion.

The management of metastatic spine lesions ranges from the simple to the complex. Experience, personal philosophy, and the patient are, at times, the only guides to this type of lesion, the most difficult of orthopedic problems.

Neurogenic Tumors of the Thoracolumbar and Lumbar Region

Spinal cord tumors are traditionally classified as extradural, intradural-extramedullary, and intradural-intramedullary (inside the spinal cord). They are all extremely rare.

Extradural

The extradural tumors are the metastatic and primary bone tumors that have been discussed in previous sections.

Intradural-Extramedullary

The two most common tumors in this classification are benign meningiomas (Fig. 4.42) and schwannomas (Fig. 4.43). They usually occur with symptoms of slowly progressive radicular pain. Late in the process, a Brown-Séquard cord lesion may occur. The diagnosis is made on MRI, and treatment is surgical excision.

An arteriovenous malformation of the cord is predominantly an extramedullary lesion that also exhibits radicular or cord symptoms and signs. A characteristic of this lesion is aggravation with exercise that increases the blood flow through the malformation, or steals blood away from the lesion. Exercise-induced quadriparesis is the hallmark of an arteriovenous (A-V) malformation. The diagnosis is confirmed by MRI. For surgical planning, angiography is necessary to define the extent of the malformation and its feeding vessels. Tedious microsurgical removal of the malformation with bipolar coagulation is the method of treatment.

Intradural-Intramedullary

Most intramedullary tumors are either benign astrocytomas or ependymomas. There are a number of other miscellaneous intramedullary tumors, gliomatous in nature, which are too infrequent to describe here.

The presentation is usually characteristic (in retrospect), with vague pain at the level of the lesion, usually without radicular distribution. The sensory and motor loss is significant at the level of the lesion and out of proportion to the minimal pain. Long tract findings, such as a spastic gait, are late to develop and usually follow upper extremity LMNL. Bladder and bowel symptoms are the last symptoms to appear.

The MRI scan is essential for diagnosis; it allows differentiation of syringomyelic cysts from solid tumors (Fig. 4.44).

Figure 4.42 *Meningioma at the cervical-thoracic junction (arrow) on a T1 sagittal full body scan.*

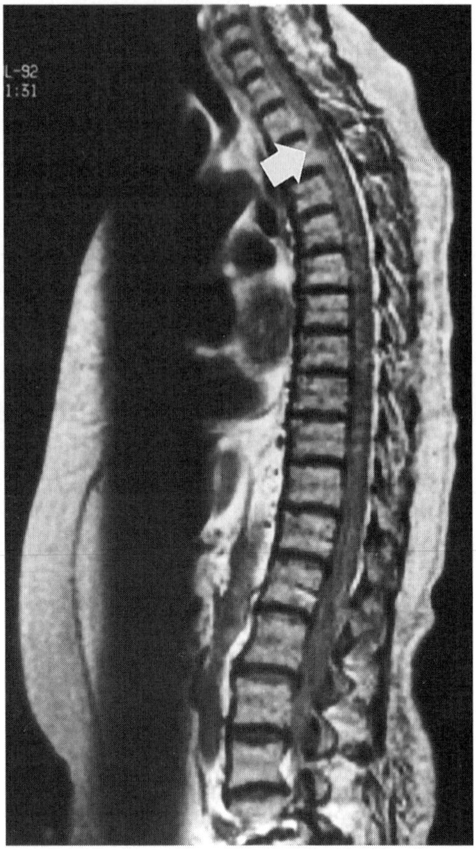

Figure 4.43 *Schwannoma completely filling the spinal canal (T1 sagittal with gadolinium enhancement).*

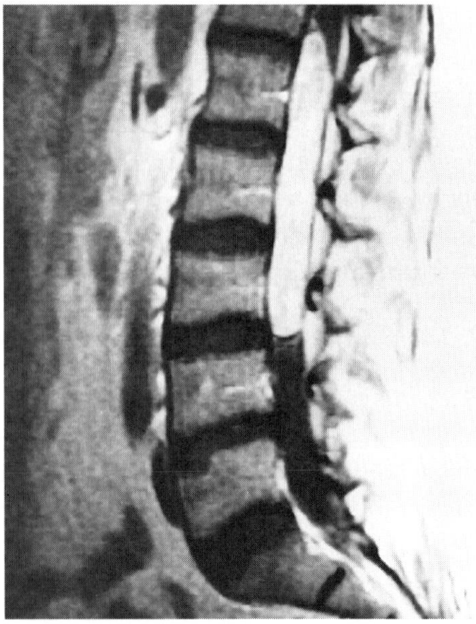

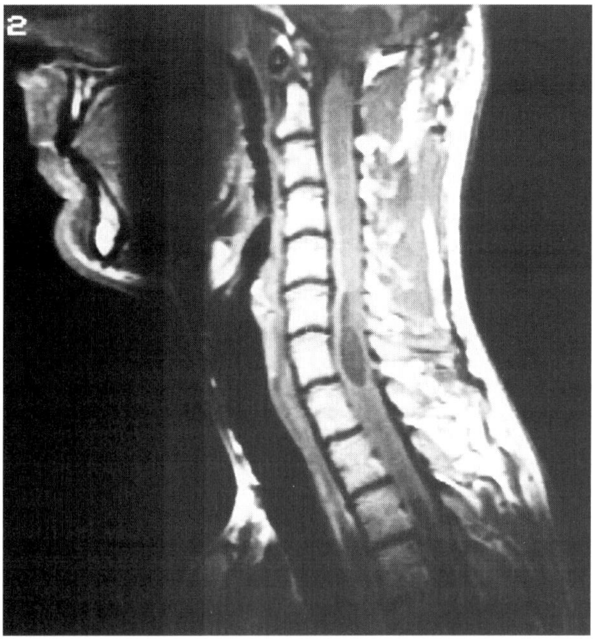

Figure 4.44 *MRI of a syringomyelia (gradient-echo sagittal showing decreased signal intensity from fluid-filled cyst).*

Treatment is surgical excision using tedious microsurgical techniques to preserve as much neurological function as possible. This is often possible with the well-circumscribed ependymoma, but rarely possible in the more diffuse astrocytoma.

METABOLIC BONE DISEASE: OSTEOPOROSIS

There are many metabolic bone diseases, but in the adult, the most common by far is osteoporosis.(11) The dynamic model of bone mass is founded on a balance between bone deposition and bone resorption. In osteoporosis, bone resorption is more extensive than bone deposition. The major impact of decreased bone mass is on thin cancellous bone (increased porosity of trabeculae) more than cortical bone (decreased cortical thickness), which weakens skeletal structures to the point where fractures occur with minimal trauma. The susceptible areas are the femoral neck, radius, ribs, and axial skeleton. Osteoporosis affects the axial skeleton through the occurrences of microfractures or gross fractures, which cause back pain.(3)

Osteoporosis may be considered as primary or secondary (Table 4.4). Primary osteoporosis is classified into postmenopausal (Type I), senile (Type II), and idiopathic (juvenile or adult).

Postmenopausal Osteoporosis

This is obviously a condition affecting women after menopause (50+ years). It affects 15–20 million Americans, resulting in 1.5 million fractures per year.

Although all women, and a few men, are susceptible to osteoporosis, there are very definite risk factors that increase the severity and consequences of osteoporosis (Table 4.5). The effect is primarily on trabecular bone, and the resulting fractures are predominantly to the vertebrae and distal radius.

Table 4.4. A General Classification of Osteoporosis

Regional	Disuse (immobilization) Post-traumatic osteodystrophy Migratory Inflammatory
General	
Congenital	Osteogenesis imperfecta Homocystinuria
Acquired Primary	Postmenopausal (Type I) Senile (Type II) Idiopathic (adult or juvenile)
Aquired Secondary	Nutritional Poor Ca^{2+} intake Poor Ca^{2+} absorption Endocrine Hyperthyroidism (thyrotoxicosis) Hyperadrenocorticism (endogenous or exogenous) Acromegaly Hypogonadism Prolonged use of steroids Neoplastic Multiple myeloma and leukemia Bone metastases Hormone-producing tumors Myeloproliferative Sickle cell anemia Thalassemia
Drug Induced	Heparin Anticonvulsants
Compound	Associated with hyperparathyroidism and some cases of osteomalacia

Table 4.5. Factors Increasing Risks of Osteoporosis

Females > Males (4:1)	
Caucasions and Asians	
Small body size	
Positive family history	
Surgically initiated estrogen deficiency (oopherectomy)	
Life-style factors:	Smoking
	Alcohol consumption
	Coffee (excessive)
	Decreased physical exercise
	Poor nutrition

Senile Osteoporosis

Senile osteoporosis decreases both trabecular and cortical bone mass. It affects both sexes who are 70 years of age or older, but the incidence is higher in women compared with men (2:1). Add the effects of senile osteoporosis to postmenopausal osteoporosis, and older women are very vulnerable to fractures.

Idiopathic Osteoporosis

Idiopathic juvenile osteoporosis is a rare condition affecting children between the ages of 8 and 12. It runs a 2- or 3-year course and then regresses spontaneously. Idiopathic osteoporosis of adults is more common in men. It usually becomes clinically evident at 40 years of age, and the symptoms may persist for 5 to 10 years. The causes of secondary osteoporosis are legion (Table 4.4).

Cause

In postmenopausal and senile osteoporosis, although both formation and resorption of bone are diminished, the rate of resorption exceeds the rate of formation. Many theories have been expounded to explain this curious phenomenon. It has been postulated that estrogen deficiency renders one more susceptible to the action of parathyroid hormone. Predictably, it has been suggested that a long-standing calcium deficiency in the diet leads to secondary hyperparathyroidism and bone resorption. Finally, lack of exercise in the older patient is said to be a contributing cause.

Clinical

The presenting symptom of vertebral osteoporosis is backache. The pain is spondylogenic in nature, being aggravated by general and specific activities and relieved to some extent, but not completely, by recumbency.

The pain has been ascribed to trabecular buckling or fractures. This is an untenable hypothesis in view of the fact that trephine biopsies of the vertebral bodies can be performed painlessly. When considering the cause of pain, it must be remembered that, although the bone mass has been markedly diminished, the size of the vertebral body remains the same. If the quantity of bone has been decreased, the other contents of the vertebral body must increase: the marrow, the fat, and the blood lakes. The fat content of an osteoporotic vertebral body does not increase primarily. Therefore, it must be presumed that the volume of the blood lakes must be greater. This implies venous stasis. The intraosseus venous pressure of a normal vertebra is approximately 28 mm Hg. The intraosseus venous pressure of an osteoporotic vertebral body is approximately 40 mm Hg. It is known that intraosseous venous stasis is seen in juxta-articular bone in osteoarthritis and that this is reversed after osteotomy. The decrease in venous pressure after osteotomy and forage of the hip joint for osteoarthritis probably accounts for the relief of pain experienced in the immediate postoperative period. It is probable that venous stasis in the vertebral bodies plays a significant role in the production of the dull, nagging, constant, boring pain about which these patients so commonly complain.

Although trabecular fractures do not play a role in the reproduction of symptoms, crush fractures of a vertebral body are common and are associated with the sudden onset of severe pain.

Fractures of the vertebral column are usually first noted in the thoracic region. Involvement of several upper thoracic vertebral bodies over a course of time may produce an increasing kyphosis, sometimes referred to as a "dowager's hump." Fractures in the upper thoracic spine may occur without a significant increase in discomfort, because of the support afforded by the rib cage; however, when crush fractures involve the lower thoracic or upper lumbar vertebrae (the usual location), severe pain may result.

Characteristically, the pain has a wide referral over the back, and is not localized to the fracture level. This is probably due to widespread muscle spasm.

At physical examination, it is usual to locate the acutely fractured vertebrae with local pressure or percussion on the spinous process. Neurological changes (radicular or myelopathic) are not present, and if so should alert you to some other cause, such as osteoporosis secondary to multiple myeloma.

The patient, then, will present with the history of a grumbling debilitating back pain punctuated on occasion with one or more episodes of severe incapacitating pain. These episodes of severe pain are usually initiated by some minor mechanical event, such as a slip or lifting. When the history is prolonged, the patients may also relate progressive loss of height and rounding of the upper thoracic spine. At examination, the thoracic kyphosis is noted, with a compensatory increase in the lumbar lordosis. If, over a period of time, the patient has sustained several vertebral crush fractures, the rib cage may come to rest on the iliac crest.

Radiograph

Radiographs of the spine show general loss of trabecular bone density and on closer inspection reveal lack of the horizontally disposed trabeculae. There may be ballooning of the discs into the vertebrae, which results in a fishtail appearance of the vertebral bodies. Compression fractures and endplate fractures are common (Fig. 4.12).

Secondary osteoporosis may produce an identical radiological appearance, and it is important to exclude the possibility of systemic disease before making the diagnosis of primary osteoporosis.

Laboratory

Idiopathic osteoporosis does not produce any changes in the blood chemistry. Osteomalacia and hyperparathyroidism specifically affect calcium and phosphorous metabolism. Bone activity is reflected by the elevated alkaline phosphatase level in both of these conditions. Multiple myeloma, which may be seen with back pain and a radiograph showing diffuse osteoporosis of the spine, is associated with significant changes in blood chemistry. There are alterations in the albumin and globulin ratios, and abnormal globulins can be detected. The sedimentation rate is raised, and frequently there is a significant anemia. The changes in blood chemistry of these various conditions are summarized in Table 4.6.

Measurement

Many attempts have been made to use radiographs to measure the extent of osteoporosis (Table 4.7). All such attempts have limitations and need to be applied and interpreted by someone familiar with the method. Because osteoporosis is such a slow dynamic event, it is also useful to repeat the test of choice over lengthy intervals to measure the progress of the disease and/or response to various treatment modalities.

The most widely used assessment method today is the Dual Energy X-ray Absorptiometry (DEXA) Scan. Using radiographic penetration, bone density in the lateral lumbar spine and proximal femur can be quickly assessed (10–20 minutes) with minimal radiation (less than 0.1 mrem) (Fig. 4.45). Reproducibility is sufficiently accurate to allow for serial studies in estimating calcium balance. Unfortunately, the US Health Care Financing Administration has decided that Medicare will pay a low rate for one scan per year of one

Table 4.6. Hematological and Biochemical Changes in Common Types of Osteoporosis

Change Factors	Osteoporosis	Osteomalacia	Hyperpara-thyroidism	Multiple Myeloma	Advanced Metastatic Disease
Hemogram				<10 gm %	↓
ESR	No			↑↑↑	↑
BUN/CR	Abnormal			N↑	N↑
Calcium	Values	↓	↑	N↑	↑
Phosphorus		↓	N↓	↑	↓
Alkaline phosphatases		↑	↑	↑	↑
Acid phosphatases					↑(prostate)
Uric acid			N↑	↑	↑
Protein electrophoresis				M spike	globulin
Immunoelectorphoresis				M spike	N/ABN

Key: ESR, erythrocyte sedimentation rate; BUN/CR, blood urea nitrogen/creatinine; N, Normal; ABN, abnormal.

Table 4.7. Methods of Quantifying Osteoporosis

Method	Basis	Drawback
Trabecular index	Count number of trabeculae in volume of bone (usually done in femoral neck)	Difficult to standardize
Cortical thickness	Measure cortical thickness relative to overall width of bone (usually done on metacarpal shaft)	Only measures endosteal bone resorption in cortex; difficult to standardize
Dual energy X-ray absorptiometry ie DEXA	Quantitative radiographic measurement of bone mass	Measures cancellous bone of spine and femur
Quantitative computed tomography	Using standard scanner, comparison of density of an area of bone (vertebral trabeculae) with a "phantom" of vials containing varying analogue	Expensive and time restraints; site specific, ie, if measuring spine, it will not give reliable information about extent of bone loss in femoral neck
Neutron activation analysis	Only available in a few research centers	Not familiar

site (eg, the proximal femur). This forces those providing the assessment service to do so at a loss, but the government bureaucrats could care less!(17)

Treatment

The treatment of postmenopausal or senile osteoporosis is frustratingly difficult. There is no evidence that any chemical therapy available to date or any replacement therapy reverses the metabolic change. The most recent addition to the medication regime has been Fosamax (alendronate sodium tablets) (Merck & Co., Inc., West Point, Penna.), that in well controlled clinical trials was shown to build bone. It is very new on the scene and general usage as of this writing has been very limited.

The risks of many therapeutic measures that are frequently advocated outweigh any possible advantage. Estrogens have been given for the treatment of this condition; they

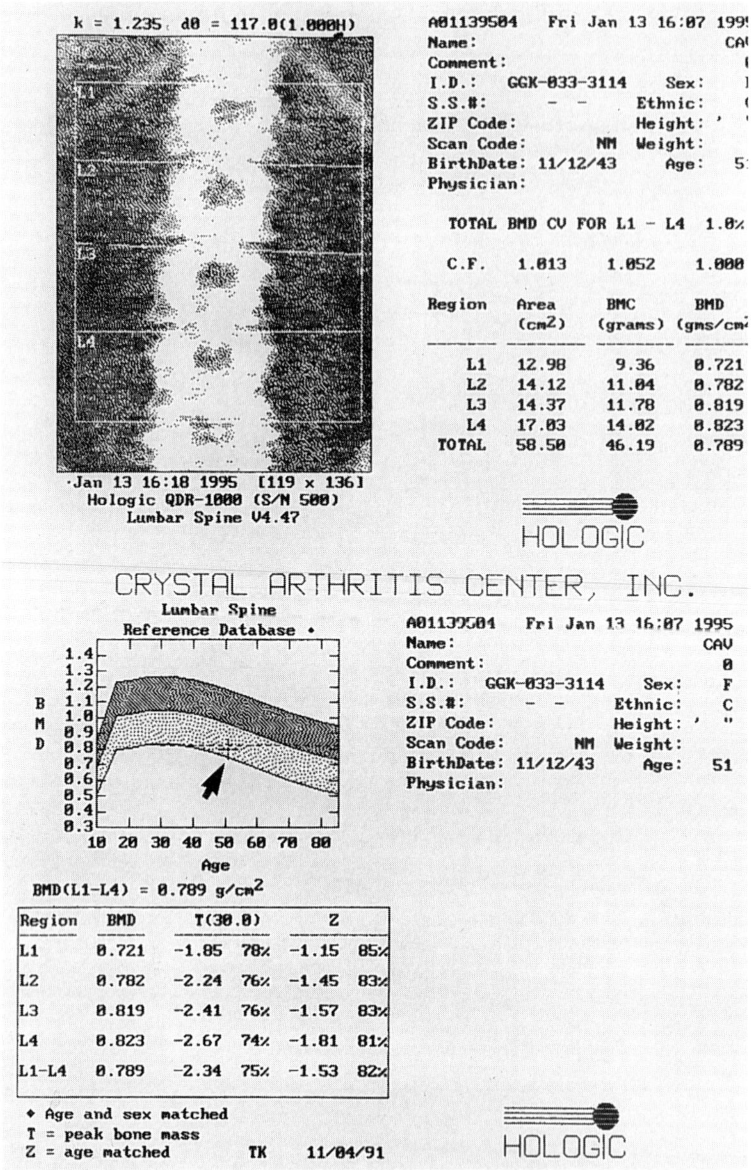

Figure 4.45 *A Dual Energy X-ray Absorptiometry scan of the lumbar spine. Top, figure and table depict the bone mineral density (BMD), which is plotted (below) as an average (cross hairs [arrow]) compared with normal (heavy stippled area).*

are associated with the nuisance of withdrawal bleeding and the increased risk of endometrial or breast malignancy. Estrogen therapy does not reverse the calcium imbalance. Androgens and anabolic steroids are more likely to increase muscle bulk than bone bulk. The administration of fluorides is sometimes associated with some subjective improvement and an apparent, albeit slight, increase in bone density on radiograph. This may be an artifact occasioned by the fact that fluoride salts are more radiopaque. The side effects of fluorides (gastrointestinal upset, ulceration, and joint stiffness) have limited their usefulness.

Treatment can be divided into two phases:

Prevention Any disease is best prevented. The treatment of osteoporosis should be directed at young women who are at risk and be designed to eliminate as many risk factors as possible (Table 4.5). The basis of prevention is threefold: hormonal substitute when osteoporosis risk is high (eg, oophorectomy at a young age and menopause); adequate calcium intake (minimum 1000 mg/d); and regular exercise. Other life-style changes such as elimination of excessive intake of alcohol and coffee should also be encouraged.

Treatment of Established Osteoporosis If serial DEXA scans or quantitative CT scans show advancing osteoporosis or the patient suffers an osteoporotic fracture, active treatment of osteoporosis should be instituted. This includes:

Treatment of the Fracture Obviously, fractures of the radius, femur, or vertebral body must be treated according to established principles. Most important, rest, which decreases bone mass, should be kept to a minimum. Vertebral compression fractures should be initially braced for comfort, and the patient should be quickly ambulated. (12) Treatment of vertebral compression fractures will extend to 3 or 4 months.

Hormonal Therapy Of the female sex hormones, estrogen is the basis of hormonal treatment. The combination with progesterone likely decreases the chance of endometrial hyperplasia and the increased risk of uterine cancer. The effect of estrogen is to reduce bone resorption, thus slowing the rate at which bone loss occurs.

Chemical Therapy Two drugs are available for the treatment of osteoporosis (7):

Calcitonin Calcitonin is a hormone produced by the thyroid gland that suppresses bone resorption. Unfortunately, its effect is most pronounced with intermuscular injection, a fact that strains patient compliance.

Diphosphonates (Etidronate) This drug, like estrogen and calcitonin, also inhibits bone resorption. There are limits to its use as well, including a 4-hour curtailment of food ingestion before and after oral ingestion of the drug. Recently, an advisory committee to the US Food and Drug Administration recommended against approving the use of etidronate in the treatment of osteoporosis. The basis of this decision was the failure of scientific studies to show a reduction in the incidence of spinal fractures in a large study population.

Nutritional Therapy It seems rather fruitless to prescribe hormonal and chemical treatment of osteoporosis if the patient has poor intake or absorption of calcium. The use of calcium supplementation (1000 mg/day) along with a regular diet is advisable. Vitamin D from a multivitamin is also useful to increase the gastric absorption of calcium. Abstinence from excessive alcohol and all smoking further enhances these nutritional steps.

Exercise The single most important fact in osteoporosis prevention and treatment is regular exercise to increase the stimulus to bone formation. If every postmenopausal woman would take a brisk 3-mile walk every day (15–20 minute mile), there would be much less osteoporosis to trouble us.

Summary

This chapter has presented much information on trauma, tumors, infection, and osteoporosis. Obviously, the information is mainly of summary value, but also serves as a reminder that when a patient presents with back pain, there are literally hundreds of diagnoses to consider.

REFERENCES

1. Bohlman HH. Treatment of fractures and dislocations of the thoracic and lumbar spine. J Bone Joint Surg 1985;67A:165–169.
2. Calvé JA. Localized affection of spine suggesting osteochondritis of vertebral body, with clinical aspects of Pott's disease. J Bone Joint Surg 1925;7:41–46.
3. Cohen LD. Fractures in the osteoporotic spine. Orthop Clin North Am 1990;21:143–150.
4. Denis F. The three column spine and its significance in the classification of acute thoracolumbar spinal injuries. Spine 1983;8:817–831.
5. Frankel H, Hancock DO, Hyslop G, et al. The value of postural reduction in the initial management of closed injuries of the spine with paraplegia and tetraplegia: i. Paraplegia 1969;7: 179–192.
6. Fraser RD, Osti OL, Vernon-Roberts B. Discitis following chemonucleolysis: an experimental study. Spine 1986;11:679–687.
7. Frost HM. Treatment of osteoporosis by manipulation of coherent bone cell populations. Clin Orthop 1979;143:227–244.
8. Huvos AG. Bone tumors: diagnosis, treatment and prognosis. Toronto: WB Saunders; 1979.
9. Johnsson R, Herrlin K, Hagglund G, et al. Spinal canal remodelling after thoracolumbar fractures with intraspinal bone fragments. Acta Orthop Scand 1991;62:125–127.
10. Knight RQ, Stornelli DP, Chan DP, Devanny JR, Jackson KV. Comparison of operative vs. non-operative treatment of lumbar burst fractures. Clin Orthop 1993;293:112–121.
11. Lane JM (ed). Symposium of metabolic bone disease. Orthop Clin North Am 1985;15:596–790.
12. Lukert BP. Vertebral compression fractures: how to manage pain, avoid disability. Geriatrics 1994;49:22–26.
13. Marcove RC, Weiss LD, Vaghaiwalls MD, et al. Cryosurgery in the treatment of giant cell tumors of the bone. Cancer (Philadelphia) 1978;41:957–969.
14. McAfee PC. The unstable burst fracture. Spine 1982;7:365–373.
15. McAfee PC, Yuan HA, Frederickson BA, et al. The value of computed tomography in thoracolumbar fractures. J Bone Joint Surg 1983;65A:461–473.
16. Modic MT, Feiglin DH, Piraino DW, et al. Vertebral osteomyelitis: assessment using MR. Radiology 1985;157:157–166.
17. Sartoris DJ. Coding and reimbursement issues for dual-energy x-ray absorptiometry. AJR 1994;163:137–139.
18. Weinstein JN, Collalto P, Lehmann TR. Long-term follow up of non-operatively treated thoracolumbar spine fractures. J Orthop Trauma 1987;1:152–159.
19. Weinstein JN, McLain RF. Primary tumors of the spine. Spine 1987;12:843–851.

5

Spondylolysis/Spondylolisthesis

"False facts are highly injurious to progress of science, for they often endure long; but false views, if supported by some evidence do little harm, for everyone takes a salutary pleasure in proving their falseness."

— Charles Darwin

INTRODUCTION

Scoliosis, spondylolysis, and spondylolisthesis are the major structural changes in the spine that may, on occasion, give rise to low back pain. Scoliosis is a topic in itself and therefore, is mentioned only when discussing the differential diagnosis of low back pain. Spondylolysis/spondylolisthesis is more directly related to the various low back pain syndromes and, therefore, merits a more detailed description.

SPONDYLOLYSIS

With the significant increase in sporting effort in high school athletes ("My son is the best linebacker in his high school's history!"), there is an epidemic of spondylolysis. Up until recently, we have considered this condition a routine problem. More recently, with the use of computed tomography (CT) scanning and single photon emission computed tomography (SPECT) scanning, it has been found that the condition is far from routine, and it is difficult to be dogmatic with regard to the criteria for diagnosis and treatment.

Etiology of Spondylolysis

The classic teaching of causation for spondylolysis has been that an individual is born with a weakness in the pars interarticularis, and at approximately age 6, a fatigue injury occurs that breaks the pars.(11) Kids will be kids, and the event often goes unreported. Later, in high school, with the weight lifting and contact stresses of football or the extension stresses of gymnastics or wrestling, the latent fracture is irritated and becomes symptomatic.

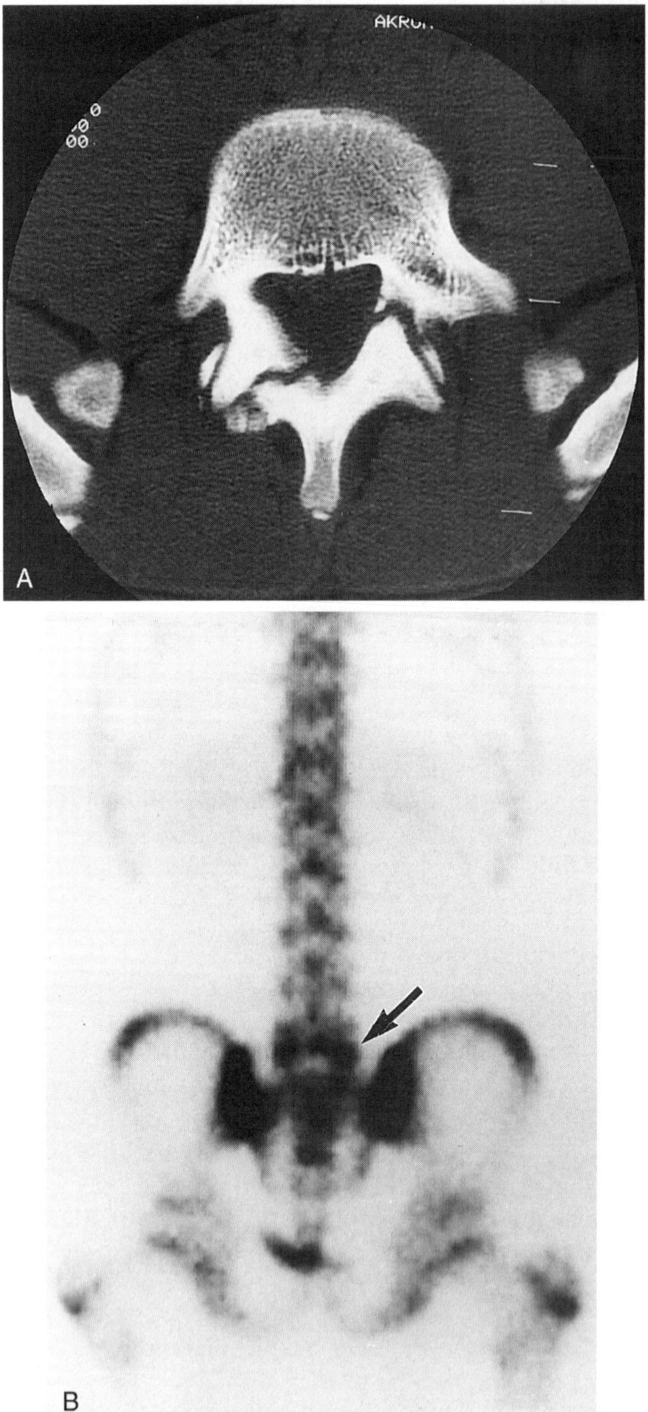

Figure 5.1 **A.** *Axial CT of spondylolysis, L5.* **B.** *Bone scan in same patient showing bilateral "hot" pars interarticularis (arrow).*

Another group of teenagers exists who present with an acute lesion. They have no history of injury, and they suffer a significant hyperextension injury or compressive force to their lumbar spine, which is followed by the immediate and sudden onset of very severe low back pain. Radiographs reveal a fresh fracture, and these patients have a very hot bone scan (Fig. 5.1) (14). These patients are in the minority and represent a special treatment situation.

Finally, remember that 5% of the general population walks around with a spondylolysis that is completely asymptomatic.(14) Spondylolysis may be unilateral in up to one third of these patients.

Clinical Presentation

A wide spectrum of presentations exists in these young patients, ranging from an acute disabling episode of back pain to mild low back discomfort when the patient engages in certain activities. The back pain may be dominant to one side, but more often is across the lumbosacral junction. Radiating leg pain is rare in spondylolysis, but hamstring tightness on straight leg raising testing is common. Obviously, neurological symptoms and signs are absent.

Radiographic Findings

The radiographic findings have no set pattern. Although most teenagers will have a defect that is seen on oblique radiographs (Fig. 5.2), enough negative oblique radiographs occur (Fig. 5.3) to require additional radiological investigation in a young patient with unexplained mechanical back pain.

Additional investigative steps include a SPECT scan (Fig. 5.4) and a CT scan (Fig. 5.5). Experience has shown us that there is no pattern to the findings in these three tests (oblique lumbar radiographs, SPECT scan, and CT scan). You can almost pick whichever combination you wish: for example, positive oblique radiographs / negative SPECT and CT; negative oblique radiographs and SPECT / positive CT; positive oblique radiographs, SPECT, CT; and so on. In addition, the CT scan findings are by no means uniform (Fig. 5.6).

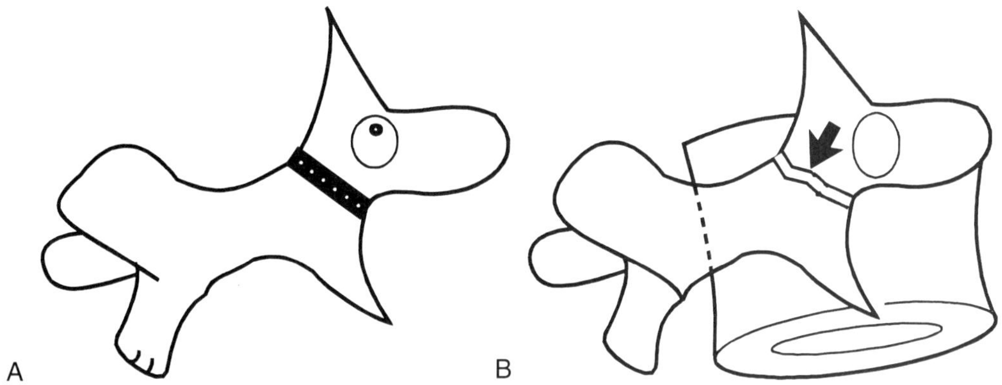

Figure 5.2 **A.** *Schematic of oblique view of spondylolysis (arrow).* **B.** *Note how lesion looks like a collar on a Scottish terrier.*

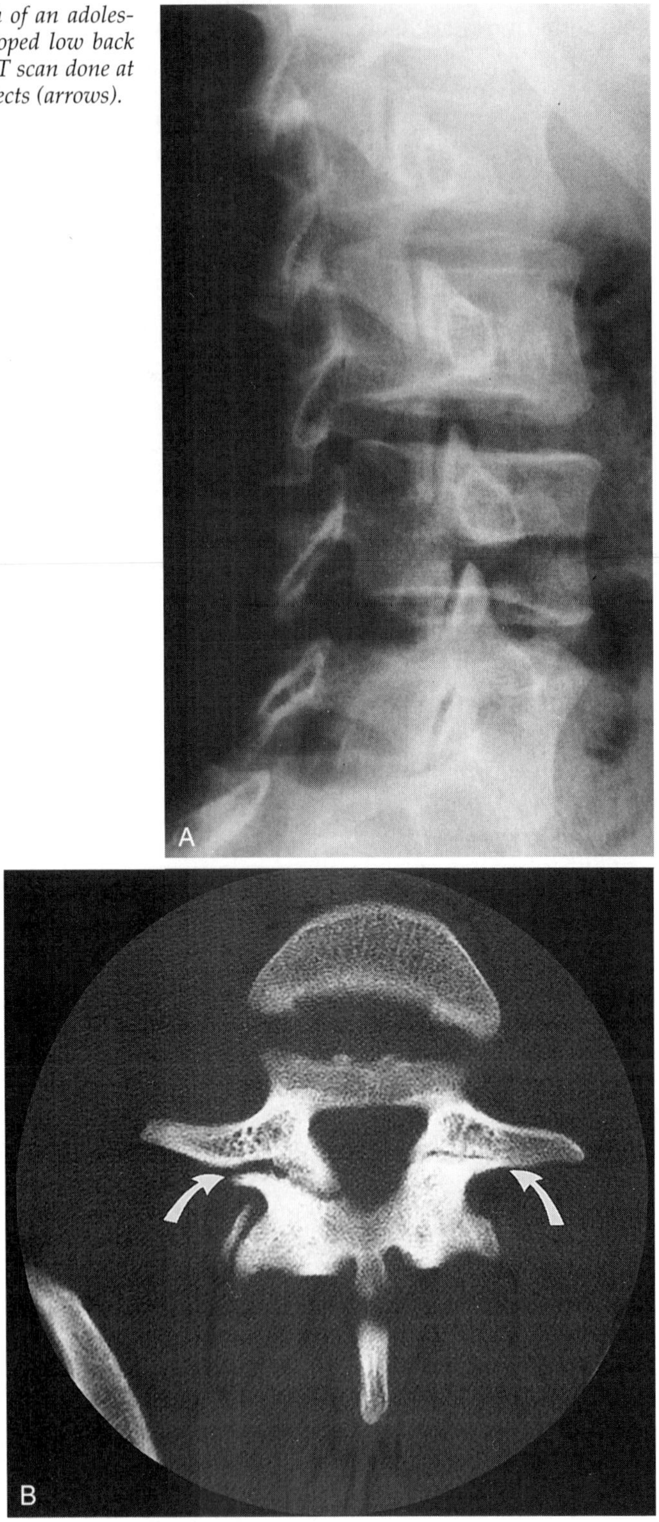

Figure 5.3 **A.** *An oblique radiograph of an adolescent who, after a football injury, developed low back pain; there is no apparent fracture.* **B.** *CT scan done at the same time showing bilateral pars defects (arrows).*

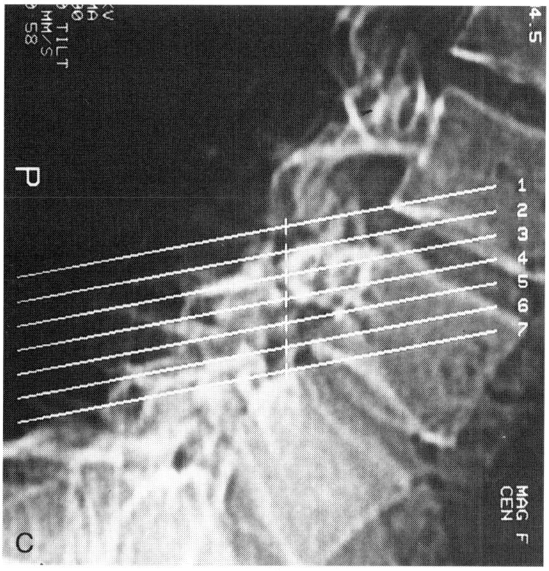

Figure 5.3 (continued) **C.** *The reverse gantry angle technique used to show defect in 5.3, B.*

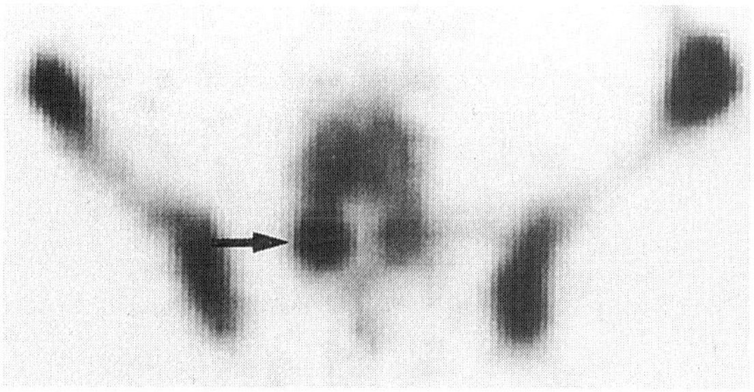

Figure 5.4 *SPECT of spondylolysis (arrow).*

Level of Lysis

The majority of spondylolytic lesions occur at L5, but a few will be present at higher lumbar levels (Fig. 5.7), a fact that sometimes leads to false-negative radiographic readings.

Treatment

After many years of programmed treatment (eg, a hot bone scan means a fresh fracture that must be immobilized), we have reduced our advice to two rules for two different groups of patients:

1. If the patient has low back pain and any one of the three tests is positive, take the patient out of the sport, put them in exercise physical therapy, and brace them. When they become asymptomatic, they join Group 2.
2. If the patient has no symptoms, do not restrict activities and do not brace them (or take them out of a brace), despite the results of radiographs, bone scan, and CT scan.

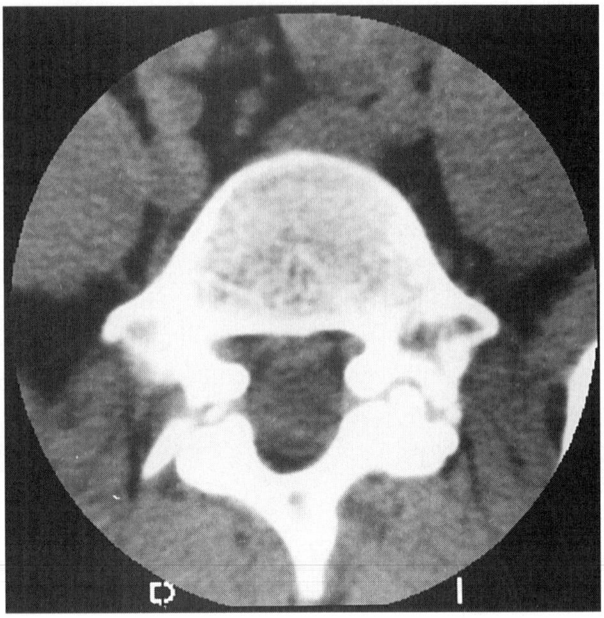

Figure 5.5 *A CT scan of an old lysis (L5 bilateral).*

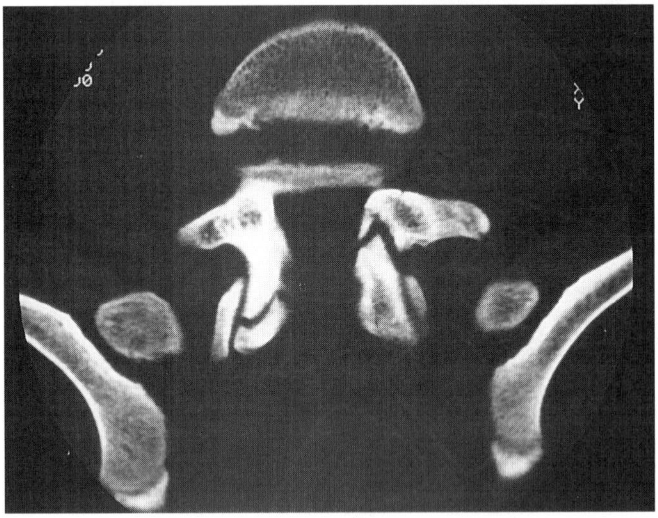

Figure 5.6 *Compare this CT of spondylolysis to Figures 5.5 and 5.3; each scan shows a different fracture pattern.*

Unfortunately, many young persons fall between these two groups and require some form of activity restriction, therapeutic exercise, and bracing. The real problem comes when trying to determine the duration of treatment. Remember, "my son is the best linebacker in his high school's history," which is a statement usually associated with an important game in the near future at which all the college scouts will be in attendance! In this pressure situation of having to treat the patient/parent team, do what is best for the patient. If the patient is asymptomatic, let them play regardless of the investigation results. If the patient is symptomatic, restrict activities (regardless of the investigation results).

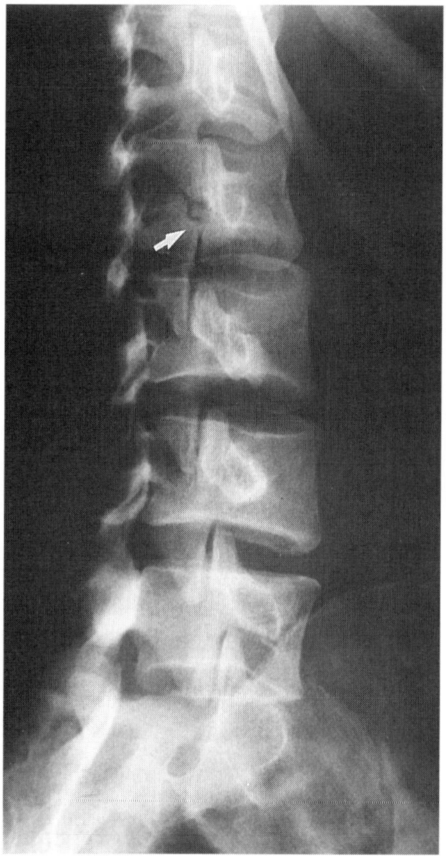

Figure 5.7 *A spondylolysis of L2 (arrow).*

Specific Treatment of Spondylolysis

Conservative Treatment

Patients are treated with modalities and a flexion exercise program. Once symptoms start to improve, a generalized conditioning program and specific equipment-based exercises are instituted to strengthen the low back. During this program, the patient is abstaining from the aggravating activity (sport), which in itself may be the most important treatment step.

On relief of symptoms, the patients gradually return to sports. The most difficult aspect of judging the rate of return to sports is to balance what a stoical teenager who wants to "mix it up" with his/her peers is telling you about ongoing symptoms with what you, the treating physician, observes on examination.

Surgical Treatment

It is rare that a young patient cannot improve with conservative treatment. In these situations, direct surgical repair of the defect can be considered. Figure 5.8 shows the various ways of accomplishing this repair.

Follow-up

On follow-up, plain radiograph, and CT scan, we have seen a minority of these lesions heal despite the patient becoming asymptomatic (Fig. 5.9). We simply follow up these patients every 6 months to a year with a standing lateral lumbar spine radiograph. If they start to develop a slip (spondylolisthesis), we become more aggressive with treatment intervention.

SPONDYLOLISTHESIS

Herbineaux,(4) a Belgian obstetrician, noted in 1782 that occasionally a bony prominence in front of the sacrum constituted an obstruction to labor. It has always been assumed that

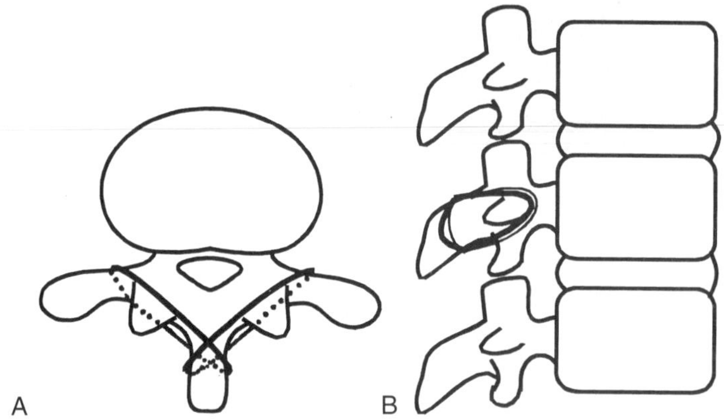

Figure 5.8 **A.** *Axial view of repair of spondylolysis with wire around spinous process and transverse processes.* **B.** *Sagittal view of the same repair.*

Figure 5.9 *This is the CT scan of the same patient in Figure 5.3, 5 months later; the patient experienced no pain and was playing sports. The pars interarticularis fractures are still obvious.*

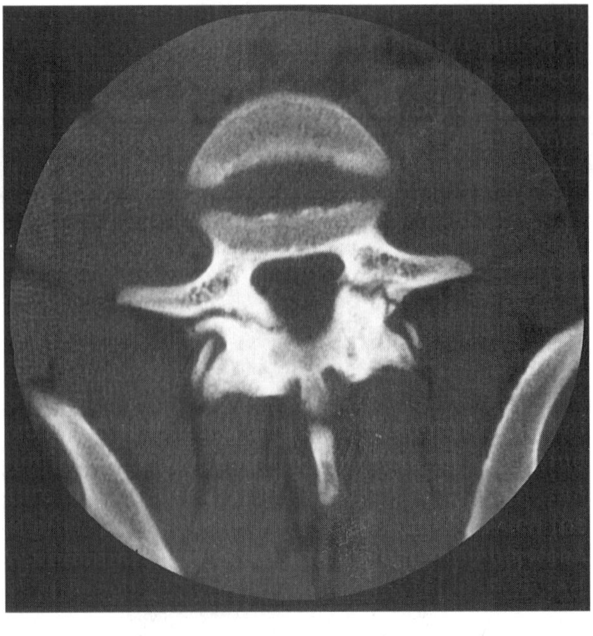

the condition he was describing was a complete spondylolisthesis: a spondyloptosis. Herbineaux is regarded as the first person to describe this lesion. Killian,(8) who coined the term spondylolisthesis, believed that the lesion was due to a slow subluxation of the posterior facets. However, Robert(8) theorized that the slip could not occur without a defect in the neural arch. The lesion was demonstrated 30 years later by Lambl.(8) Neugebauer (8) recognized the fact that the slip could occur with or without a defect in the neural arch. His work, unfortunately, was largely forgotten, and subsequent interest became focused on the neural arch defect. The discussions on the nature, etiology, age of onset, and radiological appearance of the defect obscured the fact that spondylolisthesis can, and does, occur with an intact neural arch.(6) The management of painful spondylolisthesis obviously must depend on the type of lesion present; therefore, before discussing treatment, it is necessary to describe in detail the various types of spondylolisthesis.

Forward slip of the fifth vertebra is resisted by the bony locking of the posterior facets, the intact neural arch and pedicle, normal bone plasticity preventing stretch of the pedicle, and the intervertebral discs bonding the vertebral bodies together (Fig. 5.10). Breakdown of this normal locking mechanism occurs with articular defects and defects in the neural arch. These pathological defects produce five recognizable clinical groups of spondylolisthesis (10) (Tables 5.1 and 5.2): dysplastic, isthmic, degenerative, traumatic, and pathological.

Description of Spondylolisthesis on Radiograph

Before describing the various types of spondylolisthesis, it is best to understand the terms used to measure the extent of the vertebral body slip.

The classic measurement of the slip degree has been that of Myerding,(7) an obstetrician who described 4 degrees of slip (Fig. 5.11)(Grade 1 = 25%, Grade 2 = 25 to 50%, Grade

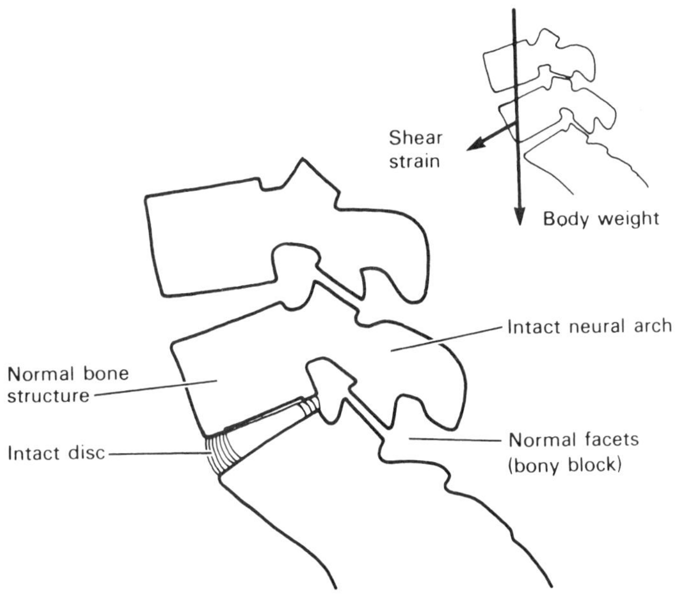

Figure 5.10 *The normal locking mechanisms resisting forward displacement of the fifth lumbar vertebral body. From Macnab I: Backache. Williams & Wilkins, Baltimore (1977), p. 45.*

Table 5.1. Working Classification of Spondylolisthesis

Bony Location of Defect	Etiology: Congenital	Etiology: Acquired
Pars	Isthmic (fatigue fracture)	Traumatic fracture
Facet joint	Congenital absence or dysplasia	Degeneration of facet joint
Bone	0	Weak or 'plastic' bone

Table 5.2. Commonly Accepted Clinical Classification of Spondylolisthesis

Type	Classification	Description
I	Dysplastic	Congenital abnormalities of upper sacrum or arch at L5
II	Isthmic	Lesion in pars interarticularis
		Lytic—fatigue fracture
		Elongated but intact pars
		Acute fracture
III	Degenerative	Facet joint degeneration
IV	Traumatic	Fractures in areas of arch other than pars
V	Pathological	Secondary to generalized or localized bone disease

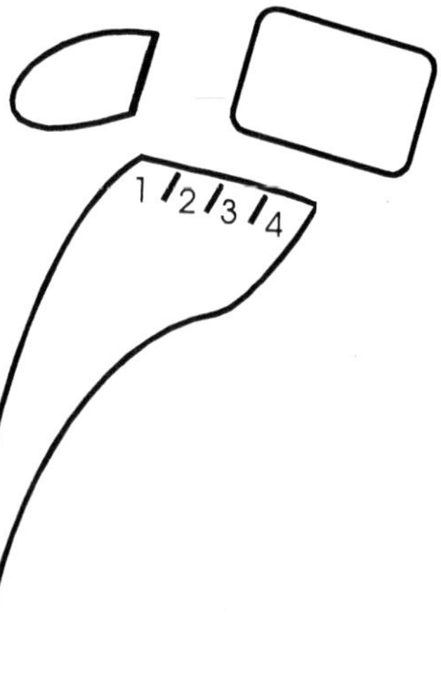

Figure 5.11 *Myerding(7) classification of slip grades, which divides the sacrum into "quarters." This is a drawing of a Grade II slip.*

3 = 50 to 75%, and Grade 4 = 75 to 100% slip). A complete dislocation of L5 on S1 (Fig. 5.26) was called a spondyloptosis.

More recently, Wiltse and Winter (12) proposed a more sophisticated group of measurements (Fig. 5.12). The reason for this was to separate the tangential movement in the low-grade slips (Grades I and II) from the angular/tangential slips that occurred in the higher levels of slip. In fact, this more complete classification has served to point out that the low-grade slips behave like degenerative disc disease, and the high-grade slips are

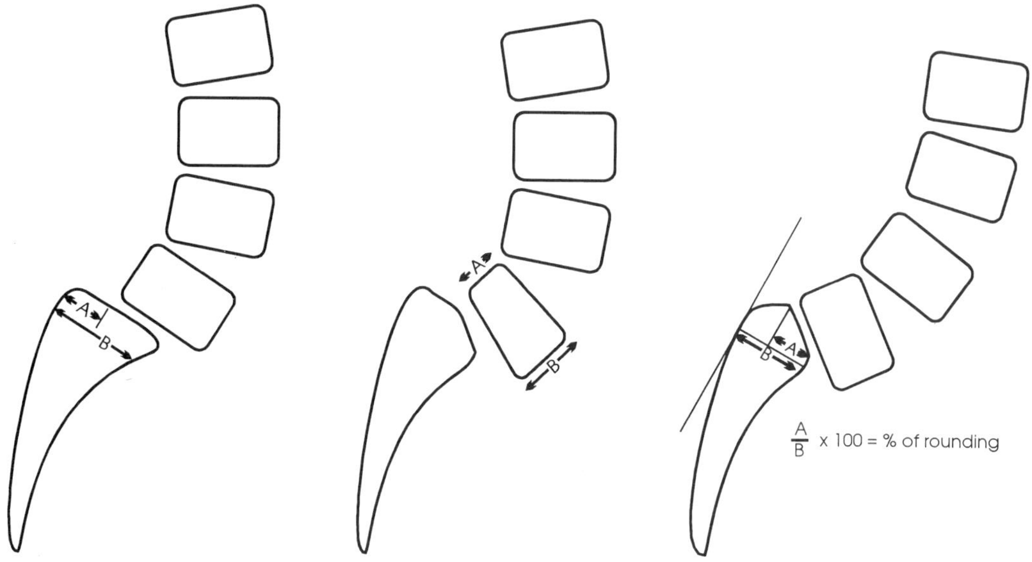

Figure 5.12 *The Wiltse-Winter nomenclature. Left: The degree of slip is expressed as the percentage* **A** *is of* **B.** *Middle: Vertebral wedging—again, what percent* **A** *is of* **B.** *Right: sacral rounding.*

more like a spinal deformity that requires a whole new set of management principles. This distinction will be covered in the following sections.

TYPE I CONGENITAL OR DYSPLASTIC SPONDYLOLISTHESIS

Congenital spondylolisthesis with forward displacement of a vertebral body at birth is a clinical curiosity. The spinal defect is usually only one of multiple congenital anomalies, and the clinical problem presented is not the management of the spondylolisthesis, but the management of the associated congenital scoliosis.

In a true dysplastic spondylolisthesis, the lesion may be either dysplasia of the upper sacrum, specifically in the facet joints (Fig. 5.13), or an attenuation of the pars interarticularis that gets pulled out and thinned as though it were made of a malleable plastic (Fig. 5.14). As the slip increases, and as the pars interarticularis becomes increasingly stretched, it may eventually break; but this break is secondary to the slip and is not the cause of the slip. This concept represents a slight deviation from the Wiltse-Newman- Macnab classification,(10) the reason for which is explained in the legend of Figure 5.13. 0n occasion, there may be a subluxation of the posterior joints between L5 and the sacrum due to a lack of development of the first sacral arch, with absence or dysplasia of the superior articular facets of the sacrum. The only structure preventing forward slip of the fifth lumbar vertebra is the lumbosacral disc. When this breaks down, the fifth lumbar vertebra slips forward, with the inferior facets gliding over the rudimentary superior articular facets. The spinous process of L5 eventually comes to rest in the fibrous defect in the first sacral arch (Fig. 5.13). However, this by itself would not allow a very marked slip. Further slipping must involve attenuation and elongation of the pars interarticularis.

In this form of spondylolisthesis, slipping occurs early in life and is permitted by virtue of detachment of the hyaline cartilage plate. The degree of slip is usually quite marked.(2)

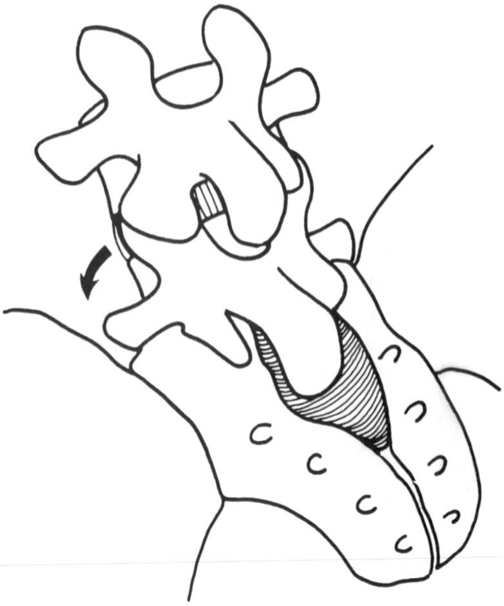

Figure 5.13 *Dysplastic spondylolisthesis. This lesion is frequently associated with rudimentary superior articular facets of the sacrum. With degeneration of the lumbosacral disc, the fifth lumbar vertebra is displaced forward in relation to the sacrum.*

The spinous process of L5 eventually comes to rest in a fibrous defect usually present on the dorsal aspect of the first sacral arch. This represents the purest form of dysplastic spondylolisthesis. From Macnab I: Backache. Williams & Wilkins, Baltimore (1977), p. 47.

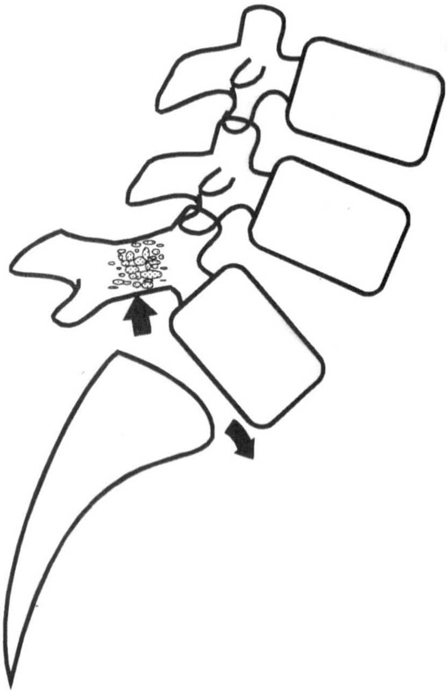

Figure 5.14 *An elongated pars may allow for a spondylolisthesis.*

In severe degrees of slip, the basic pathology is frequently overlooked because when severe degrees of slip are noted on radiograph, it has always been assumed that there must be a defect in the pars interarticularis. The fact that the defect may not be shown on the radiograph has been ascribed to difficulties in radiological techniques. The important clinical feature of the lesion is the fact that often there is lack of a defect in the pars interarticularis. Because there is no defect, the neural arch comes forward with the slipping vertebra, and the cauda equina may be compressed between the laminae of L4 and L5 and the dorsal area of the first sacral body. Lane (8) in 1893 described a young woman who had the misfortune to be the serving maid of a man who suffered from the delusion that life was all cricket. He would frequently strike her in the rear with a cricket bat that he always carried around with him. She gradually became paraplegic. Lane, describing his operative findings, stated that the neural arch was intact, and as the arch had slipped forward, it had compressed the dura mater of the cauda equina. According to Lane, the spinous process of L5 lay in the fibrous defect of the dorsal sacrum. This is a beautiful description of the pathology of dysplastic spondylolisthesis. Although examples of cauda equina compression are sometimes seen with this type of spondylolisthesis, the attenuation and elongation of the isthmus that inevitably occur usually prevent any significant distortion of the cauda equina (Fig. 5.15). In fact, the majority of patients present without any evidence of nerve root irritation at all.

The average age of symptom onset may be very young but is most often 14 in girls and 16 in boys (± 4 years), the final growth spurt age. The onset may be quite sudden and dramatic and is aptly termed a "listhetic crisis." The patient experiences a sudden onset of backache and, on examination, characteristically presents with a rigid lumbar spine that is commonly associated with a spastic or functional scoliosis. The pelvis is rotated anteriorly, giving rise to a flat sacrum; hamstring spasm is frequently seen, which makes the patient walk with bent knees (Fig. 5.16).

The reason for differentiating this group of spondylolisthesis from the others is that the indications for surgery are much more clear-cut than in the next group, isthmic spondylolisthesis. If a dysplastic spondylolisthesis progresses to the stage of producing severe symptoms before the age of 21, with or without signs of nerve root irritation, it is unlikely that the patient will make a complete recovery without surgical intervention. Patients presenting with a first- or even second-degree slip will probably continue to slip more if seen in their early teens. Evidence has substantiated the view that fusion performed at this stage will prevent further slip.

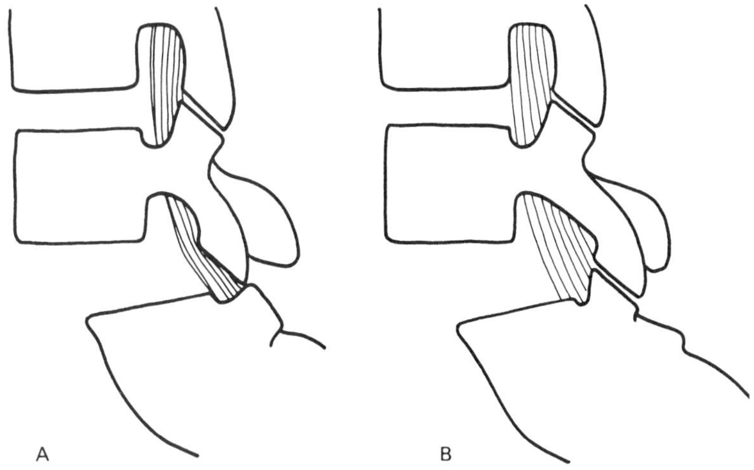

Figure 5.15 *Dysplastic spondylolisthesis. In the presence of a normal pars interarticularis, forward dislocation of the fifth lumbar vertebra in relation to the sacrum is likely to produce compression of the cauda equina* **(A).** *The elongation of the pars interarticularis associated with the forward displacement of the fifth lumbar vertebra in dysplastic spondylolisthesis maintains the diameter of the spinal canal and obviates compression of the cauda equina* **(B).** *From Macnab I: Backache. Williams & Wilkins, Baltimore (1977), p. 48.*

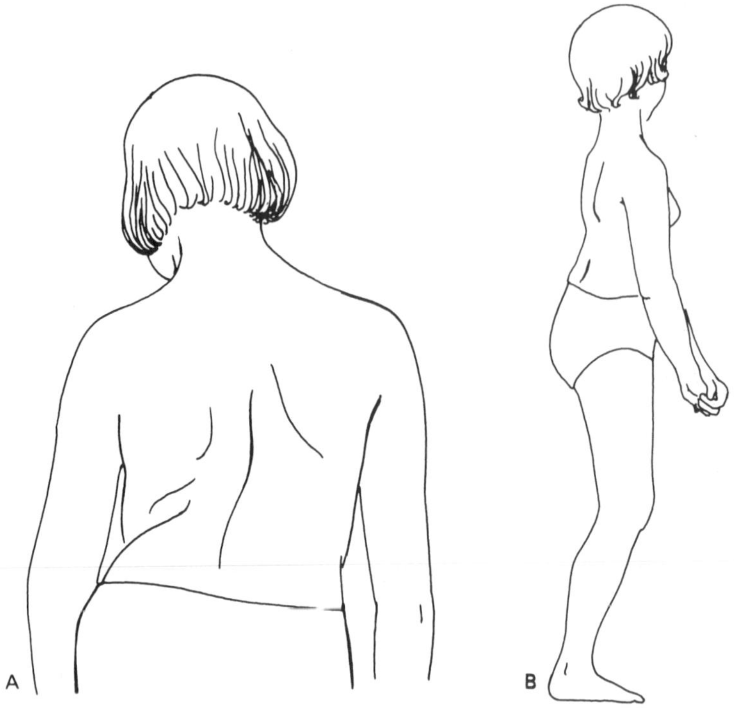

Figure 5.16 *A "listhetic crisis" is frequently associated with a functional scoliosis* **(A).** *Hamstring spasm is common despite anterior rotation of the pelvis, and the patient frequently stands and walks with bent knees* **(B).** *From Macnab I: Backache. Williams & Wilkins, Baltimore (1977), p. 49.*

In the surgical management of this condition, the following points must be borne in mind: It is unwise to attempt to reduce the slip. Even if the slip is successfully reduced, it is most unlikely that the reduction will be held and, even so, nothing much has been achieved. Patients who present evidence of root tension or impairment of root conduction will require laminectomy and, on occasion, decompression of the involved root or roots. All patients will require stabilization, and the best method of fusion devised to date is the ala transverse fusion (Fig. 5.17).

Isthmic Spondylolisthesis

Lytic: Fatigue Fracture of Pars

In isthmic spondylolisthesis, the basic lesion is a defect in the pars interarticularis of the neural arch (Fig. 5.18). The etiology of this lesion is unknown, but Wiltse et al (10) and others postulate that it is a fatigue fracture of the pars. This lesion likely occurs in a congenitally weakened pars.(13) The neural arch defects occur most commonly between the ages of 5 and 7. Forward slipping of the vertebral body occurs most frequently between the ages of 10 and 15 and rarely increases after age 20.

Despite the uncertainty relating to the etiology of the neural arch defect, the radiological appearance is well known. The patient with low back pain presents an irksome problem for the orthopedic surgeon. The diagnosis is usually obscure or cannot be proved.

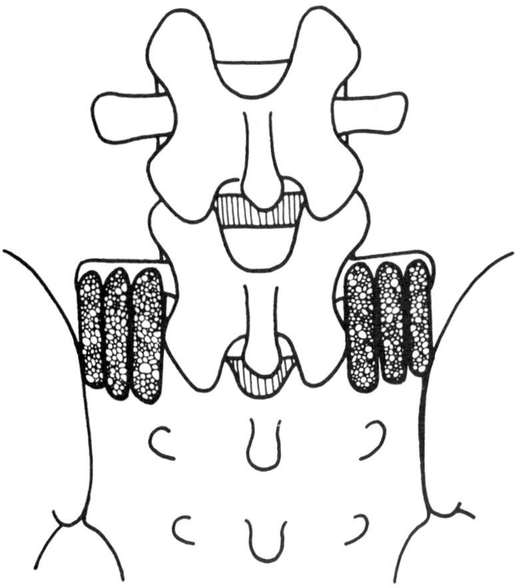

Figure 5.17 *Ala transverse fusion using corticocancellous grafts bridging the gap between the transverse process of L5 and the ala of the sacrum. From Macnab I: Backache. Williams & Wilkins, Baltimore (1977), p. 50.*

Treatment perforce is empirical, and the results of treatment, in many instances, are unrewarding. Therefore, the demonstration on radiograph of a gross abnormality of this type is generally greeted with a sigh of relief: Here is a recognizable cause of backache; here is an easily understood and treatable lesion. However, a word of caution must be interjected. Severe degrees of slip may be present in patients who engage in very vigorous activities, and yet they never suffer from backache.(3)

Because there is no doubt that lytic spondylolisthesis can, and does occur without producing symptoms, the mere radiological demonstration of the defect in a patient with back pain does not indicate that the source of the symptoms has necessarily been demonstrated. Other anatomical variants have in the past been thought to be a cause of backache. It is now generally accepted that none of these anatomical variants is, by itself, a cause of low back pain. The question must arise, therefore, as to whether a neural arch defect, with or without a slip of the vertebral body, is yet another example of an anatomical variant incorrectly blamed as a cause of low back pain.

In examining this question further, it is important to take the following points into consideration. Stewart (9) has shown that in some Eskimo communities the incidence of neural arch defects may rise as high as 50%. It is most unlikely that 50% of the Eskimos in these communities are severely handicapped by low back pain. The incidence of spondylolysis in the white population of the North American continent is about 6%. If neural arch defects were a common cause of low back pain, the incidence of such defects in the backache population should be very much higher than 6%. However, when Macnab analyzed 996 adult patients with low back pain seen over the course of 1 year, he found an incidence of neural arch defects of only 7.6%. This incidence is not significantly greater than that of the population as a whole. The analysis as it presently stands raises doubts as to whether neural arch defects are ever a source of symptoms. However, it is not unusual that patients with spondylolisthesis may become completely symptom free after a successful spinal fusion. In trying to explain this apparent contradiction, many years ago Dr. Macnab divided patients with back pain into three age groups (under 25, 26–39, and over 40), and the incidence of spondylolisthesis was studied in each group (Table 5.3) Over age

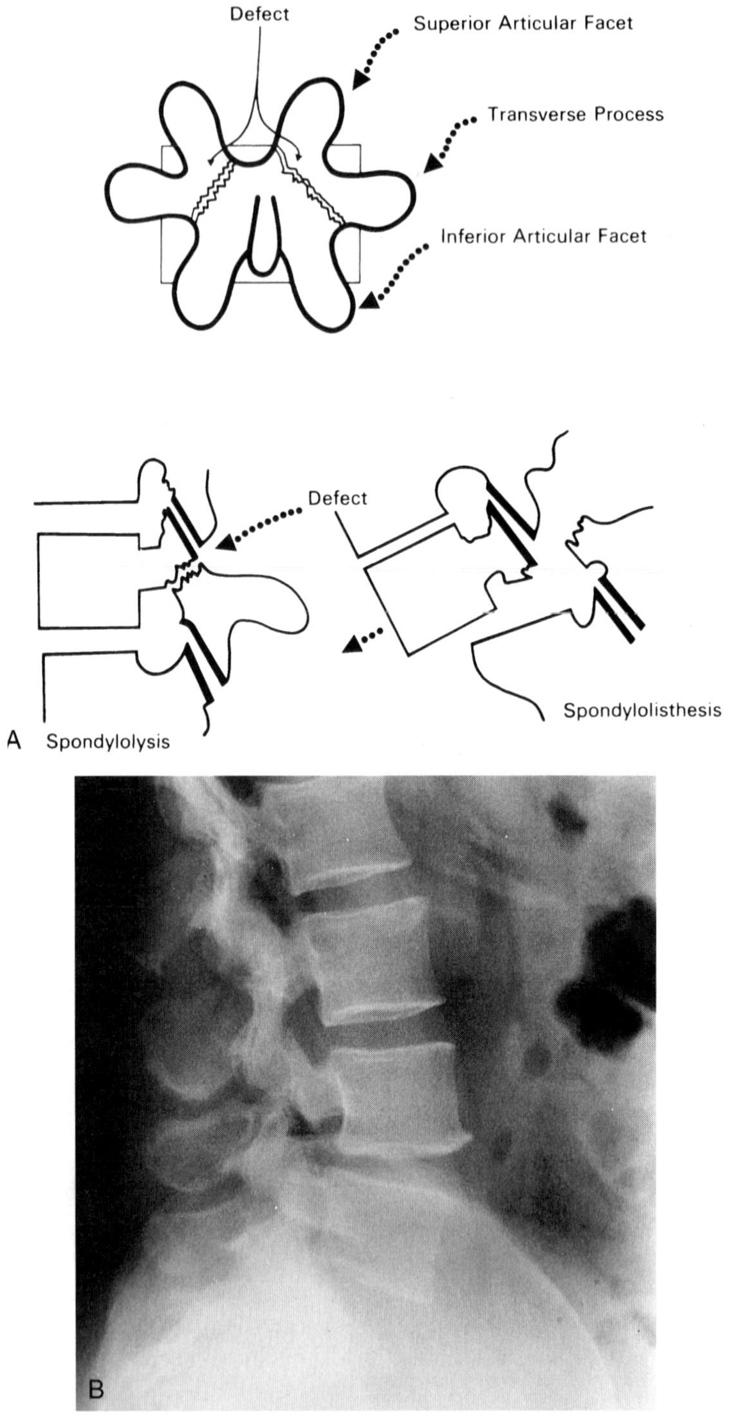

Figure 5.18 **A.** *Isthmic spondylolisthesis. The basic lesion is a defect in the neural arch across the pars interarticularis. When degenerative changes occur in the subjacent disc, the vertebral body will displace forward carrying with it the superimposed spinal column and leaving behind the inferior articular facets, lamina, and spinous process. From Macnab I: Backache. Williams & Wilkins, Baltimore (1977), p. 51.* **B.** *Lateral radiograph of spondylolisthesis at L4–5.*

Table 5.3. Incidence of Spondylolisthesis

Age	No. of Patients	Arch Defects	Percentage
Under 26	116	22	18.9
26–39	350	26	7.6
Over 40	530	28	5.2
Total	996	76	7.6

40, the incidence was approximately the same as the population as a whole, whereas under age 25, nearly 19%, a significant number, showed the defect. From these findings, it can be said that if the radiograph of a patient with back pain shows a lytic spondylolisthesis, and the patient is under 26, the defect is probably the cause of the symptoms; between ages 26 and 40, the defect is only possibly the cause; and over age 40, it is rarely, if ever, the sole cause of symptoms. In the management of lytic spondylolisthesis associated with neural arch defects, the age of the patient, therefore, is of prime importance.

When considering the pathogenesis of symptoms in this group, the following points must be remembered. The lesion may be asymptomatic. If the syndesmosis firmly bonds the two halves of the neural arch together, there is no mechanical instability and probably no mechanical reason for pain. If, however, the syndesmosis is loose, separation occurs on flexion (Fig. 5.19), and a strain is applied to the fibrous syndesmosis and the supraspinous ligament as well. Repetitive strains of this nature could give rise both to local and referred pain in a sciatic distribution.

Root irritation is not uncommon. With forward slip of the vertebral body, the intervertebral foramen is generally enlarged, and the nerve root may not be encroached upon because the neural arch is left behind as the vertebral body slips forward. However, nerve root compression can occur in the following circumstances. On occasion, when the vertebral body slips forward, the neural arch will rotate on the pivot formed by its articulation with the sacrum and may encroach upon the foramen (Fig. 5.20). A second form of root

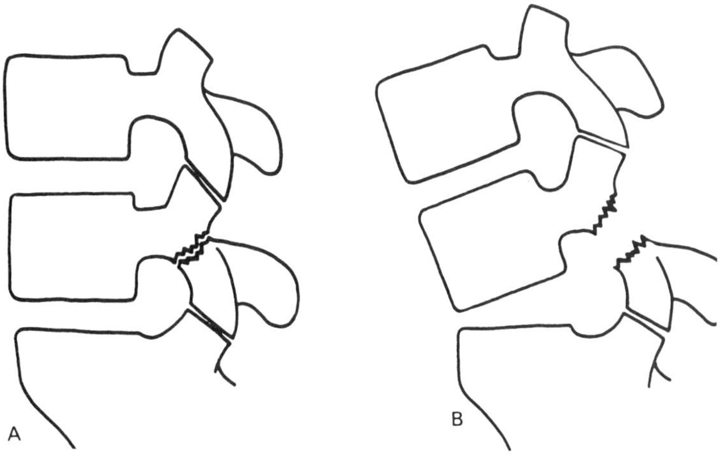

Figure 5.19 *In isthmic spondylolisthesis, although the defect may be closed when the patient holds the spine in extension* **(A)**, *separation may occur to a marked degree on flexion* **(B)**. *From Macnab I: Backache. Williams & Wilkins, Baltimore (1977), p. 52.*

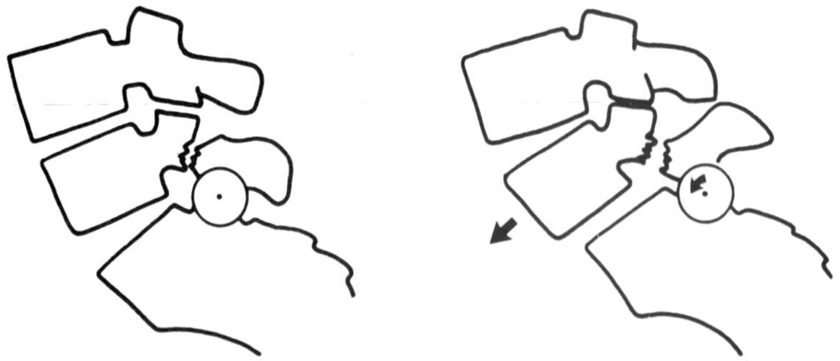

Figure 5.20 *When the vertebral body slips forward, the traction applied to the free neural arch may cause it to rotate on the pivot formed by its articulation with the sacrum. When this occurs the anterior aspect of the neural arch defect may encroach upon the foramen and compress the emerging nerve root. From Macnab I: Backache. Williams & Wilkins, Baltimore (1977), p. 53.*

encroachment is a small hook frequently found on the proximal edge of the isthmic defect that engages the nerve root (Fig. 5.21). The likelihood of foraminal entrapment of the nerve root is increased if disc space narrowing occurs, which allows the pedicle to guillotine the nerve root (Fig. 5.21). The fibrocartilaginous contents of the pars interarticularis defect may also encroach on the nerve root (Fig. 5.22). The least common cause of root involvement is disc rupture at the slip level (Fig. 5.23) or a different level.

The nerve root, after it has emerged through the intervertebral foramen, is more or less fixed as it courses through the large muscle masses. With spondylolisthesis, the vertebral body glides forward and downward along the inclined plane of the superior surface of the vertebral body below. This downward drop is particularly marked at L5–S1. With this movement of the vertebra, the pedicles descend on the nerve roots and kink them as they emerge through the foramen (Fig. 5.21).

Forward slipping will not occur without some degenerative changes occurring in the underlying disc. This generally takes place as a slow attrition of the disc, but sometimes the disc collapses and bulges out around the periphery of the vertebral body just like squashed putty. The nerve root may get buried in this bulging mass after it has emerged from the foramen.

There is a strong ligamentous band that runs from the undersurface of the transverse process to the side of the vertebral body, the corporotransverse ligament (Fig. 5.24). At L5, the fifth lumbar nerve root runs between the ligament and the ala of the sacrum. With marked forward slip and downward descent of L5, the ligament comes down like a guillotine on the fifth lumbar root and may entrap it against the ala of the sacrum. Kinking of the nerve root by the pedicle and extraforaminal entrapment of the nerve all encroach on the nerve emerging through the foramen at the site of the slip. With slipping of the fifth lumbar vertebra, it is the fifth lumbar root that is involved. A possible cause of fifth lumbar root compression in a patient with an L5–S1 slip is, of course, a disc herniation at L4–L5. However, in a patient with an L5–S1 slip who shows L5 root signs, if the myelogram does not reveal any defect, pedicular kinking of extraforaminal compression must be considered as the possible source of the clinical signs. This is not a problem in diagnosis when CT and magnetic resonance imaging (MRI) are used for investigation.

Spondylolysis predisposes to premature disc degeneration in the subjacent disc, and spondylolisthesis eventually causes disc degeneration. These degenerative changes may

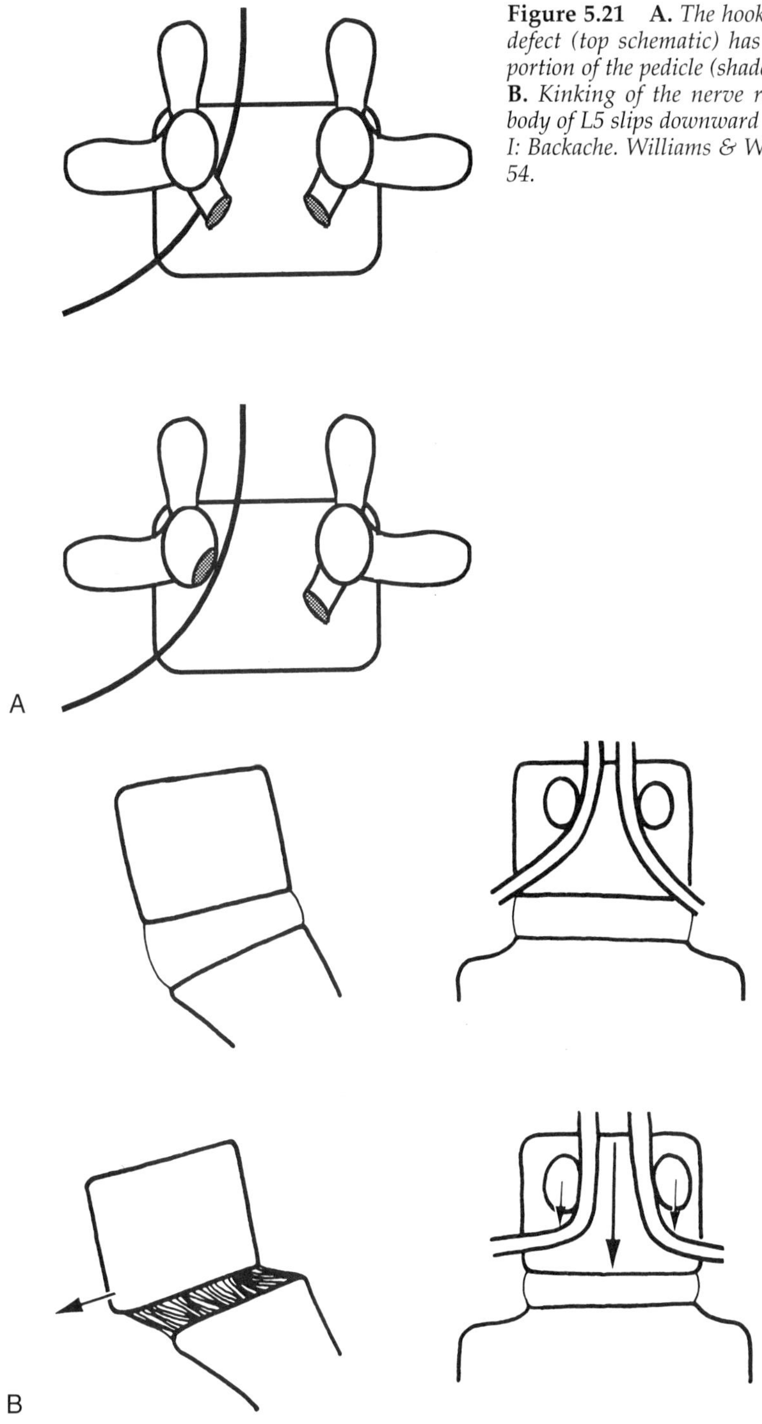

Figure 5.21 **A.** *The hook on proximal portion of the defect (top schematic) has been excised along with a portion of the pedicle (shaded) in the bottom schematic.* **B.** *Kinking of the nerve roots by the pedicles as the body of L5 slips downward and forward. From Macnab I: Backache. Williams & Wilkins, Baltimore (1977), p. 54.*

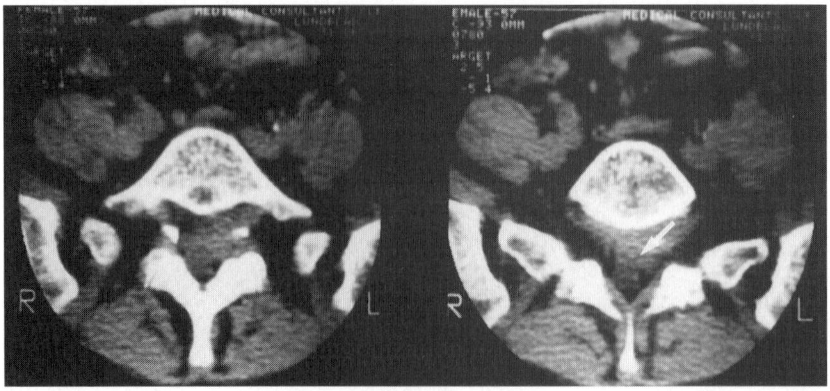

Figure 5.22 *A lytic spondylolisthesis with ossified portion to fibrocartilaginous contents of defect. This small ossicle of bone is often lying on the nerve root to cause compressive symptoms. Did you notice the large herniated nucleus pulposus on the left in the axial slice to the right (arrow)?*

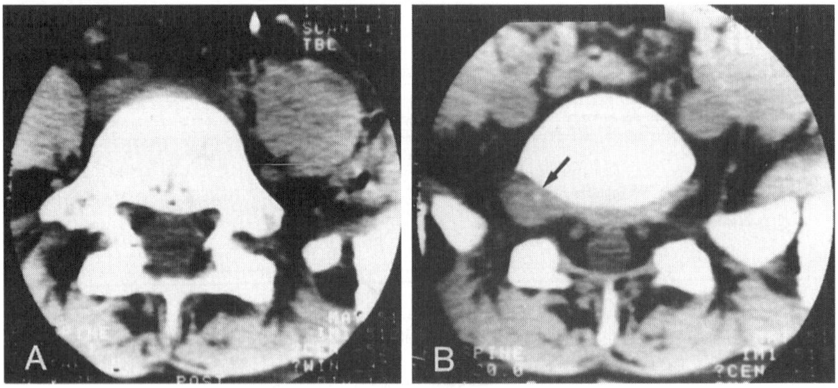

Figure 5.23 **A.** *A CT scan (unfortunately a soft tissue window) showing a lytic spondylolisthesis.* **B.** *The next slice caudally shows the reason for the severe right leg pain in this patient—a large foraminal herniated nucleus pulposus of the slip level (L5-S1) (arrow).*

of themselves be painful, giving rise to local or referred pain in sciatic distribution without root irritation.

Therefore, the local causes of pain in spondylolysis, with or without a slip, are instability, foraminal encroachment of the nerve root, extraforaminal entrapment of the nerve root, and disc degeneration.

Over the age of 30, other sources of pain become increasingly common, and these must of course influence treatment. A disc rupture may occur in association with spondylolisthesis. Although the rupture may occur at the disc involved in the slip (Figs. 5.22 and 5.23), much more commonly it is seen at the disc above the slip (Fig. 5.25). When a disc rupture occurs at the segment above the slipping vertebra, one has to accept the fact that the patient's symptoms may be stemming solely from the herniated disc and that the spondylolisthesis may be asymptomatic. In some instances, discectomy alone is sufficient to give complete relief of symptoms. This is particularly true in patients who have never experienced any back disability previously.

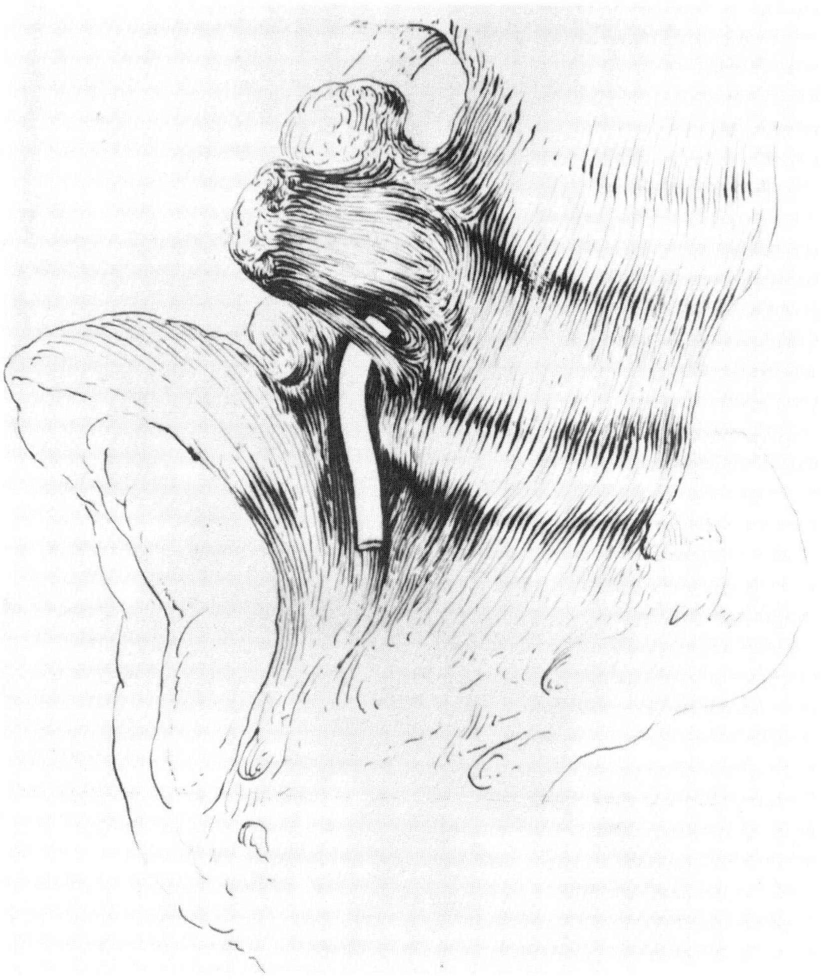

Figure 5.24 *The relationship of the fifth lumbar nerve root to the corporotransverse ligament. From Macnab I: Backache. Williams & Wilkins, Baltimore (1977), p. 55.*

Symptomatic disc degeneration, as distinct from disc herniation, may occur above the level of the slip. This may produce local pain or referred leg pain.

Unlike dysplastic spondylolisthesis, in which severe slips are associated with pelvic rotation and flattening of the back, in lytic spondylolisthesism, a forward slip of more than 50% is frequently associated with hyperlordosis above the slip and a kyphosis at the slip level. These high-degree slips (Grades 3, 4, and 5 [spondyloptosis]) (Fig. 5.26) are, in essence, kyphotic deformities of the lumbosacral junction causing as much, or more, deformity than backache. Extensive discussion of these deformities can be found in other texts.(1, 2) When this occurs, the hyperlordosis, by itself, may cause part or all of the symptoms complained of, and the symptoms derived from this source will, of course, persist after a spinal fusion.

With long-standing lumbosacral pathology, the lumbodorsal junction becomes the site of maximal movement, and in patients over age 35, degenerative changes of a marked degree are frequently seen in the discs and posterior joints in this area. Patients with degenerative

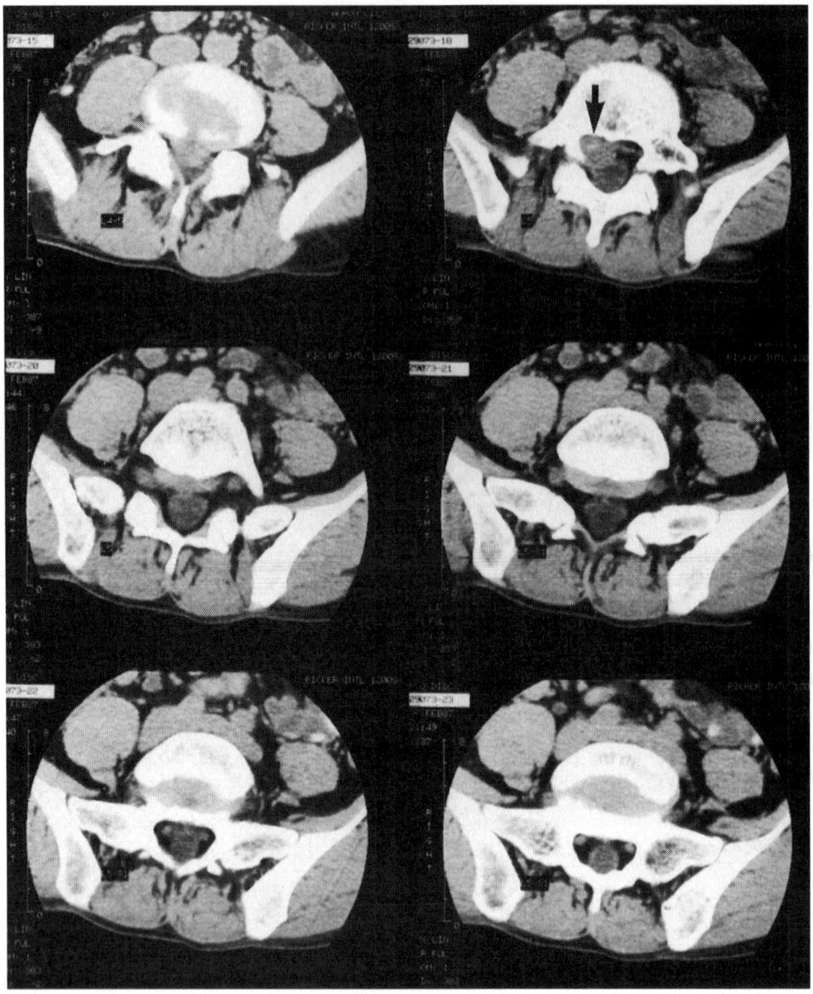

Figure 5.25 *CT scan showing a lytic spondylolisthesis (L5-S1) with large herniated nucleus pulposus, L4-5, right (arrow).*

changes in this region may present with low back pain as the sole symptom. The fact that changes at the lumbodorsal junction play a role in the production of the patient's low back pain can be demonstrated on clinical examination. With the patient lying on his/her side, with hips and knees flexed to flatten the lumbar curve, the examiner applies firm lateral pressure to the spinous processes of the vertebrae at the lumbodorsal junction. If there is disc instability at this region, and pressure is applied to the spinous processes and maintained for a moment, the patient will experience pain referred down to the lumbosacral region.

It must always be remembered that a spondylolisthesis may be asymptomatic; consequently, the possibility of other sources of back pain must never be forgotten.

In summary, when a patient with low back pain demonstrates a spondylolisthesis on radiograph, it is important to remember that the spondylolisthesis may be asymptomatic, and the back pain may stem from causes outside the spine.

If the pain is indeed spinal in origin, it may be due to instability at the defect, root

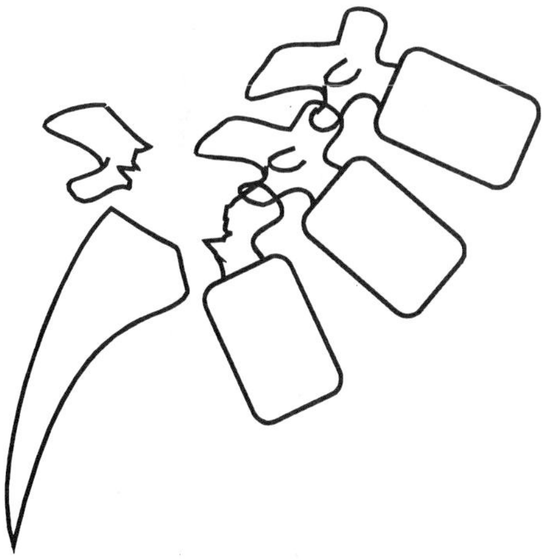

Figure 5.26 *Spondyloptosis: the back of the slipped vertebrae (L5) is in front of the sacrum.*

pressure due to disc herniation above or below the slip, foraminal encroachment of the nerve root, or extraforaminal entrapment of the nerve root. The pain, however, may arise elsewhere in the spine, being due to disc degeneration above the slip, hyperlordosis, or thoracolumbar disc degeneration. Finally, the pain may stem from an entirely unrelated cause, such as a metastatic malignancy in the spine.

Treatment

Even if the patient's symptoms are indeed due to the spinal lesion, the mere radiological demonstration of a spondylolysis or spondylolisthesis does not indicate that operative intervention is mandatory. There are, of course, certain unusual instances in which operative intervention is unavoidable, such as evidence of cauda equina compression, or evidence of unresolving or increasing impairment of root conduction. Apart from such examples, primary treatment should be conservative. Unlike dysplastic spondylolisthesis, further slipping is unlikely to occur in the older age group, and surgery, therefore, is not indicated to prevent further forward displacement. Continuing disabling pain constitutes the sole indication for surgery in this group of patients.

The type of surgical intervention required demands very careful evaluation of the patient. If the patient presents evidence of root tension or impairment of root conduction, the level of the lesion must be determined by clinical examination and confirmed by CT or MRI. In instances of foraminal encroachment of the root, diagnostic root sleeve infiltration is a very useful ancillary measure. The technique of nerve root infiltration is described in Chapter 11. When the patient's complaints are mainly of pain of a sciatic distribution due to foraminal encroachment of the fifth lumbar root, a foraminotomy may be all that is required. If the patient has an acute unilateral radicular syndrome due to a disc herniation, with no back pain, all that is required is disc excision. This will be needed, obviously, at the level of the disc rupture—L4–5 more frequently than L5–S1. The decision to fuse the spine is determined by a history of repeated episodes or continuing back pain of incapacitating severity. If the discs above the level of an L5–S1 slip are normal on T2 MRI (Fig. 5.27), a localized lumbosacral fusion is all that is required. The most reliable method of obtaining a single segment fusion in slips up to 50% is to fuse the transverse process of L5 to the ala of the sacrum (Fig. 5.28).

Figure 5.27 *A T2 sagittal MRI with normal discs above and below an L4–5 slip.*

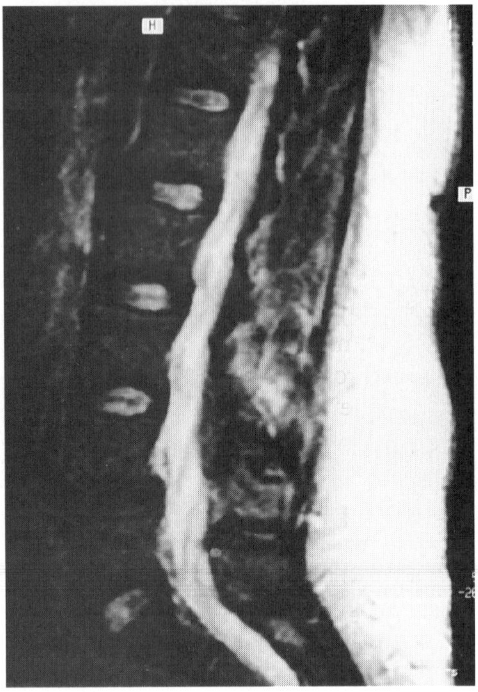

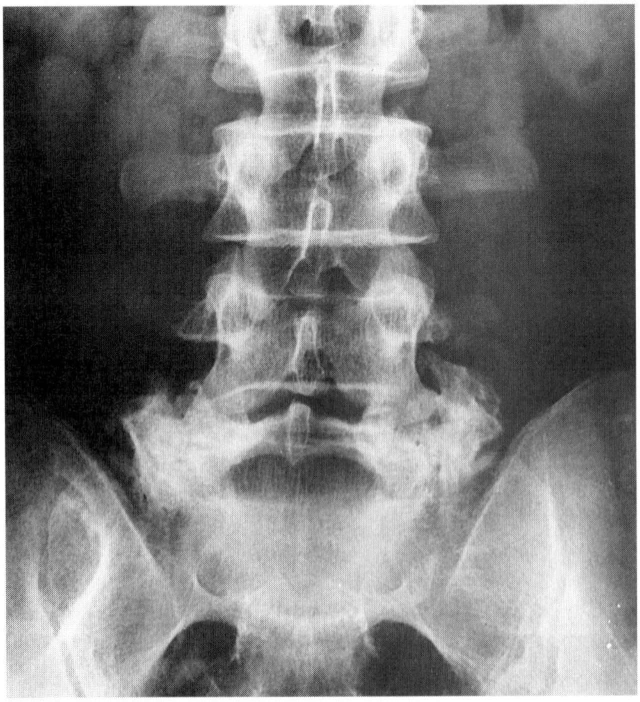

Figure 5.28 *An anteroposterior radiograph of an L5-S1 fusion for spondylolisthesis.*

When the forward displacement is more than half of the width of the sacrum, or when T2 MRI reveals degenerative changes at the L4–L5 disc, the accepted method of treatment is a fusion extended up to the transverse process of L4. Some authors skilled in deformity surgery have advocated reduction of the high-grade slips through anterior and posterior combined approaches (Fig. 5.29).(1)

The necessity for a three-segment fusion arises from time to time, for example, a spondylolysis of the last three lumbar segments. A similar problem is presented by an L5–Sl slip with symptomatic degenerative changes at L3–L4 and L4–L5, an L4–L5 slip with disc degenerative changes at the segments above and below the slip, or an L3–L4 lesion with symptomatic degenerative changes in the subjacent discs. Reviews of three-segment fusions for disc degeneration reveal a pseudarthrosis rate of 40%. To avoid this high pseudarthrosis rate, these cases are probably best treated by instrumentation; the various pedicle screw systems are the preferred choice.

Type IIB Elongated

Isthmic spondylolisthesis with an elongated pars (Type B) represents repeated microfractures of the pars that later heal in the elongated position. It is an acquired lesion with no congenital facet changes, which serves to distinguish it from the orphan mentioned under the discussion of dysplastic spondylolisthesis. This condition rarely causes significant back pain.

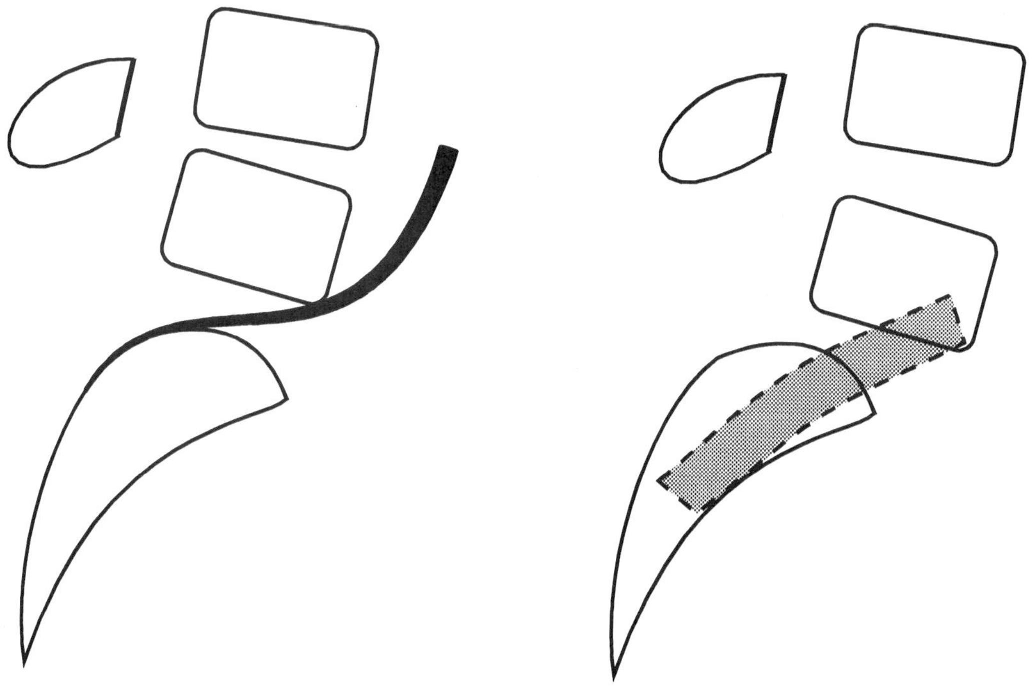

Figure 5.29 *A reduction of the spondylolisthesis through an anterior approach (left), followed by a fusion (right).*

Type IIC Traumatic

This condition was discussed in the opening section on spondylolysis. A neural arch defect across the pars interarticularis may also occur on rare occasions as a result of trauma, either from a forced hyperextension or from a forced flexion strain. Here again, the problem always arises as to whether the defect resulted from the accident or whether the patient had the defect before the accident. The sites and types of defects are frequently unusual. Healing of the lesion on immobilization is irrefutable evidence of the traumatic origin of the lesion.

Type III Degenerative Spondylolisthesis

In 1930, Junghanns(5) reported 14 cases of spondylolisthesis found in autopsy specimens without any defect in the neural arch (Fig. 5.30). He coined the term pseudospondylolisthesis. The lesion remained in the background to lytic spondylolisthesis until Macnab published his landmark paper on the subject in 1950.(6) The slip is never very great (Fig. 5.31), and most commonly it occurs at the L4–5 interspace. The L4–L5 segment of the lumbar spine is normally the site of the greatest mobility. In an L4–L5 degenerative spondylolisthesis, it is this excessive mobility (Fig. 5.32), combined with a

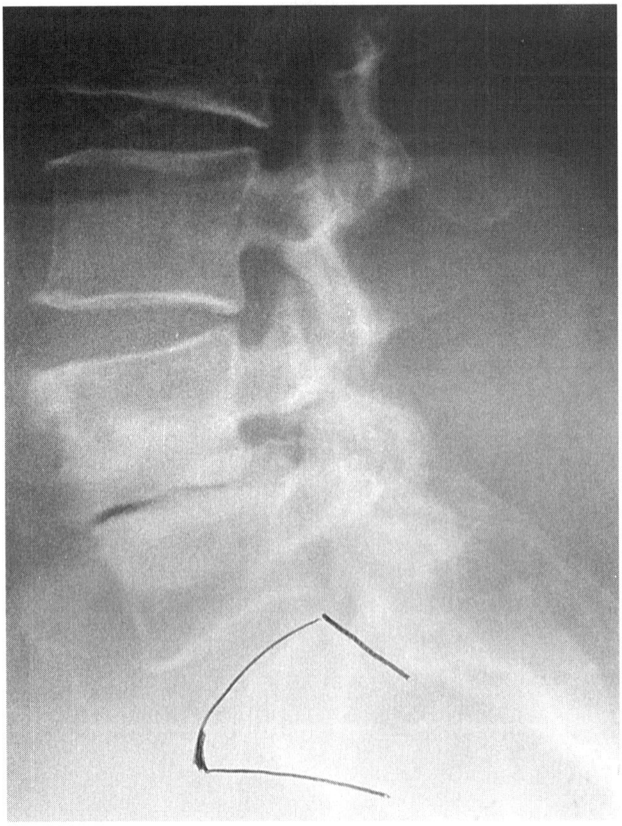

Figure 5.30 *A degenerative spondylolisthesis (L4–5) with associated severe degenerative disc disease.*

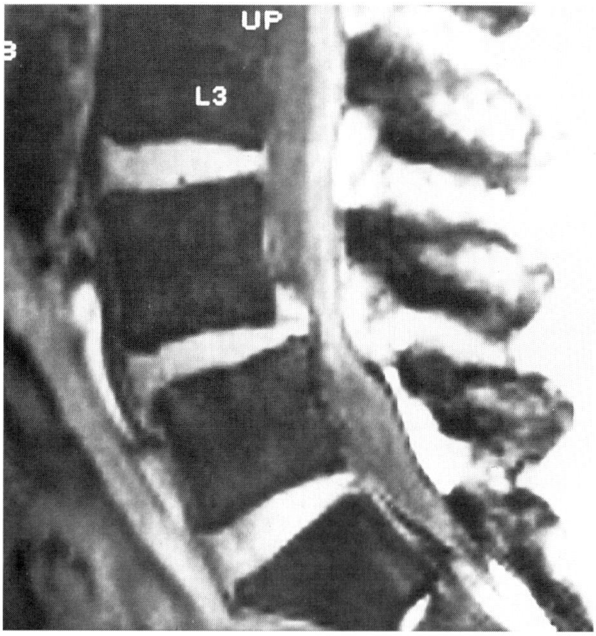

Figure 5.31 *A gradient echo sagittal MRI showing a low-grade slip in degenerative spondylolisthesis with associated encroachment on the common dural sac.*

more sagittal alignment of the facet joints, that results in the lesion. Excessive movement is postulated to cause the breakdown in the posterior joints, which results in the slip. This condition predominantly affects women, with the age of onset of symptoms usually more than 50 years of age. This form of spondylolisthesis is really a manifestation of disc degeneration that may produce back pain because of the gross segmental instability and associated posterior joint damage. The usual patient presentation is bilateral neurogenic claudication due to root entrapment. This may be produced by a combination of a diffuse annular bulge at the level of the slip, shingling of the laminae, and buckling of the ligamentum flavum (Fig. 5.33). The spinal canal is further narrowed by subluxation of the posterior joints, which are enlarged by osteophytic outgrowths. All of these factors combine to produce entrapment of the nerve roots as they course through the spinal canal or the subarticular gutters. Degenerative spondylolisthesis with narrowing of the spinal canal or lateral zone is the most common form of spinal canal stenosis and is discussed in detail in Chapter 17. In summary, the nature and pathogenesis of the lesion make it obvious that the management of degenerative spondylolisthesis is indeed not unlike the management of degenerative disc disease with or without nerve root irritation.

TYPE IV TRAUMATIC SPONDYLOLISTHESIS

Forward slipping of a vertebral body may occur as the result of a dislocation of the posterior joints, or because of a fracture of a spinous process extending into the lamina at the pars interarticularis. These are really examples of fracture dislocations of the spine and are classified as traumatic spondylolisthesis. A fracture through the pars interarticularis (Type IIC) with forward slip of the vertebral body, a true traumatic spondylolisthesis, is rare. When a patient who has been involved in a severe accident

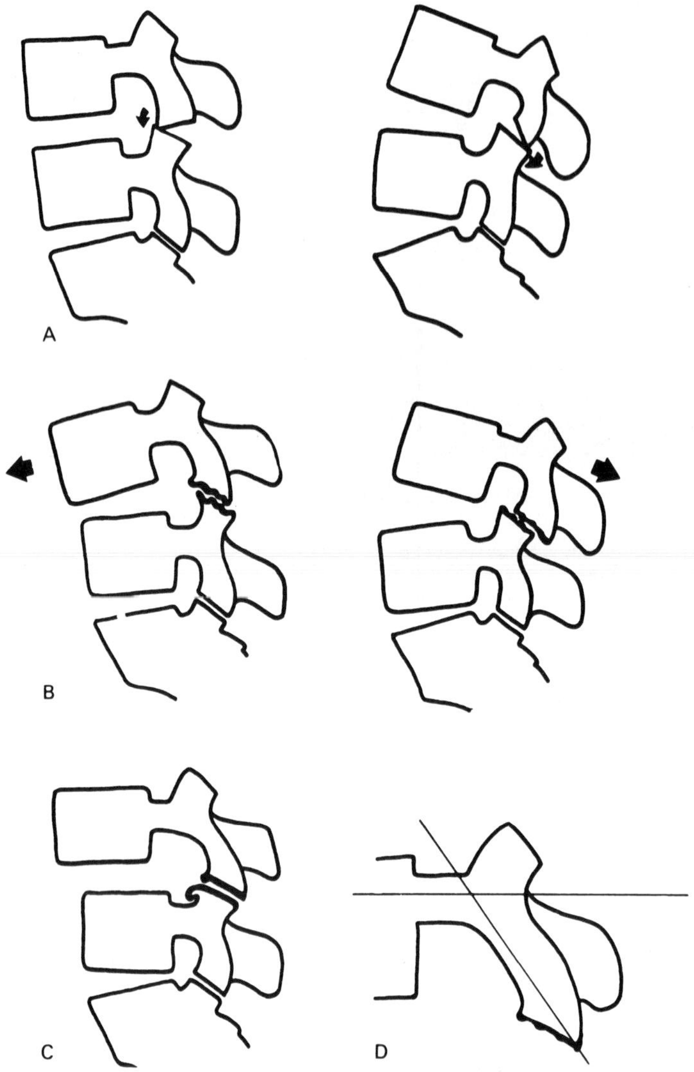

Figure 5.32 *Mechanical insufficiency of an intervertebral disc permits excessive movement on flexion and extension* **(A).** *The posterior joints undergo degenerative changes because of this abnormal movement and with increasing breakdown permit forward and backward gliding of the involved vertebral bodies* **(B).** *Subluxation of the arthritic zygapophysial joints permits forward displacement of the vertebral body* **(C),** *and the displacement becomes fixed because of an increase in the angle between the pedicle and the inferior processes* **(D).** *From Macnab I: Backache. Williams & Wilkins, Baltimore (1977), p. 61.*

demonstrates a spondylolisthesis on radiograph, it is difficult to say whether or not the patient had a pre-existing spondylolisthesis. Clearly defined fracture edges of the pars of L5 and a sharply pointed anterior margin of the sacrum are both suggestive of an acute lesion. A positive bone scan (SPECT scan) will resolve the legal issues. In contradistinction to spondylolytic and isthmic spondylolisthesis, an acute traumatic slip can be openly reduced and maintained in the reduced position with the use of instrumentation and fusion.

TYPE V PATHOLOGICAL SPONDYLOLISTHESIS

On occasion, generalized bone disease such as osteogenesis imperfecta, osteomalacia, achondroplasia, or a localized bony change such as a secondary deposit or Paget's disease may allow attenuation of the pedicles and thereby permit the vertebral body to slip forward. It is to be noted that, unlike the other types of spondylolisthesis (except Type IIB), forward displacement of the vertebral body in pathological spondylolisthesis is permitted by elongation of the pedicle (Fig. 5.34). Obviously, the management of the local lesion in

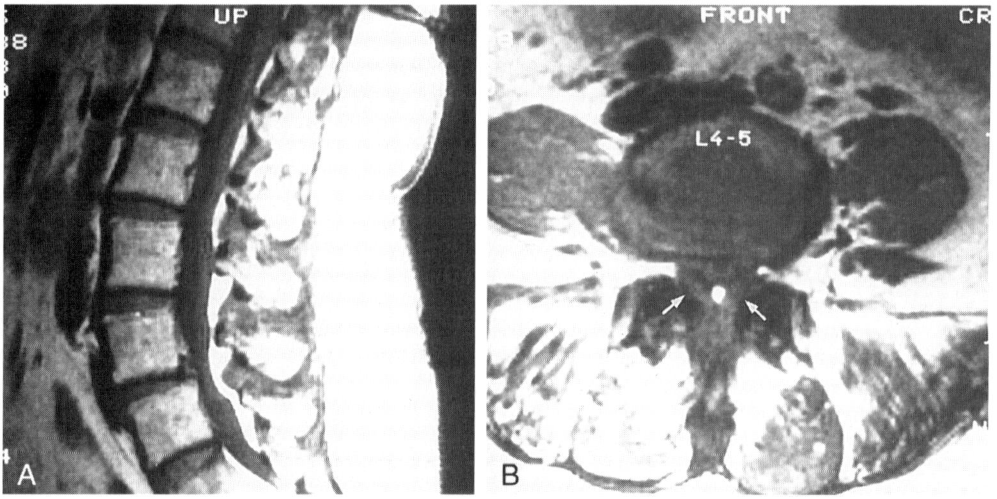

Figure 5.33 **A.** *MRI (T1 weighted sagittal) of spinal canal stenosis at L4–5 due to ligamentum flavum hypertrophy from behind and annular bulging in front.* **B.** *MRI (T1 weighted axial) of spinal canal stenosis in same patient showing extent of ligamentum flavum encroachment (arrows) on common dural sac.*

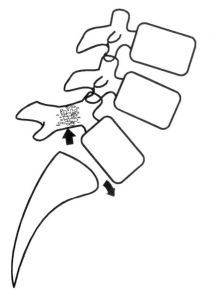

Figure 5.34 *Pathological spondylolisthesis (curved arrow) due to softening and elongation of bone in pars interarticularis (straight arrow).*

this group of cases depends on the management of the cause of the primary disease. This particular problem is rare in clinical practice.

IATROGENIC SPONDYLOLISTHESIS

Spondylolisthesis secondary to aggressive surgical intervention that destabilizes a spinal segment is not included in the Wiltse-Newman-Macnab classification. It occurs most commonly in spinal stenosis decompression without fusion, when too much (or all) of a facet joint is removed, which allows for a later slip at the surgical level. It is likely that many of these patients had a subtle, unrecognized slip at the time of surgery that simply became worse (and obvious) at a later date. A variant of iatrogenic spondylolisthesis is spondylolisthesis acquisita, a vertebral body slip above a lumbar fusion. This is simply a degenerative spondylolisthesis that occurs because a solid fusion transfers motion to the segment above. The increase in facet joint and disc forces may result in degeneration and a subsequent spondylolisthesis.

SUMMARY

Although spondylolisthesis presents a dramatic picture on radiograph, it may be asymptomatic and remain asymptomatic for the lifetime of the patient. When the lesion does indeed produce symptoms, the pathogenesis of the symptoms (instability, root compression, and so on) must be established before treatment is instituted.

REFERENCES

1. Bradford DS. Spondylolysis and spondylolisthesis in children and adolescents. In: Bradford DS, Hensinger RN, eds. Pediatric Spine. New York: Thieme and Stratton; 1985.
2. Bradford DS, Lonstein JE, Moe JH, Ogilvie JW, Winter RB. Moe's Textbook of Scoliosis and Other Spinal Deformities. Philadelphia: WB Saunders; 1987.
3. Eisenstein SMC. Spondylolysis. A skeletal investigation of two population groups. J Bone Joint Surg 1973;60B:488–494.
4. Herbineaux G. Traite sur Divers Accouchments Laborieux, et sur les Polypes de la Matrice Jl. Brussels: DeBoubers; 1782.
5. Junghanns H. Spondylolisthese. Bruns' Bietr Klin Chir 1930;148:554.
6. Macnab I. Spondylolisthesis with an intact neural arch— the so-called pseudospondylolisthesis. J Bone Joint Surg 1950;32B:325–333.
7. Myerding H. Spondylolisthesis: Surgical treatment and results. Surg Gynecol Obstet 1932; 54:371–377.
8. Neuwirth MG. Spondylolysis and spondylolisthesis in children and adults. In: Camins MB, O'Leary PF, eds. The Lumbar Spine. New York: Raven Press; 1987, pp 257–273.
9. Stewart TD. The age incidence of neural arch defects in Alaskan natives, considered from the standpoint of etiology. J Bone Joint Surg 1953;35A:937–950.
10. Wiltse LL, Newman PH, Macnab I. Classification of spondylolisthesis. Clin Orthop 1976; 117:23–29.
11. Wiltse LL, Jackson DW. Treatment of spondylolisthesis and spondylolysis in children. Clin Orthop 1976;117:92–98.

12. Wiltse LL, Winter RB. Terminology and measurement of spondylolisthesis. J Bone Joint Surg 1983;65A:768–772.
13. Wynne-Davis R, Scott JHS. Inheritance and spondylolisthesis: a radiographic family survey. J Bone Joint Surg 1979;61B:301–305.
14. Yu C, Garfin SR. Recognizing and managing lumbar spondylolisthesis. J Musculoskeletal Med 1994:55–63.

6

Lesions of the Sacroiliac Joints

"Who is this that darkeneth counsel by words without knowledge."

— Job 38:2

INTRODUCTION

The sacroiliac (SI) joint is an enigma. It is obviously an important set of joints that anchor the pelvis to the sacrum, which in turn act as a supporting "door frame" for the mobile lumbar spine and even more mobile legs. So why shouldn't the resultant concentration of forces cause pain in this joint? Chiropractic, osteopathic, and physical therapy practitioners believe and promote the SI joint "dysfunction" as a source of low back pain,(5) whereas physicians are reluctant to accept this proposal. The problem in understanding SI joint sprains, strains, and injuries is the lack of scientific evidence to support the manual therapists' proposal of this joint as a source of pain to be corrected by their particular brand of administrations.

STRUCTURE AND FUNCTION OF THE SI JOINT

The SI joint is a combination of a synarthrodial and diarthrodial joint—a unique joint in the body. The major portion of the joint is a syndesmosis (diarthrodial) joint and is characterized by a very irregular topography, strong fibrous connections within the joint, and strong extra-articular supporting ligaments. The message from study of joint morphology is that this joint moves very little. The inferior portion of the joint is synovial, but it offers up no increased mobility. The joint is said to move 2 to 3° in any one direction,(4) a phenomenon that decreases with aging changes that stabilize the joint. These aging changes start by age 30 and obviously decrease movement in the joint, just as patients enter the decades of backache (30 to 60 years of age).

THE SACROILIAC JOINT SYNDROME (SIJS)

The SIJS is said to have a classic presentation (5):

1. There is pain over the SI joint.
2. The SI joint is locally tender to palpation (hard enough pressure can make any SI joint tender!).

3. The pain may be referred to the groin, trochanter, and buttock.
4. The pain is aggravated by provocation tests.
5. There is clinical evidence of increased movement or asymmetry of the SI joint.
6. There is no other apparent cause of the patient's SI joint pain localization (if it is not ...., therefore it must be sacroiliac joint syndrome!).

SACROILIAC SPRAINS

The concept of a "sacroiliac sprain" as a common cause of backache and sciatica was introduced by Goldthwaite (1) in 1905. To this day, little scientific evidence exists to support the fact that sacroiliac joint sprain or strain is a symptom-producing condition. A common finding in patients suffering from mechanical backache is pain situated over the sacroiliac joint and tenderness in this region. This does not mean that the SI joint is the source of pain. Rather, this finding is usually a manifestation of the confusing phenomenon of referred pain. Mechanical lesions of the lumbosacral junction associated with disc degeneration frequently give rise to pain referred to the sacroiliac region, and such patients will exhibit local tenderness that region. It is understandably tempting to ascribe these findings to a pathological lesion in the underlying sacroiliac joint. However, the true source of this SI joint pain can be demonstrated by experimental reproduction of the pain by hypertonic saline injection of the supraspinous ligaments at the lumbosacral junction, and by reproduction of the pain by discography of the L4–L5 and L5–S1 discs.

The anatomical configuration of the components of the sacroiliac joint makes the joint extremely stable (Fig. 6.1), and this inherent stability is reinforced by the powerful, massive posterior interosseus ligaments and by the strong accessory ligaments—the iliolumbar, the sacrotuberous, and the sacrospinous ligaments.

Over the age of 35—the backache years—in 30% of the population, the anterior capsule of the sacroiliac joint is ossified and, in these patients at least, the sacroiliac joints may be exonerated from the blame of backache. Under the age of 35, minimal sliding and rotary movements occur, but considerable force, such as that generated by falls from heights or motor vehicle injuries, is required to push the sacroiliac joint beyond its physiologically permitted range, either dislocating or fracturing the joint. This leads to true post-traumatic painful osteoarthritic degeneration of the joint that has an unequivocal clinical presentation.

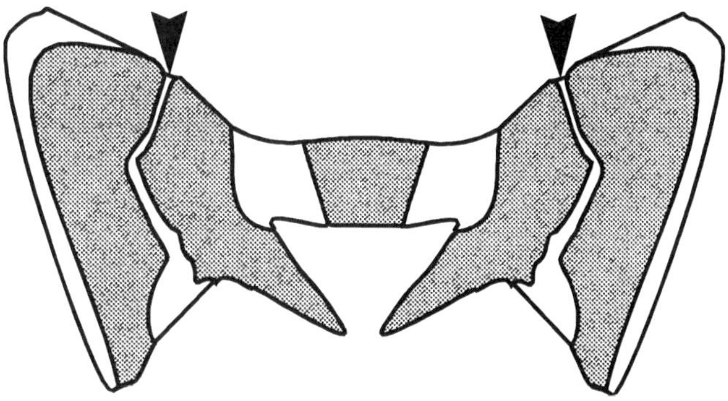

Figure 6.1 *The SI joints (arrows) are very stable joints simply by their construct.*

POST-TRAUMATIC PAINFUL OSTEOARTHRITIC DEGENERATION OF THE SI JOINT: SI JOINT INSTABILITY

Violence severe enough to injure the SI joint will usually be associated with a fracture of the pelvis but, in the unusual circumstances in which the whole brunt of the blow is absorbed by the supporting ligamentous structures of the sacroiliac joint, the findings are specific and pathognomonic:

1. There is tenderness over the lower third of the sacroiliac joint below the posterior inferior iliac spine.
2. The pubic symphysis is tender on palpation. The pelvis is a closed ring and cannot undergo stretching at one site only. In the absence of a fracture of the pelvic ring, if the sacroiliac joint is displaced, the symphysis pubis must also suffer some disruption (Fig. 6.2).
3. The symptoms experienced clinically may be reproduced by stressing the sacroiliac joint with any of the following maneuvers:
   a. Lateral manual compression of the iliac crest (Fig. 6.3).
   b. Resisted abduction of the hip joint. When the gluteus medius contracts to abduct the hip, it pulls the ileum away from the sacrum. With sacroiliac joint lesions, abduction against resistance is painful (Fig. 6.4).
   c. Hyperextension of the hip on the affected side against a stabilized pelvis. Although this maneuver, Gaenslen's test (Fig. 6.5), was originally described for eliciting sacroiliac joint pain, the test is not specific.(3) Hypertension of the hip performed in this manner will also be painful in the presence of pre-existing hip disease (a positive Ely's test), and patients suffering from irritation of the fourth lumbar nerve root may experience anterior thigh pain on this form of hyperextension of the hip (a positive femoral stretch test).
   d. Forced external rotation of the affected hip in the supine position (Patrick's test, or fabere sign) (Fig. 6.6) causes pain in the SI joint.
4. Patients with painful sacroiliac joints may develop gluteal inhibition, with a resulting Trendelenburg lurch when walking (Fig. 6.7).
5. There are often accompanying degenerative changes in the symphysis pubis.

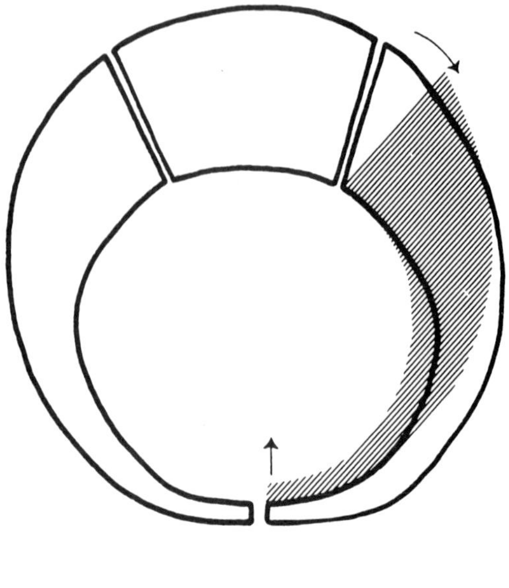

Figure 6.2 *Diagram showing that any movement of the sacroiliac joint must be associated with corresponding displacement at the symphysis pubis. From Macnab I: Backache. Williams & Wilkins, Baltimore (1977), p. 65.*

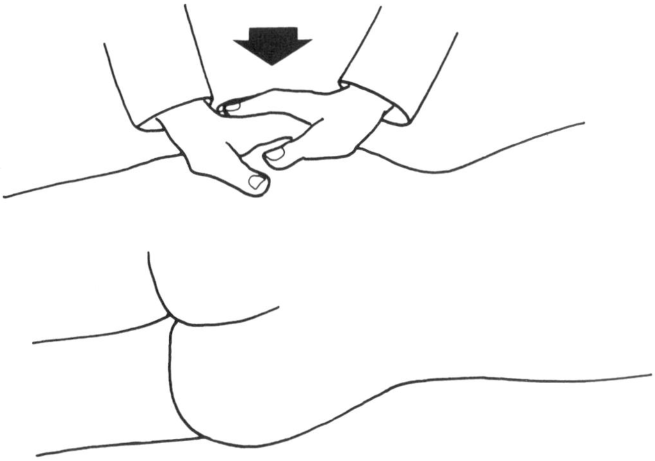

Figure 6.3 *With the patient lying on his/her side, the sacroiliac joint can be stressed by manually applying compression to the pelvis. From Macnab I: Backache. Williams & Wilkins, Baltimore (1977), p. 66.*

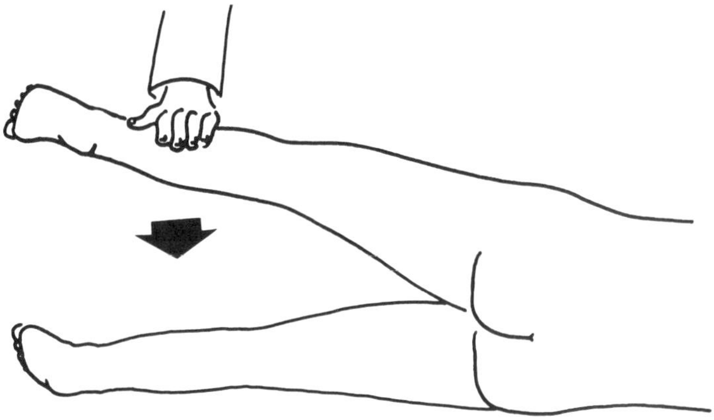

Figure 6.4 *In the absence of hip joint disease, pain experienced over the sacroiliac joint on resisted abduction of the leg is highly suggestive of a sacroiliac joint lesion. From Macnab I: Backache. Williams & Wilkins, Baltimore (1977), p. 66.*

In addition to post-traumatic osteoarthritic degeneration of the SI joint, there is another obvious source of SI joint pain—pregnancy.

THE PAINFUL SI JOINT OF PREGNANCY

During the latter months of pregnancy, the supporting ligaments of the sacroiliac joints become "relaxed" to allow enlargement of the birth canal. At this time, and during parturition, the joints are indeed susceptible to strain as a result of trivial trauma. Patients complain of pain localized to the involved sacroiliac joint, and the pain radiates around the greater trochanter and down the anterolateral aspect of the thigh. Patients exhibit, on examination, the specific physical findings previously described.

The symptoms of true sacroiliac sprains generally subside rapidly with bed rest, analgesics, and anti-inflammatory medications. The use of a trochanteric belt can give relief while walking and can obviate the antalgic gait (Fig. 6.8). In a few patients whose symptoms persist, administration of intra-articular steroids may be necessary.

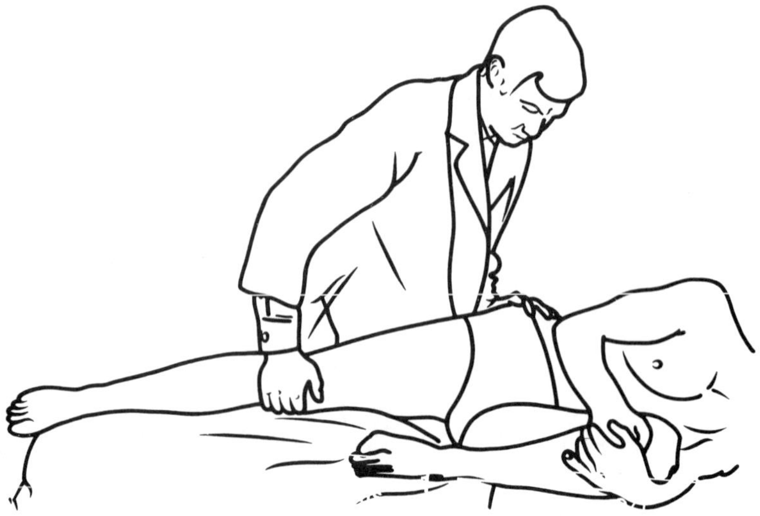

Figure 6.5 *Gaenslen's test. From Macnab I: Backache. Williams & Wilkins, Baltimore (1977), p. 67.*

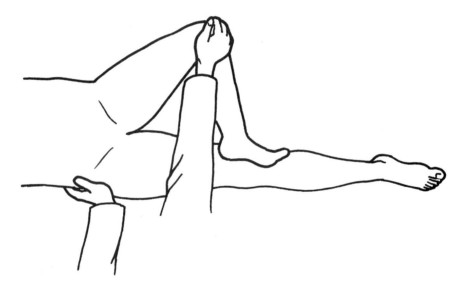

Figure 6.6 *Faber test, also known as the Patrick test, is done with the hip on the test side in flexion (f), abduction (ab), and external rotation (er), (thus faber). Downward pressure on the knee while fixing the opposite side of the pelvis will stress the left SI joint.1*

Osteitis Condensans Ilii

Osteitis condensans Ilii is a condition of mild-to-moderate SI joint pain occurring in postpartum women 30 to 40 years of age. The major problem with this disease is its confusion with ankylosing spondylitis. The cause is unknown, but its very high prevalence in women suggests some relationship to the laxity of the SI joint late in pregnancy and delivery being the cause.

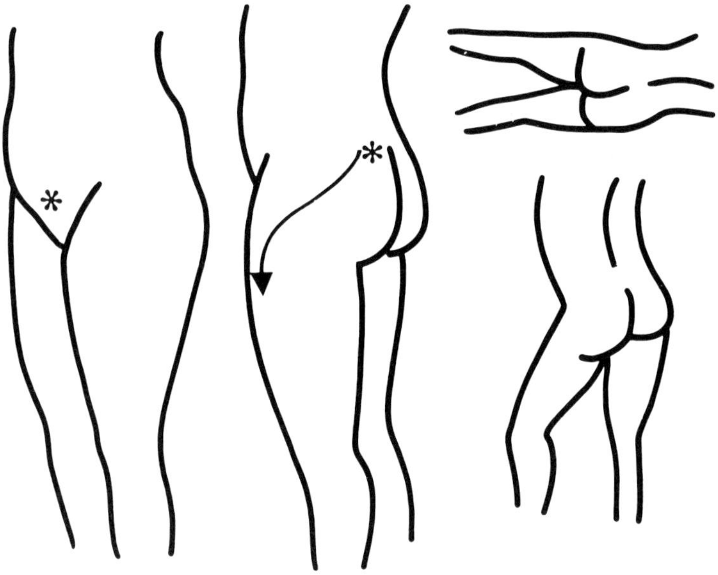

Figure 6.7 *Summary of findings in sacroiliac joint disease. Tenderness can be elicited not only over the sacroiliac joint but over the symphysis pubis as well. The pain usually radiates over the lateral aspect of the great trochanter and down the front of the thigh. The patients exhibit pain on abduction of the hip on the affected side and walk with a Trendelenburg lurch. From Macnab I: Backache. Williams & Wilkins, Baltimore (1977), p. 67.*

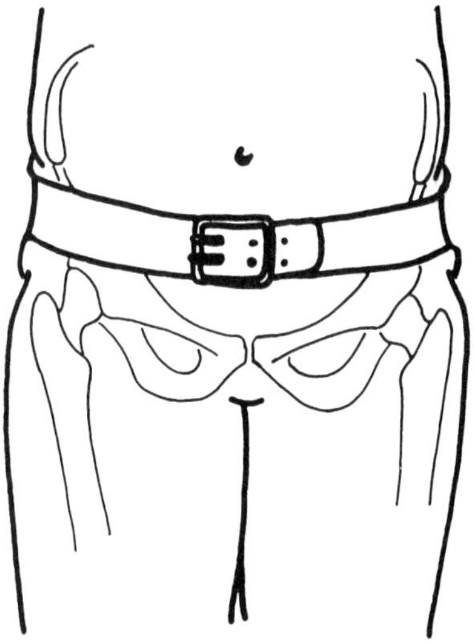

Figure 6.8 *Trochanteric cinch. From Macnab I: Backache. Williams & Wilkins, Baltimore (1977), p. 68.*

The symptoms are rarely severe, and the radiographic presentation is classic (Fig. 6.9). The triangular sclerosis is confined to the iliac side of the SI joint, with no evidence of the destruction of the SI joint that occurs in ankylosing spondylitis.

The course of osteitis condensans Ilii is almost always benign. Treatment consists of an explanation to the patient of the benignity of the problem and simple measures such as heat or ice and mild analgesic/anti-inflammatory medicine. With time, the symptoms almost always disappear.

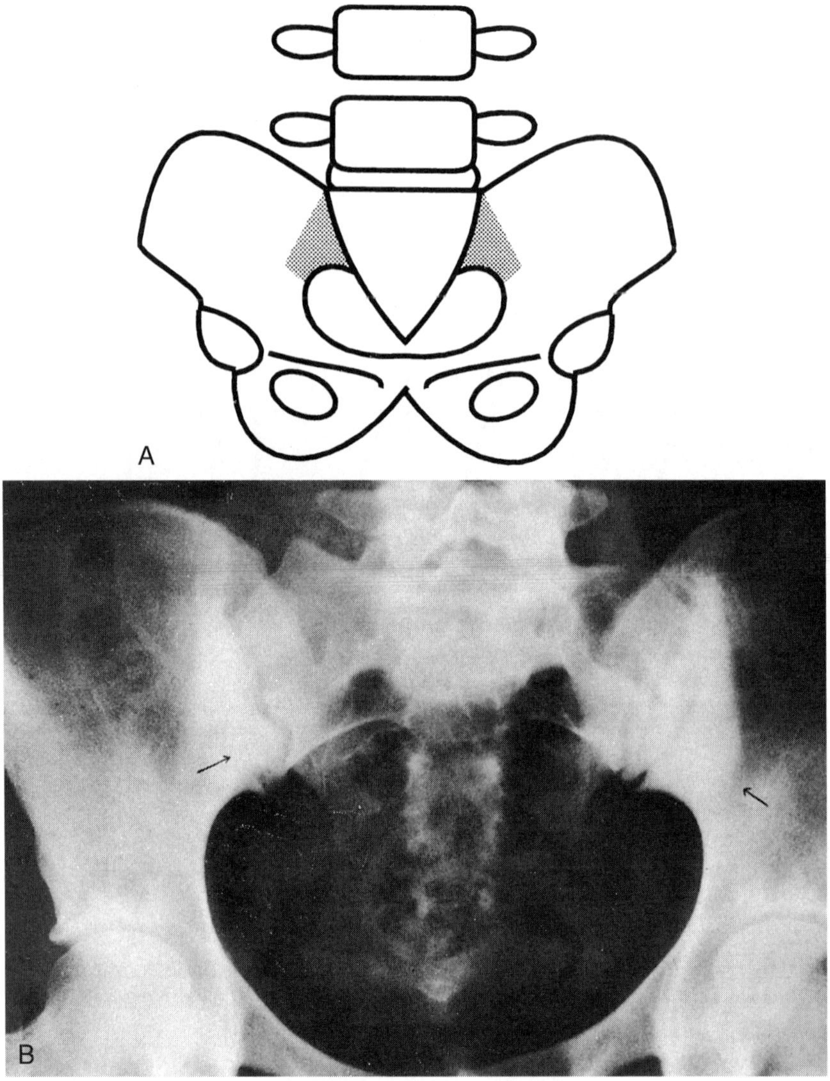

Figure 6.9 **A.** *Osteitis condensans ilii is represented schematically.* **B.** *Osteitis condensans ilii. Note that the area of bone sclerosis is confined to the iliac side of the sacroiliac joint. From Macnab I: Backache. Williams & Wilkins, Baltimore (1977), p. 70.*

SUMMARY

In summary, it is worth repeating that sacroiliac strains, apart from those following parturition, are excessively rare, although commonly diagnosed. The concept of a sacroiliac strain is yet another example of how the phenomenon of referred pain and tenderness has clouded and confused the recognition of the pathological basis of spondylogenic pain. The sacroiliac region is a common site for referred pain and tenderness derived from segmental discogenic backache. The mere complaint of pain over the sacroiliac joint and the demonstration of local tenderness do not justify the diagnosis of a sacroiliac sprain.

After decades of injection of and manipulation of the SI joint, it is time for prospective scientific studies on the natural history, clinical presentation, and treatment of the SI joint

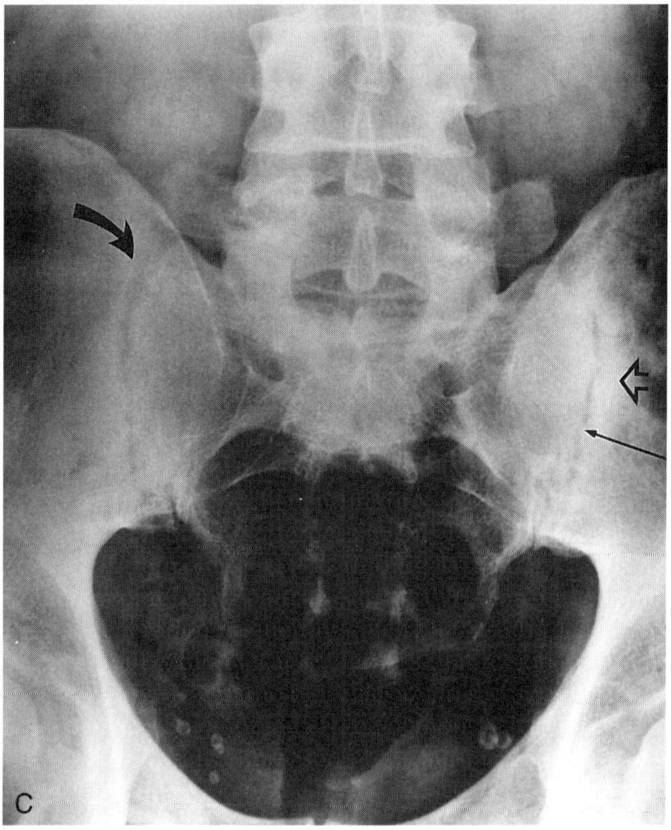

Figure 6.9 (continued) C. *In ankylosing spondylitis there are simultaneous erosions (pseudo-widening of the joint) (curved arrow), subchondral sclerosis on each side of the joint (open arrow), and transarticular bony bridges (ankylosis) (long arrow).*

syndrome. Failure of those practitioners in the manual therapy fields to pursue these studies will only discredit the sacroiliac sprain diagnosis.

Inflammatory Lesions of the Sacroiliac Joint

With a clearer understanding of the clinical syndromes affecting the lumbar spine, sacroiliac strains become less of a viable diagnosis on which to base treatment decisions. The flip side of the coin is to have blinders on and see degenerative conditions of the lumbar spine in every patient presenting with low back pain only to miss the very real, and not uncommon, sacroiliitis due to an inflammatory lesion. These are the so-called seronegative spondyloarthropathies that include ankylosing spondylitis, Reiter's syndrome, psoriatic arthritis, and enteropathic arthropathy. They are overlapping entities, likely of a common pathogenesis. The most commonly recognized inflammatory lesion of the sacroiliac joint is ankylosing spondylitis.

Ankylosing Spondylitis

At one time ankylosing spondylitis (AS) was regarded as the spinal variant of rheumatoid arthritis. It is now known that these two diseases are distinct entities. The name is derived from the Greek roots ankylos (bent, or fusion) and spondylos (spinal vertebrae).

Epidemiology

With the standardization of criteria for the diagnosis of AS,(2) better epidemiologic studies have been completed. Initially, AS was thought to be a disease predominantly affecting men (M:F = 10:1), but more recent studies suggest that women are affected quite commonly, although with a milder form of the disease. AS usually has its insidious onset during the ages of 20 to 35 years and is rare in onset after the age of 40 years.

The progress of the lesion and its major pathological features are well demonstrated on repeated radiographic examinations. Because the disease does not have a clear clinical presentation, a criteria approach to diagnosis is used (Tables 6.1 and 6.3).

Etiology

The cause of AS is unknown, except that individuals who have inherited the human leukocyte antigen (HLA)-B27 gene are predisposed to develop the syndrome. The overall incidence of AS in North American Caucasians is 0.1 to 0.2%, whereas the incidence of AS in Caucasians with the HLA-B27 gene is 10 to 20%. There is a 20-times greater incidence of AS among relatives of persons with ankylosing spondylitis. These relatives have a much higher incidence of HLA-B27 than the normal population. Whether the B27 gene/antigen is the primary cause or whether it acts as a receptor for an infective and/or environmental agent that triggers the disease is unknown.

Pathology

AS affects both synovial and fibrous joints; the pathological changes take the form of chronic synovitis. The chronic synovitis is followed by cartilage destruction, erosions, sclerosis of underlying bone, and finally, fibrosis and ankylosis of the affected joints. The sacroiliac joints are involved 100% of the time; the intervertebral discs, symphysis pubis, and manubriosternal joints are frequently involved. Two categories of extra-articular involvement are characteristic:

1. Inflammatory lesions of articular capsule and ligament insertion into bone occur (enthesitis).
2. Extraskeletal lesions may occur in the eye (uveitis [25–30%], aortic root [1–4%], and pulmonary tree) (Table 6.2).

Table 6.1. Natural History of Ankylosing Spondylitis[a]

The onset is insidious.
There are exacerbations and remissions.
Morning stiffness becomes a dominant symptom.
Spinal movement limitation and deformity are progressive.
If peripheral joints are involved, it happens early.
Iritis is early and recurrent.
A more severe course has an earlier onset.
The course in women is milder than in men.

[a]Adapted from Little H. The natural history of ankylosing spondylitis. (Editorial). J Rheum 1988; 15:1179–1180.

Table 6.2. Less Common Symptoms in Ankylosing Spondylitis

Constitutional symptoms, such as fatigue and weight loss.
Chest pains from costosternal involvement.
Eye symptoms (acute iritis).
Extra-articular bony tenderness (enthesopathy, enthesitis).
Heart and ascending aorta lesions.
Apical fibrosis of lung.

Clinical Features

The usual presentation is in a young (adolescent or early adulthood) man who reports the insidious onset of grumbling low back pain. Characteristically, there are remissions and exacerbations over the months. The pain may refer to the buttocks and upper thigh and may even be unilateral, leading readily to confusion with the diagnosis of a ruptured disc. Typical of AS is the absence of neurological symptoms and the presence of good straight leg raising, which should make the diagnosis of a disc rupture immediately suspect. The next most prevalent complaint is stiffness of the lumbosacral area, especially in the morning, with a hot shower and/or the morning's activity alleviating this complaint. Prolonged periods of inactivity worsen the back pain and stiffness. At times, back pain may awaken the patient at night, and often this pain is at the thoracolumbar junction as well as the low back. Eventually, the pain and stiffness affect the entire spine, causing clinically detectable loss of range of movement. Spread to the peripheral skeleton occurs and most often affects the shoulders and hips. Other symptoms are listed in Table 6.2.

Physical Findings

Early in the disease, there is little to find on clinical examination, which leads to a delay in diagnosis. Probably the two most commonly mistaken diagnoses are to label the patient as having "fibrositis" or to mistake unilateral sacroiliac pain for a disc rupture. To the careful examiner, there will be detectable loss of lumbar motion in all three planes: flexion, extension, and lateral flexion. This is in contrast to a patient with a herniated nucleus pulposus, who usually has limited flexion, good backward extension, and limitation of lateral flexion to one side more pronounced than the other (determined by the location of the disc fragment on the nerve root). In AS, there may be pain on direct pressure on the sacroiliac joint, and various tests that stress the sacroiliac joint may increase the pain.

As the disease progresses, there is loss of lumbar lordosis and a decrease in ability to expand the rib cage. Contrary to other reports, these two changes occur early in the natural history of the disease. (3) The loss of chest cage mobility occurs because of involvement of the posterior costovertebral and costotransverse articulations and the anterior costochondral junctions. The normal chest expansion (measured at the level of the fourth rib) is reduced from more than 5 cm to under 2 cm.

The final stage of advancement in the disease is ankylosis of the spine, and if this occurs in a poorly supervised or poorly motivated patient, severe flexion deformities of the spine may occur. (Fig. 6.10)

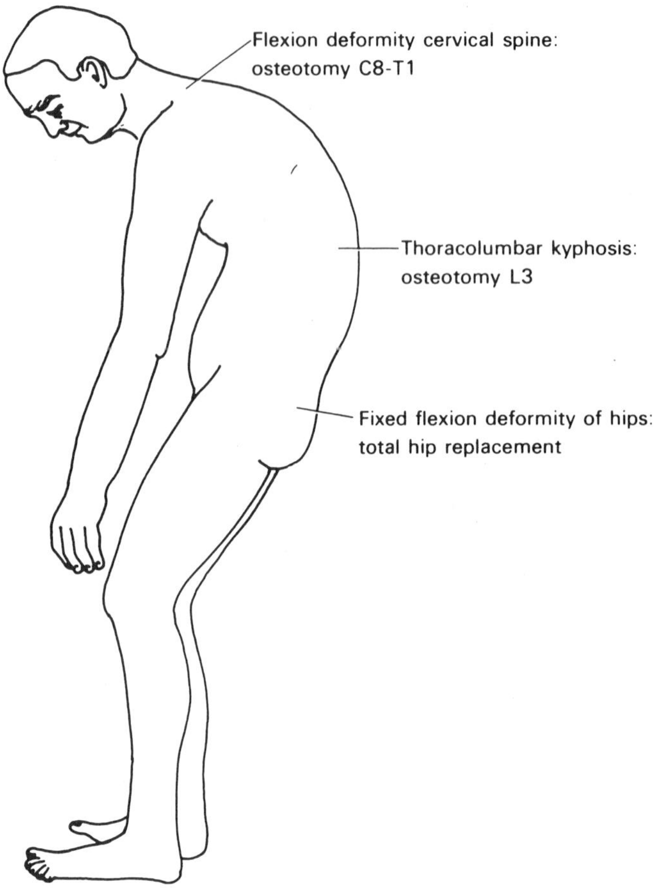

Figure 6.10 *The surgical correction of the fixed flexion deformities associated with ankylosing spondylitis is dependent on the type and site of the maximal deformity. From Macnab I: Backache. Williams & Wilkins, Baltimore (1977), p. 76.*

Early in the disease, the enthesopathy may present as tenderness over bony prominences of the ischial tuberosity, greater trochanter, calcaneus, spinous processes, and other bony prominences.

The course of AS is unpredictable. Women tend to have a less severe form of involvement, as do men with later onset. The most severely involved tend to be younger men, but the variability in progression is striking. With proper supervision and an exercise regimen, even the most severely affected can maintain long-term, gainful employment.

Aside from severe extraskeletal involvement of the aorta and pulmonary tree (fortunately rare), the most limiting symptoms come from ankylosis of the hips (25%), a spondylodiscitis causing severe back pain, or an atlantoaxial subluxation causing severe neck pain.

The patient with AS is very susceptible to accidents causing fractures of the spine. These fractures are more common in the cervical spine but can occur anywhere in the ankylosed spine. The trauma is usually minor, and the fracture is often missed on initial examination. If a neurological lesion (paraplegia/quadriplegia) occurs at the time of the spinal fracture, the prognosis for recovery is dismal.

Laboratory Tests for AS

Ninety percent of symptomatic patients have positive blood test results for HLA-B27. The incidence of HLA-B27 in the normal Caucasian population is 6 to 8%. Most patients will have some elevation in the erythrocyte sedimentation rate, although this elevation is rarely dramatic. There is no association with rheumatoid factor and antinuclear antibodies; thus, the designation "seronegative spondylarthropathies."

Radiographic Findings

The diagnosis of AS is made by radiograph. The characteristic involvement of the sacroiliac joints in the presence of several of the clinical criteria listed in Table 6.3, confirm the diagnosis.

Stages of Radiographic Changes in the Sacroiliac Joints (The radiographic involvement is usually symmetric despite lateralization of symptoms.)

Early Stages (Fig. 6.11)

- Blurring of the joint margins.
- Erosions and sclerosis of bone.

Both of these changes may occur throughout the SI joint but are seen earliest in the lower two thirds (the synovial portion) of the SI joint. The erosions eventually leave the appearance of widening (pseudowidening) of the SI joints.

Late Changes (Fig. 6.11)

- With disease progression, calcification and interosseous bridging of the SI joints occur.

These radiological changes (early) must be distinguished from osteitis condensans Ilii. In this lesion, almost invariably found in multiparous women, there is a wedge-shaped area of sclerosis confined to the iliac side of the joint (Fig. 6.9, B).

Development of Syndesmophytes

Initially, there is inflammation of the annulus fibrosus and the corners of the vertebral bodies. With subsequent erosions of the corners of the vertebral bodies, the anterior aspect of the vertebral body appears squared (Fig. 6.12). This is soon followed by ossification of the

Table 6.3. Clinical Criteria Suggesting Ankylosing Spondylitis*

1. insidious onset of discomfort
2. age less than 40 years
3. persistence for more than 3 months
4. association with morning stiffness
5. improvement with exercise

*from Primer on the Rheumatic Disease, Pg. 145, Ninth Edition, 1988.

annulus fibrosus, which bridges the disc space (syndesmophytes)(Fig. 6.13). The ultimate fate is ossification of all ligaments of the spine and the complete fusion of the vertebral column (bamboo spine) (Fig. 6.14).

Other Skeletal Radiographic Changes

Characteristic changes may occur in the manubriosternal joint (Fig. 6.15). Bony erosions and whiskering at sites of osseous-tendon attachments may be seen on ra-

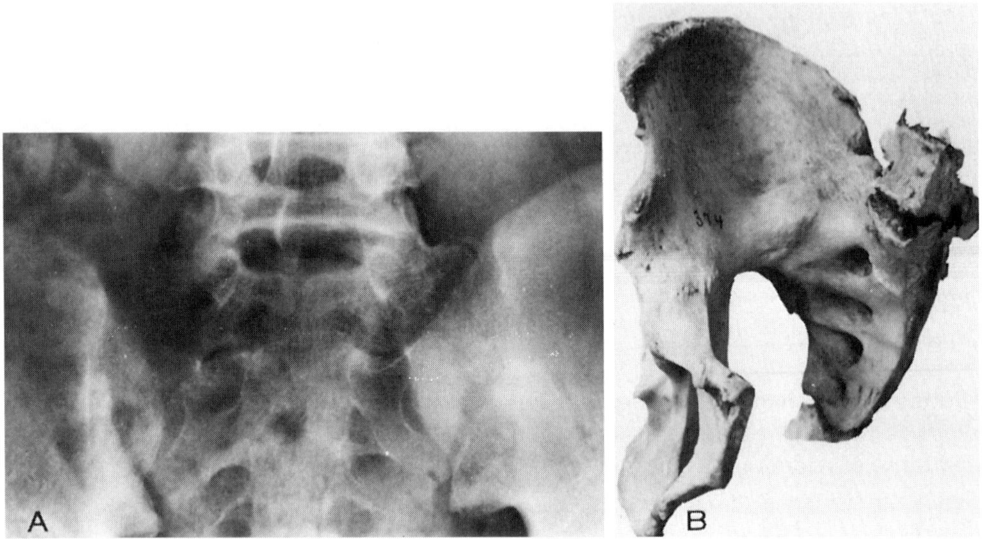

Figure 6.11 **A.** *X-ray demonstrating the irregular definition ("fuzziness") of the sacroiliac joints commonly seen in the early stages of ankylosing spondylitis.* **B.** *In the later stages of the disease, the sacroiliac joint is completely obliterated by a bony ankylosis as shown in this specimen.*

Figure 6.12 **A.** *The lateral view of a normal lumbar vertebral body presents a slight concavity anteriorly.* **B.** *In the early stages of ankylosing spondylitis, this concavity is filled in with the result that the vertebrae appear to be "squared off." From Macnab I: Backache. Williams & Wilkins, Baltimore (1977), p. 72.*

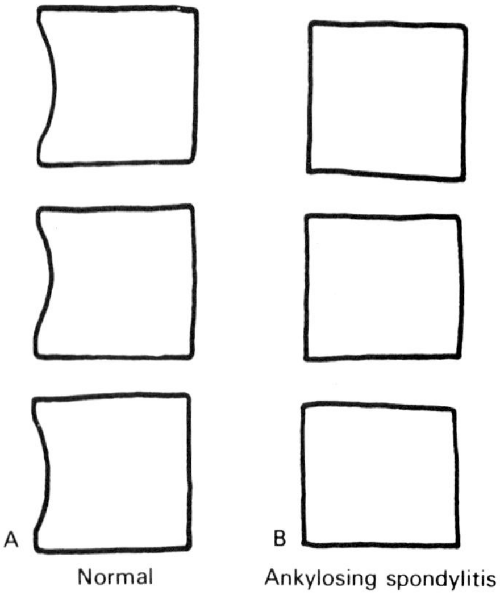

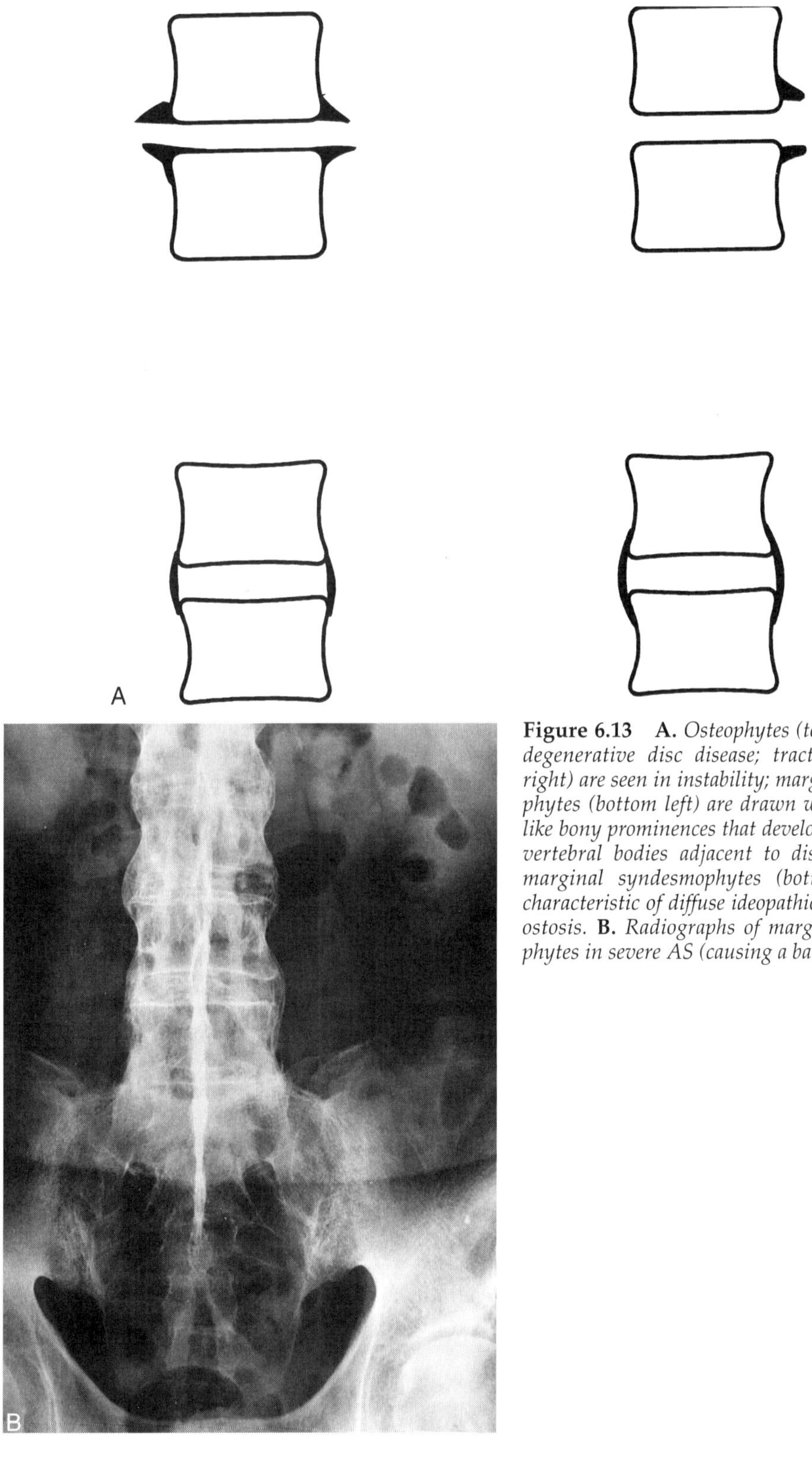

Figure 6.13 **A.** *Osteophytes (top left) occur in degenerative disc disease; traction spurs (top right) are seen in instability; marginal syndesmophytes (bottom left) are drawn with other spur-like bony prominences that develop on the edge of vertebral bodies adjacent to disc spaces; nonmarginal syndesmophytes (bottom right) are characteristic of diffuse ideopathic skeletal hyperostosis.* **B.** *Radiographs of marginal syndesmophytes in severe AS (causing a bamboo spine).*

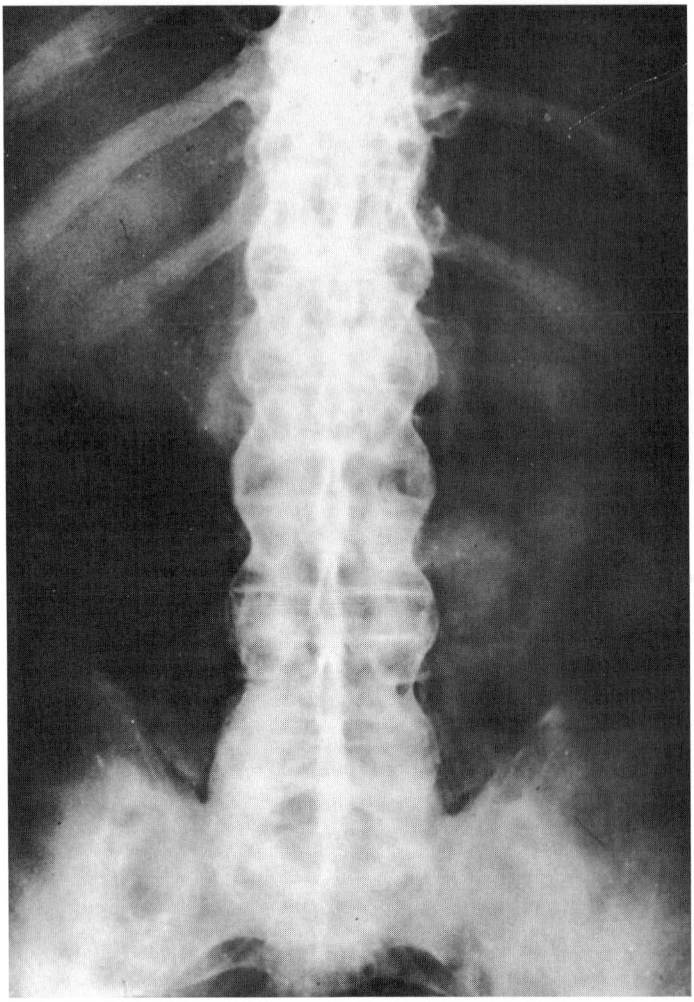

Figure 6.14 *The "bamboo spine." From Macnab I: Backache. Williams & Wilkins, Baltimore (1977), p. 73.*

diograph (Fig. 6.16). Figure 6.17 summarizes the clinical and radiographic findings in AS.

Diagnostic Choices Early in the Disease

The clinician who sees many patients with low back pain is usually very sensitive to diagnosing AS. When AS is suspected clinically, but not supported by plain radiographic films of the sacroiliac joints, what radiographs should be done? It has been suggested that the following radiographic studies are useful: special views of the SI joints, bone scans of the SI joints, and computed tomography (CT) scans of the SI joints.

The yield of useful information with these tests is so low that when balanced against the financial cost of routine use, it is probably not worth doing the tests. Providing other disease entities have been ruled out, the most reasonable choice is to treat the patient as having suspected AS and repeat the plain radiographs in a number of months, rather than chasing down the diagnosis with expensive tests.

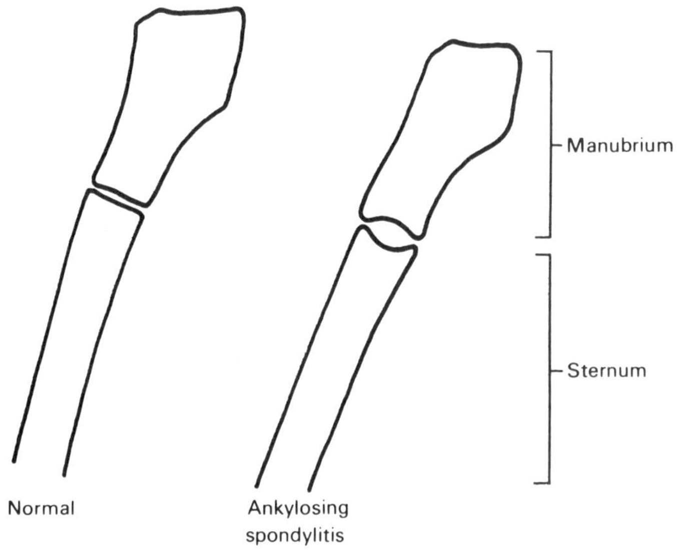

Figure 6.15 *In ankylosing spondylitis the manubriostructural joint may present a biconcave appearance on x-ray. From Macnab I: Backache. Williams & Wilkins, Baltimore (1977), p. 74.*

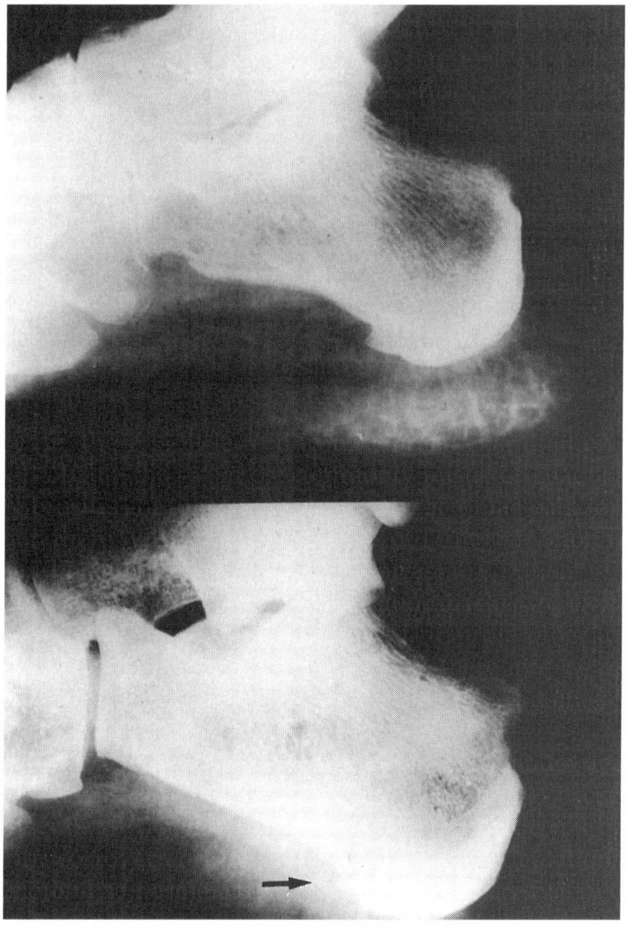

Figure 6.16 *Enthesopathy—whiskering along inferior border of os calcis (arrow).*

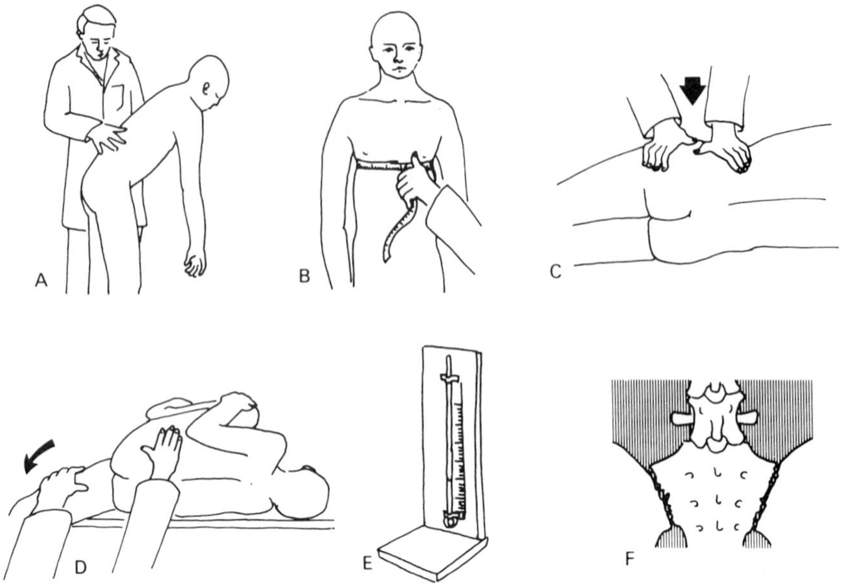

Figure 6.17 *Summary of major findings in ankylosing spondylitis.* **A.** *Rigidity of lumbar spine on forward flexion;* **B.** *Decrease in chest expansion;* **C.** *Pain on side-to-side compression of the pelvis;* **D.** *Pain on Gaenslen's test;* **E.** *Elevated sedimentation rate; and* **F.** *"Fuzziness" of sacroiliac joints on x-ray. From Macnab I: Backache. Williams & Wilkins, Baltimore (1977), p. 75.*

Treatment of AS

No specific treatment of a curative nature presently exists. The role of the physician is diagnostic awareness of the disease, amelioration of the symptoms with the carefully controlled use of anti-inflammatory medications, patient education, attention to the possibility of spinal deformities, and management of peripheral joint arthropathies.

It is essential for the patient to understand the natural history of the disease in order that he/she understands the need for reasonable rest and a continuing program of postural education and exercises.

The exercise program is designed to maintain a straight spine or to attempt to increase lumbar lordosis. Every attempt must be made to maintain the already reduced respiratory excursion.

Occasionally, despite anti-inflammatory medication and excellent continued physical therapy, the spinal deformities progress relentlessly and inexorably to a stage at which the patient can only see a few feet in front of him/her when standing and may have difficulty in sitting and eating. In such instances, surgical correction of the deformities must be considered. Operative correction is undertaken at the site of the maximal deformity, taking into full account the serious surgical hazards of respiratory problems and the danger of producing irreversible neurological damage (Fig. 6.10).

Spondylitis Associated with Chronic Inflammatory Bowel Disease: Enteropathic Arthritis

It has been found that spondylitis and a peripheral seronegative arthritis occur in 5 to 20% of patients suffering from regional enteritis and chronic ulcerative colitis.

The etiology and pathogenesis of the peripheral arthropathy are unknown. Several distinguishing features have been noted: the gradual onset, involvement of weight-bearing joints, a migratory pattern, and a short-lived course. The spondylitis is clinically and roentgenographically indistinguishable from idiopathic ankylosing spondylitis. In this regard, it is interesting to note that nearly 80% of the patients with spondylitis associated with inflammatory bowel disease are HLA-B27 positive.

If a patient being treated for Crohn's disease or ulcerative colitis subsequently develops a grumbling backache, the possibility of sacroiliitis with spondylitis must be suspected. One must be aware that spondylitis can occur before the onset of intestinal disease and does so in at least one third of cases. Whereas the severity of the arthropathy correlates with the activity of the bowel disease, the spondylitis appears to progress independently of the primary lesion, and medical and surgical treatment of the bowel disease does not alter progression of the spondylitis.

Spondylitis Associated with Psoriasis

Almost identical radiological changes in the sacroiliac joints and lumbar spine may be seen in patients suffering from psoriatic arthritis. The age of onset of psoriatic arthritis is generally in the second or third decade, with women equally afflicted as men. The etiology and pathogenesis have not been clarified. It is interesting to note that, on tissue typing, 60% of patients with psoriatic arthritis, 90% of patients with psoriatic sacroiliac joint arthritis, and 100% of patients with psoriatic spondylitis have an HLA-B27 antigen.

The clinician must always be mindful of the fact that the skin lesion of psoriasis does not protect patients from developing simple mechanical backache. Not every patient with psoriasis and back pain is suffering from spondylitis; nevertheless, if the patient has a peripheral arthritis, the possibility of a psoriatic sacroiliitis or spondylitis must be suspected, and appropriate radiographs should be ordered.

Spondylitis Associated with Reiter's Syndrome (Reactive Arthritis)

Back pain may be the presenting symptom of Reiter's syndrome (RS). It is difficult to define Reiter's disease precisely. Historically, it was considered to be a triad of nonbacterial urethritis, arthritis, and conjunctivitis, but this rigid classification inhibited an understanding of the complexity of the disease. After much debate,(6) RS is now defined as an episode of peripheral arthritis of more than 1 month's duration, occurring in association with urethritis and/or cervicitis. Other clinical situations that may coexist are conjunctivitis, mucous membrane lesions, and other cutaneous lesions. The onset is most common between the ages of 20 and 40, with men predominantly affected. Episodes of extramarital sexual intercourse may precede attacks, and the patients tend to be "sexual giants." The etiology of the disease is unknown, but evidence tends to point to an infectious agent.

Any one of the clinical manifestations may be the presenting symptom, although urethritis is by far the most common initial feature. The arthritis is marked by acute onset and asymmetrical involvement of a few joints. The large weight-bearing joints, the joints of the midfoot, and the metatarsophalangeal and interphalangeal joints of the toes are the most commonly afflicted.

A high percentage of patients with Reiter's syndrome show radiographic evidence of sacroiliitis, but it is only a small percentage that develop a spondylitis. When spondylitis occurs, it is late in the disease evolution and is noted, therefore, as an association rather than a presenting finding.

INFECTIONS OF THE SACROILIAC JOINTS

In the past, tuberculosis was the most common cause of infective arthritis of the sacroiliac joints. Recently, an increasing frequency of pyogenic involvement has been noted, especially in children. The clinical picture is unfortunately vague. There are pain and tenderness over the sacroiliac joints, and the erythrocyte sedimentation rate is raised. With pyogenic infections, the patient may be febrile, but there is very little else to define the nature of the underlying lesion. The damage to the sacroiliac joint may not be apparent for several weeks, and it is understandable that definitive diagnosis may, therefore, be delayed for a long period of time. If the clinician is very suspicious of the diagnosis, a bone scan may demonstrate a "hot spot," and the associated bony changes can then be defined by tomography. It must be remembered, however, that this area of the skeleton always takes up more technetium on a routine scan than other portions of the pelvis.

On occasion, a fluctuant abscess will form. Under such circumstances, confirmation of the diagnosis and isolation of the organism can be achieved by needle biopsy. If aspiration proves impossible, with the presumptive diagnosis provided by the overall clinical picture, the bone scan, and the CT scan, open biopsy is mandatory in order that appropriate antibiotic therapy can be instituted.

Ewing's sarcomata have a predilection for the pelvis and, when occurring adjacent to the sacroiliac joint, may mimic the radiological appearance of destructive pyogenic arthritis. On occasion, the differentiation from septic arthritis in such instances can only be established by open biopsy.

Because of the rarity of septic arthritis of the sacroiliac joint as a cause of backache and because of the nonspecific nature of the clinical picture, the diagnosis may be missed easily.

In summary, the patient does not look well and complains of pain in the sacroiliac region, with tenderness on palpation. He/she is febrile and usually is seen with an elevated erythrocyte sedimentation rate and, in instances of pyogenic arthritis, an elevated white blood cell count. The radiographs may not show significant abnormality initially, but continued concern over the possibility of the diagnosis should prompt the request for a bone scan and computerized axial tomography.

SUMMARY

Affections of the sacroiliac region may present as backache. The anatomical characteristics of the joint and the natural history of ankylosis should prevent the occurrence of the so-called sacroiliac sprains.

Pelvic instability is an infrequent but definite hazard of taking a bone graft from the posterior superior iliac crest and is related to the inadvertent division of the iliolumbar ligament.

The introduction of the use of histocompatibility antigen studies may lead to a redefinition of ankylosing spondylitis as a broader disease process. At present, radiographic changes in the sacroiliac joints are essential to a firm diagnosis.

The sophistication of today's bone scanning techniques minimizes the delays in diagnosis so prevalent with infection and neoplasm involving the sacroiliac joint region.

REFERENCES

1. Goldthwaite JE. Essentials of Body Med. Philadelphia: JB Lippincott, 1937.
2. Little H. The natural history of ankylosing spondylitis (editorial). J Rheum 1988;15:1179–1180.
3. Potter NA, Rothstein JM. Intertester reliability for selected clinical tests of the sacroiliac joint. Phys Ther 1985;65:1671–1675.
4. Stuvesson B, Selvik G, Uden A. Movements of the sacroiliac joints: A Roentgen stereophotogrammetric analysis. Spine 1989;14:162–165.
5. Walker JM. The sacroiliac joint: a critical review. Phys Ther 1992;72:903–915.
6. Wilkens RF, Arnett FC, Bilter T, et al. Reiter's syndrome. Evaluation of preliminary criteria for definite disease. Arth Rheum 1981;24:844–849.

7

Spondylogenic Backache: Soft Tissue Lesions

"Knowledge of structure of the human body is the foundation on which all rational medicine and surgery is built."

— Mondini de Luzzi

INTRODUCTION

By far, the most important soft tissue syndromes to be described in this chapter are lesions of the disc:disc degeneration with or without disc rupture, and the secondary phenomenon of root encroachment. But no discussion of soft tissue lesions would be complete without including "fibrositis" and "myofascial pain syndromes." When you read Chapter 12, you will note that these syndromes are included in the psychosomatic classification of nonorganic pain and have been given the descriptive term of "the orthopaedic ulcer."

The major factor that has clouded and confused the diagnosis of soft tissue lesions of the back is the phenomenon of referred pain.(27) When a deep structure is irritated, either by trauma, disease, or the experimental injection of an irritating solution, the resultant pain may be experienced locally, referred distally, or experienced both locally and radiating to a distance. The classic example is the patient experiencing myocardial ischemic pain who may report discomfort, numbness, heaviness, and/or a sensation of swelling in the arm along with referred pain to other sites, such as the neck and jaw or the shoulder. It is important to recognize that tenderness may also be referred to a distance. The injection of hypertonic saline into the lumbosacral supraspinous ligament may give rise to pain radiating down the leg as far down as the calf, and the pain may also be associated with tender points commonly situated over the sacroiliac joint and the upper outer quadrant of the buttock (Fig. 7.1).

The complaint of pain and the demonstration of local tenderness may obscure the fact that the offending pathological lesions are centrally placed and may lead the clinician to believe erroneously that the disease process underlies the site of the patient's complaints. This erroneous belief may apparently be confirmed by the temporary relief of pain on injection of local anesthetic into the site of the referred pain. These points must be borne in mind when the clinician considers soft tissue lesions giving rise to low back pain.

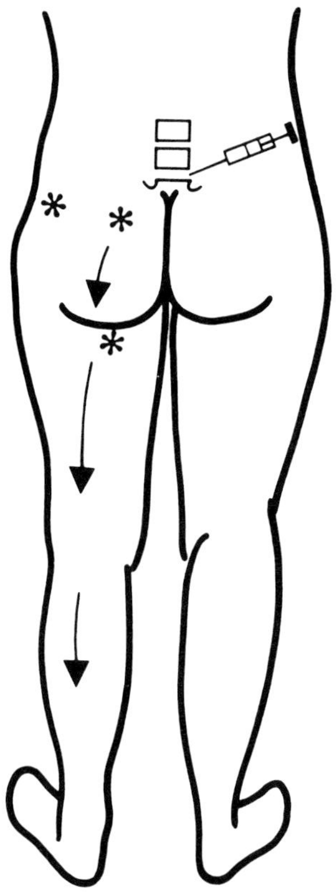

Figure 7.1 *The injection of hypertonic saline into the supraspinous ligament between L5 and S1 will give rise to local pain and pain referred down the back of the leg in sciatic distribution. In addition to this, there will be areas of tenderness produced in the lower limb most commonly at the sites noted by the asterisks. From Macnab I: Backache. Williams & Wilkins, Baltimore (1977), p. 81.*

THE NEUROPHYSIOLOGY OF PAIN AND REFERRED PAIN

Pain is a complex neurophysiological phenomenon, initiated peripherally, appreciated centrally, and in between modified by a complex relationship of fiber tracts.(21) Chronic pain carries with it the burden of past experiences and emotional and socioeconomic reactions.(21) Is it any wonder that scientists have not solved the puzzle of pain? Add to that the fact that patients cannot describe pain, and we have a foundation of quicksand on which to construct an understanding and treatment of one of the most common presenting complaints in medicine: low back pain. The nociceptors and fiber tracts that modulate pain will be discussed in Chapter 12, but are summarized here.

Let us try to follow pain from its origin to a patient's response to the painful stimulus:

Peripheral Modulation

Step 1

Nerve endings of many different types (encapsulated or free nerve endings) detect the painful stimulus. These nerve endings that detect pain are known as nociceptors.

Step 2

The impulse message of pain travels through afferent sensory nerves in large (fast conduction myelinated α fibers) and smaller and slower conduction nonmyelinated fibers.

Step 3

The dorsal ganglion (Fig. 7.2) contains the cell bodies for the conduction axons in Step 2. Here, a synapse occurs, and the messages continue on to the dorsal horn of the spinal cord. There is some consideration that a threshold of stimulus has to be reached before the impulse message of pain makes it through the synapse in the dorsal root-ganglion. This represents the first of the various gates that painful impulses have to traverse.(27)

Step 4: The Dorsal Horn—The Gate

From the dorsal root-ganglion, impulses travel to the dorsal horn substantia gelatinosa (Fig. 7.3). This is where Wall and Melzack have erected their primary gate construct.(27) They have postulated the presence of a sorting-out center in the dorsal horns of the spinal cord. These sorting-out centers act to increase or decrease the flow of nerve impulses from the peripheral fibers to the central nervous system (CNS). How the gate behaves is determined by a complex interaction of distal afferent stimulation and descending influences from the brain. There is a critical level of pain information that arrives in the dorsal horn and that will stimulate and open the gate and allow for higher transmission (Fig. 7.3)

The dorsal (sensory) afferent fibers travel in the dorsal root entry zone for one or two segments before entering the dorsal horn (Fig. 7.3). The dorsal horn is made up of six lamina. Which lamina a sensory fiber synapses in is determined by the fiber size:

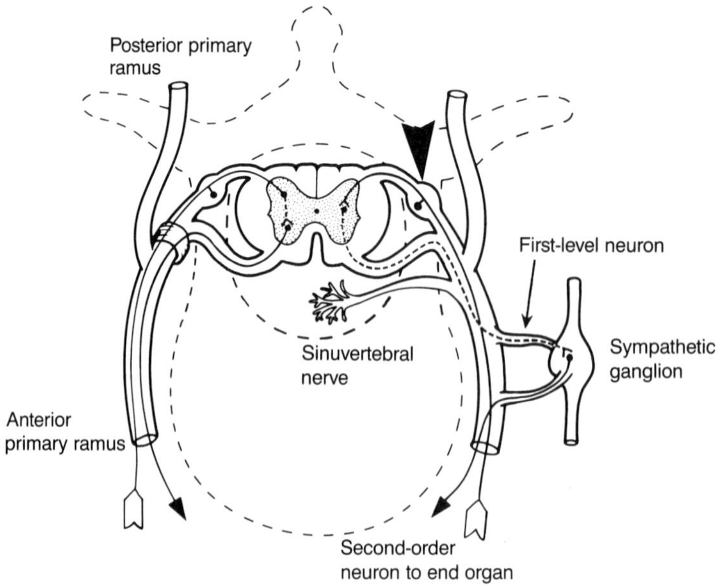

Figure 7.2 *The proximal origins of the peripheral nerve fiber tracts. The dorsal root-ganglion is designated by the arrowhead on the right.*

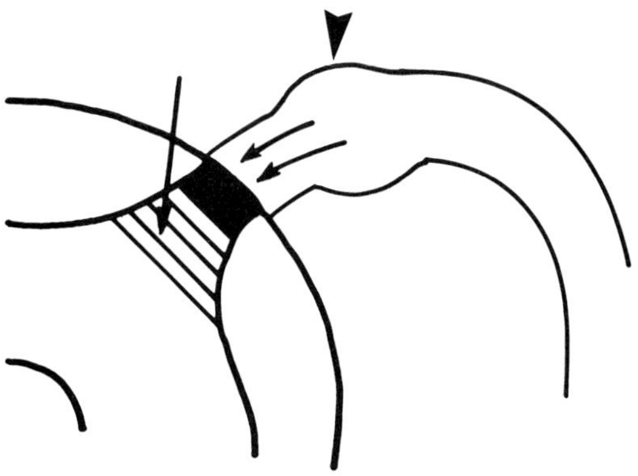

Figure 7.3 *The gate control theory of pain: sensory fibers (double arrows and dorsal root-ganglion designated by arrowhead) arrive in lamina of dorsal horn. Higher centers (single arrow) influence whether or not "gate" opens for transmission of pain impulses to higher centers.*

- C fibers terminate in laminae 1 and subsequently, in lamina 2.
- A δ fibers terminate in laminae 2 and 5.

Like computers, these laminae simulate the information delivered, pass it back and forth, and receive descending modulation impulses. It is after this computerized analysis of the information that the pain impulses are ready for collection and discharge up the spinal cord pathways. This section of the dorsal horn is the gate center for pain modulation.

It is thought that activity in the nonmyelinated C fibers tends to inhibit transmission and thus closes the gate; conversely, small myelinated A δ-fiber activity facilitates transmission and opens the gate.

From a clinical point of view, trigger zones in the skin and muscle are postulated to keep the gate open. Anxieties, depression, life situation pressures, and past memories of pain can all serve to keep the gate open and increase the appreciation of pain. Local anesthetic/steroid trigger injections are used to negate this phenomenon. Likewise, transcutaneous electrical nerve stimulation units are used to stimulate the C fibers and close the gate to transmission of pain impulse to higher centers. The most common "gate closers" are obviously analgesics.

Step 5: The Spinal Cord Tracts (Transmission Pathways)

Now, things really get complicated. What is known for sure is that from the dorsal horn, pain fibers cross to the opposite side to ascend in the spinothalamic tract (Fig. 7.4)

Within the human spinal cord, there are approximately five ascending pathways for the pain impulses:

1. Spinothalamic tract;
2. Spinoreticular tract;
3. Spinomesencephalic tract;
4. Spinocervical tract; and
5. Second-order dorsal column tract.

These tracts are not independent pathways to higher centers but instead, have many cross-connections. In fact, the spinoreticular and spinomesencephalic tracts are considered one and the same by some neurobiologists.(8) They are probably "brain-stem" tracts, carrying an altering message to the reticular formation that pain is something with which the body is going to have to contend. These tracts end in the brain-stem reticular zones of the medulla and pons.

The last two listed tracts are more theoretical than real and are simply mentioned for completeness.

By far, the most important afferent pain pathway is the lateral spinothalamic tract, which is located in the anterolateral column of the cord and carries crossed pain fibers from the contralateral side of the body. After the afferent fibers leave the dorsal horn gray matter zone, they cross the midline to enter the spinothalamic tract. More caudal fibers are displaced laterally as more cephalad fibers enter the tract from the opposite side (Fig. 7.5).

Pathways for temperature sense travel in close association with the lateral spinothalamic tract. It is the lateral spinothalamic tract that is transected during percutaneous cordotomy for the control of pain.

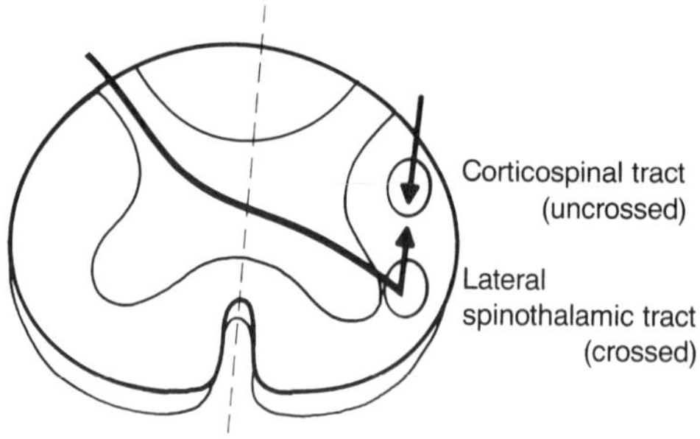

Figure 7.4 *Pain fibers cross (in the same segment or one or two cord segments higher) to enter the lateral spinothalamic tract on the opposite side.*

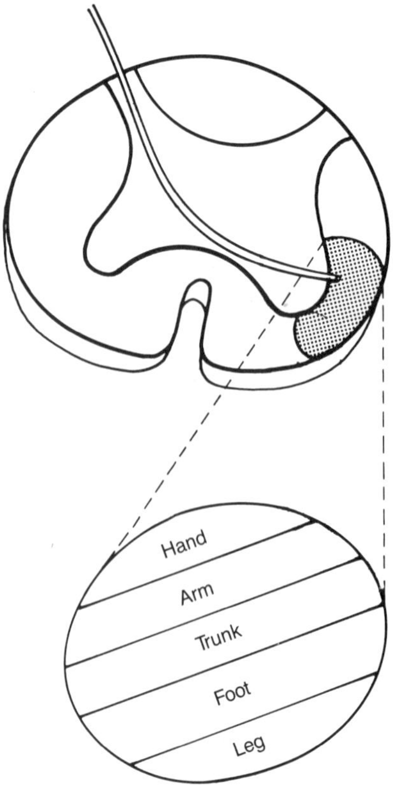

Figure 7.5 *The lamination of fibers in the lateral spinothalamic tract (lower) is such that the later entering (upper extremity) fibers displace the earlier entering (lower extremity) fibers to the periphery.*

Step 6: The Higher Centers

Higher Centers for Receipt of Pain Fibers As higher levels in the central nervous system are observed, the discrete sensory tract blends into many other CNS pathways. To say exactly where every pain pathway goes at this higher level is impossible. Only the most basic concepts are mentioned here:

1. Fibers from the spinothalamic tract go to the thalamus, from whence they are distributed to many higher centers.
2. Other afferent sensory tracts end in the brain-stem reticular formation.
3. Fibers from the thalamus going on to higher cortical centers travel through the internal capsule.
4. Many of these fibers will end up in the postcentral gyrus of the cortex, which is considered to be the predominant sensory area of the cerebral cortex.

Summary of Concepts Presented When trying to understand the nervous system pathways for pain, one is struck by the multidimensional character of pain:

1. There are multiple nociceptors activating multiple neural systems.
2. There are multiple ascending tracts.
3. There are multiple CNS receptors.

Step 7: The Psychological Aspects of Pain

The greatest gray area in trying to understand pain lies in the obvious psychological modulation of pain that occurs in every human being. As clinicians, we are aware of patients in whom the slightest amount of pain seems to cause significant disability, and we are also aware of patients in whom a significant amount of pain is accompanied by little alteration in acts of daily living. The reason for this discrepancy and range of pain response lies in understanding the psychological aspects of pain, which is best depicted in Figure 7.6.(14)

The nociception circle is the actual injury. The pain response is the result of the injury. Without any psychological modification, a patient would suffer with the pain.

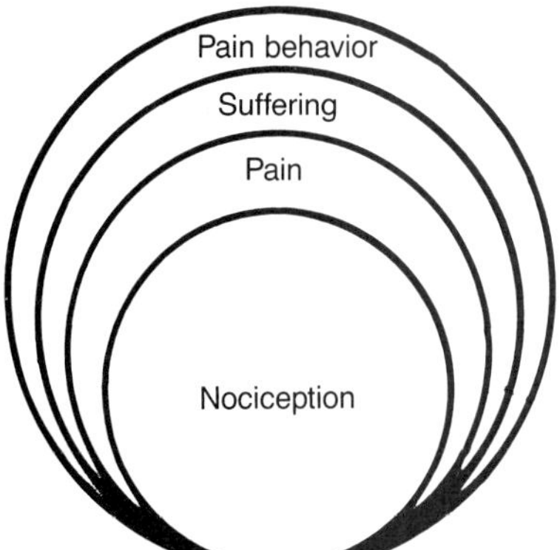

Figure 7.6 *The staging of pain originating with the painful stimulus (received by the nociceptors).*

The difficult part of this diagram is the pain behavior circle. This is what is manifested by the patient and what doctors and relatives observe in a patient experiencing pain. Pain behavior is wrapped up into the theories of primary and secondary pain and may include moaning, grimacing, limping, excessive talking, excessive silence, refusing to work, seeking health care, and taking medications. The clinician can only conclude that pain is always accompanied by a display of emotions. These emotions are in the form of anxiety, fear, depression, anger, aggression, and so forth, and manifest themselves as pain behavior. Waddell and co-workers (26) have enhanced this concept with their Glasgow illness model (Fig. 7.7), which is more applicable to the back pain sufferer—plied and enticed by such societal phenomena as accidents, lawyers, courts, and financial awards.

The emotional intensity and pain behavior of the patient are significantly related to genetic makeup, cultural background, and interpretation of past events. It is an extremely complex cognitive process beyond the scope of this book.

From the six previous steps and multiple "hoop jumps," let us try to construct a theory of referred pain!

REFERRED PAIN

From the original work of Kellgren (12) to the more recent work of Mooney and Robertson,(19) the concept of referred pain has enjoyed wide support among spine surgeons. Whether this support is correct remains to be seen in light of new work that must be done in this field. The most confusing position has been stated by Bogduk and Twomey,(2) which states that if pain traveling down the leg is not associated with neurological symptoms or signs, it is not true radicular pain. This is obviously incorrect, because many patients with sciatica, especially those in the younger age group, present exclusively with leg pain and marked reduction of straight leg raising (SLR), with little in the way of neurologic symptoms or signs. On investigation, they are found to have a disc herniation; when the disc herniation is treated, these symptoms abate. To conclude that these patients had referred sclerotomal or myotomal pain rather than true radicular pain is obviously an error.

At the other end of the spectrum, there are those in the field who state that any pain that does not go below the knee is referred pain and that any pain that travels below the knee is radicular pain. This also is incorrect because there are many young patients who present with a disc herniation manifested only by high iliac crest or buttock discomfort.

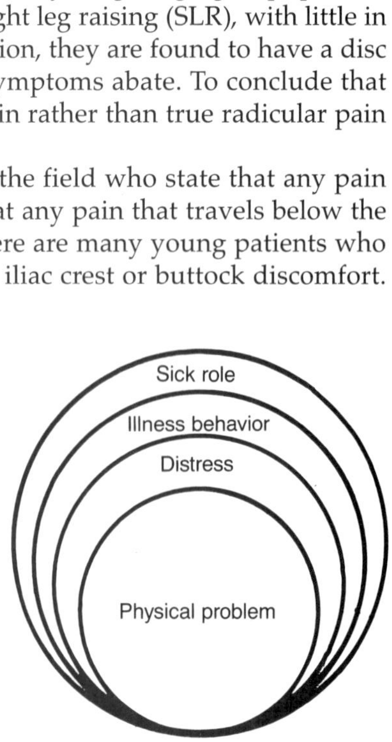

Figure 7.7 *Waddell has modified the conceptual model of pain to a more clinically useful model of illness: "an operational model for clinical practice." (Reprinted with permission from Waddell G. A new clinical model for the treatment of low back pain. Spine 1987;12:632–644.)*

On investigation, they are found to have a disc rupture; when the disc rupture is treated, their pain disappears (see Chapter 15).

Finally, there are patients who have radiating pain down the leg, full SLR, and no neurologic changes and who are also thought to have referred extremity pain. Some of these patients are in the older age group and, on computed tomography (CT) scanning and magnetic resonance imaging (MRI), are found to have various degrees of encroachment in the lateral zone. When these encroachment phenomena are relieved microsurgically, the pain disappears and, obviously, they have had radicular rather than referred discomfort.

For all of these reasons, it is time to repeat the work of Kellgren (12) and Mooney and Robertson (19), knowing exactly the pathology that lies at each segment as documented on CT scan and MRI. It is predicted that many of the patients who have previously been tagged with the label "referred pain" will, in fact, have radicular pain due to the direct involvement of a nerve root.

Many experts would accept patients as having referred pain when they present with a very diffuse sensation in their legs, which is bilateral in nature and not associated either with any radicular pattern or any root tension irritation or compression findings. Provided that those patients do not have spinal stenosis on CT scan or MRI, they probably have referred pain.

The concept of referred pain is one of two types of discomfort. Either it is a deep discomfort felt in a sclerotomal or myotomal distribution, or it may be superficial in nature and felt within the skin dermatomes. The fact that gallbladder pain can be felt in the shoulder obviously supports the fact that referred pain is a phenomenon that does occur.

In theory, somewhere in the nervous system is a convergence and summation of nerve impulses from the primary painful area. This is probably lamina 5 in the dorsal horn. The stimulation of this lamina opens a gate and allows central dispatch of the pain message and distal referral of other sensations that indicate referred pain. The essential feature of the relationship between the site of the pain and the distal referral is the common segmental origin of the sensory innervation for both the origin and the distal referral site. Some of that commonality may occur in the complicated ascending pathways in the spinal cord. You can increase the painful sensation by touching the sites of referred pain. These areas are known as trigger zones, and through various methods of stimulation and anesthetization, referred pain can be altered.

In summary, the concepts of referred pain are likely to be alerted with today's sophisticated investigations in the form of CT scanning and MRI. With these tools in hand, it is time to go back and repeat the outstanding work of Kellgren (12) and Mooney and Robertson (19) in an attempt to further understand the concept of referred pain.

MYOFASCIAL SPRAINS OR STRAINS

Partial tears of the attachment of muscles may occur, giving rise to local tenderness and pain of short duration. There is always a history of specific injury. The pain and tenderness are always away from the midline. This is a young person's injury occurring in strong muscles that are guarding a healthy spine. A similar injury sustained by an older man, with weaker muscles and degenerated disc, is much more likely to result in a posterior joint strain.

The lesions heal quickly with the passage of time despite, rather than because of, treatment. Injections of local anesthetic (with or without the addition of local steroids) into the areas of maximal tenderness certainly afford temporary relief of varying duration, but it is doubtful whether they speed the resolution of the underlying pathology.

The symptoms may persist for approximately 3 weeks, during which time the patient is well advised to avoid provocative activity. If symptoms persist beyond this period of time, the problem should be carefully reassessed lest some more significant underlying lesion has been overlooked.

FIBROSITIS (FIBROMYALGIA) AND MYOFASCIAL PAIN SYNDROMES

The name "fibrositis" was first introduced by Sir William Gowers (7) in 1904, when he coined the word to denote nonspecific inflammatory changes in fibrous tissue that he felt were responsible for the clinical syndrome of "lumbago." Fibrositis is now the most common cause of chronic, widespread, nonarticular, musculoskeletal pain in general practice. To date, the underlying pathological lesion has never been demonstrated histologically and probably does not exist. The so-called "fibrositic" nodules, or tender points, which are palpable over the iliac crest, are usually localized nodules of fat. These "trigger points" are considered to be one of the hallmarks of fibrositis. Never mind that the examiner forgot to test the skin overlying these trigger points for tenderness, or that the point locations have not been submitted to rigid scientific testing to determine validity.

The tender points are situated in an area that is a common site of referred tenderness derived from an underlying spinal lesion and they, along with the overlying skin, may be tender on pressure. The demonstration of a tender nodule associated with back pain and the occasional relief of symptoms by the injection of local anesthetic has lent weight to this clinical concept. Surgical exploration of the nodules has revealed their questionable anatomical nature.

The concept of fibrositis becoming the most common cause of back pain in general practice for nearly half of a century is a classic example of how the phenomenon of referred pain and tenderness have clouded the recognition of the pathological basis of low back pain derived from soft tissue disorders. There is no reason why the term should not be retained to describe the clinical syndrome: "low back pain of undetermined origin associated with tender points." However, it must be remembered that the term does not denote a specific pathological process. Rather, it describes a perfectionist or anxiety-laden personality, with diffuse chronic pain, in whom the bones, joints, bursae, and nerves are normal. These patients complain of musculoskeletal pain; nothing can be found on physical examination or investigation (except the tender points), so these patients are lumped into the nebulous category of fibrositis. If their syndrome is localized to one area of the body, such as the low back, there is a tendency to label the entity "myofascial pain syndrome" rather than "fibrositis." This hair splitting does little to help us understand the problem.

Much of what we are describing throughout this text conforms to the traditional medical model of disease:

1. A rational collection of symptoms and signs.
2. A probable diagnosis.
3. Verification of the diagnosis through investigation.
4. Resolution through scientifically proven treatment regimens.

Fibrositis does not fit this model. Although it is a recognizable collection of symptoms (with few signs) (Table7.1), it fails the remaining tests of the traditional medical model. By the time the diagnosis is made, you have a despondent patient and a frustrated primary care physician.

Table 7.1. Clinical Characteristics of Fibrositis

Pain: chronic, changing, widespread, deep
Associated stiffness, weakness (nonmeasurable)
Trigger points: numerous, throughout body
Aggravation: by internal (eg, fatigue) and external (eg, cold) stimuli
Sleep: nonrestorative sleep pattern

There is little question that the syndrome can be modified by psychosocial and economic factors.(23)

Treatment of fibromyalgia patients is less than gratifying because the syndrome cannot be cured. Those clinicians with the "patience of Job" can do a great deal to ameliorate symptoms and lead patients to a better quality of life.

Effective methods of treatment have included some or all of the following:

1. Reassure the patient of the benign nature of the problem.
2. Do not reinforce through excessive investigation or treatment that the problem is serious.
3. Provide extensive education to the patient: make the patient the center of the solution and encourage him/her to take control of the symptoms through:
   a. Behavioral modification.
   b. Loss of weight.
   c. Improved physical fitness.
   d. Abstinence from smoking and excessive alcohol intake.
4. Judiciously use drugs such as mild analgesia/anti-inflammatories and antidepressants.
5. Limit the repetitive use of trigger point injections.
6. Control unlimited use of manipulation, modalities, biofeedback, and so forth, until the patient has a clear understanding of the nature of fibrositis and the non-curative nature of these interventions.
7. Discourage politicians and bureaucrats from liberalizing compensation and Social Security regulations that encourage this syndrome through financial reward.

All too often, the doctor-patient relationship follows two extremes concerning fibrositis: 1. "The condition doesn't exist; all of the patients are crazy and I will not care for them." 2. "The patients are sick and require extensive investigation and treatment," which some clinicians would describe as overservicing. The best road to follow with these patients is the middle road, helping the patient to understand the psychosomatic nature, placing them in a vigorous self-supervised exercise program and, on occasion, providing low doses of Elavil (Stuart Pharmaceuticals, Wilmington, Del) to help with the sleep disorder.

Piriformis Syndrome

The piriformis muscle has taken on a high profile as a cause of sciatica. A number of patients with pain down their leg in a sciatic distribution will arrive in the clinician's office with the latest "newspaper clip" describing how the piriformis muscle (Fig. 7.8) has trapped the sciatic nerve deep in the buttock. This entrapment, theoretically, causes pain radiating down the leg in a sciatic distribution and up into the back. The presentation is identical to lumbosacral root encroachment problems, such as disc herniations and lateral zone encroachment (Chapters 15 and 16). A variant of this syndrome is the carrying of a fat wallet in one's hip pocket, which in turn puts pressure on the piriformis muscle and irritates the sciatic nerve.

Proponents of this syndrome as a cause of sciatic pain say they can diagnose and treat the condition by stretching the hip into internal rotation (Fig. 7.9). Modalities such as ultrasound and massage to the piriformis area of the buttock have been proposed to reduce muscle spasm and inflammation.

The problem with this diagnosis and treatment is the lack of scientific testing of the parameters. Until appropriate studies on the clinical presentation and effective treatment are provided, it is best to see this diagnosis as a low level possibility in a patient who probably has sciatica due to a disc rupture or subarticular root encroachment.

KISSING SPINES: SPRUNG BACK

Approximation of the spinous processes ("kissing spines"), and the development of a bursa between them, have been indicated as a cause of low back pain. "Sprung back" is a term used to describe rupture of the supraspinous ligament after a sudden flexion strain applied to the spine with the pelvis fixed, as in falling on the buttocks with the legs out

Figure 7.8 *The piriformis muscle (arrow) exiting the sciatic notch, with the sciatic nerve (*) in close proximity. Spasm of the piriformis muscle may irritate the nerve.*

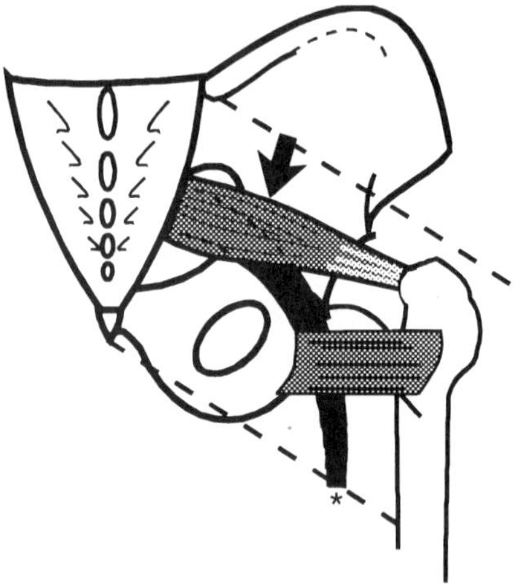

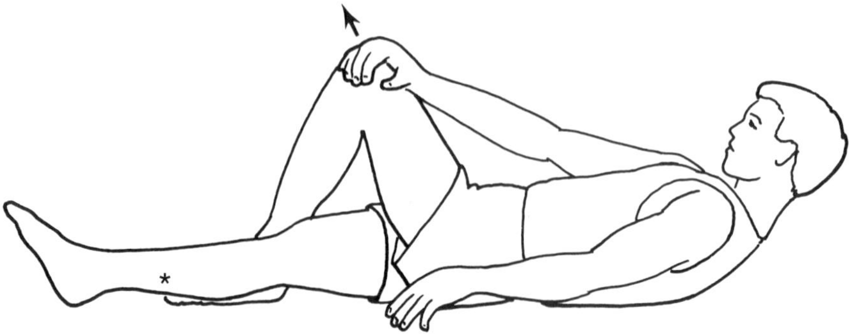

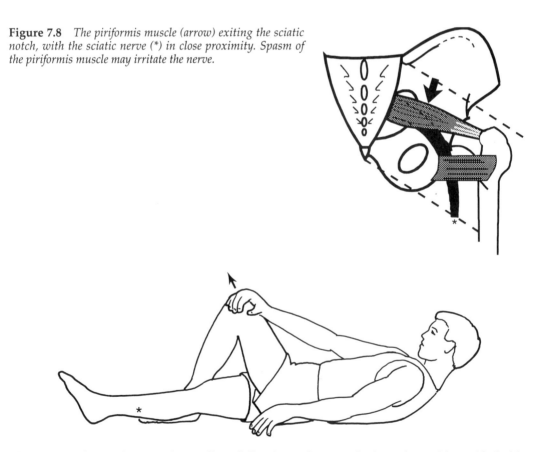

Figure 7.9 *The stretching exercise to relieve piriformis muscle spasm. In the supine position, with the hip and knee flexed and the foot crossed, (*) the hip is adducted (arrow).*

straight. It is doubtful whether either of these entities are, in and of themselves, a cause of low back strain (Fig. 7.10).

SACRALIZATION OF A LUMBAR VERTEBRA (BERTOLOTTI'S SYNDROME)

Bertolotti (1), in 1917, described attachment between the transverse process of L5 with the sacrum and associated this attachment with low back pain (Fig. 7.11). Whether or not the radiographic change that Bertolotti noted is associated with an increased incidence of back pain has been hotly debated since 1917. Although it is possible that some unilateral assimilation between the transverse process of L5 and the sacrum can result in mobile

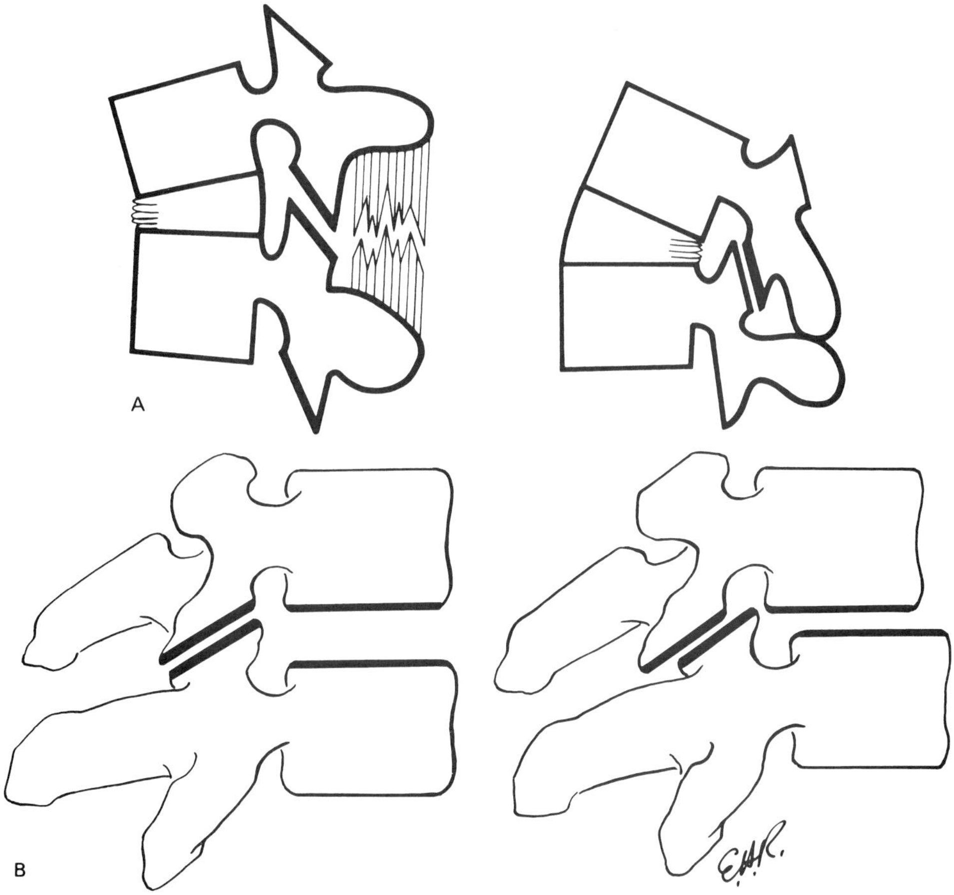

Figure 7.10 **A.** *The radiological demonstration of apposition of the spinous processes has been referred to as "kissing spines." This anatomical disposition of the spinous processes cannot occur in the absence of an unstable disc segment. In the balance of probabilities, it is the associated disc degeneration rather than the bony apposition of the spinous processes that is the cause of the patient's symptoms. From Macnab I: Backache. Williams & Wilkins, Baltimore (1977), p. 83.* **B.** *As the intervertebral discs lose height and the vertebral bodies approach one another, the posterior joints must override and assume the position normally held in hyperextension. It is to be noted that owing to the inclination of the posterior joints, as the upper vertebral body approaches the vertebral body beneath it, it is displaced backward producing a retrospondylolisthesis. This posterior displacement of the vertebral body, indicative of posterior joint subluxation, is readily recognizable on routine x-ray examination of the lumbar spine. From Macnab I: Backache. Williams & Wilkins, Baltimore (1977), p. 88.*

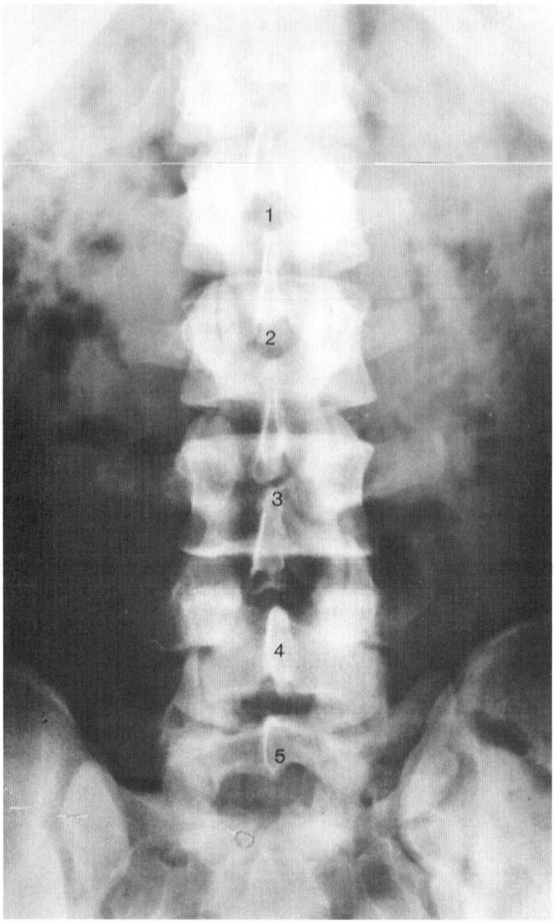

Figure 7.11 *Bertolotti's syndrome. Some surgeons would describe these segments as partial sacralization of L5; others would be tempted to number the segments differently (see Chapter 1 for a discussion of congenital lumbosacral anomalies).*

articulations that can develop degenerative changes (Fig. 7.12), it is rare that these changes are symptomatic,(4) and even rarer that they should be corrected surgically.

DISC DEGENERATION

In order to understand the pathogenesis of symptoms derived from degenerative disc disease, it is necessary to have a clear concept of the mechanical changes that may arise from breakdown of an intervertebral disc.(30)

The functional components of the intervertebral disc are described in Chapter 1, where it is indicated that the combination of the annulus (fibrous), nucleus pulposus (gelatinous), and hyaline cartilage plate makes for a very efficient coupling unit, provided all of the structures remain intact.

The natural aging process, with or without repeated minor episodes of trauma (the heavy worker), results in loss of the nuclear jelly (because of failure to reproduce the

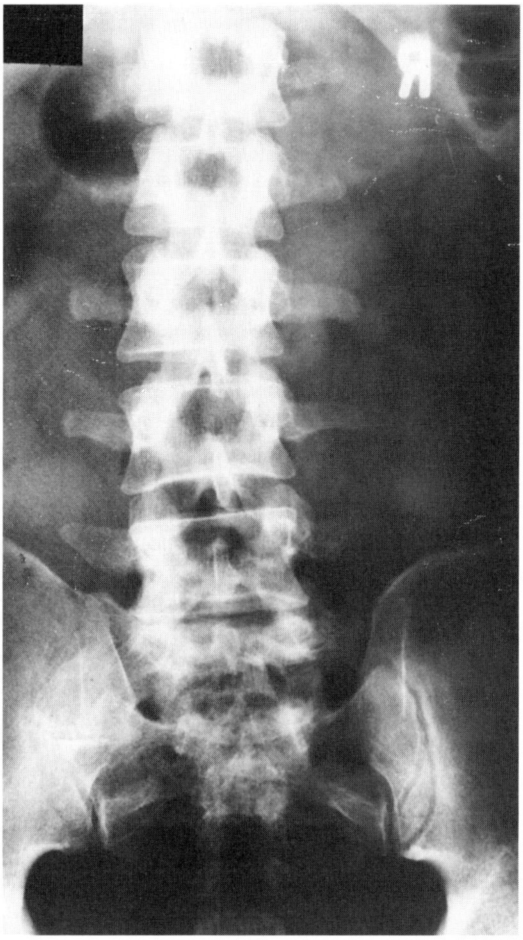

Figure 7.12 *Bertolotti's syndrome with apparent degenerative changes in articulation.*

degradated proteoglycans) and weakening of annular support (because of failure of the collagen linking).(11) This stage has been labeled by Kirkaldy-Willis et al as the phase of dysfunction.(13) With advancement of these degenerative changes, any one of the components of the disc loses its biomechanical integrity due to changes such as inspissation of the nucleus pulposus, a tear in the annulus, or a rupture of the hyaline cartilage plate. At this point, a cascading series of events occurs:

1. Fibroblasts fail to reproduce new collagen to replace degradated collagen in the annulus.
2. Chondrocytes fail to reproduce new proteoglycan to replace degradated proteoglycan in the nucleus.
3. Nutritional flow of glucose, O2, and sulfates to the disc is decreased.
4. These factors (in number 3) change disc metabolism negatively and likely decrease the pH within the disc.
5. The decrease in pH gives the upper hand to degrading enzymes (proteases), which further increases disc degeneration.

Swelling Pressure

Normally, the nucleus pulposus can take on water (swell) or release water (shrink), which allows for the balancing of mechanical loads (Fig. 7.13). With the cascading degenerative changes, the ability to move water in and out of the nucleus is impaired, and swelling pressures can no longer absorb the mechanical load. The balancing act (cushioning) of the disc is upset.

Disc stability or the smooth roller action is lost, and the movement between adjacent vertebral segments becomes uneven, excessive, and irregular. This is the stage of segmental instability, a term first proposed by Harris and Macnab,(9) and subsequently relabeled the dysfunctional stage by Kirkaldy-Willis.(13) Excessive degrees of flexion and extension are permitted, and a certain amount of backward and forward gliding movements occur as well.

Normally, on flexion of the spine, the discal borders of the vertebral bodies become parallel above the level of L5. This is the maximal movement permitted. In the stage of segmental instability, excessive degrees of extension and flexion are permitted, and a certain amount of backward and forward gliding movement occurs as well (Fig. 7.14).

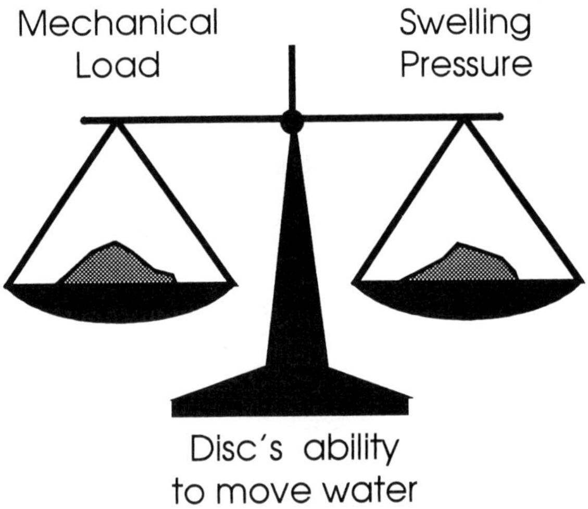

Figure 7.13 *A balancing act exists between mechanical load and swelling pressure; that is, when mechanical pressures increase, the disc gives up water to absorb the load; the reverse occurs when loads decrease (eg, at night when sleeping).*

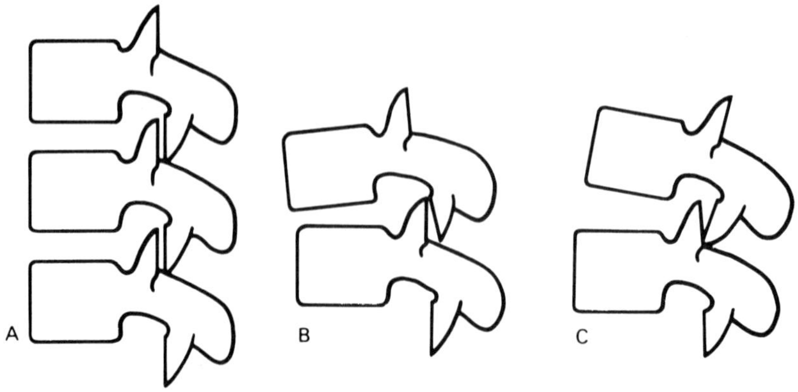

Figure 7.14 **A.** *In the early stages of degenerative disc disease, excessive degrees of flexion and extension are permitted at the involved segment. This abnormal mobility is associated with rocking of the posterior joints* **(B and C).** *From Macnab I: Backache. Williams & Wilkins, Baltimore (1977), p. 85.*

This abnormal type of movement can be shown by radiographs taken with the patients holding their spines in full extension and flexion. One problem posed by motion studies is the fact that, when a patient is in pain, the associated muscle guarding does not permit adequate flexion and extension radiographs to be taken. However, there are two radiological changes that are indicative of instability, Knuttson's phenomenon of gas in the disc (Fig. 7.15) and the "traction spur" (Fig. 7.16).

The traction spur differs anatomically and radiologically from other spondylophytes in that it projects horizontally and develops approximately 1 to 2 mm above the vertebral body edge.(15) It owes its development to the manner of attachment of the annulus fibers. In Chapter 1, the mode of attachment of the outermost fibers to the undersurface of the epiphysial ring is described. With abnormal movements, an excessive strain is applied to these outermost fibers, and it is here that the traction spur develops. It is the

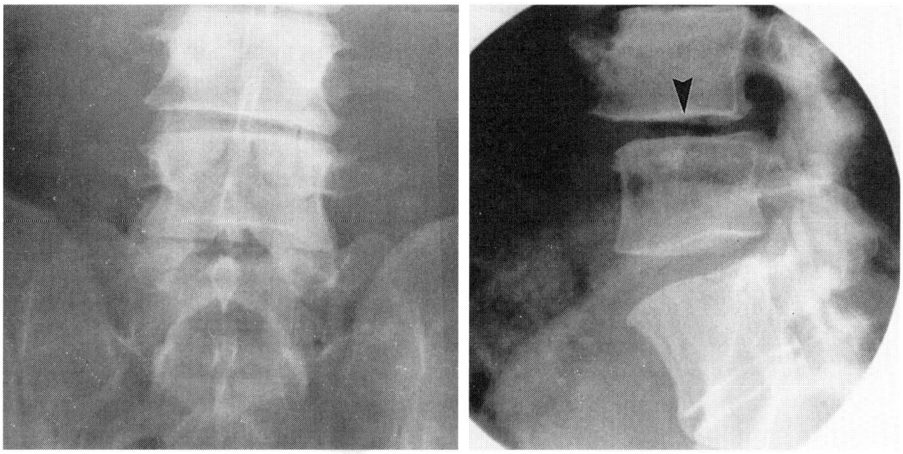

Figure 7.15 *Knuttson's phenomenon at a degenerative spondylolisthesis level.*

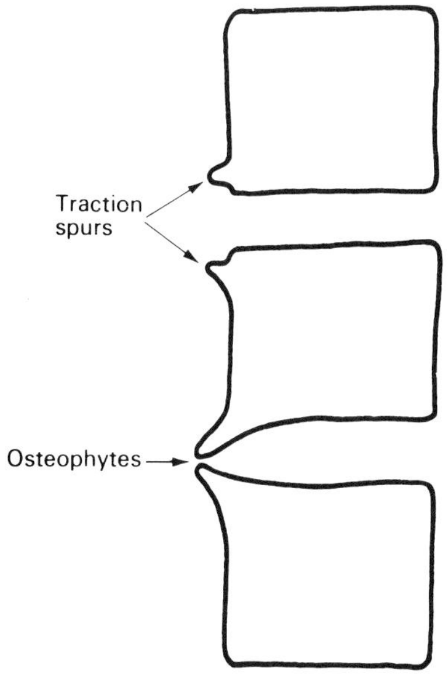

Figure 7.16 *The traction spur projects horizontally from the vertebral body about 1 mm away from the discal border. From Macnab I: Backache. Williams & Wilkins, Baltimore (1977), p. 86.*

small traction spur that is clinically significant in that it is probably indicative of present instability. The large traction spur indicates that this segment has been unstable at some time in the past, but it may be stable now because of fibrotic changes occurring within the disc.

Segmental instability, by itself, is probably not painful, but the spine is vulnerable to trauma. A forced and unguarded movement may be concentrated on the wobbly segment and produce a posterior joint strain or subluxation. Repeated injuries produce secondary degenerative changes in the capsule and cartilaginous surfaces of the facet joints.

The next stage of disc degeneration is segmental hyperextension. Extension of the lumbar spine is limited by the anterior fibers of the annulus. When degenerative changes cause these fibers to lose their elasticity, the involved segment or segments may hyperextend (Fig. 7.17).

A similar change may be seen in the next stage of disc degeneration, disc narrowing. As the intervertebral discs lose height, the posterior joints must override and subluxate, and vertebral body shifts occur (Fig. 7.18). In both segmental hyperextension and disc narrowing, the related posterior joints in normal posture are held in hyperextension, and this postural defect is exaggerated if the patient has weak abdominal muscles and/or tight tensors and is overweight.

When the posterior joints are held at the extreme of their limit of extension, there is no safety factor of movement, and the extension strains of everyday living may push the joints past their physiologically permitted limits and thereby produce pain. Eventually, the posterior joint may subluxate.

Repeated damage to the posterior joints, especially when associated with subluxation, will lead to degenerative changes. This is true osteoarthritis of the spine. Gross lipping to the vertebral bodies, often erroneously referred to as osteoarthritis of the spine, is merely a manifestation of disc degeneration (Fig. 7.19). Gross lipping may be present without associated degenerative changes in the posterior joints.

Figure 7.17 *When the anterior fibers of the annulus lose their elasticity, the involved segment falls into hyperextension permitting subluxation of the related posterior joint. From Macnab I: Backache. Williams & Wilkins, Baltimore (1977), p. 87.*

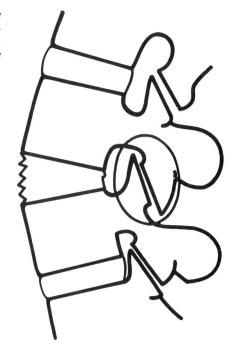

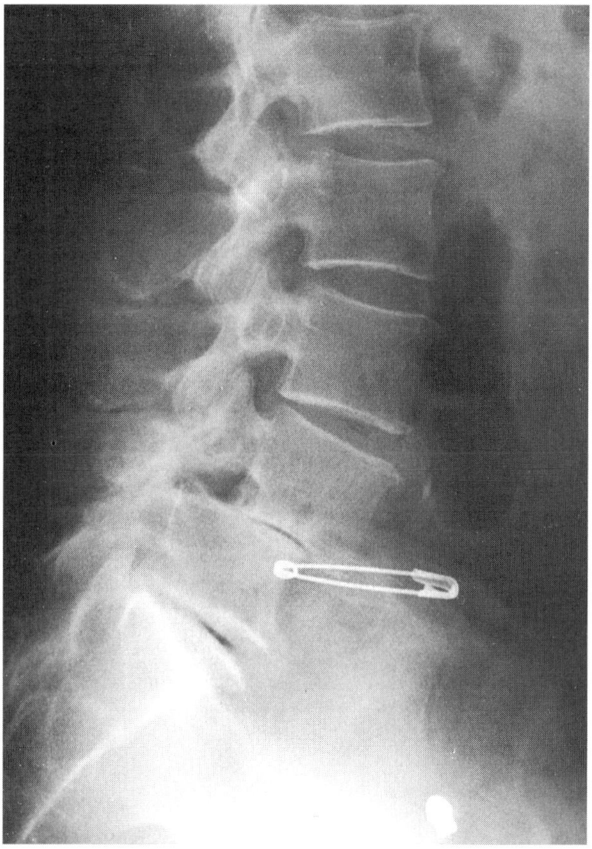

Figure 7.18 *At the level of the safety pin, there is a forward "slip" of L4 on L5 due to degenerative changes in the facet joints. (The safety pin was a radiologic marker, not a form of fixation for the slip!)*

So much for the morbid anatomical changes associated with disc degeneration. What is the relationship of these changes to the pain experienced? In attempting to answer this, some clinical observations must be noted.

Scoliosis (exclusive of secondary disc degeneration) rarely gives rise to significant back pain, even if left untreated, yet the lesion is associated with very gross posterior joint subluxation at many levels (except in mild idiopathic lumbar scoliosis).

On the premise that the majority of backaches have their first occurrence before the age of 40, the radiographs of 300 40-year-old laborers, who had been engaged in heavy work all their lives, were reviewed by Dr. Macnab. Of these, 150 had no history of low back pain, and 150 were under treatment for backache at the time of the review. A careful statistical analysis of the radiographs showed no difference in the incidence of anatomical variant and degenerative changes in the two groups studied. Indeed, some of the patients who had been employed in strenuous occupations all their lives without a twinge of back pain showed very marked degenerative changes on radiograph.

If every radiological sign of disc degeneration is given a numerical rating, and these numbers are added together to give an arbitrary "degenerative index," it can be shown that, although radiological evidence of degenerative disc disease shows a linear increase with advancing years, the incidence of backache has a peak at 45 and thereafter tends to decline (Fig 7.20).

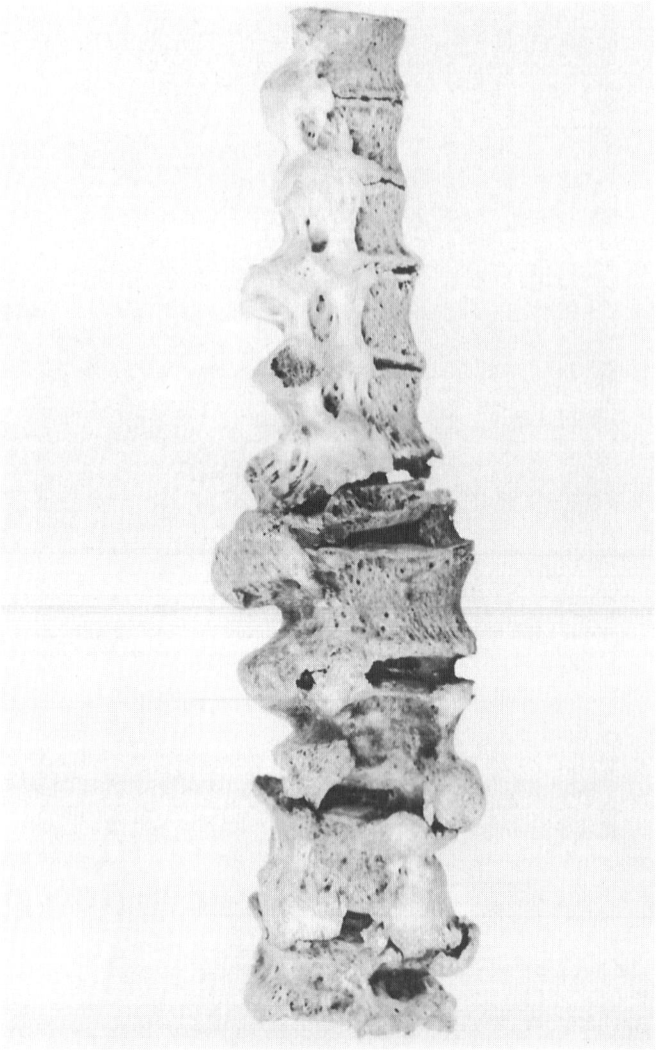

Figure 7.19 *Photograph of an excised lumbar spine showing the various bony outgrowths that are associated with disc degeneration. These bony outgrowths are correctly referred to as "spondylophytes." From Macnab I: Backache. Williams & Wilkins, Baltimore (1977), p. 89.*

A patient may be seen with severe low back pain, and radiographs taken may show evidence of disc degeneration with segmental instability and posterior joint subluxation. After a period of conservative therapy, the patient's pain subsides, and the he/she returns to heavy work. Follow-up radiographs show identical changes, even though the patient is completely symptom free. This observation serves as more evidence to show that the clinician should assess and treat patients' symptoms and not their radiographs.

On the other hand, it has been the experience of many clinicians that a patient previously incapacitated by low back pain, with radiological evidence of mechanical insufficiency of the spine due to disc degeneration, can, after a successful spinal fusion, return to

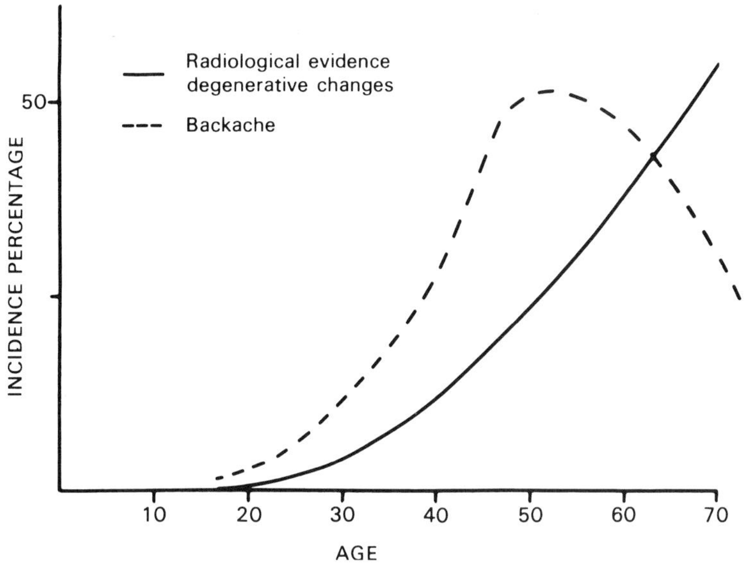

Figure 7.20 *Note from this graph that although the incidence of radiologically demonstrable degenerative changes in the lumbar spine increases with age, the maximal incidence of backache has a peak at 45 and thereafter tends to decline. From Macnab I: Backache. Williams & Wilkins, Baltimore (1977), p. 90.*

strenuous activities without pain. In such an instance, mechanical instability was surely the cause of the original disability.

With our present stage of knowledge, only the following may be stated: (1) Disc degeneration does occur as part of the aging process and often remains asymptomatic. (2) Disc degeneration may be associated with changes within the disc itself that may be productive of pain. (3) Disc degeneration may give rise to mechanical instability that renders the spine vulnerable to trauma, as a result of which pain may arise from ligamentous or posterior joint damage.

The pain experienced may remain localized to the back, or there may be both local pain and referred pain, or referred pain only. The experimental injection of hypertonic saline into the supraspinous ligament between D12 and L1 may give rise to pain referred to the low back and both buttocks and as low as the greater trochanter. A similar injection into the supraspinous ligament between L5 and S1 may give rise to buttock pain and pain referred down the leg. The pain referred down the leg in a sciatic distribution rarely goes below the knee, although on occasion it may extend to the ankle. Patients suffering from degenerative changes at the lumbodorsal or lumbosacral junction may present with pain referred in a similar manner.

Posterior joint damage produced by degenerative changes of the L4–L5 disc may also produce pain referred to the groin. It is important to emphasize the fact that pain down the leg associated with degenerative disc disease may indeed be referred pain, and the patient's complaint of "sciatica" does not necessarily mean that a nerve root is being compromised.

Degenerative disc disease may lead to nerve root compression under the following circumstances: disc ruptures, bony root entrapment, ligamentous root entrapment, and adhesive radiculitis.

Why Does Disc Degeneration Cause Pain?

The pain of spinal origin can be divided into two groups:

1. Pain originating from the bony column: specifically, its three-joint complex of disc and facet joints.
2. Pain arising as a consequence of direct involvement of the spinal nerve root (which will be discussed in the next section of this chapter). Other low back pains, such as those referred from the prevertebral visceral spaces, are not discussed in this chapter.

There continues to be controversy as to whether free nerve endings have a functional presence in spinal structures such as the annulus. Everyone would agree that the deeper annular-nuclear portion of the disc is not innervated. It is well established that the posterior longitudinal ligament is richly supplied with nociceptor fibers from the sinuvertebral nerve. More recently, Yoshizawa et al (30) and Malinsky (16) have solved the controversy by very definitely demonstrating various types of encapsulated and unencapsulated pain receptors in the outer aspect of all of the annulus. The sources of these fibers have been further documented by Malinsky (16) and include the sinuvertebral nerve, the ventral rami, and the sympathetic gray rami communicantes (Fig. 7.2).

Because it has been extremely difficult to demonstrate nerve fibers in the outer annulus, it is likely that the annulus is reinnervated as the body grows older and as the process of disc degeneration occurs. It is well known that a disc is avascular during most of its adult life, but the disc does become vascularized as it degenerates. Perhaps a similar reaction occurs with nerve supply to the annulus.

Free nerve endings are also present in (1) the fibrous capsule of the facet joint, (2) the sacroiliac joints, (3) the anterior aspect of the dura, (4) the periosteum, (5) the vertebral bodies, and (6) the blood vessel walls. Theoretically, the presence of these nociceptors implies that a stimulus to these areas will be transmitted as a pain impulse. Although this appears to be a simple conclusion, it is not supported by any surgeon who has operated on the spine under local anesthesia and who has palpated the annulus without reproducing pain. In addition, discography can be done in a normal disc, with tremendous pressures placed on the disc, and yet no appreciation of pain on the part of the patient. Thus, the simple presence of these nociceptors does not explain how pain arises in a spinal segment. Further work has to be done with regard to: (1) chemical changes that occur with disc degeneration, and (2) the influence of abnormal movement.

DISC RUPTURES

In 1934, Mixter and Barr (18) suggested that sciatic pain could result from irritation of a lumbar nerve root by a prolapsed intervertebral disc. Although skeptically received at first, this concept soon became universally accepted and founded the "dynasty of the disc," during which time the complaint of sciatic pain tended to become uncritically equated with the diagnosis of disc herniation. Surgical exploration of patients with evidence of lumbar root irritation had revealed the fact that there are indeed several sources of nerve root compromise, of which a ruptured intervertebral disc is but one example.

The term "herniated disc" tends to be used so loosely now as to lose much of its clinical significance and, indeed, there has been confusion in terminology (Table 7.2). Sometimes, the operative note will state with disarming simplicity, "a disc was found." The height of absurdity was the introduction of the term "concealed disc" (5) to describe a herniated disc that could not be demonstrated at operation. One can imagine the confusion that would result if the term "concealed appendix" was considered an adequate explanation of a negative laparotomy. To avoid further confusion, therefore, it is perhaps advisable to define the pathological state implied by the term "disc rupture."

The exact mechanism of a disc rupture has not been demonstrated, but it is a common misconception that a disc rupture consists of an extrusion of nuclear material through an annular defect much like toothpaste exuding through a hole in the side of a toothpaste tube. Operative experience belies this impression. It is unusual at surgery to find a disc herniation consisting solely of extravasated nuclear material exuding through a defect in the annulus. The protrusion, extrusion, or sequestration always consists of a varying amount of nucleus, annulus, and cartilage plate.

In an attempt to avoid the confusion of terminology, it is suggested that the following classification be considered. Disc ruptures can be defined as a focal distortion of the normal anatomical configuration of the annulus. Two major pathological states are to be distinguished: contained disc protrusions and noncontained disc herniations (Table 7.3) (Fig. 7.21). Throughout this discussion you will note we move back and forth between the terminology "ligamentous" (eg, transligamentous) and "annular" (eg, subannular). In fact, at L4–5 and L5–S1, the posterior longitudinal ligament is very narrow, and the structures that contain nuclear material are the annular fibers.

Contained Disc Protrusions

Normally, the annulus fibrosus forms a smooth, continuous ring confining the nucleus pulposus. A protrusion is a localized or focal disc bulge with the annular fibers still continuous and maintaining their Sharpey's fiber attachments to the vertebral body (Fig. 7.22).

This "focal" alteration of disc architecture is to be distinguished from disc collapse (degeneration), with the annulus circumferentially bulging beyond the peripheral rim of the vertebral bodies (Fig. 7.23). The appearance is as though the disc has been made of putty

Table 7.2. Synonyms for 'Herniated Disc'

Herniated disc	Protruding disc
Prolapsed disc	Bulging disc
Sequestrated disc	Ruptured disc
Soft disc	Extruded disc
Slipped disc	'Disc'

Table 7.3. Types of Disc Herniations

Contained
1. protrusions
2. subligamentous (subannular) extrusion

Noncontained
3. transligamentous extrusion
4. sequestered

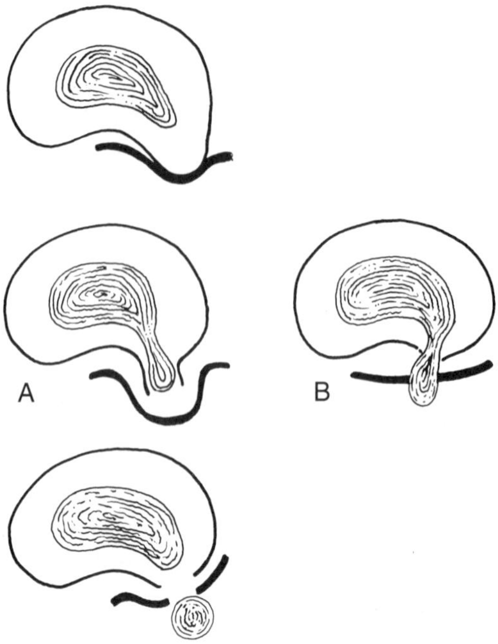

Figure 7.21 *There are two basic types of disc herniations, contained and noncontained. Top row: protrusion (contained); middle row:* **(A)** *Extrusion: subannular (contained);* **(B)** *Extrusion: transannular (noncontained); bottom row: sequestered (noncontained).*

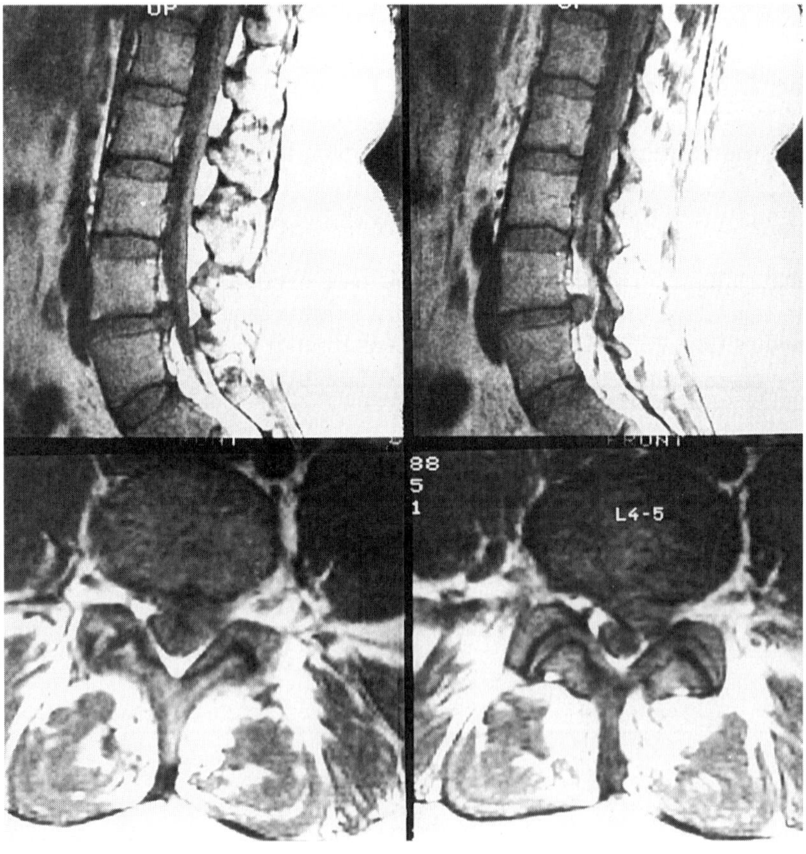

Figure 7.22 *MRI of a disc protrusion. These views are all from a T1 protocol, with two adjacent sagittal slices (top) and two adjacent axial slices (bottom) showing an apparent contained disc herniation in the first story of the 4th anatomic segment. Note the "focal" prominence of the disc herniation.*

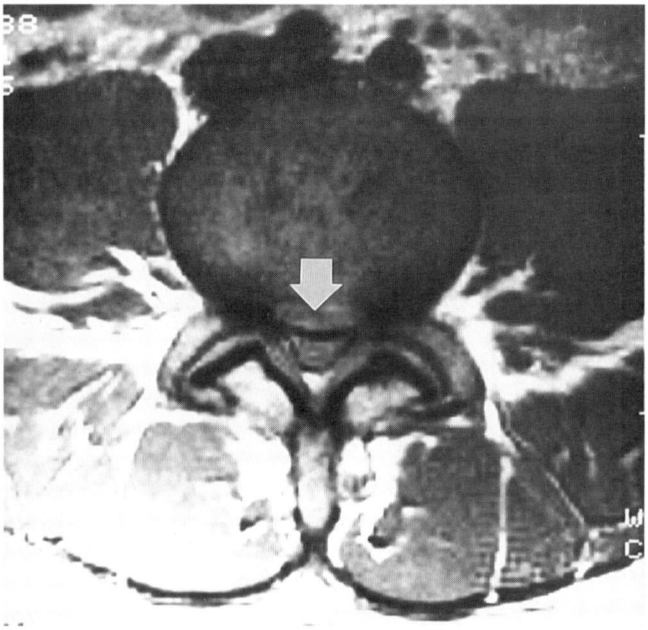

Figure 7.23 *A diffuse annular bulge on T1 axial MRI (arrow) adds to a spinal stenosis of L4–5.*

and the vertebral bodies have been compressed together: the middle-aged spread of a middle-aged disc. The annular fibers remain intact, and at surgery, when a square window is cut in the former, (focal protrusion), the nucleus will spontaneously extrude, whereas in non–focal, diffuse annular bulging, an annular window will not be followed by spontaneous expulsion of disc material.

Subligamentous (Subannular) Extrusion

The displaced nuclear material is still confined by a few of the outermost fibers of the annulus and, if not appreciated beforehand, these fragments can be missed at surgery. The disc herniation has traveled up behind the vertebral body or down behind the vertebral body below (Fig. 7.24). The most common migratory pattern for a disc extrusion is caudally to lie behind the vertebral body below. Disc herniations that rupture in a cephalad direction are more often sequestered than extruded fragments.

Noncontained Disc Herniations

Disruptions of the annular fibers, whether in their body or at the attachment to the vertebral body margin, will permit extrusion, or sequestration, of nuclear material. In an adult practice, the most common material to herniate is the nuclear material, but as mentioned earlier, annulus and endplate may be included in the ruptured fragment (Fig. 7.25). The inclusion of endplate usually occurs in younger patients and is typical of a juvenile type of disc rupture. After detachment of a segment of the cartilage plate and/or disruption of the posterior annular fibers, a portion of the annulus, along with nuclear material, may be displace posteriorly. Two types of noncontained disc herniations can be

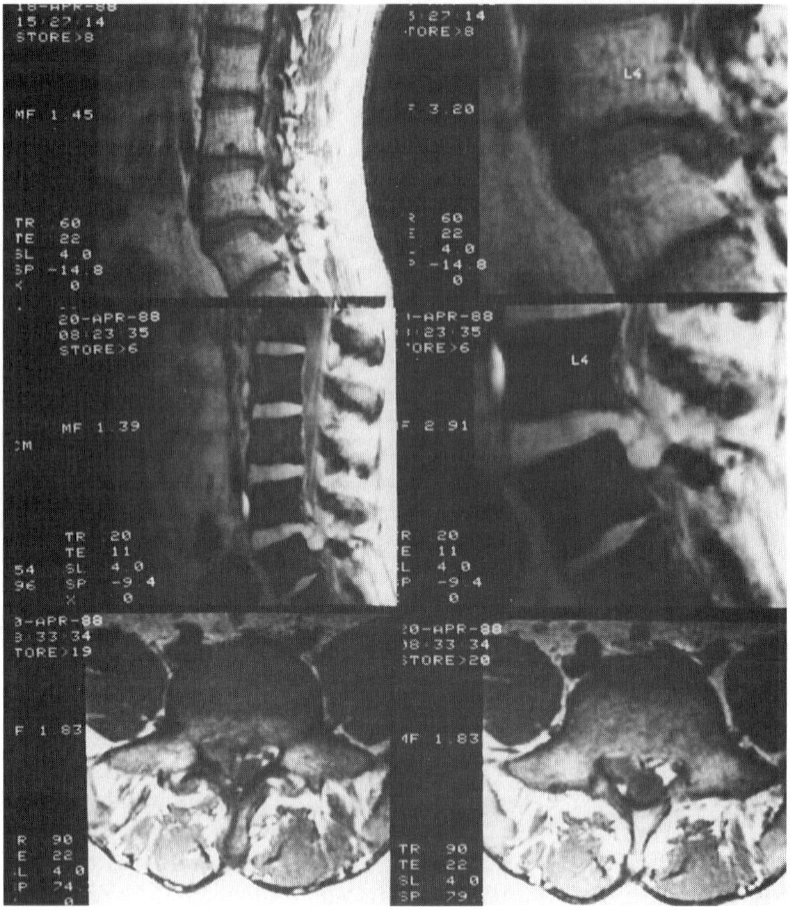

Figure 7.24 *MRI showing a subligamentous disc extrusion from L4-5 to lie in the third story of L5.*

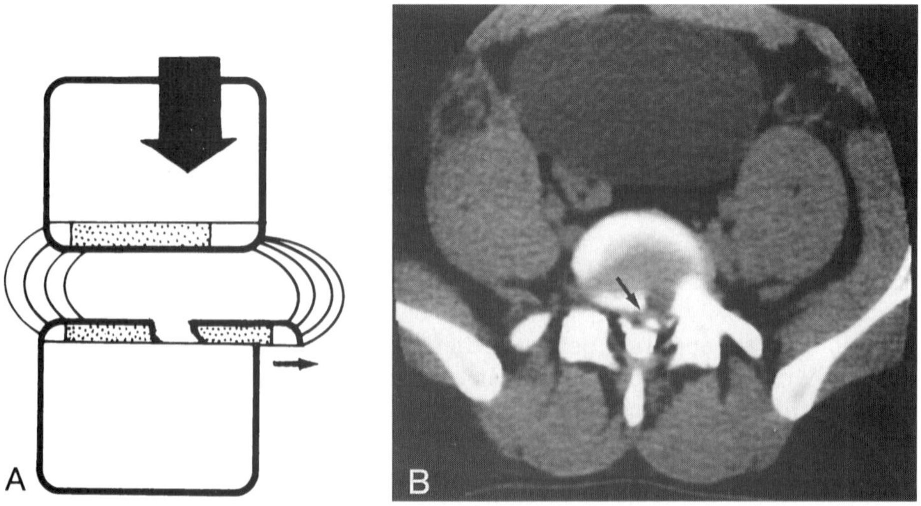

Figure 7.25 **A.** *Disc rupture with piece of endplate included (arrow).* **B.** *CT showing fragment of endplate (L5-S1, left).*

recognized, depending on the extent of the displacement of the nuclear material and where it lies relative to the annular/posterior longitudinal ligament complex.

Transligamentous (Transannular) Extrusion

In this lesion, the displaced nuclear material has burst through the posterior fibers of the annulus and the posterior longitudinal ligament to lie in the spinal canal (Fig. 7.26). However, there is still a connection between this extruded discal material and the disc space cavity. If the extrusion remains in its abnormal position long enough, a very thin membrane may form over it, in the body's attempt to separate the discal material from the neurological structures. This flimsy membrane is not to be confused with annular fibers or posterior longitudinal ligament.

Sequestered Intervertebral Disc

Nuclear material has not only ruptured through the annular/posterior longitudinal ligamentous complex, it has completely separated itself from the nuclear cavity, and the discal fragment lies free in the spinal canal. Characteristically, these disc herniations are either extremely large or have migrated away from the disc space. Discal material can travel posteriorly to lie posterior to the nerve root. Sequestered disc herniations can also travel caudally to lie behind the vertebral body below (Fig. 7.27). A sequestered disc herniation is a common description in surgical pathology; in fact, it does not occur as commonly as disc extrusions. On occasion, the freed portion of the disc may erode or burst through the dura. This is more likely to happen in a patient who has had a previous surgery for a disc herniation and who suffers a sudden rerupture of the same disc on the same side. Because of the scarring of the dura around the root to the disc space, a transdural discal herniation may occur.

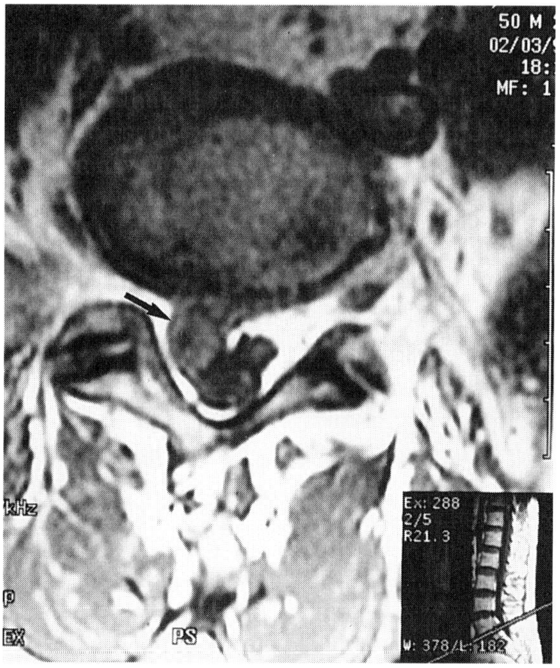

Figure 7.26 *A transannular (or pedunculated) disc rupture (arrow) on T1 axial at L5–S1.*

Figure 7.27 *A sequestered disc lying behind the vertebral body of L2 (arrow). Did you see anything else on the T1 sagittal MRI? (Do not tell us you missed the degenerative spondylolisthesis at L4–L5?)*

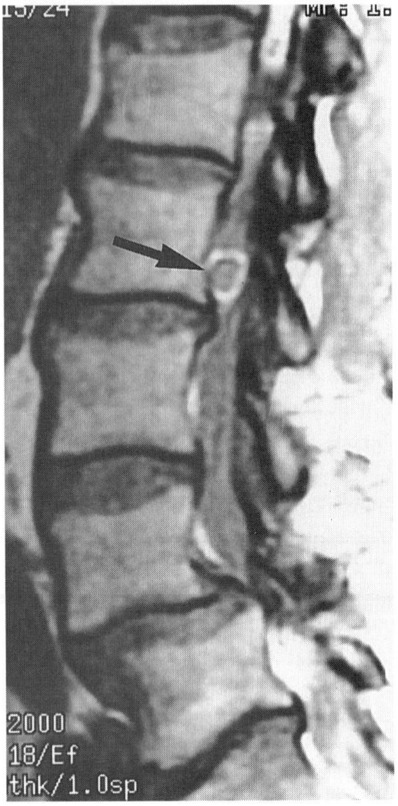

Intradiscal Rupture (Internal Disc Disruption)

This is largely a theoretical concept. It is believed that on occasion the innermost fibers of the annulus will rupture, with degeneration of nuclear material producing an autoimmune reaction within the disc space. This distention within the nuclear space may produce pain. Unfortunately, this condition is revealed by discography, and when found, can lead to surgery.

Nature of Ruptured Disc Material

Of equal importance to the location of a disc fragment is the nature of the fragment (Table 7.4). Disc protrusions tend to be more proteoglycan-like disc herniations, just as sequestered discs are almost always collagenous fragments of discal material. In between, the extruded disc herniation can have various combinations of proteoglycan and collagen, although the predominant makeup is collagenous in nature).

Table 7.4. Nature of the Herniated Nuclear Fragment (Fig. 7.33)

Mass of nuclear material
Distention (by proteoglycan and water) within the mass
Inflammation between the mass and nerve root

Clinical Presentation of the Sequestered/Extruded Disc

After consecutively reviewing 50 patients who had surgically documented sequestered or extruded discs, the senior author (JM) found no clinical pattern by history or physical presentation that allows for the prediction of a sequestered/extruded disc. It has become obvious that the diagnosis of a sequestered/extruded disc is more a neuroradiological assessment based on the following four radiological criteria:

1. Size: A disc herniation that occupies more than 50% of the spinal canal in any one direction (usually sagittal) has a high likelihood of being sequestered (Fig. 7.28).
2. Shape: A pedunculated disc herniation (long sagittal dimension and narrow coronal dimension) has a high likelihood of being sequestered/extruded (Fig. 7.26).
3. Location: A disc herniation that lies behind the vertebral body, above or below the disc space, or out in the foramen, is likely to be a sequestered/extruded disc (Figs. 7.27 and 7.29).
4. Artifact: A disc herniation that contains air (nitrogen gas) is likely to be a sequestered/extruded fragment (Fig. 7.30).

PATHOGENESIS OF SYMPTOMS RESULTING FROM DISC RUPTURES

There is no clear, single explanation as to why a disc rupture causes sciatica. Some disc ruptures remain asymptomatic. Many years ago, it was noted that on routine screening of the lumbar spine when performing myelography for disease elsewhere, 37% of patients were shown to have a significant defect in the lumbar spine.(10) Most myelographic defects were at L4–5, and all were asymptomatic. More recent CT and MRI studies have bolstered this concept.(3, 29)

In trying to understand the back and leg complaints of a patient with a herniated nucleus pulposus (HNP), a few things are clear. The patient's major complaint is pain. Yet, physical pressure on a peripheral nerve does not produce pain; it produces paresthesia. In examining this problem further, at the conclusion of routine laminectomy for HNP, Macnab instituted placement of a Fogarty catheter underneath the emerging nerve root of a segment above. When the patients had regained consciousness, and before they had been

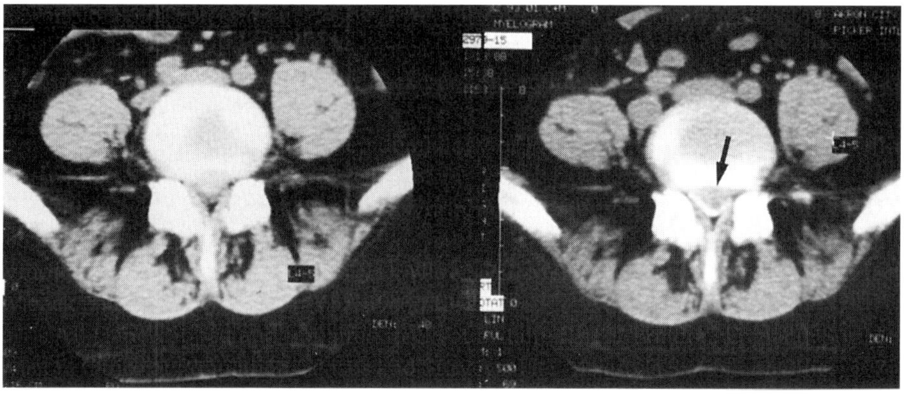

Figure 7.28 *CT/myelogram showing HNP fragment occupying more than 50% of canal (arrow)—a high likelihood that the disc is sequestered/extruded.*

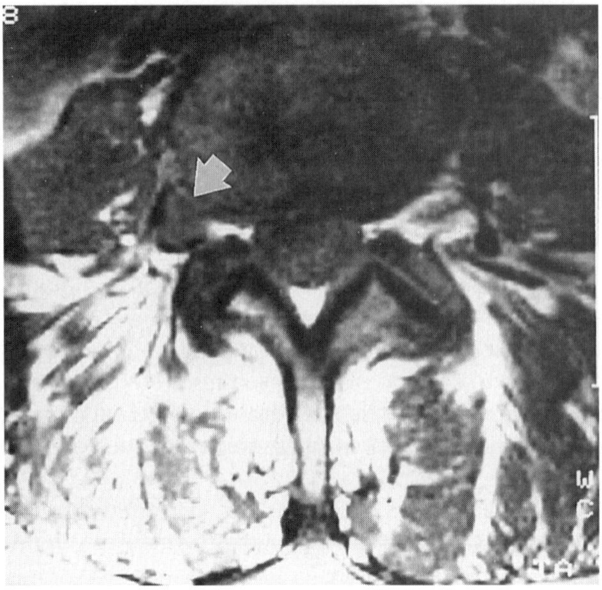

Figure 7.29 *A foraminal disc herniation (white arrow) on T1 axial MRI.*

Figure 7.30 **A.** *CT/myelogram showing HNP with "air" in fragment (arrow).* **B.** *CT/myelogram, next slice down, showing larger fragment in the third story of L5 with "air" present in fragment (arrow) almost certainly an extruded or sequestered disc.*

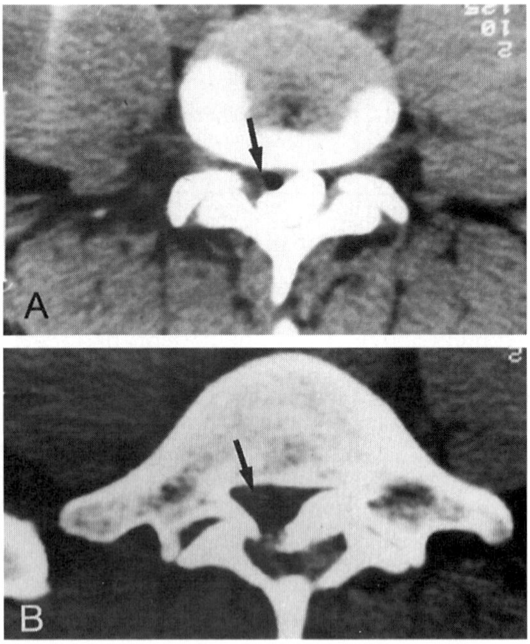

given any analgesics, the catheters were distended. It was found that although distention of the catheter underneath an involved, angry, red, inflamed nerve root reproduced the sciatic pain, distention of the catheter underneath the normal nerve root produced paresthesia only.

It is likely that no one neuromechanical theory can explain the mechanism of symptom production in an HNP.(6) In the routine consideration of simple sciatica, there are many clinical observations that are not easy to explain:

1. The description of sciatica from patient to patient is so variable that there are obviously many factors involved in the production of symptoms.
2. In the early phases of a disc herniation (a few hours to a few days), a patient may report only back pain immediately after the "snap" sensation heralding the disc rupture. During this time, leg pain is absent as a symptom; root tension (straight leg raising [SLR] reduction) is present as a sign; and the results of the CT or MRI, if done, will be positive.
3. Some patients in the early phases of sciatica will report only paresthesia, which gives rise to an irritating, diffuse, ill-localized numbness in the lower leg and foot.
4. Patients with an HNP have more pain and more SLR reduction than those patients with lateral zone stenosis, yet the latter group of patients have more root encroachment. Rupture a piece of disc into a root that is already squashed in a narrowed subarticular gutter, and you have a patient with incredible leg pain, reasonable SLR ability, and neurological symptoms and signs (Fig. 7.31).
5. Young patients with an HNP have a lower incidence of neurological findings than the average 40-year-old patient with an HNP.
6. The average 40-year-old patient with an HNP is more likely to have neurological changes than the older patient with lateral zone stenosis whose nerve root is usually severely compromised in the subarticular zone.
7. A patient with a foraminal disc herniation has the most severe pain of all; this phenomenon raises the question as to the mechanism of pain production when a disc herniation lies on the dorsal root-ganglion.(28)
8. It has been documented that patients undergoing myelography, CT, or MRI, after bed rest has relieved sciatica, may still have a positive study results. This phenomenon had been reported up to 15 months after sciatica has disappeared.(6)
9. In some patients undergoing successful chemonucleolysis, the CT scan defect has persisted despite relief of symptoms and recovery from nerve root tension and compression (19) (Fig. 7.32).
10. Infrequently, a patient presents with the sudden onset of severe leg pain, which is quickly followed by a profound neurological lesion (eg, drop foot), followed by an

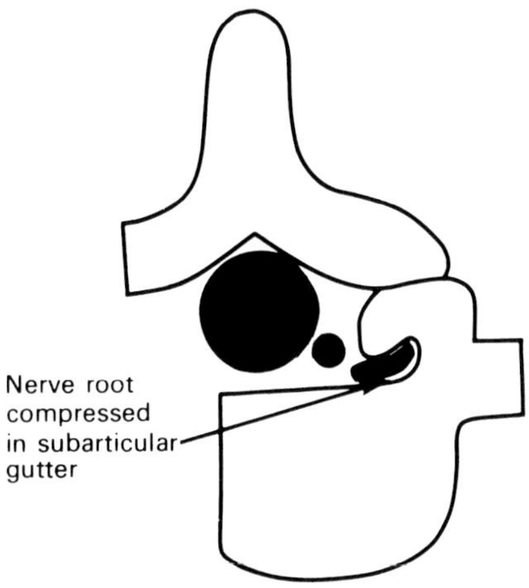

Figure 7.31 *The nerve root as it courses through the subarticular gutter may be compressed between a hypertrophied arthritic posterior joint and the dorsum of the vertebral body. From Macnab I: Backache. Williams & Wilkins, Baltimore (1977), p. 100.*

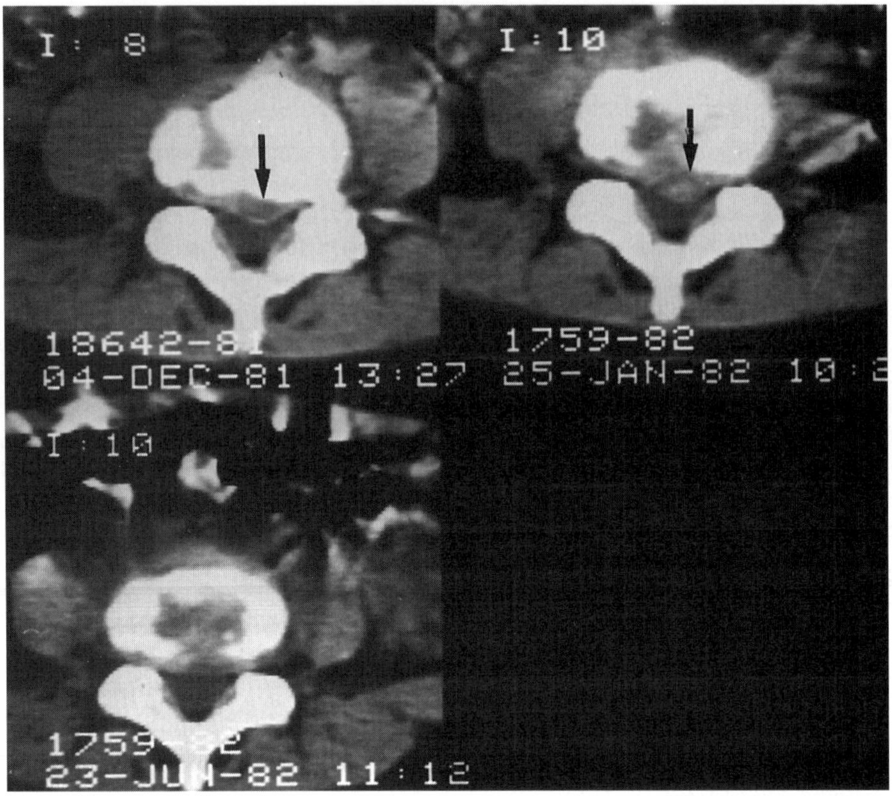

Figure 7.32 *CT before and after chemonucleolysis: Top left, before chymopapain. HNP, L4-5, left (arrow). Top right, 1 month after chemonucleolysis. Leg pain has been relieved but the CT scan defect is still evident (arrow). Bottom left, 6 months after chemonucleolysis. No further treatment, no further symptoms; the defect has gone.*

equally dramatic disappearance of pain and root tension in a few hours to a few days. Prolonged observation of these patients often reveals a significant degree of neurological recovery.

11. Pain is an unpleasant emotional state. So much depends on past experiences of the patient and his/her emotional state and needs at the time of discomfort (see Chapter 12).
12. If a patient with diabetes is unfortunate enough to also develop an HNP, the degree of pain experienced is often so much more than usual. Are the diabetic patient's nerves extra sensitive to compression factors?

Although it is impossible to answer all of these questions, many research attempts are being made to try and explain the pathogenesis of sciatica. There are a number of factors involved, but three major factors have to be considered:

1. The nature of the compression by the disc herniation on the nerve root structure.
2. Where on the root-ganglion the compromise is occurring.
3. The ultimate pathological changes that occur in the nerve root, which in turn depend on pre-existing conditions (eg, an osteophyte, and the patient's age).

Nature of the Herniated Nuclear Fragment

Three subfactors need to be considered: (1) the presence of a mass adjacent to the nerve root, (2) the distension within that mass, and (3) the inflammatory interface produced by the distended mass lying adjacent to the nerve root (Table 7.4; Fig. 7.33).

Mass

As evidenced by the human experiment with the Fogarty catheter, the simple presence of a mass is not enough to produce sciatica. If the mass is present long enough, it is likely that it will set up an inflammatory reaction in the interface between the ruptured discal material and the nerve root.

Distention within the Mass

If you had your choice between a cotton ball or a hard golf ball pressing on your nerve root, you would surely pick the former because of the softness and diffuseness of the pressure. However, distend the mass with proteoglycans binding water, and in your mind you can just feel the pain increasing. The proteoglycan-water distending nature of the disc herniation serves as a hydraulic piston increasing and decreasing its pressure on the nerve root according to mechanical stimulation. At surgery, we have exposed a large disc protrusion and have noted the glistening sheen of distention present. We have then injected these discs with chymopapain, before annular incision, and the sheen of distention immediately disappears; the mass of disc protrusion, although still present, is obviously less distended and softer on palpation. Further, we have observed patients in a number of documented cases in which after chemonucleolysis symptoms and signs have been totally relieved, yet a mass still persists on CT scan (17) (Fig. 7.32). This is no different from the persistence of a myelographic defect reported by Falconer et al (6) 47 years ago and represents the "cotton ball" mass pressing on a nerve root that may be minor enough not to cause symptoms.

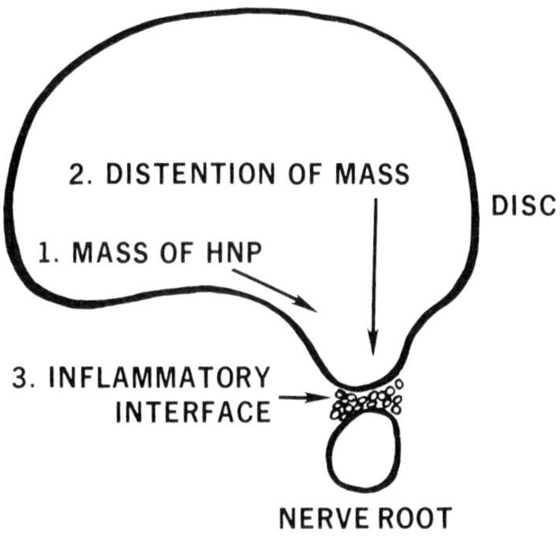

Figure 7.33 *The three local factors responsible for nerve root compression and irritation: 1, mass of HNP; 2, distention within mass; 3, the inflammatory interface between disc herniation and nerve root.*

Inflammation

Nachemson (20) has shown that the pH at the interface between a disc herniation and a nerve root is abnormal; Weinstein (28) has stated that others have isolated noxious chemicals from the area. All of these abnormal factors serve as early indicators that there is some alteration in the chemistry of the region as a direct consequence of disc material lying adjacent to nerve roots. Evidence of this inflammatory component is the reddened, inflamed nerve root seen at surgery.

Anatomical Location of the Pressure on the Root-Ganglion

The potential anatomical locations for pressure of an HNP are:

1. Cauda equina.
2. Single root.
   a. Motor.
   b. Sensory.
3. Sympathetic fibers.
4. Dorsal root-ganglion (28)

Two things are apparent. First, patients who have a foraminal disc herniation with implied direct pressure on the dorsal root-ganglion tend to have more severe pain than do patients with any other type of disc herniation. Second, many patients describe a change in temperature with their sciatic discomfort, which implicates some upset in vascular tone that is almost certainly due to stimulation of the sympathetic nervous system (some experts might argue that the sympathetic chain ends at L1–L2, and there are no sympathteic fibers in the lower lumbar roots. The frequent occurrence of "coldness" as a symptom in disc ruptures signifies that some sympathetic fibers in the area are being irritated).

Dorsal Root-Ganglion

There is a very large potential role for an irritated dorsal root-ganglion to modulate pain in low back disorders. The effect may arise through direct irritation from an HNP or indirect stimulation through some unknown mechanism. Weinstein (28) has called the dorsal root-ganglion the "brain" of the motion segment.

The net effect of ganglion irritation is the release of neuroactive peptide (eg, substance P) (24) that has long been identified as a resident compound of the dorsal ganglion. Only recently has an increase in retrievable substance P been documented upon vibratory stimulation. (28) This phenomenon is secondary to stimulation of unmyelinated and thinly myelinated fibers.

Ultimate Pathological Changes

Obviously, the compression of nerve tissue by a disc rupture upsets normal neural function and thus produces symptoms. Nerve function is dependent on the adequate supply of oxygen and other nutrients by way of the intraneural microcirculation. It is most likely that one of the significant events in the pathogenesis of sciatica is the primary upset in vascular supply to a nerve root, with the secondary phenomenon of interference with nerve root nutrition, both of which upset neurophysiological function.

Nerve roots are different from peripheral nerves in two respects (22):

1. Nerve roots do not have the protective connective tissue covering of a peripheral nerve; for example, the dura substitutes for epineurium, the cerebrospinal fluid substitutes for perineurium.
2. The microcirculation of a radicular nerve is provided through surface arteries. Radicular nerves come from both a proximal and distal direction, with an anastomotic zone that is vulnerable to a decrease in blood flow. Using the vital microscope and direct observation, Rydevick et al (24) have shown that compression and tension of a nerve root decreases its blood supply. This results in changes in intraneural blood, an increase in vascular permeability that results in edema, and an upset in axonal transport. If these changes are long-standing, intraneural fibrosis ultimately occurs.

Myelinated fibers are more susceptible to this distortion; these fibers demonstrate wallerian degeneration if enough pressure for enough time has been brought to bear upon a nerve root.

Neurophysiology

In the end, there is a decreased capacity of the nerve root to transmit impulses. There may also be hyperexcitability and generation of ectopic activity. This results in the numerous symptoms that occur in sciatica, including pain, tingling, pins and needles, and weakness.

Summary

Considering that: (1) ruptured nuclear material may compress motor, sensory, and sympathetic fibers, or the dorsal root-ganglion; (2) the effect of an HNP on a nerve root can be compression, tension, or inflammation, separately or together; and (3) with time, the pathological changes in a nerve root can be inflammation, edema, intraneural fibrosis, demyelination, axonal degeneration and regeneration; it is thus easy to understand that there is no one cause of sciatica nor is there one classic presentation of sciatica. Sciatica due to an HNP has many faces.

Other Modes of Nerve Root Compression

A ruptured intervertebral disc is not the only cause of nerve root irritation in association with disc degeneration in the lumbar spine. Clinicians gradually became aware of the fact that bony overgrowth in the lumbar spinal canal or lateral recess can produce compression of the emerging nerve roots. Verbiest (25) coined the term "spinal stenosis." Soon, like the earlier "dynasty of the disc" theory, this diagnosis became indiscriminately employed as a pathology garbage can to describe the pathogenesis of any form of leg pain not attributable to a disc rupture.

Spinal stenosis is defined as a narrowing of the spinal canal that may produce a bony-soft tissue constriction of the cauda equina and the emerging nerve roots. This bony-soft tissue encroachment may in turn produce symptoms. The bony-soft tissue constraint can be considered anatomically as being either lateral in the canal (giving rise to compression of the emerging nerve roots), or midline (giving rise to compression of the cauda equina), or both simultaneously. These constraints may be congenital (developmental) or acquired in origin. Most cases are probably a combination of the two etiologies. This condition is described in great detail in Chapter 17.

Bony compression of the emerging nerve roots may arise as a result of subarticular entrapment, pedicular kinking, or foraminal impingement due to posterior facet joint subluxation.

Subarticular Entrapment

The nerve roots course downward and outward, passing underneath the medial border of the superior articular facets before they swing around the pedicle to emerge through the foramen. Hypertrophy of the superior articular facet may compress the nerve root between the facet and the dorsal aspect of the vertebral body (Fig. 7.34).

Pedicular Kinking

When advanced intervertebral disc degeneration is associated with marked asymmetric narrowing of the disc, the tilting of the vertebral body may on occasion kink the emerging nerve root (Fig. 7.35). Commonly, however, the nerve root is seen to be compressed in a gutter formed by a diffuse lateral bulge of the disc and the pedicle above (Fig. 7.36).

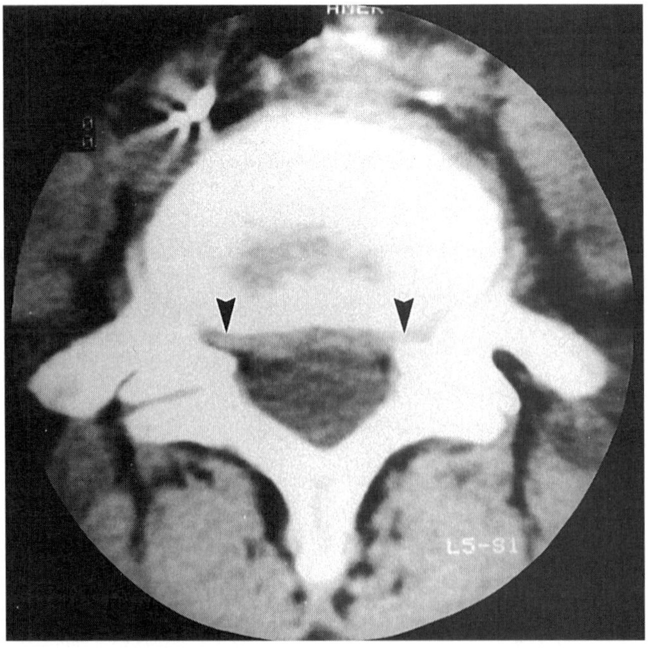

Figure 7.34 *A CT scan showing bilateral subarticular stenosis at L5–S1 (arrows).*

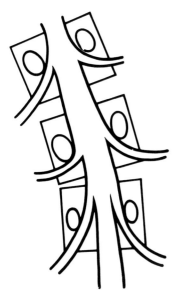

Figure 7.35 *With asymmetrical collapse of the disc and tilting of the vertebral body, the nerve root may be kinked by the pedicle giving rise to severe compression. From Macnab I: Backache. Williams & Wilkins, Baltimore (1977), p. 100.*

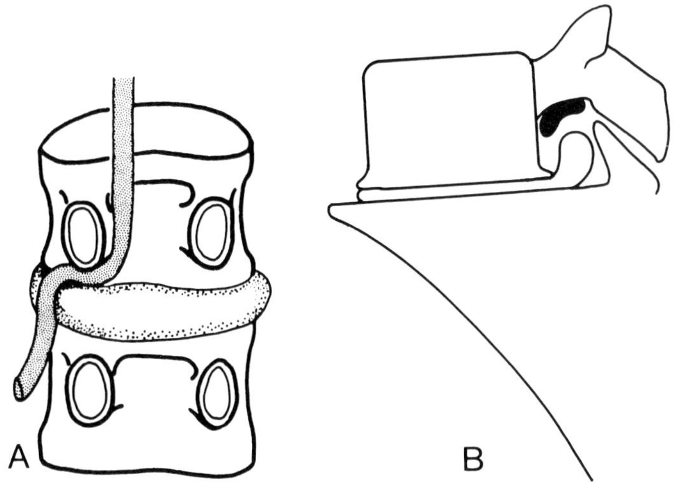

Figure 7.36 **A.** *In patients suffering from pedicular kinking of the nerve root, it is very common to find at operation that the nerve root is trapped in a gutter formed between a diffuse lateral bulge of the disc and the pedicle above. From Macnab I: Backache. Williams & Wilkins, Baltimore (1977), p. 101.* **B.** *Sagittal schematic of fig. 7.22A, depicting disc space narrowing, lateral and superior bulging of disc to compress the nerve root in the lateral zone.*

Foraminal Encroachment

As the root emerges through the foramen, it lies in close relation to the tip of the superior facet of the vertebra below. As the intervertebral disc narrows, the posterior joint overrides, and the root may, on occasion, be compressed by the superior articular facet (Fig. 7.37).

Midline Compression

Midline compression may be a sequel of disc degeneration when, after narrowing of the intervertebral disc, the spinal canal is constricted by the presence of a diffuse annular bulge, anterior buckling of the ligamentum flavum, and shingling of the laminae posteriorly. This constraint may be further aggravated by overgrowth of the arthritic posterior joints that may, indeed, also encroach on the midline (Fig. 7.38).

Forward displacement of the laminae seen in degenerative spondylolisthesis and the thickening of the lamina seen in certain pathological states, such as fluoridosis and occasionally Paget's disease, may produce a posterior encroachment of the spinal canal. Any technique of spinal fusion that involves decortication of the laminae, with or without the addition of a bone graft, may produce a diffuse hypertrophy of the posterior elements, which leads to constriction of the spinal canal. Postfusion spinal stenosis is, of course, more likely to occur if, before surgery, the patient was suffering either from a congenital

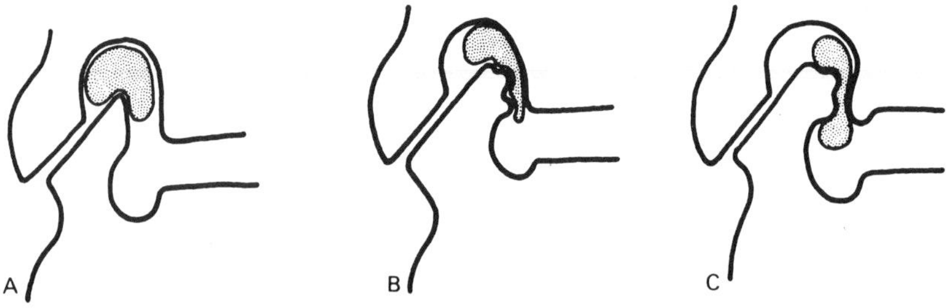

Figure 7.37 *The nerve root may be trapped in the foramen. It may be compressed between the tip of a subluxated facet and the pedicle above* **(A)**; *it may be compressed by osteophytic outgrowths on the superior articular facet* **(B)**; *or it may be compressed between the facet and the dorsal aspect on the vertebral body* **(C)**. *From Macnab I: Backache. Williams & Wilkins, Baltimore (1977), p. 101.*

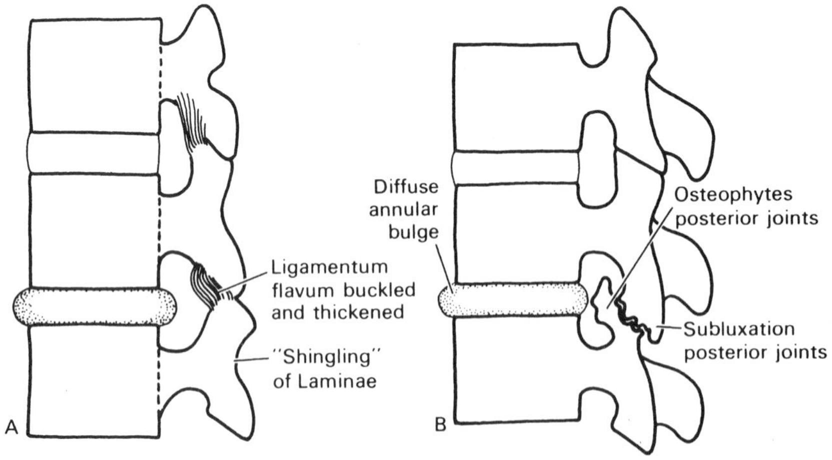

Figure 7.38 *In degenerative spinal stenosis, the spinal canal is narrowed by shingling of the laminae and by bucking of the ligamentum flavum. The arthritic posterior joints may hypertrophy and also encroach on the midline giving rise to further compression of the cauda equina. The emerging nerve roots are commonly compressed as they course through the narrow subarticular gutter. From Macnab I: Backache. Williams & Wilkins, Baltimore (1977), p. 102.*

narrowing of the spinal canal or a narrowing produced by degenerative change of the type previously described. This is most commonly seen at the L4–L5 level.

Various combinations and permutations of laminar and apophyseal compression are seen. For example, the 5th lumbar nerve root may be compressed as it courses under the superior articular facet of L5 (Fig. 7.34). Although laminar compression may occur by itself at times, it is frequently associated with lateral recess or apophyseal root entrapment that may arise at the same segment, or the laminar and apophyseal compressions may be at different segments (Fig. 7.39).

Role of HNP in Bony Encroachment

The compression produced in the subarticular gutter by hypertrophy of the facet joints may be aggravated by a localized protrusion of the annulus, and a diffuse annular bulge may critically occlude a segment with a congenital narrowing of the spinal canal. However, although these spatial disc changes augment the degree of compression present, it is important to emphasize the fact that they are not the sole source of compression, and discectomy alone will not relieve the symptoms entirely.

Bony root entrapment, then, results from narrowing of the spinal canal. This narrowing may be apophyseal and may compress the nerve roots at their point of emergence at one or more segments. The compression may be in the midline and produced by the lamina, or the root compression may be the result of a combination of both of these mechanism at the same level or at different segments. It is important to emphasize that the most common cause of symptoms in spinal stenosis is compression of a nerve root by osteophytic overgrowth of facets and ligamentum flavum infolding and hypertrophy.

The resulting radicular pain mimics the radicular pain due to a disc rupture. However, the sciatic pain due to a bony root entrapment frequently presents a claudicant character. In contradistinction to the intermittent claudication of vascular insufficiency, the symptoms do not abate on standing still. The patient will report that, if the pain strikes while walking down the road, he/she will lean forward and rest his/her hands on the knees to keep the spine in flexion in order to relieve the symptoms. The claudicant nature of the sciatic pain produced by apophyseal compression of a nerve root differentiates it from sciatica due to a disc rupture.

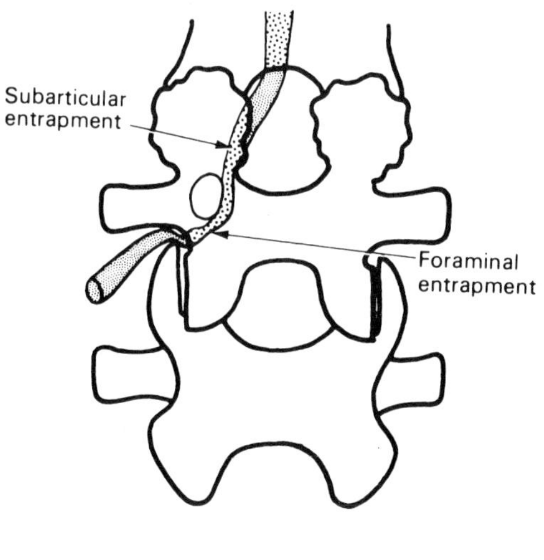

Figure 7.39 *In apophysial stenosis an emerging nerve root may be compressed at two sites. For example, as in this diagram, it may be compressed as it passes through the subarticular gutter and it may also be trapped in the foramen by the tip of the superior articular facet. From Macnab I: Backache. Williams & Wilkins, Baltimore (1977), p. 102.*

There are, in addition, several other features that differentiate bony root entrapment and compression from disc herniation. The first important difference is the age incidence. Root entrapment by bone is more common over age 50, whereas disc ruptures are more common under age 50. Patients with bony root entrapment will usually have a history of long-standing backache, with the recent gradual onset of sciatica. On examination of a patient with a neurogenic claudication, despite severe sciatic pain, one of the remarkable findings is that SLR is rarely significantly restricted. The bowstring sign and the crossed SLR are negative. Neurological changes are minimal but, when present, often incriminate more than one root. A true disc rupture, with extrusion of nuclear material, very rarely occurs at more than one segment simultaneously. This fact is not sufficiently recognized.

Conclusion

It is obvious that the pathogenesis of sciatica is multifactorial and not easily explained. The nature of the pressure of the discal fragment of the nerve root-ganglion complex, the location of the root-ganglion complex, and the resulting pathology determine the multifaceted nature of sciatica discomfort. Less important, but also bearing on the patient's symptom complex, is the age of the patient and thus, the age of the nerve root and the presence of other diseases that might decrease the resistance of the nerve root to these compressive changes.

A herniated nucleus pulposus represents not just a story of pain down the leg. A herniated nucleus pulposus is not just a defect on myelography, CT scan, or MRI.

REFERENCES

1. Bertolotti M. Contributo alla conoscenza dei vizi differencazione regionle del rachid con speciale riguardo all'assimilazione sacrale edlla v lombare. La Radiologia Medica 1917;4:113–144.
2. Bogduk N, Twomey LT. Clinical Anatomy of the Lumbar Spine. Melbourne, Edinburgh, London and New York: Churchill Livingstone; 1987.
3. Boden SD, Davis DO, Dina T, Patronas HJ, Wiesel SW. Abnormal magnetic resonance scans of the lumbar spine in asymptomatic subjects. J Bone Joint Surg 1990;72A:403–408.
4. Castellvi AE, Goldstein LA, Chan DPK. Lumbosacral transitional vertebrae and their relationship with lumbar extradural defects. Spine 1984;9:493–495.
5. Dandy WE. Concealed ruptured intervertebral disks. JAMA 1941;117:821–826.
6. Falconer MA, McGeorge M, Begg CA. Observations on the cause and mechanism of symptom production in sciatica and low back pain. J Neurol Neurosurg Psychiatr 1948;11:13.
7. Gowers WR. Lumbago. Its lessons and analogues. Br Med J 1904;1:117–121.
8. Guyton AC. Textbook of Medical Physiology. Philadelphia: WB Saunders; 1986.
9. Harris RI, Macnab I. Structural changes in the lumbar intervertebral discs. J Bone Joint Surg 1954;36B:304–322.
10. Hitselberger WE, Witten RM. Abnormal myelograms in asymptomatic patients. J Neurosurg 1968;28:204–210.
11. Holm S. Pathophysiology of disc degeneration. Acta Orthop Scand (suppl 251) 1993;64:13–15.
12. Kellgren JH. On the distribution of pain arising from deep somatic structures with charts of segmental pain areas. Clin Sci Mol Med 1939;4:35–46.
13. Kirkaldy-Willis WH, Wedge JH, Yong-Hing K, Reilly J. Pathology and pathogenesis of lumbar spondylosis and stenosis. Spine 1978;3:319–328.

14. Loeser JD. Concepts of pain. In: Chronic Low Back Pain. Stanton-Hicks M, Boas RA, eds. New York: Raven Press; 1982.
15. Macnab I. The traction spur: an indication of segmental instability. J Bone Joint Surg 1971; 53A:663–670.
16. Malinsky J. The ontogenetic development of nerve terminations in the intervertebral disc of man. Acta Anat 1959;38:96–113.
17. McCulloch JA. Computed tomography before and after chemonucleolysis. In: Computed Tomography of the Spine. Post MJD, ed. Baltimore: Williams & Wilkins; 1984, pp 460–470.
18. Mixter WJ, Barr JS. Rupture of the intervertebral disc with involvement of the spinal canal. N Engl J Med 1934;211:210–215.
19. Mooney V, Robertson J. The facet syndrome. Clin Orthop 1976;115:149–156.
20. Nachemson AL. The lumbar spine: an orthopaedic challenge. Spine 1976;1:59–71.
21. Noordenbos W. Prologue. In: Textbook of Pain. Wall PD, Melzack R, eds. Edinburgh, Scotland: Churchill Livingstone; 1984.
22. Parke WW, Gammell K, Rothman RH. Arterial vascularization of the cauda equina. J Bone Joint Surg 1981;63A:53–62.
23. Reilly PA, Travers R, Littlejohn GO. Epidemiology of soft-tissue rheumatism: the influence of the law. J Rheumatol 1991;18:1448–1449.
24. Rydevick B, Brown M, Lundborg G. Pathoanatomy and pathophysiology of nerve root compression. Spine 1984;9:7–15.
25. Verbiest H. A radicular syndrome from developmental narrowing of the lumbar vertebral canal. J Bone Joint Surg 1954;36B:230–237.
26. Waddell G. Morris EW, DiPaola MP, Bircher M, Finlayson D. A concept of illness tested as an improved basis for surgical decisions in low-back disorders. Spine 1986;11:712–719.
27. Wall PD, Melzack R: Textbook of Pain. Edinburgh, Scotland: Churchill Livingstone; 1984.
28. Weinstein J. Mechanisms of spinal pain: the dorsal root ganglion and its role as a mediator of low-back pain. Spine 1986;11:999–1001.
29. Wiesel SW, Tsourmas N, Feffer HL, Citrin CM, Patronas N. A study of computer-assisted tomography: i. The incidence of positive CAT scans in an asymptomatic group of patients. Spine 1984;9:549–551.
30. Yoshizawa H, O'Brien JP, Smith WT, et al. The neuropathology of intervertebral disc removed for low back pain. J Pathol 1980;132:95–104.

8

Epidemiology and Natural History of Spondylogenic Backache

INTRODUCTION

Although backache (with or without sciatica) is a benign, often self-limiting condition, it drains up to $60 billion per year (7) from the American government's health care budget. The cost of both time lost from work (with loss of productivity) and medical care, as well as the cost of litigation and disability claims, make back pain an industry unto itself. Competing for attention for this "cash flow" are members of all manners of disciplines, each claiming to have the "answer."

FACTS AND FACTORS

Epidemiological studies generate two sets of statistics:

1. Facts: The incidence (new cases per period of time) and the prevalence (all cases) as a measure of the natural history of the disease.
2. Factors: Environmental (especially industrial) and individual factors that affect the incidence of low back pain and can be altered to decrease morbidity.

Facts

Low back pain is a high-profile symptom in industrialized societies. A study in England (8) revealed that 2% of the population annually sought medical care for back pain. Frymoyer et al (9) have shown that during a lifetime, 70% of men will have an episode of low back pain.

Further facts that reveal the extent of low back pain as a problem for society are as follows:

1. In the United States, 2.5 million workers are injured per year.(14)
2. Each year, 2% of all employees have a back injury.(14)
3. Each year, 28.6 days per 100 workers are lost (14) (this amounts to 17 million work days per year in the United States).
4. At any one time, there are 1.2 million low-back-disabled adults in the United States.(14)
5. In the United Kingdom, one man in 25 changes his job each year because of a low back injury.(10)

In the industrial commission field, Snook and Jensen (24) have pointed out how difficult it is to calculate the cost of low back pain, because there are so many sources of payment to an injured worker. These include: (1) wages that are paid during the waiting period before compensation from workmen's compensation insurance, (2) group and individual health insurance plans, and (3) Social Security benefits. The direct cost of back injuries to the industrial commissions in the United States totals $11 billion per year.(24) Back injuries account for 20% of all compensable injuries but incur one third of the cost per year. It is estimated that the average cost per case is $6,000.00 and that within the category of low back pain, 25% of the injuries account for 90% of the costs.

Low back pain accounts for a considerable annual volume of surgery in the United States. Approximately 150,000 patients undergo a simple laminectomy for removal of a herniated disc, and another 150,000 per year undergo spine surgery for some other degenerative condition.(5) As the number of specialists who call themselves spine surgeons increases, so does the number of operations. To date, no investigator has been able to determine if Americans are better off as a result of the increase in back-spine specialists!(23)

Factors Affecting Incidence of Lumbar Disc Disease

(Disc Degeneration and Disc Herniation)

Age

Low back pain is most prevalent between the ages of 35 and 55. However, most patients in this age group have had a prior episode of back pain before age 35. Most operations for low back degenerative conditions occur between the ages of 35 and 55: younger patients usually undergo operations at the L5–S1 level, whereas surgery for the older patient usually involves the L4–L5 level.(13)

A herniated nucleus pulposus is more likely to occur between the ages to 30 and 40 years,(13, 22) at which time the disc is on its way to degeneration through a decrease in its water content. Under the age of 30, the resilience of the disc protects it from herniation; over the age of 40, a disc has developed some degree of inherent stability through fibrous changes that occur with the loss of turgor.(14) However, there are so many exceptions to these age rules that they serve as little more than general guidelines.

Sex

In the general population, the incidence of low back pain appears to be equally distributed between men and women. It is well known that workers exposed to heavy work, especially twisting and lifting, have a higher incidence of back pain. A female worker is more exposed to injury through these forces, but since there are so many more men in the heavy work force, the incidence of back injury in the working population is heavily weighted toward men.(13)

Body Build (Anthropometry)

There does not appear to be any strong correlation between height, weight, body build, and the occurrence of low back pain.(6)

Posture

Postural deformities such as scoliosis, kyphosis, hypo- and hyperlordosis, and leg length discrepancy do not predispose to low back pain.

Spine Mobility and Strength

After injury there is a decrease in low back strength and mobility.(21) There is some question as to whether this strength decrease is primarily responsible for the injury or secondary to the injury. Numerous studies are being undertaken now in order to determine if there is any predictive value in measuring the mobility and strength of a worker engaged in heavy-duty activity before injury. Studies have shown that the risk of back injury is increased if strength requirements on the job are greater than the isometric strength requirements measured in job simulation.(16) On the other hand, Bergquist-Ullmann and Larsson (2) have shown that there is no difference in the rates of recovery from acute low back pain when fit individuals are compared with unfit individuals.

Smoking

One fact is certain: if you smoke, your chances of developing low back pain are greatly increased.(6,9) Nothing has yet been proved about the causative factors related to this increased incidence, but theories abound:

- Smoking induces osteoporosis.
- Smoking induces coughing, which may cause microfractures in thinned trabeculae as well as increased intradiscal pressure.
- Smoking impairs blood flow, which is already very limited to a disc; this impairment in turn interferes with disc nutrition.
- Smoking decreases the O2 carried by hemoglobin, which may interfere with cell survival within a disc.

Occupational Low Back Pain

Approximately one third of back injuries occur at work and are the result of lifting and twisting accidents.(4) Another third of low back injuries also occur at work but are the result of slips and falls. The final third of low back injuries are not related to any particular work incident but instead, occur spontaneously outside the work environment.

There is no uniform agreement on the type of job that is most likely to precipitate a low back injury.(18) The injury rates and severity rates appear to be increased when heavy objects have to be lifted, especially from the floor level, and especially when a twisting component is involved.(11) Bulky objects and objects requiring frequent lifting also increase the incidence of low back complaints.(15)

Individuals who have to drive as an occupation have a higher incidence of low back complaints.(12) Some of this is likely related to the vibratory forces that are part of the job. Wilder and co-workers (30) have pointed out that the vibratory frequencies found in certain truck seats are a particular problem for truckers. Anyone who spends more than 50%

of their time sitting at their job also has a threefold increase in the incidence of a disc herniation.(12)

The cost to industry for low back problems is staggering, exceeding that spent on all other industrial injuries combined.(25) Adding to the incalculable cost is the fact that injury usually strikes in the peak productive years of ages 35 to 55.(1)(26)

Snook (24) made the following observation on cost:

- One third of the cost per industrial claim goes to medical care, and two thirds goes to disability payments.
- Ninety percent of the compensation costs are consumed by 25% of the injury claimants.

Further evidence of the serious impact of low back pain in industry is the fact that workers with back complaints who are absent from work for longer than 6 months have only a 50% chance of returning to productive employment.(20) Extending the work absence to 2 years virtually wipes out any chance that those workers will return to gainful employment. When exhorting an individual to work harder at physical therapy, remember that a return to work is inhibited more by whether or not the worker likes his boss and / or job than by his / her physical capacities.

Emotional State

Although much is said and written about low back pain, stress, and mental health, there is no body of scientific study suggesting that those individuals with emotional illness have an increased incidence of low back pain and sciatica.(3) It is more likely that low back pain and emotional illness can coexist independently for a short time, but eventually (and occasionally immediately) emotional lability will increase the degree of disability, sometimes beyond the bounds of the clinician's reason. Most studies (1,3,9) tend to show that the chronically back-injured worker is of poor intellectual capacity, with less ability to establish emotional contact and less in the way of a philosophical attitude toward injury. Whether this mental status precedes or results from the low back injury is open to question. Everyone would agree that worker dissatisfaction is high on the list of factors that make a worker vulnerable to a low back disability. Chapters 12 and 18 (which discusses the differential diagnosis of low back pain and sciatica), feature an extensive discussion on this aspect of low back disability.

Radiographic Factors

Back pain is more frequent in persons with multilevel degenerative disc disease.(28) Individuals with a spondylolysis or spondylolisthesis also have an increased incidence of back pain, especially when asked to do heavy work.(29)

Most studies suggest that congenital lumbosacral anomalies do not increase the incidence of low back pain.(27) The incidence of these anomalies across the general population appears to be approximately 5%; yet when one looks at studies on low back pain sufferers, the incidence of congenital lumbosacral anomalies on radiological examination approaches 10%. This doubling of the incidence of congenital lumbosacral anomalies compared with the incidence of low back pain in the general population requires further study before anyone can dismiss these radiological changes as being insignificant.

THE NATURAL HISTORY OF SPONDYLOGENIC LOW BACK PAIN

Waddell (29) has rightly pointed out that so many people suffer from low back pain at one time or another in their life, that perhaps we should see this as normal, and designate those who do not suffer from back pain as being abnormal! If spondlylogenic back pain is so common, why aren't the hospital wards and doctors' office full of the afflicted? Why should a disease, second only to the common cold in disabling those under age 45, consume up to $60 billion per year in America. Waddell has again hit the nail on the head in stating that in those countries where there are no caregivers for low back pain (eg, Africa), there is no back disability!

The most important statement we can make in this book is: **Spondylogenic low back pain is a self-limiting symptom (not a disease) that should require low cost for care.**

Ninety percent of patients with low back pain improve after 2 months.(2) Those patients who recover face a 60% recurrence rate during the following 2 years.

Kirkaldy-Willis et al (17) has provided us with the framework for understanding the natural history of spondylogenic low back pain (Fig. 8.1). He divided the spectrum of degenerative disc/facet joint disease into three phases.

Phase I: Dysfunction

Minor pathology causes limited abnormal function in the disc and/or facet joints, which leads to pain.

Phase II: Instability

This is the intermediate phase, where continuing microtrauma leads to further degeneration in the disc and facet joints, producing laxity of the annulus and facet joint capsules. The resulting instability leads to more prolonged episodes of back pain.

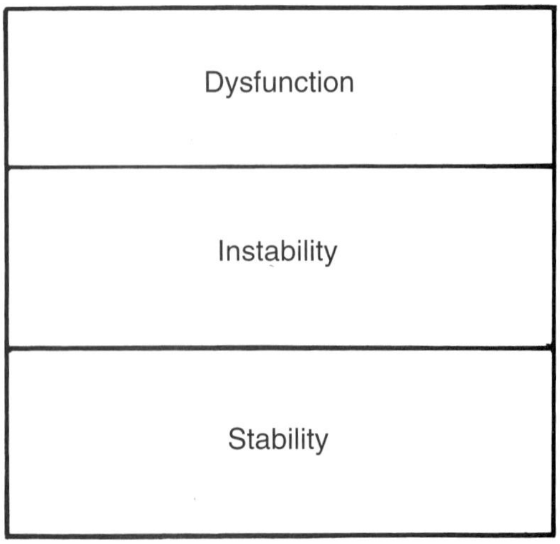

Figure 8.1 *The three phases of disc degeneration as depicted by Kirkaldy-Willis.*

Phase III: Stabilization

This is the final stage that not all patients reach. Fibrosis of the nuclear-annular complex and the facet joint capsule, along with osteophyte formation, represents the body's attempt to stabilize the motion segment. Narrowing of the disc and settling of the facet joints probably adds further mechanical stability to the segment. Many patients, as they age, will volunteer that they are not as flexible as they used to be. It is fortunate for them, because this protects them from symptoms!

SUMMARY

Low back pain is an epidemic, and more and more studies are bringing this fact to our attention. There is a greater understanding of low back pain and of the facts and factors that result in the significant cost to society of treating this condition. Fortunately, the majority of sufferers have a propensity for spontaneous resolution of symptoms. Unfortunately, a subset of patients become long-term, disabled individuals and extract a significant number (billions) of dollars from the medical care system. These factors are now coming under more scrutiny from the medical community and those paying for patient care. Change in the way we handle low back pain from degenerative conditions of the spine is upon us.

REFERENCES

1. Anderson GBJ. Epidemiologic aspects on low-back pain in industry. Spine 1981;6:53–60.
2. Bergquist-Ullmann M, Larsson U. Acute low back pain in industry. Acta Orthop Scand (suppl) 1977;170:1–117.
3. Bigos SJ, Battie MC, Spengler DM, et al. A prospective study of work perceptions and psychological factors affecting the report of back injury. Spine 1991;16:1–6.
4. Brown JR. Factors contributing to the development of low back pain in industrial workers. J Am Ind Hyg Assoc 1975;36:26–31.
5. Commission on Professional Hospital Activity of Ann Arbor, Michigan: Hospital Records Study. Ambler, Pennsylvania: IMS America Ltd; 1978.
6. Deyo RA, Bass JE. Lifestyles and low back pain: the influence of smoking, exercise, and obesity. Clin Res 1987;35:577A.
7. Deyo RA, Tsui-Wu YJ. Descriptive epidemiology of low back pain and its related medical care in the United States. Spine 1987;12:264–268.
8. Dillane JB, Fry J, Katon G. Acute back syndrome—A study from general practice. Br Med J 1966;2:82–84.
9. Frymoyer JW, Pope MH, Clements JH, Wilder DG, McPherson B, Ashikaga T. Risk factors in low back pain. J Bone Joint Surg 65A:1983:213–218.
10. Harris AI. Handicapped and Impaired in Great Britain, Part I. London, England: Social Survey Division, Office of Population Census and Surveys. Her Majesty's Stationary Office; 1971.
11. Kelsey JL. An epidemiological study of the relationship between occupations and acute herniated lumbar intervertebral discs. Int J Epidemiol 1975;4:197–205.
12. Kelsey JL. An epidemiological study of acute herniated lumbar intervertebral disc. Rheumatol Rehabil 1975;14:144–159.

13. Kelsey JL, Ostfeld AM. Demographic characteristics of persons with acute herniated lumbar intervertebral disc. J Chronic Dis 1975;28:37–50.
14. Kelsey JL, White AA. Epidemiology and impact of low back pain. Spine 1980;5:133–142.
15. Kelsey J, White A, Pastides H, Brobee G. The impact of musculoskeletal disorders on the population of the United States. J Bone Joint Surg (abstract) 1979;61:959–964.
16. Keyserling WM, Herrin GD, Chaffin DB. Isometric strength testing as a means of controlling medical incidents on strenuous jobs. J Occup Med 1980;22:332–336.
17. Kirkaldy-Willis WH, Wedge JH, Yong-Hing K, Reilly J. Pathology and pathogenesis of lumbar spondylosis and stenosis. Spine 1978;3:319–328.
18. Magora A. Investigation and relation between low back pain and occupation. Scand J Rehabil Med 1975;7:146–151.
19. Magora A, Schwartz A. Relation between the low back pain syndrome and x-ray findings. Scand J Rehabil Med 1976;8:115–125.
20. McGill CM. Industrial back problems: a control program. J Occup Med 1968;10:174–178.
21. McNeill T, Warwick D, Anderson GBJ, Schultz A. Trunk strengths in attempted flexion, extension, lateral bending in healthy subjects and patients with low back disorders. Spine 1980; 5:529–538.
22. Miller JA, Schmaalz C, Schultz AB. Lumbar disc degeneration: correlation with age, sex and level in 600 autopsy specimens. Spine 1987;13:173–178.
23. Nachemson AL. The lumbar spine—an orthopedic challenge. Spine 1976;1:59–71.
24. Snook SH, Jensen RC. Cost. In: Pope MH, Frymoyer JW, Anderson G, eds. Occupational Low Back Pain. New York: Praeger; 1984, pp 115–121.
25. Spengler DM, Bigos SJ, Martin NA, et al. Back injuries in industry: a retrospective study. Overview and costs analysis. Spine 1986;11:241–245.
26. Svenson HO, Anderson GB. Low back pain in forty- to forty-seven-year-old men, work history and work environment factors. Spine 1983;8:272–276.
27. Tilley P. Is sacralization a significant factor in lumbar pain? J Am Osteopath Assoc 1970; 70:238–241.
28. Torgerson BR, Dotter WE. Comparative roentgenographic study of asymptomatic and symptomatic lumbar spines. J Bone Joint Surg 1976;58:850–853.
29. Waddell G. 1987 Volvo Award in Clinical Sciences. A new clinical model for the treatment of low back pain. Spine 1987;12:632–644.
30. Wilder DG, Woodworth BB, Frymoyer JW, et al. Vibration and the human spine. Spine 1982; 7:243–254.

9

The History

"A doctor who cannot take a good history and a patient who cannot give one are in danger of giving and receiving bad treatment."

— Anonymous

When taking an adequate history, patience is not only a virtue, it is a vital necessity, as the following verbatim report of the first part of a prolonged consultation reveals:

Doctor: "Well, Mrs. Jones, what can I do to help you today?"
Patient: "I sure hope you can cure it."
Doctor: "Well, I'll try. Have you any pain?"
Patient: "Of course I have, I wouldn't be here if I didn't have any pain. I'm not the sort of person that keeps running to doctors with nothing wrong with them. I know you're all very busy and if..."
Doctor: "Where is the pain?"
Patient: "Haven't you looked at my radiographs?"
Doctor: "I will look at your radiographs after I have taken your history and completed an examination. Please tell me where your pain is located."
Patient: "The same place it's always been."
Doctor: "Where is that?"
Patient: "In my back, of course."
Doctor: "Where in your back—in the low back?"
Patient: "I don't know whether you would call it low or high. All I can say is it's sure a bad pain."
Doctor: "Could you point to the pain? Ah, I see. How long have you had this?"
Patient: "Ever since I tripped on the stairs."
Doctor: "When was that?"
Patient: "Didn't my doctor send you my history? His nurse promised me she'd mail it to you. Oh, this is terrible. I don't see any point in coming here if you don't know anything about me. I wonder why..."
Doctor: "When did you have the accident on the stairs?"
Patient: "In June."
Doctor: "What year?"
Patient: "Why, this year of course. I'm so sorry my doctor didn't send you my history!"
Doctor: "Have you had pain every day since then?"
Patient: "Sometimes."
Doctor: "You mean the pain is intermittent?"

Patient: "No. I mean sometimes I have the pain, and sometimes I don't."
Doctor: "When you have the pain, what aggravates it?"
Patient: "How do you mean aggravates?"
Doctor: "Does anything make the pain worse?"
Patient: "No, it's worse all the time."
Doctor: "Does lifting make the pain more severe?"
Patient: "No."
Doctor: "You can lift anything you want without hurting your back?"
Patient: "No, I can't lift anything."
Doctor: "Why?"
Patient: "Because of my back."
Doctor: "Let's just think of some things you do in your house. Vacuum cleaning, bed making, doing the laundry; do any of these things make it worse?"
Patient: "If I could do all of those things I wouldn't be here. I don't believe in running to the doctor with the least little thing. I can take a lot of pain, more than most people. You ask my husband. I can't even sit down because of the pain."
Doctor: "Does anything relieve your back pain?"
Patient: "No."
Doctor: "What do you do when the pain is bad?"
Patient: "I lie down."
Doctor: "Does lying down make the pain better?"
Patient: "No. It's just as bad when I get up."
Doctor: "When you are actually lying down, is the pain any easier?"
Patient: "Yes, but I can't spend my life lying down."
Doctor: "Does the pain stop you from doing anything you want to do?"
Patient: "I can't play golf with my husband."
Doctor: "Do you get a lot of pain in your back every time you play golf?"
Patient: "Yes."
Doctor: "When did you last play golf?"
Patient: "Eight years ago."
Doctor: "Why haven't you tried to play golf again?"
Patient: "My doctor told me not to."

INTRODUCTION

It is easy to describe a color, a sound, a taste, or a smell because these are sensations that can be shared. "I went down to the beach later that evening, when the setting sun had turned the sea into a vivid red, and all that could be heard was the plaintive cry of the sea gulls and the gentle splashing of the waves against the rocks." Statements such as this make a clear impression in the mind of the listener. It is more difficult, and yet more important, to interpret the statement, "I have this uncomfortable feeling in my back—I wouldn't call it a pain really," or, "I was paralyzed with pain that felt like red hot rivers rushing down my legs." Is the second patient exaggerating, or does he/she have more serious back trouble?

When taking a history, it is not good enough to find out that patients have "back pain" or that they have pain in the right leg or left leg. It is essential to obtain a description of the pain in meticulous detail. Having obtained a clear description of the discomforts from which the patient is suffering, it is then necessary to find out as much as you can about the personality of the patient and his/her activities in order to try to correlate the pain to the disability about which the patient is complaining. The majority of patients do not come because of pain; they come because of the disability it produces. "I've got this backache and I can't play badminton." The patient can do everything else; he/she wants you to overcome the "disability" and make him/her able to play badminton again.

You have to obtain a clear picture of the pain. From this, you must assess the possible source of pain. You have to obtain an equally clear picture of the patient who has the pain. From these facts, you have to assess why the pain is causing the complained-of disability.

Before you go any further, remember:

1. After listening to the patient's story, there is an 80% chance you will know the diagnosis (you will improve the odds another 10% by doing the physical examination, and another 5% by ordering fancy, expensive tests).
2. If after a history, physical examination, and review of tests you are still not sure of the diagnosis, go back and repeat the history! A few minutes of good history taking can save thousands of dollars in expensive testing.

Now, you can close the book and know that all you need to do in assessing a patient with back pain (and any other complaint in most of medicine) is to listen to your patients! Can you imagine how hard it is to be a good veterinarian!

PICTURE OF THE PAIN

Site of the Pain

When patients state that they have "back pain," they may mean anywhere from the base of the neck to the buttocks. It is not good enough to ask patients where they feel the pain; they must demonstrate it. A patient's grasp of anatomy is understandably vague. When patients say that they have pain in their backs, they may be referring to the interscapular region of the back, and even when they state that they have pain in the "small of the back," they may be referring to the lumbodorsal junction. When patients describe pain in the "hip," they generally mean pain in the buttock. It is necessary always to get the patients to point to where they have the pain. Let us slip in a little word about pain over the greater trochanter, so often called "trochanteric bursitis." More often it is pain referred to the region from the lumbar area. Injecting the area with local anesthetic and cortisone can often have a placebo effect and mislead you into accepting the erroneous diagnosis of trochanteric bursitis.

The method the patient chooses to demonstrate the site of pain is instructive. The emotionally stable patient generally places the palm of the hand at the site of maximal pain and moves it across the body to demonstrate the route of radiation. The psychologically troubled patient generally points out the area of the pain with his/her thumb (Fig. 9.1). He/she never touches the painful area. The pain, so to speak, is outside his/her soma.

Spread of pain to the leg is an important symptom, and patients should be asked to demonstrate the distribution of the pain. It is important to you, as the examiner, to know what constitutes the leg (Fig. 9.2). To a patient, a leg is a leg, and most will not volunteer any information as to whether the pain radiates down to the knee, or whether it goes

Figure 9.1 *Patients who are suffering from a significant emotional overlay will frequently point to the area of pain in the lower back with their thumbs. They never actually touch their body. From Macnab I: Backache. Williams & Wilkins, Baltimore (1977), p. 109.*

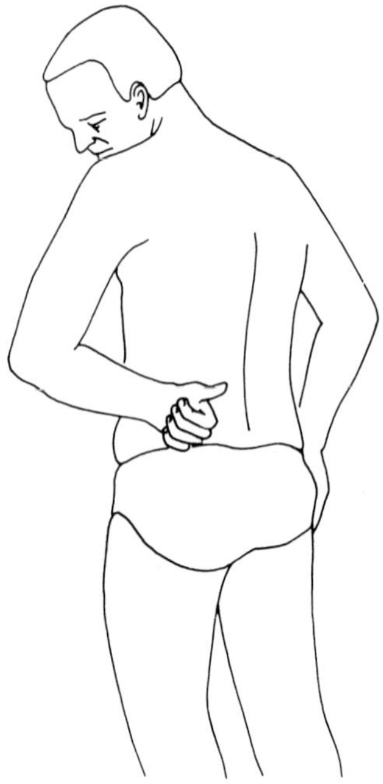

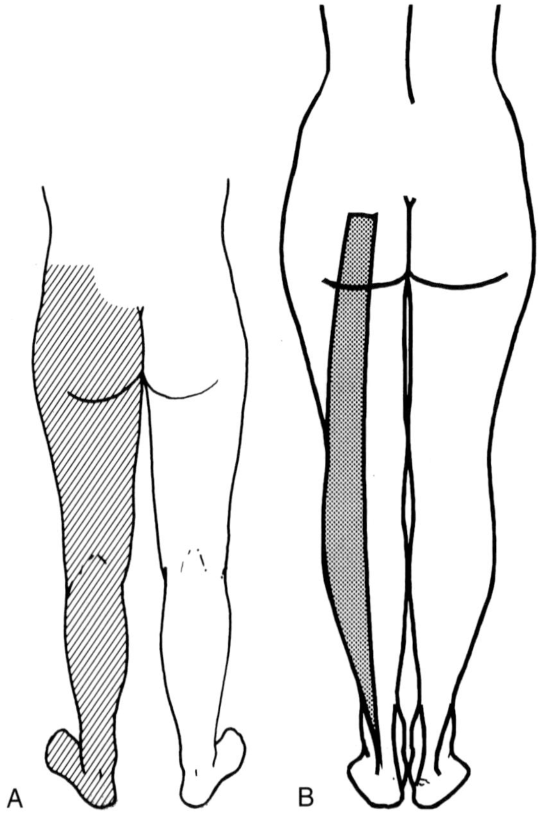

Figure 9.2 **A.** *The "leg" includes the buttock as its proximal extension.* **B.** *Radicular pain in the leg will follow a more "linear" radicular distribution.*

below the knee. The examiner needs to know this when trying to determine whether the patient is suffering from referred pain or whether the pain in the leg is due to root irritation and, if so, which root. By having patients point with their fingers, the distribution of the leg pain will be clear (Fig. 9.3).

Referred pain is rarely felt below the knee, whereas pain due to root irritation may spread to the calf or even into the foot. Pain resulting from compression of the third and fourth lumbar roots radiates down the front of the thigh. Pain from first and second lumbar root involvement is easily confused with hip disease because it concentrates around the groin.

Paresthesia

You are aware that the symptom of a sensory change is a paresthetic complaint, and the associated sign is numbness. Pain due to root irritation is frequently associated with a paresthetic sensation, and its location is a key to anatomical localization of root involvement. Paresthesia involving the lateral border of the foot is usually indicative of an S1 lesion, and a patient with an L5 lesion may describe numbness over the dorsum of the foot and even into the big toe. The location of the pins and needles or paresthetic discomfort in the shin indicates fourth lumbar root involvement; the knee cap location is third root involvement; and the lateral thigh represents second lumbar root involvement (Fig. 9.4).

The presence of these symptoms is helpful in making the diagnosis of root irritation and localizing the level of involvement. The patient does not usually volunteer this information; it must be asked for specifically. Table 9.1 outlines the two historical criteria important to the diagnosis of the acute radicular syndrome.

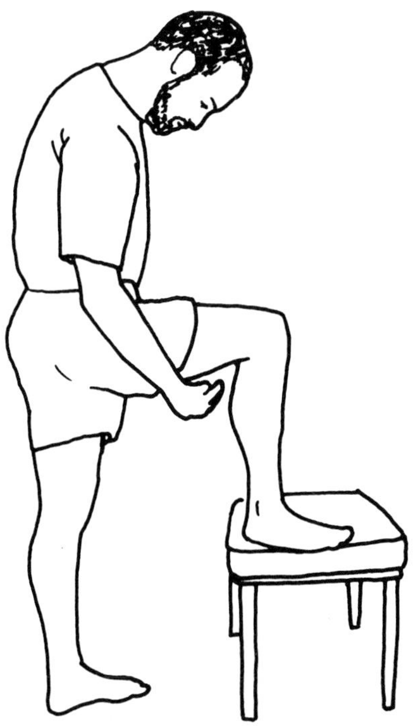

Figure 9.3 *Ask the patient to put his foot on a chair and point to the location of the leg pain: he is drawing a "road map" of the radicular distribution of the pain.*

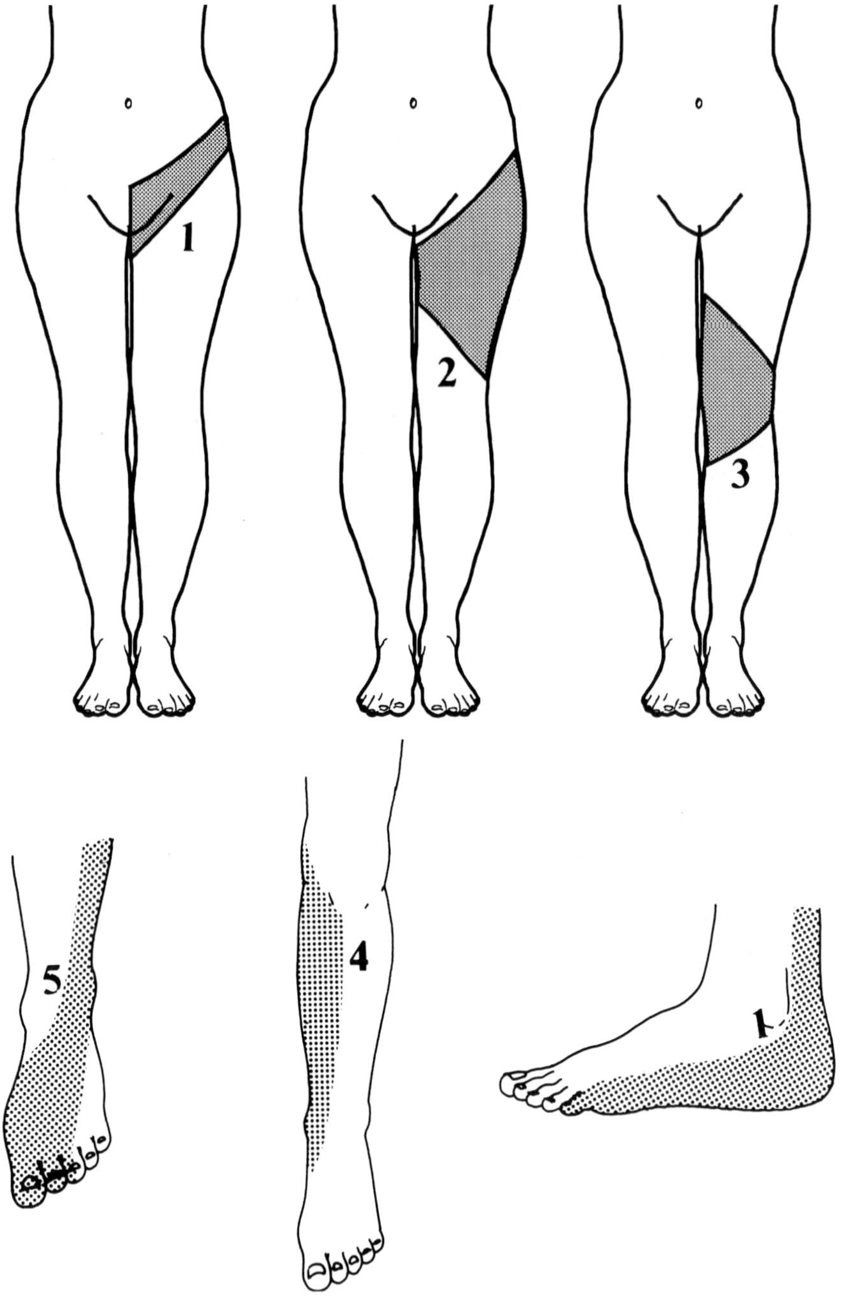

Figure 9.4 *The dermatomes of L1 to S1 are outlined and numbered.*

What Symptom Are You Hearing?

Remember, degenerative conditions of the spine cause pain. If the patient has a history of any other symptoms, be careful. Morning stiffness is a symptom of ankylosing spondylitis and some neurological conditions. It is also a classic symptom for lumbar degenerative disc disease. Parkinson's disease in its earliest phase may present with back

Table 9.1. Historical Criteria Important to the Diagnosis of an Acute Unilateral Radicular Syndrome (Usually Due to a Herniated Nucleus Pulposus

1. Leg pain is the dominant symptom when compared in severity with the back pain.
   - It dominates at the onset of the symptoms ("I've never had any back pain.").

     or
   - It dominates at the time of patient presentation.

     or
   - At some time during aggravating activity, the patient states that the main complaint is leg (and buttock) pain.
2. Paresthesias (and occasionally numbness) in a typical dermatomal distribution, for example:
   - Lateral foot and heel for S1 root.
   - Lateral calf and/or dorsum of foot and/or big toe for L5 root.
   - Medial shin for L4 root.
   - Kneecap for L3 root.

stiffness, legs that do not function properly, and a diffuse aching buttocks sensation.

Is the leg symptom predominantly weakness or sensory upset? If there is sensory upset, then there is a very high likelihood that you are dealing with a neurological disorder such as a cord myelopathy or cauda equina tumor, a neuropathy, or motor neuron disease. Lumbar spine doctors are pain doctors. Cervical spine doctors may hear about leg symptoms, but rather than symptoms of leg pain, these symptoms will be gait disturbances. The English expression for a cervical myelopathic symptom is a patient "going off their legs."

Even domination of the history by pain does not assure a diagnosis of a degenerative disc or disc rupture. Tumors of bone and neurological tissues, as well as intra-abdominal conditions, can cause pain. But the pain of these conditions is nonmechanical; that is, present at rest.

Influence of Activities

Specific questions must be asked to determine the factors that influence the pain. Backache due to a mechanical breakdown of the spine is almost always aggravated by general and specific activities and is relieved by rest. There are, or course, some exceptions to this general rule, but on the whole, it is fairly reliable. Backache due to a penetrating duodenal ulcer is not aggravated by activities, nor does it ease if the patient lies down. Patients with a neurofibroma involving a nerve root frequently report a history of having to get up at night to walk around to "get away" from the pain, and patients with a secondary deposit in the spine commonly report the story of sudden cramps of pain in their back even when lying down. A few patients with disc degeneration find that their pain is worse lying in bed, but this is most unusual. Patients who complain of pain in bed may sleep face downward, a position which, by extending the lumbar spine, aggravates discogenic pain. Constant pain in bed is also seen in the emotionally distraught.

When trying to find out whether activities increase pain, it is best to ask the following specific questions: "Does lifting hurt?", "Is your pain worse when you bend over the washbasin?", "Can you make beds?", "Can you use the vacuum cleaner?", and "Is the pain made worse by walking or climbing stairs?" Discogenic pain is frequently increased by maintaining one posture over a period of time: prolonged walking, prolonged sitting, or prolonged standing. Sudden jars to the body will aggravate any form of mechanical pain.

The history of pain shooting down the leg as a result of coughing or sneezing is highly suggestive of root compression. This is due to the Valsalva maneuver, which increases the pressure transmitted through the spinal fluid, further aggravating nerve root compression.

Many patients are confused by the question, "Is your pain better when you lie down?" They will frequently answer, "No," in the belief that the question implied that the act of lying down completely cured their backache for a period of time. They may answer, "No, it is not made better by lying down; it is just as bad as ever when I get up." It is probably better to ask them, "What do you feel like doing when the pain is very bad?" Although some patients may regard this question as being absurd, most will tell you they would like to lie down, or sit down, if they could. A classic position of comfort is lying on a hard floor with the hips and knees flexed, with the calves resting on a chair or a sofa (Fig. 9.5).

Although it may be tedious at times, it is imperative to learn from the patient what aggravates and relieves his/her symptoms.

Duration and Progression of Symptoms

It is important to have a clear knowledge of the onset, duration, and progression of the symptoms. How did the pain start? Gradually, or suddenly? Spontaneously, or with an accident? If it started with an accident, is there a lawyer involved? Is there some "commercial" value to the symptoms? Did it follow provocative activity? Has the pain been continuous or intermittent?

The sudden onset of pain after provocative activity with an intermittent course subsequently is highly suggestive of a mechanical basis for the symptoms. The sudden onset of severe back pain with a simple twisting movement is very suggestive of pathological fracture. In a man more than 50 years of age, this latter presentation may also be the presenting symptom in multiple myeloma.

Is the pain getting worse? If the patient feels that his/her symptoms are getting progressively worse, is this because the attacks are more frequent, more severe, and more prolonged, or is it because the patient has lost all tolerance and is fed up with this bothersome burden?

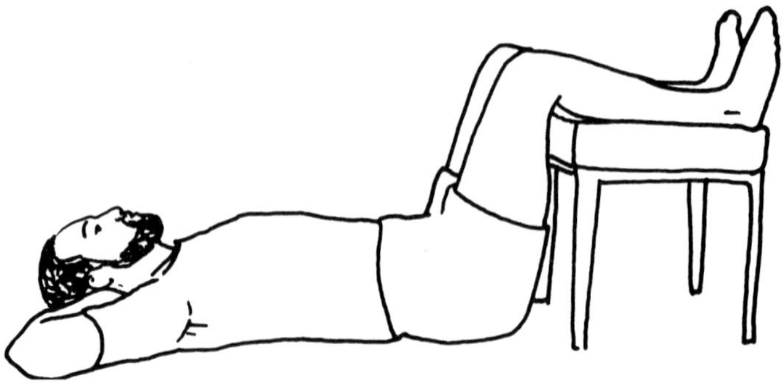

Figure 9.5 *A position of comfort for a patient with sciatica is lying on the floor with his feet up on a chair or sofa.*

What is the Functional Limitation?

A patient who has had to take to bed because of severe leg pain has a much different disability than the individual who cannot swing a "nine iron" because of back pain. The type of symptoms and the functional limitations allow you to decide if the disability is mild, moderate, or severe; a classification that allows for rational treatment decisions.

Are There Any Associated Symptoms?

Specifically, you are interested in whether there are any intra-abdominal symptoms that suggest a source of referred back pain. You are interested in that patient as a person. Is he/she anxious, depressed, or is the patient taking a rather belligerent or indifferent approach to his/her symptoms? Throughout this book, there is ceaseless referral to the patient with nonorganic spinal pain. There is good reason: the non-organically disabled patient is common, and the cost of missing this diagnosis amounts to multimillions of dollars each year in misspent investigations and ill-conceived surgery. We are sorry to keep raising the issue, but once more, you should commit to reading Chapter 12.

Most important, you would like to know if there is any serious effect of the disc pathology on urinary or bowel function. Urinary retention, with or without overflow incontinence, is an ominous symptom. Even more ominous is the association of perineal numbness signifying compression of the cauda equina. Any doubt about the presence or absence of a cauda equina syndrome requires emergency investigation (see Chapter 1).

At this state of the history, it is a good time to inquire about the patient's general health through a functional inquiry, past history, and family history. In today's age of drug addiction and immunocompromised states, all kinds of unusual low back pain will present, more often than not, due to disc space infections. Watch out for peripheral neuropathy associated with diabetes.

What Treatment Has Been Administered?

Excluding the failed back surgery patient who is discussed in Chapter 19, what conservative treatment modalities have been tried? Table 9.2 summarizes the classes of conservative treatment commonly administered to low back pain sufferers. If a patient has tried bed rest, physical therapy, and appropriate medication, it is senseless to suggest that they all be tried again. Once adequate conservative treatment modalities have failed in a patient with a moderate or severe disability, it is time to consider surgery. The last item listed in Table 9.2 is Time. Has enough time elapsed for the natural historical course of the symptoms and disease to occur? It is not necessary to rush a patient into the operating room until nature has taken its course. Obviously, bladder and bowel involvement and an advancing neurological lesion are exceptions to this rule.

ANATOMICAL BASIS OF THE PAIN

It must be remembered that back pain is a symptom and not a disease and that its source may lie outside the spine. It is essential, therefore, to include in the history a general

Table 9.2. Conservative Treatment Modalities

Rest
Bed rest, brace, weight reduction, job modification
Medication
Analgesic, anti-inflammatory, muscle relaxant
Temperature change
Heat and cold
Exercise
Flexion, extension, isokinetic
Manipulation
Miscellaneous
Acupuncture, biofeedback, transcutaneous electrical nerve stimulation, relaxation therapy
Time

functional inquiry. For example, the history of dorsolumbar pain relieved by the ingestion of food raises the possibility of a penetrating duodenal ulcer. The history of difficulty in micturition demands further inquiry to rule out prostatic cancer with secondary lesions in the spine. A family history of diabetes raises the possibility of diabetic neuropathy. A diabetes diathesis, by itself, markedly intensifies the pain of root compression. A chronic cough or a history of unexplained weight loss cannot be ignored.

It cannot be overemphasized that spondylogenic back pain is aggravated by general and specific activities and is relieved, to some extent, by recumbency.

CONCLUSION

Take time to listen to the patient. If you are a music lover, you will instantly recognize Beethoven's Symphony No. 5 in C Minor. Even the casual classical listener can recognize Tchaikovsky's 1812 overture. Listening to a patient with a complaint of pain in the back presents the same opportunities for recognition.

A patient with a herniated nucleus pulposus paints a different historical picture than a patient with mechanical instability due to degenerative disc disease. A malingerer tells a classic story in a typical manner. In fact, the history is so important that most low back pain diagnoses are known before the examiner begins the physical examination.

10

Examination of the Back

"More mistakes are made from want of proper examination than for any other reason."

— Russell Howard

"The examining physician often hesitates to make the necessary examination because it involves soiling the finger."

— William Mayo

INTRODUCTION

The purpose of this chapter is to give a general outline of a routine clinical examination of a patient suffering from significant back pain. Specific findings will be alluded to again when the examination and treatment of common clinical syndromes are discussed in later chapters. It is important to emphasize that accurate records of the history and examination should be made. These must include exact measurements and not vague terms such as "good," "poor," "limited," and so on. Good records are necessary for case analysis and comparison, and, on case reviews, for assistance to a consulting physician, and, at times, for legal purposes.

The examination of the back should be conducted in an orderly, predetermined manner. Examination of the patient should not be directed solely at eliciting signs of a specific disease suggested by the history, nor should individual systems be examined serially: neurological examination, abdominal examination, vascular examination, and so on. The examination must be conducted in an orderly manner so that all possible physical findings may be evaluated. When you finish examining each patient, you must know as much about his/her physical state as the last patient and every patient you have seen or will see.

The first prerequisite is that the patient must be undressed. To some practitioners, this is an absurd statement, because patient undressing is a routine; to clinicians who see alot of patients in a short amount of time, patient undressing is an inconvenience. A cursory examination is worse than no examination at all, because it may give the false hope that the lesion is minor.

STEP 1

Watch the patient walk. Is there an antalgic gait that suggests hip or knee disease? Is there a shuffling gait that suggests a neurological disorder of rigidity or spasticity? Does the patient walk slightly flexed, which suggests a spinal canal stenosis? Gait observation reveals alot of secrets. Not infrequently, it is difficult to decide if a patient's back and hip pain is due to pathology in the back or in the hip. More often than not, watching the patient walk the length of the hall will make the diagnosis, especially if the patient has the spastic gait of myelopathy or the antalgic limp of hip disease (Fig. 10.1).

STEP 2

By looking at the patient from the side and behind, gross postural changes will be evident. It is best to think of these postural changes as being in the sagittal plane (Fig. 10.2) or the coronal or frontal plane (Fig. 10.3).

Frontal Plane Asymmetry

There are three basic causes of frontal plane asymmetry as shown in Figure 10.3. To separate a structural scoliosis (eg, idiopathic) from a sciatic scoliosis, make the following observations:

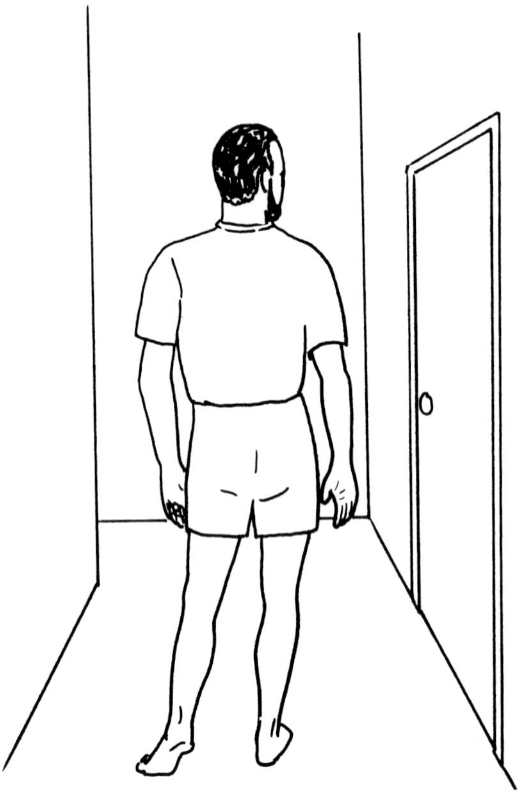

Figure 10.1 *At some point during the physical examination, it is important to watch the patient walk.*

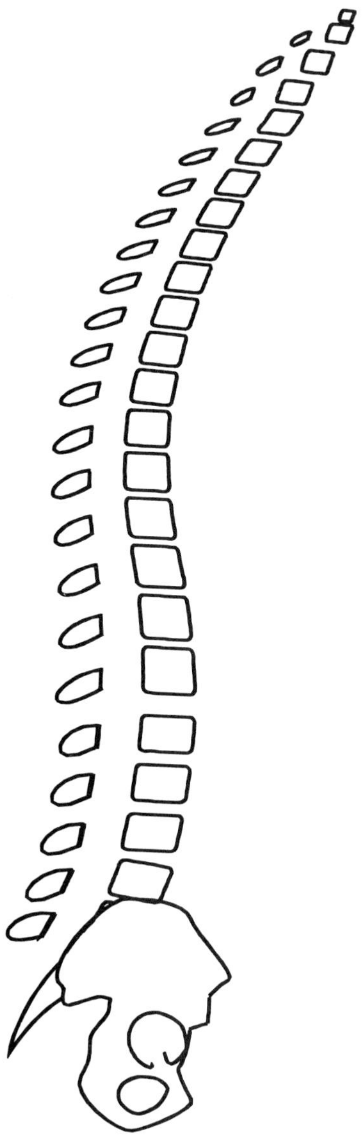

Figure 10.2 *Sagittal plane malalignment: kyphosis.*

Structural Scoliosis

1. The curve is fixed and does not change on forward flexion.
2. The common right thoracic idiopathic curve has a rib hump that becomes more obvious on flexion.
3. The curve does not reduce on recumbency.

Sciatic Scoliosis

1. Sciatica scoliosis is a more diffuse curve that does not have a rib hump.
2. On forward flexion, the curve changes, usually becoming worse, but it may even reverse its direction.

Figure 10.3 *Coronal plane malalignment: scoliosis.*

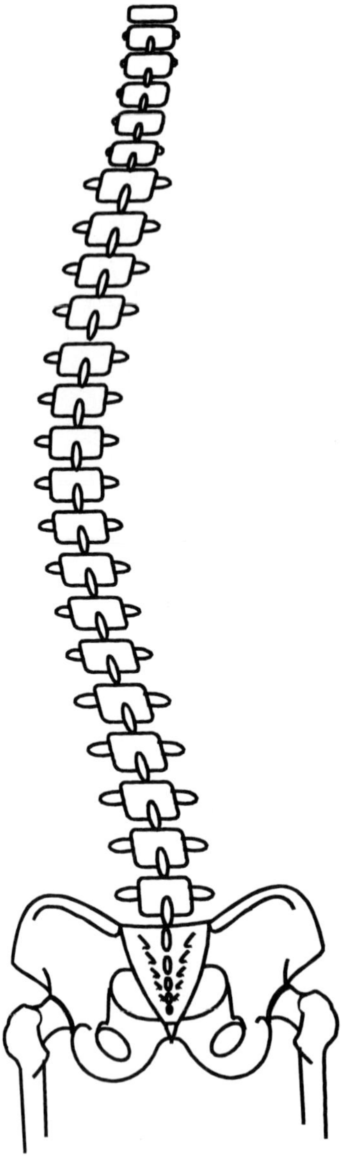

3. Forward flexion in sciatic scoliosis is much more limited than that in structural scoliosis.
4. Sciatic scoliosis usually disappears on recumbency.

Other observations to be made when examining the patient from behind are as follows:

1. Look for skin crease changes in the lumbosacral regions that might indicate a step-off of a lytic or degenerative spondylolisthesis (see Chapter 5, "Steps" of spondylolisthesis [Fig. 10.4]).
2. Skin markings: look for café–au–lait spots, a hallmark of neurofibromatosis. Other masses such as fatty tumors or hairy patches in the lumbosacral region may indicate deeper skeletal lesions such as spina bifida with or without associated tumors of or in neurogenic tissues.

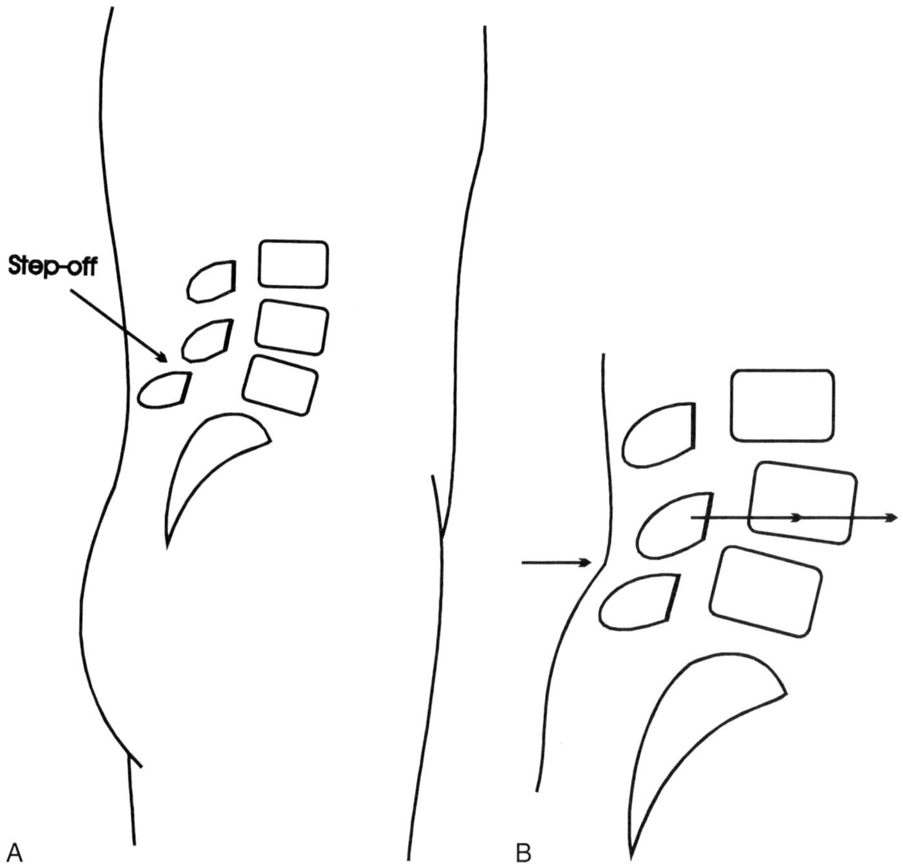

Figure 10.4 *The "steps" in spondylolisthesis.* **A.** *In a lytic spondylolisthesis (most common at L5–S1), the spinous process of L5 is left behind, that is, the step is palpable between the L4 spinous process that has moved forward and the L5 spinous process.* **B.** *In a degenerative spondylolisthesis (most common at L4–L5), a similar situation exists, except the slip vertebrae is one level higher, and the L5 spinous process is also left behind.*

STEP 3

The range and rhythm of spinal movement are tested next. The range of forward flexion is recorded by noting how far the hands come toward the floor. The rhythm of forward flexion is observed by placing the fingertips on the spinous process and noting how far they separate on flexion of the spine (Fig. 10.5).

Extension is recorded by noting how far the patient can lean backward before the pelvis tilts. Lateral flexion is measured by noting how far the patient can slide the hand down the thigh toward the knee (Fig. 10.6). Rotation can be tested by getting the patient to stand with his/her feet wide apart and rotate with hands on hips (Fig. 10.7). Also, do the simulated rotation test demonstrated in Chapter 12.

During the examination, observe any specific abnormalities; for example, look for marked limitation of the range of forward flexion without lumbar movement, as occurs in root irritation due to disc herniation. These patients frequently show deviation to the painful side on forward flexion. The rigidity of the whole spine in the later stages of ankylosing spondylitis is characteristic. Reversal of normal spinal rhythm on attempting to re-

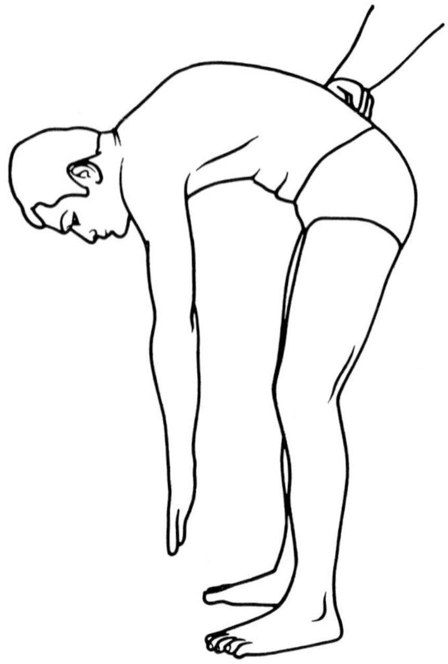

Figure 10.5 *When the patient is asked to bend forward, not only should the range of movement be noted, but the ability of the spinous processes to separate should also be recorded. This is best done by placing the fingertips over the spinous processes in the lumbar spine.*

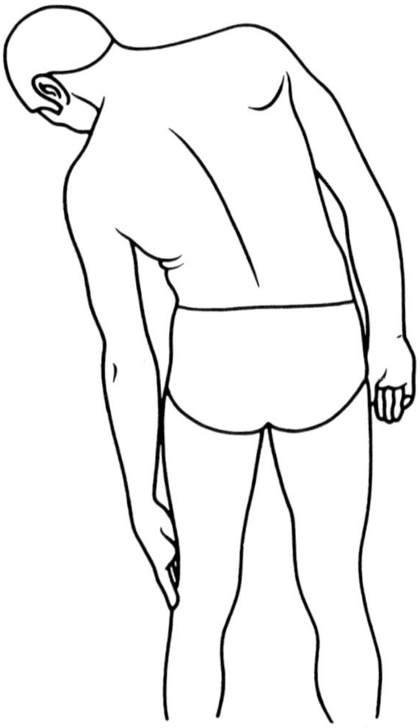

Figure 10.6 *Lateral flexion is recorded by noting how far the patient can slide his/her hand down the thigh toward the knee.*

gain the erect posture after forward flexion is characteristic of disc degeneration associated with a posterior joint lesion. To avoid putting an extension strain on the posterior joint, the patient tucks the pelvis under the spine to regain the erect position. When getting up from forward flexion, he/she will start to extend the spine, but this movement is uncomfortable. To avoid this, he/she will slightly flex the hips and knees in order to tuck the pelvis under the spine and then regain the erect position by straightening the legs (Fig. 10.8).

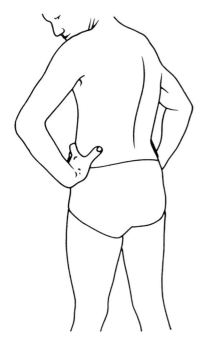

Figure 10.7 *Rotation is recorded by asking the patient to place his/her hands on the hips. The elbows then act as the arms of a goniometer and the degree of rotation permitted can be measured.*

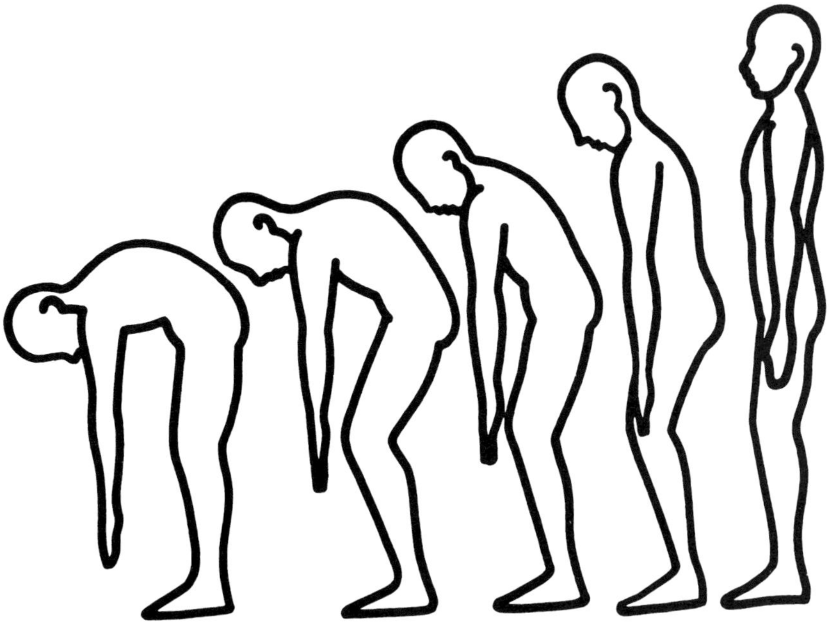

Figure 10.8 *Reversal of spinal rhythm. On attempting to regain the erect position from forward flexion, the patient will bend the knees and tuck the pelvis underneath the spine in order to stand erect. This type of movement is very characteristic of segmental instability.*

With the patient still standing, the strength of the gastrocnemius is determined by testing the ability to stand on tiptoe (Fig. 10.9). Lesions involving the 1st sacral root such as lumbosacral disc herniation may produce weakness of tiptoe raising and diminution of the ankle jerk, which can be tested with the patient kneeling on a chair. The examiner

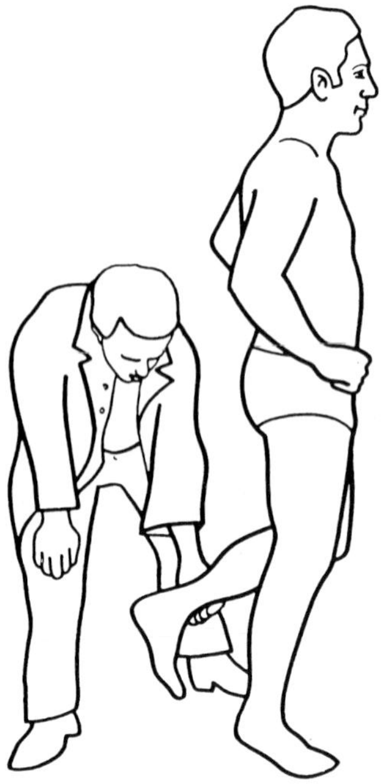

Figure 10.9 *The strength of the gastrocnemius is best tested by asking the patient to rise on tiptoe repetitively and rapidly. You are looking for fatigability, and therefore the patient must be asked to rise on tiptoe a minimum of 10 times.*

must remember that if a patient has a weak quadriceps, his/her leg will tend to buckle on attempting to rise on tiptoe. This is a diagnostic trap for the unwary.

STEP 4

Two examinations are conducted with the patient sitting on the edge of the examining table. First, examine the knee and ankle reflexes. This is usually the most comfortable position for a back pain patient and allows for reflex examination without painful posturing, something that will distort the reflex examination. Every now and then, a patient will have such a great degree of sciatica that he/she cannot sit without lifting the buttock (and thus the painful sciatic nerve) off the bed, which may falsely suppress the knee reflex. Reflexes can also be altered by a patient visually watching the reflex examination. This can be negated by reinforcement (Fig. 10.10).

The next reflex to be tested is the superficial plantar-flexor response (see Fig. 10.10). One feature of the plantar response is a reflex contraction of the tensor fascia femoris. This portion of the withdrawal response is lost with lesions involving S1.

Oh, by the way! Go back to Figure 10.10 and observe the position of the leg during the sitting Babinski's test. This is a way of examining straight leg raising in the sitting position (the so-called flip test; see Chapter 12 for a further explanation).

STEP 5

Strength Testing

Strength testing is best done with the patient in the supine position. The dorsiflexors of the ankles may become weak with lesions involving the 5th lumbar nerve root such as herniation of the disc between the 4th and 5th lumbar vertebra.

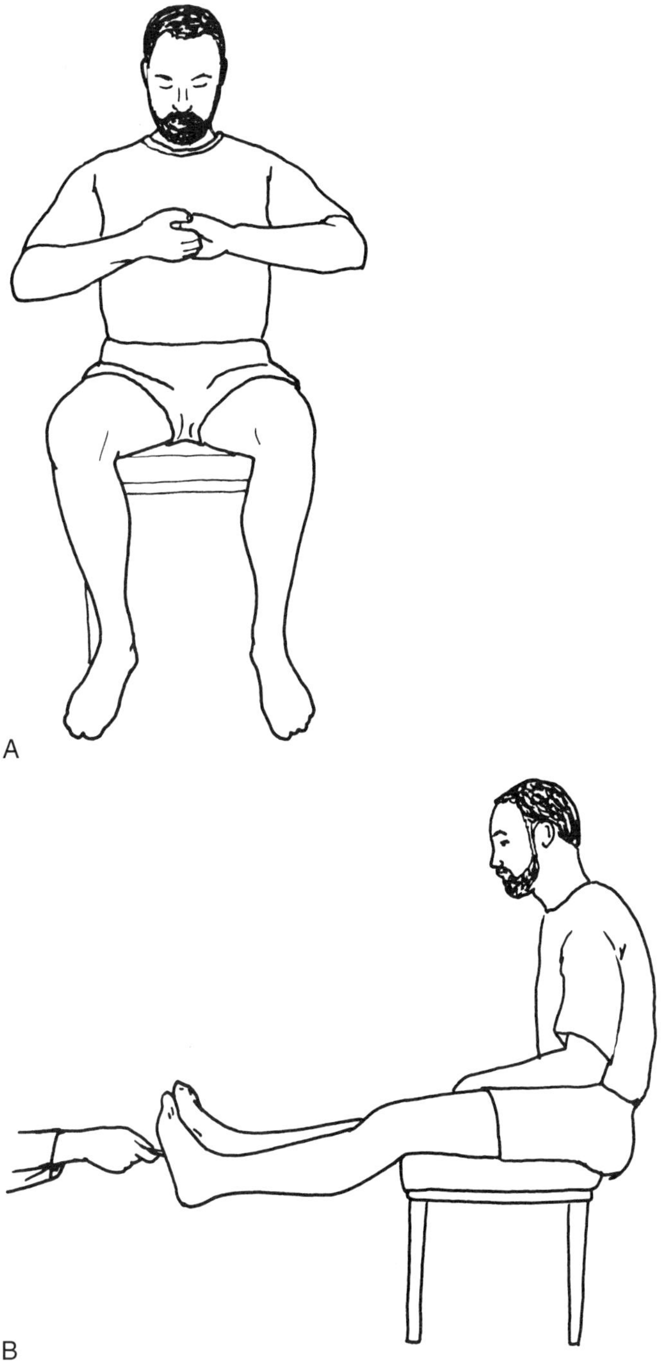

Figure 10.10 **A.** *Asking the patient to grasp and pull on the hands serves as reinforcement of reflexes.* **B.** *Sitting Babinski's test: the straight leg raising (SLR) test can be done in the sitting position while doing other tests such as that to test Babinski's reflexes.*

The strength of the dorsiflexors should not be tested with the knee extended, because if the patient has significant sciatic pain, any attempt by the patient to resist forced plantar flexion of the ankle will be painful, and a false impression of weakness may be obtained. The knee should be flexed, and full body weight pressure should be applied against the dorsum of the foot to assess the strength of the dorsiflexors (Fig. 10.11). Lesions involving the 5th lumbar root may cause weakness of the extensor hallucis longus before any significant weakness of the dorsiflexors of the ankle is apparent (Fig. 10.12). Similarly, with an S1 lesion, the flexor hallucis longus may become detectably weak before there is any noticeable weakness of the gastrocnemius. Sometimes, this can be dramatically demonstrated by asking the patient to claw or flex the toes, whereupon it may be noted that the patient can flex the big toe on one side but not on the other. Many examiners use the heel-toe walking test to examine L5 and S1 root weakness (see Fig. 10.12).

The quadriceps may be weak with lesions of the 3rd and 4th lumbar nerve root. The strength of the muscle is best tested with the patient lying on his/her back, with the hips slightly flexed and the knee placed over the examiner's forearm. The patient then tries to extend the knee against the resistance of the examiner's other hand.

Diffuse weakness of all muscle groups, particularly the psoas, is highly suggestive of an emotional breakdown. Functional or emotional weakness is characterized by jerky relaxation of the muscles regardless of what force is applied. Quite frequently, these patients will be able to resist breakdown of a fixed position, but will be unable to initiate movement of a joint against weak resistance. This is the so-called discrepant motor weakness. In gross emotional disturbances, there may be diffuse, unreasonable weakness of many muscle groups. Characteristically, these patients will be unable to extend the terminal interphalangeal joint of the thumb against the slightest resistance and will not be able to hold their eyes closed tightly shut when the examiner tries to push the eyebrow up.

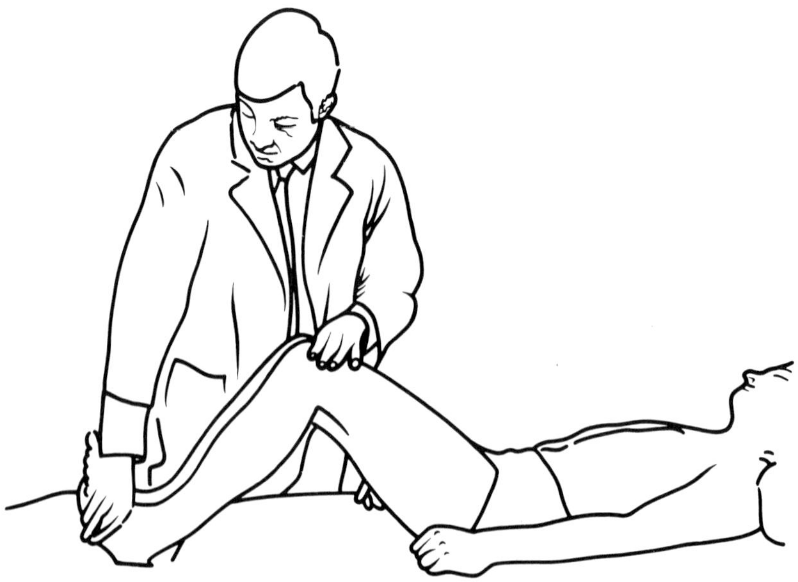

Figure 10.11 *The power of the dorsiflexors of the ankle should be tested with the patient lying on his/her back, with hips and knees flexed. The patient holds the ankle in full dorsiflexion and attempts to resist the maximal force that the physician can apply to the dorsum of the foot.*

Muscle strength test results should be graded according to the standard method of a 0–5 scale (Table 10.1). The 4th grade (movement against gravity and resistance) is usually subgraded into the following levels:

- 4+ Significant weakness (but not grade 3)
- 4++ Moderate weakness
- 4+++ Almost normal but weak

At all times, be cognizant of the effect pain has on the patient's ability to carry out the strength testing. Some patients have so much back or leg pain that despite trying to cooperate with you, they cannot participate in strength testing maneuvers. Some of the patients assume the appearance of pain and inability to cooperate, but other aspects of the history and physical examination will point you toward considering the nonorganic reactions described in Chapter 12.

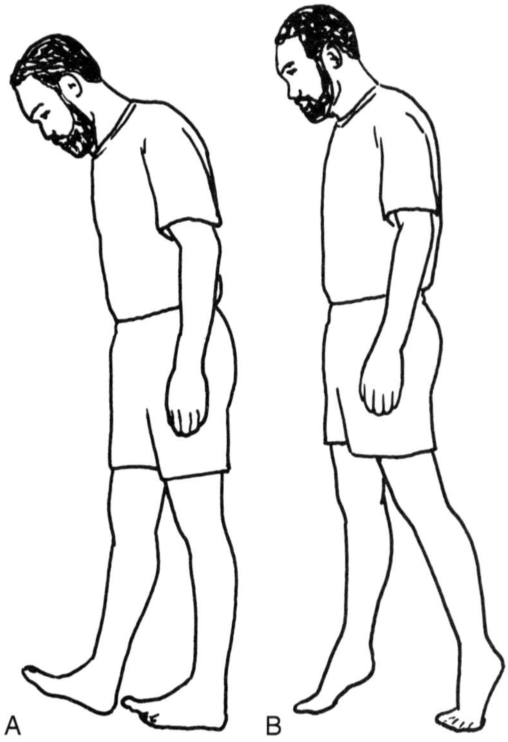

Figure 10.12 **A.** *The patient is walking on the heels: test of L5 motor function.* **B.** *The patient is walking on the toes: test of S1 motor function.*

Table 10.1. Grading of Muscle Strength

0—No movement of muscle unit
1—Flicker of tendon movement
2—Some muscle/tendon movement of joint only if gravity removed
3—More movement of joint against gravity and some resistance
4—Movement against gravity with reasonable resistance, but still weakness evident
5—Normal strength

STEP 6

Nerve root irritation is commonly associated with specific muscle tenderness. With 1st sacral root irritation, the calf becomes tender. With 5th lumbar root irritation, the anterior tibial muscles become tender; with 4th lumbar root irritation, the quadriceps are tender. Tenderness over the subcutaneous surface of the tibia is seen when emotional overtones play a large part in the clinical picture. Specific muscle tenderness is a very important physical sign of root irritation.

With the patient still supine, appreciation of pinprick can be tested, thus comparing the sensibility of the same areas in both legs. Dermatome areas are well localized. S1 supplies the sole and the outer border of the leg and foot. L5 supplies the dorsum of the foot and the anterior aspect of the lower leg; L4 supplies the anteromedial aspect of the shin (Fig. 10.13); L3 supplies the kneecap region; and L2 supplies the lateral thigh (see Fig. 10.13). The correct evaluation of sensory appreciation demands, strangely enough, a meticulous technique. Only gross changes can be detected by the perfunctory jab of a pin. When minor changes are sought, it is important to remember that sensory appreciation is dependent on summation of stimuli. Because of this physiological phenomenon, 10 pinpricks applied to a partially denervated area of the skin may be appreciated as readily as one or two pinpricks on the opposite leg. For accurate evaluation, the "stimulus" applied should be the same in both areas under comparison. The most tedious and uncomfortable part of the examination for the patient is being pricked with a pin (make sure it is not the same safety pin that has jabbed a patient before). Patients want to get the pinprick test over with quickly and are apt to agree to any suggestion of the examiner, just to get that portion of the examination over.

Vibration sensibility below the knees is not as acute in patients more than 50 years of age, and the same applies to temperature appreciation. It must be remembered that the demonstration of a "stocking" type of diminished appreciation of pinprick does not necessarily indicate that the pain is hysterical in origin. It may merely indicate that the patient is demonstrating a hysterical exaggeration of signs derived from a significant organic lesion. The significance of such a demonstration of sensory loss must be evaluated with all other symptoms and signs presented by the patient.

STEP 7

Signs of root tension may now be evaluated. Root tension is a term reserved to denote reproduction of extremity pain by stretching a peripheral nerve. When testing the sciatic nerve, the leg must never be raised suddenly by lifting the heel, because so much pain may be evoked by this maneuver as to make all other examinations useless. The leg should be raised slowly, with the knee maintained in the fully extended position by the examiner's hands (Fig. 10.14). It is important to record the range through which the leg must be raised before leg or buttock pain is experienced. Reproduction of back pain in this manner does not necessarily indicate root tension, of course. With any painful lesion of the back associated with hamstring spasm, straight leg raising will rotate the pelvis and irritate the lumbosacral region, giving rise to pain. However, reproduction or aggravation of sciatic pain by forced dorsiflexion of the ankle at the limit of straight leg raising is highly suggestive of root tension, and this impression is confirmed if the patient admits relief on bending the knee. If a patient still has pain after the knee has been flexed, and if the pain is increased on further flexion of the hip (bent leg raising), then

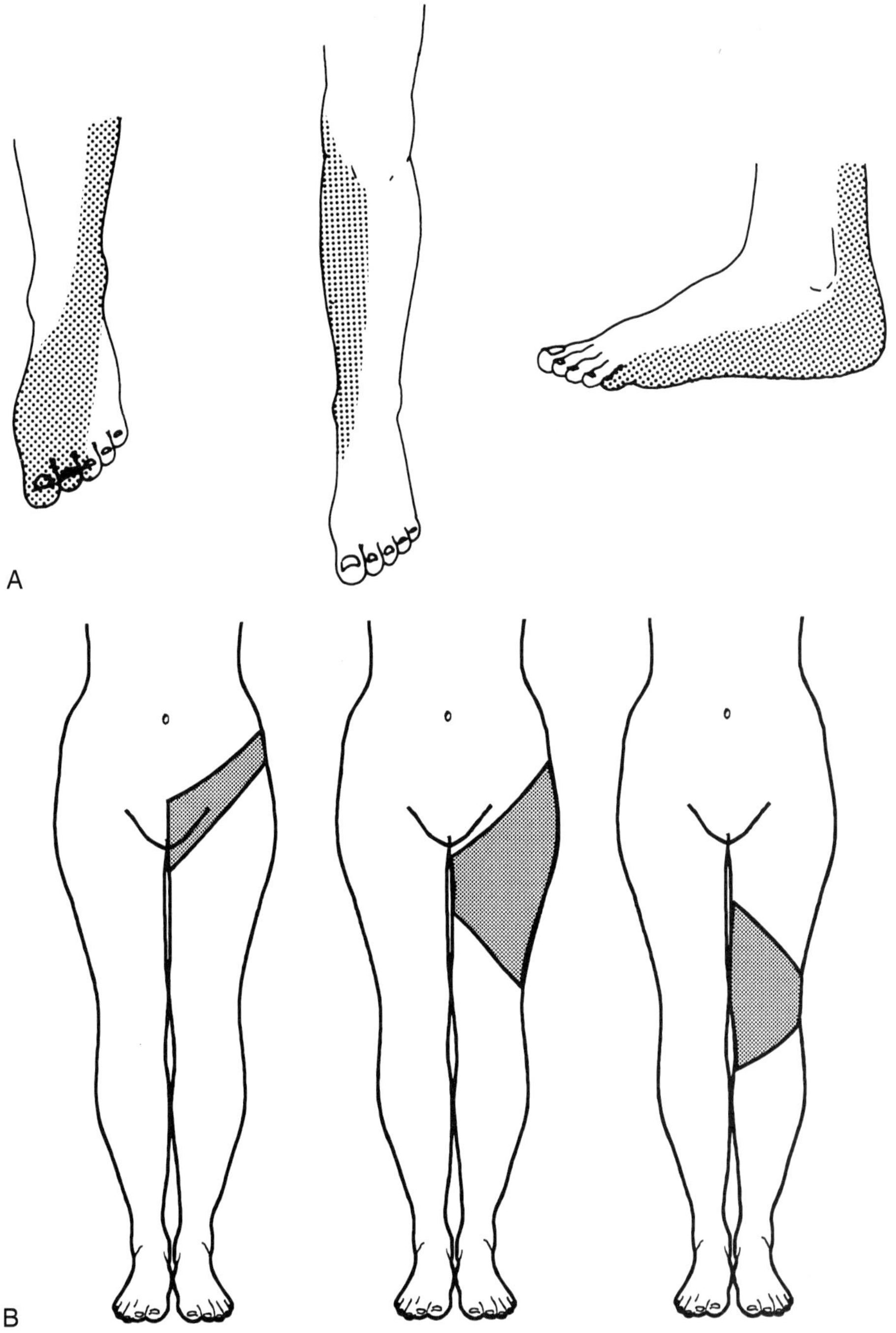

Figure 10.13 **A.** *The distribution of sensory dermatomes for lumbar roots L4 and L5 and sacral root S1 (left, L5; middle, L4; right, S1). It is unusual for a sensory loss to be dense throughout the complete dermatome; rather, the deficit may appear spotty throughout the dermatome. It is not unusual, especially in younger patients, to hear a classic story of a paresthetic discomfort in a typical dermatomal distribution, yet find no numbness on physical examination.* **B.** *L1, L2, L3 dermatomes: the stippled areas, left to right.*

the examiner should be concerned that he/she is dealing with a patient suffering from a significant emotional breakdown, or else there may be a lesion of the hip joint presenting as sciatic pain.

Straight leg raising of the opposite leg, the symptom-free leg, that gives rise to an exacerbation of pain in the affected extremity is known as crossover pain and is suggestive of a disc herniation lying in the axilla or medial to the root (Fig. 10.15).

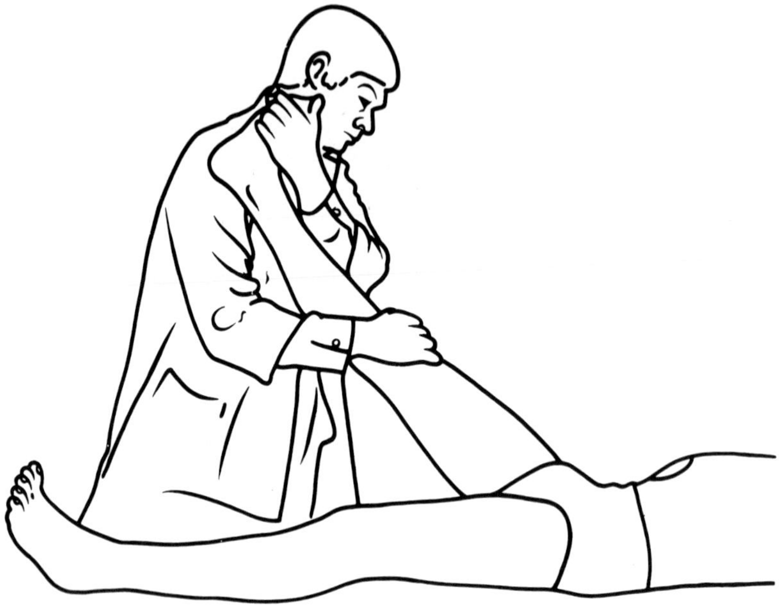

Figure 10.14 *When carrying out the straight leg raising test, it is important to remember that the leg should be raised slowly, and during this movement, the knee must be maintained in the fully extended position by the examiner's hand.*

Figure 10.15 *A disc herniation is present in the axilla of the right nerve root. SLR on the left will not only move the asymptomatic left root, but also pull the right root against the disc rupture. This will produce pain into the symptomatic right buttock, a phenomenon known as crossover pain.*

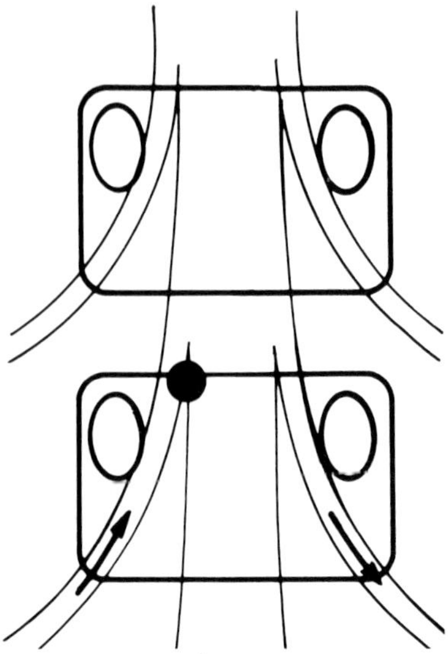

The most reliable test of root tension is the bowstring sign. In this test, straight leg raising is carried out until pain is reproduced. At this level, the knee is slightly flexed until the pain abates. The examiner rests the limb on his/her shoulder and places the thumbs in the popliteal fossa over the sciatic nerve. If sudden firm pressure on the nerve gives rise to pain in the back or down the leg, the patient is almost certainly suffering from significant root tension (Fig. 10.16). An excellent audit of the value of this test is to use the hamstring (see Fig. 10.16). Two sets of situations can exist: (1) Pressure over the medial hamstrings tendon causes no pain; pressure over the tibial nerve causes radiating pain; pressure over the lateral hamstring tendon causes no pain; pressure over the lateral peroneal nerve causes radiating pain. (2) pressure over the medial hamstring tendon causes pain; pressure over the tibial nerve causes pain; pressure over the lateral hamstring causes pain; pressure over the lateral peroneal nerve causes pain. The patient in the first situation has an obvious organic syndrome; the patient in the second situation may be an emotional cripple.

In a patient with weak abdominal muscles and disc degeneration, attempts to perform bilateral active straight leg raising are painful because the weight of the legs rotates the pelvis, causing hyperextension of the lumbar spine (Fig. 10.17).

Flexion of the hip with the knee flexed should not aggravate a mechanical back pain, but patients with emotional breakdowns frequently complain bitterly during this maneuver.

With lesions involving the 3rd and 4th lumbar roots, the patient will experience pain on stretching the femoral nerve. This test can be performed with the patient lying face downward. The hip is then extended, with the knee maintained in a slightly flexed position. This test is only of significance if the patient experiences pain radiating down the front of the symptomatic thigh (Fig. 10.18), and not down the thigh of the asymptomatic leg.

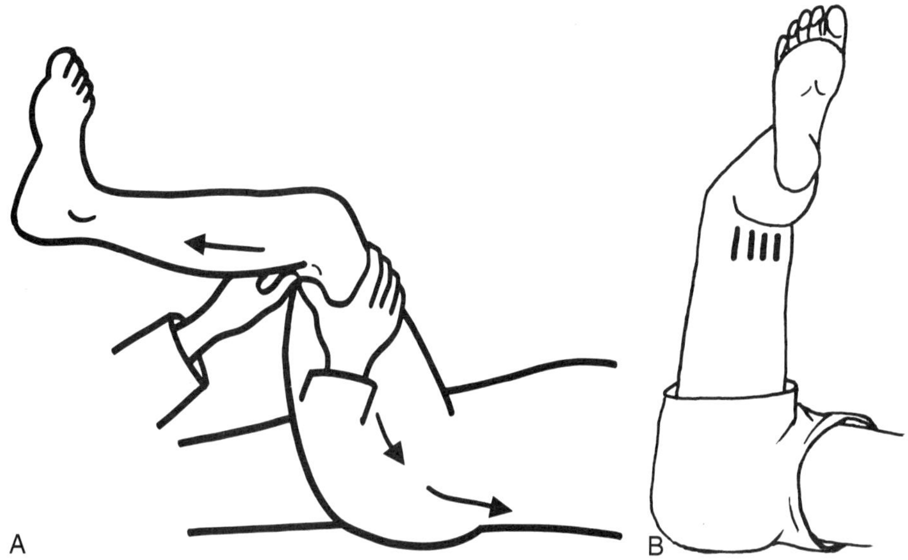

Figure 10.16 **A.** *When eliciting the bowstring sign, the patient's foot should be allowed to rest on the examiner's shoulder, with the knee very slightly flexed at the limit of straight leg raising. Sudden firm pressure is then applied by the examiner's thumbs in the popliteal fossa. Radiation of pain down the leg or the production of pain in the back is pathognomonic of root tension.* **B.** *An audit of the bowstring test: the four "cords" behind the knee are the medial and lateral hamstrings and the tibial and peroneal nerves; the latter two will be tender. The hamstring tendon pressure should not elicit pain.*

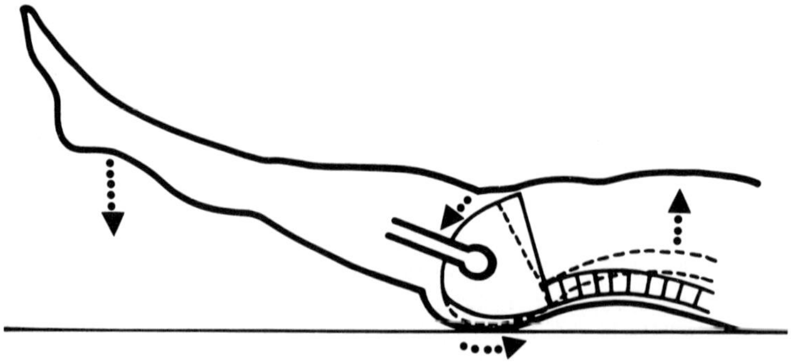

Figure 10.17 *When the patient carries out bilateral active straight leg raising, the weight of the leg causes the pelvis to rotate and thereby hyperextends the lumbar spine. Hyperextension of the lumbar spine in the presence of disc degeneration gives rise to pain. This is probably the most useful test to demonstrate the presence of painful segmental instability.*

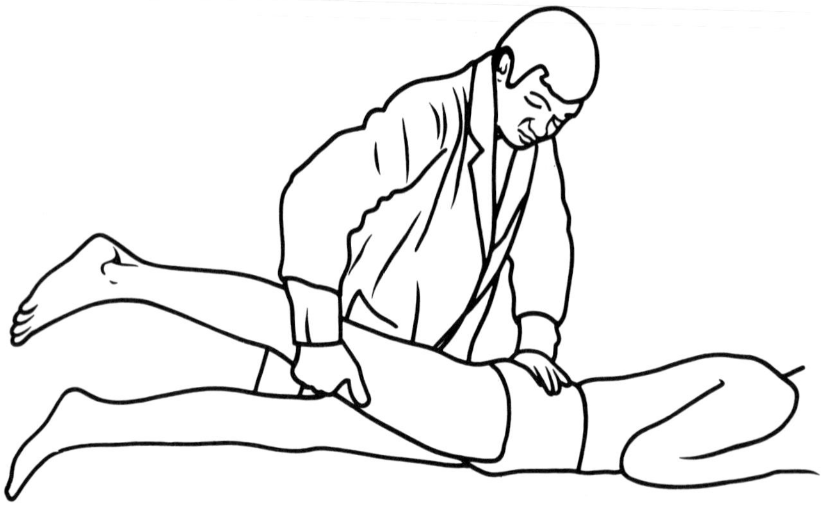

Figure 10.18 *When the fourth lumbar nerve root is compromised, the patient experiences pain radiating down the front of the thigh. This pain will be aggravated if the hip is extended with the knees slightly flexed. It is to be noted that this test may give rise to back pain by virtue of hyperextending the spine, but this finding is not of diagnostic significance.*

Care must be taken not to confuse the femoral nerve stretch test with Ely's sign (Fig. 10.19). The test for Ely's sign was designed to demonstrate contracture or shortening of the rectus femoris. The rectus femoris spans both the hip joint and the knee joint, flexing the hip and extending the knee. When the knee is fully flexed, the rectus femoris is stretched. If there is any contracture of the muscle (ie, due to hip disease), passive stretching in this manner will cause the hip to flex. This can be easily demonstrated by fully flexing the knee with the patient lying face downward; the resulting flexion of the hip is shown by the fact that the buttock rises off the bed. This is Ely's test. This test is frequently positive in patients of mesomorphic build. In some patients suffering from 4th lumbar root irritation, this maneuver gives rise to severe quadriceps pain.

STEP 8

At this stage of the examination, the full range of hip joint movements should be assessed. Osteoarthritis of the hip joint may give rise to symptoms and signs mimicking 4th lumbar root compression: pain down the front of the thigh, weakness and atrophy of the quadriceps, tenderness on palpation of the quadriceps, and pain on the femoral nerve stretch test. This confusion arises from a perfunctory examination. Always assess hip joint motion fully by: (1) watching the patient walk, (2) testing internal rotation, and (3) noting if there is any flexion deformity (Fig. 10.20).

STEP 9

Next, examine the peripheral pulses for signs of impairment of arterial circulation. Hair distribution and other atrophic changes, such as in the nails, will give some indication of vascular insufficiency. Impairment of venous outflow should also be noted. With the patient still supine, the abdomen is palpated for evidence of intra-abdominal masses, and the peripheral pulses are palpated for evidence of vascular insufficiency.

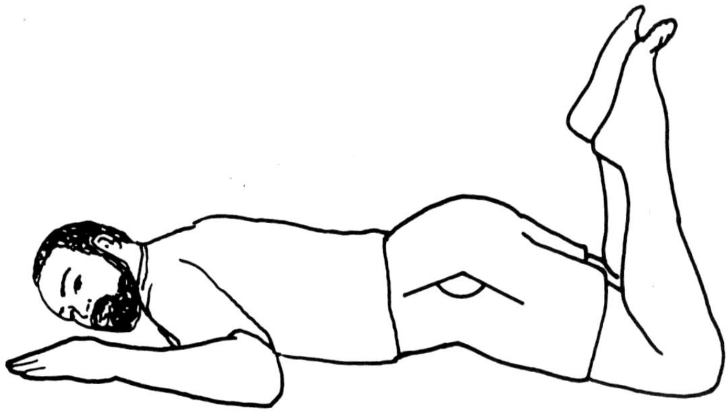

Figure 10.19 *Ely's sign: In the prone position, flexion of the knees should not normally cause flexion of the hips, as in this schematic.*

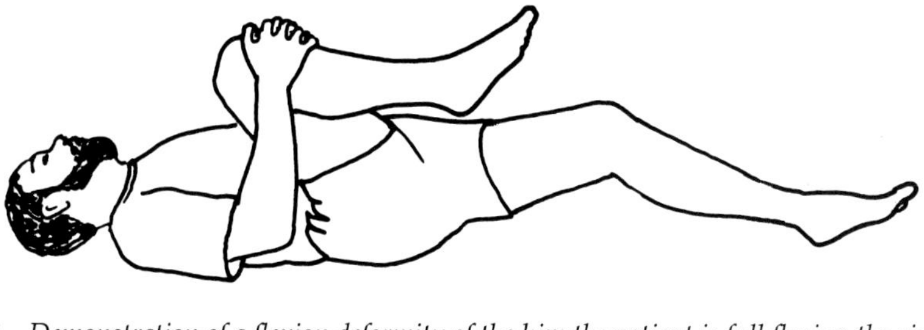

Figure 10.20 *Demonstration of a flexion deformity of the hip: the patient is full flexing the right hip; a normal left hip would allow the left leg to rest flat on the bed. A flexion deformity of the left hip with this test would not allow the left leg to rest on the bed.*

STEP 10

The patient is then turned on his/her side. The ability to abduct the leg against resistance is tested. When this movement is performed, the glutei must contract vigorously and should tend to pull the pelvis away from the sacrum. A patient with a sacroiliac strain or any sacroiliac disease will find this movement painful.

The sacroiliac joint can also be tested by applying a rotary strain. The unaffected hip joint is flexed, and the thigh is held firmly against the chest by the patient in order to lock the lumbar spine. The uppermost hip is now extended to its limit. When the hip is pushed beyond its limit of joint extension, a rotary strain is applied to the sacroiliac joint, which is a movement that causes pain when sacroiliac diseases are present (Fig. 10.21). If a sacroiliac joint lesion is present, lateral compression of the pelvis when the patient is lying on his/her side sometimes gives rise to pain.

Miscellaneous Steps

It is frequently convenient, because the patient is already on his/her side, to carry out a rectal examination at this stage. The patient is turned face downward, and the buttocks and thighs are palpated for tumors involving the sciatic nerve.

At some point during the examination leg lengths should be measured. The maximal girth of the calf is compared on the two sides, and the circumference of the thigh is measured on both sides at a fixed distance from the tibial tubercle. The patient is then asked to sit on the side of the couch so that chest expansion can be determined. A decrease in chest expansion is an early change in ankylosing spondylitis.

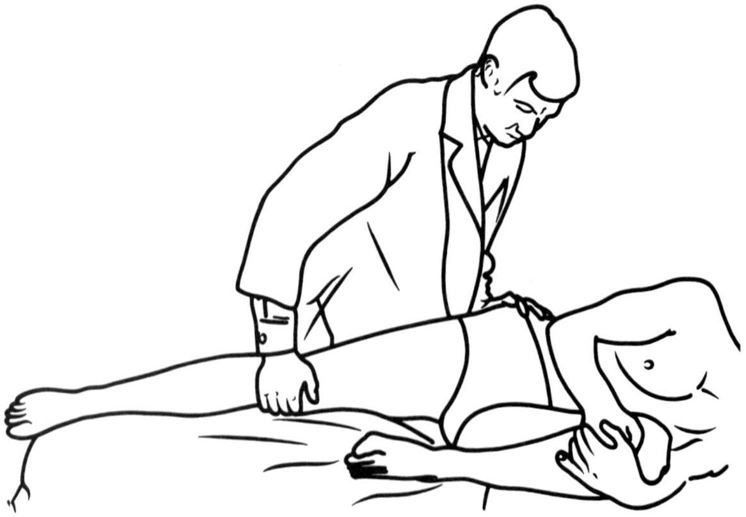

Figure 10.21 *Gaenslen's test. The patient lies on his/her side and holds the lumbar spine rigid by flexing the lowermost hip and pulling the knee against the chest. The uppermost hip is now extended by the examiner. At the limit of hip joint extension, any further extension strain applies a rotary strain to the pelvis and tends to rotate one-half of the ilium against the sacrum. With sacroiliac joint lesions, this maneuver is painful.*

This test can also be performed with the patient lying on his/her back holding the knee flexed against the chest and a hyperextension strain can be applied to the hip by allowing the leg to drop over the side of the table. From Macnab I: Backache. Williams & Wilkins, Baltimore (1977), p. 128.

The patient is then asked to step down from the couch and drape him-/herself over its edge, resting the abdomen on a pillow. This position is usually comfortable and brings all the spinous processes into prominence. An area not expected to be tender is tested first. Firm pressure applied to the spine may be uncomfortable. The patient must be able to differentiate between the expected discomfort of such pressure and the abnormal discomfort when the damaged segment is palpated. Each spinous process is palpated separately, with firm pressure being exerted anteriorly and in a lateral direction (Fig. 10.22). Examination of the back for tenderness is probably the most poorly administered part of the examination, mainly because the examiner fails to assess the patient for superficial tenderness and tenderness over the sacrum. Tuck this in the back of your mind because you will meet the concept again in Chapter 12.

Although the specific findings on examination of patients suffering from nonorganic spinal pain are discussed in detail in Chapter 12, physical signs of emotional overtones are so commonly overlooked that they cannot be overemphasized and should be separately tabulated at this point. Table 10.2 summarizes the historical and physical characteristics that suggest a nonorganic component to the patient's disability.

SUMMARY

When you leave the examining room to look at the patient's radiographs (good spine clinicians will never look at radiographs before they look at the patient!), you will be able to say the following:

1. I heard the patient's story (I listened to the music of their history), and I suspected a diagnosis.
2. I not only verified the diagnosis on physical examination, I know the anatomical level of spinal involvement (Table 10.3).
3. I also know everything there is to know about the lower extremity systems other than the neurological system, that is, the locomotor system and the vascular system.

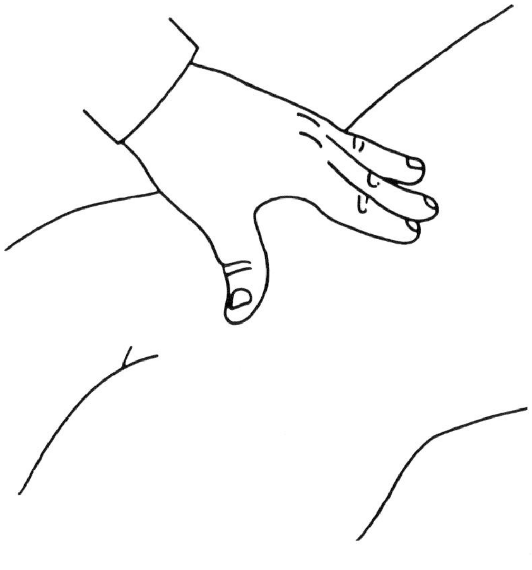

Figure 10.22 *Pain on direct pressure over a spinous process may reflect nothing more than referred tenderness. More information can be obtained if the examiner places his/her thumb against the side of the spinous process and applies pressure not only in a forward direction but in a lateral direction as well, thereby applying a rotary strain to the segment. Reproduction of the clinically experienced pain by this maneuver is of great diagnostic significance. From Macnab I: Backache. Williams & Wilkins, Baltimore (1977), p. 130.*

Table 10.2. Symptoms and Signs Suggesting a Nonorganic Component to Back Disability

Symptoms

1. Pain is multifocal in distribution and nonmechanical (present at rest)
2. Entire extremity is painful, numb, and/or weak
3. Extremity gives way (as a result, the patient carries a cane)
4. Treatment response
   a. No response
   b. "Allergic" to treatment
   c. Not receiving treatment
5. Multiple crises, multiple hospital admissions/investigations, multiple doctors

Signs

1. Tenderness is superficial (skin) or nonanatomical (eg, over body of sacrum)
2. Simulated movement tests are positive
3. Distraction test is positive
4. Whole leg is weak or numb
5. "Academy Award" performance

Table 10.3. Potential Neurological Findings in Root Lesions

	Root		
Change	**L4**	**L5**	**S1**
Motor weakness	Knee extension	Ankle dorsiflexion: EHL	Ankle plantar flexion: FHL
Sensory loss	Medial shin to knee	Dorsum of foot and lateral calf	Lateral border of foot and posterior calf
Reflex depression	Knee	Tibialis posterior	Ankle
Wasting	Thigh (no calf)	Calf (minimal thigh)	Calf (minimal thigh)

Key: EHL = extensor hallucis longus; FHL = flexor hallucis longus.

Now I am ready to review the radiographs and verify that the structural lesion that I suspect, because of the history and physical examination, is indeed present. I will look at the radiographs and other investigations with a commitment to a perfect marriage between what I suspect on clinical assessment and what I see on radiograph. If I do not have that perfect marriage just described that results in determining not only the structural lesion, but also the anatomical level, then I have made a mistake. Either my history and physical examination are in error or my interpretation of the investigation is wrong. It is then time to return to the drawing board of medicine, the patient's bedside, and start over.

11

The Investigation

"Seek, and ye shall find...."

— Matthew 7:7

INTRODUCTION

When you are seeing patients with low back pain (and other spinal pain) day in and day out, you quickly realize how easy it is to miss or err in diagnosis (Tables 11.1 and 11.2). As a clinician, you start to "build a better mousetrap" so you do not make these errors.

A Fail-Safe System (see Chapter 18)

Rather than remember all of the various diagnoses listed in Tables 11.1 and 11.2, take a very pragmatic approach to the diagnosis regarding the cause of the patient's back complaints and ask the following questions:

1. Is the pain a true physical disability, or is there a setting and a pattern on history and physical examination to suggest a nonphysical or nonorganic problem? (Also refer to Chapter 3.)
2. Is the pain a diagnostic trap (Tables 11.1 and 11.2)?
3. Is the pain a mechanical low back problem and, if so, what is the syndrome (Table 11.3)?
4. Are there clues to an anatomical level on history and physical examination before I look at the investigation?
5. After reviewing the results of the investigation, what is the structural lesion, and does it fit with my clinical syndrome (Table 11.4)?

Although these questions may not be answered sequentially during the history and physical examination, they ultimately must be answered sequentially before arriving at a diagnosis and prescribing a treatment program. That is to say, do not answer Question 5 (ie, look at a radiograph) and plan a treatment program until you have satisfactory answers to each of the preceding questions. Probably the biggest pitfall is to answer Question 3 before you have satisfactorily answered Questions 1 and 2. The answers to Questions 1 and 2 should routinely be made outside of the hospital and before computed tomography (CT), myelogram, magnetic resonance imaging (MRI), and other sophisticated investigative

Table 11.1. Differential Diagnosis of Nonmechanical Low Back Pain

Causes of Nonmechanical Low Back Pain
Referred pain (eg, from the abdomen or retroperitoneal space)
Infection
Bone
Disc
Epidural space
Neoplasm
Primary (multiple myeloma, osteoid osteoma, and so on)
Secondary
Inflammation: arthritides such as ankylosing spondylitis
Miscellaneous metabolic and vascular disorders such as osteopenia and Paget's disease

Table 11.2. Differential Diagnosis of Sciatica

Intraspinal causes
Proximal to disc: conus and cauda equina lesions (eg, neurofibroma, ependymoma)
Disc level
Herniated nucleus pulposus
Stenosis (canal or recess)
Infection: osteomyelitis or discitis (with nerve root pressure)
Inflammation arachnoiditis
Neoplasm: benign or malignant with nerve root pressure
Extraspinal causes
Pelvis
Cardiovascular conditions (eg, peripheral vascular disease)
Gynecological conditions causing sacral plexus pressure
Orthopedic conditions (eg, osteoarthritis of hip)
Sacroiliac joint disease
Neoplasms (invading or compressing lumbosacral plexus)
Peripheral nerve lesions
Neuropathy (diabetic, tumor, alcohol)
Local sciatic nerve conditions (trauma, tumor)
Inflammation (herpes zoster)

modalities are used. The classic trap is to ignore Questions 1 and 2 and admit a patient with a complaint of low back pain to the hospital, seek pathology with sophisticated investigative tools, and then prescribe a treatment plan based on false-positive findings.

Question 1

Is this a true physical disability, or is there a setting and a pattern on history and physical examination to suggest a nonphysical or emotional problem? By now, you realize the importance of this question!

This question will be addressed in its entirety in Chapter 18, and readers are referred to that chapter for a discussion of the investigation useful to the resolution of this question.

Question 2

Is this clinical presentation a trap? It is so easy, when trying to arrive at a mechanical diagnosis, to fall into the many traps in the differential diagnosis of low back pain. Examples are the young man in the early stages of ankylosing spondylitis who presents with vague sacroiliac joint pain and mild buttock and thigh discomfort and is thought to have a disc herniation. The patient with a retroperitoneal tumor invading the sacrum or sacral plexus may present with classic sciatica and also be diagnosed as having a disc herniation. It is not uncommon that patients with pathology within the peritoneal cavity will refer pain to the back. To avoid missing these various diagnostic pitfalls, always ask yourself the second question: is this clinical presentation a trap?

Two broad categories of disease are included in this question.

1. Back pain referred from outside the spine may come from within the peritoneal cavity (eg, gastrointestinal tumors or ulcers), or from the retroperitoneal space (genitourinary conditions, abdominal aortic conditions, or primary or secondary tumors of the retroperitoneal space). These patients can be recognized clinically on the basis of two historical points. First, the pain is often nonmechanical in nature and troubles the patient more at rest than it does with activity. Second, the pain in the back often has the characteristics of the pain associated with the primary pathology, that is, if the primary condition is colicky, the referred pain will be colicky.
2. Painful conditions arising from within the spinal column, including its neurological content, constitute the second group of disorders. This group is subdivided into the differential diagnosis of low back pain or lumbago and the differential diagnosis of radicular pain or sciatica (Tables 11.1 and 11.2).

These patients have nonmechanical back pain or a pain more characteristic for the primary pathology. Radiating extremity pain is not common unless neurological territory has been invaded by the disease process, a happening that usually occurs late in the disease. Unfortunately, many of these conditions are not obvious on history and physical examination and are often missed on reviewing plain radiographs. The following laboratory tests are useful as a screening mechanism:

- Hemoglobin, hematocrit, white blood cell count, differential, and erythrocyte sedimentation rate.
- Serum chemistries, especially calcium, acid and alkaline phosphatase, and serum protein electrophoresis.
- HLA-B27 antigen.
- Bone scan.

It is a good routine to agree to do the hematological tests and serum chemistries in the following individuals: all older patients (over age 55), all patients who have a significant nonmechanical component to their pain, any patient with an atypical pain pattern or distribution, and all patients who do not respond to standard conservative treatment directed at the mechanical causes of low back pain.

Although some would consider this overinvestigation of the patient, the conditions so uncovered represent a broad spectrum of medical conditions that are apt to appear in any family practice office.

Questions 3, 4, and 5 are answered in the various chapters in this book and summarized in Chapter 18. They are also summarized in Tables 11.3 and 11.4. The reasons for deciding to investigate a low back pain patient are twofold:

1. Failure of a mechanical syndrome to respond to conservative care (the most common reason).
2. The suspicion of a serious diagnosis such as infection or tumor.

Beyond plain radiographs that are shown throughout this text, the choices for investigation are:

Bone scanning (scintigraphy).
Myelography.
CT scan.
CT/myelogram.
Discography and CT/discography.
MRI.
Nerve root infiltration test.
Electromyography/nerve conduction tests.

Table 11.3. Syndromes in Mechanical Low Back Disorders[a]

Lumbago: back pain (mechanical instability)
Sciatica: radicular pain
Unilateral acute radicular syndrome
Bilateral acute radicular syndrome
Unilateral chronic radicular syndrome
Bilateral chronic radicular syndrome

[a]These syndromes are described in detail in Chapters 14, 15, 16, and 17.

Table 11.4. Structural Lesions That Cause the Syndromes in Mechanical Low Back Pain

Instability
Intrinsic to disc
Degenerative disc disease (DDD)
Extrinsic to disc
Facet joint disease (FJD)
Spondylolisthesis/spondylolysis
Soft tissue lesions
Muscle spasm
Ligamentous strain
Herniated nucleus pulposus (HNP)
Narrowing of spinal canal
Spinal canal stenosis (SCS)
Lateral zone stenosis (LZS)

BONE SCANNING (SCINTIGRAPHY)

Since the first edition of this book in 1977, bone scanning has come a long way. From whole body scanning for metastases with strontium, a tracer element that is difficult to work with and results in a high radiation dose to the patient, we are now to a stage of selective regional imaging using the workhorse radionuclide of nuclear medicine, technetium-99m-labeled phosphorus (^{99m}Tc).

Indications for Bone Scan

The location of metastatic bone lesions remains the most common indication for bone scanning, and this technology has virtually displaced the radiographic skeletal survey in the adult (except for multiple myeloma). The second most common reason for considering the use of bone scintigraphy is for early detection of bone infection, days before regular radiographic changes occur. Bone scanning is also being used in detection of osteonecrosis, the study of failed joint prostheses, the investigation of unexplained bone pain (especially in the high-powered athlete who may suffer a stress fracture), and the dating of fracture age.(2, 3)

For the purpose of this book, a brief summary of bone scanning techniques in today's world is given. The reader is advised to keep a finger on the pulse of imaging advancement; the ride will be exciting, washing away today's standards. Imaging techniques are changing dramatically, and the time period from 1980 to 2000 will be seen as a time of great change in radiography, as significant to medicine as the original observations of Wilhelm Konrad Röntgen.

Technetium-99m-Labeled Phosphorus (^{99m}Tc)

^{99m}Tc is currently the most frequently used radionuclide in nuclear medicine.(7) This predominance exists because the radionuclide is readily available and cheap, and has an ideal biological behavior pattern. This includes easy incorporation in bone, timing of incorporation that suits hospital procedures, and a low radiation dose to the patient.

So that it will target the bone cell, ^{99m}Tc has to be linked to phosphorus before being injected intravenously. Over the years, the pharmaceutical agent to which ^{99m}Tc was linked has been changing to improve image quality. Today, technetium is largely used in a linkage to diphosphonates (organic phosphates). Linkage to other compounds will change its specificity to other parts of the body (eg, when linked to macroaggregated albumin, the radionuclide will be deposited in the capillary beds of lung for lung scanning). The fact that ^{99m}Tc in phosphorus quickly incorporates in bone within 15 minutes of intravenous (IV) injection points to its mechanism of action. The exchange occurs at the interface of bone and extracellular fluid where active mineralization is taking place. The ^{99m}Tc-labeled phosphorus incorporates into bone by becoming one or more of the inorganic components of hydroxyapatite. From there, it emits gamma rays that are detectable by a gamma camera. The faster the bone turnover (the faster the mineralization of osteoid), the greater the ^{99m}Tc in deposit and the more gamma radiation is emitted by the site. This is the basis of the "hot spot" (Fig. 11.1).

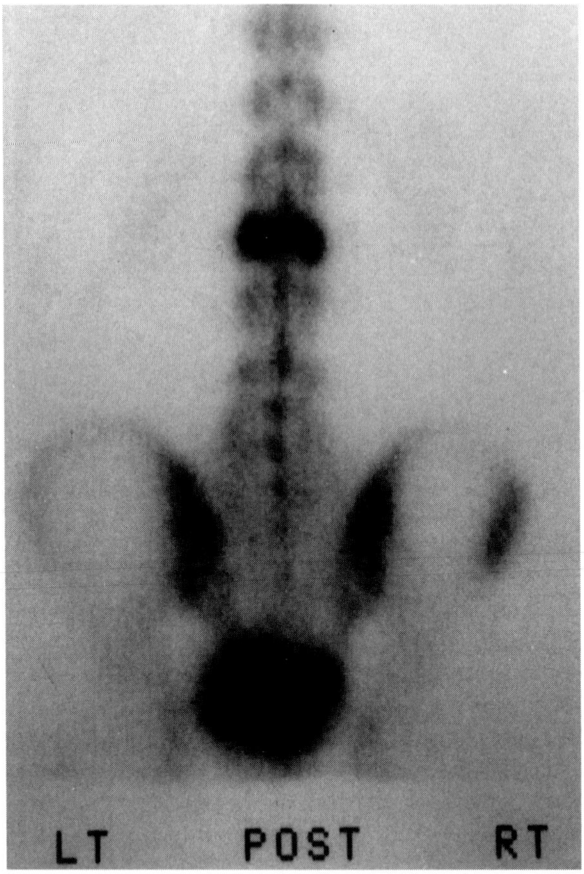

Figure 11.1 *Bone scan (Tc-99m) showing a hot spot in L2—a metastatic tumor.*

Technique

^{99m}Tc is shipped in a parent form of molybdenum-99, which in its container spins off ^{99m}Tc. The container, depending on volume of usage, will deliver useful product for approximately a week. The phosphorus-labeled compound is injected intravenously, and three phases of scans are completed (4):

Phase I The perfusion scan (flow study) is done within 1 to 2 minutes after IV injection to show whether the area of interest has a vascular supply. This scan is also known as the nuclear angiogram. It is of little use in spinal scanning but is often mentioned in the literature.

Phase II The blood pool scan is done 5 to 10 minutes after the Phase I scan and will show the internal vascular status of the lesion. Higher counts signify a vascular lesion; lower counts signify a less vascular lesion. This scan is of limited use in spinal scanning, as well.

Phase III The delayed bone image scan is done 2 to 4 hours after injection, at which time bone incorporation of the tracer isotope onto the bone hydroxyapatite crystal is maximum, and background tracer has been excreted by the kidneys. The half-life of ^{99m}Tc is 6 hours, and by this time the gamma count is becoming too low to be a useful measure.

Phases I and II scans are rarely used in nuclear scanning of the spine.

Technetium-99-labeled phosphorus is deposited where bone turnover is greatest (ie, the hydroxyapatite crystals that are the most immature). These sites are normally located in growing bones at the epiphysis, metaphyseal regions of long bones, and the sacroiliac joints (a fact that limits the usefulness of bone scanning in ankylosing spondylitis). Abnormal (faster) bone turnover occurs in tumors, infections, and fractures, as well as bone–soft tissue junctions where increased metabolic activity is occurring. Sites with decreased bone activity, such as osteonecrosis or highly destructive tumors (multiple myeloma), will show no activity change (normal bone scan) or a "cold spot" (decreased tracer activity compared with surrounding normal bone). Examples of scans are shown in Figures 11.2 and 11.3.

Dose

The usual dose of ^{99m}Tc is 10 to 20 mCi. Radiation doses administered to various tissues of the body are well within acceptable levels.(1) The greatest exposure (500–1000 mrad) occurs in the bladder and is best handled by good patient hydration before and after the scan. The height of kidney excretion and bladder exposure occurs 3 hours after injection

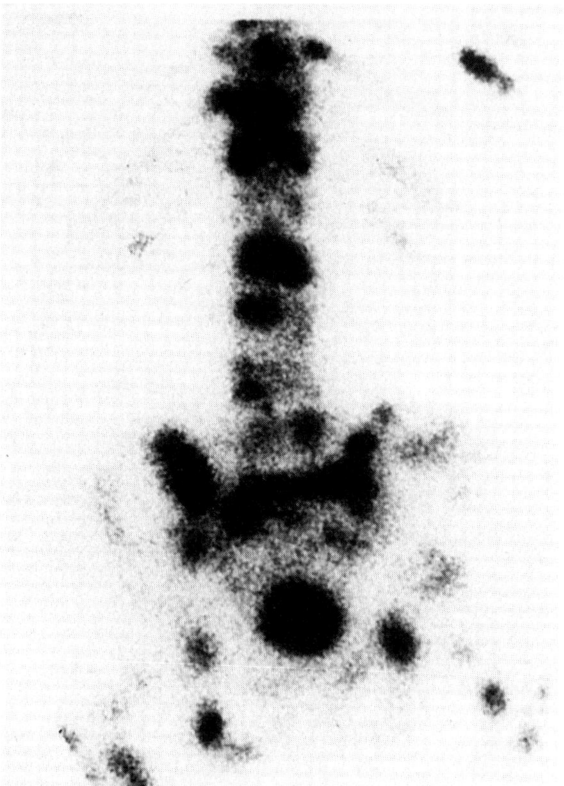

Figure 11.2 *Bone scan (Tc-99m) done 3 hours after injection, showing multiple hot spots in metastatic disease.*

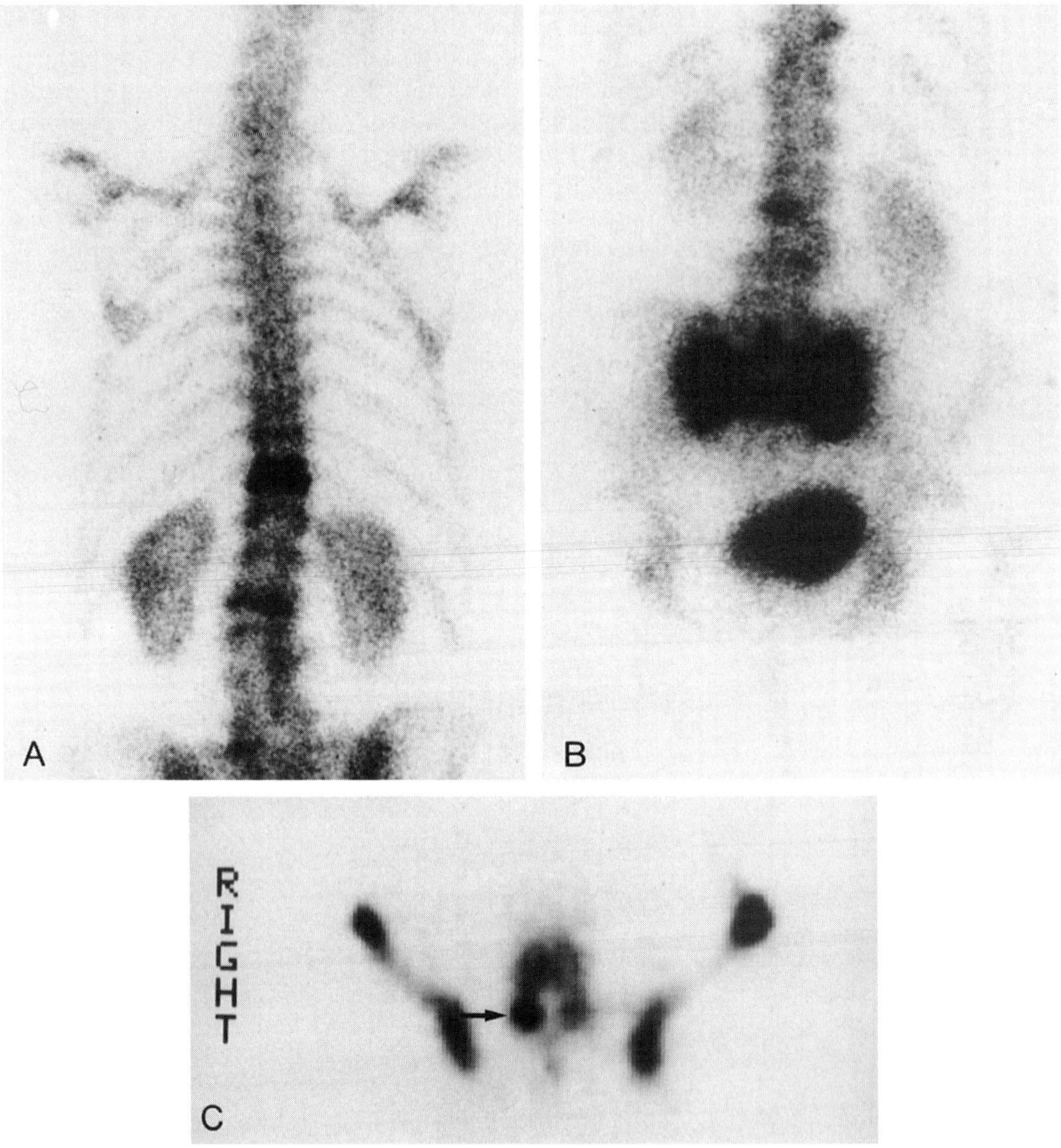

Figure 11.3 *Bone scans (Tc-99m) in:* **A,** *compression fracture;* **B,** *sacral fracture;* **C,** *spondylolysis (right, L5) (arrow).*

when at least one third of the amount of tracer injected has been cleared by the kidneys. At that time, 30 to 40% of the tracer is bound in bone, 10 to 15% is bound in other tissue, and 5% is bound in blood.

Gallium Scanning

^{99m}Tc-labeled phosphorus scanning identifies areas of increased bone turnover and is nonspecific for infection. This led to the search for compounds that would specifically bind to sites of infection, the most popular (until recently) being gallium 67 citrate (^{67}Ga). This tracer binds to transferrin and other proteins associated with inflammation and infection. Unfortunately, it emits four gamma rays (photons) ranging from low to high energy, which cause more patient exposure to radiation while at the same time making the scan less clear.

Gallium is slowly excreted through the kidneys and bowel such that the optimal time of scanning (that time when concentration in the area of interest is potentially highest, and background contamination by blood and soft tissue content is lowest) is 48 hours. This has the potential for: contaminating other scanning efforts, such as ^{99m}Tc; taxing the scheduling efforts of a large hospital department; and testing patient compliance.

More recently, a number of reports on the limited accuracy of gallium scanning, especially in low-grade infections, are appearing in the literature.(5, 6)

The value of gallium scanning appears to be enhanced by doing ^{99m}Tc and gallium 67 citrate scanning sequentially and comparing the uptake of the two scans. A hot ^{99m}Tc bone scan with increased ^{67}Ga activity is suggestive of a bone infection (Fig. 11.4).

The disadvantages of the gallium scan are a high radiation dose, poor spatial resolution, and the 48 to 72 hours of waiting between injection and imaging. As a result, ^{67}Ga scanning is not used on a regular basis.

Indium-111-Labeled Leukocytes (Fig. 11.5)

Because of the limited accuracy of ^{67}Ga scanning, further research has led to the proposal that indium-111-labeled leukocytes have a greater specificity for musculoskeletal (and other) infective foci.

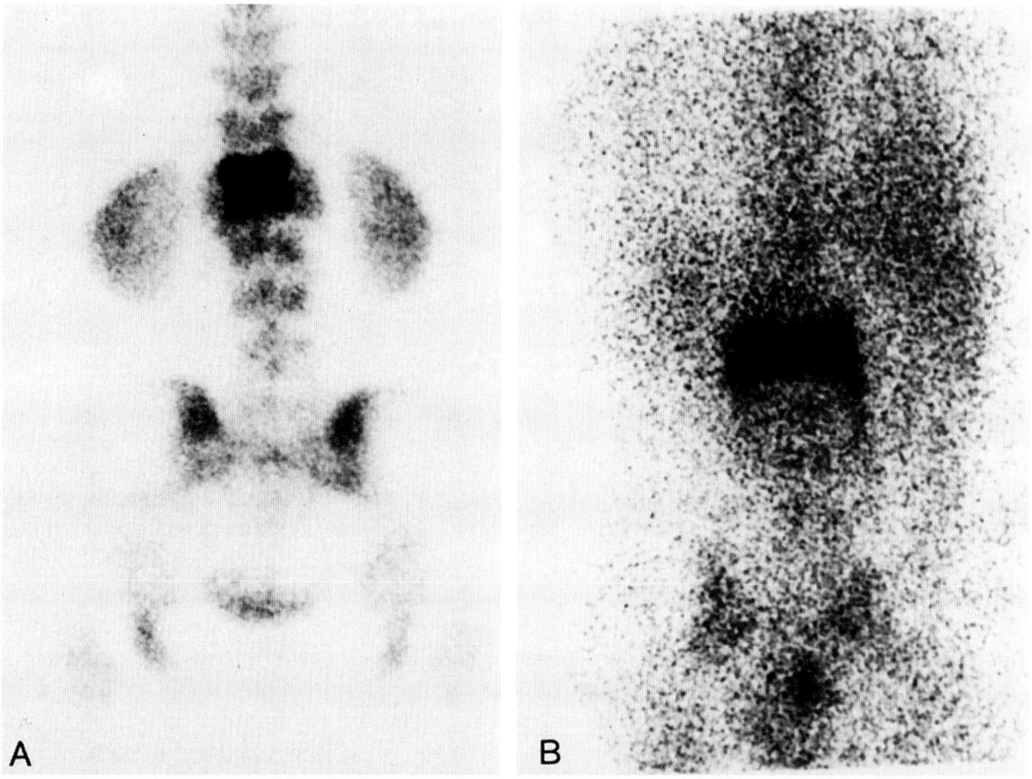

Figure 11.4 *^{99m}Tc* **(A)** *and Ga-citrate scan* **(B)** *in a patient with increasing pain after a fracture. She subsequently developed osteomyelitis.*

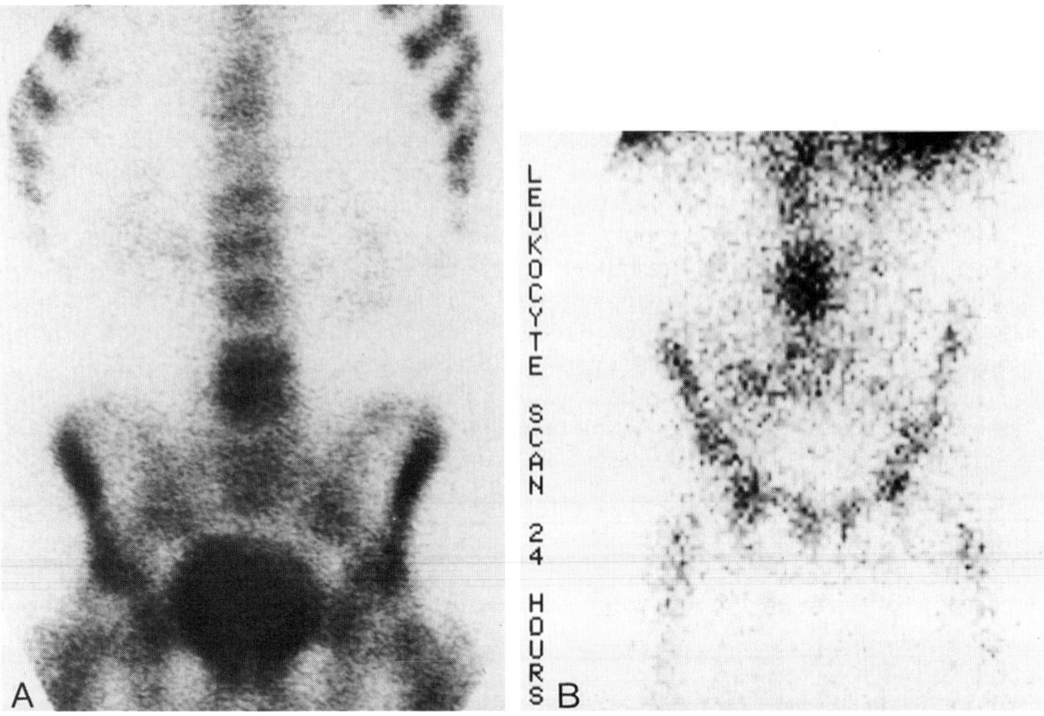

Figure 11.5 **A.** *PA lumbar spine bone scan in a middle-aged man who presented with severe back pain and a severe febrile illness. Note the increased tracer uptake at L3-4.* **B.** *An indium scan in the same patient supporting the diagnosis of a vertebral column infection that was subsequently proven on a percutaneous biopsy.*

Technique

After harvesting the patient's own blood, the WBCs are separated (by centrifuge and chemical means) and labeled with the radioactive tracer indium 111. These labeled leukocytes are resuspended in the patient's plasma and re-injected to seek out foci of infection. Twenty-four hours later, gamma activity is measured with a gamma radiation detection camera.

The higher sensitivity and specificity for indium scanning appears to be well established in the literature. Other advantages of indium scanning include a maintenance of this accuracy in the presence of low-grade chronic infection and in patients receiving antibiotics and steroids. The fact that scanning can be done 24 hours after injection facilitates hospital scheduling, although the front end load of harvesting and labeling the leukocytes is offsetting.

It would appear that the results of indium-111 scanning, when interpreted in light of clinical findings (fever) and laboratory findings (WBC count and erythrocyte sedimentation rate [ESR]), are more accurate for the detection of musculoskeletal infections than gallium 67 citrate scanning.(5, 6) ^{99m}Tc/indium-111 scanning is probably the scintigraphy method of choice for investigating a patient suspected of having increased bone turnover from tumor or infection. In the absence of the clinical suspicion of infection, ^{99m}Tc scanning alone is sufficient.

Single Photon Emission Computed Tomography (SPECT)

Normal nuclear imaging is recorded on only two planes (anteroposterior [AP] and posteroanterior and/or lateral) of the three-dimensional skeleton. The significant overlapping of anatomic structures can blur the localization of radionucleotides in the posterior elements of the lumbar spine. With more sophisticated camera systems and the principle of rotating the gamma camera 360°, multiplanar images of the spine, similar to CT, can be obtained (Fig. 11.3, C). The rotation of the more sensitive cameras minimizes the superimposed activity from over- or underlying structures that occurs in planar imaging. The principles of "slicing" tissue planes into thin wafers that is discussed later in the CT sections applies to SPECT scanning.

The usual indications for a SPECT scan are:

1. An equivocal or negative scan in a patient with no known diagnosis and significant back pain.
2. A young patient with a suspected posterior element lesion, for example, spondylolysis.

The usual format is to complete a high-resolution planner (regular) bone scan in the anterior and posterior projections and then, if indicated, to complete a SPECT scan. This routine will increase the sensitivity of bone scanning in pinpointing spondylolysis, discitis, facet joint problems, and slow-growing (benign) bone tumors.

Conclusion

Although bone scintigraphy is commonly used today, major changes in nuclear imaging are occurring and will change the indications for use of bone scintigraphy. An example is SPECT, a newer imaging technique just discussed.

PLAIN RADIOGRAPHS

In the assessment of routine mechanical low back pain, the question always arises, "Should a radiograph be taken?" A radiograph is not harmful, but it is about as illogical to take a radiograph of every patient who has a backache as it is to order a barium study on every patient who has a touch of indigestion. A radiograph on the first attendance of a patient with back pain is, however, indicated under the following circumstances:

- Severe back pain after significant trauma.
- Incapacitating back pain.
- A history suggestive of vertebral crush due to osteoporosis or malignancy. These patients, usually more than 50 years of age, report a history of pain coming on without provocative injury, punctuated by sudden cramps of pain in the bank.
- The excessively anxious patient. In such people, a radiograph is an essential part of treatment. These patients cannot be reassured by clinical examination alone.
- Patients in whom the history and examination are suggestive of ankylosing spondylitis. A specific request should be made for views of the sacroiliac joint.
- Patients with a clinically apparent spinal deformity.
- Patients with significant root tension and those presenting evidence of impairment of root conduction. In these patients, a radiograph is of importance to exclude the possibility of malignancy.

- If severe pain persists despite treatment for more than 2 weeks, a radiograph is indicated, not only to exclude the possibility of some obscure spinal abnormality but also to reassure the patient that he/she is not suffering from a serious progressive disease.

Radiographs have limited function in diagnosis and treatment. In diagnosis, the main function of a radiograph is to exclude serious disease, such as infections, ankylosing spondylitis, and neoplasms. If radiographs of the spine show disc degeneration, this radiological change merely demonstrates a segment that is vulnerable to trauma. Such a demonstration, however, does not necessarily indict this segment as the cause of the presenting symptoms. Treatment is determined by clinical assessment, not by the radiological findings.

Radiological examination of the spine carries with it certain dangers. Anatomical abnormalities demonstrated on radiograph may simply stop the physician from thinking any further about possible diagnoses. These abnormalities are rarely the cause of back pain but are a frequent cause of anxiety in patients who are told of their presence. Even the statement, "your radiographs showed degenerative discs" may induce unpleasant misapprehension in the patient.

The term "degeneration" implies to the average patient a type of "rotting away," like bad cheese. A patient should never be presented with the bald statement, "the radiographs of your spine show arthritis." First, this is rarely true. The presence of osteophytes or, more correctly, "spondylophytes" on the vertebral bodies does not denote arthritis. Second, the term "arthritis" carries with it an evil connotation for the patient. Given this diagnosis, the patients frequently foresee a progressive restriction in their way of life leading eventually to a wheelchair existence.

Detailed assessment of radiological findings indicative of mechanical insufficiency of the spine is only of value in the preoperative assessment of a patient. At this time, a thorough analysis of the radiographic findings is of importance in determining whether surgical intervention is feasible and, if so, the type of operative correction required.

In reading plain radiographs (Fig. 11.6), look at the nonskeletal areas first. Review the retroperitoneal area with specific regard to the kidneys and ureters, and the abdominal aorta. Be sure that the psoas shadows are intact. After reviewing the nonskeletal part of a lumbar spine radiograph, consider the skeleton. Look at the sacroiliac joints, survey the pedicles and vertebral bodies for erosions, and finally consider the structural defects that may have a potential for causing the patient's syndrome. Such observations as narrowing of the disc space and translation of vertebral bodies should be noted, and may turn out to be important. Various measurements on plain radiographs are not helpful in assessment of canal or recess narrowing (see Chapters 16 and 17).

MYELOGRAPHY, COMPUTERIZED AXIAL TOMOGRAPHY, AND MAGNETIC RESONANCE IMAGING

The assessment of routine mechanical low back pain becomes less routine if the patient's disability persists despite treatment. Fortunately, most low back problems resolve with routine care, and no further investigation is needed. Occasionally, low back disability will persist despite treatment efforts, and the question of further testing arises.

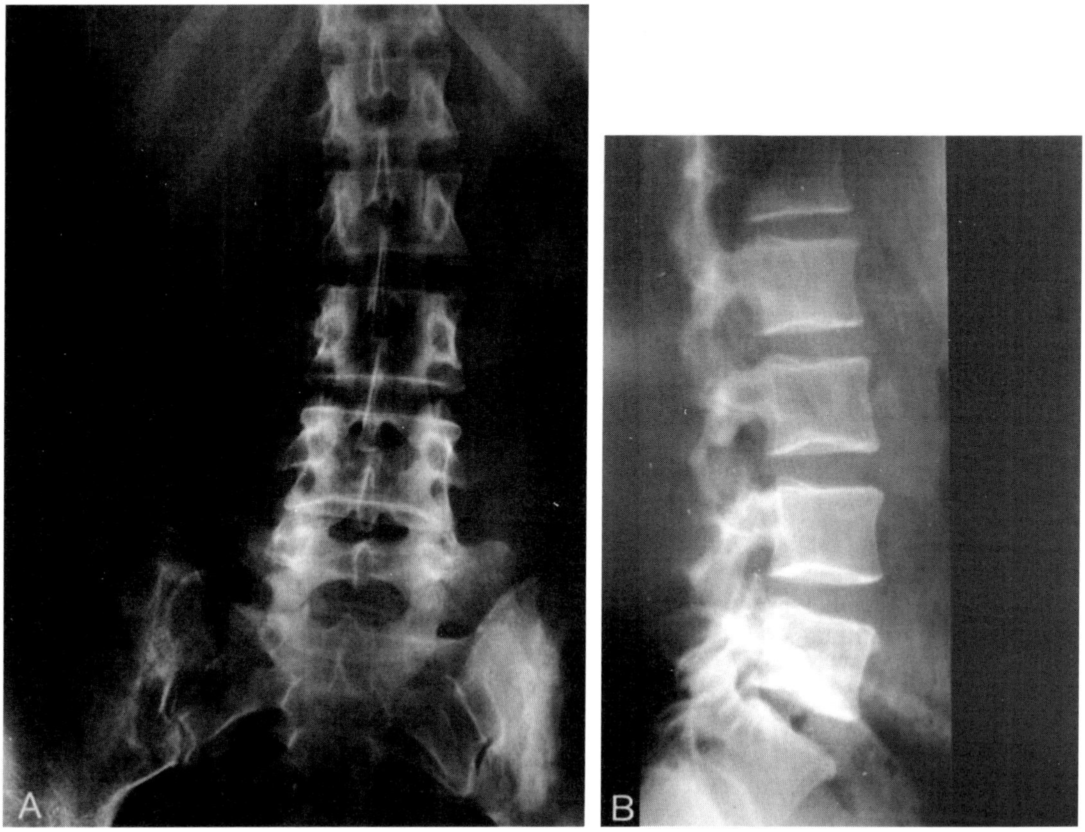

Figure 11.6 **A.** *Standard AP with psoas shadows evident, no abnormal kidney shadows, no calcification in aorta, and normal joints. Note the congenital lumbosacral anomaly.* **B.** *Lateral showing good disc space integrity and no vertebral body translations ("slips").*

At this stage, it is prudent to quickly review Questions 1 (Am I dealing with a real physical disability?) and 2 (Have I fallen into a trap, such as missing a bone tumor?). Most often, you will conclude that these questions have been satisfactorily answered, and it is time to determine, with myelography and/or CT scanning and/or MRI, what ails the patient and the possibility of preparing for a lumbar spine operation.

The demands of lumbar spine surgery require a precise definition of not only the nature of the lesion but also the location of the offending pathology. This can be provided only by CT scanning or magnetic resonance imaging. It is getting more difficult to meet the requirements of precise surgical technique with myelography alone, which results in an increased use of CT scanning and MR imaging. At the time of this writing, magnetic resonance imaging is assuming a primary role in patient assessment because it has the potential to deliver all of the necessary information on which to base a surgical game plan. In this milieu of change in imaging technique, myelography is assuming a less important place in investigation.

Before discussing the use of these newer, highly expensive imaging modalities, it is worthwhile to further explore the philosophy of investigating a patient with lumbar disc disease.

Philosophy of Investigating a Patient with Lumbar Disc Disease

The cornerstone of diagnosis of lumbar disc disease is the history and physical examination, not the investigation.

CT and MRI are ordered for two reasons: (1) almost always to verify the clinical diagnosis as correct and at the same time to plan a surgical approach to the problem, and (2) infrequently to solve a differential diagnosis problem.

Investigative procedures used to resolve a differential diagnostic problem may fall short of helping to plan surgery. An example is the water-soluble myelogram, which was the "gold standard" for diagnosis of lumbar disc disease. It is valuable in differential diagnosis, such as ruling out a conus tumor, but it fails to provide all of the necessary information to plan a surgical procedure, especially one with limited exposure.

When viewing the investigation, do so in light of the clinical information. You are seeking answers to Question 4 (What is the anatomical level?) and Question 5 (What is the structural lesion?). If there is not a perfect marriage between the clinical presentation, anatomical level, and the investigation, something is wrong. To proceed with surgery at this stage sets the stage for a poor outcome.

Consider the following clinical information and respective implications:

- A patient with an acute radicular syndrome with significant straight leg raising (SLR) reduction and S1 neurological symptoms and signs should have an unequivocal lesion involving the S1 nerve root on CT scan or MRI.
- A patient with anterior thigh pain and a positive femoral stretch with a decreased knee reflex should not be accepted as having a herniated nucleus pulposus (HNP) at L4–L5 unless it extends into the foramen to involve the 4th root.
- A patient with a long history of back pain and claudicant leg pain should have a clear-cut stenotic lesion on investigation before making the diagnosis of spinal stenosis.

The potential for false-negative and false-positive investigative findings is great.(12) CT scans and MRIs are so sensitive that it is possible to show pathology in almost every patient. CT scans show only what is scanned. If a conus tumor is present, and the scan is confined to L3 to the sacrum, the lesion will be missed. MRI covers this CT deficiency but at the same time introduces many false-positive results because of overinterpretation. Beware of the clinical diagnosis lacking substance and borderline investigative findings.

There is a "comfort" level with old and a "discomfort" level with new tests. Most surgeons are comfortable with the myelogram, more are becoming comfortable with CT scanning, and today many would base a surgical decision solely on the basis of MRI. It is important to train oneself to evaluate the newer investigative modalities to achieve a level of comfort in relying on these tests to plan surgery.

A poor quality investigative test is no good to anyone. An extradural myelogram cannot be interpreted, a poorly done electromyograph (EMG) is misleading, a blurred CT scan is useless, and a patient rushed through an MRI machine will result in a bad MRI scan. It is essential for clinicians to keep the pressure on our radiological colleagues to deliver the best quality images possible to reduce the risk of operative misadventure.

There is a tendency in the United States to order major spine investigative procedures too early in the progress of disc disease. Tests such as myelography, CT scanning, and MRI are part of an operative procedure; they are not routine radiographs to be ordered without hesitation. If a clinician is in trouble with spine differential diagnosis to the point where frequent myelograms or myelogram/CT scans and MRI are part of the practice routine, then a careful clinical examination is missing. If a significant number of tests ordered by a clinician are negative, the indications for ordering such radiologic tests are too broad and need to be reassessed. Almost every myelogram, CT scan, or MRI examination of the lumbar spine should be positive and followed by an operation. If this is not the case, indiscriminate early ordering of these tests is occurring.

Myelography

Myelography is no longer the "gold standard" of investigation in lumbar disc disease. It has been supplanted by CT/myelography and MRI.

Before "throwing out myelography with the bath water," it is essential to reflect on how valuable an investigative modality it has been in the development of lumbar spine surgery.

History

"Myelography" was introduced in 1922 by Sicard,(10) using iodized poppy seed oil (Lipiodol) injected into the epidural space. Difficulty aspirating the material and complications limited the use of epidural myelography as a replacement procedure for air myelography. By the mid 1930s, intrathecal oil myelography with Lipiodol gained favor, but again complications in the form of meningismus and late arachnoiditis led to a search for other compounds.

Steinhausen and his co-workers (11) at the University of Rochester introduced iophendylate in 1940, and Pantopaque remained the medium of choice for years. The difficulty in using large needles necessary to introduce the viscous fluid, the necessity of poststudy removal of the contrast material sometimes injuring nerve roots, late arachnoiditis, and other complications (7) led to the incongruous situation of many surgeons ordering the test, yet few themselves prepared to submit to the procedure. Obviously, Pantopaque was not a great medium for myelography, which stimulated the search for better agents. By the mid 1970s, water-soluble contrast agents had virtually eliminated Pantopaque for lumbar myelography, and since the late 1980s we have had available relatively nontoxic, cheap, water-soluble agents; these newer myelographic agents have been developed all in time to see myelography being surpassed as the procedure of choice by better CT scanning and newer MR imaging.

The object of the myelographic exercise is to:

1. Place contrast material in the subarachnoid space (Fig. 11.7).
2. Place the contrast material as close to the lesion as possible, yet not at the level of the lesion, for example, lumbar myelograms are best done through lumbar, not cervical (C1–C2), punctures.
3. Assure that contrast material is not injected in an extra-arachnoid or extradural manner (which will render the myelogram uninterpretable).
4. Use an agent that has a low viscosity and is thoroughly miscible with cerebrospinal fluid (CSF).
5. Use an agent that is easy to use, cheap, rapidly excreted, and of limited toxicity.
6. Use an agent that consistently produces radiographic images that are useful.
7. The dose of contrast material should be between 180–240 mg/cc in 10.0 to 14.0 cc of fluid.

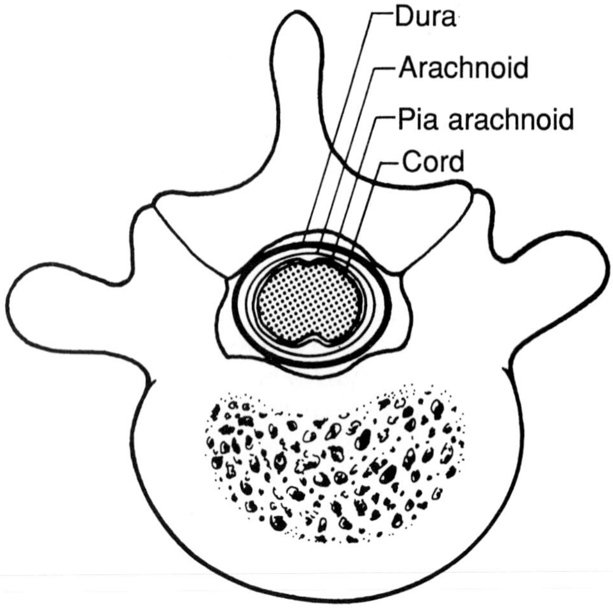

Figure 11.7 *The subarachnoid space is between the arachnoid and pia arachnoid.*

Choice of Contrast Media

The agents of choice for lumbar myelography are the water-soluble nonionic (low-osmolar) preparations. Two agents are popular today: iohexol (Omnipaque), and iopamidol (Isovue).

In the past few years, metrizamide, one of the original water-soluble contrast agents, has been replaced by iohexol and iopamidol because: (1) these compounds come premixed (unlike metrizamide, which has to be mixed just before use); (2) they are cheaper; and (3) most important, they are less toxic than metrizamide, producing 50% fewer side effects.(2, 4, 6)

Technique

Introduction of the contrast material can be done with the patient prone or in the lateral decubitus position, with the head slightly raised. A 22-gauge spinal needle is the choice because the water viscosity of the contrast material does not require anything larger puncturing the dura. The needle insertion is best at L2–L3, a site below the conus, yet close enough to most of the lumbar pathological sites at L5–S1, >L4–L5, >>L3–L4.1 After cerebrospinal fluid backflow documents the subarachnoid placement of the needle, a small amount of contrast is injected. A diffuseness to the initial injection verifies that the injected contrast is mixing with the CSF. A sharpness to the margins of this contrast injection indicates a subdural or extradural injection and trouble.

Films

Most clinicians prefer the following myelographic views: a spot lateral with the needle in place, cross-table lateral, upright lateral, thoracolumbar view, AP, and both obliques to show nerve roots.

Dynamic Examination

Some radiologists use flexion/extension films to accentuate midline stenotic lesions. Patients with spinal stenosis aggravate their symptoms in extension and are likely to show more of a myelographic defect in this position.

Cisternal or C1–C2 Puncture

Occasionally, it is not possible to do a lumbar puncture, and it becomes necessary to use the C1–C2 interspace or the cisternal space to instill the contrast material (Fig. 11.8). This is not as effective as lumbar puncture for lumbar lesions.

The following conditions may support the use of cisternal puncture: long fusion of L2–S1; a lumbar infection; severe arthritis in the lumbar spine; complete blocks at multiple levels, making lumbar puncture impossible; a patient with spinal instability who is not to be moved. The puncture is usually done in the prone position, with the needle tip directed posterior to the cord at the C1–C2 interval. Aspiration of CSF is not to be attempted at this level for fear of damaging vital neurological structures.

Basic Considerations in Myelography

There are two basic considerations in myelography:

1. What is the image quality?
2. What is the cost in adverse reactions?

Image Quality

As an indirect method of detecting canal encroachment, myelographic images must be clear and not distorted by artifact or other errors in technique. Most clinicians are comfortable with myelography, and this is reinforced by the ability of myelography to show intradural lesions, such as tumors, arteriovenous (AV) malformations, and arachnoiditis. As well, the instillation of myelogram contrast material allows for examination of the entire canal, especially the thoracolumbar junction.

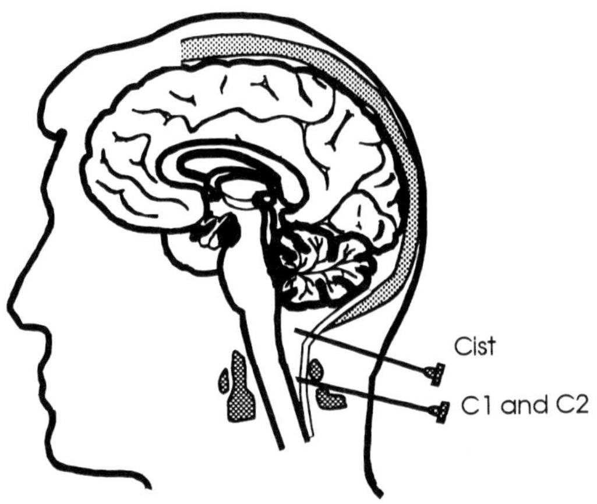

Figure 11.8 *A cisternal puncture (Cist) and a C1/C2 puncture of the subarachnoid (CSF) space.*

Adverse Reactions to Myelography

Severe adverse reactions to the instillation of contrast material occur in approximately 1:35,000 procedures. They can be divided into adverse neurological,(8) anaphylactoid reactions, and renal toxicity.

Anaphylactoid reactions are rare, especially with the newer water-soluble contrast materials. Screening of patients historically, corticosteroid and antihistamine pretreatment when indicated, and in some cases refusing to do myelography in a sensitive patient have reduced the incidence of anaphylactoid reactions to a minimum.

Renal toxicity from the doses of contrast material used for lumbar myelography are much rarer compared with the use of the higher doses of these agents that are used for vascular studies. There is a possibility that a patient with pre-existing renal disease can have a toxic reaction from intrathecal water-soluble contrast agents.

Adverse neurological reactions (2, 4, 6, 9) are the reactions that concern myelographers. They include, most frequently, headache, nausea, and vomiting; less frequently, the following reactions occur: increased pain, seizures, myoclonic spasms, psychomotor disturbances, fever, vertigo, and urinary retention.

Mechanism of Toxicity

The fact that these reactions are more common with one agent (metrizamide) than another (iohexol) and directly related to dose suggests that they are toxic in origin rather than sensitivity reactions. Because there is no barrier between the CSF space and the central nervous system (CNS) tissue, there is unhindered diffusion of water-soluble contrast material into the extracellular space of the CNS. This direct contact between contrast agent and neurons results in upset of metabolism and neuronal mechanisms, which results in the toxic effects.

The half-life of metrizamide in the subarachnoid space is approximately 4 hours, during which time it is absorbed through the arachnoid villi into the blood. From there, the dye is excreted through the kidneys within 6 to 12 hours of injection.

Most adverse reactions, specifically headaches, will occur within 4 to 8 hours of the procedure, reach their maximum by 24 hours, and be gone in 48 hours. Iohexol/iopamidol have displaced metrizamide because of a 50% reduction in side effects, both in occurrence and severity (Table 11.5).

Table 11.5. Incidence (%) of Adverse Reactions (Averaging from Literature)[a]

	Metrizamide	Iopamidol/Iohexol
Headache	30–60	50% less
Nausea	25–40	↓
Vomiting	5	

[a]Data from: Badami JP, Baker RA, Scholz FJ, McLaughlin M. Outpatient metrizamide myelography: prospective evaluations of safety and cost effectiveness. Radiology 1985;158:175–177; Neurotoxicity of metrizamide (editorial). Arch Neurol 1985;42:24–25; Eldevik OP, Nakstad P, Kendall B, Hindmarsh T. Iohexol in lumbar myelography: preliminary results from an open noncomparative multicentered clinical study. AJNR 1983;4:299–301; Kuuliala IK, Goransson HJ. Adverse reactions after iohexol lumbar myelography: influence of post-procedural positioning. AJR 1952;149:389–390; Meador KI, Hamilton WJ, El Gammal TAM, Demetropoulos KC, Nichols FT. Irreversible neurologic complications of metrizamide myelography. Neurology 1984;34:817–821.

The more serious side effects of seizures and other psycho-organic complaints, although rare with properly administered metrizamide, are further reduced with iohexol and iopamidol. Most centers are using iohexol or iopamidol because these second-generation nonionic, low-osmolality, water-soluble contrast agents are premixed, cheaper, and less toxic when compared with metrizamide. They still have the potential for side effects that can be further reduced by:

1. Properly hydrating patients before the procedure to help with renal clearance (3);
2. Keeping the dose of the contrast material within manufacturers' recommended levels;
3. Using a small needle;
4. Avoiding spillage of contrast material into the skull during the examination;
5. Reducing the dose of contrast material if a complete block is present;
6. Ensuring that patients are not receiving drugs that lower the seizure threshold, for example, phenothiazines, monoamine oxidase inhibitors, and other psychoactive drugs.

Patients prone to adverse effects are: the older patient, the patient with a previous reaction, and the long-term psychoactive drug user; extra precautions are needed with these patients. Most important, it is necessary to identify these patients with a careful pre-injection history.

Patient Positioning During and After the Myelogram

Most radiologists would agree on two points with regard to patient positioning:

1. Ensure, through neck extension, that contrast material does not spill into the skull during the examination.
2. After the examination, keep the patient's head elevated 45°. More radiologists (6) are accepting immediate ambulation after myelography (eg, bathroom privileges), because this maintains the cranium above the spine and prevents spillage of residual contrast material into the brain cavity.

Myelogram Changes

Figure 11.9 demonstrates a normal myelogram. Abnormalities in myelography indicative of an HNP are:

1. Defects in the sac alone. The most difficult defects to interpret involve the dural sac alone. A double density (Fig. 11.10) is usually indicative of a disc herniation toward the midline, but still eccentric enough to produce the typical defect. On occasion, an HNP fragment will migrate up or down from a disc space and produce a defect on the sac alone (Fig. 11.11). Simple, smooth midline defects are not to be interpreted as HNP (Fig. 11.12). These defects are known as "sucker discs" and are caused by annular bulging as part of the phenomenon of degenerative disc disease. Often, they will be accompanied by degenerative changes, especially retrospondylolisthesis.
2. Defects affecting the root sleeve. The low viscosity of water-soluble contrast materials makes it possible to readily fill the root sleeves (radiculogram). The defects demonstrated can be an absent root sleeve (Fig. 11.13);

Figure 11.9 *A normal AP myelogram.*

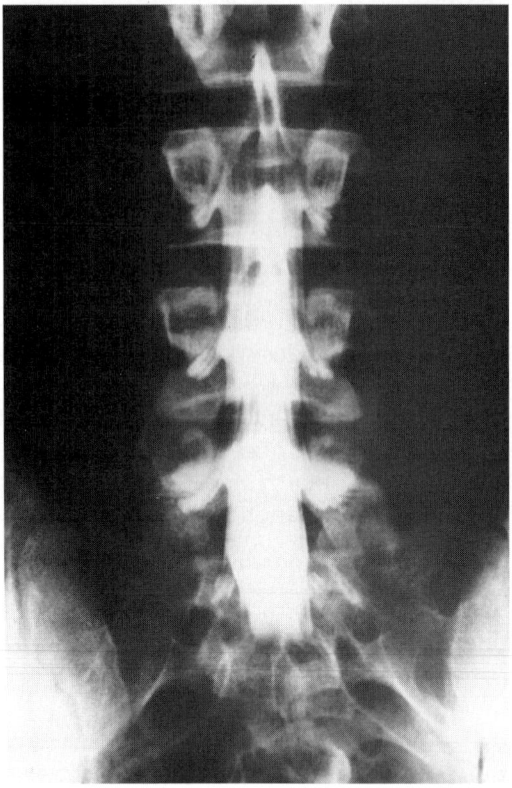

Figure 11.10 *A lateral myelogram with a double density at L5-S1 and annular bulging deforming the sac at L4-5.*

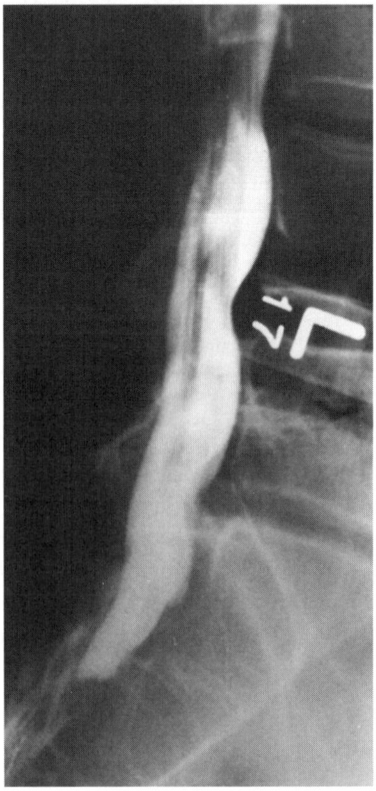

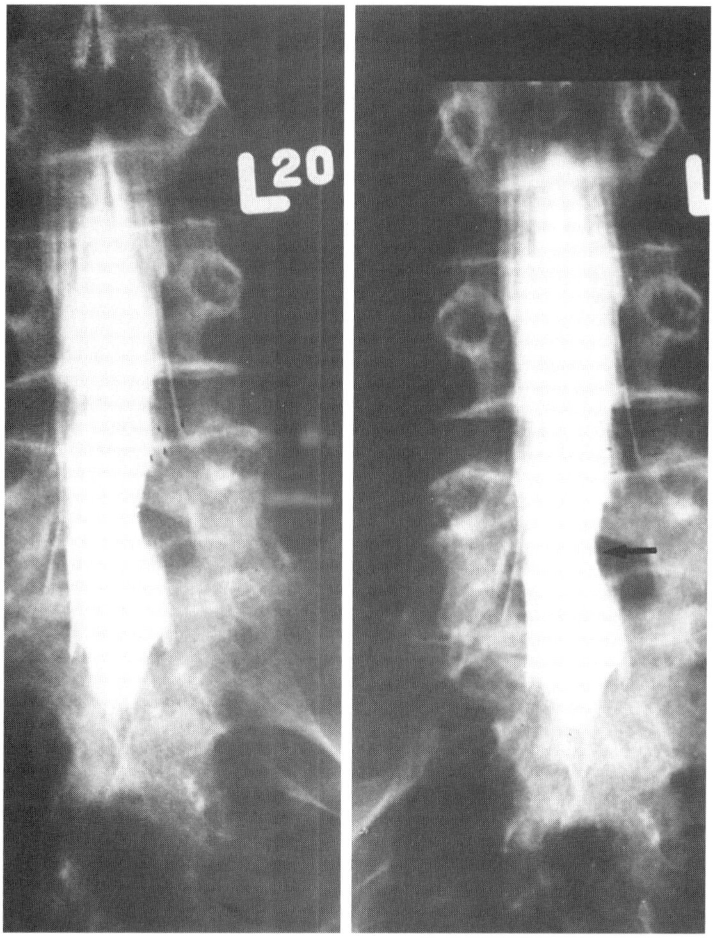

Figure 11.11 *AP myelogram showing a large HNP behind the vertebral body of L5 distorting the sac (the S1 root is also obliterated) (arrow).*

3. A root sleeve shortening or cut-off (Fig. 11.14), a root sleeve deformity (Fig. 11.15), and a swollen root sleeve (Fig. 11.16).
4. Defects affecting sac and root. These are the most obvious defects and are depicted in Figure 11.17.

Sensitivity and Specificity of Myelography

Although there are numerous reports in the literature on false-positive and false-negative myelograms,(4, 5) most reports are poor in that they do not follow up on patients to completion of treatment. Most often, the articles' conclusions are based on the statement, "The surgeons found a disc herniation at operation." Most surgeons operating on a patient for a disc herniation will find a disc bulge, no matter how small. It would be more meaningful for reports on sensitivity and specificity studies to clearly state that "not only was a disc herniation found, its removal relieved the patient of the symptoms that led to the myelogram." It is only with these studies that the true sensitivity and specificity of myelography

Figure 11.12 *Lateral myelogram showing annular bulging at L4-L5. This is the lateral of fig. 11.9, the so-called "sucker disc."*

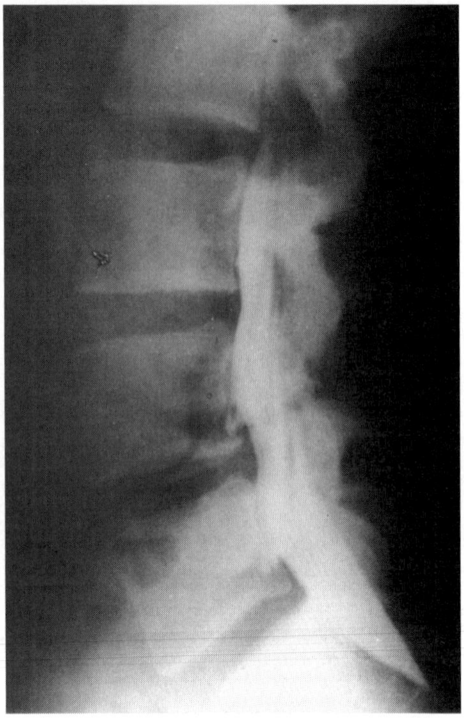

Figure 11.13 *AP myelogram showing S1 root sleeve absent on right (HNP, L5-S1, right) (arrow).*

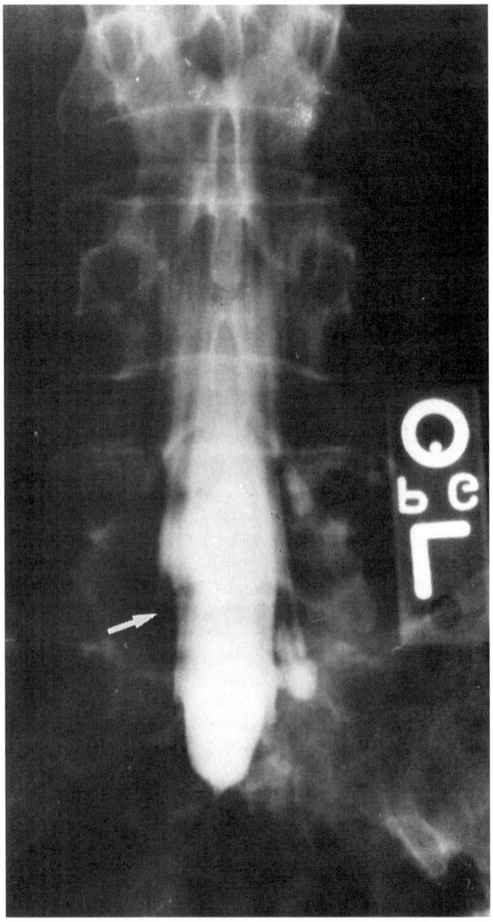

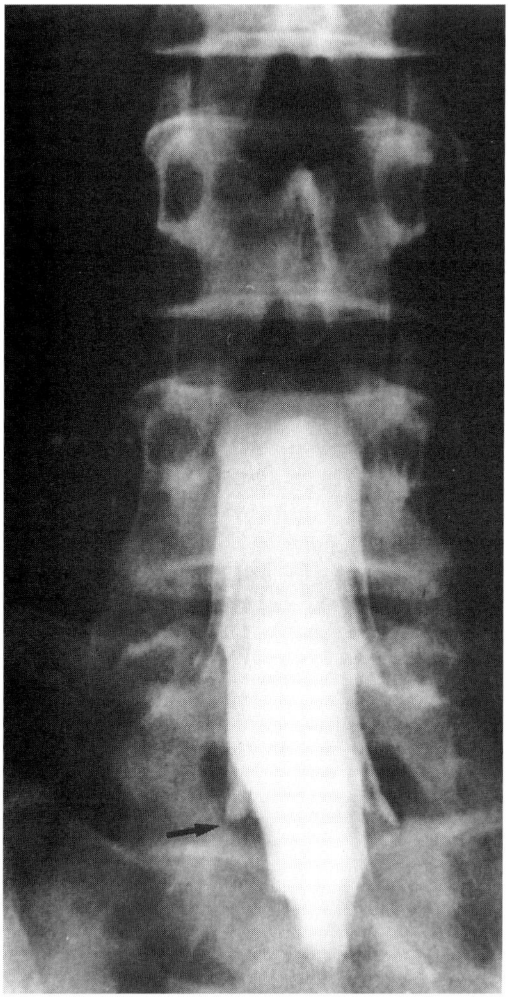

Figure 11.14 *Root sleeve shortening on AP myelogram (arrow). Compare the length of S1 root filling on the right (shorter) with the left S1 root. Now, compare the shortening of this S1 root with the absence of the S1 root in Fig. 11.13.*

will be established. It is safe to say that the incidence of false-negatives and false-positives has been reduced with the introduction of water-soluble contrast agents. False-negative myelograms can still occur with water-soluble agents in the following situations:

- Foraminal HNP (Fig. 11.18).
- Unscanned area (high lumbar disc not scanned).
- Insensitive space at L5–S1 (Fig. 11.19).
- Short or narrow dural sac at L5–S1 (Fig. 11.20).
- Conjoint nerve roots distorting the contrast column.

Outpatient Myelography (1)

With the North American desire to ration health care (contain costs), more patients are undergoing outpatient myelography. In the second edition of this book we did not support outpatient myelography. With the increasing use of low-osmolality contrast agents, outpatient myelography is most often completed without adverse patient events.

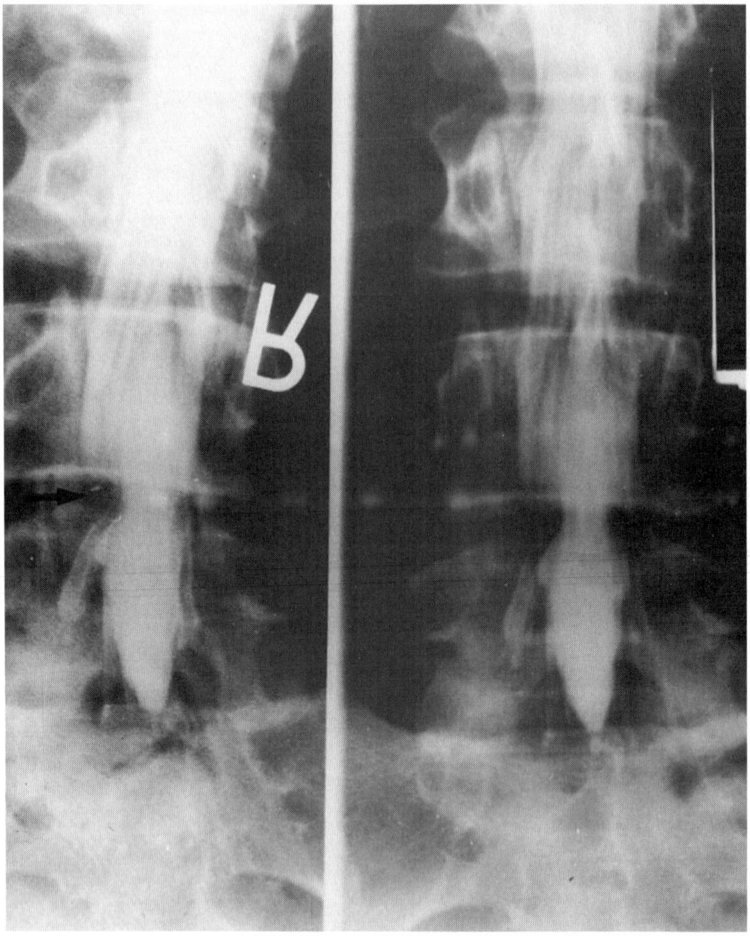

Figure 11.15 *AP and oblique myelogram showing HNP L4-L5 distorting the LS root sleeve (arrow).*

Conclusion

Having "grown up" with Pantopaque myelography and all of its technical and toxic problems, it is a relief to have newer, safer contrast agents to propose to patients. However, with the advent of CT scanning and MR imaging, the incidence of requests for myelographic examination has decreased dramatically over the last few years.

Virtually no one is doing myelography alone these days; almost all myelograms are followed by a CT examination. The issue today is whether to continue to use CT/myelography or switch to MRI as the primary investigative step before surgery. We prefer the MRI, but there are still situations where a myelogram, followed by CT, is indicated:

1. An equivocal CT or MRI in a patient who the surgeon feels has a surgical lesion.
2. An obese patient who cannot fit into the CT or MR gantries.
3. Multilevel spinal stenosis, especially with scoliosis (scoliosis interferes with proper CT or MRI "slicing" of each segment).
4. Patients in whom metal implants (eg, pedicle screws) will distort the CT scan or MRI.
5. Less than optimal MRI scanning machines (which are not that uncommon).

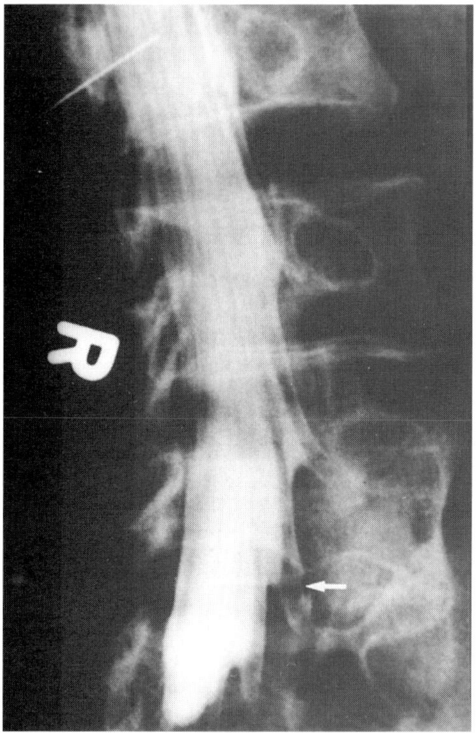

Figure 11.16 *The S1 root, left, is swollen (arrow). (Compare with the L5 root at the level above.)*

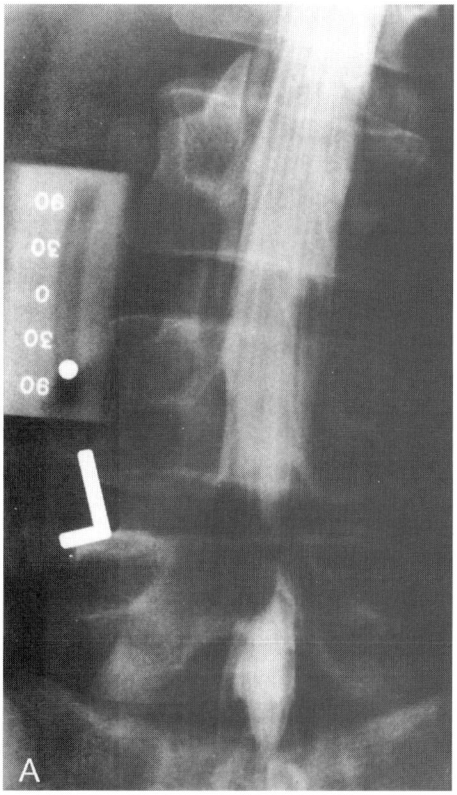

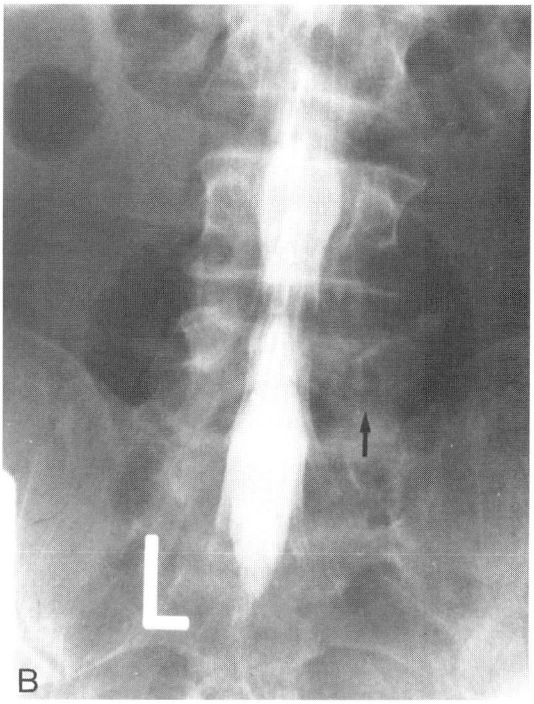

Figure 11.17 **A.** *AP myelogram showing HNP L4-L5, left, with significant distortion of sac and root. This is a large HNP that has trapped down behind the vertebral body of L5.* **B.** *Apparent defect of sac and root, L4-L5, right. Did you notice the absent pedicle, L5, right (arrow)? This was a secondary carcinoma from a lung malignancy.*

Figure 11.18 *Foraminal HNP, L4-L5, right. Arrow points to slight distortion of contrast column, a change easily missed.*

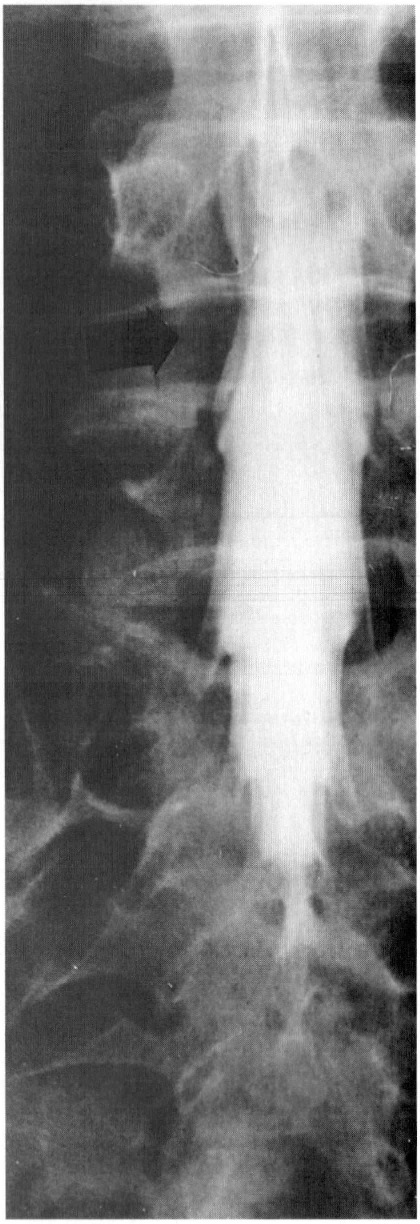

HIGH-RESOLUTION COMPUTED TOMOGRAPHY

It is becoming more difficult to plan a surgical procedure on the spine without investigation that shows not only the level, but also the precise location and nature of the pathology. Myelography is often capable of showing the level at which the pathology lies (6) but fails to show the nature of the lesion or its precise location in the anatomical segment (4, 12) (see Chapter 1). This limits the value of water-soluble myelography in surgery for lumbar disc disease, a void that is fortunately filled by CT scanning and, more recently, MR imaging.

For those surgeons who learned spine surgery in the days of Pantopaque myelography,

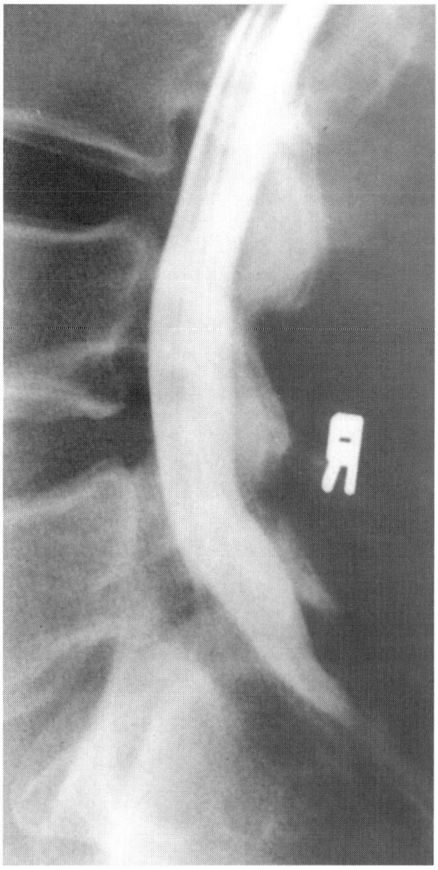

Figure 11.19 *Lateral myelogram showing wide "insensitive space" between back of L5-S1 disc space and front of "dye" column where pathology, such as an HNP, could reside and not be detected on myelography.*

the value of today's CT scanning technology is stunning.(2) From the time Hounsfield (7) introduced CT scan technology to the field, spine surgery has grown immensely.

Advantages and Disadvantages

Table 11.6 lists the advantages and disadvantages of CT scanning. The most serious problem with routine CT scanning is the ease with which the procedure can be done. With no requirement for hospitalization or injection into the body, the CT scan becomes too simple a step to take, and this procedure is capable of delivering erroneous data (17) that can lead to ill-advised surgical intervention.

Technique

For a detailed explanation of the technical aspects of CT scanning, readers are referred to other articles.(1, 3) Only those clinically relevant points will be covered in this section.

The only acceptable machines for CT scanning are the latest generation, high-resolution scanners. The authors are most familiar with the General Electric 9800, the Picker Synerview 2000, and the Siemens DRH. To perform a lumber spine scan on a scanner with technology inferior to these machines (eg, older scanners) is a disservice to patients.

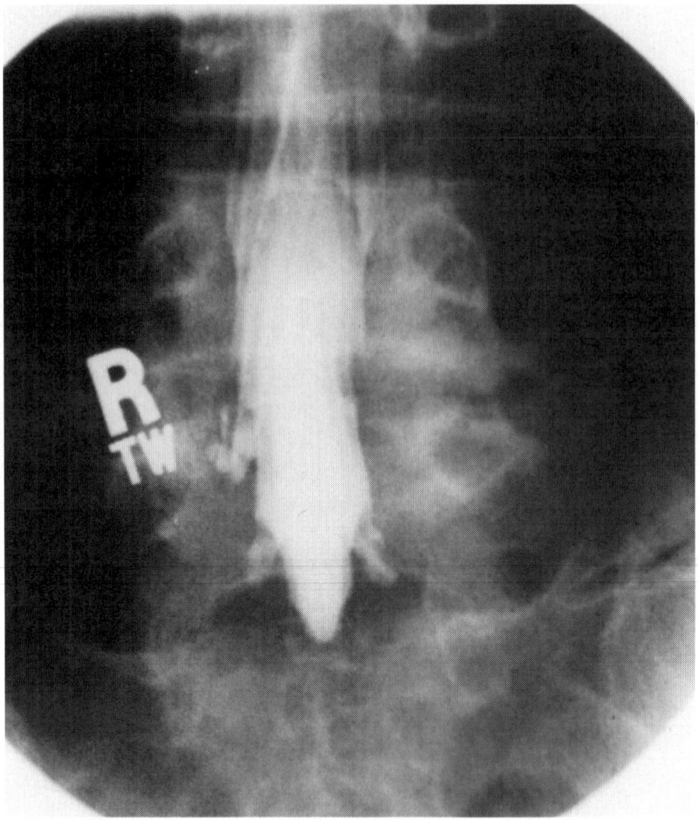

Figure 11.20 *AP myelogram showing a short dural sac, ending before it reaches the level of L5-S1. There is no hope that this myelogram would reveal an HNP of L5-S1. Fortunately, the HNP was at L4-L5, left, demonstrated by an absent root.*

It is convenient if an AP and lateral view are done at the beginning of the scan (Fig. 11.21). The inclusion of these two views on the scanner saves the logistic nightmare of trying to have all patients bring plain radiographs when they arrive for their scan. The AP view is important to alert the technician about structural problems, such as scoliosis, that will interfere with the quality of the scan. The AP scout view will show the radiologists congenital lumbosacral anomalies that will allow for the correct designation of lumbar levels.

Various scanning protocols are used in different parts of the country and world. This lack of uniformity makes it difficult for the spine surgeon reading scans from various departments and institutions. The adoption of a uniform scanning protocol is a reasonable hope for clinicians. A protocol widely used in North America (Fig. 11.22) includes:

- Two- to five-millimeter-thick sections.
- Three-millimeter intervals with overlap.
- Contiguous scans with 0-degree gantry angulation.
- Scan from midbody of L3 to midbody S1 (unless otherwise ordered), or the patient indicates on questionnaire (or pain drawing) that they have anterior thigh pain, at which time scanned levels must include the L1–L2 and L2–L3 levels.

Table 11.6. Advantages and Disadvantages of Computed Tomography (vs Myelography)

Advantages
1. Noninvasive, outpatient procedure
2. Clear picture of nature and location of pathology
3. Can see canal detail below the level of a myelographic block
4. Lower false-negative rate than myelography at L5–L1
5. Shows bone and soft tissue detail better than myelography
6. Shows paraspinal soft tissues
7. Reduced tissue radiation compared with myelography

Disadvantages
1. Poor detail in obese patient
2. Only see what you scan (higher conus pathology obviously will not be seen)
3. Too sensitive (high false-positive rate)
4. Intradural changes (arachnoiditis and tumors) not well seen
5. Radiation exposure compared with MRI (no radiation)

- Slices numbered cephalad / caudally.
- Supine patient scan.
- Axial scans only, unless there are specific indications for other formats.

Originally, most scanning protocols called for angled gantry cuts parallel to the disc space (perpendicular to the spinal canal) (Fig. 11.23). The following limitations of this approach have become evident:

1. Increased patient through-put time while the gantry angle is changed.
2. Difficulty, especially at L5–S1, to get the gantry angled parallel to the disc space.
3. Inability to do sagittal reconstructions.

The most important limitation of gantry angulation is demonstrated in Figure 11.24. It is essential to view the entire spinal canal so as not to miss portions of the third story that can harbor migrated disc fragments, spondylolysis, and the most inferior portion of the subarticular recess. For this reason, a number of departments have adopted the protocol as depicted in Figure 11.22. If a patient is scanned for an HNP, and the radiologist cannot unequivocally see the HNP on the standard scanning protocol, the gantry is angled for cuts parallel to the disc space. This latter requirement rarely occurs in our center.

Radiation Dose

Although the total dose of radiation emitted during a CT scan can be equivalent or greater than a myelogram, the collimation of the radiographic beam limits surface radiation dose to 1.6 to 2.5 rad / slice (Fig. 11.25). This results in a radiation dose to the bone marrow in the order of 0.2 to 0.4 rad, which is approximately the same marrow dose received during myelography. A full series of plain lumbar spine radiographs (AP, lateral, both obliques, and spot lateral of the lumbosacral junction) delivers approximately the same surface radiation dose as a CT scan slice.(8)

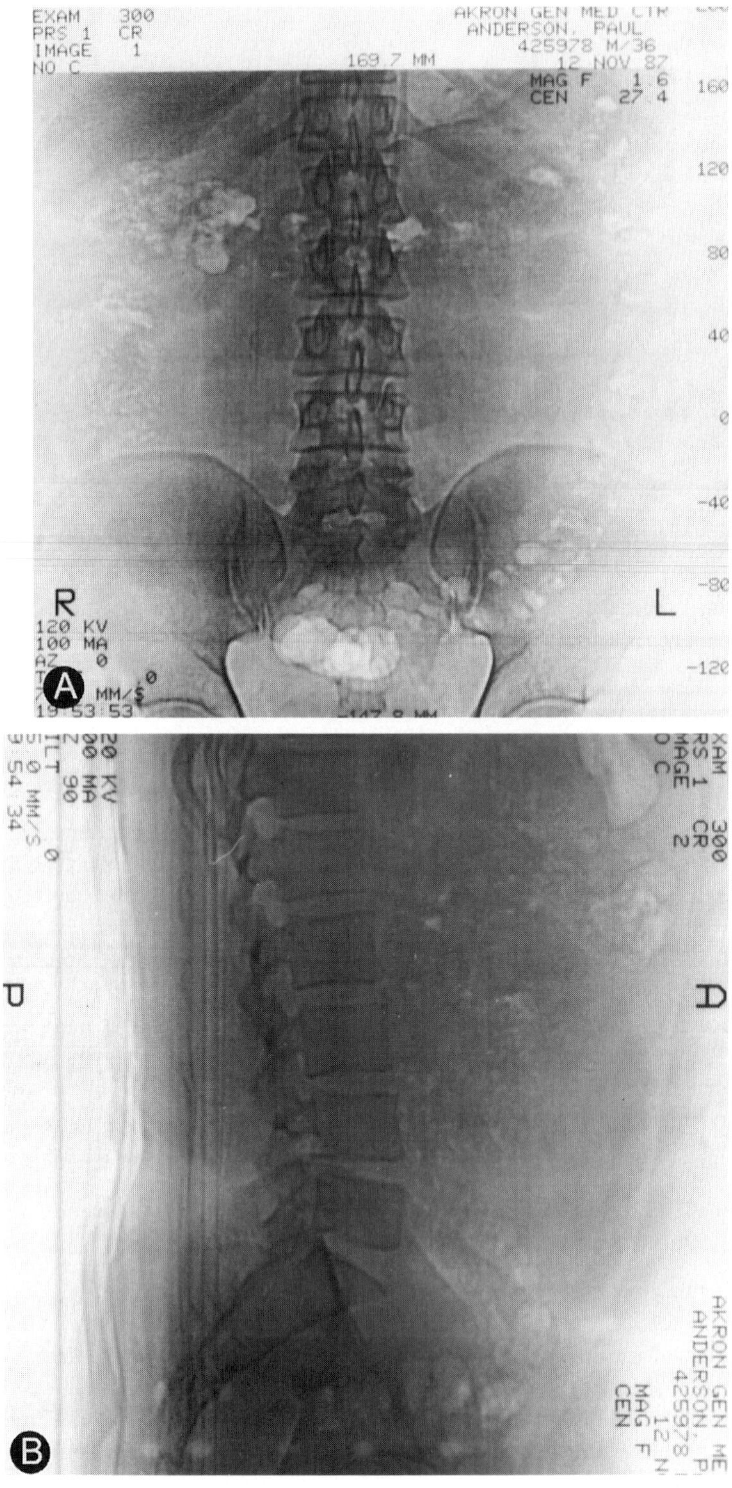

Figure 11.21 **A** *and* **B.** *AP and lateral views done at beginning of CT scan.*

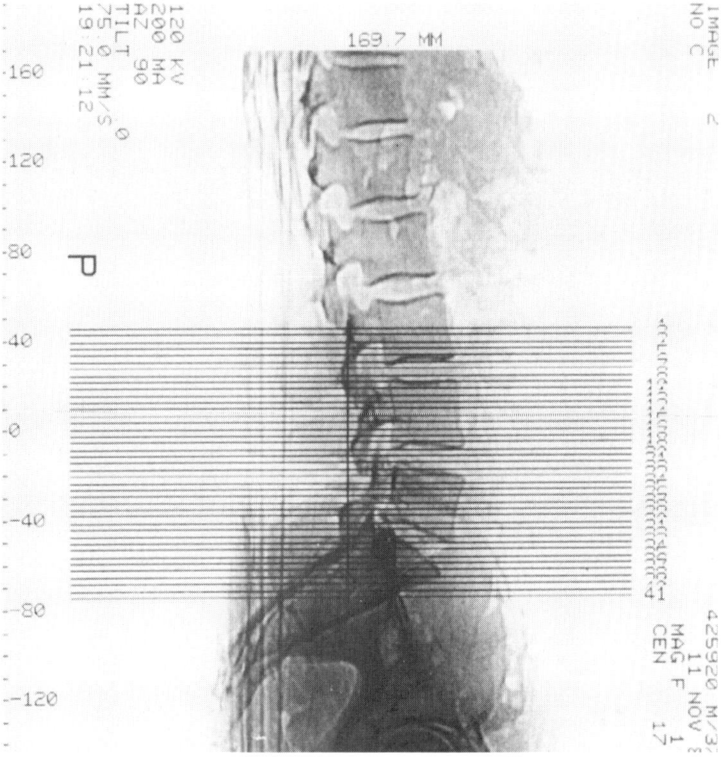

Figure 11.22 *A standard CT protocol as depicted on a lateral scout film.*

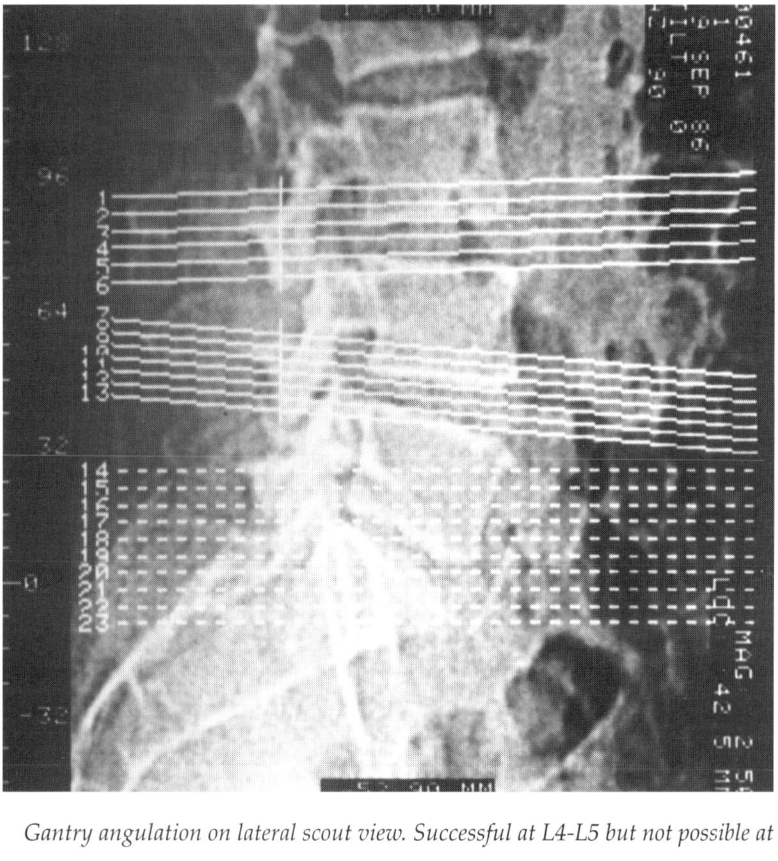

Figure 11.23 *Gantry angulation on lateral scout view. Successful at L4-L5 but not possible at L5-S1.*

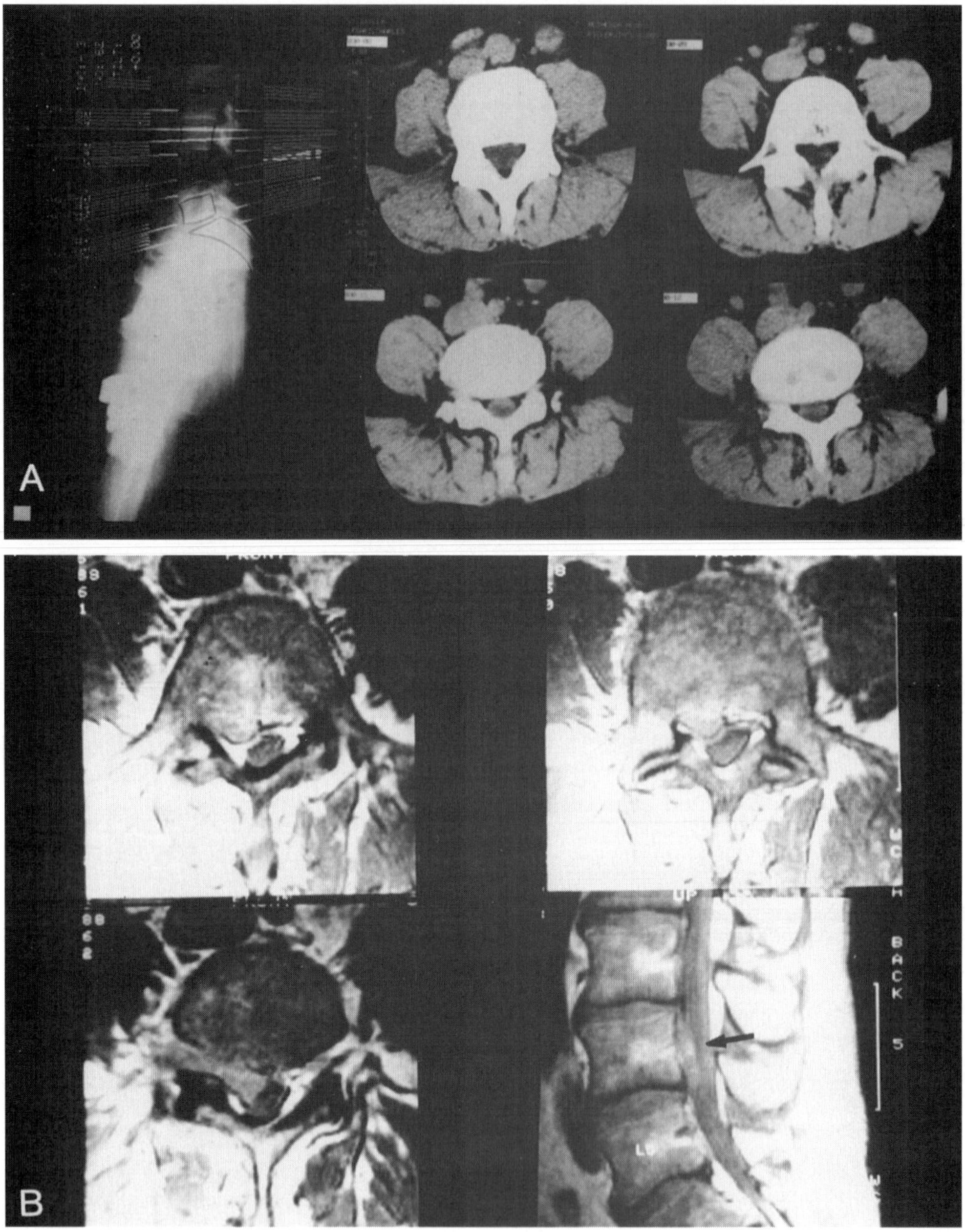

Figure 11.24 **A.** *CT showing gantry angulation and sample of axial slices. No disc herniation is to be found in this patient with significant right leg pain. Now, look at the MRI in* **B** *and see the large HNP from the L3-L4 space, trapping down behind the vertebral body of L4 (arrow). Look back at the scout view of the CT scan in* **A** *and see that the gantry angulation missed the upper* $^{2}/_{3}$ *of the spinal canal behind the body of L4 where the disc herniation lay. Unless the scout views show all of the canal (compare Fig. 11.22), the scan is not complete.*

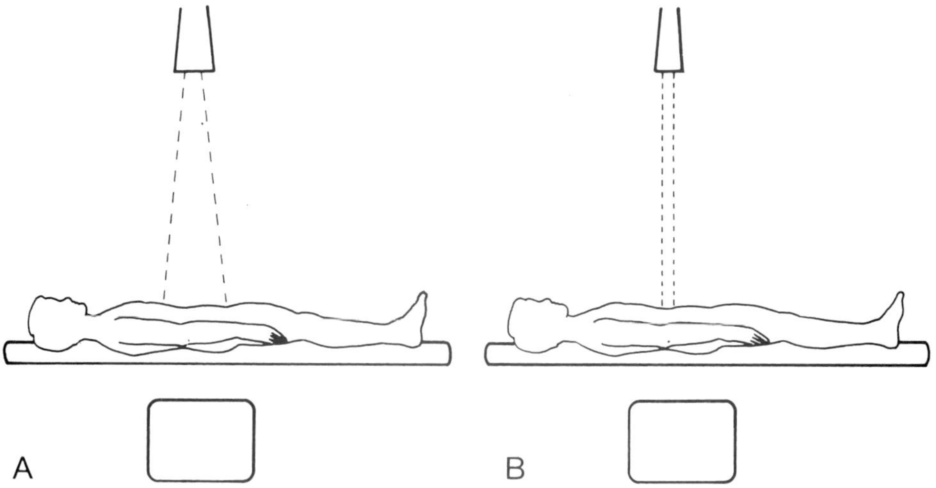

Figure 11.25 **A.** *The wider scatter to regular radiography or myelography delivers just as much total surface radiation as does the narrowed (collimated) CT scan radiographic beam* **(B).**

Technical Errors

Clinicians should be aware of potential technical errors (Table 11.7). These errors are controllable, and scans demonstrating these errors should be returned to the radiology department as unsatisfactory.

Scan Degradation

Next to technical errors, scan degradation interferes the most with interpretation of the images. This occurs because of the obesity of patients; poor machine maintenance (eg, ring artifact); patient motion; and metallic clips or prostheses. Figure 11.26 demonstrates these problems.

Hounsfield Units

The computer is capable of measuring attenuation coefficients of the various tissue densities on the scan and assigning a numerical value. These values are quoted as Hounsfield (H) units and represent gradations of gray.

air	water	bone
-1000 H units	0 H units	+1000 H units (dense cortical bone)

Most values of significance are on either side of the 0 Hounsfield units of water. An HNP is denser than the dural sac (50–100 H units), and this fact has been used to try and differentiate disc, conjoint nerve roots, and scar tissue. The margin of error has been too broad to make this technique reliable.

Table 11.7. Potential Technical Errors in Computed Tomography Scanning

Improper marking of level
Missed congenital lumbosacral anomalies (see Chapter 1)
Movement of patient causes blurring of scan slices
Improper positioning of the patient on the scanner table, resulting in an oblique cut of the disc space

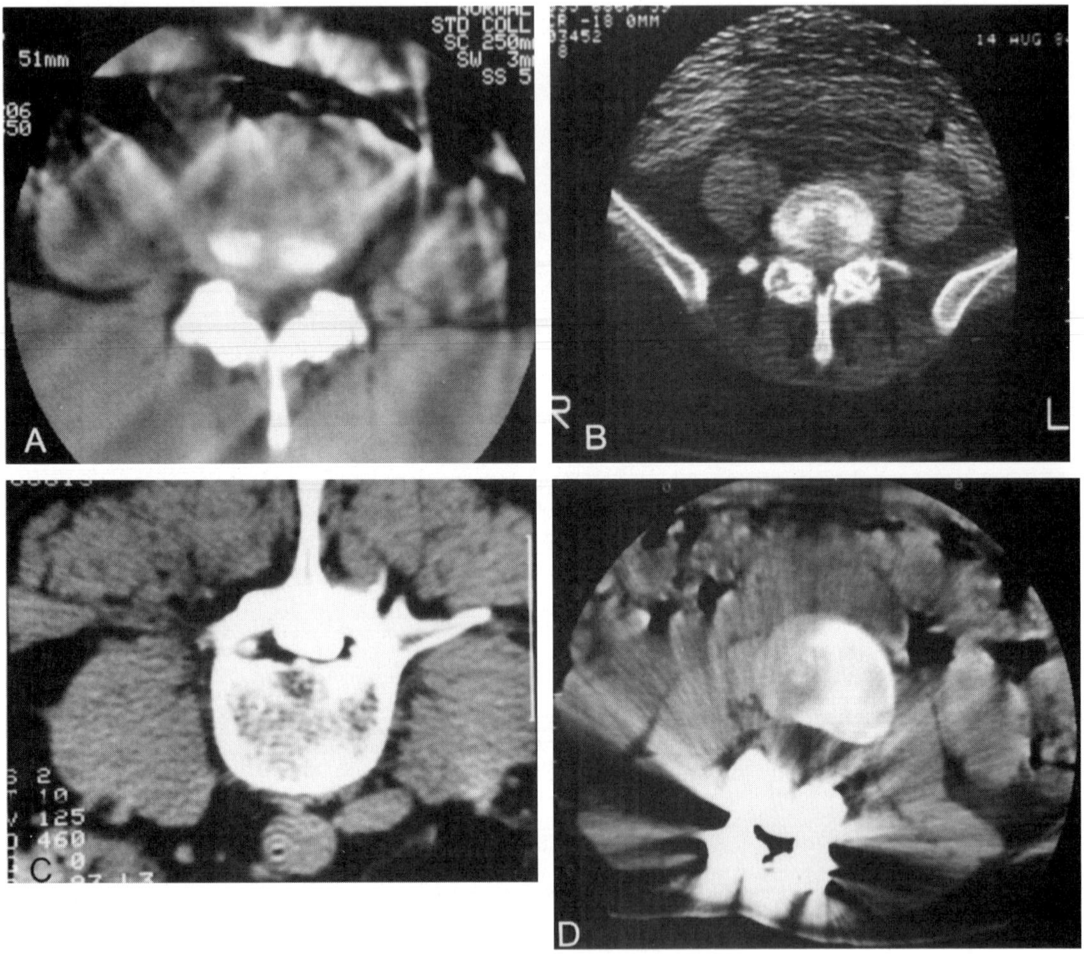

Figure 11.26 *Scan degradation, making scan interpretation difficult and dangerous:* **A.** *Poor scanner.* **B.** *Obese patient.* **C.** *Ring artifact.* **D.** *Metallic implants.*

Normal CT Scan

A clinician can relate to a CT scan film in a number of ways:

1. Listen exclusively to the radiologist and not look at the scan.
2. Look exclusively at the scan and not talk to the radiologist.
3. Look at the scan pictures with a radiologist, enlightening the radiologist with regard to the patient's clinical presentation.

Obviously, a conjoint effort between the clinician and the radiologist, reviewing the scan together, will maximize the value of the investigation.

Abnormal CT Scan

Herniated Nucleus Pulposus

The recognition of an HNP on scan is usually apparent but at times can be elusive.(18) Consider HNP recognition in three steps: the obvious, the associated changes, and the difficult.

The Obvious Figure 11.27 shows an obvious L4–L5 HNP. Note:

1. The focal protrusion of the disc distorting the normal configuration of the margin of the annulus.
2. Obliteration of the epidural fat (a change not as obvious at higher levels because of less epidural fat).
3. Deformity of the dural sac.
4. Displacement (posteriorly) of the nerve root.
5. The swollen nerve root.

Remember that scanning reproductions include many cuts, and the preceding figures are of only one slice. It is unusual for a clinically significant HNP to appear on only one slice; rather, it will be present to some degree on adjacent slices.

Other obvious features of an HNP that should be determined are size, shape, and location of the fragment. Figure 11.28 depicts significant CT findings relative to size, shape, and location of the fragment.

Abnormal Densities (Associated Changes) There are three artifactual changes in HNP material that should be recognized (Fig. 11.28): calcification, endplate displacement (see Fig. 7.25), and gas in the fragment (Fig. 11.29).

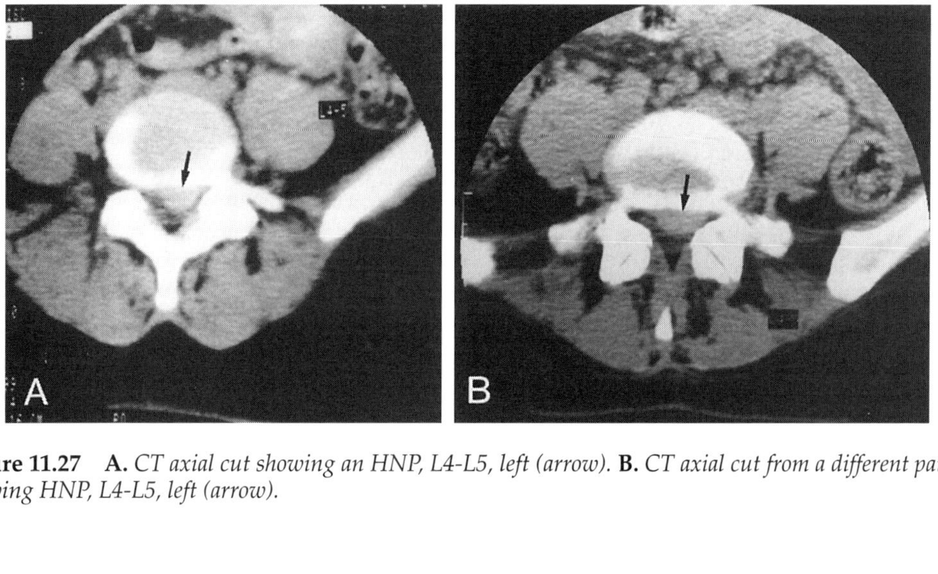

Figure 11.27 **A.** *CT axial cut showing an HNP, L4-L5, left (arrow).* **B.** *CT axial cut from a different patient showing HNP, L4-L5, left (arrow).*

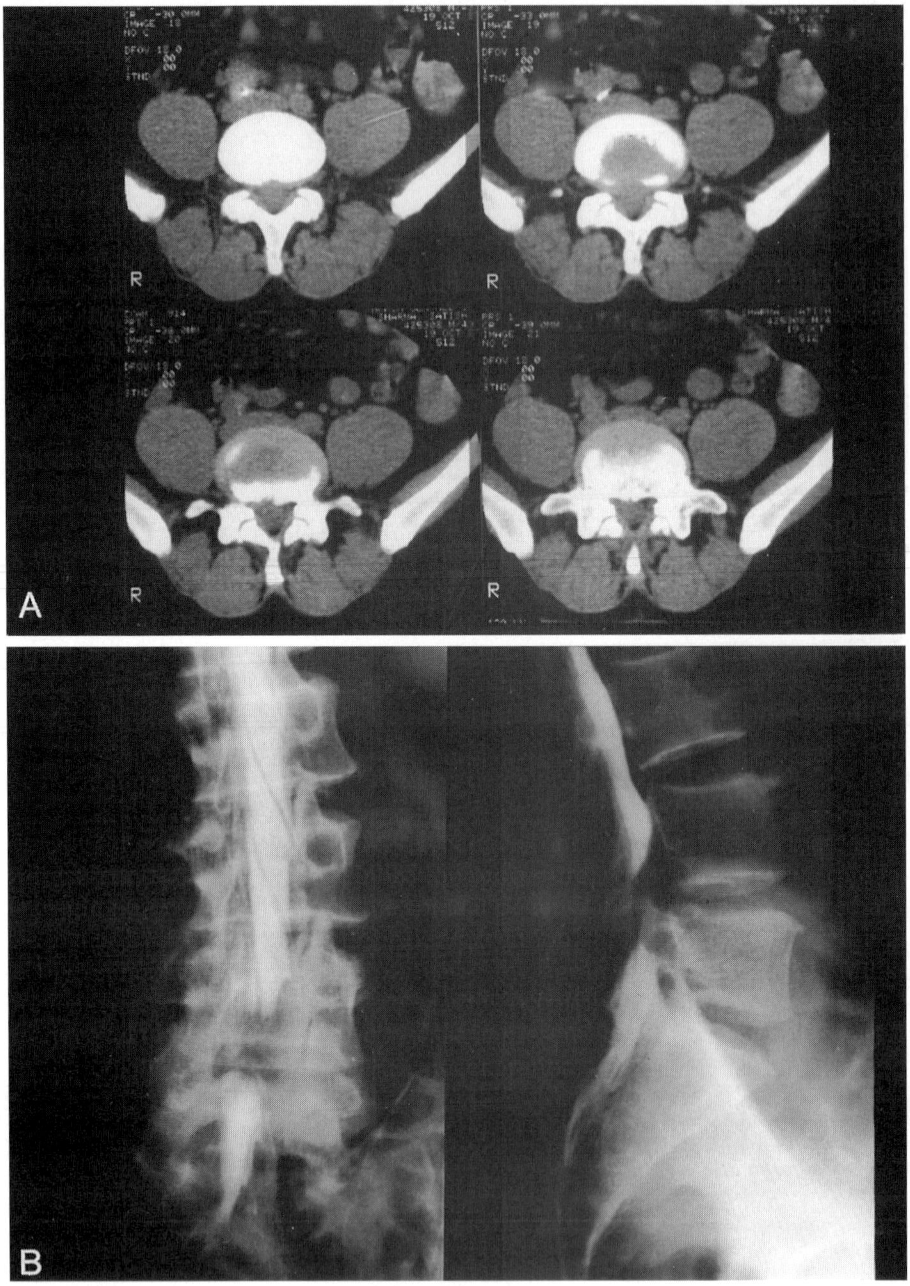

Figure 11.28 **A.** *CT scan that some might consider normal.* **B.** *Myelogram in the same patient showing a very large HNP, L4-L5.*

The Difficult to Recognize HNP There are times when the clinician feels an HNP is the source of the patient's complaints, but this is not obvious on CT scan. Aside from recurrent disc herniations in patients who have had previous surgery (Chapter 15), these problems of recognition usually occur because of associated degenerative changes or bony abnormalities (Fig. 11.30).

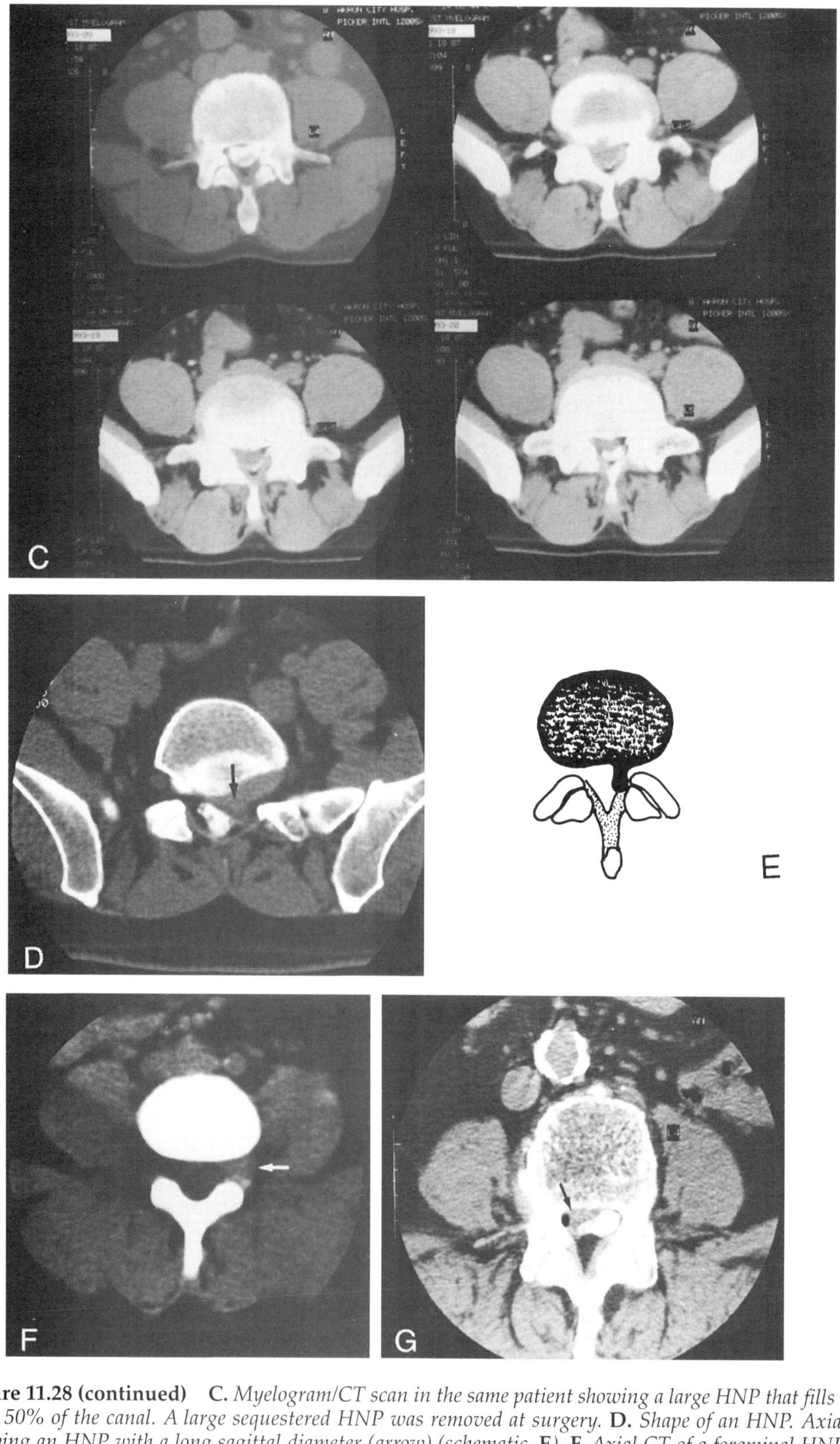

Figure 11.28 (continued) **C.** *Myelogram/CT scan in the same patient showing a large HNP that fills more than 50% of the canal. A large sequestered HNP was removed at surgery.* **D.** *Shape of an HNP. Axial CT showing an HNP with a long sagittal diameter (arrow) (schematic,* **E***).* **F.** *Axial CT of a foraminal HNP, L4, left (arrow).* **G.** *Axial CT of a pedicle disc herniation, L4, right (arrow). Also note the gas (nitrogen) in the fragment.*

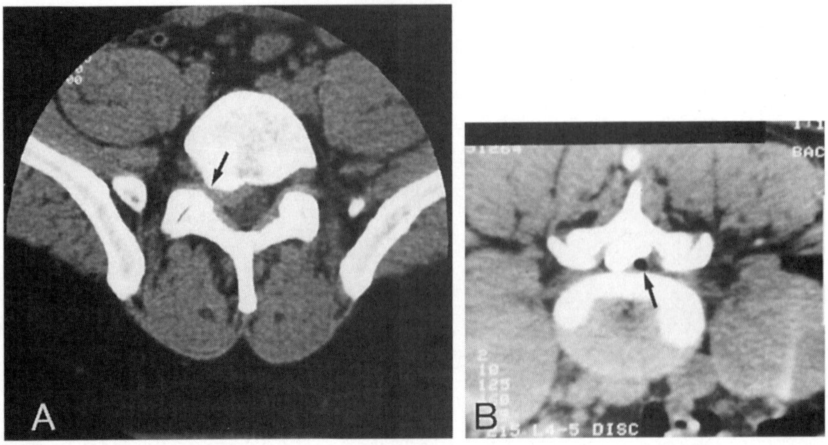

Figure 11.29 **A.** *Axial CT of HNP, L5, right, with calcific base (arrow) and soft tissue cap.* **B.** *Axial CT of an HNP containing gas (arrow).*

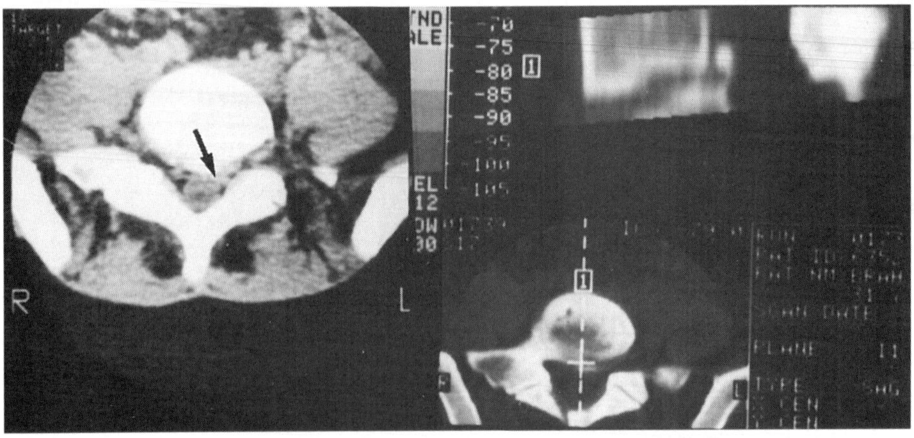

Figure 11.30 *Axial CT, L5-S1, in a patient with left sciatica. Despite a good CT, including reconstruction, the disc rupture (arrow), which was obvious at surgery, is not evident because of degenerative changes.*

Midline HNP

There is no more CT scan diagnosis fraught with a higher rate of false-positive readings than the diagnosis of a midline HNP. (10) MRI will rescue us from this dilemma, but today's technology dictates that we address the issue of the midline HNP on CT scan.

Problem 1: Volume Averaging The single cut viewed on a CT scan film is not a representation of tissue equivalent to the wafer thin radiographic film on which it is printed. Rather, it represents the "gray" average of all of the tissues the computer detected in the width of the cut (Fig. 11.31). If the slice thickness is 5 mm, all tissues 2.5 mm on either side of the scout view marking line are registered by the computer and represented by one average shade of "gray." It is this phenomenon that resulted in a protocol calling for angulation of the gantry to reduce the distorting effects of volume averaging.

Problem 2: Annular Bulging (2, 4, 19) Aging of a disc, with annular bulging, is a fact of life. The longer one lives, the more degeneration will occur in a disc, resulting in a high rate of annular bulging evident in the older patients undergoing CT scanning (Fig. 11.32). Add to these degenerative changes a forward slip (spondylolisthesis) or backward subluxation (retrospondylolisthesis), and annular bulging becomes even more pronounced (Fig. 11.33).

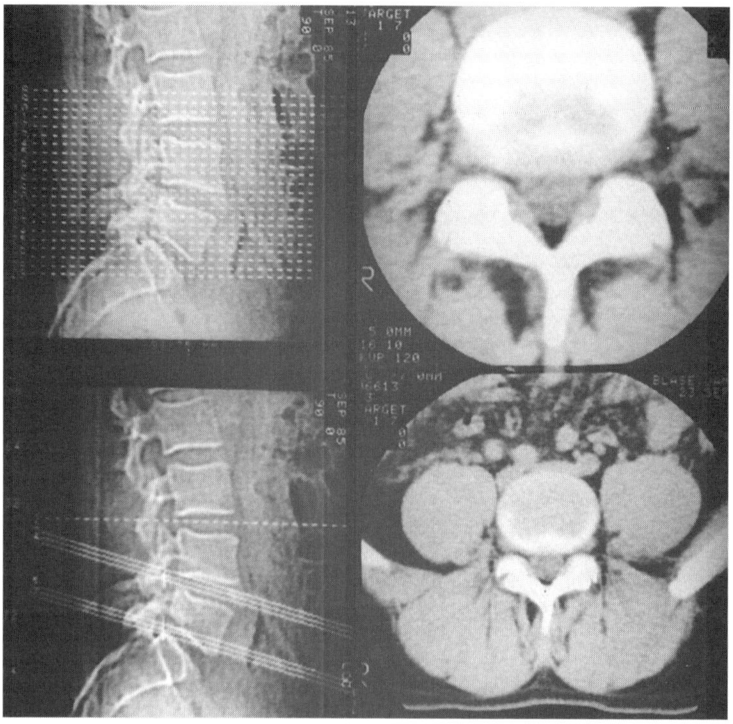

Figure 11.31 *Volume averaging: (L4-L5) The top row shows the unangled gantry and all of the tissue averaged, suggesting a large midline HNP; the bottom row shows how gantry angulation in the same patient removes the effect of volume averaging.*

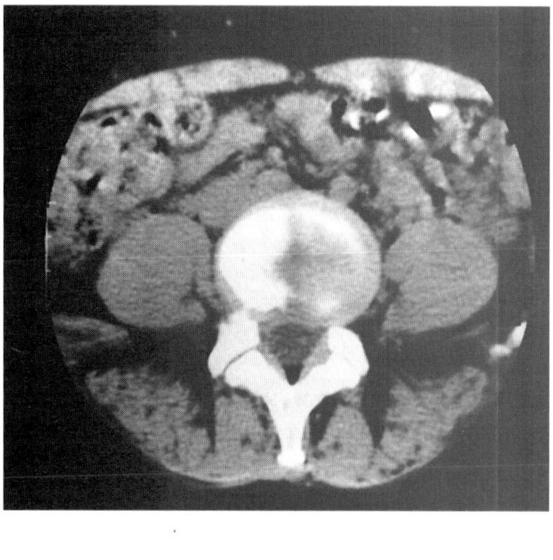

Figure 11.32 *Axial CT showing annular bulging.*

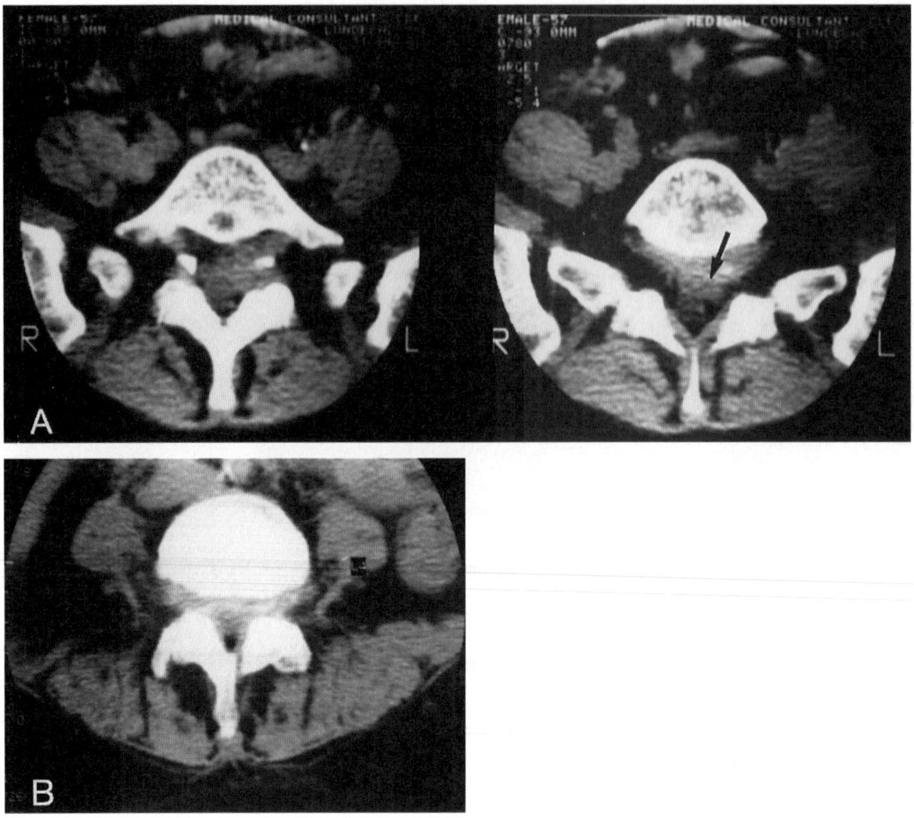

Figure 11.33 **A.** *Axial CTs in a patient with severe left sciatica. Image on right suggests annular bulging, but image on left shows mass in lytic defect on left (arrow) that is not present on right. This was a sequestered fragment of disc.* **B.** *Axial CT in degenerative spondylolisthesis with diffuse disc bulge.*

With the advent of MRI, the "problem" of the midline disc herniation has been resolved (12) (Fig. 11.34). It is important to recognize the rare midline disc herniations because:

1. Remove a midline HNP from a patient with bilateral leg symptoms due to direct root irritation, and the patient will be made better.
2. Remove a "midline disc bulge" (shown on CT scan) from a patient with back pain (with or without referred leg pain) due to lumbar segmental instability, and the patient will be made worse.

In the days of both Pantopaque myelography and water-soluble myelography, and to this day with CT scanning, annular bulges are being removed surgically to the detriment of the patient's good health. The "sucker disc" lives on!

Solution

The first step in the solution is to accept that it is possible to have direct root irritation from a midline HNP and that the resulting bilateral leg symptoms can be relieved by a simple disc excision. The next step is to realize that the syndrome is rare compared with the more common posterior lateral HNP with unilateral radicular pain.

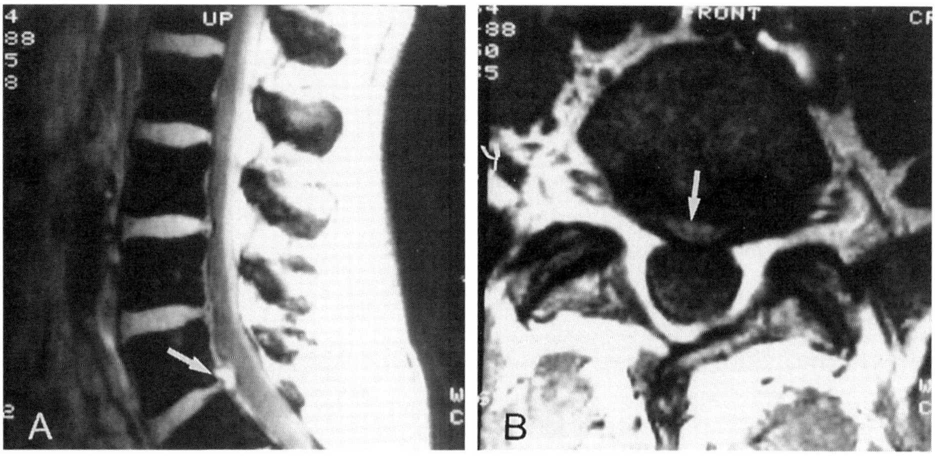

Figure 11.34 **A.** *Sagittal MRI showing midline HNP, L5-S1 in a patient with predominant back pain (arrow).* **B.** *Axial MRI of same patient showing midline HNP, L5-S1 (arrow).*

Bilateral Radicular Syndrome Due to a Midline HNP

The massive central disc herniation, with bilateral leg pain and bladder and bowel involvement, is: most often a large sequestered disc, always a surgical emergency, and excluded from the designation of "midline HNP."

The syndrome of bilateral leg pain due to midline disc herniation has the following clinical characteristics:

1. It occurs in the younger age group (25 to 40 years).
2. It becomes a diagnosis of consideration only after a number of disabling episodes.
3. At the height of a disabling episode, the patient will complain of:
   a. Dominant back pain.
   b. Both legs are affected by a radicular-like pain, either alternating from one leg to the other during the single acute episode or from one episode to the next.
   c. Occasionally, a paresthetic discomfort in the foot will be present.
   d. If the patient is examined during an acute episode, the following findings will be noted:
      - Bilateral SLR reduction due to back pain.
      - Possibly bowstring discomfort.
      - No, or minimal, neurological signs.
      - Inability to flex forward because of bilateral leg (buttock) and/or back pain, yet good backward extension with little pain.
4. Between episodes, the patient is close to being asymptomatic and capable of normal activities. A patient with back pain due to segmental instability as a result of degenerative disc disease has a more consistent history of back pain, that is, for months or years activity aggravates the back pain.

CT Scan Diagnosis of a Midline HNP

The foundation of all CT diagnosis of an HNP is "focally dominant" extension of disc material beyond the normal peripheral limits of an intervertebral disc (into the epidural space). The "midline disc herniation" is no exception. Figure 11.35 is an example of a midline HNP. An important clue to the diagnosis is the patient's statement to the effect that although both legs are symptomatic, one leg dominates in its affliction over the other. If the midline HNP can be shown to be eccentric to that dominant side on CT scan, this is support for the diagnosis.

The final support for the diagnosis of a bilateral radicular syndrome due to a midline HNP lies in the successful relief of symptoms with removal of the HNP, a criterion often not met or even discussed in this syndrome.

Degenerative Disc Disease (Disc Degeneration)

With the demonstration of a focal protrusion of disc material into the spinal canal (HNP), there is a reasonable chance that the patient had symptoms, has symptoms, or will have symptoms due to that pathology. Just the reverse is true in disc degeneration in the lumbar spine. Like graying of the hair and wrinkling of the skin, disc degeneration occurs as part of the aging process. Whether that causes symptoms and whether disc degeneration (a pathological state) becomes degenerative disc disease (the symptomatic state) are topics separate from the CT scan diagnosis of degenerative disc disease.

The clinical importance of recognizing disc degeneration on CT scan is:

1. If a patient with back pain has these changes confined to one level, there is a possibility of surgical assistance (stabilization procedure) when conservative care fails.
2. The aging process has afflicted the spine if degenerative changes are noted at multiple levels. In these patients, surgical intervention at one level, although initially affecting symptoms, is unlikely to reverse the aging process, and thus unlikely to prevent subsequent symptoms due to aging occurring at another level.
3. If one level of degenerative disc disease is present, the perusal of adjacent CT scan levels, looking for early signs of disc degeneration, is useful.

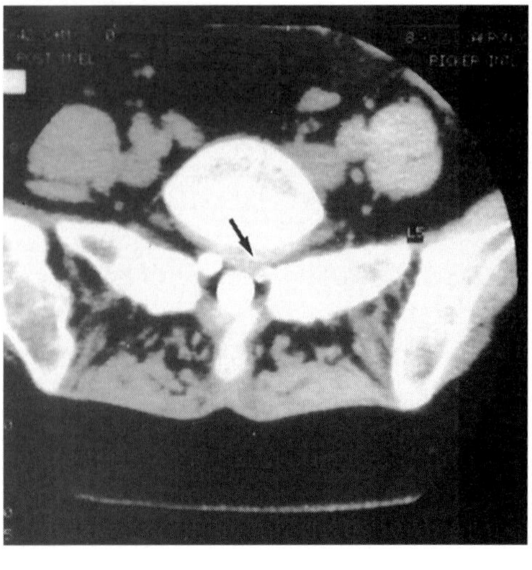

Figure 11.35 *An axial CT showing a midline HNP at L5-S1; the disc herniation and symptoms were eccentric left (arrow).*

Lateral Zone

The lateral zone of the spinal canal is outlined in detail in Chapters 1 and 16. In summary, the zone is defined (Fig. 11.36) as subarticular, foraminal, and extraforaminal, and its CT scan pathology is demonstrated in Figure 11.37.

Central Canal

Aside from an HNP, central canal neurological territory can be encroached upon by degenerative or congenital changes (8, 16). Spinal canal stenosis due to degenerative changes is by far the most common and is depicted in Figure 11.38.

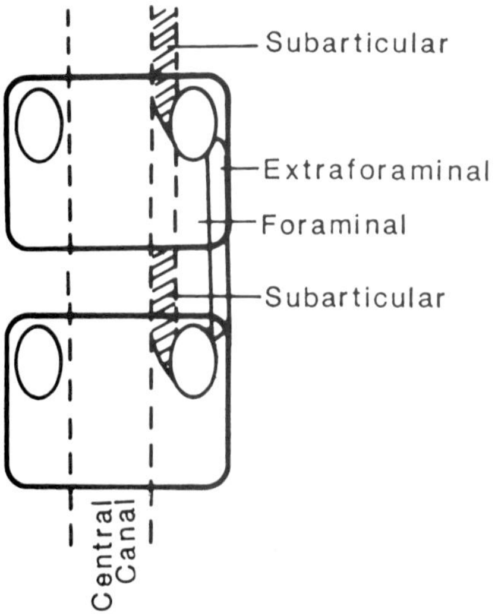

Figure 11.36 *Schematic depicting the three regions of the lateral zone.*

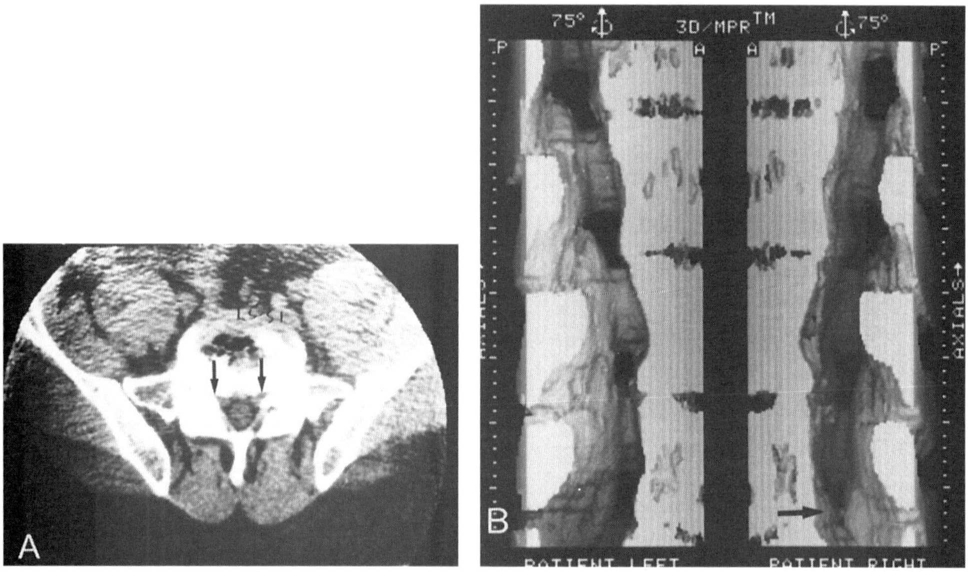

Figure 11.37 **A.** *Subarticular stenosis on axial CT (arrows).* **B.** *Foraminal stenosis (L5 foramen, right) on sagittal CT (arrow).*

Facet Joints

Degenerative facet joint changes are akin to degenerative disc changes: their presence does not necessarily mean the patient is having symptoms. The changes are common and are shown in Figure 11.39.

Spondylolisthesis

In an adult spinal surgical practice, lytic and degenerative spondylolisthesis is the common CT scan change seen. This condition's appearances was shown in Figures 5.3, 5.5, and 5.6.

CT Scan Appearance of Conjoint Roots (5, 15)

Figure 11.40 shows conjoined nerve roots. The nerve root tissue is isodense, with the cauda equina compared with an HNP that is denser (whiter) than nerve tissue. Reviewing

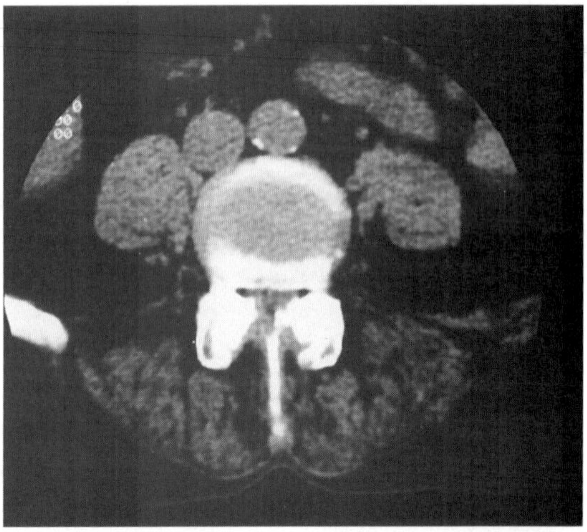

Figure 11.38 *Axial CT showing significant canal stenosis.*

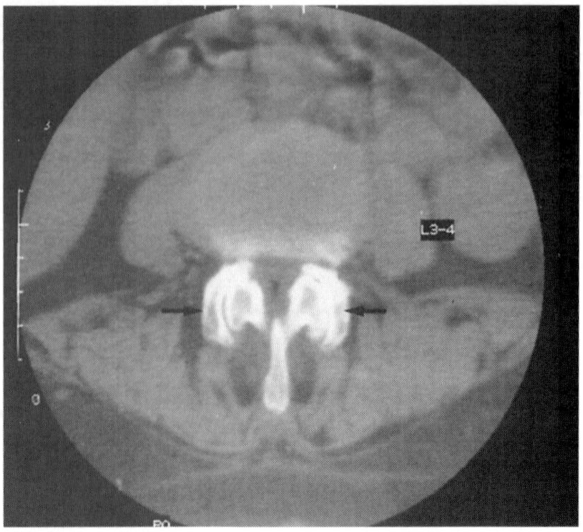

Figure 11.39 *Axial CT showing degenerative facet joints (arrows) and significant canal stenosis.*

scan slices from proximal to distal will reveal that the conjoint roots are closely related to the dural sac proximally, and separate distally, in preparation for their exit through the neural foramen.

The bony canal changes that usually accompany conjoined nerve roots have been well described by Helms and co-workers (5) and are shown in Figure 11.40.

Conclusion

The conjoined nerve root is easily observed on myelography (Fig. 11.41), which makes the diagnostic exercise easy. But with more surgery being based on MRI or CT scanning without myelography, conjoined nerve roots are important to recognize preoperatively.

A good test of the value to neuroradiology, CT scanning, and surgical intervention occurs in the patient who has sciatica due to an HNP and at the same level has a conjoined nerve root and lateral zone stenosis. Fortunately, the occurrence is rare because the diagnosis is difficult, and the surgery is tedious.

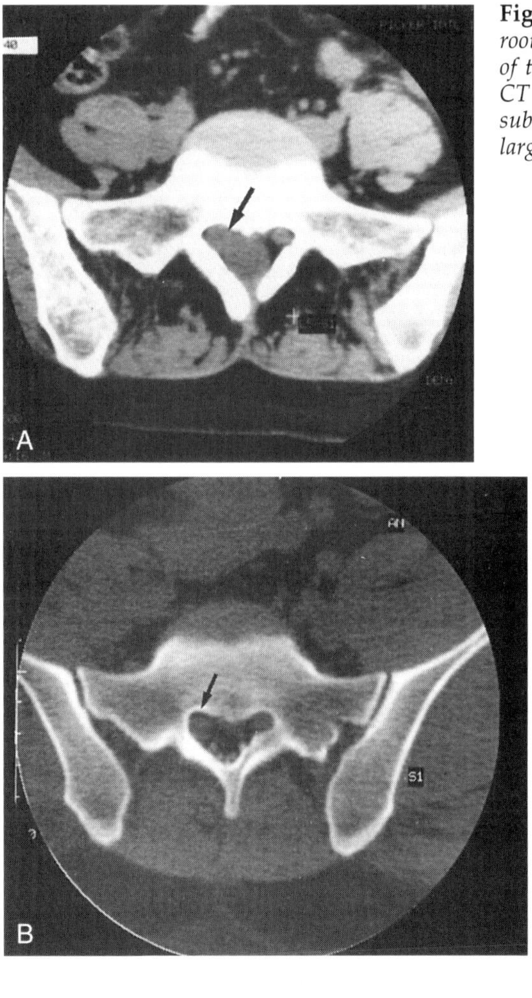

Figure 11.40 **A.** *Axial CT showing conjoined nerve root (S1, right) (arrow). Note the difference in the shape of the "root canal"—it is larger on the right.* **B.** *Axial CT (bone window) showing congenitally larger bony subarticular zone on right (arrow) to accommodate larger sized conjoined root.*

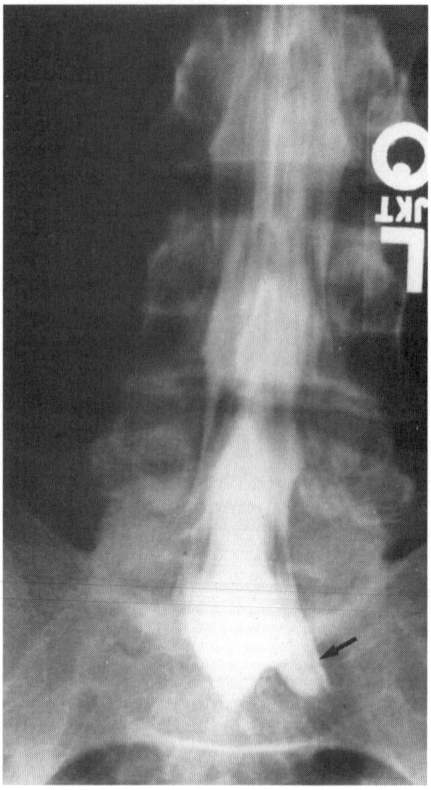

Figure 11.41 *An AP myelogram showing obvious conjoined root at S1 level on left (arrow).*

Sagittal Reconstructions/Three-Dimensional Reconstruction and Helical (Spiral) CT

Most CT scanning machines sold today are capable of spiral scanning (Fig. 11.42). Although the technique has many advantages in other parts of the body (lung, brain), it is of limited use in the spine. To date, the only known advantage is faster scanning of the cervical spine in polytrauma patients. Its use in the lumbar spine is limited because the time (and number of spirals) to scan from L3–S1 is so long that the radiograph tube overheats. The only proposed use of the spiral CT scan in the lumbar spine has been for sagittal reconstruction and three-dimensional reconstruction of the lumbar spine in difficult cases such as failed back surgery (20) (Fig. 11.42). The strength of CT over MRI has always been the superior depiction of bony detail. Add to this the even more superior resolution of helical CT with three-dimensional reconstruction, and you are better able to see residual bony encroachment, especially in the foramen.

CT/Myelograms (9)

There was an initial reluctance on the part of the surgeon to give up the gold standard of myelography while traveling the learning curve of CT scanning. This led to the use of pre-CT subarachnoid-injected, water-soluble contrast material: the CT/myelogram (Fig. 11.43).

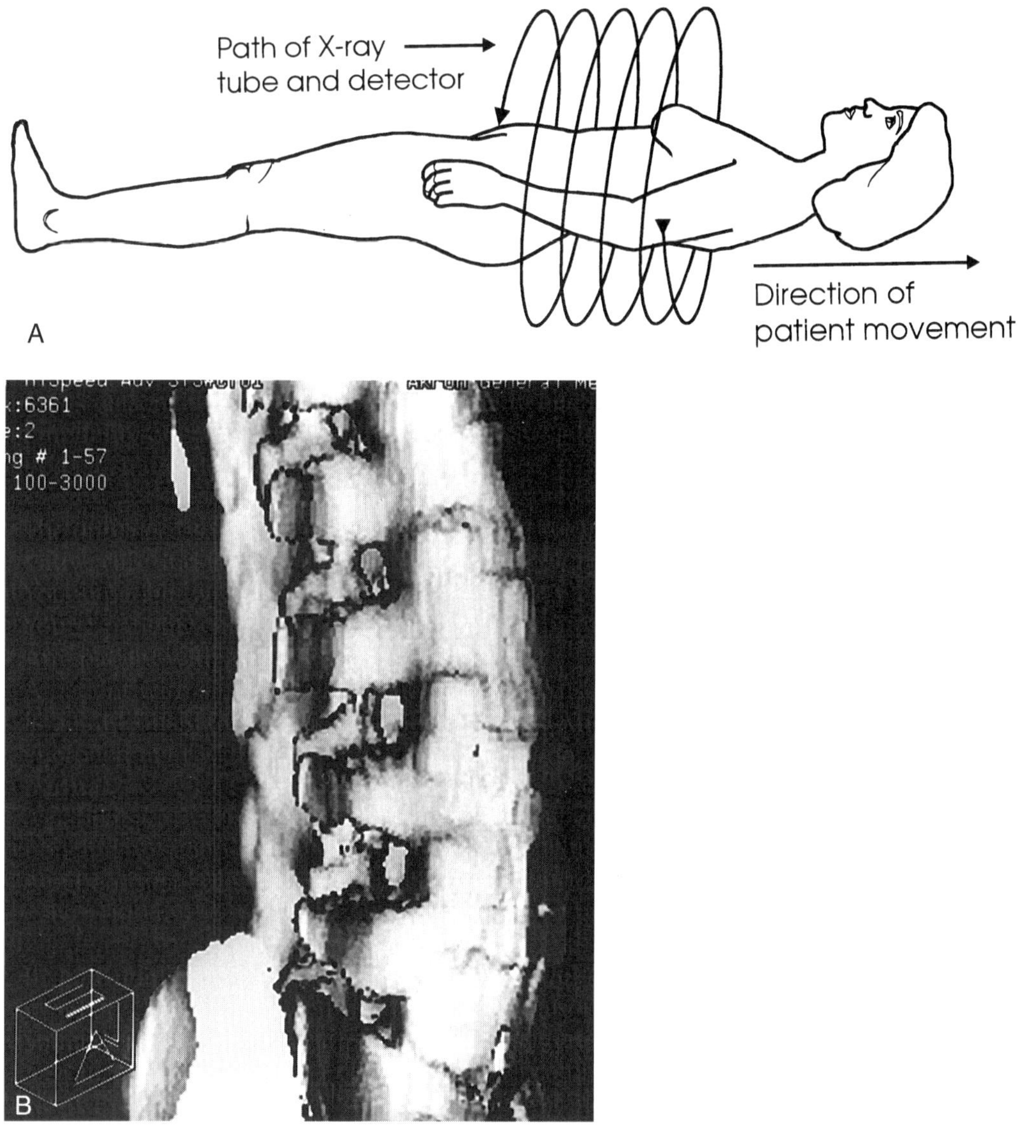

Figure 11.42 **A.** *The spiral scan technique.* **B.** *A spiral scan technique was used to obtain this three-dimensional image of the foraminal zone.*

With improved CT scanning hardware and software resulting in clearer images, the necessity for subarachnoid instillation of contrast material has waned. The final step in relegating myelography to an infrequent procedure has been the increasing use of MRI as the primary diagnostic test in lumbar disc disease.

At present, CT/myelography is not routine in our center, but this procedure is useful for:

1. An obese patient, in which case scanning images are anticipated to be of poor quality.
2. Anticipation of a difficult differential diagnosis that might include higher lumbar lesions.

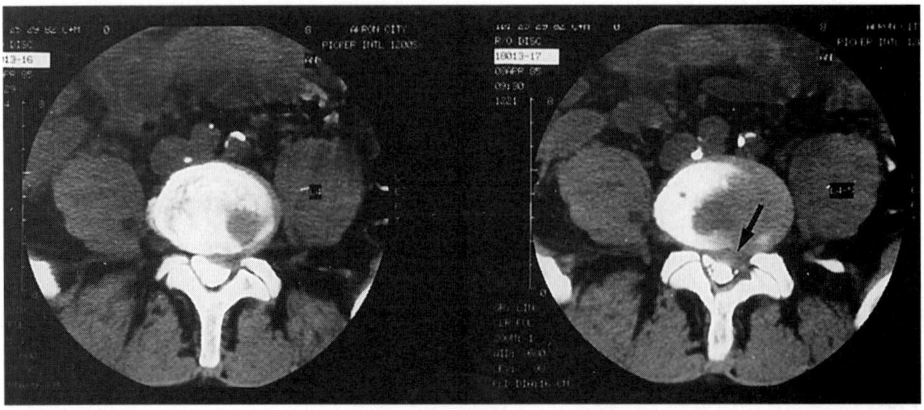

Figure 11.43 *A CT myelogram showing HNP, L4-L5, left (arrow). With increasing familiarity by clinicians for the increasing imaging capabilities of CT and MRI, the myelogram and CT/myelogram will largely disappear.*

3. The older patient with spinal stenosis symptoms and:
   - Proximal leg symptoms suggesting a high lumbar lesion.
   - Scoliosis on plain radiograph.
   - A questionable diagnosis (eg, high erythrocyte sedimentation rate, positive bone scan). (A patient with classic spinal stenosis symptoms and no associated abnormal tests can be investigated adequately with MRI scanning alone.)
4. A young patient with a suspected midline HNP used to be an indication for CT/myelography, but MRI has supplanted this need.
5. A confusing CT scan due to a perineural cyst,(14) conjoined nerve roots, and so on.

The decreasing use of CT/myelography in the face of improved CT and MR imaging is a trend supported in the literature.

Intravenous-Enhanced CT Scan

The use of IV-enhanced (Conray 60) (Fig. 11.44) CT scanning was useful in the assessment of a patient with recurrent symptoms, after previous spinal surgery. Now, with the advent of gadolinium-enhanced MRI, very few clinicians would consider the use of enhanced CT for the assessment of the symptomatic patient who has had previous lumbar spine surgery.

Discography and CT/Discography

Because discography is a test almost exclusively used for the assessment of degenerative disc disease, we have moved its description and discussion to Chapter 14. We are not very supportive of the use of discography for the assessment of any lumbar spine problem.

A number of articles (11, 13) have appeared in the literature describing CT/discography (Fig. 11.45) as a method of assessing patients with lumbar symptoms. We have performed more than 10,000 discograms and remain unimpressed with the value of discography as a basis for surgical decision making. To extend this technique to CT exam-

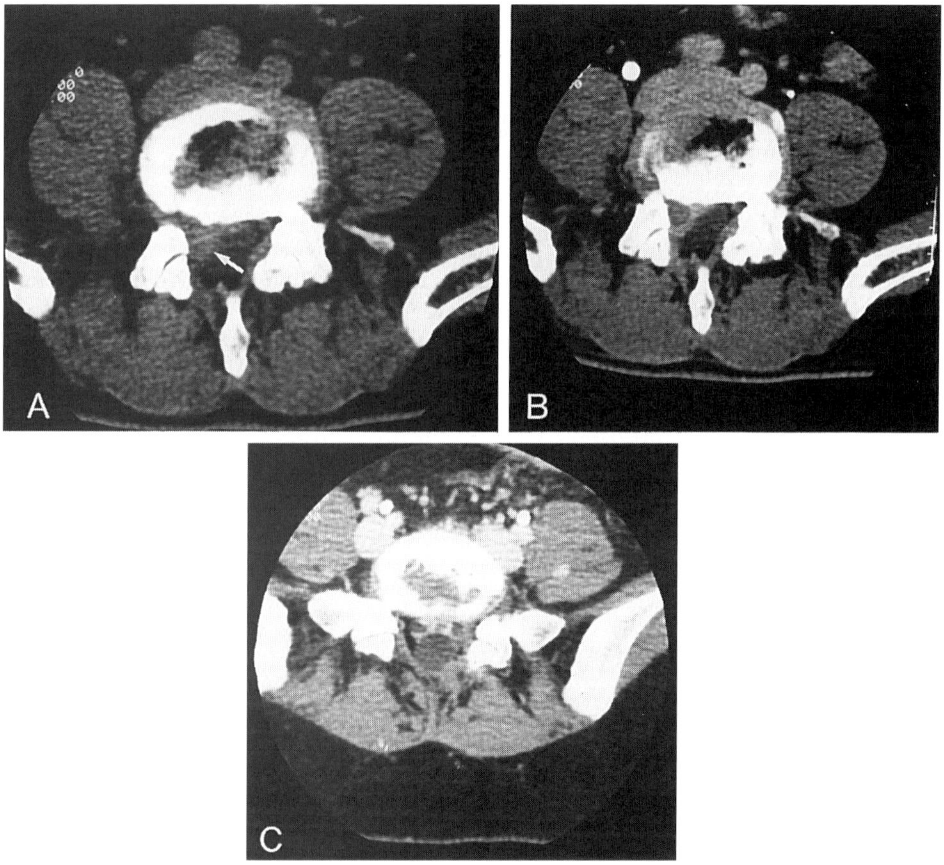

Figure 11.44 *IV-enhanced CT scan.* **A.** *Postoperative patient with recurrent right sciatica. Note the homogeneous mass of scar, L4-L5, right (arrow).* **B.** *After an IV injection of Conray 60, the scar tissue enhances, and the recurrent avascular disc fragment does not.* **C.** *A patient with continuing postoperative symptoms. IV Conray injection shows no residual or recurrent disc fragment.*

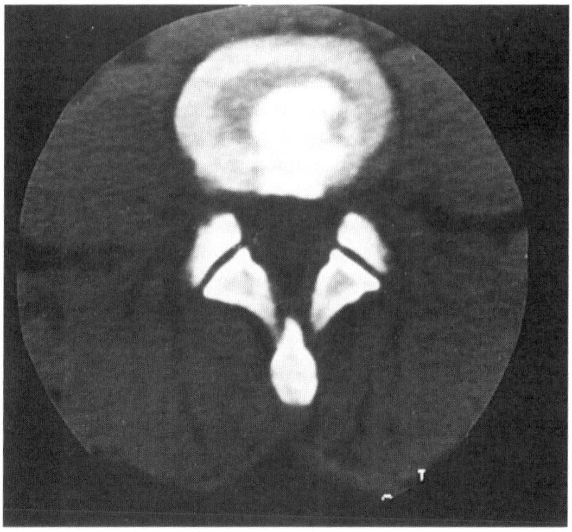

Figure 11.45 *A CT/discogram.*

ination of instilled contrast material increases the risk of false-positive findings and improper surgery. Until further studies on the scientific validity of CT/discography appear in the literature, their routine use for surgical decision making is to be discouraged.

Conclusion

There is no question that spine surgical practice has been immensely enhanced by CT scanning technology. Understanding the strengths and weaknesses of any investigation or technique will only help the procedure grow and become even more useful. The final missing link in this growth potential for CT is an increased joint effort for neuroradiologists to deliver quality images and clear diagnoses, and for clinicians to relate the clinical material to this effort. This should result in more collaborative studies on surgical outcomes appearing in the radiological literature. The difficulty in obtaining an unbiased intraoperative determination of normal, bulging, or herniated disc can be balanced only by independent surgical follow-up: The radiologist made a diagnosis. The surgeon operated. Did the patient get better?

A satisfactory patient outcome is the only way to verify that the radiological diagnosis was firm. Simple observation at surgery is no longer good enough.

MAGNETIC RESONANCE IMAGING

Magnetic resonance imaging is the major medical imaging development of the century. Its effect on the practice of medicine will be even more profound than Röntgen's original proposal for the use of radiographs to view internal structures. We said in the second edition of this book that MRI developments are coming so quickly that by the time the chapter was published, it would likely be out of date. Things have not changed in MRI; there is still rapid change. The rate of advancement is bewildering, and it is important that the clinician grasp the basics now and hang on for the ride.

For years (1, 12), molecular biologists and chemists used magnetic resonance spectroscopy for the laboratory study of molecular and pharmacological structures. It was not until 1971 (2) that MRI was proposed for human use, and it was in 1981 (3) (only 15 years ago!) that the first high-quality image of the brain was generated at Hammersmith Hospital in London, England. Today, clinicians are getting high-quality images of spinal structures, yet the radiological scientists have only scratched the surface. MRI has become the imaging modality of choice for investigation of degenerative conditions of the spine, with CT scan and myelography assuming a secondary role.

Physics

A clinician's chance of understanding the physics of MRI is remote. However, a grasp of the basic physics is helpful in appreciating the potential for growth in MRI. These basics will be presented in point form.

Point 1

The following definitions apply:

Magnetic There are two magnets essential to MRI:

1. The external magnet.(1) That is, the magnet that is part of the imaging machine. Its strength is described in tesla (T) units, and the most common sizes are 0.5, 1.0, and 1.5 tesla, the strongest magnets in the world. Work is ongoing with 2 tesla and 4 tesla units as experimental magnets (not FDA approved). As of this writing, the strongest commercially available magnet is 1.5 tesla.
2. The internal magnets (zillions), that is, the miniature magnet of the hydrogen atom contained in the body.

Resonance A resonating system is a system "in sync," that is, all the violins are on the same wavelength to produce a nice sound for the audience. Resonance in MRI-talk is the matching of the frequency of the radiowaves (the violins) used for excitation with the frequency of the spinning hydrogen atoms (the audience) in the magnet field. Like an audience that leaves a concert with renewed vigor, the hydrogen atoms absorb energy from the radiowave, which changes the magnetic vector. Some audience members fail to get excited during a concert (some even fall asleep!) because the resonating sound from the stage simply did not excite them. Similarly, hydrogen atoms have to be resonated with the correct frequency, or they will not respond (fortunately, the hydrogen atoms are much more predictable than a symphony audience!).

Point 2

An atom is the smallest unit of a chemical element that retains its chemical identity. It is composed of a nucleus around which electrons orbit (Fig. 11.46). The nucleus comprises almost all of the mass of an atom, but because of the orbiting electrons, comprises less of the actual size of an atom. A nucleus is made up of protons, with a single positive electrical charge, and neutrons, with no charge. The number of protons in the nucleus is the atomic number of the atom or element. Nuclei with uneven atomic numbers are 1 (H), 23 (Na), and 31 (P). The nuclei have spin and charge, giving them angular momentum, so that they act like small magnets.

Point 3

The atom used for MRI is the hydrogen (1H) atom because it is abundant in the body and capable of giving off a strong signal when excited. Hydrogen is a simple element with one proton in the nucleus, no neutrons, and no orbiting electrons. This atom is everywhere in

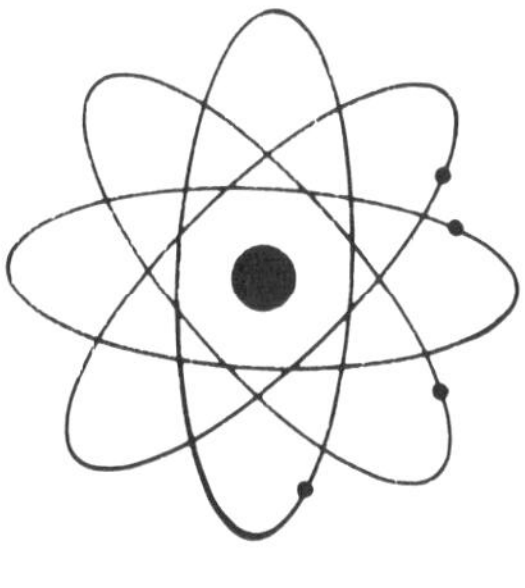

Figure 11.46 *An atom = nucleus + orbiting electrons.*

the body: water, lipids, proteins, and nucleic acids. It is the hydrogen ion in water that is available for excitation. To a lesser extent, the hydrogen ion of lipids will contribute to the MRI signal, with protein and nucleic acid H ions offering nothing to the signal.

The hydrogen atom is positively charged and possessed of spinning or angular movement. This movement produces an internal minimagnetic field around each of the multitude of hydrogen atoms in the body. Normally, at any one moment, the hydrogen ions are randomly oriented in the body with a net neutral magnetic effect.

Point 4

The hydrogen atom magnets are randomly oriented in the body, but when placed in an external magnetic field, some will align themselves parallel to the magnetic field, producing a net magnetic vector.

Technique of Performing Magnetic Resonance Imaging

Step 1

Place the patient in the magnetic coil of the scanner and turn on the magnet. (The magnet is, in fact, constantly turned on.) The magnetic field across the body will cause some of the hydrogen (and other magnetic atoms) to line up with the external magnetic field, producing the net magnetic vector (Fig. 11.47).

Step 2

Broadcast a radiofrequency wave into the body tissue (Fig. 11.48). The pulsating radiofrequency wave will be of a predetermined frequency, such that its most significant effect will be on the hydrogen atom. The predetermined frequency is called the "resonant frequency." Some of the hydrogen magnets will absorb some of the energy from the series of radiowave energy and tilt over (Fig. 11.49). The "excited" hydrogen atoms have absorbed the energy from the radiofrequency (RF), and in their tilted position are said to be at a higher energy level, which results in an overall change in direction of the net magnetic vector.

The series of the RF pulse are repeated in cycles of finite time known as "repetition time" (TR).

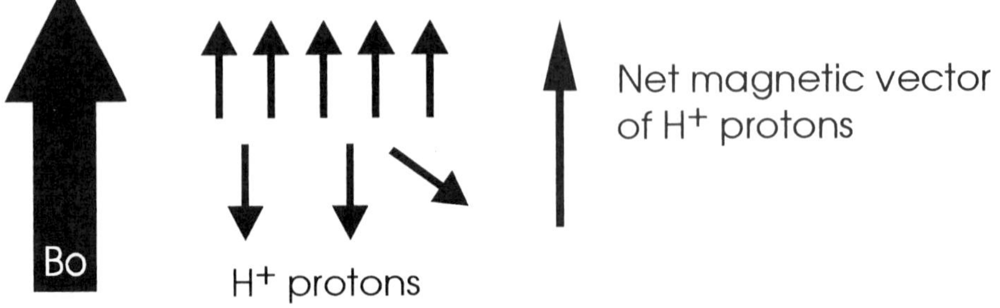

Figure 11.47 *The hydrogen protons of the body, when placed in the main (external) magnetic field (Bo) will line up as shown.*

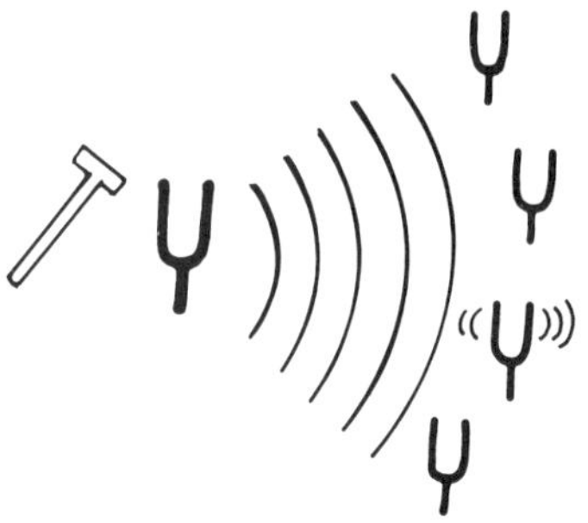

Figure 11.48 *The preselected broadcast frequency will have its most significant effect on the hydrogen ion just as a vibrating tuning fork will have an effect only on a tuning fork of the same frequency, leaving other tuning forks of different frequencies relatively unaffected.*

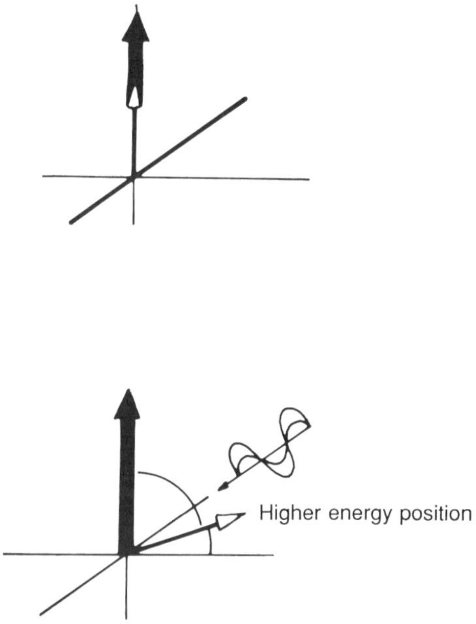

Figure 11.49 *The hydrogen ion, so affected by the specific frequency, absorbs the energy of that frequency as it deflects into a higher energy position (bottom vector). (Reprinted with permission from Young SW: Nuclear Magnetic Resonance Imaging Basic Principles, Raven Press, New York, 1984.)*

Step 3

During a gap in the pulsatile RF wave, the hydrogen magnets (atoms) will try and reorient themselves in the magnetic field, returning the net magnetic vector to its original position. In doing so, the hydrogen atoms will release energy by rebroadcasting the RF signal they absorbed on deflection. This rebroadcasted radiofrequency wave can be picked up with an antenna just as a car radio picks up a broadcast signal. By "tuning in" to a particular frequency, the echo of the RF signal can be picked up. The time in the gap in the RF wave when "tuning in" is done is known as the echo time (TE). The TE can be altered by altering the time when the detection antenna is turned on.

Step 4

As the net magnetic vector returns to its original position, the rebroadcasted signal is detected by an antenna in the form of a surface coil applied to the patient's spine. (The patient is actually lying on the coil.) As explained later, the use of surface coils in spinal imaging has resulted in much improved images. Different RF signals from different regions of the sam-

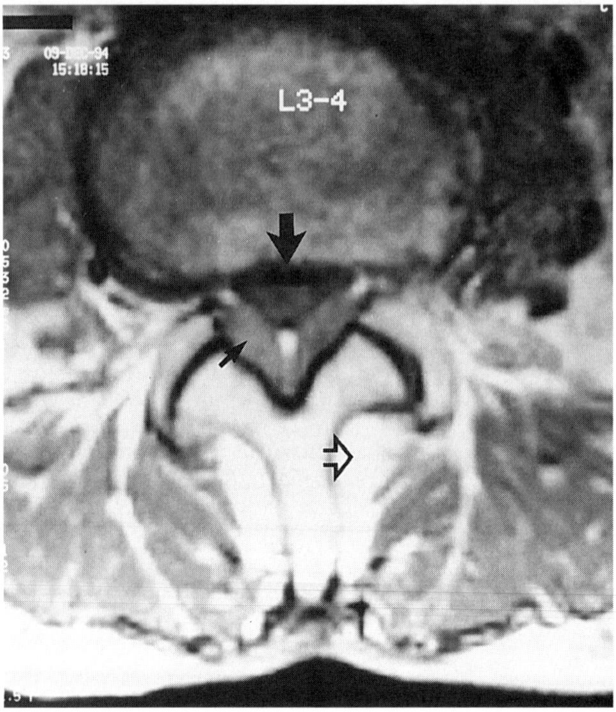

Figure 11.50 *An axial T1-weighted MRI showing the various shades of gray: a dark CSF space (heavy arrow), a less dark ligamentum flavum (small arrow), and white fat (open arrow).*

ple are recorded as digital data by the computer. The computer, in turn, converts this digital data into varying shades of gray to produce an image. The image is easily transferred to a film just like a CT scan image. If there is high signal intensity (ie, lots of hydrogen atoms talking back to you), the gray scale will be white (Fig. 11.50). If there are no hydrogen atoms (protons) talking back, the gray scale will be black (Fig. 11.51).

Images Available in MRI

The varying shades of gray produced in CT depend on the varying densities of the tissues absorbing the radiation. Thus, only one parameter, electron density of different tissues, determines the image in CT.

MRI density information is based on four independent components (one physical, and three biochemical):

1. Density of the nuclear species being measured. Presently, hydrogen atoms are being studied, but in the future other nuclear species (atoms) such as phosphorus and sodium will be measured at the same time. They can then be superimposed, through computer interpretation (eg, color) and added to the present images. The possibilities are endless.
2. Relaxation time T1
3. Relaxation time T2

> determined by inherent properties of compounds and adjacent compounds. By varying TR/TE, you can accentuate T1 or T2 characteristics (ie, weighted).

4. Motion or flow of materials (eg, blood).

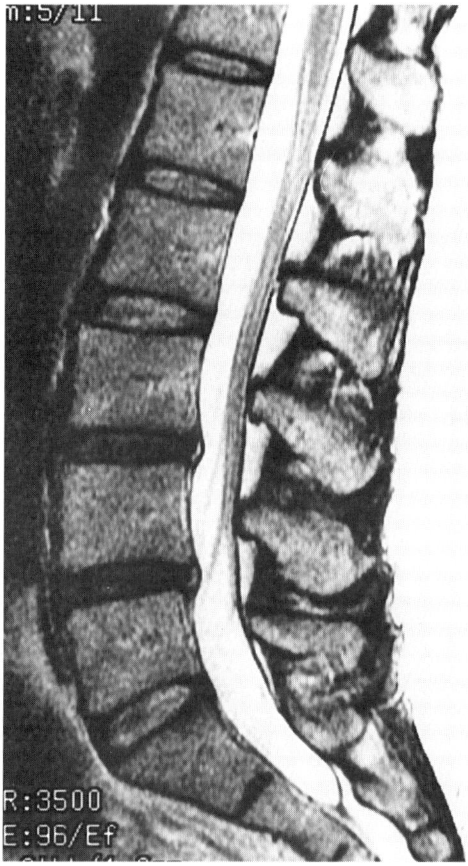

Figure 11.51 *A fast spin ECHO sagittal showing high signal intensity (white) CSF, gray marrow of vertebral bodies, and blackened (degenerative) discs, especially at L3–L4 and L4–L5.*

Images can be formed in axial, sagittal, and coronal planes by varying the direction of the magnetic gradients across the patient. The type of image formed depends on the computer detection of the parameters as listed previously, that is, signal strength; relaxation time (T_1); relaxation time (T_2); and state of motion of protons (blood flow, because of its motion, gives no signal, ie, black, unless the computer converts it to white).

The signal received, like a light bulb, is either bright (white) or dim (black), with many shades of gray (brightness) in between. The exact shade of gray is determined by the H ion concentration of the various tissues scanned and the T_1 and T_2 characteristics of the tissues imaged.

Each study represents a set of characteristics predetermined by the computer software and ordered up by the radiographic technician. Most scanners reproduce three separate studies: sagittal T_1-weighted, sagittal T_2-weighted, and axial (T_1>) images.

Technical Details

It is at this level of imaging physics that the clinician will get lost trying to understand what the MRI machine can do. It is important to recognize that MR technology is changing rapidly and is very dependent on a radiologist being constantly on top of these changes. This makes it fruitless for clinicians to think they can own or operate an MRI without a radiologist. Further, the production of quality MR images is very operator dependent. It is possible, but unexpected, that an average radiographic technologist can produce a poor radiograph or CT image. It is easy for an average technologist to produce a poor MR image.

It is important that supervision provide direction on the appropriate coil, imaging plane and matrix, slice thickness, number of excitations, pulse sequence parameters (TR), and echo time (TE), all terms with which clinicians are not familiar.

Field Strength MRI machines are built with varying magnet sizes measured in tesla. The strength of the magnet is many times the earth's gravitational pull and is capable of twisting aneurysm clips, pulling hair pins out of the head, moving wheelchairs, and decoding credit cards. Magnet sizes commonly used in medicine today are 0.5T, 1T, and 1.5T. It is not necessarily true that the bigger magnet is better, but imaging of difficult areas, such as the posterior fossa and base of the brain, is better with the higher field strengths. Although the manufacturers state that it is possible to get good spinal images from the lower field strength machines, the authors' early and continuing experiences would suggest that the most consistently good spinal images come from the machines with the highest field strength.(7) The quality of MRI images varies between manufacturers, with the GE Signa unit producing consistently good quality spinal MR images. Most of the MRI scans in this book have been produced by a Siemans Magnetom unit, which is the scanner used in the senior author's (JM) hospital.

Pulse Sequence In reading about MRI, clinicians will see the term "pulse sequence" mentioned often. There are three types of pulse sequences commonly used today: One (spin echo) was used exclusively for clinical imaging of the spine in the original protocols; a second (gradient echo) acquisition of a new pulse sequence has recently been introduced to speed up image acquisition time and give more contrast between CSF and its surrounding tissues. The latest pulse sequence to come along is "fast spin-echo," which simply reduces image acquisition times without significant loss of image quality, a particularly useful tool in the acquisition of T_2 spin-echo images (Fig. 11.51).

Spin-Echo Pulse Sequence A combination of 90° and 180° radiofrequency waves result in hydrogen ion magnet deflecting out of its magnetic position, where it spins like a top. The resulting signal is called the spin echo.

Gradient-Echo Pulse Sequence (GRASS, FLASH) Gradient-echo (GE) sequences were introduced to shorten image-gathering time compared with spin-echo pulse sequences. GE sequences use less radiofrequency power, which results in less angle deflection of H + ion, and these sequences require less time for recovery of magnetization. The result for the patient is a shorter time between excitation of the hydrogen atom and recovery of the digital information necessary to produce the image.

Fast Spin-Echo Fast spin-echo (FSE) imaging techniques deliver exactly what is implied in the term: faster image acquisition (Fig. 11.50). From the moment MRI was introduced to clinical medicine in 1982, it was apparent that this mode was a slow imaging technique. The routine acquisition of sagittal and axial T_1-weighted and T_2-weighted images of the spine would take 30 to 45 minutes and sometimes longer. This is a long time for a patient, especially with pain, to lie still in the gantry. Speeding up image acquisition time without sacrificing image quality would be a winner.

FSE is that apparent winner. Using MRI physics too complicated to explain, multislice image acquisition is completed such that the T_2 examination time is less than 5 minutes. Conventional spin-echo (CSE) techniques acquire images one at a time, which explains the slowness of conventional SE T_2 when TR is 2000 to 3000 milliseconds per slice. With relatively cheap hardware and software updates to the MRI machine, FSE images are obtainable.

The images have a high signal-to-noise ratio and high resolution and are every bit as good as CSE T_2-weighted pictures. The imaging method is known as "rapid-acquisition, relaxation enhanced." It is beyond the scope of this book to explain the physics: just remember that you can get T_2 SE images in less than 5 minutes. The only difference between CSE and FSE is the increased signal intensity from fat, which results in somewhat poorer spatial resolution between CSF and cord. Nerve roots are seen better in the CSF, and supposedly the decreasing signal intensity with increasing disc degeneration is unchanged.

FSE techniques will probably replace most gradient-echo protocols because of the better spatial resolution.

Other Terms

Echo Time (TE) This measurement is the time between the initial pulse, which deflects the hydrogen atom 90 degrees, and the middle of the spin echo production when the antenna "listens in" to detect the amount of signal.

Repetition Time (TR) This measurement represents the period of time between one radiofrequency pulse and the next. By varying TE and TR, various tissue relaxation times are produced, and different tissue contrasts can be produced. The differences in the strengths of the primary magnetic field (0.5 to 1.5 tesla) also change tissue relaxation times, a factor to be aware of when reviewing scans from different centers.

Relaxation Times This is the intrinsic property of tissue, after being magnetized and struck with radiofrequency waves. It is determined by the behavior of atoms in a magnetic field and can be used to produce images of varying tissue contrast. By varying TR and TE, two basic types of tissue contrast are produced. The two types of relaxation mechanisms are:

- T_1 Relaxation time (T_1-weighted images) (spin lattice or longitudinal relaxation time). Produced by using a short TR/TE, it is the time required for spinning atoms to realign themselves with the externally applied magnetic fields after displacement with radiofrequency waves.

A good analogy would be the length of time it takes a regiment of soldiers, briefly at ease and talking to one another, to "present arms."

- T_2 Relaxation time (T_2-weighted images) (spin-spin or transverse relaxation time). Produced by longer TR/TE times, it represents the time required for the loss of signal caused by interaction of adjacent nuclei.

The analogy here would be giving the regimental soldiers a little more time to intermingle and then let them go home, their disappearance being the signal (Table 11.8).2

Each tissue, be it normal or abnormal, has characteristic T_1 and T_2 relaxation times, dependent upon chemical composition. This composition determines the signal intensity and thus the ultimate image produced.

Signal Intensity The ranges of signal intensity are low (a black image) to high (a white image) (Table 11.9).

Those tissues that give off a high intensity signal (high hydrogen ion concentration that can be affected by the magnet and the radiofrequency wave) are water, fat, marrow, and nerve tissue. Intermediate signal intensity comes from muscle and articular cartilage. Low signal intensity (black) structures are cortical bone, ligaments, tendons, and menisci. Because of the flow of blood (ie, the hydrogen ions will not stand still long enough to be counted), no signal intensity is produced by blood vessels that appear black.

Signal-to-Noise Ratio (S:N) The signal is what the antenna wishes to record; the noise is the interference from other structures that are not of interest. The higher the S:N ratio, the better the image. With the introduction of surface coils as the antenna to pick up the signal, two things happened in spinal (8) (and other) imaging:

1. The antenna was placed close to the signals that were to be detected, increasing the signal intensity.
2. Signals of no interest (noise) were eliminated, resulting in a high S:N ratio and a better image.

The MRI Gray Scale

The varying shades of gray produced in CT and other radiographic studies are determined by one factor: the different densities of the tissues (to be exact, the density of the orbiting electrons of each atom). The varying shades of gray produced on MRI are based

Table 11.8. T_1 and T_2 Values of Various Tissues (Midfield Strength Magnet)

Tissue	T_1(ms)	T_2(ms)	
CSF (water)	2000	250	Long
Fat	150	150	↓
Muscle	450	64	Short

Table 11.9. The Gray Scale

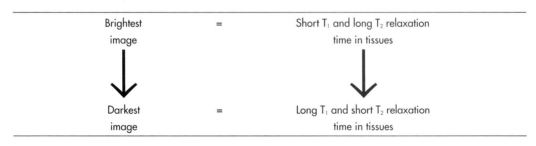

Brightest image	=	Short T_1 and long T_2 relaxation time in tissues
↓		↓
Darkest image	=	Long T_1 and short T_2 relaxation time in tissues

on four independent components of tissue, one physical (proton density) and three biochemical (relaxation time T_1, relaxation time T_2, and motion or flow of materials).

Proton Density

For now, let us consider proton density to introduce the gray scale; proton density is not a frequently used "menu" in MRI, but will help to understand the gray scale. The signal intensity or brightness from resonated tissues depends on the mobile protons in water and fat. Exclusive of T_1 and T_2 relaxation times, proton density image brightness (whiteness) and darkness (black) are simply determined by the number of free, mobile hydrogen protons in this tissue. The more protons, the brighter the signal and the whiter the shadow on the image. Materials with high proton density include fat, CSF, blood, and other fluids. Materials with low proton density, which thus give off little or no signal (ie, produce a black shadow on the image), are calcium, air, cortical bone, and fibrous tissue (Figs. 11.52 and 11.53).

T_1, T_2, and the Gray Scale

By using a long TR and a short TE, the T_1 and T_2 tissue characteristics are dampened, and the signal becomes dependent solely on the number of mobile protons: the more protons, the brighter (higher) the signal intensity and the whiter the image. This physical property of tissue response to MR is no different than electron density determining the gray scale in CT. The superior soft tissue depiction comes not from proton density but from $T_1$and T_2 relaxation effects. This is because many substances with similar proton and electron densities will emanate different signal intensities on MR due to the marked differences in T_1 and T_2 values (Fig. 11.52). (3) Note that water (CSF) has the longest T_1 and T_2 relaxation times, whereas fat protons have short T_1 and intermediate T_2 relaxation times. These relaxation times can easily be altered by binding the H+ proton with protein macromolecules; that is, fluids (water) can have a variety of signals (appearances) based on their protein content.

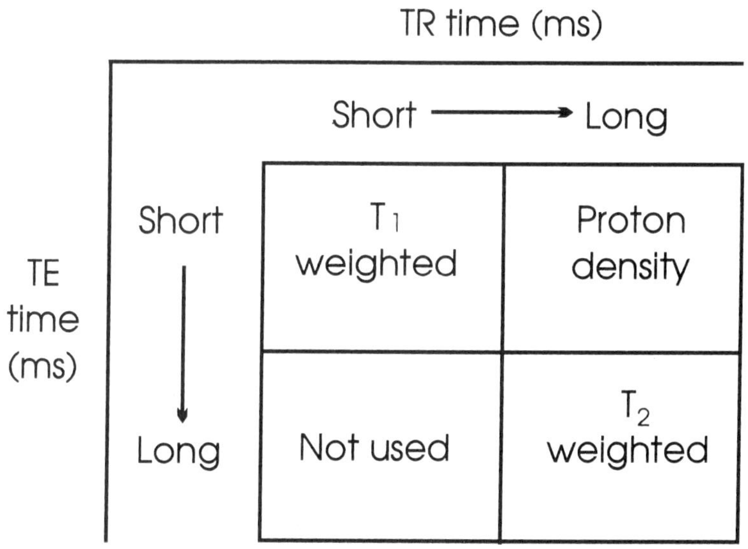

Figure 11.52 *A short TR/TE is a T1-weighted image; a long TR/TE is a T2-weighted image.*

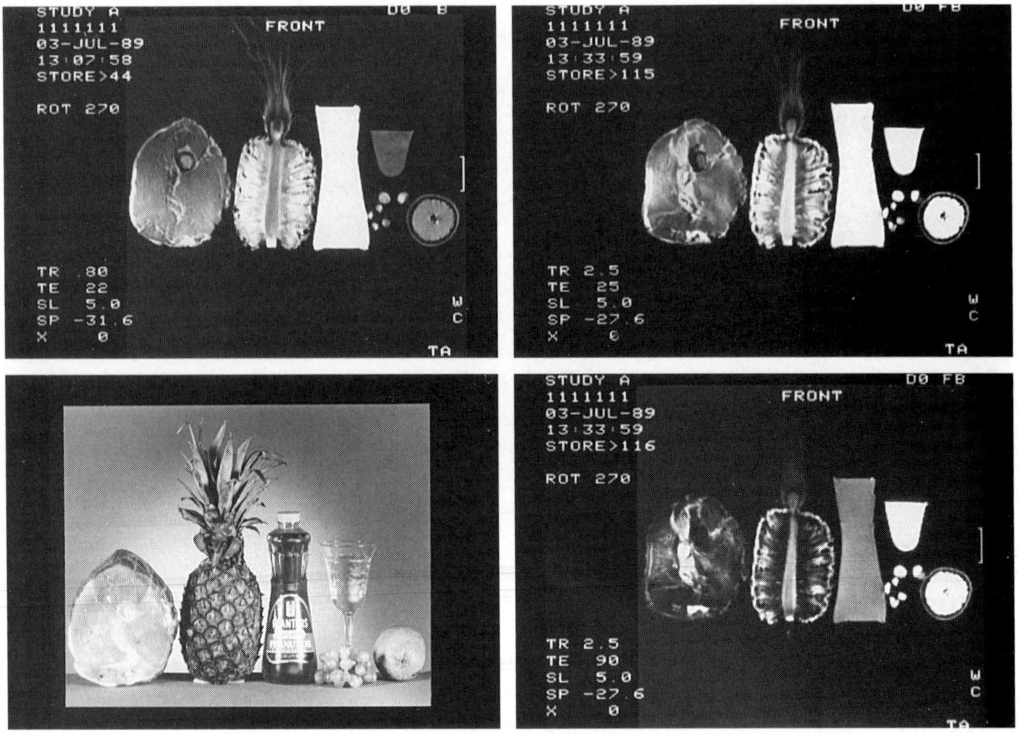

Figure 11.53 *The gray scale. (Bottom left). A ham (muscle), pineapple (fiber), peanut oil (fat), grapes (water), water, orange (water). (Top left) T1. (SE 800/22). Compare fat and water to the T2 image (Bottom right). On T1 weighting, fat has a high (white) signal intensity, while water is intermediate. Next, look at muscle (ham), which is also intermediate signal. Bone has no signal on T1 and is black. The only other high signal intensity (like fat) comes from the external surface of the ham. Although parts of the pineapple have whiter or higher signal intensity than water, it is still not equivalent to fat. (Bottom right). T2 (SE 2500/90). Now, fat (oil) has an intermediate signal intensity, and water is brighter. Compare the orange and the grapes: they have followed water in signal intensity or whiteness, that is, they are predominantly water. The part of the pineapple that has the most water (whiteness) is its skin! Bone is still black, with no signal intensity at all. These three figures show how to use the gray scale to determine tissue composition. (Exercise courtesy of Dr. Edward Bury, Neuroradiologist, Akron City Hospital, Akron, Ohio.)*

It should be noted that:

- Substances with the shortest T_1 relaxation time give off the brightest signal (fat, lipid-containing molecules or proteinaceous fluid).
- Substances with the longest T_1 relaxation time (edema, CSF, pure fluid, tumors [benign and malignant]) give off a low signal and appear grayer (Fig. 11.54 and Table 11.9).

By selecting a scanning protocol with a short TR and TE, the image is weighted to emphasize these T_1 characteristics, but weighting too heavily will ruin the image by invoking other physics equations that affect signal-to-noise ratios, scan time, and so on, a subject far beyond this chapter. Just the correct amount of TR and TE is needed to produce a useful T_1 image.

A protocol that lengthens both TR and TE (Table 11.9) is called a T_2-weighted image, in which the reverse signal characteristics occur: that is, the longer the T_2 relaxation time, the brighter the signal (remember, the longer the T_1 relaxation time, the grayer the picture) (Fig. 11.55).

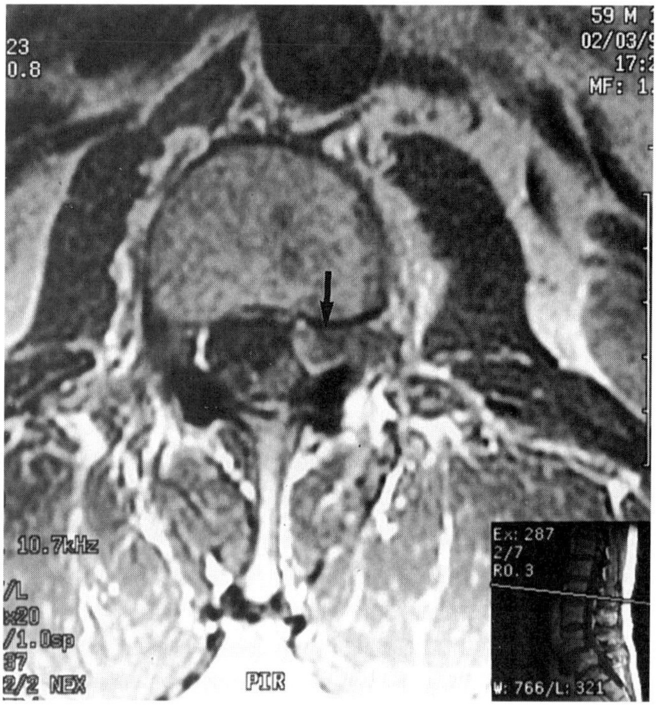

Figure 11.54 *An axial T1-weighted MRI to show gray scale: note signal intensity from water (CSF), mu-cle, fat. An arrow points to a disc herniation.*

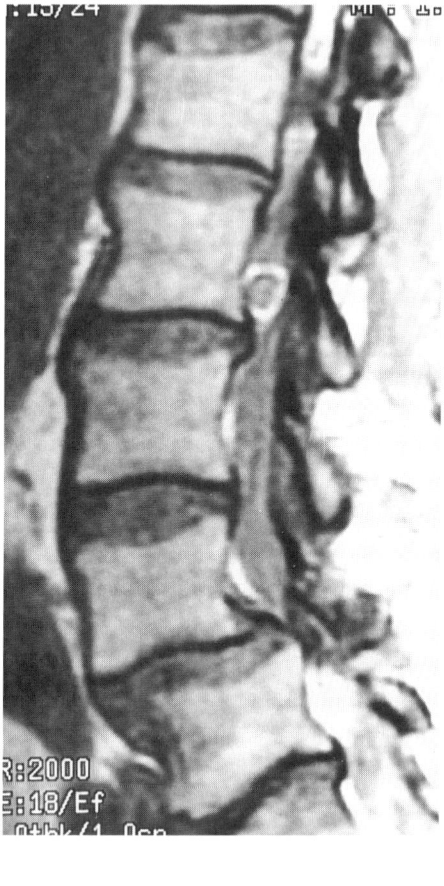

Figure 11.55 *A sagittal proton density (refer to Fig. 11.52) showing the same disc herniation behind the vertebral body of L2.*

Substances with a short T_2 relaxation time include muscle and tendons. Substances with a long T_2 (brighter image) include water and CSF and edematous and inflamed tissue. Thus, many common disease processes become conspicuous on T_2-weighted images because the increased free water of edema and inflammation gives a brighter (whiter) signal.

The T_1- and T_2-weighted images are summarized in Tables 11.9 and 11.10.

Today's MRI Routine

At the time of writing of this text, our MRI machines are still set up with the following technical details (9):

T_1 Weighted	T_2 Weighted
TR = 600 milliseconds	TR = 2000 milliseconds
TE = 30 milliseconds	TE = 60/90 milliseconds
Slice Thickness (SL) = 4 to 5 mm	SL = 4 to 5 mm

We thought that at the time of writing the second edition, these values would likely be out of date, but they continue to be reasonable.

Images Produced by MRI

Most protocols for the spine produce one axial and two sagittal images. Advantages of each image are: Sagittal T_1 (Fig. 11.56) depicts the following:

Root canals (foramina).
Facet joints.
Vertebral bodies.
Spinal cord.

Sagittal T_2 (Fig. 11.57) brightens (whitens) fluid (H_2O)-containing structures, and thus boundaries:

Table 11.10. The Gray Scale in Various Tissues

Tissue	T1-weighted	T2-weighted
CSF	Black	White
Gray matter	Gray	White
White matter	White	Gray
Marrow	Gray	Whiter
Disc nucleus	Gray	White
Disc annulus	Less gray	Black
Fat	Bright	Gray
Subacute hemorrhage	Bright	Gray
Gadolinium-enhanced tissues	Very white	Gray
Muscle	Gray	Gray

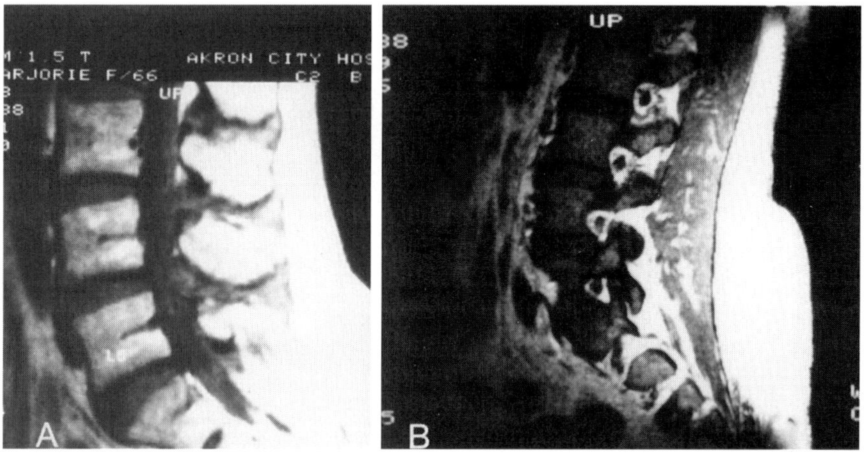

Figure 11.56 *Sagittal T_1 MRI:* **A.** *Midline;* **B.** *Lateral, showing neural foramina.*

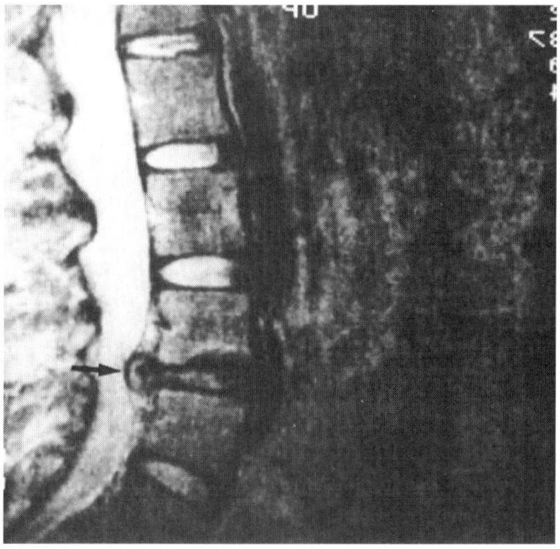

Figure 11.57 *Sagittal T_2 MRI. Note the large midline HNP at L4-L5 (arrow) and the whiteness of the CSF and nucleus.*

CSF.
Internal structure of disc.
Osseous structures are poorly seen on T_2-weighted image.

Axial T_1 (Fig. 11.58) depicts:

Facet joints.
Ligamentous flavum.
Foramina.

Advantages of MRI over CT

1. MRI does not require the use of ionizing radiation (which also means that the quality of the MR images is not affected by patient size).
2. MRI produces excellent sagittal sections, that is, images at 90° to axials.

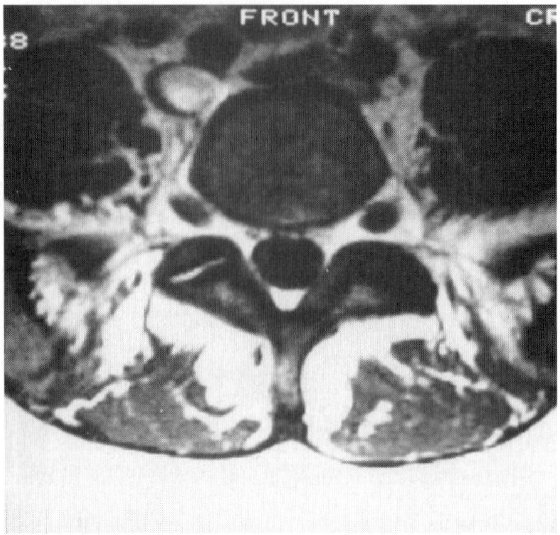

Figure 11.58 *Axial (T_1) MRI. Note facet joint and foraminal detail.*

3. MRI produces excellent soft tissue detail. In fact, clinicians trying to travel the MRI learning curve are struggling to contend with the superior (exaggerated) detail as they try to avoid a high incidence of false-positive MRIs.
4. MRI will detail intradural lesions such as tumors, syrinx, and arachnoiditis.
5. MRI signal is not impeded by bone, which results in better images in the posterior fossa and the base of the brain.
6. MRI does not produce artifact from nonferromagnetic metals in surgical clips and prostheses.

Disadvantages of MRI

1. The gantry for MRI is smaller and longer than the CT gantry and is more prone to producing a claustrophobic feeling for the patient.
2. The scan time is longer for MRI, and a patient in pain may find it difficult, if not impossible, to be still for the time required.
3. Patients with ferromagnetic materials in their body cannot be scanned if the following conditions apply:
   - Cerebral aneurysm clips will be torqued by the magnet.
   - Pacemakers will be converted to a fixed rate.
   - Transcutaneous electrical nerve stimulation units will be drawn into the magnet.
   - Ocular metallic foreign bodies may be moved and result in damage to vision.
   - Metallic cardiac valves are at risk.
   - Life support devices are at risk.

Fortunately, most orthopedic implants are not ferromagnetic and thus do not affect image quality, unless directly in the field, for example, pedicle instrumentation.

4. The MRI machine is more costly to purchase and install in a specially shielded room. This high initial capital cost transfers into the necessity for a higher fee for MRI compared with CT. In the future, both hardware and software changes will hopefully lead to reduced costs.
5. MRI does not image bone as well as CT, resulting in somewhat poorer delineation of

calcified discs or osteophytes. Changes in the MRI protocol are likely to result in improved bone images.

6. MRI is very operator dependent: If the radiologist does not keep on top of the changing technology, or if the technologist does not operate the equipment properly, poor images will result.

Today's Indications for MRI (for Degenerative Spine Conditions)

The title of this section is "Today's Indications" because tomorrow's will be different. There is reasonable expectation today in many leading centers that MRI will be the imaging modality of choice for all spinal problems.

Today's indications are:

- The only necessary investigation of a patient with a disc rupture who has failed conservative care and is being considered for surgery.
- Young patient with a suspected midline HNP!
- Young patient with a suspected HNP!
- Any patient with an HNP (7)!
- A patient with single level degenerative disc disease and no radicular symptoms who is being considered for a single level fusion. An MRI will verify: (1) There is no root encroachment within the canal or lateral zone; and (2) the discs above or below are normal.
- A patient with a classic story of spinal stenosis, with no unusual neurological presentation and no scoliosis.
- A patient suspected of having arachnoiditis.
- Recurrent HNP.

In addition, MRI has been very useful for other spinal problems, such as tumors, trauma, and infection, and it has been extremely useful for assessment of a host of intraspinal lesions, such as multiple sclerosis and syrinx.

Patient Preparation

Most imaging centers will give patients preparatory instructions that include such things as:

- Do not wear metal items to the examination (eg, belts, hairpins, metal arched high-heeled shoes, jewelry, zippers).
- Do not wear eye makeup, some of which contains iron or cobalt.
- Do not bring credit cards that all contain a magnetized code.
- Do not wear a dial-type wrist watch.

It is unnecessary for a patient to fast before an MRI.

Weight Restrictions

There is a patient weight restriction of approximately 300 lb. This has as much to do with the size of the gantry (tunnel) as with the ability of the table to carry a heavy patient. Taller patients a little heavier than 300 lb may fit into the tunnel and shorter patients weighing less than 300 lb may not fit into the tunnel. Open, low field strength permanent magnet units are available to accommodate the very large patient. We are not impressed that the images from these scanners are suitable for surgical planning. This statement introduces an important consideration in MRI. If you are looking for a diagnosis in lumbar spine problems, do a careful history and physical examination, do not order an expensive MRI. If you do need an MRI for diagnosis, any old clunker of a machine, along with a radiologist's familiarity, has a reasonable chance of getting you that diagnosis. You will not even need to go and look at the MRI, just read the radiologist's report. If you are trying to plan a surgical procedure (especially with a limited exposure), you need to read your own MRI, and it needs to be of superior quality. This creates a gap in understanding between radiologists and surgeons: radiologists fulfill their job description and make a diagnosis on the basis of average scans, but surgeons cannot plan surgery with anything other than a high-quality series of MRI images.

Abnormal MRI

Figs. 11.59 to 11.68 show examples of degenerative spine problems.

Newer Techniques

Contrast-Enhanced MRI

The word "contrast" in radiograph (eg, myelography) implies a direct effect of a compound on the image produced. Contrast-enhancement in MRI is purely an indirect effect of a pharmaceutical on signal intensity.(11) These pharmaceuticals are in the form of three paramagnetic compounds known as gadolinium chelates; Magnevist, Prohance, and Omniscan. When administered intravenously, they are deposited in tissues with high water content, providing there is a good blood supply. These compounds will not deposit in tissues with poor blood supply (eg, disc material). Within edematous tissues,

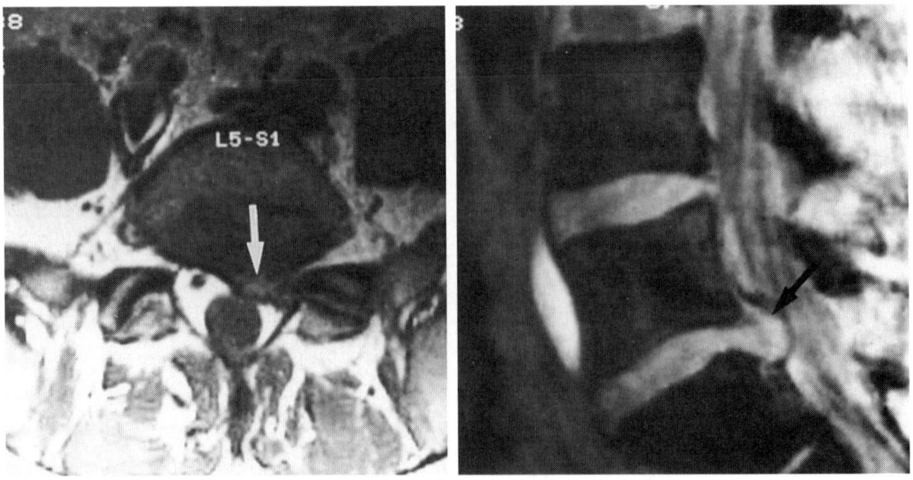

Figure 11.59 *Axial T_1 weighted showing HNP, L5-S1, left (arrow). Sagittal gradient echo showing same HNP (arrow).*

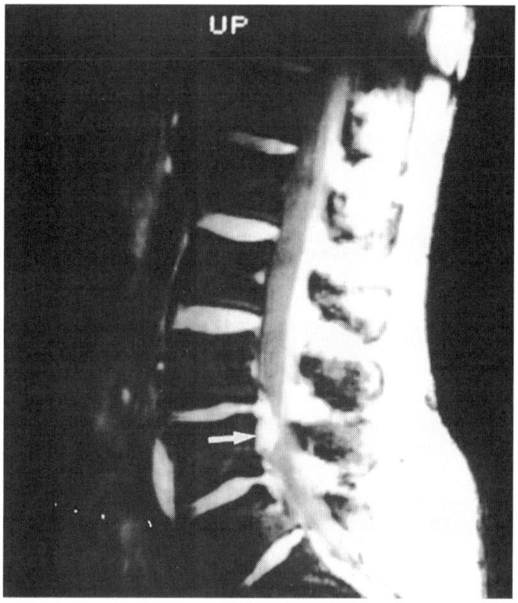

Figure 11.60 *Sagittal gradient echo image showing HNP, L3-L4, trapping down into third story of L4 (arrow).*

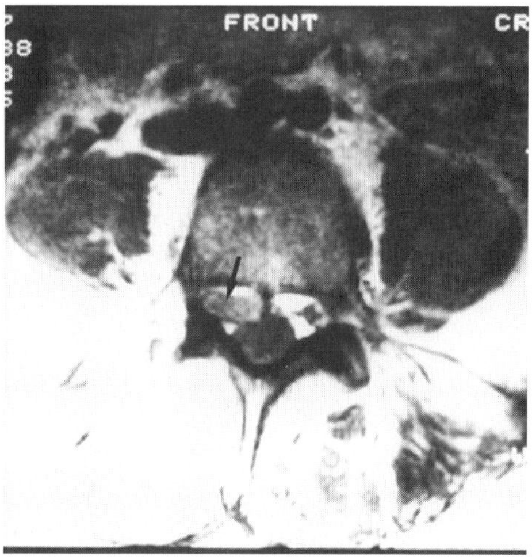

Figure 11.61 *Free fragment of disc material well down into third story of L4, right (T_1 axial) (arrow).*

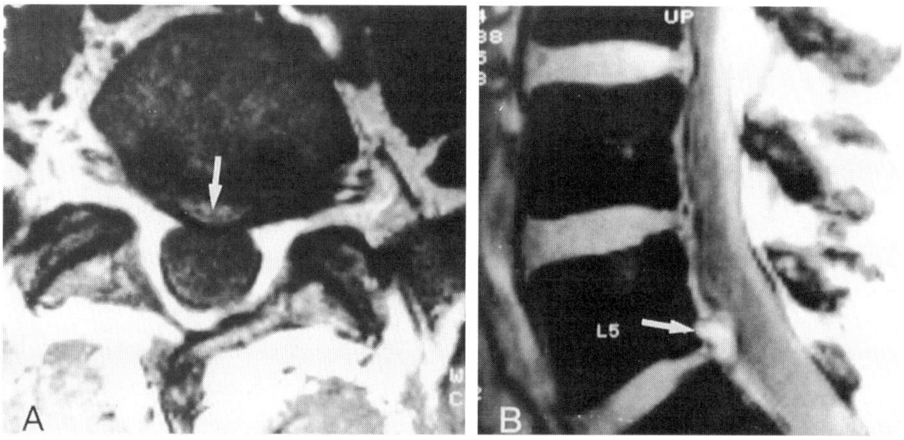

Figure 11.62 *Midline HNP (L5-S1);* **A,** *axial T_1 (arrow);* **B,** *sagittal gradient echo (arrow).*

Figure 11.63 *Sagittal T_1—foraminal HNP, L2 (arrow).*

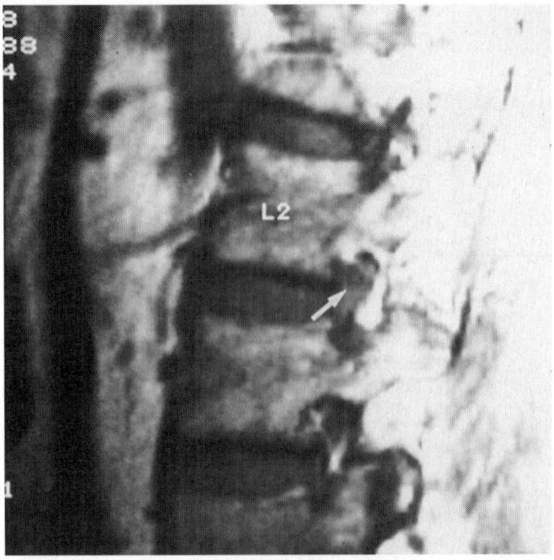

Figure 11.64 *HNP, L5, left, second story, on T_1 axial (arrow).*

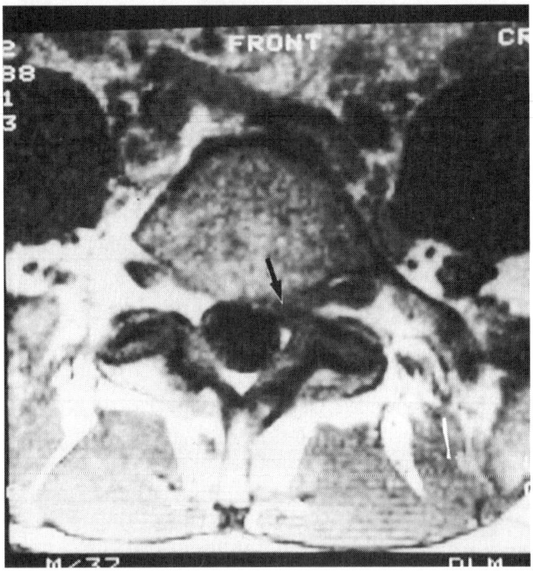

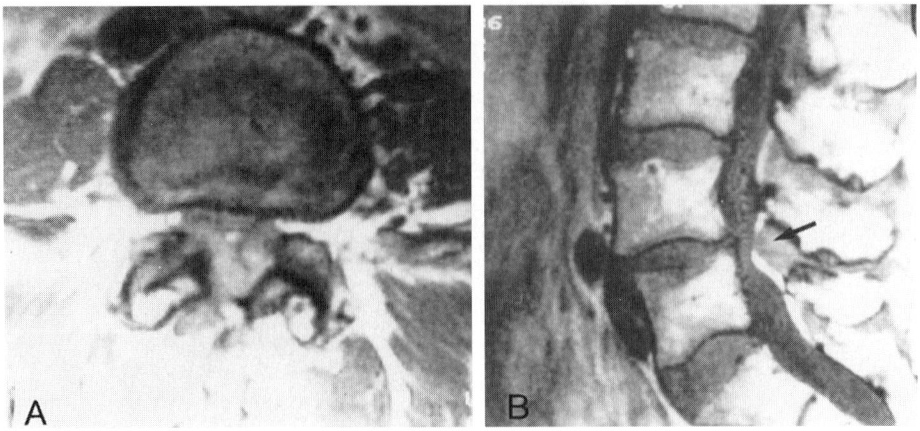

Figure 11.65 *Spinal canal stenosis (at degenerative spondylolisthesis level, L4-L5:* **A,** *axial T_1;* **B,** *Sagittal T_1 (arrow).*

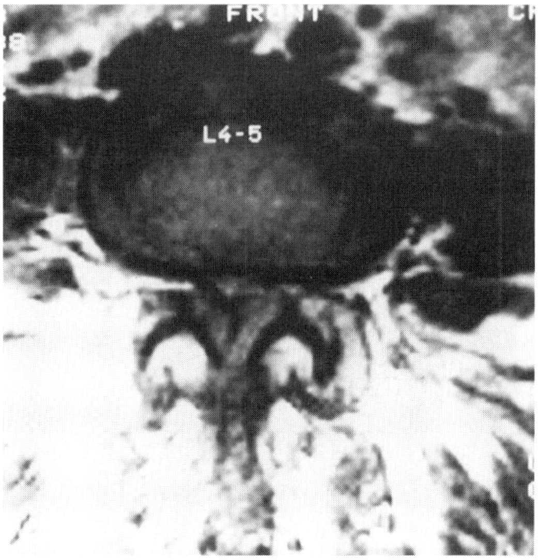

Figure 11.66 *Spinal canal stenosis (L4-L5)—axial T[1].*

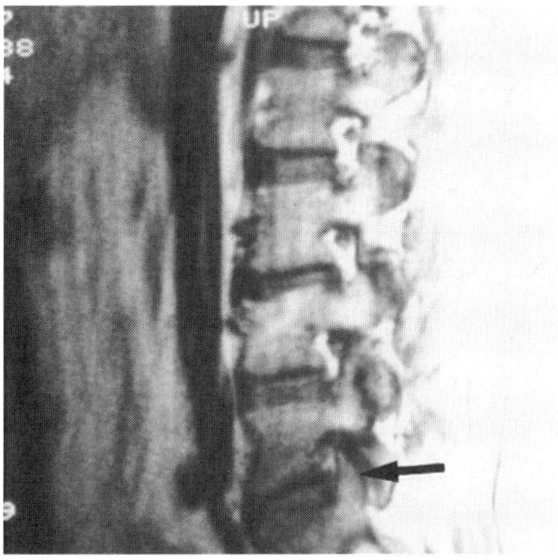

Figure 11.67 *Spinal stenosis, lateral zone, L5 foramen on axial T_1. Note the subluxed superior facet of S1 filling the L5 foramen (arrow).*

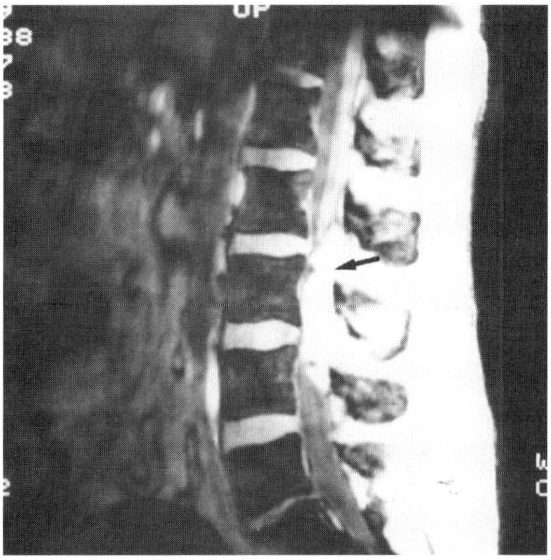

Figure 11.68 *Extradural tumor (lymphoma), L2 to L4 (arrow), on gradient echo image, sagittal slice in midline.*

these paramagnetic compounds lower T_1 relaxation values and increase their signal intensity. Thus, scar in the lumbar spine enhances, whereas recurrent disc ruptures do not enhance (Fig. 11.69). The enhancement of scar tissue is more pronounced on high field strength magnets.

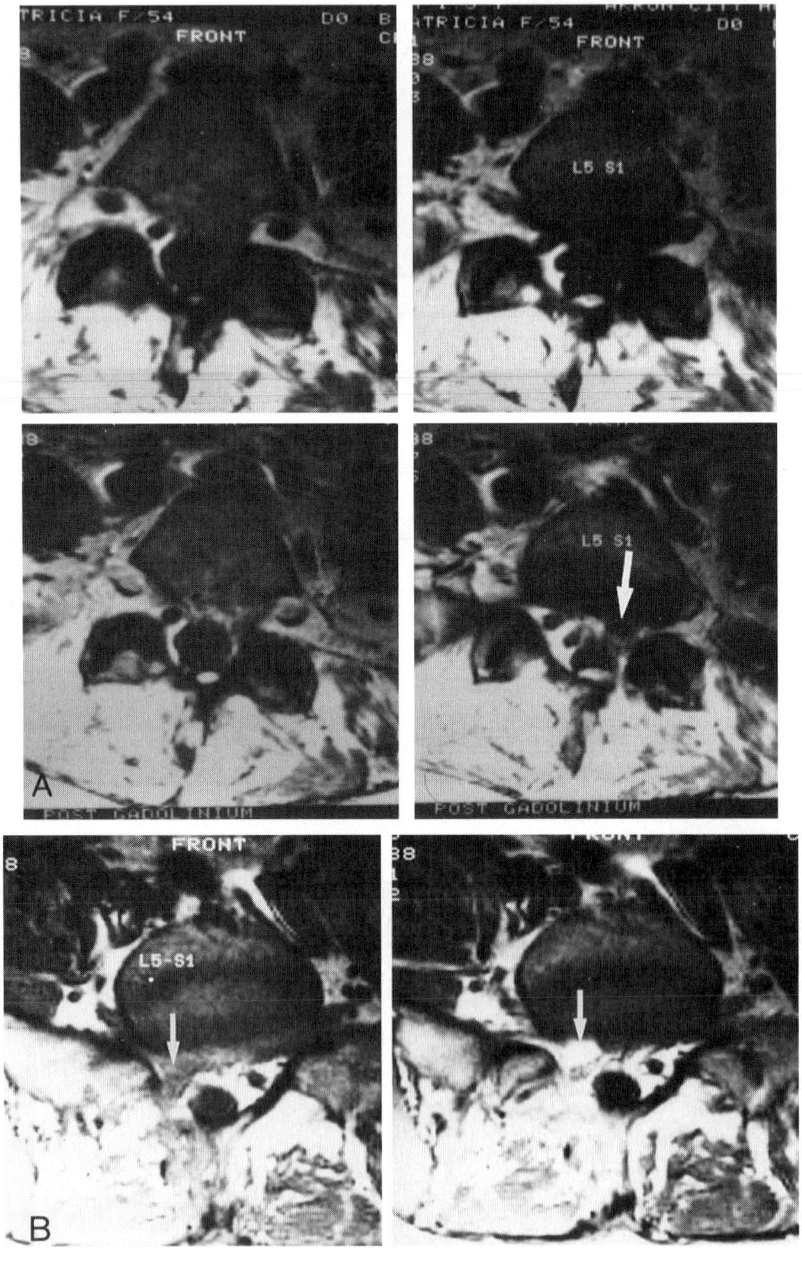

Figure 11.69 **A.** *Top row: axial MRI (T_1) of patient with recurrent leg pain 15 years after L5-S1 discectomy, left. Bottom row: axial MRI (T_1) after injection of gadolinium-DTPA. Scar, lit up by the gadolinium-DTPA, is evident on the left; a nonenhanced recurrent disc herniation is evident in the lower right cut (L5-S1, left) (arrow).* **B.** *A young doctor, 6 weeks after operation, had continuing right leg pain. An enhanced MRI shows bright scar tissue and no recurrent HNP (arrows).*

Fat-Suppression Techniques

The spine is surrounded by a lot of fat: the marrow spaces, the epidural space, and the neural foramina. This is useful on T_1 images because it improves contrast between the normal fatty marrow and the pathological tumor or infection that is replacing the marrow (Fig. 11.70). On infusion of contrast material (gadolinium), the fat has a tendency to obscure the enhancement of the tumor or edema. By suppressing the high intensity of the fat signal on T_1-weighted images, the contrast enhancement of pathology is more evident (Fig. 11.70). For inflammatory and neoplastic diseases of the spine, fat suppression plus gadolinium contrast material helps to demonstrate early lesions of the posterior elements and disease extension into the epidural space. In failed spine surgery, the technique also increases conspicuousness of epidural fibrosis, nerve roots individually and within the common dural sac (eg, demonstration of arachnoiditis) (Fig. 11.71), and helps distinguish ganglia from disc fragments.

Nothing in life is free. Fat-suppression techniques decrease spatial resolution because of a decreased signal-to-noise ratio, that is, the images just are not as sharp.(5) The images take longer to acquire, and sometimes the fat suppression is uneven. Despite these drawbacks, fat suppression of T_1 gadolinium-enhanced MRI images is a useful sequence to have available when looking for tumors and infections and when trying to assess scar tissue in the postoperative lumbar spine.

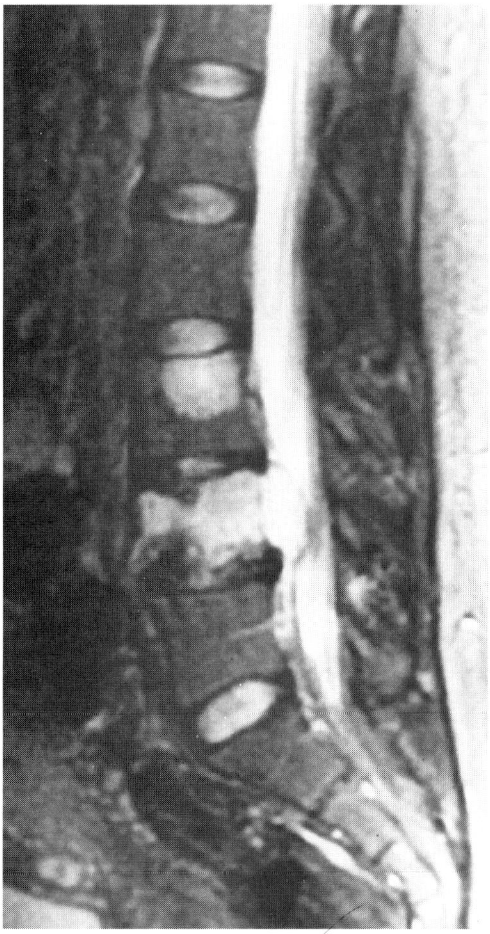

Figure 11.70 *The fat suppression technique has obliterated the marrow fat to reveal metastatic carcinoma of lumbar vertebral bodies 3 and 4.*

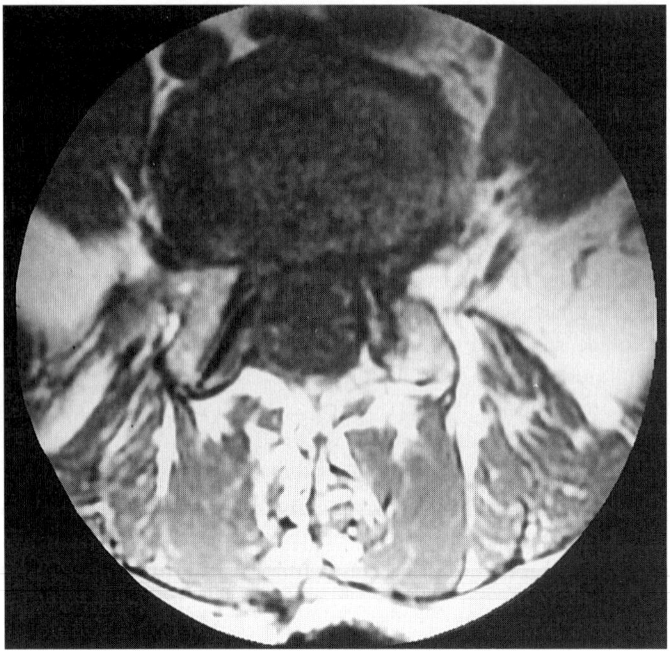

Figure 11.71 *Arachnoiditis without the fat suppression technique: note the clumping of the nerve roots around the periphery of the common dural sac in this postoperative patient.*

Conclusion

To date, the MRI has been used to substitute for CT, but Haughton (6) believes that the future use of MRI will expand to include the study of the following pathological and chemical changes:

- Disc bulge versus disc herniations.
- Water content and disc degeneration.(10)
- Annular tears.
- Intervertebral disc pH measurements relative to degenerative disc disease.
- Scars and adhesions.
- Pulsations and movement of the CSF in such conditions as spinal stenosis (4).

From the first brain images in 1982 to the excellent spine images today, MRI has made dramatic advances. Even more rapid changes are in store for the clinician, making it essential to stay close to the science. Failure to do so may result in MRI technology running away from clinical science. In spine surgery, at least, MRI diagnoses must be audited by surgical outcomes.

Nerve Root Infiltration Test

Nerve root infiltration is an investigative procedure that involves blocking the anterior primary ramus of a single nerve root. It is usually the 5th lumbar or 1st sacral nerve roots that are blocked, but any root can be blocked. It is an investigative procedure that is useful only when one is sure that a radicular syndrome is present but unsure of which nerve root is affected. This procedure is of no value in trying to separate referred pain from radicular pain, or a herniated nucleus pulposus from lateral recess stenosis. Most often, the procedure is used in the chronic unilateral radicular syndrome (due to lateral zone stenosis) when structural lateral zone stenosis lesions are noted at the level of the 5th lumbar and the 1st sacral nerve roots, and there are no clinical clues as to the anatomical level. The second indication for a nerve root infiltration is in the presence of scarring or arachnoiditis when trying to decide which root is the most symptomatic.

The technique is accomplished with the patient in the prone position under image intensifier control. A paraspinal approach is used to place the needle in the 5th lumbar nerve root, catching it just as it exits under the pedicle of lumbar vertebrae4 5 (Fig. 11.72). The S1 nerve root is blocked through the posterior 1st sacral foramen. Under image intensifier control, a long needle is slowly advanced toward the nerve root. When the nerve root is encountered, radiating discomfort down the leg will result. Usually, this radiating discomfort is typical enough that the block can then be accomplished with 3 mL of .5 or .75% Marcaine long-acting anesthetic agent. On occasion, the radiating discomfort will not be striking, and water-soluble contrast material is given by injection to be sure of needle placement.

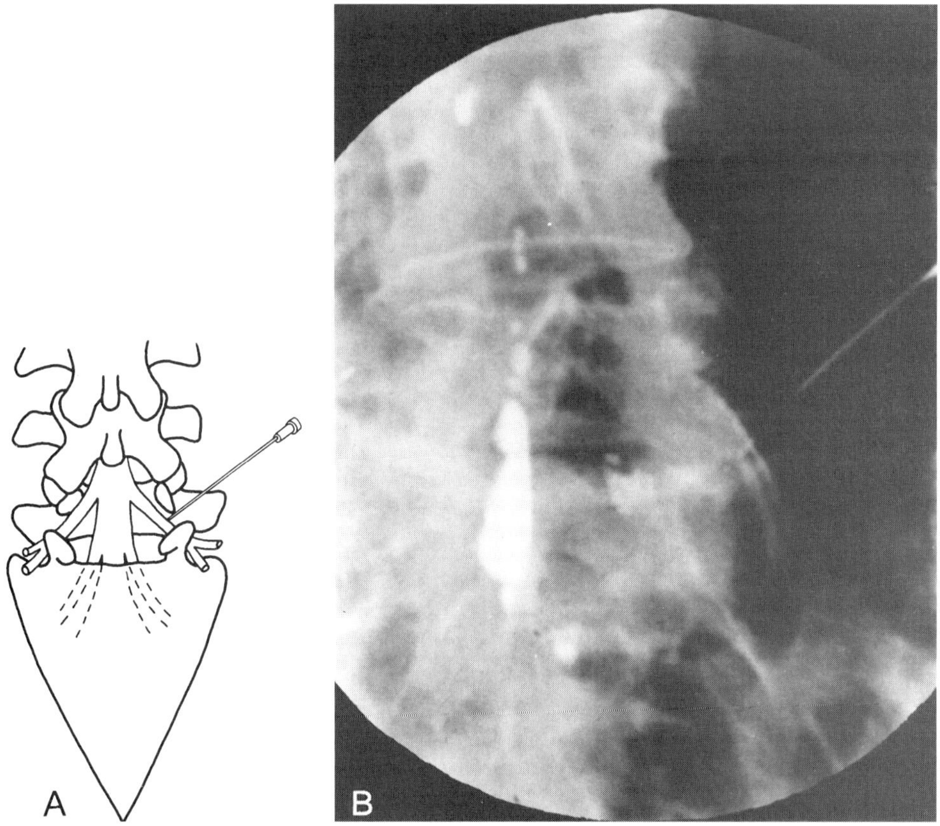

Figure 11.72 **A.** *Schematic of nerve root injection (L5).* **B.** *AP radiograph showing contrast in the L5 root, left.*

Although a radiograph is used to assist in accomplishing a nerve root infiltration, the procedure is not a radiographic evaluation procedure. The first principle of nerve root infiltration is to obtain a good root block. That is to say, if a 5th lumbar nerve root is blocked, the patient should have a drop foot and numbness over the dorsum of the foot when the procedure is finished. Similarly, if the 1st root is blocked, the patient should have numbness to pinprick sensation along the lateral border of the foot and weakness of plantar flexion. Once a good nerve root block is obtained, the patient is then asked to participate in the activity that was most aggravating. Usually, the patient needs a cane for support because of the profound nature of the root block. Long-acting anesthetic agents last 4 to 6 hours, and at the end of that time, the patient should record the impressions of relief or lack of relief of symptoms with the root block. If you suspected the 5th lumbar nerve root as the culprit, and a good 5th lumbar nerve root block relieves the patient's pain, the procedure has satisfactorily pinpointed the 5th lumbar nerve root as the source of symptoms. The appropriate surgical procedure can then be carried out with confidence.

DISCOGRAPHY

There is no subject in spine surgery that is more controversial. Its appearance as a topic of conversation can turn friends into acquaintances and reduce scientific meetings to chaos. Why should such a commonly performed procedure excite such emotion? Mainly because there is no body of science to support the use of discography as a decision-making procedure in low back disability. Inserting a needle in a patient's disc, distending that disc with test material, and reproducing pain does not assure that you have located the source of symptoms ("the pain generator"). There are so many variables involved in proper needle placement, proper testing standards, proper ways to ask for patient response, and acceptable ways for patients to respond that discography has yet to pass the test of scientific scrutiny. Imagine yourself as a patient lying on the radiograph table, needle in disc, and a doctor trying to reproduce your pain. How many times will you let him or her try before you agree to whatever leading question is asked? In our practices, discography was largely limited to the demonstration of a normal disc at the level above a proposed fusion. T_2 sagittal MRI has now displaced this only remaining indication for discography. Stretching the indication for discography to verify the levels that need to be fused is the area of controversy and is discussed in Chapter 14 relative to the role of lumbar fusion in the treatment of degenerative disc disease.

THERMOGRAPHY

Thermography, once a promising diagnostic test, has largely been dropped from clinical use because of the lack of scientific support.

ELECTROMYOGRAPHY/NERVE CONDUCTION TESTS

The neuromuscular system is an electrical circuit board, and its activity can be measured with appropriate equipment. The electrophysiological tests used are electromyography and nerve conduction tests. Other electrical testing methods that are being used in spine problems include somatosensory-evoked potentials and motor-evoked potentials. These are beyond the interests of this book, and readers are referred to other texts.

Electrical physiological testing is used to study two basic groups of problems:

1. Orthopedic—nerve root lesions.
   —Overuse and entrapment syndromes.
   —Plexus injuries.
2. Neurologic—neuropathies.
   —Myopathies.
   —Spinal cord (UMNL) mixed with lower motor neuronal lesions such as amyotrophic lateral sclerosis, multiple sclerosis, and Friedreich's ataxia.

The two basic ways of studying these problems are:

1. Nerve conduction tests (NCT).
2. Electromyography (EMG).

Nerve Conduction Tests

Nerve conduction tests are used to evaluate nerve entrapment syndromes. As such they are not particularly valuable in assessment of low back problems unless you have a differential diagnostic problem such as an L5 nerve lesion that could be due to a root lesion (disc rupture) or entrapment neuropathy in the pelvis or around the knee. NCT are very valuable in cervical disc/upper extremity entrapment neuropathies, where differential diagnosis can be very confusing.

A nerve conduction test is shown in Figure 11.73. After stimulating proximally and measuring the action potential distally (usually no more than 8 to 10 cm away from stimulation), the duration to travel the distance can be calculated as follows:

$$\text{Nerve Conduction Time} = \frac{\text{Distance Action Potential Traveled}}{\text{Time Taken}}$$

The NCT can then be compared to the standard tables (eg, normal limit for conduction along peroneal nerve around fibular head is 41.65 msec). If the NCT is longer than what the tables say it should be, there is a delay in nerve conduction time, that is, an entrapment between the stimulation site and the recording site. By moving proximally and distally along the nerve, sites of entrapment can be localized.

Electromyography

Electromyography is a method of studying the intrinsic electrical activity of individual motor units of muscle. After inserting a needle electrode into muscle (Fig. 11.74), both spontaneous and volitional electrical impulses can be recorded on an oscilloscope. EMG is largely a study of lower motor neuron phenomena and is useful for diagnosing neuropathies and myopathies.

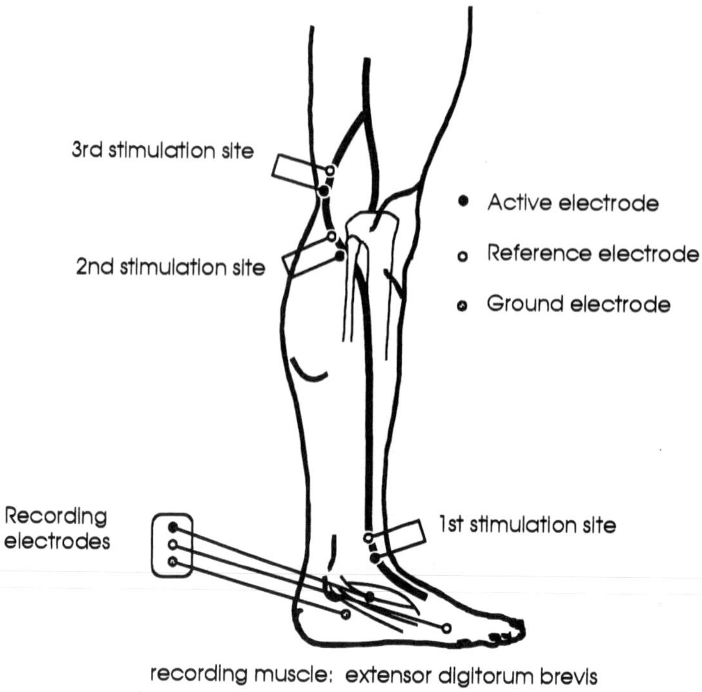

Figure 11.73 *A nerve conduction test of the peroneal nerve showing the various locations for stimulation and the sight of recording in the extensor digitorum brevis.*

Five parameters of electrical activity are studied (Fig. 11.75):

1. Voltage: the amplitude of the wave from peak to peak (normal is up to 4 or 5 thousand microvolts).
2. Duration: how long the wave lasts (normal is 8–12 msec).
3. Waveforms: how many dips in waveform (normal is a bi- or triphasic wave).
4. Frequency: number of waves/second (normal is 1–60/sec).
5. Sound: the actual sound the waves make on the oscilloscope.

These normal values change from muscle to muscle (eg, flexors vs extensors) and from young to old. Electrical potentials are examined on insertion of the needle electrode, with the muscle at rest and with the patient providing maximum contraction of the muscle being examined.

EMG can be used to localize the level of lumbar nerve root involvement. Healthy, normally innervated muscle is electrically "silent" at rest, and the insertion of an electromyographic needle does not produce sustained electrical discharges. However, in the presence of a nerve root lesion, a series of involuntary electrical discharges can be recorded. These are characterized by a shortened potential and reduced amplitude (fibrillation potentials) or by altered waveforms (positive waves). The positive waveforms are produced only on needle insertion, but the fibrillation potentials can be recorded all of the time (Fig. 11.75).

On voluntary contraction of a normal muscle, the motor unit action potentials evoked are biphasic or triphasic in form. With partial denervation, the quantity of motor units recording is decreased, and polyphasic waves are seen (Fig. 11.76).

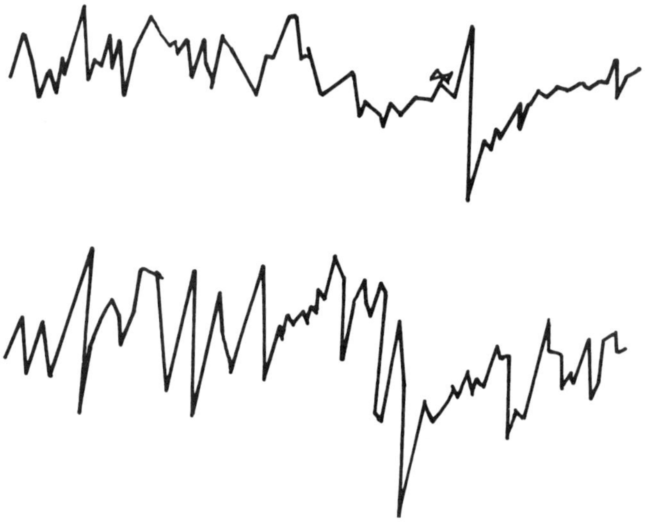

Figure 11.74 *EMG volitional motor unit activity.*

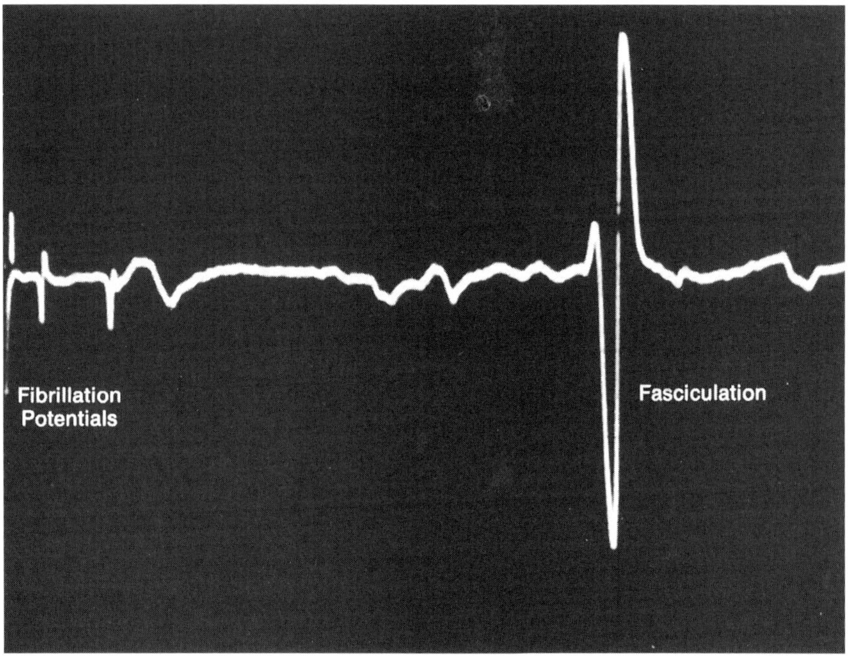

Figure 11.75 *A drawing of normal and abnormal EMG changes.*

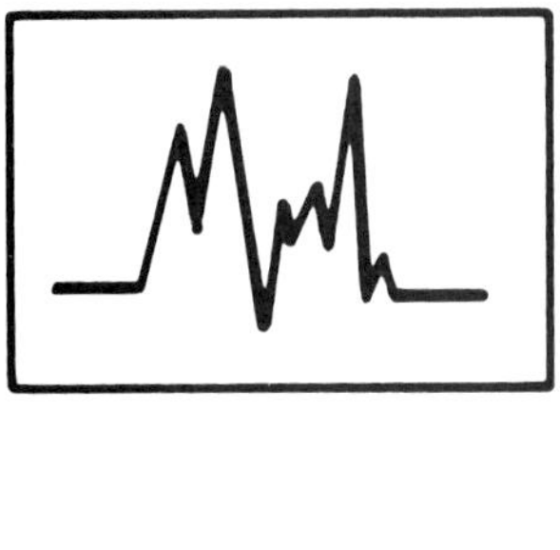

Figure 11.76 *Abnormal polyphasic potentials.*

The paraspinal muscles are supplied by the posterior primary rami of the emerging lumbar nerve roots. In the electromyographic examination of a patient suffering from nerve root compression, the electrical activity of the paraspinal muscles at rest and on voluntary activity is observed. Lesions producing interference of root conduction will demonstrate the electromyographic changes described.

In addition to testing the paravertebral muscles, the muscles in the lower limbs innervated by the lumbar nerve roots must also be assessed. In S1 lesions, the examination can be broadened to include the sensory limb of the sciatic nerve. It is possible to stimulate the afferent limb of S1 with an electrode in the popliteal fossa and to measure the time required to travel to the dorsal root, pass through the reflex arc, travel down the efferent limb, and eventually produce a contraction of the gastrocnemius. This is Hoffmann's reflex, sometimes referred to as the H-reflex. With S1 root involvement, the time between the sensory stimulus and the motor response will be prolonged, and the pattern of the evoked potential may be abnormal. The H-reflex is only useful in the evaluation of the S1 root.

In summary, the major electromyographic changes associated with nerve root compression are fibrillation potentials and positive sharp waves at rest, and a decrease in the number of active potentials on voluntary activity associated with the presence of polyphasic waves. In S1 lesions, a prolonged latency or absence of the H-reflex is of great diagnostic significance.

Electromyographic examination may demonstrate root lesions at several levels. This may be seen with spinal stenosis, but it is also seen in metabolic disorders such as diabetes and in subclinical neuropathies. Electromyography is of great value in the assessment of hysterical paralysis.

Despite the apparent science of EMG, it takes great skill and a lot of subjective input on the part of the electromyographer to arrive at a suitable conclusion. This explains why some electromyographic reports are more useful than others. In addition, the evaluation of electrical activity of muscle to determine nerve root involvement is loaded with pitfalls:

1. Acute nerve root lesions take at least 14 days to show up as EMG changes; performing an EMG in the lesion too early can be misleading.
2. So many root lesions are irritative and non-compressive (especially in young patients) and will show no EMG changes.
3. Many root lesions are incomplete and will show delayed EMG changes and/or mixed electrical evidence of both denervation and reinnervation.
4. Even though EMG may document a root lesion (eg, L5), it still does not give you the anatomical level of involvement; an MRI is needed for that.
5. Patients will often complain that the test was very painful.

With the availability of MRI and CT to accurately demonstrate anatomical levels of nerve root involvement, the use of EMG in the evaluation of obvious nerve root lesions is not needed. However, if you have a differential diagnostic problem, for example, a diabetic patient presenting with an acute radicular syndrome who may have diabetic neuropathy and not a disc herniation, EMG is very valuable; diabetic mononeuropathy will spare the paraspinals, and despite its label, will show signs of denervation in more than one nerve root distribution.

Summary

After 25 years of practice, the authors are awed by the sophistication of investigation available to evaluate a patient with low back pain. After a careful history and physical examination, it is possible with the appropriate choice of investigation to be fairly certain of the diagnosis. When planning a surgical procedure for degenerative disc disease problems (eg, a ruptured disc), an MRI will so precisely localize the nature of the problem and the anatomical level that very limited surgical procedures can be planned. These investigations have become the "eyes" of the surgeon, allowing for precise surgery, only when a problem is clearly identified on testing.

REFERENCES

Bone Scanning (Scintigraphy)

1. Freeman LM, Blaufox MD. Physicians' Desk Reference of Radiology and Nuclear Medicine. Oradell, New Jersey: Medical Economics; p 101, 1979.
2. Holder LE. Radionuclide bone imaging in the evaluation of bone pain. J Bone Joint Surg 1982;(64A):1391–1396.
3. Kirchner PT, Simon MA. Current concepts review, radioisotopic evaluation of skeletal disease. J Bone Joint Surg 1981;(63A):673–681.
4. Krishnamurthy GT, Tubis M, Hiss J, Blahd WH. Distribution pattern of metabolic bone disease. A need for total body skeletal image. JAMA 1977;237:2504–2506.
5. Magnusson JE, Brown ML, Hauser MF, Berquist TH, Fitzgerald RH, Klee GG. In-111-labeled5 leukocyte scintigraphy in suspected orthopedic prosthesis infection: comparison with other imaging modalities. Radiology 1988;168:236–239.
6. Merkel KD, Brown ML, Dewanjee MK, Fitzgerald RH. Comparison of indium-labeled leukocyte imaging with sequential technetium-gallium scanning in the diagnosis of low-grade musculoskeletal sepsis. J Bone Joint Surg 1985;(67A):465–476.
7. Subramanian G, McAfee JG. A new complex of 99mTc for skeletal imaging. Radiology 1971;99:192–196.

Plain Radiographs and Myelography

1. Badami JP, Baker RA, Scholz FJ, McLaughlin M. Outpatient metrizamide myelography: prospective evaluations of safety and cost effectiveness. Radiology 1985;158:175–177.
2. Neurotoxicity of metrizamide (editorial). Arch Neurol 1985;42:24–25.
3. Eldevik OP, Nakken KO, Haughton VM. The effect of dehydration on the side effects of metrizamide myelography. Radiology 1978;129:715–716.
4. Eldevik OP, Nakstad P, Kendall B, Hindmarsh T. Iohexol in lumbar myelography: preliminary results from an open noncomparative multicentered clinical study. AJNR 1983;4:299–301.
5. Hindmarsh T, Ekholm SE, Kido DK, Sahler L, Sands M. Lumbar myelography with iohexol and metrizamide. A double blind clinical trial. Acta Radiol Diagn 1984;25:365–368.
6. Kuuliala IK, Goransson HJ. Adverse reactions after iohexol lumbar myelography: influence of post-procedural positioning. AJR 1952;149:389–390.
7. Mason MS, Raaf J. Complication of pantopaque myelography: case report and review. J Neurosurg 1952;19:302–305.
8. Meador KI, Hamilton WJ, El Gammal TAM, Demetropoulos KC, Nichols FT. Irreversible neurologic complications of metrizamide myelography. Neurology 1984;34:817–821.

9. Nakstad P, Helgetveit A, Aaserud O, Ganes T, Nyberg-Hansen R. Iohexol compared to metrizamide in cervical and thoracic myelography. Neuroradiology 1984;26:479–484.
10. Sicard JL. Roentgenologic exploration of the central nervous system with iodized oil (Lipiodol). Arch Neurol Psychiatry 1926;16:420–426.
11. Steinhausen TB, et al. Iodinated organic compounds as contrast media for radiographic diagnoses. Radiology 1944;43:230–235.
12. Wiesel SW, Tsourmas N, Feffer HL, Citrin CM, Patronas N. A study of computer-assisted tomography: I. The incidence of positive CAT scans in an asymptomatic group of patients. Spine 1984;9:549–551.

CT Scanning

1. Dorwart RH. Fundamentals of computed tomographic evaluation of lumbar disc disease. In: Genant HK, ed. Spine Update 1984. Radiology and Research and Education Foundation, UCSF; 1983.
2. Fries JW, Abodeely DA, Vijungco JC, Yeager VL, Gaffey WR. Computed tomography of herniated and extruded nucleus pulposus. J Comput Assist Tomogr 1982;6:874–887.
3. Genant HK. Computed tomography of the lumbar spine: technical considerations. In: Genant HK, Chaftez N, Helms CA, eds. Computed Tomography of the Lumbar Spine. San Francisco: University of California; 1982.
4. Haughton VM, Eldevik OP, Magnaes B, Amundsen P. A prospective comparison of computed tomography and myelography in the diagnosis of herniated lumbar discs. Radiology 1982;142:103–110.
5. Helms CA, Dorwart RH, Gray M. The CT appearance of conjoined nerve roots and differentiation from a herniated nucleus pulposus. Radiology 1982;144:803–807.
6. Hitselberger WE, Witten RM. Abnormal myelogram in asymptomatic patients. J Neurosurg 1968;28:204–207.
7. Hounsfield GN. Computerized transverse axial scanning (tomography). Part I: description of system. Br J Radiology 1973;46:1016–1022.
8. John V, Ewen K. Vergleichende Untersuchungen zur Strahlenexposition des Patienten bei des spinalen Dunnschicht. Computertomographie Strahlentherapie. 1983;159:180–183.
9. Ketonen L, Gyldensted C. Lumbar disc disease evaluated by myelography and postmyelography spinal computed tomography. Neuroradiology 1986;28:144–149.
10. Macnab I. Negative disc exploration—an analysis of the cause of nerve root involvement in sixty-eight patients. J Bone Joint Surg 1971;(53A):891–903.
11. McCutcheon ME, Thompson WC. CT scanning of lumbar discography. Spine 1986;11:257–259.
12. Modic MT, Masaryk T, Boumphrey F, Goormastic M, Bell G. Lumbar herniated disc disease and canal stenosis: prospective evaluation by surface coil MR, CT and myelography. AJNR 1986;7:709–717.
13. Sachs BL, et al. Dallas discogram description: a new classification of CT/discography in low-back disorders. Spine 1987;12:287–294.
14. Tarlov IM. Spinal perineural and meningeal cysts. J Neurol Neurosurg Psychiatry 1970;33:833–843.
15. Torricelli P, Spina V, Martinelli C. CT diagnosis of lumbosacral conjoined nerve roots. Neuroradiology 1987;29:374–379.
16. Verbiest H. The significance and principles of computerized axial tomography in idiopathic development stenosis of the bony lumbar vertebral canal. Spine 1979;4:369–378.
17. Wiesel SW, Tsourmas N, Feffer HL, Citrin CM, Patronas N. A study of computer-assisted tomography. I: the incidence of positive CT scans in an asymptomatic group of patients. Spine 1984;9:549–551.

18. Williams AL, Haughton VM, Daniels DL, Grogan JP. Differential CT diagnosis of extruded nucleus pulposus. Radiology 1983;148:141–148.
19. Williams AL, Haughton VM, Meyer GA, Ho KC. Computed tomographic appearance of the bulging annulus. Radiology 1982;142:403–408.
20. Zinreich SJ, Long DM, Davis R, Quinn CB, McAfee PC, Wang H. Three-dimensional CT imaging in post-surgical "failed back" syndrome. J Comput Assist Tomogr 1990;14:574–580.

Magnetic Resonance Imaging (MRI)

1. Bloch F, Hansen WW, Packard ME. Nuclear induction. Phys Rev 1946;69:127–135.
2. Damadian R. Tumor detection by nuclear magnetic resonance. Science (Washington, DC). 1971;171:1151–1153.
3. Doyle FE, Gore JC, Pennock, et al. Imaging of the brain by nuclear magnetic resonance. Lancet 1981;2:53–57.
4. Enzmann DR, Rubin JB, De La Paz R, Wright A. Cerebrospinal fluid pulsation: benefits and pitfalls in MR imaging. Radiology 1986;161:773–778.
5. Georgy BA, Hesselink JR. MR Imaging of the spine: recent advances in pulse sequences and special techniques. AJR 1994;162:923–934.
6. Haughton VM. MR imaging of the spine. Radiology 1988;166:297–301.
7. Jenkins JPR, Hickey DS, Zhu XP, Machin M, Isherwood I. MR imaging of the intervertebral disc: a quantitative study. Br J Radiology 1985;58:705–709.
8. Modic MT, Masaryk T, Boumphrey F, Goormastic M, Bell G. Lumbar herniated disc and canal stenosis: prospective evaluation by surface coil MR, CT and myelography. AJNR 1986; 7:709 –717.
9. Modic MT, et al. Magnetic resonance imaging of intervertebral disc disease: clinical and pulse sequence considerations. Radiology 1984;152:103–111.
10. Panagiotacopulos ND, Pope MH, Krag MH, Bloch R. Water content in human intervertebral discs: part 1. Measurement by magnetic resonance imaging. Spine 1987;12:912–917.
11. Peterfy CG, Linares R, Steinbach LS. Recent advances in magnetic resonance imaging of the musculoskeletal system. Radiol Clin North Am 1994;32:291–311.
12. Purcell EM, Taurry HC, Pound RV. Resonance absorption by nuclear magnetic moments in a solid. Phys Rev 1946;69:37–46.

12

Pain

"It is as important to know as much about the man who has the pain as it is to know about the pain the man has."

— Numerous Great Physicians and Surgeons

INTRODUCTION

It is virtually impossible to place this chapter in its correct location in the book. In the first edition (1977), the topic was mentioned throughout the book, but there was no chapter designated to the subject. In the second edition (1990), we decided to dedicate a complete chapter to this troublesome aspect of back pain evaluation. We thought it was important enough that we put it right at the front of the book after anatomy and a classification of back pain. Now, in the third edition, the chapter is sliding toward the back of the book. It is even after the Investigation chapter; if you are investigating a low back patient with fancy and expensive tests, and you have not considered this chapter, you are in trouble! It is probably the most important chapter in the book, and hopefully someday we will figure out where it belongs!

That medicine should concern itself with the whole person is often stated but frequently ignored. The hallmark of a good clinician is the ability not only to diagnose disease but also to assess the "whole patient." No test of the art of medicine is more demanding than the identification of the patient with a nonorganic or emotional component to a back disability.

To start, recognize the disability equation:

$$\text{Disability} = A + B + C$$

where A = the physical component (disease); B = the patient's emotional reaction; C = the situation the patient is in at the time of disability (ie, compensation claim, motor vehicle accident).

Each patient presenting with a back disability may have some component of each of these entities entwined in their disability. For example, the presentation of a collection of symptoms with no physical disability evident on examination should lead the clinician to think of the other aspects of the equation and look for emotional disability or situational reactions.

PAIN

Back pain has been around for as long as history has been recorded. With the advent of compensation legislation in the 19th century, the concept of pain was attached to the inability to function and initiated the rising tide of "spine disability."

In an attempt to clarify the issues, this chapter is divided into the following sections:

1. Pain.
2. Non-organic syndromes.
3. Psychological assessment.

Then, in Chapter 21, assessment of impairment and disability is addressed. When and if you finish all of this book, you will still be stuck with one unanswered question: "What is pain?"

PAIN

As musculoskeletal physicians and surgeons, we spend the majority of our time dealing with pain. Each of us has our own view of pain, based on training, experience, and, ultimately, biases. As time goes by, we lose contact with general theories on pain and develop a narrow tubular view of the patient with pain. The purpose of this chapter is to review the various pathophysiological theories that affect a patient's pain appreciation.

Definition of Pain

The International Association for the Study of Pain (8) defines pain as "an unpleasant sensory and emotional experience, associated with actual or potential tissue damage, or described in terms of such damage."

As such, pain is a perception rather than a sensation. Like vision, hearing, and other senses, there are well-documented pain pathways through the nervous system. Unlike those other senses, pain is a complex set of actions and reactions, modified by intellect, emotion, and many other factors. Pain is unpleasant to the point that the body is motivated to do something to stop the sensation; this situation is very different from the positive motivation of pleasant sounds and sights.

Types of Pain

Pain can be divided into acute or chronic pain. Acute pain is of short duration, arises from specific trauma or disease, and has associated pain behavior and closely reflects and parallels the stimulus; that is, a small painful stimulus is associated with a small amount of acute pain. Acute pain usually responds to traditional treatment methods such as analgesia, immobilization, and surgery.

Chronic pain occurs once the initial causes of pain have faded. Other non-nociceptive phenomenon have then interceded, such as culture, family, emotion, situation, and drug use. Chronic pain is associated with many subjective symptoms. It fails to respond to the usual treatment measures, especially those for acute pain as just mentioned.

The following discussion is predominantly centered around the concepts of acute pain; set chronic pain aside for now.

Categorization of Pain (10)

There are four main categories of pain:

Category 1: Pain due to External Events

- Involves skin receptors.
- Is precise in location.
- Usually precipitates withdrawal.

Category 2: Pain Due to Internal Events

- Organ pain that does not involve skin.
- Is less specific in its identification.
- Cannot be handled by withdrawal.

Category 3: Pain Associated with Lesions of the Nervous System (eg, Herniated Nucleus Pulposus [HNP])

- Prolonged pain that does not directly involve skin but may refer to skin.
- Cannot be handled by withdrawal; the identification of this kind of pain is usually more specific than the pain due to internal events.

Category 4: Pain Associated with Psychological, Environmental, and Other Factors

Research usually centers around pain due to external events. Unfortunately, it is easy to move concepts from this category in an attempt to explain the pain of Category 3. There is no proof that a pain concept can be moved from Category 1 to Category 3 pain.

Morphological Anatomy of Pain Receptors and Pathways

End Organs

End organs for pain are know as nociceptors, that is, receptors sensitive to a noxious (tissue damaging) or potentially noxious stimulus.

General Discussion The body contains many different sensory receptors that register changes around, adjacent to, and within the body. The specialized sensory organs, to a certain extent, are stimulus specific and are the end organs of the different nerve fibers. After end-organ stimulation, the information is transmitted as an impulse along the sensory nerve.

A Classification of End Organs (3)

Teleceptors These end organs record stimuli from a distance. Examples are the receptors in the eyes and in the ears.

Enteroceptors, Visceroceptors, and Proprioceptors These end organs provide information about the position and movement of joints and also provide information regarding other phenomena such as tension within a muscle or tendon. Other receptors that record sensations from within the body are chemoreceptors and baroreceptors.

Exteroceptors These record stimuli from the skin. They can be subdivided into mechanoreceptors (which record touch and pressure sensation), thermoceptors (which record cold and heat changes), and nonciceptors (which record painful stimuli).

Pain receptors can be further classified into: (1) free nerve endings and (2) encapsulated end organs.

Free nerve endings cover the entire body and transmit pain and temperature impulses.

Encapsulated end organs are of many morphological types:

1. Meissner's corpuscles (touch),
2. Pacini's lamellar corpuscles (pressure),
3. Krause's corpuscles (cold), and
4. Ruffini's corpuscles (warmth).

Currently, the specificity of stimulation on these nerve endings is in doubt. However, they do exist, and perhaps excessive stretch or pressure activates them; massage, manipulation, acupuncture, and transcutaneous electrical nerve stimulation (TENS) have been used in an effort to modify pain, through stimulation of these end organs. Wall and Melzack (14) have postulated that damage to tissue may directly excite nerve endings by:

1. Mechanical effect,
2. Thermal effect, and
3. Chemical effect (effects on nerve membrane).

The authors (14) have divided skin receptors basically into two types.

1. High threshold mechanoreceptor units. These receptors respond only to strong pressure. They do not respond to heat and chemicals. They are thought to be the nerve endings of A delta fibers.
2. Polymodal nociceptors. These receptors respond to pressure, heat, and chemicals. They are thought to be the origin of the C fibers.

Chemical Mediators of Pain

Chemists have identified non-neurogenic mediators of pain (prostaglandin, bradykinin, and so on) and neurogenic mediators of pain (substance P, vasoactive intestinal peptide, and so on). The neurogenic mediators are thought to originate in the dorsal root ganglion.(17) The proteolytic enzymes are produced in response to injury or degeneration and are capable of acting in many ways to introduce pain into what should be a quiet (painless) motion segment. It is thought that the C fibers are constantly "tasting" the metabolic state of tissues and that, by way of impulses and transfer of the chemicals just mentioned, the C fibers assist in modulating pain.

Tracts

Peripheral Nerves

A peripheral nerve contains thousands of nerve fibers (axons) that are myelinated or nonmyelinated. Myelin acts as fiber insulation and, along with interspersed nodes of Ranvier, facilitates fast conduction. All nerve fibers, myelinated or nonmyelinated, are surrounded by sheaths of Schwann, which, in turn, are enveloped by a connective tissue sheath known as endoneurium. Several bundles of nerve fibers are, in turn, enveloped by epineurium to form a peripheral nerve (Fig. 12.1).

Fiber Types Peripheral nerve fibers can be classified according to (1) nerve fiber diameter, (2) degree of myelination, or (3) conduction velocity (Tables 12.1 and 12.2). It is postulated that pain perception is a combination of firing of A delta (fast) and C (slow) fibers. This is evident by the "after burn" of putting your foot in very hot bath water. The immediate pain and withdrawal of the foot (A fibers) is followed by a second sensation of a diffuse wavelength discomfort (C fibers) that follows the original, more sharp painful sensation. Modalities such as TENS are partially founded on the basis of manipulation of C-fiber impulses.(14)

Proximal Nerve Tracts

The proximal peripheral nerve fiber tracts, to and from the lumbar spine and extremities, are four in number (Fig. 12.2):

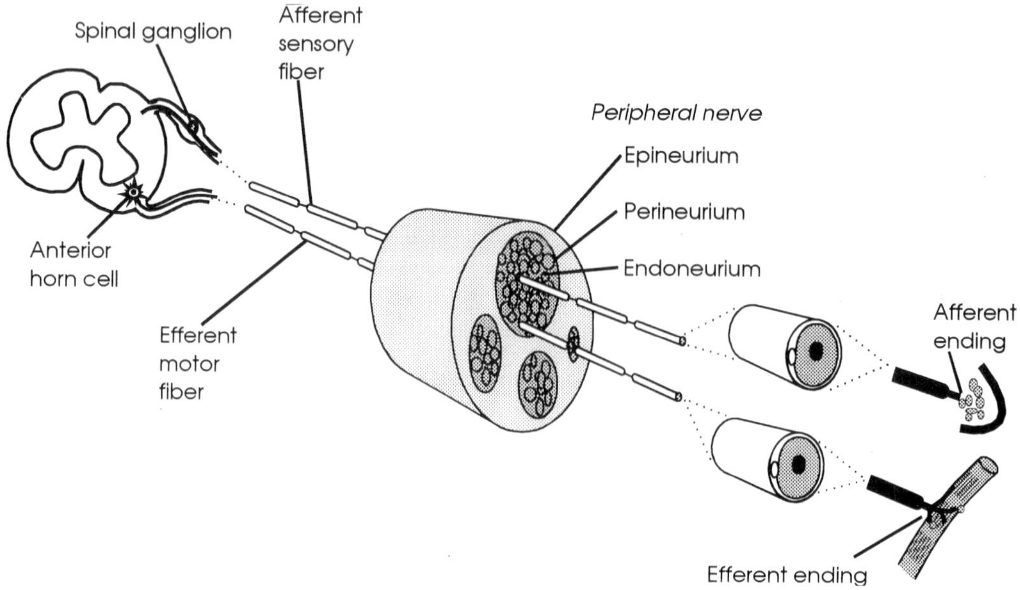

Figure 12.1 *A cross-section of a peripheral nerve from the spinal cord to the end organ.*

Table 12.1. Types of Peripheral Nerve Fibers

Classification	Fiber Size	Myelin Coverage	Conduction Velocity (m/sec)
Group A (motor and sensory)	Large (2–20 m)	Significant	15–100
Group B (visceral sensory)	Intermediate (2 μm)	Much less	2–15
Group C (automatic and some pain, temperature, heavy touch)	Small (1 μm)	No myelin	0.5–2

Table 12.2. Subdivisions of Group A Peripheral Nerve Fibers

Class	Fiber Size (μm)	Conduction Velocity (m/sec)	Peripheral Organ	Receptor Organ	Function
A_α	12–20	70–120	Muscle	Annulospiral, Golgi	Proprioception
A_β	12–20	70–120	Muscle	Same as above	Same as above
A_γ	5–12	30–70	Muscle and skin	Touch and pressure receptors	Touch, pressure, vibration
A_δ	2–5	12–30	Muscle and skin	Pain receptors	Pain and temperature

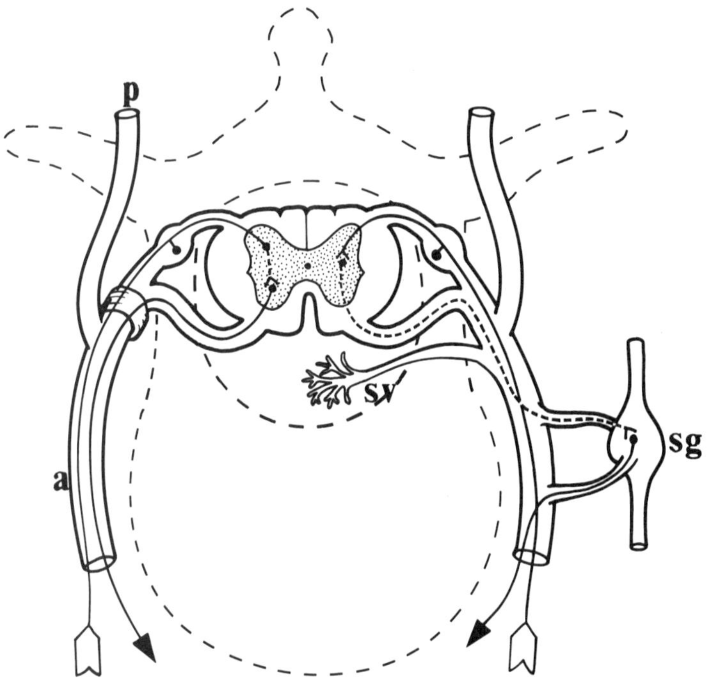

Figure 12.2 *The anterior* **(a)** *and posterior primary rami* **(p)** *are shown, along with the sympathetic ganglion* **(sg)** *and the sinuvertebral nerve* **(sv)**.

1. Anterior (ventral) ramus;
2. Posterior (dorsal) ramus (medial and lateral branches);
3. Sinuvertebral nerve (recurrent nerve of Luschka); and
4. Sympathetic fibers (gray rami communicans).

The types of nerve fibers and distribution of the tracts are as follows:

1. Anterior (ventral) ramus.
   a. Types of fibers.
      i. Motor and sensory (afferent).
      ii. Sympathetic: are present only above L2; below L2, there are no sympathetic fibers in the ventral ramus (Fig. 12.3).
   b. Distribution.
      i. Limbs.
      ii. Lateral annulus fibrosus.
2. Posterior (dorsal) ramus.
   a. Types of fibers.
      i. Motor and sensory (afferent).
      ii. Sympathetic.

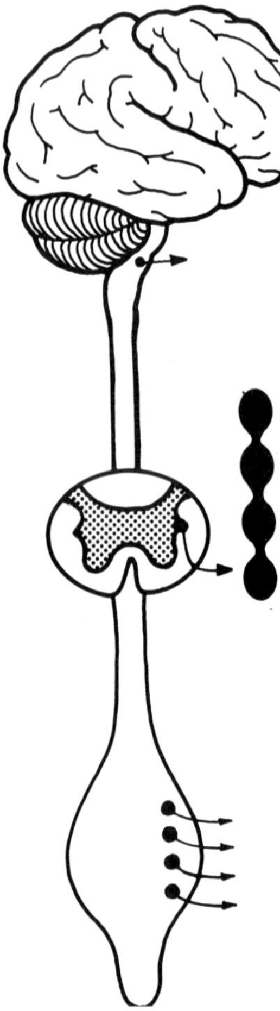

Figure 12.3 *The sympathetic system is considered the thoracolumbar outflow system, and the parasympathetic system is considered the cervical-sacral outflow system (arrows).*

   b. Distribution to the skin and to the muscles of the back (medial and lateral branches): medial branch goes to the facet joints; lateral branch supplies the paraspinal muscles and skin.
3. Sinuvertebral nerve (recurrent nerve of Luschka or meningeal ramus).
   a. Types of fibers.
      i. Sensory (afferent) branch from the ventral ramus.
      ii. Sympathetic fibers.
   b. Distribution.
      i. Posterior longitudinal ligament.
      ii. Ventral aspect of dural sac (the dorsal aspect of the dural sac does not have nerve supply).
      iii. Blood vessels of the spinal canal.
4. Gray rami communicans (sympathetic fibers).
   a. Types of fibers.
      i. Unmyelinated postganglionic.
   b. Distribution.
      i. Lateral and anterior annulus.
      ii. Anterior longitudinal ligament.

The role of the sympathetics in pain is poorly understood. It is thought that they have some modulating effect on the pain receptors. It is known that blocking the sympathetic ganglion, such as a stellate ganglion block, will alter pain appreciation.

Spinal Cord Transmission Pathways

Within the human spinal cord, there are approximately five ascending pathways (Fig. 12.4) for the pain impulses:

1. Spinothalamic tract (the most significant);
2. Spinoreticular tract;
3. Spinomesencephalic tract;
4. Spinocervical tract; and
5. Second-order dorsal column tract.

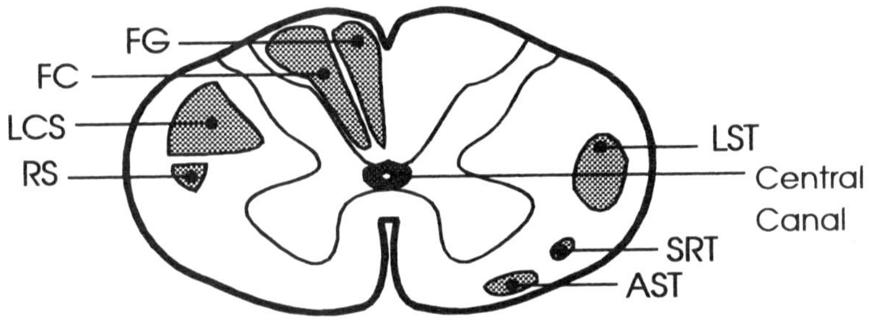

Figure 12.4 *Tracts in the spinal cord: the two important tracts are the lateral spinothalamic (LST) and the lateral cortical spinal (LCS). The dorsal columns are labeled FC and FG. RS = rubrospinal tract; SRT = spinal reticular tract; AST = anterior spinothalamic tract.*

These tracts are not independent pathways to higher centers but, instead, have many cross-connections. In fact, the spinoreticular and spinomesencephalic tracts are considered to be one and the same by some neurobiologists.(14) They are probably "brain-stem" tracts, carrying an alerting message to the reticular formation that pain is something with which the body is going to have to contend. They end in the brain-stem reticular zones of the medulla and pons.

The last two listed tracts (4 and 5) are more theoretical than real and are simply mentioned for completeness.

By far, the most important afferent pain pathway is the lateral spinothalamic tract. It is located in the anterolateral column of the cord and carries crossed pain fibers from the contralateral side of the body. After leaving the dorsal horn gray matter zone, pain fibers cross the midline to enter the spinothalamic tract. More caudal fibers are displaced laterally as more cephalad fibers enter the tract from the opposite side (Fig. 12.5).

Pathways for temperature sense travel in close association with the lateral spinothalamic tract. It is the lateral spinothalamic tract that is transected during the percutaneous cordotomy for the control of pain.

The Dorsal Horn

With their gate control theory of pain, Wall and Melzack (14) have called much attention to the dorsal horn. This is discussed later in the chapter, but an introductory description at this stage is in order.

The concepts and diagrams of the gate control theory of pain are attacked on all sides by the purists, but to the pragmatists they represent the groundwork on which to seek new understanding of pain mechanisms.

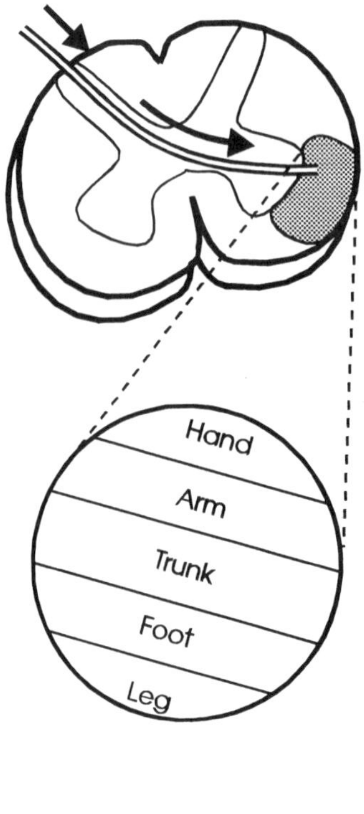

Figure 12.5 *Note the lateral displacement of sensory (and motor) fibers by the more proximal fibers, such that the fibers to the hand are more centrally positioned.*

The dorsal sensory afferents travel in the dorsal root entry zone for one or two segments before entering the dorsal horn (Fig. 12.6). The dorsal horn is made up of six lamina. Which lamina a sensory fiber synapses in is determined by the fiber size, for example:

- C fibers terminate in lamina 1, and subsequently in lamina 2.
- A delta fibers terminate in laminae 2 and 5.

Like a computer, these laminae simulate the information delivered, pass it back and forth, and receive descending modulating impulses. It is after this computerized analysis of the information that the pain impulses are ready for collection and discharge up the spinal cord pathways. This section of the dorsal horn is the gate center for pain modulation (Fig. 12.7).

Higher Centers for Receipt of Pain Fibers

As one goes higher in the central nervous system (CNS), the discrete sensory tract blends into many other CNS pathways. To say exactly where every pain pathway goes at this higher level is impossible. Only the most basic concepts are mentioned:

1. Fibers from the spinothalamic tract go to the thalamus, from whence they are distributed to many higher centers.
2. Other afferent sensory tracts end in the brain-stem reticular formation.
3. Fibers from the thalamus going on to higher cortical centers travel through the internal capsule.
4. Many of these fibers will end up in the postcentral gyrus of the cortex, which is considered to be the predominant sensory area of the cerebral cortex.

Summary of Concepts Presented

When trying to understand the nervous system pathways for pain, one is struck by the multidimensional character of pain:

1. There are multiple nociceptors activating multiple neural systems.
2. There are multiple ascending tracts.
3. There are multiple CNS receptors.

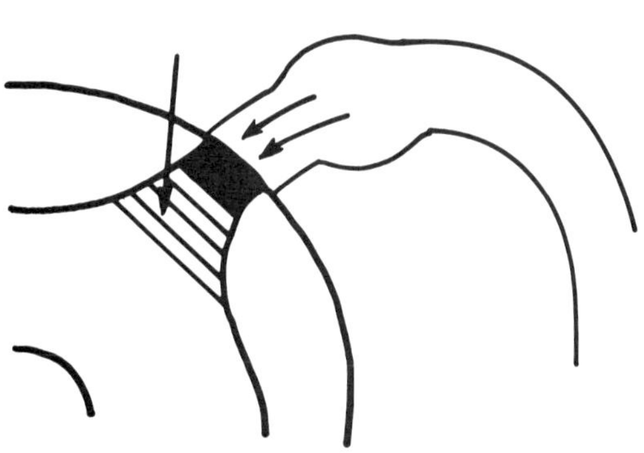

Figure 12.6 *The dorsal root entry zone: striped area.*

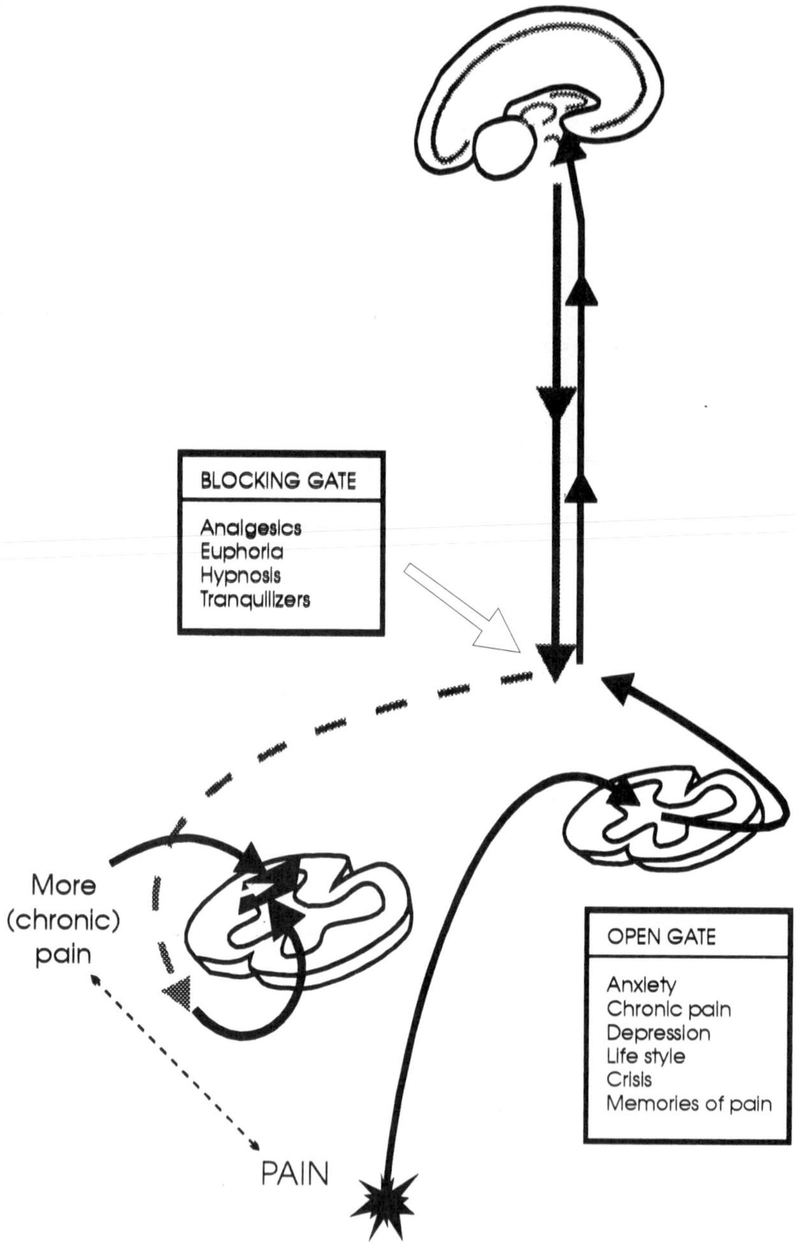

Figure 12.7 *The gate control mechanism: the blocking agents close the gate (white arrow) to decrease painful impulses.*

PSYCHOLOGICAL ASPECTS OF PAIN

The greatest gray area in trying to understand pain lies in the obvious psychological modulation of pain that occurs in every human being. As clinicians, we are aware of patients in whom the slightest amount of pain seems to cause significant disability, and we are also aware of patients in whom a significant amount of pain is accompanied by little alteration in acts of daily living. The reason for this discrepancy and range of pain response lies in understanding the psychological aspects of pain. This is best depicted in Figure 12.8.(5)

The nociception circle is the actual injury. The pain response is the result of the injury. Without any psychological modification, a patient would suffer with the pain.

The difficult part of this diagram is the pain behavior circle. This is what is manifest by the patient and what the doctors and relatives observe in a patient experiencing pain. It is wrapped up into the theories of primary and secondary gain and may include moaning, grimacing, limping, excessive talking, excessive silence, refusing to work, seeking health care, and taking medications. One can only conclude that pain is always accompanied by a display of emotions. These emotions are in the form of anxiety, fear, depression, anger, aggression, and so on, and manifest themselves as pain behavior. Waddell (13) has enhanced this concept with his Glasgow illness model (Fig. 12.9), which is more applicable to the back pain sufferer, plied and enticed by such societal phenomena as accidents, lawyers, courts, and financial awards.

The emotional intensity and pain behavior of the patient is significantly related to the genetic makeup, cultural background, and interpretation of past events. It is an extremely complex cognitive process beyond the scope of this book.

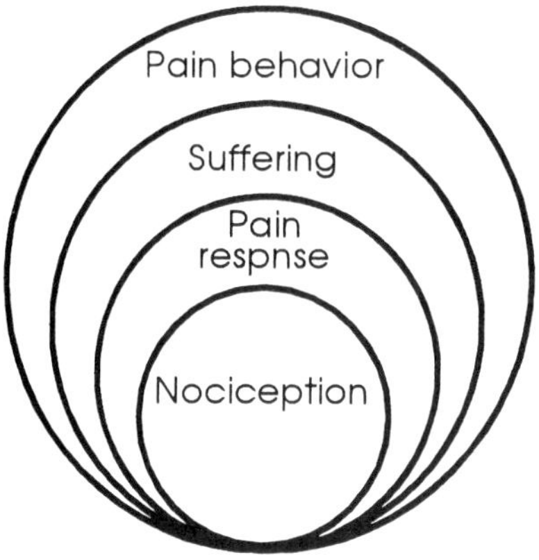

Figure 12.8 *The circles of expanding pain and disability.*

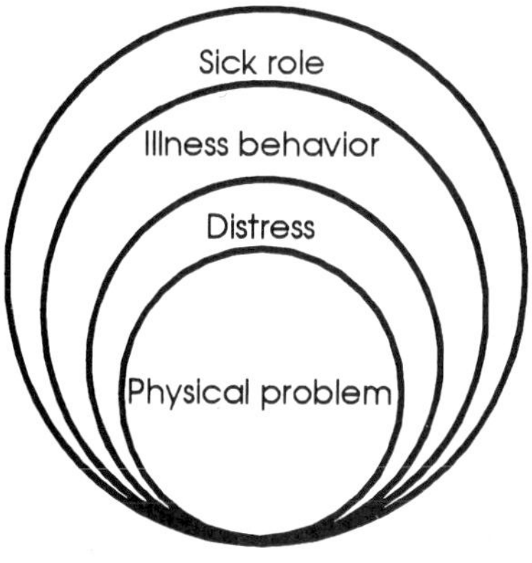

Figure 12.9 *The Glasgow illness model.*

Theories of Pain Transmission

There is no one theory that is universally accepted to explain how pain is appreciated. At one time or another, the following theories have enjoyed support.

Specificity Theory

This is the traditional theory of pain, which states that excitation of a specific nerve ending sends pain impulses along a specific nerve, which travel through specific pathways in the spinal cord to the pain center in the brain. In addition to a pathway for pain, there is also a pathway for temperature and touch. Support for this concept lies in the fact that there are various morphologies for nerve endings, so they must obviously have various functions. In addition, there are specific peripheral nerve fibers such as A delta, and there are specific pathways in the spinal cord.

Pattern Theory

This theory states that pain perception and response depend on the stimulus intensity. That is to say, varying intensities of stimulation produce varying patterns of pain. The concept of phantom limb pain has been explained with this theory, which states that a central summation of pain impulses must occur before the suffering and pain behavior is evident.

Affect Theory

This theory states that pain is strictly a sensory modality like vision and hearing. The ultimate appreciation of pain is strictly an emotional event based on those factors that are discussed in the section on psychology. This was one of the earliest theories of pain but no longer enjoys support.

Gate Control Theory (14)

As mentioned earlier, this is the theory advanced by Wall and Melzack, who are today's most widely read pain researchers. Their theory postulates the presence of a sorting-out center in the dorsal horns of the spinal cord. These sorting-out centers act as a gate, controlling the pain impulses. The gate can act to increase or decrease the flow of nerve impulses from the peripheral fibers to the central nervous system. How the gate behaves is determined by a complex interaction of distal afferent stimulation and descending influences from the brain. There is a critical level of pain information that arrives in the dorsal horn and that will stimulate and open the gate and allow for higher transmission (Fig. 12.7).

It is thought that activity in the nonmyelinated C fibers tends to inhibit transmission and thus closes the gate; conversely, small myelinated A-delta-fiber activity facilitates transmission and opens the gate.

From a clinical point of view, it is postulated that trigger zones in the skin and muscle keep the gate open. Local anesthetic/steroid trigger injectors are used to ablate this phenomenon. Likewise, TENS units are used to stimulate the C fibers and close the gate to transmission of pain impulses to higher centers.

Referred Pain

From the original work of Kellgren (4) to the more recent work of Mooney and Robertson,(9) the concept of referred pain has enjoyed wide support among spine surgeons. Whether this support is correct remains to be seen in light of new work that must be done in this field. The most confusing position has been stated by Bogduk and Twomey (1) to the effect that if pain traveling down the leg is not associated with neurological symptoms or signs, it is not true radicular pain. This is obviously incorrect because many patients with sciatica, especially in the younger age group, present exclusively with leg pain and marked reduction of straight leg raising (SLR), with little in the way of neurologic symptoms or signs. On investigation, these patients are found to have a disc herniation; when the disc herniation is treated, their symptoms abate. To conclude that these patients had referred sclerotomal or myotomal pain rather than the true radicular pain is obviously an error.

At the other end of the spectrum, there are those who state that any pain that does not go below the knee is referred pain, and that any pain that travels below the knee is radicular pain. This is also incorrect, because there are many young patients who present with a disc herniation manifested only by high iliac crest or buttock discomfort. On investigation, these patients are found to have a disc rupture; when the disc rupture is treated, their pain disappears (see Chapter 15).

Finally, there are patients who have radiating pain down the leg, full SLR, and no neurologic changes who are also thought to have referred extremity pain. Some of these patients are in the older age group and, on computerized tomography (CT) scanning and magnetic resonance imaging (MRI), are found to have various degrees of encroachment in the lateral zone. When these encroachment phenomena are relieved microsurgically, the pain disappears and, obviously, they have had radicular rather than referred discomfort.

For all of these reasons, it is time to repeat the work of both Kellgren (4) and Mooney and Robertson,(9) knowing exactly the pathology that lies at each segment as documented on CT scan and MRI. It is predicted that many of the patients who have previously been tagged with the label "referred pain" will, in fact, have radicular pain due to the direct irritation and/or compression of a nerve root.

Many clinicians would accept patients as having referred pain when they present with a very diffuse sensation in their legs, bilateral in nature, not associated with any radicular pattern and not associated with any root tension irritation or compression findings. Provided that those patients do not have spinal stenosis on CT scan or MRI, they probably do have referred pain.

The concept of referred pain is one of two types of discomfort. Either it is a deep discomfort felt in a sclerotomal or myotomal distribution, or it may be superficial in nature and felt within the skin dermatomes. The fact that gallbladder pain can be felt in the shoulder obviously supports the fact that referred pain is a phenomenon that does occur.

In theory, somewhere in the nervous system is a convergence and summation of nerve impulses from the primary painful area. This is probably lamina 5 in the dorsal horn. The stimulation of this lamina opens a gate and allows central dispatch of the pain message and distal referral of other sensations, including referred pain. You can increase the painful sensation by touching the sites of referred pain. These areas are known as trigger zones, and through various methods of stimulation and anesthetization, referred pain can be altered.

In summary, the concepts of referred pain are likely to be altered with today's sophisticated investigations in the form of CT scanning and MRI. With these tools in hand, it is time to go back and repeat the outstanding work of Kellgren (4) and Mooney and Robertson (9) in an attempt to further understand the concept of referred pain.

Control of Acute Pain

Intrinsic

There are descending analgesic pathways within the CNS that have the potential for modifying acute pain. The midbrain contains areas that, if stimulated, anesthetize an extremity. These areas contain many opiate receptors, and it is postulated that the distal extremity anesthetization comes about because of the release of opiate-like neuropeptides from the midbrain. These are known as endorphins. Somehow, the endorphins affect or travel down the spinal cord to the dorsal horn to modulate the pain impulse.

External

There are external methods to control pain, and these can be summarized as follows:

1. Pain can be controlled by (a) blocking the pathways with local anesthetic, (b) cutting peripheral nerves, and (c) interrupting tracts in the spinal cord.
2. Drugs can be used to (a) block receptors, (b) block the gate center in the dorsal column, (c) block brain-stem transmission of pain, or (d) dull the higher-center appreciation of pain.
3. A TENS unit can be used to manipulate the sensory side of the reflex arc. Theoretically, low level stimulation by the TENS unit selectively activates the large C fibers and closes the gate in the dorsal horn. Acupuncture also works in this fashion. Stimulation of the dorsal columns in the spinal cord provides intense stimulation to the brain stem, which supposedly inhibits the sensory appreciation from below. As fine as the theories appear with regard to the TENS unit, acupuncture, and dorsal column stimulators, in practice these theories appear to work only in those patients with chronic pain who have a significant psychological component to their pain. This raises the spectrum of placebo response, which is a fact of life for spine surgeons evaluating any treatment modality.
4. Obviously, pain can be modified by manipulating psychological factors. This can be accomplished through desensitization, hypnotic training, relaxation training, biofeedback, and behavior modification.

Pain Factors Specific to The Lumbosacral Region of the Spine

The pain of spinal origin is of the Category 3 variety (see section on categorization of pain), and it can be divided into two groups:

1. Pain originating from the bony column: specifically, its three-joint complex of disc and facet joints; and

2. Pain arising as a consequence of direct affection of the spinal nerve root.
3. Other low back pains, such as those referred from the prevertebral visceral spaces, are not considered in this chapter.

There continues to be controversy as to whether free nerve endings have a functional presence in spinal structures such as the annulus. Everyone would agree that the deeper annular-nuclear portion of the disc is not innervated. It is well established that the posterior longitudinal ligament is richly supplied with nociceptor fibers from the sinuvertebral nerve. More recently, Yoshizawa et al (17) and Malinsky (6) have solved the controversy by very definitely demonstrating various types of encapsulated and unencapsulated pain receptors in the outer aspect of the entire annulus. The sources of these fibers have been further documented by Malinsky and include the sinuvertebral nerve, the ventral rami, and the sympathetic gray rami communicans.

Because of the difficulty in demonstrating nerve fibers in the outer annulus, it is likely that the annulus is re-innervated as the body grows older and as the process of disc degeneration occurs. It is well known that a disc is avascular during most of its adult life, but that it does become vascularized as it degenerates. Perhaps a similar reaction occurs with nerve supply to the annulus.

Free nerve endings are also present in (1) the fibrous capsule of the facet joint, (2) the sacroiliac joints, (3) the anterior aspect of the dura, (4) the periosteum, (5) the vertebral bodies, and (6) the blood vessel walls. Theoretically, the presence of these nociceptors implies that a stimulus to these areas will be transmitted as a pain impulse. Although this appears to be a simple conclusion, it is not supported by anyone who has operated on the spine with local anesthesia and has palpated the annulus without reproducing pain. In addition, discography can be done in a normal disc with tremendous pressures placed on the disc, and no appreciation of pain on the part of the patient occurs. Thus, the simple presence of these nociceptors does not explain how pain arises in a spinal segment. Further work has to be done with regard to (1) chemical changes that occur with disc degeneration, and (2) the influence of abnormal movement.

Conclusion

A normal motion segment is painless. Even a normal motion segment taken to the extremes of physiological movement is painless. It is the introduction of pathological

Table 12.3. Pathological Changes That Initiate Pain

1. Within the disc
Annular tears
Disc resorption
Osteophyte formation
2. In facet joints
Synovitis
Capsular laxity
Degeneration of articular cartilage
Joint subluxation
3. Muscles and ligaments
Stretch
Tear and hematoma

changes (Table 12.3) that brings pain to the motion segment. Pain endings and pain fibers are plentiful in the spinal column, but why do some pathological changes cause pain, whereas other aging pathological changes remain asymptomatic? This is an enigma.

NON-ORGANIC SPINAL PAIN

Now, from pain theory to even more intangible concepts. A classification of nonorganic spinal pain is outlined in Table 12.4. The term nonorganic has been chosen over other terms such as nonphysical, functional, emotional, and psychogenic.

Before even considering this section, recognize that nonorganic syndromes do not occur in a void. There is always a clinical setting that supports the fact that there is a nonorganic component to the patient's disability, that is, if you make the diagnosis of psychosomatic pain, there will be a tension-producing situation in the patient's life or a patient in anxiety; if you make the diagnosis of psychogenic pain syndrome, you will find a premorbid personality or emotional state that fostered the reaction; if you make the diagnosis of situational spinal pain, a situation such as a motor vehicle accident and a lawyer or a compensation claim will exist. *Nonorganic reactions do not occur in a void.*

The following definitions are used:

1. Psychosomatic spinal pain is defined as symptomatic physical change in tissues of the spine, which has anxiety as its cause. The expression of anxiety is mediated as a prolonged and exaggerated state that eventually leads to structural change (spasm) in the muscles of the neck or low back.
2. a. Psychogenic spinal pain is defined as the conversion or somatization of anxiety into pain referred to the neck or back, unaccompanied by physical change in the tissues of these regions. The pain is variously known in the literature as conversion hysteria, psychogenic regional pain, traumatic or accident neurosis, and hypochondriasis.

   The emotional upset brings pains to the back just as it may bring tears to the eyes. The reason for the conversion is found in complex psychodynamic mechanisms beyond the scope of this chapter. The reaction represents a sincere, unconscious emotional illness that offers the patient the primary gain of solving inner conflicts, fears, and anxieties. Inherent in the conversion reaction is the concept of suggestion and hypnosis, the importance of which will become apparent later in this chapter.
2. b. Psychogenic modification of spinal pain is a sincere emotional reaction that modifies the appreciation of an organic pain. Usually, the organic pain by itself would not be disabling, but with the psychogenic modification, a significant disability

Table 12.4. Nonorganic Spinal Pain

1. Psychosomatic spinal pain
Tension syndrome (fibrositis)
2. Psychogenic spinal pain
Psychogenic spinal pain
Psychogenic modification of organic spinal pain
3. Situational spinal pain
Litigation reaction
Exaggeration reaction

ensues. No associated physical change occurs as a result of anxiety, and a conversion reaction may or may not coexist.

An example is the patient burdened with life situational pressures (mortgage payments, car payments) who, because of the physical illness, feels that he/she cannot sustain the effort necessary to meet these demands. A resulting depression may occur, and the symptoms of fatigue, loss of appetite, insomnia, impotence, constipation, and so on, so dominate the history that the underlying physical condition is missed. Other examples are patients with passive dependent personality, drug or alcohol dependence, or psychosis, who, in the face of a minor physical problem, use their illness as an excuse to step out of the demands of the real world into a life-style mode of frequent demand for mood-altering or analgesic medications.

Some obsessive-compulsive patients cannot adjust to a minor physical problem, and this personality trait leads them to feel that they have a significant disability.

3. Situational spinal pain is a reaction whereby a patient, through a collection of symptoms, maintains a situation (with potential secondary gain) through over-concern or conscious effort.

3. a. The litigation or compensation reaction is defined as overconcern by the patient for present and future health, arising out of a litigious or compensable event that initially affected the patient's health. The reaction manifests itself in a patient's complaint of continuing neck or back pain coupled with a concern that, upon formal severance from his/her claim to compensation, deterioration in health may occur. The patient with this reaction is neither physically nor emotionally ill.

This reaction is not to be confused with the ambiguous terms "litigation neurosis" or "compensation neurosis." Like "whiplash," the terms "litigation and compensation neurosis" have no medical or legal value and should be dropped from our vocabulary. If a patient has a true neurosis arising out of a litigious or compensable event (accident), then those terms listed under "psychogenic spinal pain (2a or b)" should be used for diagnostic purposes (eg, traumatic neurosis or accident neurosis). If the patient's disability appears to be based more on an awareness of the commercial value of his/her symptoms, the reaction should not be legitimized by the use of the term neurosis in conjunction with the words litigation or compensation (thus, litigation reaction).

3. b. Exaggeration reactions are attempts by the patient to appear ill or magnify an existent illness. "Malingering" is a term frequently applied to this reaction and is defined as "the conscious alteration of health for gain."

As will be described later, it is possible for the physician to detect effort to magnify, but it is not proper to assign motives (gain) to the patient. The lawyer involved is in a reversed role. He/she may raise doubts about the plaintiff's motives (gain) but not be in a position to clinically detect effort to magnify or exaggerate. The choice of the word malingering implies proficiency in two professions, which is an uncommon occurrence. For this reason, the terms malingering and conscious effort are best not used by the physician when discussing nonorganic spinal pain.

Alteration of health in order to deceive, evade responsibility, or derive gain does occur. Those who would deny its occurrence deny the existence of human nature. The patient who tries to alter or reproduce symptoms or signs of a spinal problem may do so in a number of ways:

Pretension No physical illness exists, and the patient willfully fabricates symptoms and signs. This mode occurs infrequently in the military during wartime and is a rare civilian event.

Exaggeration Symptoms and signs of a spinal disability are magnified to represent more than they really are.

Preservation Symptoms and signs that were once present have ceased to exist but continue to be described or demonstrated by the patient.

Allegation Genuine disability is present, but the patient fraudulently ascribes these to some causes associated with gain, knowing that, in fact, his condition is of a different origin.

Civilian nonorganic situational spinal pain is usually the exaggeration or preservation type. Pretension and allegation are uncommon forms of gainful alteration of health in civilian practice. Like the patient with the litigation reaction, these patients are neither emotionally ill nor physically ill. However, they differ from the litigation reaction in that they are attempting to demonstrate physical illness through the effort of exaggeration or preservation. The reason for this effort is usually, but not always, found in secondary financial gain.

Clinical Description

Before describing each of these entities, it is important to emphasize:

1. This is a simplistic classification that is useful only to the family practitioner or the spinal surgeon. It does not allow for the complex assessments done by psychologists, psychiatrists, and so on, but it does allow for a foundation on which to build clinical recognition of these entities so that the patient can be referred to others more skilled in the field.
2. One cannot rigidly define disability, because there are gray areas. However, there is a tendency for a nonorganic disability to fall largely into one category.
3. It is most important to determine whether the setting exists for one of these nonorganic disabilities.
    a. A patient who has had previous emotional problems is prone to have an emotional component to a disability. Symptoms such as fatigue, sleeplessness, agitation, gastrointestinal upset, and excessive sweating should signal that an emotional component is likely present.
    b. A patient who is in a secondary gain situation such as a motor vehicle accident claim has the potential for these nonorganic reactions. It is important to establish the presence of such circumstances early in the patient encounter. If a patient states that low back pain started suddenly with an incident, it is important to document whether the incident is a claim type of accident and whether insurance and legal factors are involved. Conversely, if there is no secondary gain detected on history, it is unusual for the clinician to arrive at a secondary gain diagnosis such as litigation reaction or magnification exaggeration reaction.
4. A vague and confusing history, a baffling physical examination, and an elusive diagnosis signal a possible nonorganic diagnosis. Reflect on this before taking the expensive step of hospital admission and sophisticated and expensive testing that has the potential to give a false-positive result.

5. A patient who quickly establishes an abnormal doctor/patient relationship has a potential nonorganic component to his disability. These abnormal doctor/patient relationships include patients who are hostile or effusively complimentary, those who have had many other doctors involved in care before your assessment, some who fail to respond to standard (physical) conservative treatment measures, and patients who are critical of other doctors.

Psychosomatic Back Pain

The psychosomatic phenomenon of muscle spasm arising out of tension states usually affects the neck but may affect the low back. It should be known as the "orthopaedic ulcer" but more often is given the label of fibrositis. Patients with this problem are overtly strained and tense, as evidenced by facial expression. They are fidgety and restless and may sit on the edge of the chairs while they wring their hands. Some of these patients will place their hands on their neck or back during the history and literally wring the area while describing the pain. They have a general feeling of restlessness and a specific feeling of a tightness in their neck with associated sensations of cracking and a constant feeling of the need to stretch out the neck and shoulder muscles. The pain is not specifically mechanical but does tend to accumulate with the day's activity, especially when that activity is carried out in the tension-producing environment (eg, work).

The pain typically responds to chiropractic or physiotherapeutic intervention, but relief is usually temporary, a fact that makes the patient tend to seek prolonged care.

Physical examination reveals a good range of movement in the back, with a complaint of pain only if movement is done too quickly or carried to extremes. The significant physical finding is the presence of firm, tender muscles when the affected part is examined in a position of rest. The patient may be able to demonstrate the "cracking" to the touch or auditory perception of the examiner.

No evidence of nerve root involvement exists in the lower extremities. Skin tenderness, the significance of which is explained later, is not an unusual finding. This condition is also described in further detail in Chapter 7.

Psychogenic Back Pain

The patient with psychogenic spinal pain is emotionally ill. These patients often have a history of past illnesses replete with emotional problems. It follows that the history of present illness contains a preponderance of emotional symptoms, and the description of the pain will not be typical of any organic condition. The patient is convinced that he/she is ill, and that conviction extends to the frequent demand for consultations with numerous doctors. Considerable financial hardship and aggravation will occur in some cases when these consultations take the patient great distances to and from major clinics or spas throughout the world. Throughout their constant demand for care, these patients notice times when their symptoms do improve. This is due to the institution of some new form of treatment that affects the patient through suggestion or hypnotism, a fact that makes placebo trial of little value in the evaluation of these problems.

It follows that because these patients are emotionally ill, no causative organic problem will be found on physical examination. The conversion reaction is associated with an upset body image appreciation such that a topographical unit (the back and leg), indifferent to matters of innervation or anatomical relationship, will contain physical findings of skin tenderness and dulled sensory appreciation (13) (Fig. 12.10). The somatization infrequently reaches the stage of weakness, with wasting and depression of all of the reflexes in the contiguous part, for example, an arm or leg.

However, the important observation on physical examination of this patient is the paucity of physical findings, which separates him/her from the magnifier and exaggerator, who by definition has many "physical" findings.

Psychogenic Modification of Organic Pain

Of all of the nonorganic causes of spinal pain, the patient who psychogenically modifies organic pain presents the most difficult diagnostic and therapeutic challenge. Sometimes, but not always, the organic problem by itself would not be disabling. Thus, the historical and physical component of the disability related to the organicity is not significant. Those findings indicative of a physical illness will be appropriate and a quantitative guide to the extent of physical illness. However, the life situational pressures or the personality of the patient modify the disability to a significant point. As well, the psychogenic reaction interferes with response to treatment and leads to persistence of the disability. In a surgical practice, this failure to respond to conservative treatment is the classic indication for operative intervention. If the surgeon fails to recognize that the failure to respond to physical treatment measures is due in this instance to a psychogenic disability, he/she will gradually build a practice containing a number of spinal surgery failures.

Psychogenic modifications are commonly seen in the patient with an inadequate personality. By definition, this patient's personality may limit advancement up the social, educational, and occupational ladder and confine him/her to the unskilled worker classification. Some of these patients can be found in the workmen's compensation board pop-

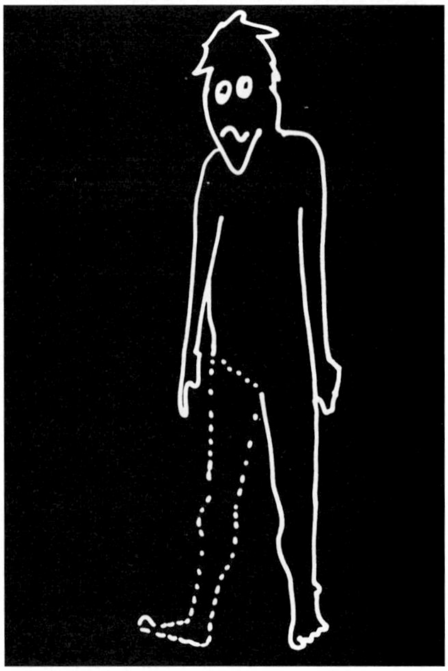

Figure 12.10 *During sensory testing, it is evident that the sensory loss extends over many dermatomes and is, in fact, a loss indifferent to matters of innervation or anatomical relationships. The whole leg appears numb.*

ulation, which may be one of the reasons for poorer results of treatment sometimes obtained in the compensation patient.

These patients are seen with a minor physical problem (eg, back strain), yet they have a total disability. All attempts at treatment fail to return the patient to the work force. Frequent office visits reinforce the disability for the patient. If the doctor fails to recognize this maladaptive reaction and reinforcement, he/she may initiate treatment that will not help the patient in any way.

Other psychogenic modifications come about through drug addiction and alcohol dependence. Occasionally, psychotic behavior will convert a minor physical problem into a prolonged disability.

Physical examination will reveal the nature and extent of the physical impairment. Usually, the physical impairment by itself would not be significantly disabling. The loss of movement in the back is minor, the limitation of SLR is minimal, and the neurological changes are of questionable significance. In the face of repeated assessments and a continuing statement of disability, the patient's minor physical problem may become magnified in the mind of the clinician who does not assess personality and life situational factors.

Situational Spinal Pain

Litigation Reactions

This patient is neither physically nor emotionally ill. Thus, few emotional symptoms will be present on historical examination. The patient is in the process of litigation or under the care of the workmen's compensation board. These patients often state that they do not care about the litigious or compensation issue, yet they also state that they are afraid to settle or return to work for fear that further illness will develop. Their continuing complaints are rather vague and would not normally be incapacitating. If they are receiving treatment, they are not improving. Physically, there may be an increased awareness of the body part in question, as manifested by skin tenderness in the affected area, but no organic illness is detectable, and there is no attempt to exaggerate or magnify a disability.

Magnification-Exaggeration Reaction

Some or most of the following historical characteristics will be obtained from this patient. The most obvious historical point is the secondary gain situation that usually has involved the fault of someone else and/or payment of financial compensation. Other secondary gain situations can occur. The initiating event is usually a trivial or minor incident. There may be a latent period of hours or days between the incident and the onset of symptoms, during which time the patient speaks to friends and relatives and learns of the commercial value of the injury.

The patient describes the pain with some degree of indifference, as evidenced by a smile or a laugh when describing the severe disability. He/she is vague in describing and localizing the pain, giving the examiner the impression of someone struggling to remember a dream. Specificity and elaboration require memory for repetition, a quality not present to a significant degree in this type of patient. The individual wishes you to believe this pain is unique and severe. This attempt to have you believe in the pain is often accompanied by a salesman-like attitude, with many examples of the disability spontaneously listed. Inability to engage in sex is usually at the top of the list.

Despite the trivial initiating event, the disability may have been present for a long time. Three types of treatment patterns occur:

1. The patient follows a "straight line" course of treatment; he/she does not respond to the standard physical treatment nor to the inherent suggestion and hypnosis of treatment, that is, he/she does not improve or gets worse.
2. The patient is not receiving treatment because he/she is "allergic" to all medications prescribed, "suffocates" in the neck or back braces, or becomes ill in a physiotherapy setting.
3. The patient is not receiving treatment because he/she has failed to seek treatment.

Certain behavior patterns become apparent after seeing a number of these patients. Some never appear for appointments despite weeks of notification. Others appear late for the appointment and do not apologize or state indifferently that the traffic was heavy. There may be an attempt to manipulate your feelings with a compliment about your reputation or your office. There may be an effort to play one doctor against another by making false statements about another doctor. Finally, hostility may appear during the assessment. A patient truly ill will not be aware or afraid of an exposé and will not be hostile unless provoked. A patient exaggerating a disability is suspicious. He/she may start out hostile, but the usual pattern is one of developing hostility as discrepancies in the history and physical examination are exposed. Examiners are advised, for obvious reasons, not to precipitate this final behavioral pattern.

The patient who is magnifying or exaggerating a disability can be exposed only through an adequate physical examination. Those physicians who do not physically examine patients will not recognize this reaction, which may explain the reluctance of the psychiatric community to accept this clinical entity.

The physical findings of magnification or exaggerated reaction are classified into those that demonstrate acting behavior, those that indicate anticipatory behavior, and those that fail to support the patient's claim to illness.

Acting Behavior Exaggerating a disability requires acting by the patient. This acting may be general in nature such as the Academy Award performances put on by some patients as they moan and groan through the examination, walk around the examining room with their eyes closed, and either reach for objects to support themselves or reach for their painful areas. The incongruity of this acting behavior may be evident when the patient mounts the examining table with considerable ease and/or dresses within minutes of the examination and smiles and waves goodbye as he/she leaves the office.

Specific examples of acting behavior are the rigid back, a condition that disappears on the examining table (Fig. 12.11); the reduction of SLR that disappears in the sitting position (Fig. 12.12); tender skin; and the paralyzed, insensitive extremity. That these findings are a result of acting can be demonstrated through the use of distraction testing (Table 12.5). Using nonpainful, nonemotional, and nonsurprising examination techniques, it is possible not only to change the acting behavior but also to demonstrate normal physical function. It is the authors' opinion that proper distraction testing that abolishes an acted physical finding and demonstrate normal physical function is a method of demonstrating magnification-exaggeration behavior. The best distraction test is simple observation of the patient as he/she gets undressed and moves about the examining room.

Varying degrees of acting behavior occur in different patients. In general, the more sophisticated the patient, the more sophisticated the acting behavior, and the more sophisticated the examination must be (Fig. 12.13).

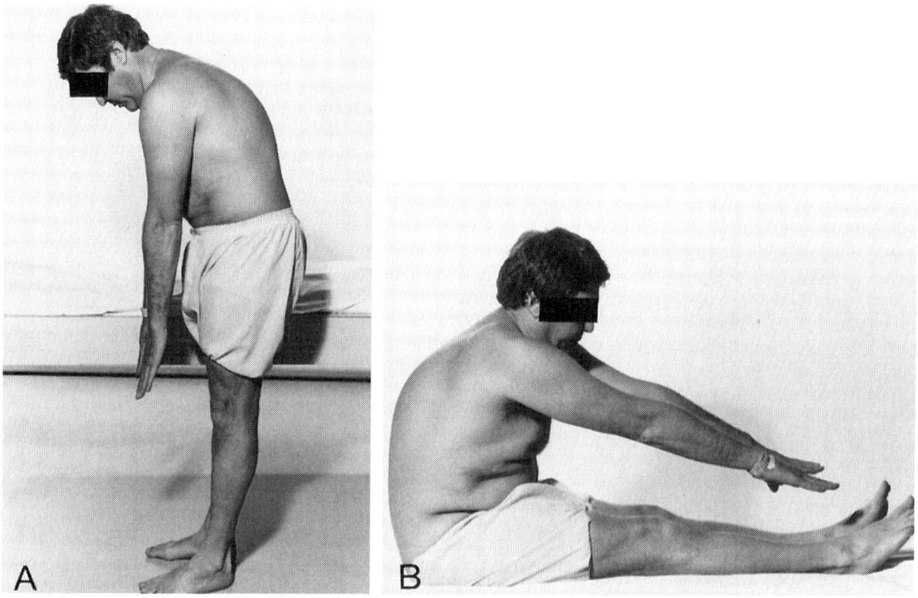

Figure 12.11 **A.** *Acting behavior. During testing of flexion, the patient pretends that very limited flexion is possible.* **B.** *Acting behavior. Later in the examination, a similar test of flexion is possible by asking the patient to sit as shown. If the patient shows not only good flexion ability, but also reverses the lumbar lordosis, no physical stiffness in the lumbar spine is evident.*

Anticipatory Behavior The second group of physical findings in this reaction represents anticipation on the part of the patient to the test situations. This anticipatory behavior leads to an appropriate response by the patient in an attempt to indicate illness. These tests are illustrated in Figure 12.14.

Contradictory Clinical Evidence

Statements by the patient to the effect that he/she is unable to work may not be supported by clinical observations. Some patients will say that they are unable to drive, yet will have driven by themselves great distances to get to the examination. Some patients will say that they require frequent medication, yet will arrive from great distances without their medication. The patient who claims to be continuously wearing a collar or a brace should show signs of this wear on the body and the appliance. If a patient carries the brace to the examination, ask him/her to put it on. It may turn out to be a friend's brace that was borrowed for the doctor visit, and it either does not fit, or he/she does not know how to put it on! Patients with calluses on their hands and knees contradict their story of a prolonged inability to work. Other evidence of work may be in the form of paint stains on the skin or a particular distribution of sunburned areas on the skin. Patients with nicotine stains on a grossly paralyzed limb should start to demonstrate similar stains on the opposite hand. Finally, those patients who attempt to demonstrate a prolonged and profound weakness in an extremity should have associated wasting of that extremity.

Just because a patient has one contradictory finding does not mean the patient should be classified as a magnifier/exaggerator or litigant reactor. It is important to stress that a collection of symptoms and signs should be present with the appropriate

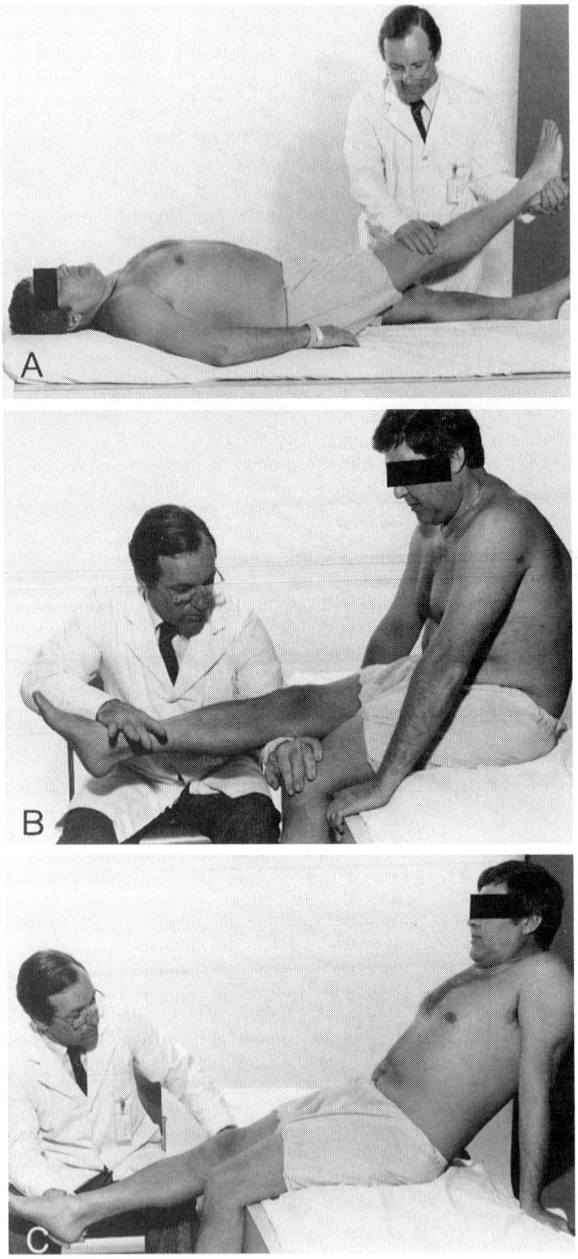

Figure 12.12 *Acting behavior. The flip test:* **A.** *The patient voluntarily demonstrates SLR reduction.* **B.** *In the sitting position, SLR to 90 degrees is possible—a discrepancy between* **A** *and* **B** *that cannot be explained on the basis of root tension from a disc herniation. Rather, this discrepancy in SLR ability can only be explained on the basis of a nonorganic reaction.* **C.** *If true root tension were present, the patient would "flip" back on sitting SLR testing.*

Table 12.5. Demonstration of Acting Behavior Through Distraction Testing

Condition	Response
Physical finding (acting behavior)	Reduction in straight leg raising
Distraction test, eg, flip test Nonpainful Nonemotional Nonsurprising	Normal straight leg raising
Result	Normal physical function

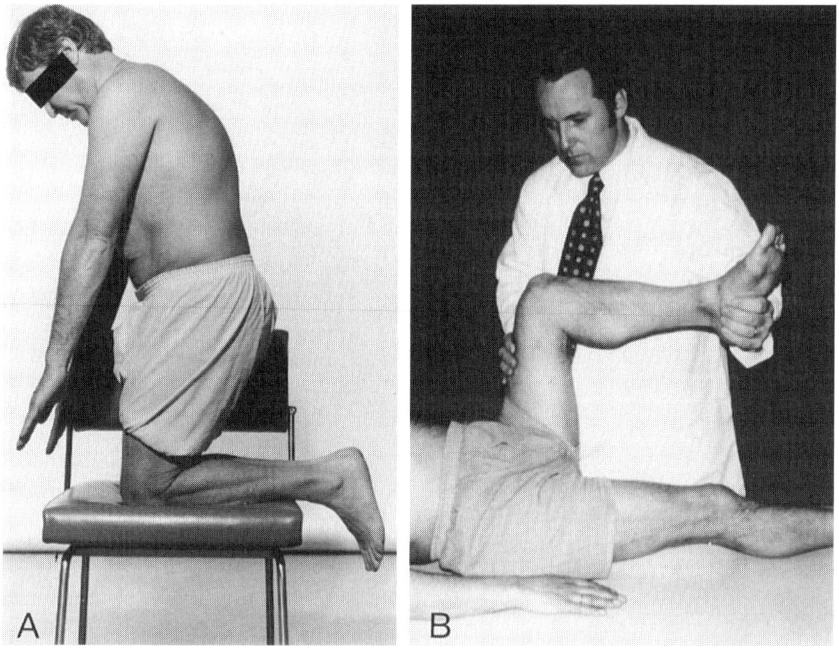

Figure 12.13 *Acting behavior.* **A.** *In the kneeling position, with the hamstrings relaxed, more lumbar flexion should be available.* **B.** *With the hip and knee flexed, the patient acts out back pain, which does not occur in organic pain.*

clinical setting to make the diagnosis of magnification/exaggeration behavior. Waddell et al (12) have documented the significant symptoms and signs that, when collected together, suggest that a nonorganic component to a disability is present. These symptoms and signs have been scientifically documented as valid and reproducible. As a screening mechanism, they are an excellent substitute for pain drawings and psychological testing (see Table 12.6).

It is one thing to have a fancy classification, and it is another to make that classification work. When interviewing the patient, try to place him/her in one of the following categories:

The Everyday, Normal Patient with Low Back Pain Fortunately, this group is by far the largest group of patients with which most of us deal. It seems, without great socioeconomic studies, that people tend to associate with kindred spirits. Turkeys prefer to flock

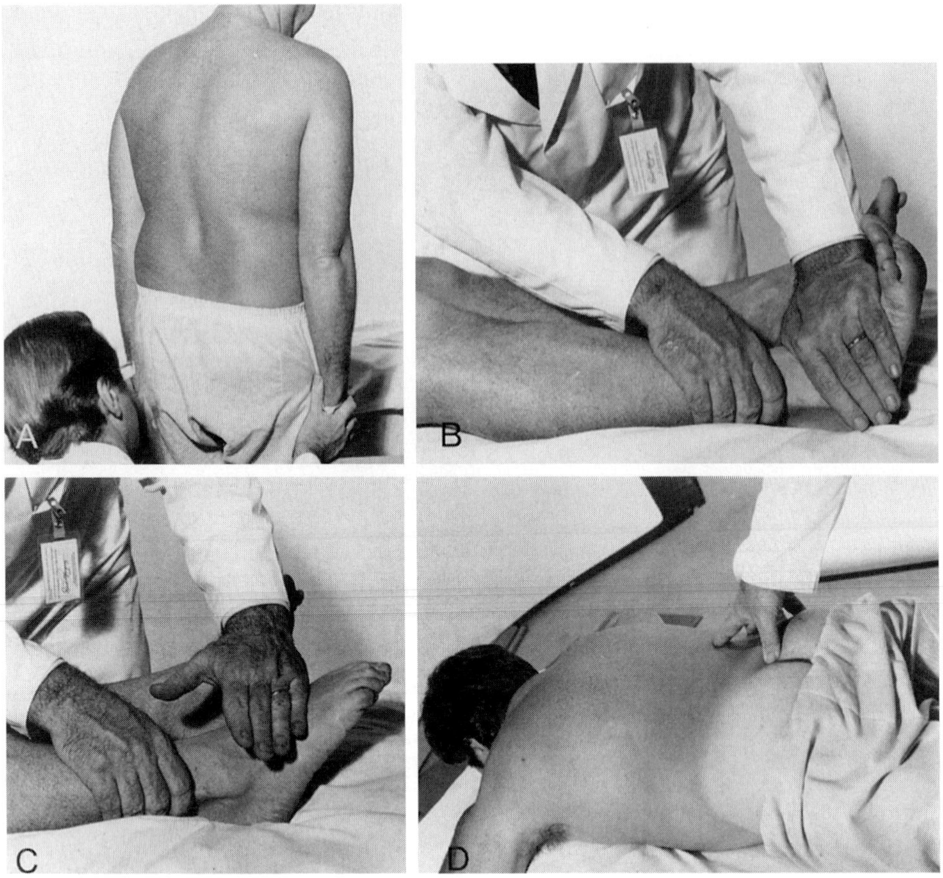

Figure 12.14 *Anticipatory behavior.* **A.** *Simulated movement: Rotate the patient's trunk through the hip joints. This should not cause pain in organic low back pain because the back is not being moved.* **B.** *Dorsiflexion testing for strength. The toes will remain extended as pressure is applied to the dorsum of the foot.* **C.** *The nonorganic patient will give way either in a cogwheel fashion or signal the onset of feigned weakness by giving way voluntarily with the toes and then the foot.* **D.** *Skin tenderness and/or tenderness over the body of the sacrum is most often nonorganic in nature.*

with turkeys, and eagles like to soar with eagles. Similarly, the hypochondriacal patient tends to associate with other anxious, tension-ridden people. If, as a practitioner, you are oversympathetic and solicitous to patients with emotional components to their disability, then soon their friends start appearing as your patients, and soon the bulk of your patient load ceases to be the normal, everyday patient with low back pain.

The Stoic This patient is usually in your office at his wife's request. When asked why he is there, the patient may state that there is a little pain present in his leg, but "not to worry, I can walk and play." Do not be misled. This patient may have no more than 5 degrees of SLR ability, no ankle reflex, and no plantar flexion power, that is, he has a significant physical problem due to the ruptured disc at L5–S1. But the patient does not have time in his busy life for illness. We have used the male designation for this example because most (but not all) of these patients are men. They are not always from "management"; many who come from the laboring segment of the economy have yet to succumb

Table 12.6. Symptoms and Signs Suggesting a Nonorganic Component to Disability

Symptoms	
	1. Pain is multifocal in distribution and nonmechanical (present at rest).
	2. Entire extremity is painful, numb, and/or weak.
	3. Extremity gives way (as a result, the patient carries a cane).
	4. Treatment response No response "Allergic" to treatment Not receiving treatment
	5. Multiple crises, multiple hospital admissions/investigations, multiple doctors.
Signs	
	1. Tenderness is superficial (skin) or nonanatomic (eg, over body of sacrum).
	2. Simulated movement tests are positive.
	3. Distraction test is positive.
	4. Whole leg is weak or numb.
	5. "Academy Award" performance.

to the financial inducements to illness behavior inherent in the various workmen's compensation systems.

The Racehorse Syndrome

The racehorse syndrome applies to the group of tense, hard driving, hyper-reactive patients. In stressful situations, they tend to hyperextend their backs and assume the "fight" position as a result of their chronic muscle spasm. Throughout their lives, they have responded to tense situations in this manner without pain. However, once they develop disc degeneration, segmental instability and muscle spasm, this allows the related posterior joints to be pushed beyond the permitted physiological range when this posture is adopted, and pain results. The pain that they experience interferes with their ability to get on with their normal way of life, and the frustrations that they feel increase the tension in the sacrospinalis muscles, thereby aggravating and perpetuating their discomfort. In the treatment of these patients, the significance of this postural change must be explained. In addition to the routine conservative treatment of discogenic back pain, these patients should be taught voluntary muscle relaxation, and they need mild sedation to take the edge off their normal tensions and anxieties. (Classification: This patient has a variety of psychosomatic pain that aggravates the organic condition of degenerative disc disease.)

The Razor's Edge Syndrome The razor's edge syndrome refers to patients who precariously trend their way through life on the razor's edge of emotional stability. These patients have hysterical personalities, and like people in show business, play their lives in high C.

Before the recent changes in sartorial habits, these patients could be spotted easily. The women loved outlandish hair styles and heavy eye makeup. They decorated themselves with large earrings and rows of necklaces. Multiple bracelets and bangles adorned their wrists, and they wore huge garish rings on their fingers. The men grew beards, and men and women wore dark glasses even indoors. In today's world, dress and hairstyle can no longer be regarded as being of diagnostic significance, but the dramatization of symptoms is characteristic. Superlatives are thrown around with gay abandon. The pain is "agonizing." "I was paralyzed with pain." "It was as though someone was tearing the muscles out of my leg." ".... like boiling water poured on my back." "I haven't had a wink of sleep in 2 months."

Examination reveals diverse corporal contortions such as twitching, turning, writhing, and rolling about, and the examiner's discovery of tender points is invariably vocally acknowledged by wails, moans, groans, and sharp intakes of breath or uncontrolled and alarming shouts.

No drug will give these patients a chemical vacation from their exhausting reaction to life. If the underlying cause of their symptoms can be recognized through the emotional smoke screen they have put up, it should be treated along routine lines. When the cause of the pain has been overcome, they will return to a way of life that is normal for them.

Hysterical reactions are common in childhood. When a child grazes the knee, he/she walks with a stiff leg. There is no need to do this; it is a hysterical response to injury: an exaggerated response for the purposes of gain, namely, attention and sympathy. In a child, this is understood and tolerated with a smile. In an adult, the same response generally irritates the physician and indeed may irritate him/her to such a degree that examination tends to be superficial, and treatment becomes perfunctory. At times, it is difficult to remember that these patients cannot control or modify their reactions: it is in their genes; they are built this way. The physician is treating a patient, not a spine, and regardless of the bizarre description of the symptoms and the histrionics on examination, the physician must accept the possibility of a physical disorder and investigate its probability, if indicated. (Classification: This patient is a psychogenic modifier: more often than not, with a minor physical problem.)

The Worried-Sick Syndrome Only a moron is totally unconcerned about the development of inexplicable symptoms. Most patients are concerned not only about the cause of their symptoms but also about their significance. Many have seen relatives in the terminal phases of malignancy whose last symptom was low back pain. Many people associate pain in the back with "arthritis," and this fear may be reinforced by being told previously that the "radiographs of the spine showed arthritic changes." To most patients, arthritis denotes a relentlessly progressive dread disease that leads eventually to confinement in a wheelchair.

These fears are common, although not commonly expressed. Above all else, the physician must reassure the patient and disabuse him/her of unfounded anxieties. If the patient has disc degeneration, he/she must never be told that the diagnosis is "arthritis of the spine."

Anxiety may be a form of intelligent concern, but in some persons who are born to worry, an almost pathological unfounded concern about their symptoms may be more disabling than the pain itself. These patients confuse the words "hurting" and "harming." Every time they do something that increases pain, they are terrified that they have done themselves irreparable damage. They treat their backs as though they are made of Dresden china, and are fearful of doing anything that may be painful. In the routine management of discogenic back pain, these patients may be told to avoid certain activities such as bending, lifting, playing tennis, or bowling. This is good advice, but they must also be told that these modifications of activity are suggested to decrease discomfort, not to prevent damage. Unless told this, patients may gradually cut themselves out of all activities until eventually they just vegetate.

"This back pain is completely ruining my life: I can't bowl, I can't ski, I can't play golf, I can't do anything," the patient may say. The doctor asks, "Do you get a lot of pain when you do these things?" The patient answers, "I don't know: I haven't done anything for 2 years." The doctor again queries, "Why haven't you tried to play a game of golf again?" The patient's answer is: "My doctor told me I shouldn't."

After weeks or months of inactivity, it will be extremely difficult to get these patients back to the business of normal living. Every increase in activity may be associated with a new twinge of pain that may frighten them back to the security of their beds. Their problems are compounded by apprehension and misapprehension, and the physician must deal firmly with both. (Classification: These patients have a variety of situational spinal pain. Although worried about their symptoms, they have not gone through complex psychodynamic mechanisms resulting in somatization. Rather, these patients simply need encouragement to deal in a more positive way with their symptoms and recognize the significant difference between hurt and harm.)

The Last Straw Factor The havoc wrought on a patient's life by back pain may destroy the patient's emotional stability; for example, look at the case of a patient who speaks little English and has no special skills, who works as a laborer in a small town and supports a wife and five children. An insecure job situation, because of industrial recession in the area, keeps him constantly concerned about his ability to keep up payments on his debts. The back pain resulting from an accident stops him from working for a few days. A recurrence without provocative trauma makes both the employer and the patient doubtful about his ability to hold down a job, and the third attack results in his unemployment. Inability to find alternative employment increases this man's debts, and articles of furniture are repossessed by the finance company. To this patient, his backache is the major disaster of his life, and his symptoms and signs may well be exaggerated beyond recognition.

This patient cannot be helped solely by measures directed at his back. His whole problem has to be alleviated, and the help of all social services has to be enlisted. (This patient not uncommonly seen can be classified as having psychogenic modification of organic spinal pain.)

The Camouflaged Emotional Breakdown Depressive states are common between the ages of 45 and 55. These patients, commonly very active when younger, find that as their energy level decreases, that is, as they move into second gear, they are increasingly unable to cope with the demands made on them. Despite the term "depression," they do not present a picture of melancholia. They demonstrate concealed or overt hostility. They are more easily provoked to anger and tears. They are increasingly critical of the faults they recognize in people around them. They are constantly tired, and sleep does not refresh them. They do not sleep well and frequently awaken early in the morning. They cannot make decisions. They do not want to go out, but they hate staying in. They lose their sense of fun. They claim that this unsociable state is the result of their wretched spine. Remember, a persistent backache seldom makes people miserable, but miserable people frequently have backache and complain loudly about it.

The back pain from which these patients suffer becomes a scapegoat to explain their inability to cope with life. "I was always a very active woman. I was president of the local parents/teachers association, I was one of the campaign organizers for the last election, and I always went with my husband on trips, but, with this backache, I am useless." These patients have an almost delusional belief in the organicity of their symptoms. They believe, and would like you to believe, that had it not been for the backache they would still be a leader in the community and, characteristically when reporting their history, they will constantly refer to this restriction in activities.

The curtailment of these patients' activities is not solely due to their backaches. If they were in better emotional health, they could cope with their discomforts, mollifying and minimizing their pain with mild analgesics and a slight modification of their daily activities. Simple therapeutic measures directed at the organic basis of these patients' complaints will not preempt them to return to normal activities. Failure of conservative treatment may lead to desperation surgery, which is nearly always attended by poor results and an aggravated deterioration in the patient's emotional health. Treatment must be directed at the patient as a whole, and psychiatric guidance must be sought early. (This mode is simply another variety of psychogenic modification.)

The "What If I Settle" Syndrome These patients bring a vague set of symptoms and little in the way of physical findings to the doctor-patient encounter. They are simply drifting in the sea of their minor symptoms, the wind in their sails sometimes provided by an unscrupulous lawyer hoping for prolonged symptoms, more investigation, and a larger "green poultice" in the end. If an unscrupulous doctor joins in the cause, the situation may never end for the patient. This unsuspecting and usually sincere patient has become a pawn of the professionals involved in his/her claim and care. A simple explanation to the patient will often bring matters to a satisfactory conclusion. (Classification: Obviously, this patient is in a litigation or compensation reaction.)

The "Head to Toe" Syndrome Although these patients rarely complain "outright" of pain from the tops of their heads to the tips of their toes, it becomes apparent during their history that there is no part of the body that does not hurt. They may represent psychogenic pain or, if secondary gain is involved, they may be magnifying their disability. As soon as the examiner recognizes that pain is present head to toe, there appears a resignation to our natural training as doctors to "give the patient the benefit of the doubt." This may be accompanied by a rather perfunctory examination, missing the historical and physical feature of magnification behavior. The charade goes on in an attempt to pump up damages to which, in the end, an unscrupulous lawyer makes substantial claim.

Rather, in this setting, the doctor should attempt to separate the patients into those who have emotional disability and are in need of counseling from those whose disability will disappear only when contentious issues are removed from their considerations (ie, settlement of the lawsuit).

It is apparent that these everyday clinical occurrences can be classified into psychosomatic, psychogenic, or situational spinal pains with or without some organic component. Once classified, treatment by the appropriate explanation and/or therapy can be intuited.

But wait! Is there any further help for assessing these patients?

ASSESSMENT OF NONORGANIC SPINAL PAIN

There are additional methods of assessing these conditions, including the pain drawing,(11) psychometric testing, and the pentothal pain study.(15) Although the orthopedic literature is full of descriptions of these various assessment methods, it is probably best that these assessment methods are conducted and interpreted by those skilled in the field. Orthopedic surgeons, by and large, are not skilled in these fields, and it is somewhat dangerous for them to be using these tests. These tests can be used to suggest the presence of a nonorganic component to the disability that results in referral of the patient to someone more skilled in the assessment of this aspect of disability. We do not use any of these ancillary assessment methods, but rather rely on history and physical examination findings described in the preceding sections. A brief description of these three assessment methods is offered.

Pentothal Pain Study

The introduction of the thiopental sodium pain assessment by Walters (15) has been of value in assessing the significance of emotional states in the production of the disability presented by the patient. The basis of this test lies in the fact that, in the state of light anesthesia, although the patient is unconscious, he/she is still capable of demonstrating primitive reactions to pain. The patient is anesthetized with thiopental in a slow fashion and then allowed to rouse until the corneal reflex returns. At this stage of anesthesia, the patient will withdraw from pinprick and will grimace when a painful stimulus is applied, such as squeezing the tendo Achillis. With the patient maintained at this level of anesthesia, maneuvers that were previously painful on clinical examination are re-evaluated. An example would be a patient who had SLR reduction of 20 degrees before induction of the thiopental sodium anesthesia. Theoretically, two extremes can occur. At one extreme, the 20-degree SLR reduction will persist under the light general anesthesia, a finding that may be taken as irrefutable evidence of significant root tension. If, on the other hand, at the stage of anesthesia when the patient will withdraw from pinprick, SLR, which was only 20 degrees on clinical examination, can now be carried out to 90 degrees without any response from the patient, the clinician may safely conclude that there is no evidence of root tension. It is likely that this patient's disability is due to an emotional reaction rather than to any organic source of pain.

If the patient previously had the diffuse, stocking-type of hypesthesia at this stage of narcosis, he will withdraw his limb when it is pricked by a pin. If, however, in addition to the hysterical response, there is a sensory loss due to root compression, then the patient will not show any response on pricking the skin over the dermatome of the root involved.

Thiopental sodium pain assessment is used in the patient with a combined nonorganic/organic disability. Its use is best confined to psychiatrists who have an interest in chronic pain, whereas the spinal surgeon relies on the symptoms and signs outlined in Table 12.6 to detect the potential for a nonorganic component to the disability.

Pain Drawing

The pain drawing (Fig. 12.15), popularized by Mooney and co-workers,(11) is a simple form of psychometric testing that can be done by the patients while in the waiting room. Patients do not mind doing a pain drawing, because they regard this as cooperating with the physician in keeping an adequate record of their symptoms. But patients have just the reverse reaction to psychometric testing. The pattern used by the patient to fill out the pain drawing weighs the disability toward an organic or a nonorganic basis. The pain drawing is based on the assumption that organic back pain will be distributed along axial (low back) or radicular structures. The reverse is true in nonorganic pain syndromes, leading patients to draw less distinct and more widespread pictures to describe their pain (Fig. 12.15).

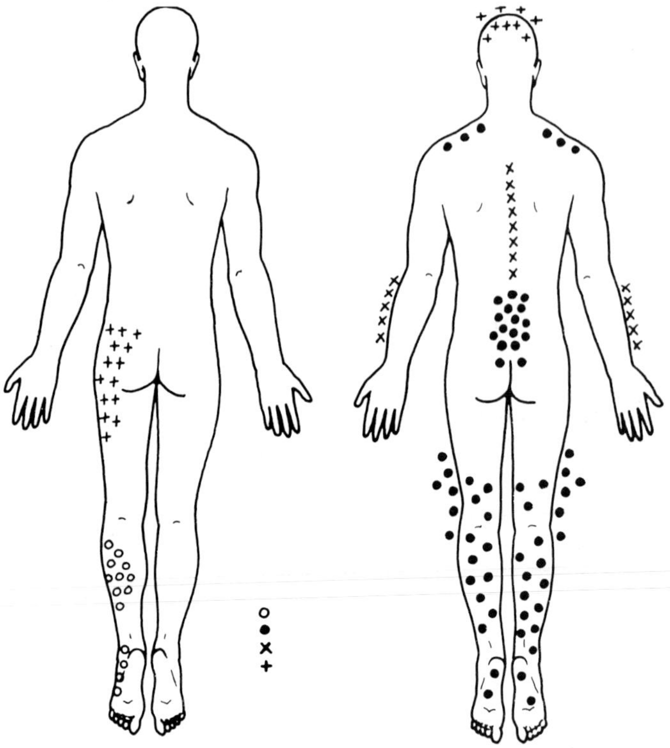

Figure 12.15 *The pain drawing. Each patient is asked to draw with +, ○, •, and x (+ = stabbing; ○ = numbness; • = pins and needles; x = burning) where they feel various pain sensations. The drawing to the left is by a patient with left sciatica. The drawing to the right is typical of a nonorganic pain patient.*

This is probably the safest assessment method for a spine surgical practice, but there are enough pitfalls in the use and interpretation of the test that it should be used by the orthopedic surgeon or neurosurgeon in a screening fashion only. Chan and co-workers (2) have demonstrated a good correlation between nonorganic pain drawings and a Waddell score (nonorganic historical and physical findings). An abnormal pain drawing should then result in referral of the patient to some other professional more skilled in the assessment of nonorganic disability.

Psychological Testing

Psychometric testing is a simple, rough guide to a patient's emotional health. The use and interpretation of these tests depend greatly on the experience of the user. Wiltse and Rocchio (16) have demonstrated convincingly that patients with a good emotional profile as shown on the Minnesota Multiphasic Personality Inventory (MMPI) studies could be confidently expected to obtain better results following chemonucleolysis than those patients in whom a psychological profile was abnormal. There are so many psychometric tests with various strengths and weaknesses that it again is suggested that the spinal surgeon who recognized the potential for a nonorganic component to the disability refer the patient to someone skilled in the use of these tests.

It has been frequently mentioned in this text that psychological testing should be conducted by individuals skilled in the field. The suggestion to a patient that you wish to explore psychological or emotional aspects of their disability (step) will often provoke hostile behavior. The basis for this is the patient's perception that this step implies that "there is nothing wrong with my back, it is all in my head." These patient referrals have to be handled with understanding and a clear statement that there is something wrong with their back, but that the step in this direction is an appropriate avenue for them to explore.

Tests the Patient May Encounter

Minnesota Multiphasic Personality Inventory (MMPI)

This is the most common psychological test used. It contains 550 true/false questions and is scored on 10 clinical scales. Scales 1 and 3, hypochondriasis (Hs) and hysteria (Hy), if high, have been associated with poor treatment outcomes.(16) Many studies have questioned the validity of these studies. Along with the fact that this test is long and tedious for patients to take, and contains many questions of a psychiatric nature, it is losing favor as a psychological test for low back pain patients.

McGill Pain Questionnaire (7)

This test is used to measure the quality of pain by asking patients to pick adjectives to describe their pain. This is a simpler test for patients and is easily scored.

There are many other tests available for psychological evaluation, and each psychologist has his/her favorites. Fortunately, there are many in the field willing to help in the evaluation of these patients.

CONCLUSION

Every human attends the school of survival. Sometimes, the lessons lead patients to modify or magnify a physical disability at a conscious or unconscious level. One word of caution: the presence of one of these nonorganic reactions does not preclude an organic condition such as an HNP. The art of medicine is truly tested by a patient with physical low back pain who modifies the disability with a nonorganic reaction such as tension, hysteria, depression, or other factors.

Low back pain is only a symptom; it will only become a chronic disease if we poorly diagnose, poorly treat, and carry out injudicious surgery. Then we are dealing with DISABILITY (see Chapter 21). The best way to prevent this expensive cascade of events is to understand the physical and non-physical aspects of back pain and help patients lead as close to normal lives as possible. Read on!!

REFERENCES

1. Bogduk N, Twomey LT. Clinical Anatomy of the Lumbar Spine. Melbourne, Australia: Churchill Livingstone; 1987.
2. Chan CW, Goldman S, Ilstrup DM, Kunselman AR, O'Neill PI. The pain drawing and Waddell's nonorganic physical signs in chronic low back pain. Spine 1993;18:1717–1722.
3. Guyton AC. Textbook of Medical Physiology. Philadelphia: WB Saunders; 1986.

4. Kellgren JH. On the distribution of pain arising from deep somatic structures with charts of segmental pain areas. Clin Sci Mod Med 1939;4:35–46.
5. Loeser JD. Concepts of pain. In: Stanton-Hicks M, Boas RA, eds. Chronic Low Back Pain. New York: Raven Press; 1982.
6. Malinsky J. The ontogenetic development of nerve terminations in the intervertebral disc of man. Acta Anat 1959;38:96–113.
7. Melzack R. The McGill Pain Questionnaire: major properties and scoring methods. Pain 1975;1:277–299.
8. Merskey R. Pain terms: a list with definitions and notes on usage. Pain 1979;6:249–252.
9. Mooney V, Robertson J. The facet syndrome. Clin Orthop 1976;115:149–156.
10. Noordenbos W: Prologue. In: Wall PD, Melzack R, eds. Textbook of Pain. Edinburgh, Scotland: Churchill Livingstone; 1984.
11. Ransford AO, Cairns D, Mooney V. The pain drawing as an aid to the psychological evaluation of patients with low back pain. Spine 1976;1:127–134.
12. Waddell G, McCulloch JA, Kummel EG, et al. Non-organic physical signs in low back pain. Spine 1980;5:117–125.
13. Waddell G, Morris EW, DiPaola MP, Bircher M, Finlayson D. A concept of illness tested as an improved basis for surgical decisions in low-back disorders. Spine 1986;11:712–719.
14. Wall PD, Melzack R. Textbook of Pain. Edinburgh, Scotland: Churchill Livingstone; 1984.
15. Walters A. Regional pain alias hysterical pain. Brain. 1961;84:1–18.
16. Wiltse LL, Rocchio PD. Preoperative psychological tests as predictors of success in chemonucleolysis in the treatment of low back syndrome. J Bone Joint Surg 1975;57A:478–483.
17. Yoshizawa H, O'Brien JP, Smith WT, et al. The neuropathology of intervertebral disc removed for low back pain. J Pathol 1980;132:95–104.

13

Treatment of Lumbar Disc Disease

"Physical pain is not a simple affair of an impulse, traveling at a fixed rate, along a nerve. It is the resultant of a conflict between a stimulus and the whole individual."

— Rene Leriche

INTRODUCTION

The symptoms of low back pain derived from disc degeneration are usually insidious in onset. A careful, detailed history commonly reveals that over a long period of time, the patient has been "conscious" of his or her back. Frequently, the patient will relate recurrent episodes of a "stiff back" or a "crick" in the back. More commonly, the patients will attribute the onset of symptoms to a specific incident; for example, "I spent a lot of time working in the garden." Occasionally, the onset is sudden, dramatic, unanticipated, and unrelated to any precipitating activity. The patient may awaken one morning with an extremely painful stiff back; during the passage of the day, the pain may radiate to the buttock and leg region, rendering the patient painfully immobile. Such episodes generally subside within 10 to 14 days with or without treatment but have an unfortunate tendency to recur. Eventually, the patient presents continuing symptoms affecting the axial skeleton and/or its neurological contents. With your knowledge of pathogenesis (Chapters 7 and 8), and the clinical examination (Chapters 9 and 10), you have established a diagnosis and can prepare for treatment.

The treatment decision in lumbar disc disease is based on a clear understanding of four factors:

1. Do you have an accurate diagnosis? Is this a soft tissue syndrome, a discogenic problem, a root encroachment problem, a cauda equina encroachment problem, or a combination of various syndromes?
2. Do you know the anatomical level?
3. Do you know your patient? Is he or she accurately reporting the disability, or is there some embellishment for medical-legal or compensation purposes?
4. What is the functional limitation? Is this collection of minor symptoms of nuisance value to the patient, or is there chronic cauda equina compression to the point that the patient needs aids for ambulation?

CONSERVATIVE TREATMENT

Choices in conservative treatment can be classified into:

1. Rest.
2. Medication.
3. Modalities.
4. Manipulation, mobilization, and massage.
5. Miscellaneous (eg, transcutaneous electrical nerve stimulation [TENS] unit, trigger point injections, and epidural steroids).
6. Exercise.
7. Education.

It is well to remember that TIME heals a lot of low back pain problems. Probably the most important treatment decision is to be patient. Do not get too aggressive, because most of the symptoms associated with lumbar disc disease are self-limiting and will go away spontaneously whether or not a doctor, physical therapist, or chiropractor is involved. How many spectacular cures have been claimed by these disciplines, when in fact the resolution of symptoms was due to the wonderful ability of the body to heal itself.

It is also well to remember that a sympathetic ear and reassurance to the patient that he/she does not have a serious problem (despite severe pain) will do more to restore the patient's good health than a wheelbarrow full of pills. It is also well to remember that the your best laid treatment plans can go astray because of unrecognized psychological and sociological problems confronting the patient.

Finally, remember that Big Brother is watching! Who is Big Brother? Big Brother is the government, the insurance company, and the managed care organizations who are paying for this treatment. They are tired (and rightfully so) of paying for unproved therapies, medical or surgical, and will bring pressure to bear that will shake out alot of what we are about to discuss.

Rest

There are many forms of rest, including bed rest, external braces, and traction. Even exercise, by rebuilding muscular strength, which in turn reduces stress on joints, can be included as a restful treatment modality.

Bed Rest

Occasionally, the pain is so severe that patients cannot cope with the daily activities of life, even with the help of analgesics, sedation, and wearing a brace. Under such circumstances, patients should be advised to go to bed. It must be remembered that the strained joints of the spine have to support the weight of the body, which can be significant. The only way to take this weight away from the posterior joints is to persuade the patient to lie down in bed.

Nachemson (24) has shown that the position that results in the greatest reduction in intradiscal pressure is supine, with appropriate pillow support (Fig. 13.1). Simply rolling over onto one's side or sitting propped up in bed defeats the purpose of bed rest. To condemn a patient to this fixed position in bed for longer than a few days has to constitute cruel and unusual punishment.

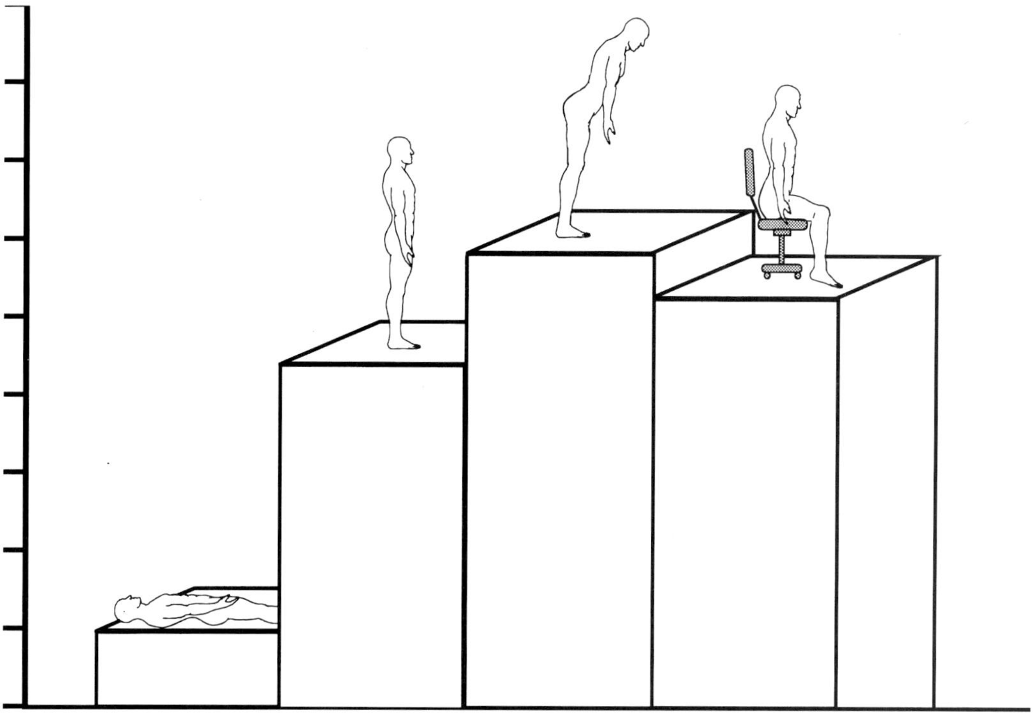

Figure 13.1 *Nachemson's disc pressure study has shown that the least pressure across the disc occurs when the patient is lying down. Sitting causes more stress on a disc than standing.*

Recent studies (6, 13, 18) suggest that the maximum amount of bed rest to be prescribed is 2 to 3 days. Bed rest beyond that period has no scientific support for being beneficial. In fact, prolonged bed rest will enforce in the patient's mind that he/she has a severe illness. While patients are building this scenario lying in bed, they will lose muscle mass, bone mass, and cardiopulmonary conditioning.(13) Add to that the economic loss of prolonged absence from work, and there is little to recommend bed rest beyond a few days.

Modification of Activities

Modification of activity can play a significant role in the management of back pain. Bending and lifting may aggravate back pain, and it may be possible to simply eliminate that activity and improve symptoms. In today's tough economic times, a suggestion to modify work too often leads to a layoff. For this reason we play down work modification unless the pain is terribly acute and requires bed rest, or the chronic pain is not resolving with other treatment measures, and there is a clearly defined work aggravation. Dr. Macnab always taught that "it is better to change a worker's job to relieve chronic back pain rather than change their back with an operation." How true that is !

Orthoses (Bracing)

Since the earliest of times, bracing has been a staple of managing low back problems. The Quebec Task Force (26) on low back pain concluded that there is little scientific evidence to support the use of corsets to treat low back pain. Why, after 2500 years of medical prescription, do the highly intelligent health care professions not have an answer to why we use braces?

Theoretically, braces are used to immobilize the lumbar spine, stabilize abnormal motion segments, maintain alignment, and correct deformity. Braces do well in treating scoliosis, but in the treatment of degenerative conditions of the spine, they do none of the previously mentioned functions. Braces may immobilize the L1–L4 motion segment, but unless they hold onto the thigh (Fig. 13.2), they may actually increase motion at L4–L5 and L5–S1, where the bulk of low back problems occur. Theory has replaced science, with more than 25% of low back pain patients being placed in an orthoses at one time or another. These various appliances are shown in Figure 13.3 . There is no doubt that they increase intra-abdominal pressure, which in turn supports the lumbar spine; also, there is no doubt that braces remind the patient that something is wrong with their back and they should be protective. Beyond that, there is little to support braces' "joint immobilization" ability or other benefits.

The routine use of orthotics in the treatment of low back pain is to be discouraged. Over the long haul, most low back pains will subside, and they do so with sustained relief if the back and abdominal muscles have not been weakened by the crutch of a brace.

Figure 13.2 *A lumbar brace with a thigh extension is the only way to immobilize a lumbar spine when the patient wishes to be ambulatory. There are very few patients who will tolerate this trial.*

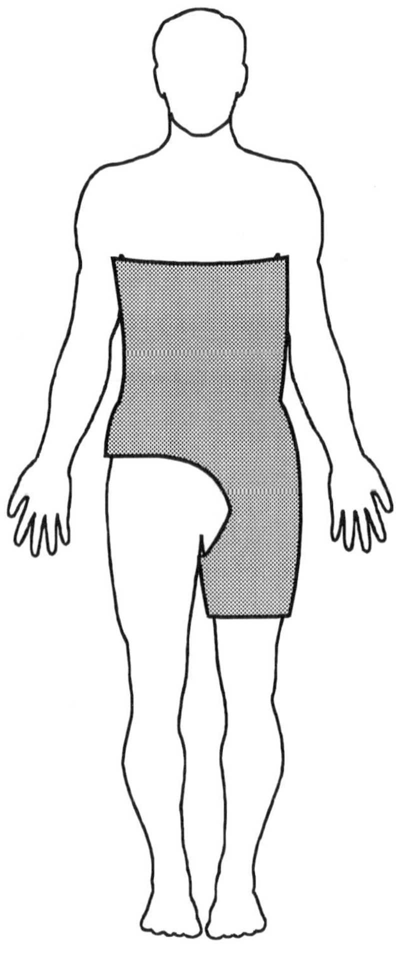

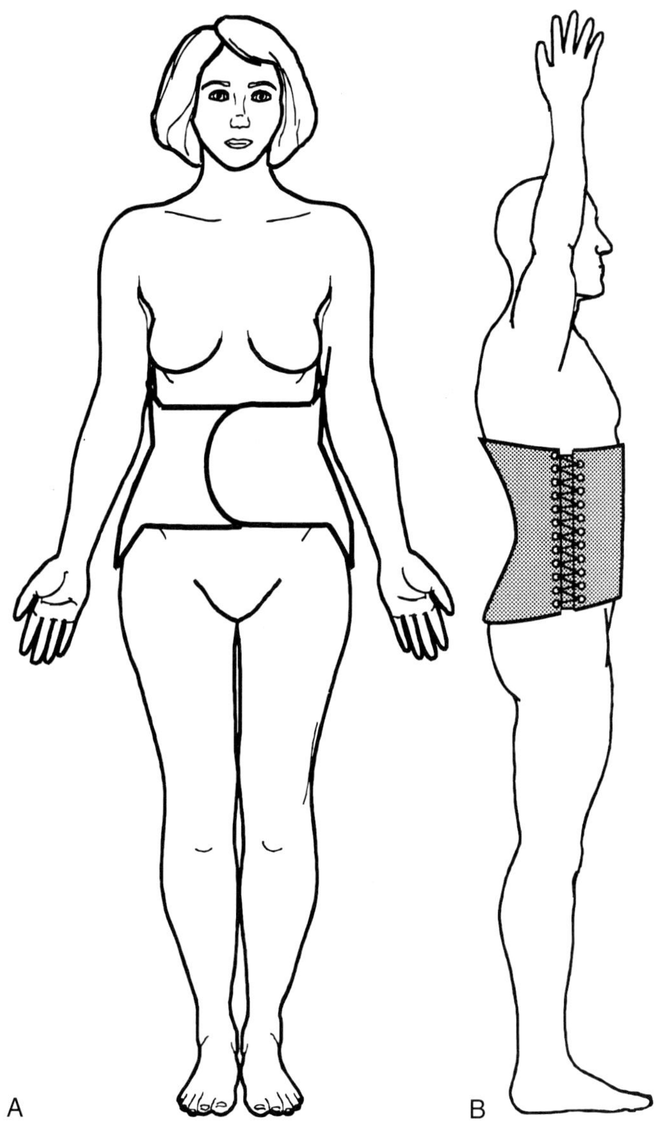

Figure 13.3 *Various lumbar corsets:* **A.** *Warm-n-form corset that has a molded insert posteriorly;* **B.** *Lace-up "Camp" corset.*

The indications for orthotic use are:

1. A patient who is recovering after bed rest and wishes to return to work quickly. In this situation, the corset becomes a "bed on the back" that allows the patient limited ambulation.
2. Postoperative support.
3. An older patient who is not a candidate for surgery, or who does not wish to consider surgery, but wishes to achieve a more comfortable level of movement for activity.

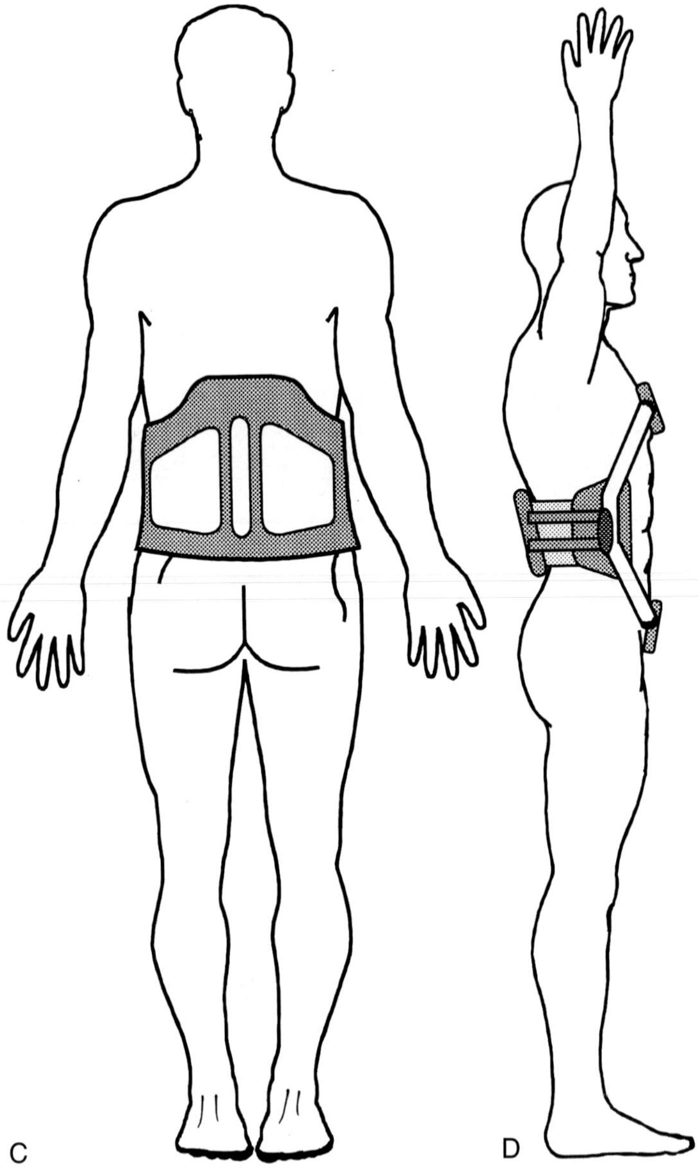

Figure 13.3 (continued) **C.** *Chair-back brace;* **D.** *A hyperextension brace (Jewett-type).*

Type of Corset Everyone has their own favorite corset or brace and a good reason for using it. Remember:

- The only way to totally immobilize a spine is to put the patient to bed.
- Most corsets and braces function as abdominal binders that in turn support the back.
- To achieve some measure of control of lumbar spine movement, it is necessary to take the orthosis well down over the iliac crests and up onto the rib cage. This results in a cumbersome corset that tests patient compliance.

The authors have no specific recommendations for particular types of corsets, except to suggest simple abdominal corsets for temporary use and more molded, individually fitted braces for more rigid support and longer use (Fig. 13.3). Do not make the mistake of using a short orthosis for a high lumbar problem, which will transfer more mobility to the level of the lesion and aggravate rather than relieve the patient's pain.

Adequate trunk muscles are the major guardians against repeated attacks. It must be remembered that the spinal column is not a self-supporting structure. If the trunk and abdominal muscles are paralyzed, such as in infantile paralysis, the spine collapses. The spine is supported by muscle action in much the same way that the mast of a ship is supported by stays (Fig. 13.4). In addition to this, the abdominal cavity acts as a hydraulic sac, dissipating loads by pressing upward on the diaphragm and downward on the pelvic floor, thereby unweighting the spine (Fig. 13.5). Because of this, the tone and strength of the abdominal muscles are of vital importance in protecting the spine against weight-bearing and extension strains.

The prolonged wearing of a corset or brace will be uncomfortable to the patient and will result in muscle atrophy and loss of function. The psychological aspects of brace wearing are largely negative. Finally, some patients will not even comply with your prescription for a corset.

Our recommendation is that orthoses be used sparingly. Certainly, they are useful in the treatment of scoliosis deformity, but in the management of low back pain they should be limited to short-term use in acute low back pain and in the postoperative patient.

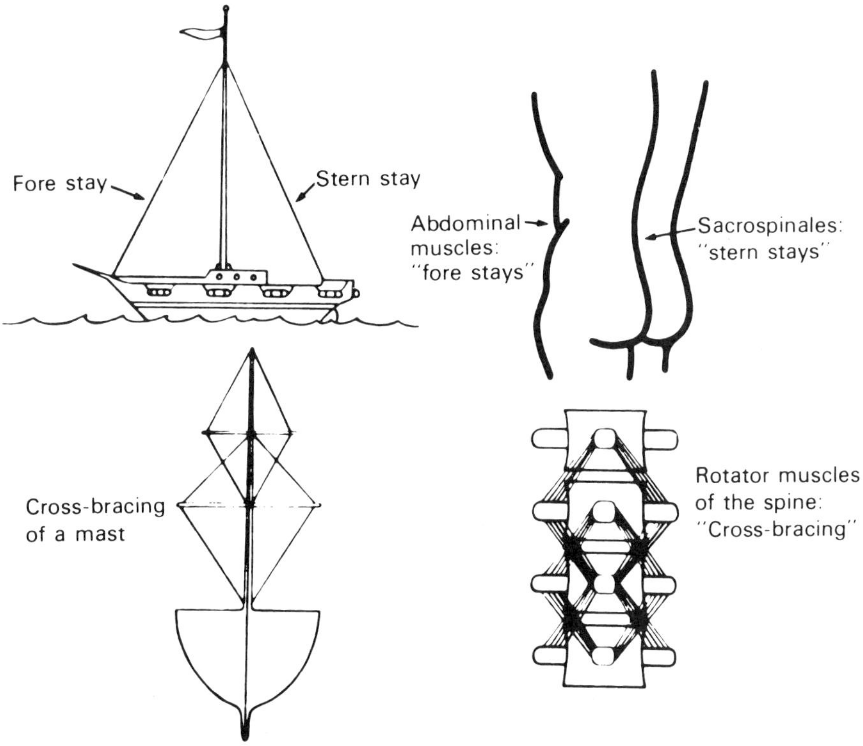

Figure 13.4 *It is interesting to note the similarity between the bracing used to support the mast of a ship and the muscular bracing of the human spine.*

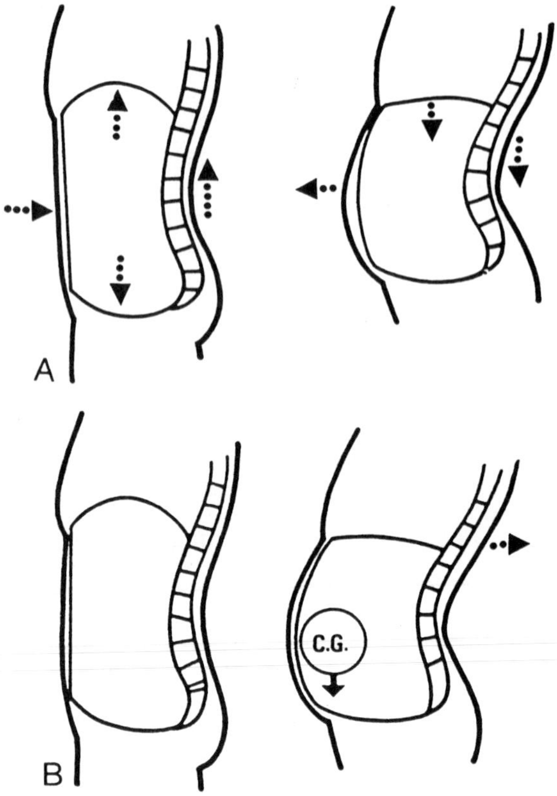

Figure 13.5 **A.** *The abdominal cavity acts in a manner similar to a hydraulic sac. By increasing intra-abdominal pressure, the diaphragm is pushed up, and the pelvic floor is pushed down. This tends to "elongate" the lumbar spine, thereby taking some of the weight off the discs and the posterior joints.* **B.** *Obesity, by pulling the center of gravity forward, causes the spine to hyperextend.*

Traction

Traction has also been used over the centuries to treat low back pain on the theory that stretching the muscles and separating the vertebrae will have a positive effect on the disc. (34) Some theorize that pulling the vertebrae apart will allow a "dislocated" disc to recede back into the disc space,(30) something yet to be shown on CT or MRI.

There are various forms of traction: continuous in hospital; intermittent in physical therapy; auto-traction (patient controlled); and gravity traction (Fig. 13.6). The amount of weight required to affect the disc space is at least 25% of body weight, which either pulls the patient to the end of the bed or is not tolerated. The Quebec Task Force (26) has concluded that traction is not effective in the treatment of acute or chronic low back pain, a conclusion with which we concur.

Medication

Analgesics

Analgesics are usually the first line medications for pain. (14) The choices are simple: use nonnarcotics (acetaminophen) or narcotic medication in increasing potency (Table 13.1) for

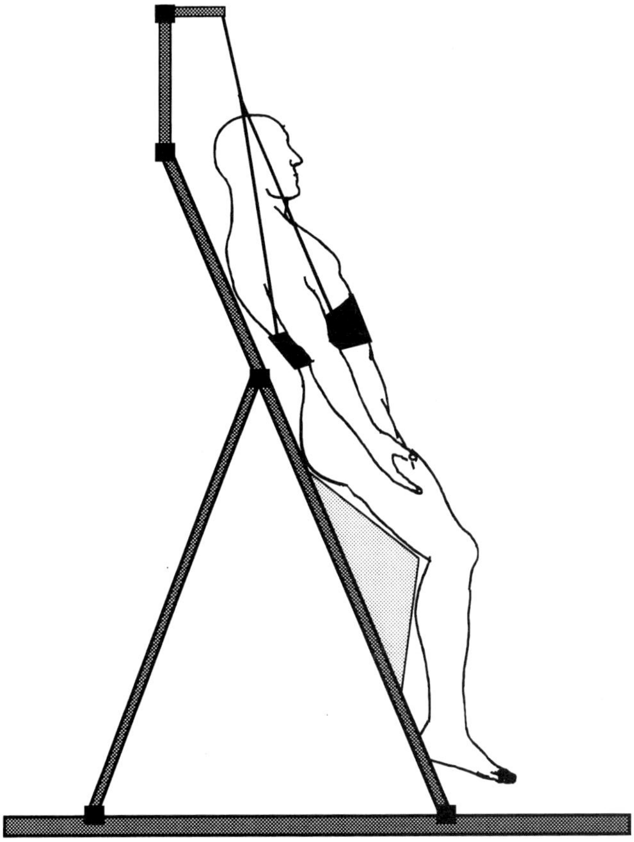

Figure 13.6 *Gravity lumbar traction.*

Table 13.1. Analgesic Medications

1. Nonnarcotic-ASA, NSAIDs
2. Narcotic analgesics
   a. Moderate pain (agonists)
      Codeine
      Hydrocodone-(Vicodin)
      Oxycodone (Percodan, Percocet, Tylox)
      Propoxyphene (Darvon)
   b. Moderate-to-severe pain (agonists)
      Meperidine (Demerol)
      Morphine
      Hydromorphone (Dilaudid)
      Levorphanol (Levo-Dromoran)
   c. Moderate pain (mixed agonists/antagonists)
      Pentazocine (Talwin)

more severe pain. There are obvious problems with the introduction of pain medication in a patient with a potentially chronic low back problem; the use of narcotics and the symptom of back pain may become chronic together.(32) For this reason, nonsteroidal anti-inflammatory drugs have become a very popular method of dealing with musculoskeletal pain.

Nonsteroidal Anti-inflammatory Drugs (NSAIDs)

Because of their analgesic, anti-inflammatory, and antipyretic actions, NSAIDs have become a popular group of drugs. (3, 18, 31) They are thought to act at the (peripheral) site of injury, rather than centrally, by blocking prostaglandin synthesis; prostaglandins supposedly sensitize free nerve endings to nociceptor impulses. The equation is simple: inflammation leads to increased prostaglandin synthesis and thus pain: anti-inflammatories decrease the prostaglandin synthesis of inflammation and thus decrease pain. At low doses, NSAIDs are analgesic and at higher sustained doses they are anti-inflammatory.

Metabolism of NSAIDs occurs in the liver, but side effects are largely confined to the gastrointestinal tract and the kidneys.(2) Indomethacin and phenylbutazone have the added toxicity of bone marrow suppression. The older patient is especially prone to these side effects from those NSAIDs with a long half-life (Dolobid [Merck & Co, West Point, PA]; Naprosyn [Syntex, Palo Alto, CA]; Clinoril [Merck & Co]; Feldene [Pratt Pharmaceuticals, New York, NY]). Doses of these drugs have to be lower in the geriatric population. Anyone with GI upset, young or old, has to either receive gastric protection (eg, H2-receptor antagonists like Tagamet [SmithKline Beecham Pharmaceuticals, Philadelphia, PA], or synthetic prostaglandins like Cytotec [misoprostol, Searle, Chicago, IL]) or have the NSAID discontinued. Because NSAIDs cause water retention, hypertensive patients need careful monitoring of their blood pressure. NSAIDs also inhibit platelet aggregation, and most surgeons ask patients to stop taking anti-inflammatory drugs for 10 days before surgery. Table 13.2 lists the commonly used NSAIDs.

Gastrointestinal complications are the most common side effects of NSAIDs and deserve special mention.(2) The chance of a patient who is receiving NSAIDs developing an ulcer (gastric or duodenal) ranges from 2 to 20%; approximately 20% to 40% of patients admitted to hospitals with acute upper GI bleeding have been receiving NSAIDs. To prevent these complications, Babb (2) recommends the following:

1. Prescribe the lowest possible dose, and avoid combinations with other NSAIDs and corticosteroids.

Table 13.2. Commonly Used NSAIDs

Class	Chemical Name	Trade Name
Salicylates	Aspirin	Numerous
	Enteric-coated ASA	Ecotrin
Salicylate substitutes	Diflunisal	Dolobid
	Salsalate	Disalcid
Propionic acid derivatives	Ibuprofen	Motrin
	Naproxen	Naprosyn
	Ketoprofen	Orudis
	Flurbiprofen	Ansaid
	Ketorolac Tromethamine	Toradol
Indoles (acetic acids)	Sulindac	Clinoril
	Indomethacin	Indocin
	Tolmetin	Tolectin
Oxicam	Piroxicam	Feldene
Pyrazolones	Phenylbutazone	Butazolidin

2. If patients especially at risk for NSAID gastropathy (the elderly, the chronically ill, and those with a history of peptic ulcer disease) have to be given an NSAID, prophylactic ulcer therapy should be considered.
3. The prevention of NSAID ulcers remains controversial. Misoprostol (Cytotec) helps to prevent gastric ulcers, but its use in duodenal ulcer prophylaxis is unclear. H2-receptor antagonists, such as ranitidine (Zantac, Glaxo Pharmaceuticals, Research Triangle Park, NC), help prevent duodenal ulcers but not gastric ulcers.

Corticosteroids

Corticosteroids are mentioned mainly to caution against their use. On occasion, an acute radicular pain is so severe that a very aggressive short-term therapy program lasting 3 to 7 days may be instituted. A Medrol (Upjohn, Kalamazoo, MI) dose pack is a convenient way to prescribe. Frequent use of this treatment modality in your practice, or prolonged use in an individual, is simply not good medical judgment.

Muscle Relaxants

The next most-used group of drugs for lumbar conditions are the muscle relaxants, and nobody can explain why. They all work on the central nervous system (CNS), with hopeful transfer of the action to the peripheral site of muscle spasm.(8) No scientific proof exists to support this transfer phenomenon. The common muscle relaxants are cyclobenzaprine (Flexeril, Merck & Co, West Point, PA); orphenadrine citrate (Norflex, 3M Pharmaceuticals, St. Paul, MN); chlorzoxazone (Parafon Forte DSC, McNeil Pharmaceutical, Raritan, NJ); methocarbamol (Robaxin, Robins Company, Richmond, VA); carisoprodol (Soma, Wallace, Cranbury, NJ); and diazepam (Valium, Roche Products, Nutley, NJ). To make them even more attractive, drug manufacturers have parceled them together with analgesics: Norflex + acetylsalicylic acid (ASA) + caffeine (Norgesic, 3M Pharmaceuticals); methocarbamol + ASA (Robaxisal, Robins Company); and carisoprodol + codeine (Soma Compound with codeine, Wallace). When the side effects of depression and a "spaced-out" feeling are combined with the potential for habituation—and in light of the cost of these drugs and the lack of scientific support for their usefulness—one has to wonder why so many muscle relaxants are prescribed.

Antidepressants

Patients who suffer from chronic pain are thought to become depressed because of, or in addition to, depletion of serotonin in the brain. Antidepressants supposedly increase serotonin production in the CNS, which in turn inhibits pain.(28, 35) Other antidepressant effects are to increase activity in the endogenous opiate system and to decrease anxiety and muscle tension. Commonly used antidepressants are imipramine (Tofranil, Geigy Pharmaceuticals, Summit, NJ); amitriptyline (Elavil, Stuart, Wilmington, DE); and doxepin (Sinequan, DuPont Pharma, Wilmington, DE, and Roerig, New York, NY).

Antidepressants have a high incidence of side effects, including frequent cross-drug reactions with antihypertensive and glaucoma medication. Unless you are prepared to closely monitor the patient for side effects, do not use these drugs.

Modalities

How often have you written a prescription for physical therapy and wondered: "What will happen to the patient in that department in the basement?" One of the common things a physical therapist does is change the temperature of the affected body part.(19)

Ice

Ice packs decrease circulation to the area of contact, which reduces swelling, spasm, and therefore pain. Ice is used in the form of massage or ice packs and is only useful in acute low back pain.

Heat

Heat may be superficial (hot packs or infrared) or deep (ultrasound or shortwave diathermy). The heat increases blood flow to the damaged or inflamed tissue, clearing away noxious metabolites and bringing oxygen to the area. Heat also increases the stretchability of collagen tissue. Because of the increased vasodilatation, heat should not be used in the acute phase of injury.

Manipulation, Mobilization, and Massage

The laying on of hands! This act alone has a significant placebo effect on patients. Controversy surrounds these modalities, yet the practitioners of these manual efforts continue to make patients better.(9, 10, 11, 16, 17, 27, 29, 33) Massage is designed to break down scar tissue and stretch local muscles. It is a very soothing therapy.

Manipulation is practiced largely by the chiropractic community, while mobilization is a tool of the physical therapist.(30) The latter practitioner feels it is safer and gentler to mobilize a painful joint by passively coaxing a joint (or joints, as in the case of the back) to its normal physiological range of movement. Chiropractic theory, on the other hand, proposes that sudden, assisted, passive joint motion—just beyond the normal range of movement—is more effective in stretching muscles, reducing subluxated joints, and increasing joint movement.(11) The trick with manipulation is to take a patient's joint(s) up to, but not beyond, the anatomical limits of movement. That is why the skill requires training (chiropractic or osteopathic school) and why the techniques are largely safe. Although the occasional serious consequence to manipulation occurs, such as a massive disc herniation and cauda equina syndrome,(12) it is with such infrequency that manipulation, in the hands of a skilled practitioner of the art, is safe.

But is this type of manipulation effective? The majority of studies that we have reviewed (11, 17, 29) support the use of manipulative techniques for acute low back pain without a major neurological deficit. However, use as a "maintenance" (prophylactic) effort or in the treatment of chronic low back pain does not appear to be beneficial.(11)

Despite the apparent effectiveness of manipulation, no one has a universally accepted theory as to why it works. The sudden thrust is supposed to reduce subluxation of lumbar joints and break down muscle spasm. Listening to the cracking that occurs during the maneuver, patients know that something has happened! Yet pre- and post-manipulation radiographic studies have failed to show "reduction" of joint subluxations, or reduction in the size of a herniated disc fragment.

Besides a yet-as-unexplained benefit of manipulation, chiropractors routinely offer a more sympathetic ear and a better explanation of the benefits of their care when compared with doctors.(17) Obviously, this reflects in outcome studies when chiropractic care is compared to other modalities. Suffice it to say, if you are in a primary care practice, a good relationship with a good chiropractor will benefit some of your patients who have acute low back pain.

Manipulation is not indicated in patients with a significant disc herniation causing neurological compression, nor should it be used in osteopenic patients or patients who are receiving anticoagulants.

Physical Therapy

Physical therapists bring a different perspective to the management of low back pain. Therapists who are interested in managing this very unique and, at times, trying patient population are a valuable asset. But therapists who have little interest in back pain or who simply apply hot packs and send a patient home with a picture of some exercises should probably be kept out of the loop of treatment.

Physical therapists are less pathoanatomy/pain oriented and are more tuned into the function that actually causes the pain. Through the design of a proper exercise program and education, therapists try to improve function primarily, which in turn reduces pain. They do this by choosing an exercise program to strengthen back and abdominal muscles and increase low back flexibility. Overall fitness and postural instructions are an important part of a therapist's re-education program for the patient.

Choice of Exercises Exercises are either localized, to strengthen back muscles or stretch shortened muscle fibers, or generalized to improve cardiovascular fitness.

The two popular low back floor exercise programs are the Williams flexion program and the McKenzie hyperextension program (34) (Figs. 13.7 and 13.8).

The Williams program is designed to strengthen abdominal muscles and reduce lumbar lordosis, which in turn opens the facet joints and widens the exiting foramen. The McKenzie program is designed to shift the nucleus pulposus forward in the disc cavity, reducing its pressure effects on the posterior annulus and nerve roots. An effective extension program "centralizes" pain, that is, reduces leg pain and increases central back pain. This transfer of pain location can then be treated with a Williams program. The Williams flexion program tends to be more effective for back pain that occurs with walking and standing, whereas the McKenzie program is more effective for leg pain that is increased by sitting. These are not hard and fast rules, which is why an effective exercise program requires supervision by a physical therapist.(5, 15) The use (and choice) of modalities before exercise is also something the physical therapist can use to maximize the effectiveness of exercise.(30)

Back School

Therapists have long recognized that helping a patient understand the anatomy of the lumbar spine, the pathology that has them disabled, and the theory behind treatment proposals will lead to better outcomes. This educational effort has been formally organized as a "Back School." There are many models throughout the world (1), but they all involve classroom instruction with appropriate visual aids and demonstration of physical do's

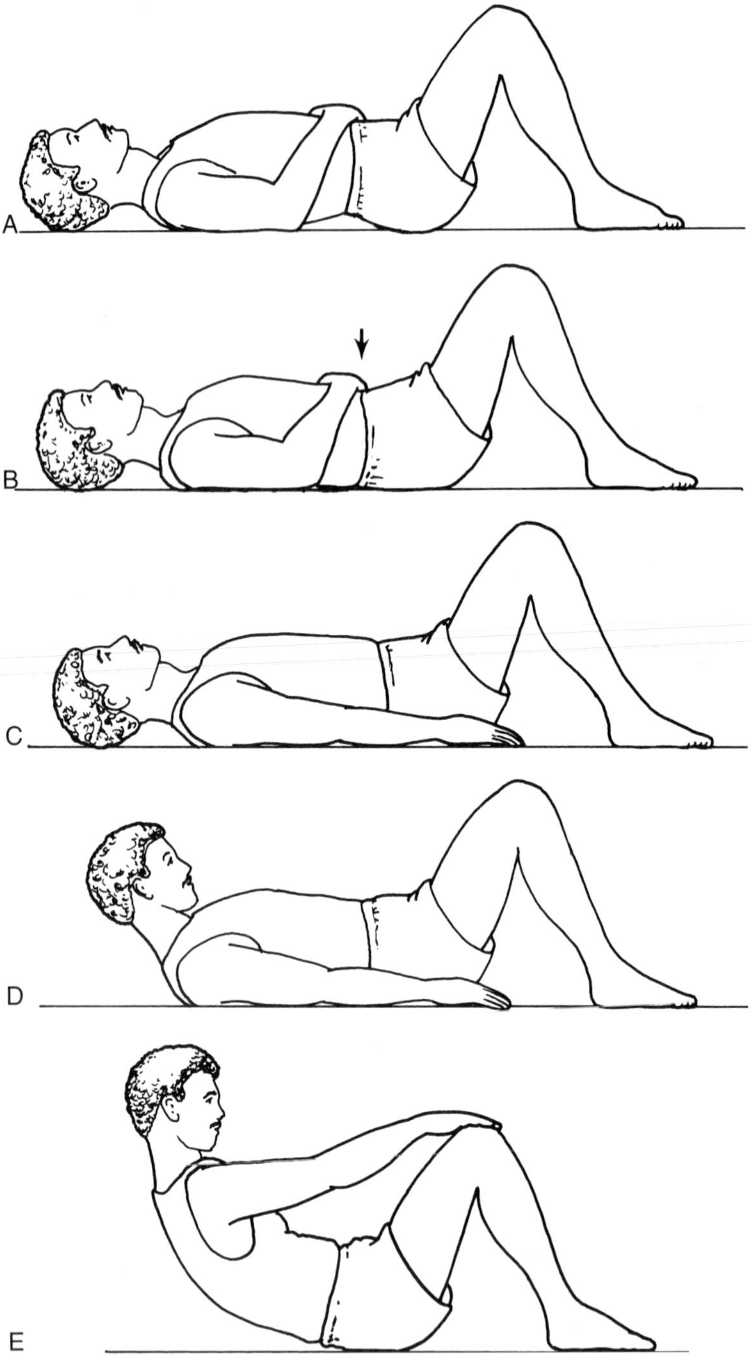

Figure 13.7 *Williams flexion exercises:* **A.** *Relaxation phase;* **B.** *Pelvic tilt by abdominal flexion;* **C.** *Relaxation phase;* **D.** *Partial sit-up;* **E.** *Full sit-up.*

and don'ts, as well as motivational or psychological support. The theory is that by helping the patient understand his/her problem, the patient is better able to take control of the pain and cope with it in a more reasonable fashion.

Back schools range from a few classroom lectures to extensive inpatient programs that are part of a comprehensive spine rehabilitation program. These programs are more suc-

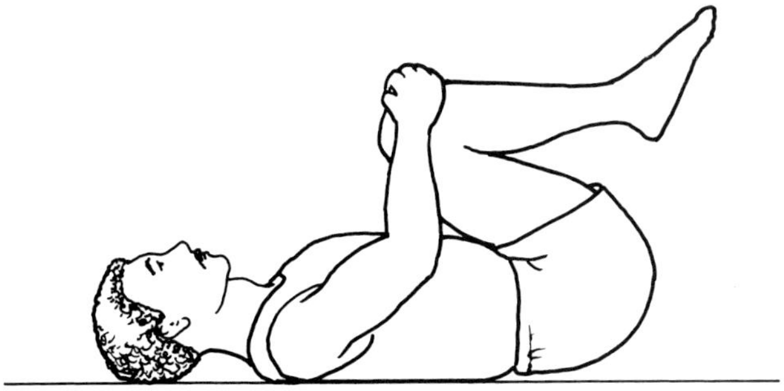

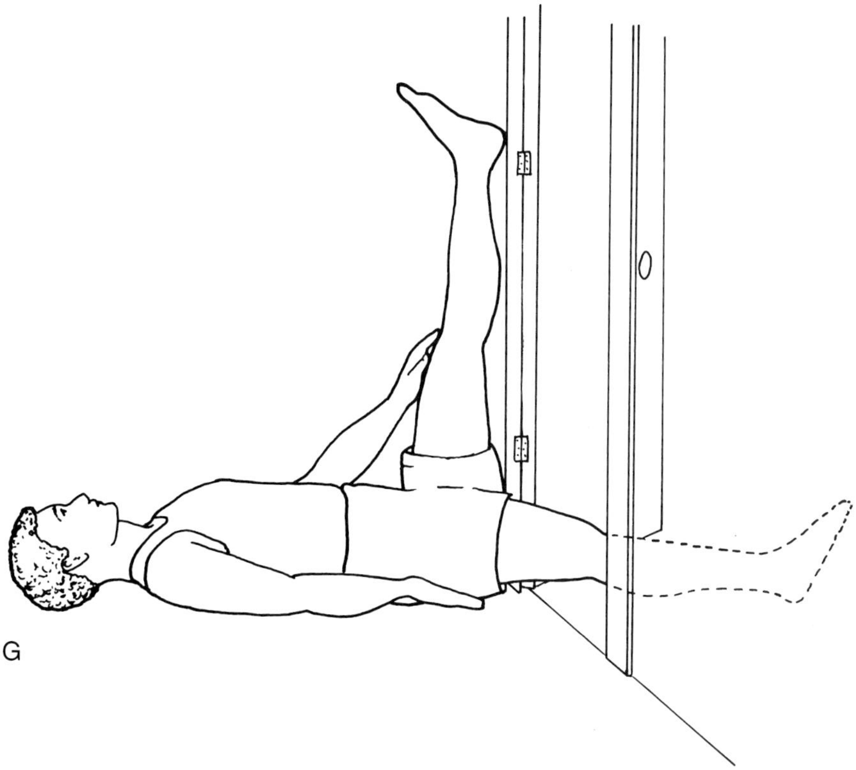

Figure 13.7 (continued) **F.** *Bilateral knee flexion roll;* **G.** *Hamstring stretch of left leg. Each exercise is done for a set time and repetition as set down by the therapist.*

cessful in the management of chronic pain, but are used in some industrial settings to try and return the acutely injured worker back to work quickly.

Work Hardening

An extension of the back school is the rehabilitation effort directed at returning a patient to heavy work. Although many patients do not need work hardening, there are a group of patients that should go through such a program. These include chronic pain patients and those postoperative patients who are facing a return to heavy work.

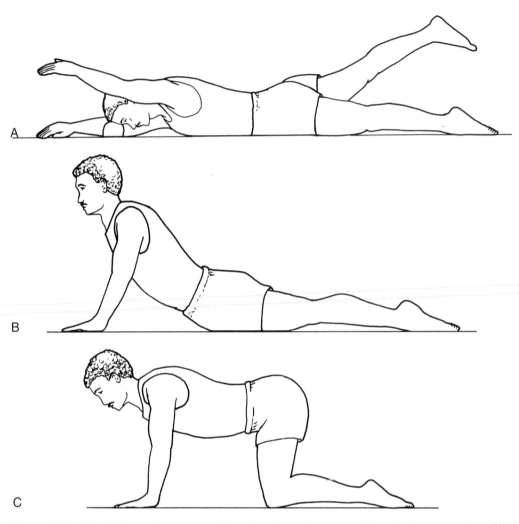

Figure 13.8 *The McKenzie Routine:* **A.** *Extension of opposite arm and leg;* **B.** *Hyperextension of back;* **C.** *Hyperextension of back in kneeling position.*

A work hardening program focuses more on a graded work simulation than on pain and increased physical activity. The multidisciplinary team builds realistic industrial settings in which the patient is encouraged to build the physical and psychological fitness to work. Through graduated steps, the patient ends up "working" a full day in a work hardening program and soon concludes he/she is capable of doing a full day's work for which he/she might as well be paid.

Miscellaneous

Injections

A number of injection therapies have been used in the treatment of low back pain. These include:

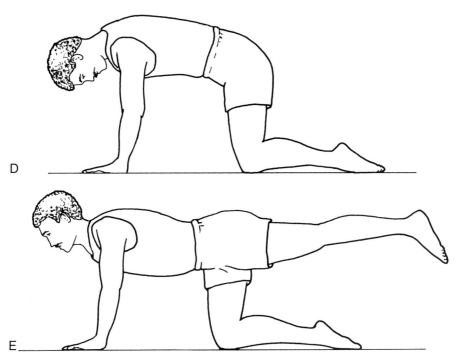

Figure 13.8 (continued) **D.** *Flexion of back;* **E.** *Extension of hip. Each exercise is done for a set time and repetition as set down by the therapist.*

1. Epidural cortisone.(4, 36)
2. Trigger point.(20)
3. Facet joint.(23)
4. Nerve blocks.(23)
5. Intramuscular injection.

Most of these injections are a combination of local anesthetics and steroids. There is no doubt that these treatments have a short-term benefit, but studies to support their long-term benefit are lacking.

Epidural cortisone, although not proved to be effective in the treatment of acute radicular pain, can be useful in the management of the chronic pain of spinal stenosis or in the postoperative patient who develops recurrent leg pain without a recurrent disc rupture that is documented on magnetic resonance imaging.

Nerve blocks, including sympathetic blocks, are useful in some of the causalgic/reflex sympathetic dystrophy pains that affect the lower extremity.

Transcutaneous Electrical Nerve Stimulation (TENS)

Live better electrically! TENS units theoretically close gates in the CNS (Fig. 13.9). By transcutaneously sending an electrical impulse into the peripheral nerve, the large (fast-conducting) myelinated A-alpha nerve fibers are stimulated such that the smaller (slower conducting) unmyelinated C fibers are blocked at the gate from transmitting their nociceptor impulses. It is sort of like the big guy beating up on the little guy so that he is not heard from! Whether this concept works is presently under serious scrutiny.(5, 7, 37)

Figure 13.9 *A TENS unit is attached to the patient's right belt line: it will stimulate electrode pads on the patient's low back and right thigh.*

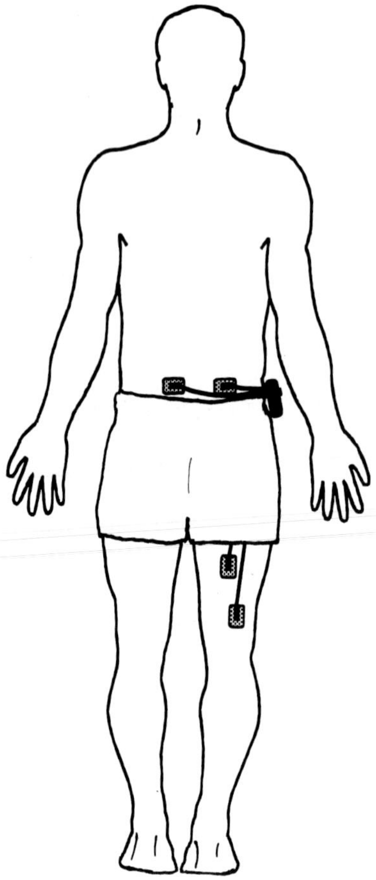

Acupuncture

Again, controversy abounds! The theory makes sense: acupuncture is a counterirritant and a stimulator of endorphin release. It is also thought to close gates and modulate the transfer of painful stimuli to higher CNS centers.(21) In North America, it is hard to find scientific evidence to support acupuncture's efficacy.(22)

Nutrition and Low Back Pain

We are often asked if there is any change that can be made in the diet to heal or prevent low back problems. Aside from the dietary recommendations for osteopenic patients, we are not aware of any study that suggests that additions to, or deletions from, a normal diet are beneficial to low back pain.

Biofeedback and Relaxation Therapy

Those proponents of biofeedback and relaxation therapy are "centralists." They believe that chronic pain leads to a depressive or vegetative state. This change in personality can change the perception of pain, and if the clinician concentrates on peripheral treatment only (injections, exercise therapy, and so on), he/she will miss the central influence of the patient's mind. Persons teaching biofeedback (the measurement of peripheral effects of muscle spasm) or relaxation techniques use the mind to positively influence the peripheral cause and the central appreciation of pain. However, few studies support this approach.(25)

Prevention of Low Back Pain

It is often said that preventing a condition from occurring is better than having to treat a condition. Unfortunately, the aging process is universal and will eventually cause some back pain in 80% of the population. Deyo's study (5) showed limited evidence to recommend exercise as a preventative tool. Further, there was no evidence to support the use of back school, mechanical supports, and/or risk factor (smoking, weight loss) modification as being useful in the prevention of low back pain.

Evaluation of Conservative Treatment Measures

It is simply amazing how treatment measures have continued to be used over decades with little or no scientific support for their efficacy. Not any more! Those paying the costs are demanding proof of usefulness. This pressure has brought to a head just how difficult it is to design adequate studies on the usefulness of conservative treatment measures to treat low back pain. Compared with studies on a fractured femur, studies on low back pain are flawed because of poorly defined diagnoses, spontaneous cures, and additional factors such as psychological and sociological pressures. Even a well-designed study requires a large number of patients: some patients will leave the study; others will add another treatment at the suggestion of a friend; and some will simply get better because they are being studied. It is all very frustrating, but fortunately we are dealing with a self-limiting disease.

Duration of Treatment

Most lumbar degenerative conditions, except for some spinal canal stenoses, are self-limiting. There is no rush to the operating room. It is recommended that a minimum of 6 weeks of conservative treatment be tried before considering investigation that may lead to surgical intervention. Before taking this step, emphasize to the patient that there is hurt, not harm, in living with back and/or leg symptoms, and only when symptoms interfere significantly with activities of daily living and fail to respond to conservative care should investigation and surgery be considered.

CONCLUSION

There are many conservative treatment measures that are available to treat the largely self-limiting affliction of low back pain. There are many professions offering "cures" for low back pain that use one or more of these modalities. To all, it is a time for science, a time for controlled studies to prove or disprove efficacy. When these studies are completed, we suspect we could shorten this chapter to one or two pages!

REFERENCES

1. Andersson GBJ. Back schools. In: Jayson MIV, ed. The Lumbar Spine and Back Pain, 3rd ed. Edinburgh, Scotland: Churchill Livingstone, pp 315–320, 1987.
2. Babb RR. Editorial: Be cautious in the use of NSAIDs. Orthop Review. 1992;21:687–688.
3. Brooks PM, Day RO. Nonsteroidal anti-inflammatory drugs: differences and similarities. N Engl J Med 1991;324:1716–1725.
4. Cuckler JM, Bernini PA, Wiesel SW, Booth RE, Rothman RH, Pickens GT. The use of epidural steroids in the treatment of lumbar radicular pain: a prospective, randomized double blind study. J Bone Joint Surg 1985;67A:63–66.
5. Deyo RA. Conservative therapy for low back pain: Distinguishing useful from useless therapy. JAMA 1983;250:1057–1062.
6. Deyo RA, Diehl AK, Rosenthal M. How many days of bed rest for acute low back pain? A randomized clinical trial. N Engl J Med 1986;315:1064–1070.
7. Deyo RA, Walsh NE, Martin DC, Schoenfeld L, Ramamurthy S. A controlled trial of transcutaneous electrical nerve stimulation (TENS) and exercise for chronic low back pain. N Engl J Med 1990;322:1627–1634.
8. Elenbaas JK. Centrally acting oral skeletal muscle relaxants. Am J Hosp Pharm 1980;37: 1313–1323.
9. Friedman LW, Galton L. Freedom from Backaches. New York: Simon & Schuster; 1973.
10. Godfrey CM, Morgan PP, Schatzker J. A randomized trial of manipulation for low-back pain in a medical setting. Spine 1984;9:301–304.
11. Hadler NM, Curtis P, Gillings DB, Stinnett S. A benefit of spinal manipulation as adjunctive therapy for acute low back pain: a stratified controlled trial. Spine 1987;12:703–706.
12. Haldeman S, Rubenstein SM. Cauda equina syndrome in patients undergoing manipulation of the lumbar spine. Spine 1992;17:1469–1473.
13. Harper CM, Lyles YM. Physiology and complications of bed rest. J Am Geriatr Soc 1988;36: 1047–1054.
14. Inturrisi CE. Narcotic drugs. Med Clin North Am 1982;66:1061–1071.
15. Jackson CP, Brown MD. Analysis of current approaches and a practical guide to prescription of exercise. Clin Orthop 1983;179:46–54.
16. Jayson MIV, Sims-Williams H, Young S, Baddeley H, Collins E. Mobilization and manipulation for low back pain. Spine 1981;6:409–416.
17. Kane RI, Leymaster C, Olsen D, et al. Manipulating the patient: a comparison of the effectiveness of physician and chiropractic care. Lancet 1983;1:411–416.
18. Lahad A, Malter AD, Berg AO, Deyo RA. The effectiveness of four interventions for the prevention of low back pain. JAMA 1994;272:1286–1291.
19. Landon BR. Heat or cold for the relief of low back pain? Phys Ther 1967;47:1126–1130.
20. McCray RE, Patton NJ. Pain relief at trigger points: A comparison of moist heat and shortwave diathermy. J Orthop Sport Phys Ther 1984;5:175–181.
21. Melzack R. Acupuncture and related forms of folk medicine. In: Wall PD, Melzack R, eds. Textbook of Pain. Edinburgh, Scotland: Churchill Livingstone, pp 691–700, 1984.
22. Mendelson G, Selwood TS, Kranz H, et al. Acupuncture treatment of chronic back pain: A double-blind, placebo-controlled trial. Am J Med 1983;74(1):49–55.
23. Murphy TM, Raj PP, Stanton-Hicks M. Techniques of nerve blocks—spinal nerves. In: Raj PP, ed. Practical Management of Pain. Chicago: Year Book Medical Publishers; pp 597–636, 1986.
24. Nachemson A. The load on lumbar disks in different positions of the body. Clin Orthop 1966;45: 107–122.

25. Nouwen A. EMG biofeedback used to reduce standing levels of paraspinal muscle tension in chronic low back pain. Pain 1983;17:353–360.
26. Quebec Task Force on Spinal Disorders. Report. Scientific approach to the assessment and management of activity-related spinal disorders. A monograph for clinicians. Spine 1987;12 (suppl 7): S1–59.
27. Paris SV. Spinal manipulative therapy. Clin Orthop 1983;179:55–61.
28. Pheasant H, Bursk A, Goldfarb J, Azen SP, Weiss JN, Borelli LL. Amitriptyline and chronic low-back pain: a randomized double-blind crossover study. Spine 1983;8:552–557.
29. Shekelle PG, Adams AH, Chassin MR, Hurwitz EL, Brook RH. Spinal manipulation for low-back pain. Ann Intern Med 1992;117:590–598.
30. Sikorski JM. A rationalized approach to physiotherapy for low-back pain. Spine 1985;10: 571–579.
31. Simon LS, Mills JS. Drug therapy: Nonsteroidal anti-inflammatory drugs. N Engl J Med 1980;302:1179–1186.
32. Stimmel B. Pain, analgesia, and addiction: An approach to the pharmacologic management of pain. Clin J Pain 1985;1:14–19.
33. Swezey RL. The modern thrust of manipulation and traction therapy. Semin Arthritis Rheum 1983;12:322–331.
34. Tan JC, Roux EB, Dunand J, et al. Role of physical therapy in the management of common low back pain. Clin Rheumatol 1992;6(3):629–655.
35. Ward NG. Tricyclic antidepressants for chronic low back pain: Mechanisms of action and predictors of response. Spine 1986;11:661–665.
36. White AH, Derby R, Wynne G. Epidural injections for the diagnosis and treatment of low-back pain. Spine 1980;5:78–86.
37. Woolf CJ. Transcutaneous and implanted nerve stimulation. In: Wall PD, Melzack R, eds. Textbook of Pain. Edinburgh, Scotland: Churchill Livingstone, pp 679–690, 1986.

14

Disc Degeneration Without Root Irritation: Acute and Chronic Low Back Pain

"It is easy to get a thousand prescriptions but hard to get a single remedy."

— Anonymous

INTRODUCTION

Low back pain is a symptom not a diagnosis. It is a very common symptom, affecting 80% of individuals during their lifetime (28) (Chapter 8). It is an expensive symptom with direct costs (for treatment) and indirect costs (due to lost time) totaling up to 50 billion dollars a year in the United States. If 80% of humans are afflicted at some time with low back pain why do we not have a "nation of cripples?" The answer is that all but a few of these symptomatic individuals get better whether or not they visit a healthcare professional. The next question is obvious: why do we spend up to 20 billion American dollars of our limited health care funds to care for this symptom? This is a question a lot of individuals and paying organizations are asking.

Low back pain is the equivalent to the neurologists headache with one major difference: there is an operation that can be done for the symptom of back pain, the lumbar fusion. The operation arose out of the observation that when a painful hip or knee was fused the pain would disappear. In today's world these painful knees and hips are treated by joint replacement to retain joint mobility. The spine surgeons are still fusing lumbar spines because there is not a viable joint replacement option.(10, 54) But are all the fusions (75,000 to 100,000 per year in the United States) needed?

DISC FUNCTION AND DYSFUNCTION

To understand the phenomenon of disc degeneration and degenerative disc disease, you need an understanding of disc function and how disease causes the disc to dysfunction.

Disc Function

Two balances occur within the disc:

1. Swelling pressure balance (Fig. 14.1) or chemical balance.

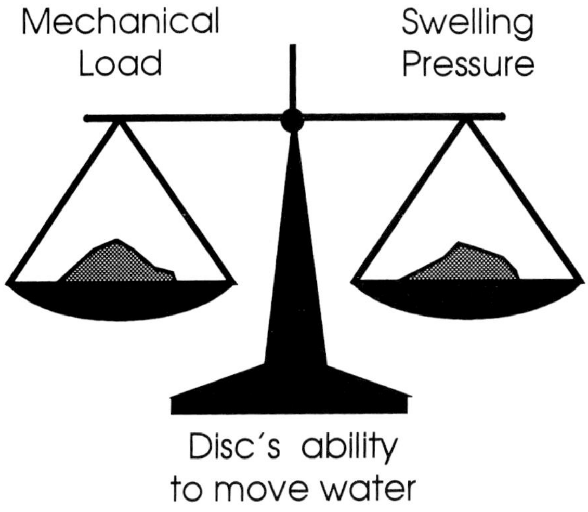

Figure 14.1 *Swelling pressure balance of a disc depends on the movement of water in and out of the nucleus; as the mechanical load increases, water moves out of the nucleus to decrease the swelling pressure to help absorb the load.*

The nucleus of the disc is composed of collagen fibers woven throughout a proteoglycan gel. The proteoglycans imbibe water and swell while the collagen tissues resist that swelling. The swelling pressure balance obviously is the contest between swelling proteoglycans and the resisting collagen fibers.

2. Mechanical balance.

When mechanical loads are applied to the disc, the nucleus absorbs the force and in turn transfers the force to the annulus. The ability of the nucleus to dissipate these forces depends on its ability to imbibe and release water, that is, its swelling pressure. If the nuclear/annular complex starts to degenerate, the swelling pressure balance is upset and the ability of the disc to absorb forces is reduced, i.e. disc mechanics are no longer balanced.(40)

Disc Dysfunction

Lumbar disc degeneration (dysfunction) is the result of deterioration of the mechanical and chemical properties of the disc. The cause is the universal phenomenon of the aging process aided and abetted by episodes of trauma throughout one's life. The deterioration in physical and chemical properties leads to the loss of low back function manifest as mechanical disorders ("my back hurts when I bend and lift") and/or neurological compressive disorders ("my leg[s] hurt[s] when I sit or walk"). We all get older and by default we all deteriorate our discs yet we are not all symptomatic.(8) It is a constant theme throughout this book that degenerative disc disease routinely occurs without symptoms, or when it does become symptomatic there is a powerful natural tendency toward self healing.

The actual physical and chemical changes that occur with aging are loss of water in the nucleus and the annulus (the conversion of a grape to a raisin!) the end stage of which is intradiscal fibrosis. The body does an autofusion with fibrous tissue replacing the nucleus and annulus reducing movement in the segment. This explains why we get stiffer as we get older and why the vast majority of individuals grow older without back pain.

The reason for these chemical changes centers around an understanding of disc nutrition (Fig. 14.2). The intervertebral disc is avascular after age 8 and receives its nutrition through transport across the cartilaginous endplate and through the annulus. With aging these vascular channels start to fail and diffusion of nutrients decreases. The result is a decrease in the number of fibroblasts and chondrocytes and a decrease in formation of collagen and proteoglycans. The end result is failure of the disc to absorb mechanical forces because of failure of the swelling pressure balance. The result is disc dysfunction. In addition to being part of the aging process, disc dysfunction is aggravated by poor health habits such as smoking and lack of exercise.

The Stages of Disc Dysfunction

Kirkaldy-Willis and Farfan (49) put it all together in 1982 when they described the three phases of disc degeneration (Fig. 14.3).

Phase 1 Disc Dysfunction

In this phase, the ability of the disc to exchange water and balance the swelling pressure starts to deteriorate. With microtrauma, annular tears appear and facet cartilaginous fissures develop, along with increased secretion of synovial fluid into the irritated facet joints.

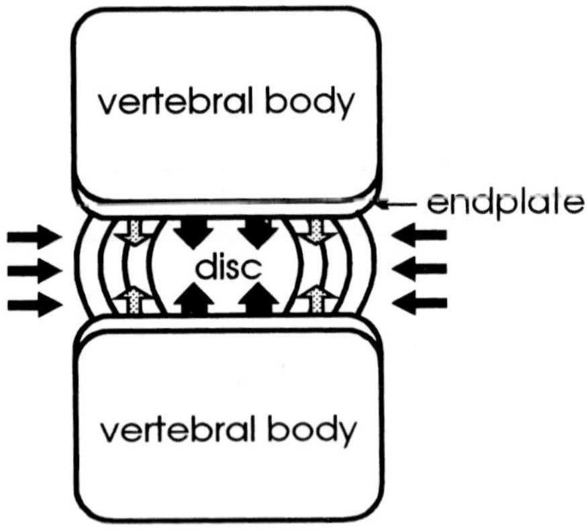

Figure 14.2 *Disc nutrition is by diffusion of nutrients across the endplate and through the annulus.*

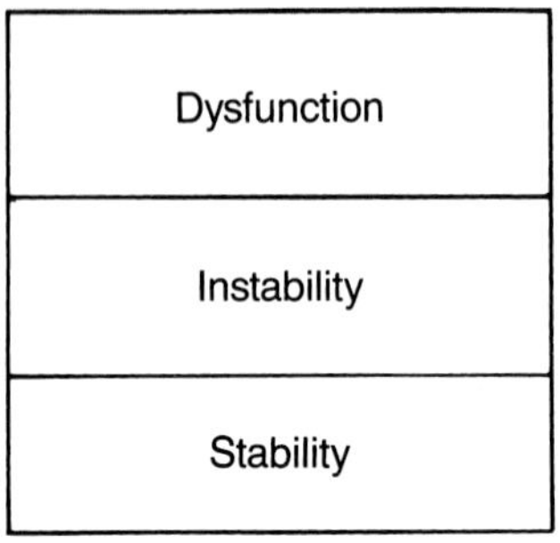

Figure 14.3 *The three stages of disc degeneration.*

Phase 2 Instability

In this phase, disc height is decreased, ligaments become lax and osteophytes form in an attempt to restabilize the functional spinal unit (FSU) (Fig. 14.4). Facet joint changes include degeneration of the cartilage and laxity of the capsule.

Phase 3 Stability

In this phase, the FSU restabilizes itself. Within the disc space, disc narrowing and fibrosis do the trick while osteophytes (Fig. 14.5) stabilize the periphery of the disc space. In the facet joint, subluxation (Fig. 14.5) and capsular fibrosis further stabilize the FSU. Unfortunately, the stabilizing osteophytes may encroach on nerve roots and interfere with root function (see Chapter 17).

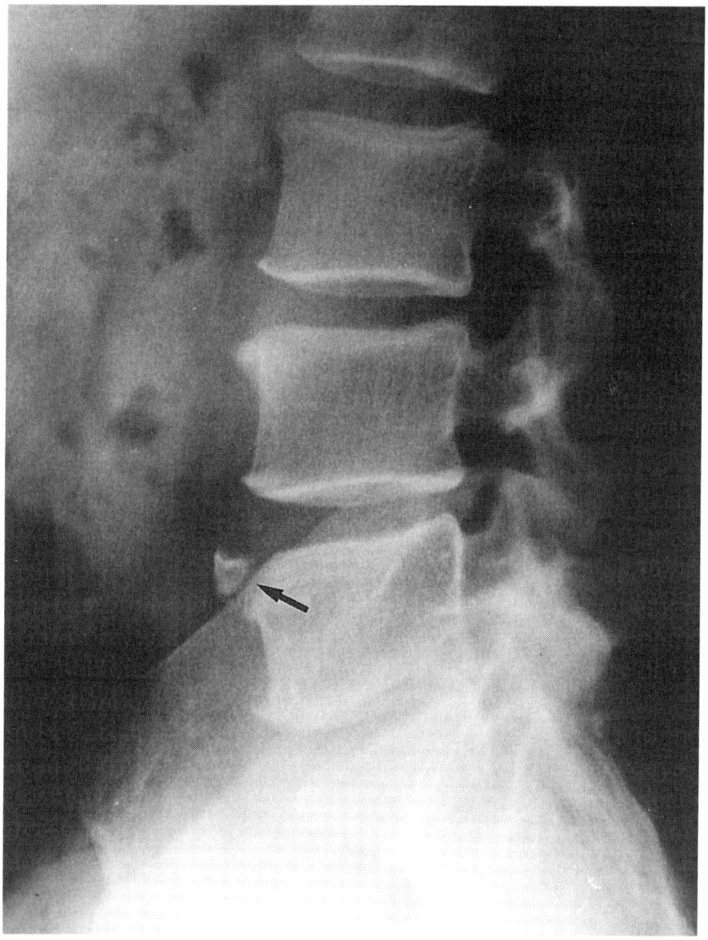

Figure 14.4 *The phase of instability: the L4–L5 disc space is narrowed, and an early retrospondylolisthesis is present. The L3–L4 space is also narrowed, and osteophytes are forming anteriorly. Note the limbus vertebrae (arrow) that is a variant of Schmorl's node; it is not a fracture.*

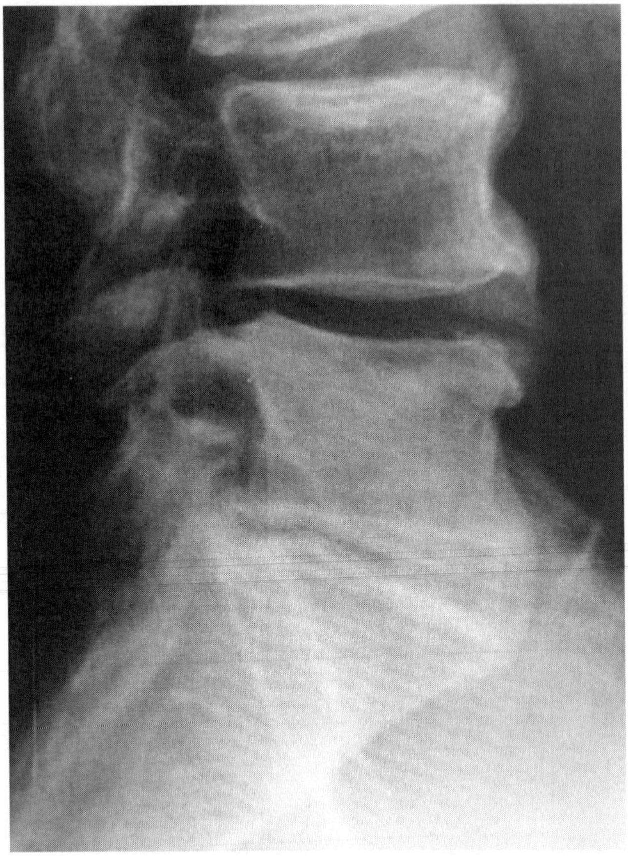

Figure 14.5 *A well-stabilized L5–S1 disc with osteophytes. The same osteophytic stabilization is occurring at the L4–L5 and L3–L4 levels.*

INSTABILITY OF THE FUNCTIONAL SPINAL UNIT

The midphase of Kirkaldy-Willis's disc degeneration is the phase of instability of the functional spinal unit (FSU) (Fig. 14.3). Instability is not a particularly difficult word to define. The problem is to come up with a clinically meaningful and useful definition. Instability in trauma (fractures) of the lumbar spine has been clearly established by White and Panjabi (98) (Fig. 14.6) and is defined as more than 4 mm of translation or 10 degrees of angulation of one vertebral body relative to its mate. These parameters are also useful for lytic and degenerative spondylolisthesis (Fig. 14.7). At the other end of the spectrum we have the obviously stable FSU (Fig. 14.7). The problem lies between these two extremes (Fig. 14.8) where obvious degenerative changes have occurred, yet no abnormal movement can be detected on radiograph.(83) There is no measurement of instability in this group of patients.

Which Tissues are the Source of Pain?

Kuslich and co-workers (52) have carried out the best clinical work in this field. While doing microdiscectomies for disc ruptures under local anesthesia in more than 700 pa-

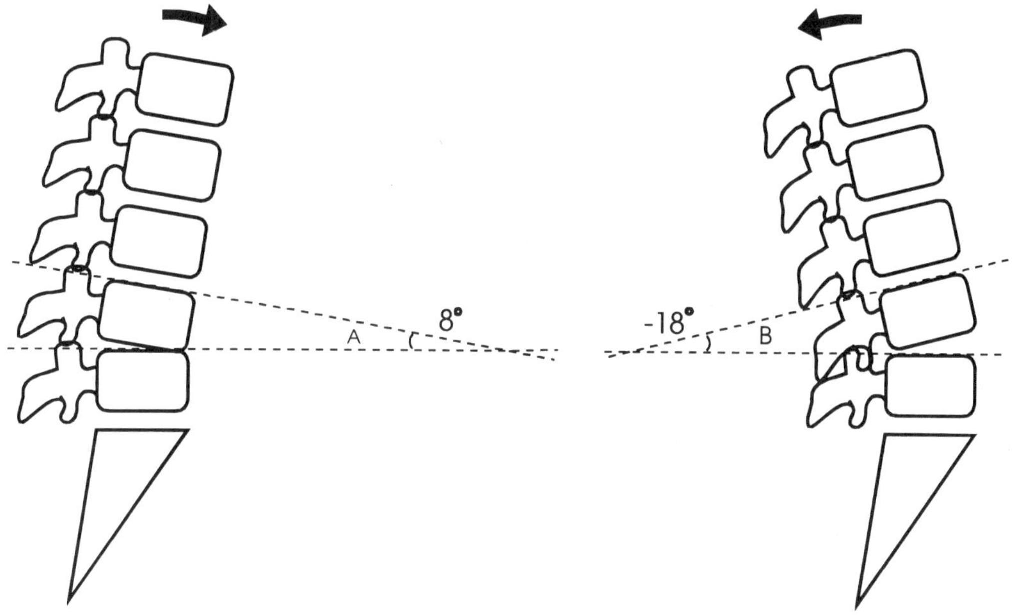

Figure 14.6 *On flexion-extension (schematic drawn from a radiograph), angulation goes from 8 degrees to -18 degrees, a change of 26 degrees, which is by definition an unstable segment.*

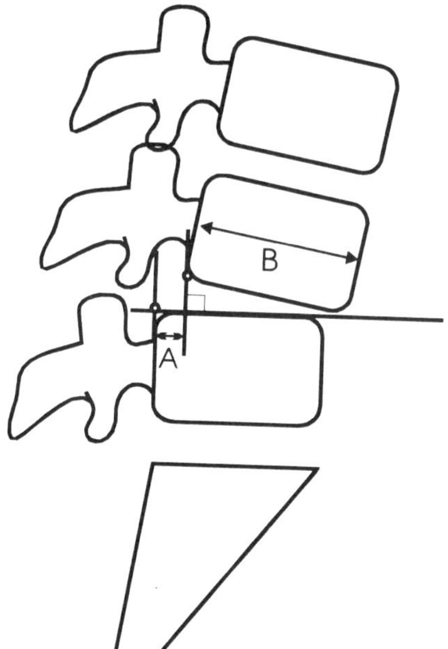

Figure 14.7 *A schematic of a degenerative spondylolisthesis showing angulation of more than 10 degrees and forward subluxation of L4 on L5 of more than 4 mm.*

tients, these researchers took the opportunity to stimulate various tissues and record the patient's response. They found that muscle, fascia, and bone were largely insensitive structures, whereas the facet joint capsule was painful in half of the patients. The outer annulus was the most consistent structure to produce back pain when stimulated. The

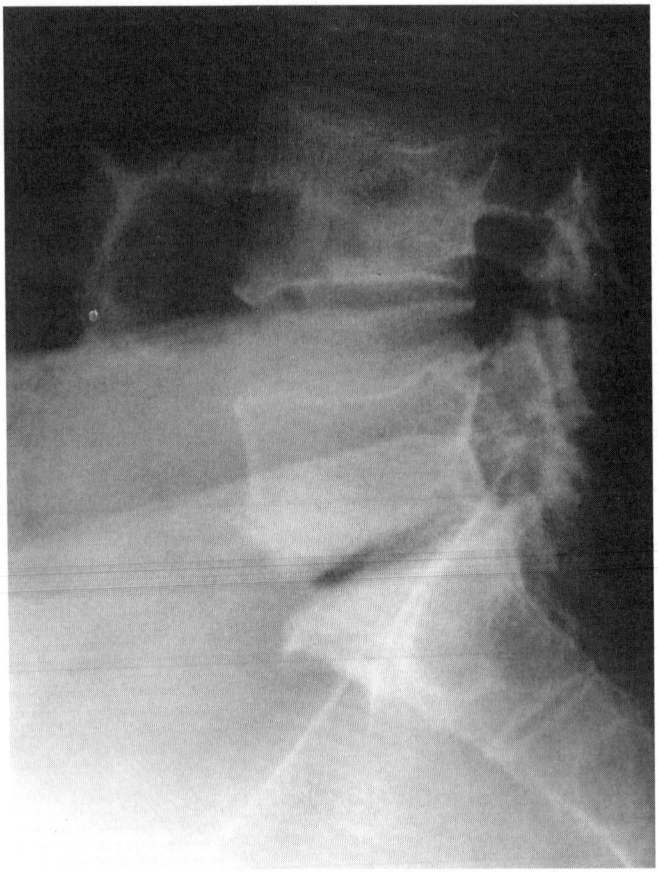

Figure 14.8 *Note the severe degenerative disc disease at L5–S1 with air (nitrogen) in the disc space (Knuttson's phenomenon).*

inner annulus and nucleus were largely insensitive structures. The surgery for the patients in this study was being done for the symptom of sciatica and the disease of disc rupture. The researchers found that stretching the already stretched, compressed, and inflamed nerve root reproduced or exacerbated the patients' leg pain.

Proof of Instability

We have shown obvious instability in the previous radiographs. In those patients where instability cannot be demonstrated on radiograph, some investigators have used provocative/ablation testing. Examples of the latter are bracing or the external fixator (22, 74) (Fig. 14.9) to see if back pain can be decreased. Bracing does not work because to immobilize the lower lumbar spine, where most instability occurs, the thigh must be included in the brace (Fig. 14.10), which severely strains patient compliance. The external fixater has been largely abandoned because it is invasive, loaded with complications and very difficult for patients to comply with for any length of time.

An example of provocative testing is lumbar discography, a discussion of which splits

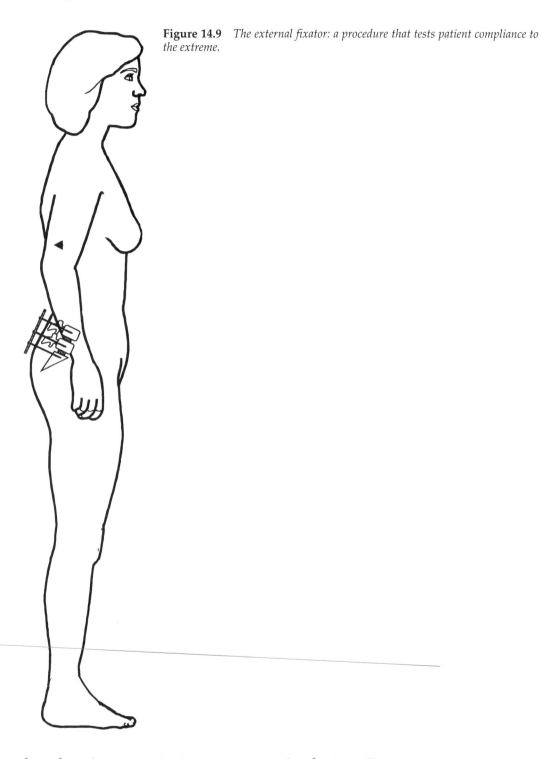

Figure 14.9 *The external fixator: a procedure that tests patient compliance to the extreme.*

the orthopedic community into naysayers and enthusiasts. For most neurosurgeons performing spine surgery there is no controversy: discography is a useless test.(43) The senior author (JM) has performed over 10,000 discograms as part of an extensive experience with chemonucleolysis and agrees with the neurosurgeons: it is a useless test.

Figure 14.10 *A brace or cast that holds onto the rib cage and one thigh.*

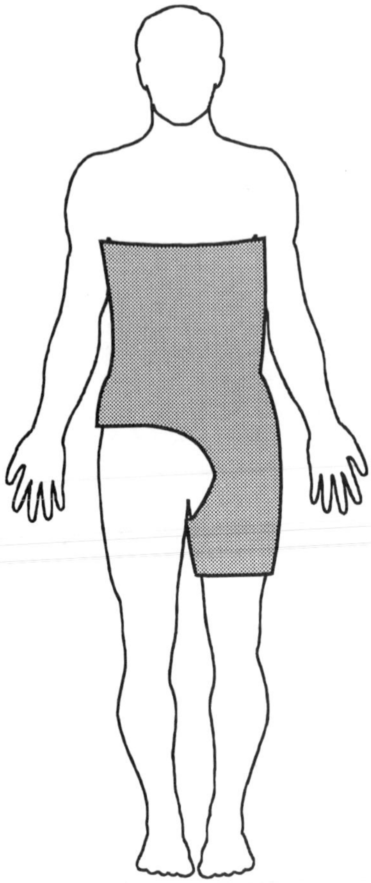

DISCOGRAPHY

Discography is the injection of contrast or other test material into the disc. Sometimes it is followed by radiographic examination and sometimes by computed tomograpghy (CT) (Disco-CT). Discography has been firmly embraced by well respected spine investigators. (11, 17, 18, 19, 87, 88, 100) Unfortunately, discography has little or no scientific basis for its continuing use. While this statement will be immediately repudiated by those surgeons who use discography to pick surgical levels, it is a statement supported in the radiological and neurosurgical communities, and by many other orthopedic surgeons. There is a significant feeling in these circles that discography is a "test looking for an operation." A number of studies completed in the senior author's chemonucleolysis population failed to show that response to discography or other parameters of discography had any bearing on the outcome of chemonucleolysis.(61) For the purpose of this discussion, we would like to first outline aspects of discography on which most supporters and detractors would agree.

Discography involves introducing a needle under radiographic control into the nucleus of an intervertebral disc and injecting contrast material. The approach used most widely is the posterolateral or lateral approach (60) (Fig. 14.11). The exact site of the tip of the needle is identified by radiographs taken in two planes. To test the integrity of the disc, a water-soluble contrast material, or water itself, can be injected. If the disc is normal, the injected contrast material is confined to the nucleus (Fig. 14.12). Although a normal disc

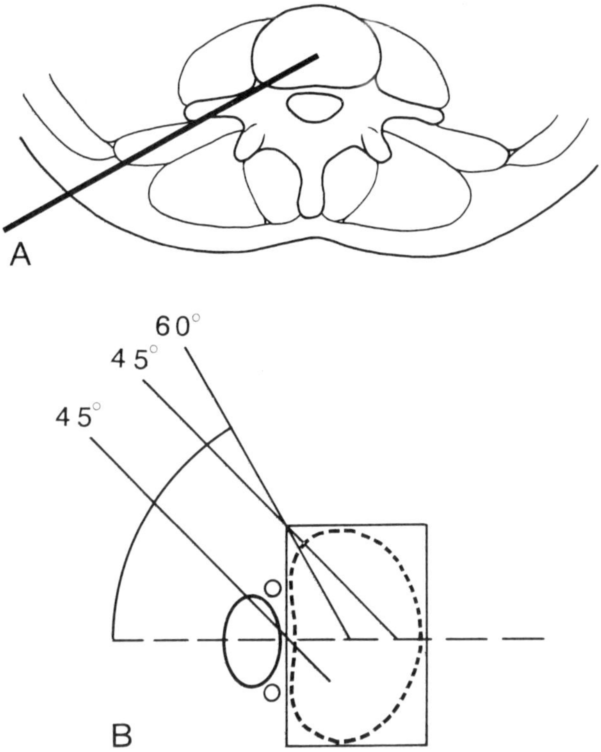

Figure 14.11 **A.** *The posterolateral approach to disc penetration.* **B.** *The various angles and distances from the midline. Ideal is 8 to 10 cm from the midline and 60-degree angulation into the disc.*

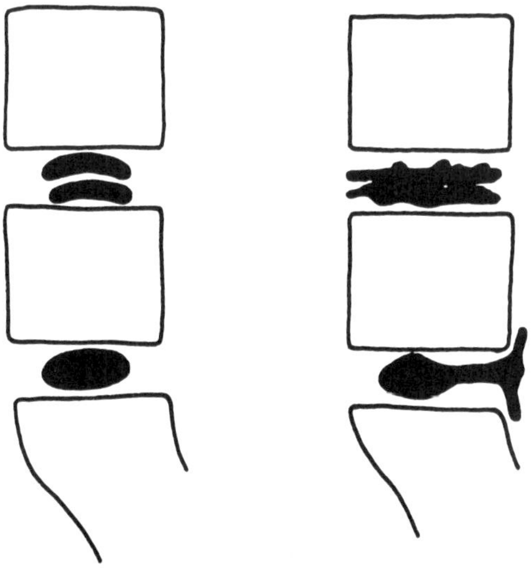

Figure 14.12 *Discography. With normal discs, the injected dye remains confined within the nucleus. The dye may present a spherical or bilobular appearance. When degenerative changes have taken place, the injected dye spreads throughout the disc and into the annulus. On occasion, the dye may be seen to spread posteriorly and run vertically underneath the posterior longitudinal ligament. This latter appearance, however, does not denote the presence of a disc rupture.*

offers considerable resistance to the injection, the resulting distention does not evoke a painful response. In the presence of disc degeneration, on the other hand, there is little or no resistance to the injection, the dye spreads diffusely through the disc, and the patient may experience pain. If you have read this slowly, you will recognize four parameters to assess in discography (Table 14.1).

At one time considerable significance was placed on the pattern of the injected dye (Fig. 14.12). Increasing clinical experience has shown, however, that the only conclusion that can be drawn from the discographic pattern is either that the disc is normal or that it shows morphological evidence of degeneration. No statement can be made that the demonstration of morphological abnormality indicates that the disc injected is the source of symptoms.

Injection into a normal disc is painless. Injection into a degenerate disc may also be painless (102) but if the degenerative changes are symptomatic, distention of the disc may or may not reproduce the patient's clinically experienced symptoms.(85) The presence or absence of pain on distention of the disc may be the important finding and the test is more accurately described as a "discometric assessment."

If this fact is acknowledged, discography is of greater value if the discs are injected first with saline or water. In contrast to the injection of radiopaque iodine compounds, the pain produced in a symptomatic degenerate disc on the injection of water is of short duration. This short duration of pain is of importance because it does not cloud and confuse the results of subsequent injection into other discs. Moreover, because of the low intensity and short duration of the discomfort produced, it permits the examiner to repeat the injection when necessary, to enable the patient to compare the pain with the clinically experienced symptoms.

The injection of contrast material is an important part of the procedure (Fig. 14.13). A very small quantity (0.5 mL) may be injected after the insertion of the needle to confirm the fact that the point of the needle is, indeed, lying in the center of the nucleus. At the conclusion of the procedure dye may be injected to demonstrate the morphological pattern of the disc thereby providing documentary evidence of a normal disc or a painless disc degeneration.

Despite this attempt at a scholarly description of the phenomenon of discography, there is not one article in the literature that addresses both the sensitivity and specificity as well as the accuracy of discography. Still, the test is used to search out painful motion segments for fusion. Unfortunately most publications of this use describe discography in the multiply operated patient, which only confuses the issue further. (47)

Acceptable Statements About Discography

Most scientists, aware of the pros and cons of discography would agree on the following points:

Table 14.1. Parameters to Assess in Discography

	Normal Disc	Disc Degeneration
1. Volume of test material	Limited (1–2 cc)	More than 4 cc
2. Resistance	Firm endpoint	Significant decrease in resistance
3. Pain reproduction	None	Often painful
4. Pattern of contrast material	Round ball (Fig. 14.12)	Diffuse (Fig. 14.12)

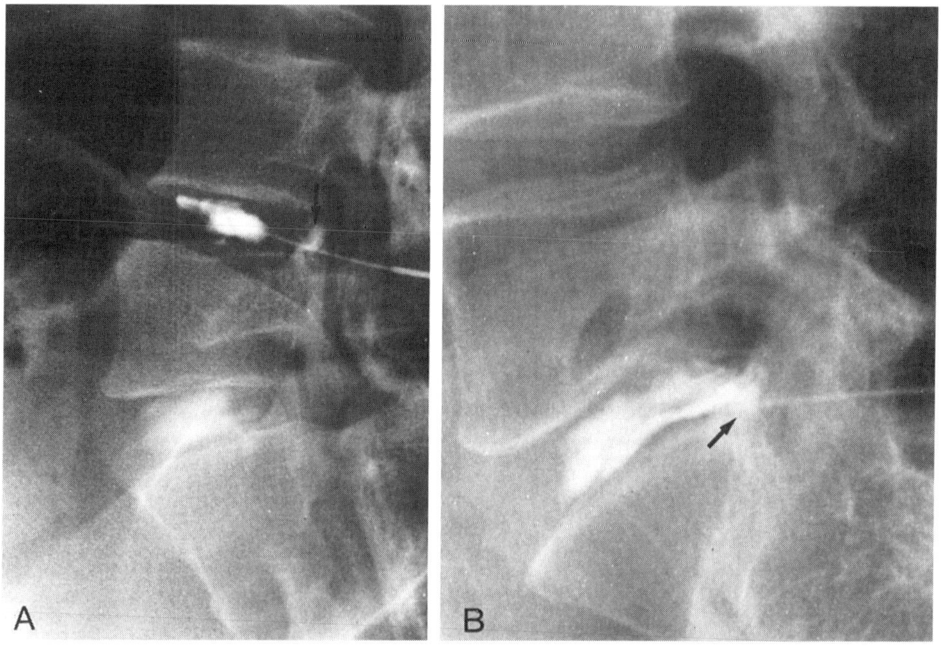

Figure 14.13 **A.** *Abnormal discogram, L4–L5, with contrast (dye) leaking to back of disc space (arrow). At L–S1 the needle has been withdrawn, but the dye pattern reveals a normal disc.* **B.** *Abnormal discogram, L5–S1 (arrow).*

1. Unlike CT and magnetic resonance imaging (MRI), discography is an invasive test. It is painful to patients and carries with it the risk of disc space infection (1–4%).(26)
2. Most discographers use the posterolateral approach (60) because it is less irritating to the patients when compared with the midline approach. At the L5–S1 level, the posterolateral approach can damage the L5 nerve root.
3. Most discographers would agree that it is necessary to evaluate both the appearance of contrast on radiographs (variously described as morphology and/or nucleogram) and the patient's pain response to the injection.(88) Those studies that have left out the evaluation of pain response are largely invalid.
4. Discography for the evaluation of cervical or lumbar radicular pain has largely been abandoned because (45): (1) it has never been proven of value; (2) CT and MRI are so much more accurate in the assessment of radicular pain. Discography is now used primarily in the assessment of axial (back) pain. The abnormal findings produced by the injection of test material indicates the so-called "contained" discogenic diseases, variously known as degenerative disc disease, and/or internal disc disruption. These patients characteristically have dominant back pain, a normal extremity exam (in regards to straight leg raising and neurological exam) and have CT and/or MRI studies which show, at most, a "bulging disc (64)."
5. Discography, for the assessment of back pain, should only be used after the decision has been made to operate, that is, to do a fusion.(100) Its sole purpose is to assist the surgeon in deciding on what levels to include in the fusion. This is a conclusion that has never been tested in a prospective scientific study.
6. The other two parameters of discography, namely volume of test material and the pressure of injections have largely been abandoned except when trying to decide if a

disc is contained (high pressure on injection) or non-contained (low pressure on injection).(16) This may or may not be a important consideration when deciding on chemonucleolysis or percutaneous discectomy.

7. The most often quoted study supporting discography is the one by Walsh and co-workers(96). This study included discograms at three levels on asymptomatic college students (average age, 22 years) and was done to determine the validity of Holt's (42) study, which showed a false-positive rate in young healthy prisoner volunteers. The authors criticized Holt's study on the following counts:
    a. Holt considered morphology only and did not evaluate pain response.
    b. The veracity of Holt's patient population (volunteer prisoners) was a few levels below that of the individuals studied by Walsh and co-workers (college students)!
    c. Holt's technique in doing discography was poor.
    d. Holt used plain radiographs rather than CT/discography.
    e. Holt used very irritating contrast material (Hypaque).

Walsh's study showed a 100% specificity for discography in young college students when pain response was added to disc morphology (nucleogram). They proved that, in asymptomatic young patients, discography would remain negative. But can you extrapolate that to the general population of patients with back pain, which would be much older? What their study did not address was the validity or sensitivity of discography, that is, the ability of discography to predict not only which level is symptomatic, but whether or not fusion of that level will relieve the patient of his/her suffering.

Problems with Discography

The major problem with discography is the lack of any sensitivity studies to support its continuing use.(63) Perhaps, the two best studies to show how poor discography is as a predictor of pathology or surgical outcomes were done by Jackson et al(45) Their first study dealt with the sensitivity and specificity of discography in predicting disc herniations in a difficult patient population referred by other orthopaedic surgeons. The study was done before MRI was generally available and concentrated on the ability to reproduce the patient's extremity pain on provocative testing. They found an 89% specificity (ability of the test to remain negative when a disc rupture was NOT present at subsequent surgery), but only a 43% sensitivity (ability of the test to be positive when a disc rupture was present). In other words, the test was reasonably good in not producing false-positives, but poor because there were a large number of false-negatives.

The second study was directed at the more frequent use of discography to assist in using it as a test to help decide fusion levels. It was a retrospective determination of discography's ability to select fusion levels in successful 1, 2, and 3 level fusions, completed 2 years after the fusion. The conclusion was that "pain reproduction by discography preoperatively is a very poor predictor of clinical outcome postoperatively in patients with solid posterolateral lumbosacral fusions."

Esses et al (22) used an external fixator to select fusion levels. All patients had provocative discography before the fixator was placed. They concluded that discography was a less sensitive predictor of surgical results than degenerative changes on routine radiograph, thus supporting the findings of Hess and Jackson.(38) Esses's study can be criticized because:

1. The majority of patients were compensation patient who had been out of work at least 30 months.
2. More than 50% of his patients had had previous surgery.
3. The successful outcome to surgery, as measured by relief of pain occurred in only 17 of 27 patients.
4. No statement was made regarding to the ultimate test of successful surgical outcomes in compensation patients: the return to work rate.

So many of the studies in support of discography can be criticized as readily as Esses's study.

1. They did not include provocation pain responses.
2. Only a few studies have used surgical outcome as the "gold standard" to assess the usefulness of discography. One study that did this was by Colhoun and colleagues (18) who prospectively reviewed the role of discography in successful surgical fusions. These researchers demonstrated that, of the 137 patients in whom discography had revealed disc disease and provoked symptoms, 89% derived significant and sustained clinical benefit from operation. Of the 25 patients whose discs showed morphologic abnormality, but had no provocation of symptoms on discography, only 52% had clinical success. The conclusions of this study are difficult to reconcile with the opposite (negative) conclusions of Jackson.(45)

Many studies (19, 96) are hard to accept in support of discography because:

1. They did not use surgical outcome as a determinant in the efficacy of discography
2. They had very low or very high surgical success rates.
3. There were so many variables in the patient population, it was impossible to draw valid conclusions about the usefulness of discography.(97)

A number of studies have attempted to show that even in the presence of a normal MRI (T2 sagittal), discography can produce an abnormal pain response and/or morphology (9, 12, 30, 105). We cannot accept their conclusions because many of the MRIs were of poor quality or were not midline cuts or did show posterior clefts in the annulus.(56) In addition, the morphology on discography revealed minor changes, compatible with some of the reproduced MRIs. The final criticisms of all of these studies is the absence of any clinical outcome criteria.(51)

The latest study to be presented has really set off the fireworks! Rhyne and Smith (81) evaluated 25 patients who had not undergone surgery and had single-level, positive discograms at an average of 4.9 years after discography. After the positive discogram and recommendation for fusion, various reasons prevented the surgery from taking place (patient's change of mind, insurance company said no, Charlie's car would not start on the morning of surgery). Seventeen (68%) were improved without surgery, two (8%) were the same and 6 (24%) were worse. Of those patients who worsened, 4 (66.7%) turned out to have a concomitant psychiatric illness. The researchers concluded that the outcomes in their study were as good as or better than those who had fusions after the discograms.

Obviously, the role of discography in surgical decision making cries out for valid clinical trials. (96) In setting up these trials, investigators will have to answer the following questions:

1. What is the source of pain on provocative volumetric testing of a degenerative disc? Is it the annulus, the endplate, the facet joints or surrounding ligaments?
2. How do you explain the production of pain on the injection of hypertonic saline into tissues of normal (asymptomatic) volunteers?
3. Why, as we get older and develop more degenerative disc disease do we see fewer patients with low back pain?
4. If response to disc space injection is most important, what are the parameters that are important to describe the response? Is it the patient's response at the beginning, in the middle, or at the end of the injection? What volume of test material is considered adequate? Should the injection be fast or slow? How many times should the test be repeated in each disc, and which response is the correct one: the response to the first, middle, or last injection? In multiple disc space testing, how long do you wait after a painful test to test again? Does pain reproduction have to be the exact same pain or just pain in the area where that patient normally has felt pain? Is a sedated patient a valid reporter of pain? If multiple discs are being examined, what is the proper order?
5. As you can see, there are so many variables in patient response to provocative testing that only the most fastidious, pedantic scientists will be able to complete the study. These qualities are usually not a major part of an orthopedic surgeon's temperament!
6. Discography is used for the assessment of fusion levels in axial pain, which by its very nature is a chronic condition before it ever arrives at a stage of fusion considerations. How can a test that produces acute pain be used to evaluate a chronic painful condition that is so often modified by intellect, emotion, culture, and environment?
7. If we are agreed that morphology is of limited value (compared with provocation of pain), how does the addition of CT (CT/discography [82, 92]) add any value to discography?

Conclusions

Nachemson (70) has called for the discontinuation of discographic studies, except for prospective studies performed in large spine centers. He proposed they only be done after the approval of human experimentation committees where the intent is to find out if they can really help in the treatment selection for the chronic low back pain patient. While this proposal might seem an unwarranted intrusion on the freedom to practice in the United States, it is a criticism and comment that is not far off the mark. As we watch the number of spine surgeries increase in a linear fashion, with the increasing number of spine surgeons that appear in a community, as we watch the number of failed spine surgeries and long term spinal disability (95) increase dramatically, someone is going to intervene in the controversy of discography. We can criticize our critics or we can start proper trials of discography based on scientific methods. If not, discography has a reasonable chance of disappearing over the abyss into clinical irrelevancy. It was very unfortunate that a number of discographers used the "bully pulpit" of the journal *Spine* to issue an unscientific "Position Statement on Discography." (72) It did little to advance the science and damaged the credibility of the journal. Discography was first introduced in 1948.(55) It is now 48 years after the fact, and a highly intelligent surgical community has not brought science to bear on the controversy. If and when this occurs, discography will likely be abandoned as a fusion-decision making test. For now (in the United States) with the unbundling of fees and the introduction of instrumentation, multilevel lumbar fusion, often discographically directed, has taken on a life of its own, for ill-defined diagnoses. The outcomes are difficult to objectively define or justify. Nachemson is right: it is time to stop looking for the "pain generator" with discography. Chronic symptomatic degenerative lumbar disc disease is a complex set of factors that cannot be resolved with a simple test.

To Summarize

Instability is a tough issue. Many great scientific minds have tackled the problem and moved it to what we have described previously.(76) But we do not have a clear understanding of the clinical aspects of instability except to say some of these patients have back pain without radiographic evidence of instability and a surprising number of patients have radiographic evidence of instability and no back pain.

It is easy enough to deal with theoretical conundrums: we do more research. It's a little more difficult to try and apply these principles to patients with back pain. It is a giant step to take unproven testing such as discography and let it be the main determining factor in whether or not to operate.

The Treatment of Instability (Back Pain)

Like anything else, the choices for treatment of instability causing back pain are either conservative or surgical. Conservative measures include short terms of bed rest, modification of activity, exercise and back school (see Chapter 13 for a discussion).

Surgical methods to stabilize the spine are most commonly accomplished by fusion (Fig. 14.14). Graf (33) has proposed we reconstitute ligamentous laxity with artificial ligaments (Fig. 14.15), and Brock (10) and Lee (54) have proposed the use of an artificial disc. These later two proposals are still in the development stage, leaving the lumbar fusion, with or without instrumentation as the only viable option. These options will be discussed later.

THE NATURAL HISTORY OF DEGENERATIVE DISC DISEASE

When deciding on treatment for back pain it is important to keep in mind the natural history of lumbar degenerative disc disease. Many studies have shown that with time, most patients' symptoms will settle and interfere little with their function. Before getting too aggressive with surgery, too prolonged with conservative treatment efforts and too enthusiastic about your claims to cure back pain, it is best to pay homage to the natural ability of the body to stiffen an unstable motion segment and ameliorate pain.

Another fundamental understanding necessary to grasp in treating a patient with low back pain is that there is often no relationship between the patient's symptoms and what is seen on radiograph (Fig. 14.16).

With these concepts in mind let us discuss some of the clinical presentations of low back pain.

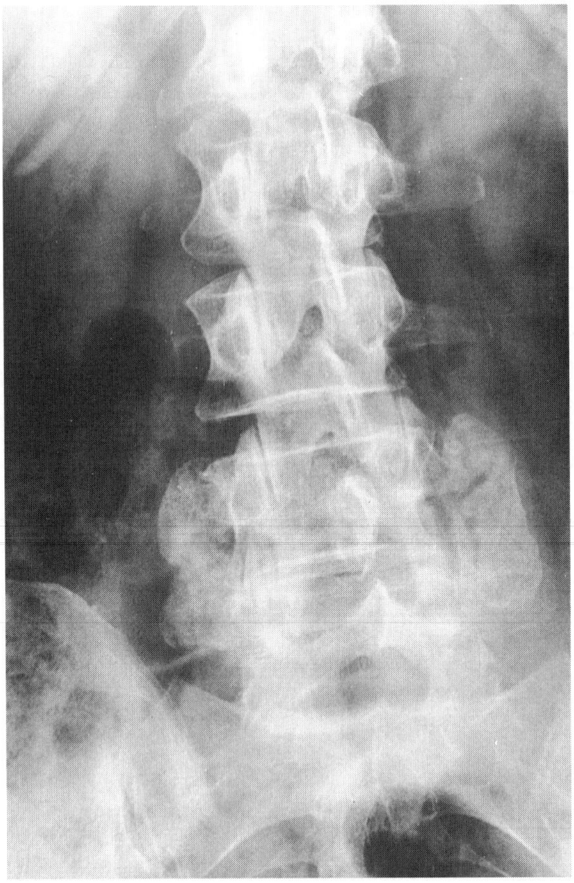

Figure 14.14 *An L4–L5 lumbar fusion in the intertransverse interval.*

Acute Incapacitating Backache: The Acute Back Strain

There are not many people who have lived for a half century who have not, at some time in their lives, been smitten by an acute episode of incapacitating backache. Perversely, this is encouraging. These people do not remain incapacitated: they get better, perhaps despite treatment rather than because of it. They are visiting with Kirkaldy-Willis' s (49) Phase 1 of spinal dysfunction.

Characteristically, the patient, while engaged in some trivial activity, is suddenly seized with back pain and cannot move. "I was paralyzed with pain." The lumbar spine is splinted rigidly and the patient can only move with painful caution, clutching his/her back and walking with the trunk leaning forward, keeping the hips and knees slightly bent.

Examination reveals that all movements of the spine are limited by pain and muscle spasm, but there is no evidence of root tension, irritation, or compression. In some of these patients, there is so much back spasm and muscle splinting that attempting to perform the straight leg raising (SLR) test will cause back pain and leave the examiner with the false impression that a disc rupture may be present. A useful examination is the sitting SLR test. Most of these patients can sit in a few moments of comfort; in this sitting position, gentle SLR testing (Fig. 14.17) will reveal good SLR.

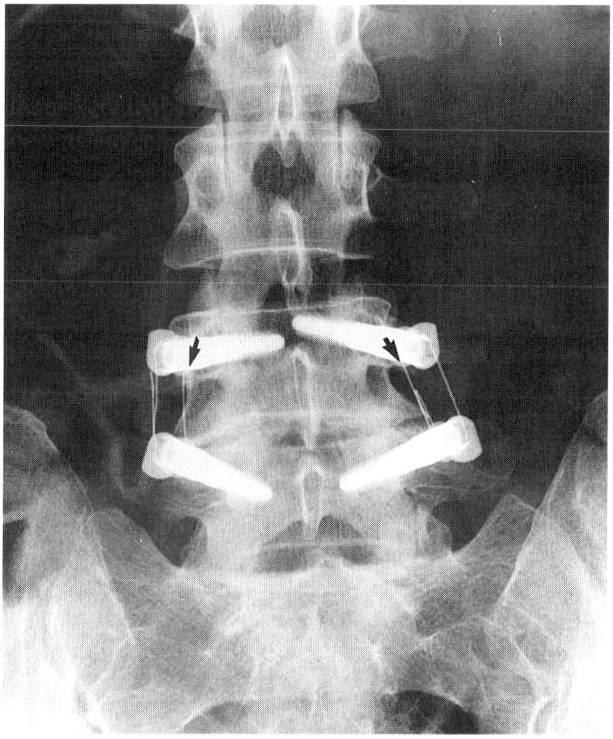

Figure 14.15 *Graf ligaments (arrows) are shown at L4–L5. No bone graft (for fusion purposes) is used. (Illustration courtesy of Mr. Michael Sullivan, Royal National Hospital, London.)*

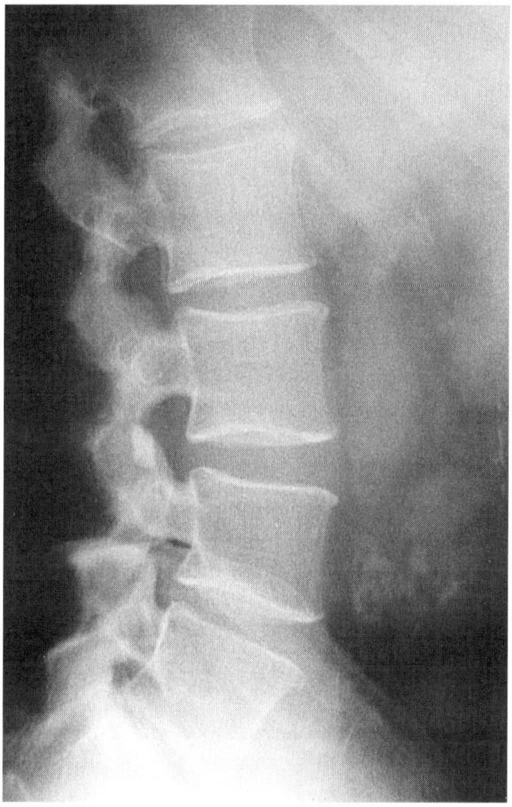

Figure 14.16 *A lateral plain film of a patient with severe back pain. Note two things: (1) the normal lumbar spine, except for degenerative disc diease at L5–S1, and (2) the large aortic aneurysm! The next time you are looking at an intravenous pyelogram and see lots of lumbar degerative disc disease, ask the patient if they have ever had back pain. The answer is likely to be "no."*

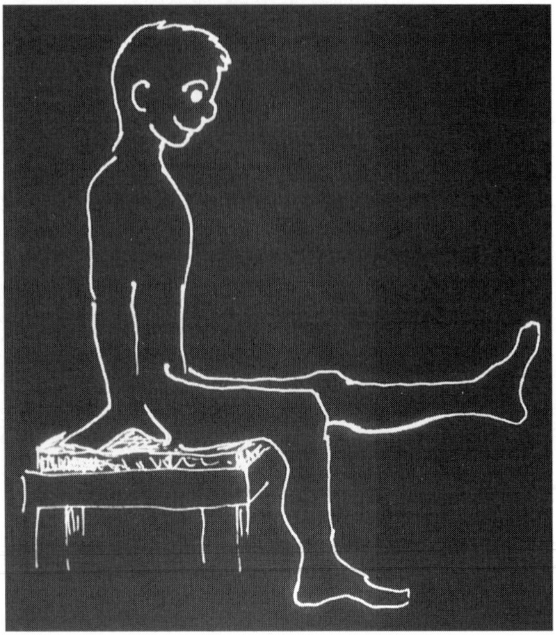

Figure 14.17 *The sitting straight leg raising test. If a patient with acute back pain can sit in this position, the ability to raise each straight leg to 90 degrees, as shown, tends to rule out a herniated nucleus pulposus.*

The clinical picture is explosively dramatic and threatening to the patient, if they have not been through a previous episode. The physician must not overreact. The physician must constantly remind him-/herself that even if the elected treatment involved rubbing peanut butter on each of the patient's buttocks, in the balance of probabilities, the patient would get well fairly quickly.

In the majority of such cases the patient is suffering from painful dysfunction of the disc space or a "sprain" of one of the zygapophyseal joints. When trying to rationalize treatment, one should compare the lesion with a severely sprained ankle in a patient who has only one leg and who is unable to wear a prosthesis. There is only one way to treat a severely sprained ankle in such a patient: the patient has to be put to bed. Theoretically, the patient with an acute severe low back strain should also be considered for bed rest. However, theoretical treatment must be tempered by reason. If your patient is a young married woman who is responsible for care of the children and getting the meals, how are these responsibilities going to be met? What about the responsibilities of functioning in the office for the dentist with acute back pain?

Let us repeat: you are treating a patient and not a spine, and the experience of the lay world is that many, in fact, the majority, will get better by just creeping around, with their pain mollified by analgesics.

Some patients, however, cannot cope. The pain is too severe. In such instances, if they cannot do their normal daily work, they should be sent to bed. A patient with pneumonia is ill and may feel defeated; that person is happy to go to bed. A patient with severe low back pain feels well except for his/her back and does not want to go to bed. This patient is hopping mad at the affliction, and your insistence on bed rest will increase the frustration, unless you take care and time to explain in detail the purpose of this apparently neglectful form of management. It is advisable to give the low back pain patient some literature explaining in detail the probable underlying pathology and the rationale of treatment by bed rest (Table 14.2). You must advise the patient regarding the use of toilet facilities. Using a bed pan at home is impractical. The use of crutches makes it easier for the patient to get to the bathroom, and the purchase of a high toilet seat is sometimes essential.

Although analgesics are rarely needed once the patient is in bed, in the majority, sedatives such as tranquilizers are essential. At present there is no specific medication to speed the resolution of the symptoms, although anti-inflammatory drugs may help some patients.(5)

The question of the role of manipulation is always raised. The "locking" of the back by spasm of the paraspinal muscles may tend to perpetuate the problem, and gentle flexion of the spine into the fetal position of rest appears to release the muscle by hyperactivity. This is best accomplished initially by getting the patient to flex the knees and hips and then use the hands to pull the knees against the chest repetitively (Fig. 14.18). Later, a passive flexion manipulation can be carried out. The patient lies on his/her back with hips and knees flexed. The heels are grasped so that feet point toward the ceiling. The feet are then pushed gently over the patient's head. The movement is repeated slowly and rhythmically. This repetitive rocking must be carried out with slow simple harmonic motion with each swing of the legs flexing the spine a little further. This rhythmical swinging is continued for approximately 2 minutes (Fig. 14.19).

This is a much more effective maneuver for the occasional manipulator than the specific manipulation of spinous processes or the commonly employed flexion rotation manipulation of the lumbosacral joint (Fig. 14.19)

Table 14.2. Instructions for Patients on the Purpose of Bed Rest

- Many patients with an acute incapacitating back pain are surprised when they are told that the only significant form of treatment is complete bed rest. This does not appear to be treatment at all. It almost seems like neglectful indifference on the part of the physician.
- You must remember that the spine is a column made of blocks of bone connected together by small joints and that an acute mechanical backache is in reality simply a severely sprained joint. It gives rise to pain in the same way that a severe sprain of the ankle gives rise to pain. With a sprained ankle, however, you can limp and continue to get around by taking the weight off the injured joint, while putting most of your weight on the other leg.
- However, if a patient with only one leg sprains his ankle, he cannot limp. He cannot take the weight off his injured foot. He cannot walk around. He must go to bed until the "inflammation" of the sprain settles down.
- The same applies to the spine. You have only one spine, and when you severely sprain the joints in your spine, the only way to take the weight and strain of activities away from the spinal canal is to lie down.
- Therefore, bed rest is rational treatment. It is the quickest way to recovery.
- Prolonged bed rest (beyond a few days) is not good for your bone strength and muscle strength. Prolonged bed rest will lead both to weaken, and extend your recovery.

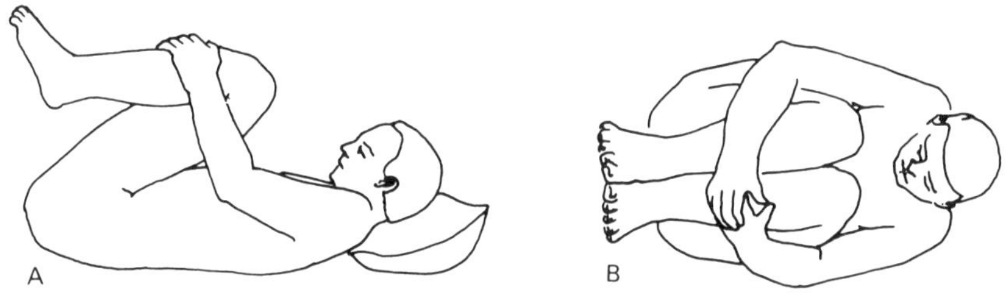

Figure 14.18 *A patient may abort an acute episode of low back pain by lying on the back and pulling the knees slowly up to the chest* **(A).** *He should maintain this position for 5 minutes. In very acute attacks with severe pain, the patient may find it easier to assume the same position lying on the side* **(B).**

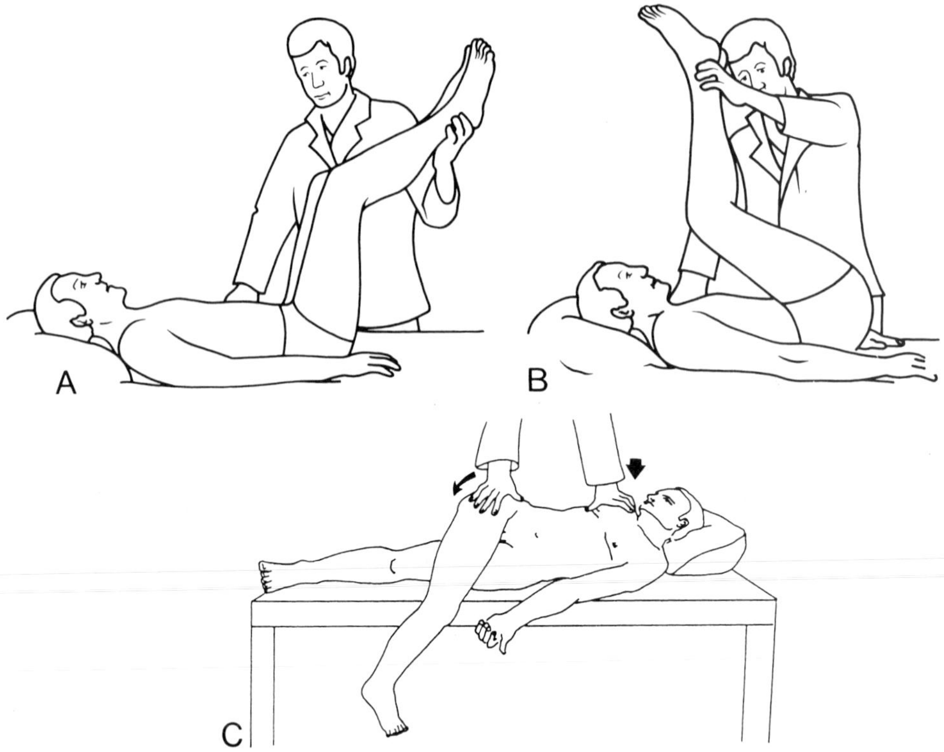

Figure 14.19 *If, on clinical examination, there is no evidence of root compression, resolution of symptoms may be speeded by a flexion manipulation. The patient lies on the back, and the physician raises the patient's legs, maintaining the knees in flexion* **(A).** *By applying pressure to the heels, the physician then pushes the patient's knees toward the shoulders* **(B).** *This movement is done very slowly, and the degree of flexion obtained is determined by the discomfort the patient experiences. This movement is then repeated slowly and rhythmically over a period of 5 minutes. In the majority of instances, the range of movement that can be achieved by this passive manipulation gradually increases. At the conclusion of the manipulation, the patient is instructed to flex his knees fully and allow his feet to come down to the bed, soles first.* **C.** *Rotation manipulation.*

To be effective, however, this manipulative therapy must continue on a daily basis and, therefore, the patient must learn how to perform these maneuvers independently. The patient should be taught specific steps. The manipulation exercises are carried out on a bed, not on the floor. The neck is kept slightly flexed by a pillow to minimize the effects of the inevitable contraction of the sternomastoids when the patient first makes an attempt to kick his/her feet up in the air.

The hips and knees are first flexed to a right angle. The legs are then raised toward the ceiling, keeping the knees slightly bent. The feet are then moved over the patient's head. This movement must not be in the form of a sudden kick. The buttocks must be raised slowly and smoothly off the bed by contraction of the trunk flexors and then, just as slowly, the legs are lowered. This movement is repeated several times, each time lowering the legs just to the starting position with the hips flexed at 90 degrees. The legs must not be lowered to the bed.

After five "kickups", the patient rests by lowering his/her legs, with the knees fully flexed, thereby putting the feet onto the bed, soles first (Fig. 14.20). This routine, at this stage in the treatment of an acute back pain, is not designed to be an exercise program. It is really an active flexion manipulation of the spine. The duration of these flexion manip-

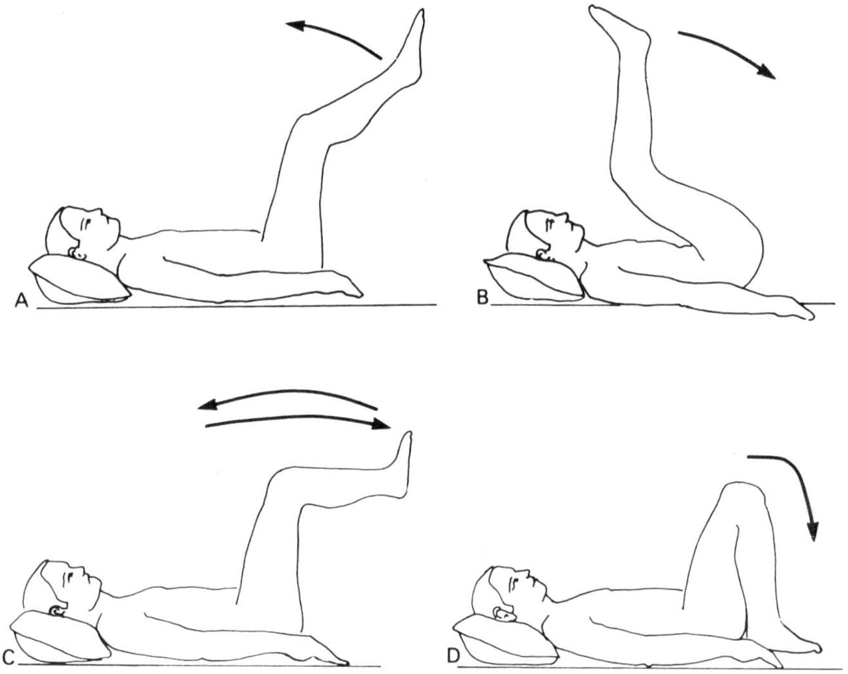

Figure 14.20 *Flexion exercise manipulation of the lumbar spine. The patient lies on the bed with the head supported by a pillow. The hips are flexed to 90 degrees, and the knees are slightly flexed* **(A).** *The patient now attempts to kick the feet over the head, raising the buttocks approximately 6 inches off the bed* **(B).** *After each "kickup," the patient returns to the starting position* **(C).** *After five kickups, the patient rests by lowering the legs with the knees fully flexed, thereby putting the feet on the bed, soles first* **(D).** *It is very important not to lower the legs with the knees fully extended, because this places a painful hyperextension strain on the spine.*

ulations should be restricted to 10 kickups only and these should be repeated three times a day.

If you are uncomfortable describing this regime to the patient and you think the patient can be driven to a professional's office, refer them to a skilled practitioner of the manipulative arts. Chiropractors are the most skilled, while many osteopaths are pursuing more "traditional" methods of medical care. Some physical therapists also include manipulation (in addition to mobilization) in their armamentarium.(31)

Bed rest should be continued until the patient can make journeys to the toilet in relative comfort without the aid of crutches (usually no more than a few days). After this period of time, the patient gradually increases activities within the limits set by his/her own tolerance of decreasing discomforts. The time of return to work is determined largely by the demands made on the patient's need to return to the job.

In the first edition of this book the use of plaster body jackets in the treatment of the acute incapacitating discogenic backache was described. This method of treatment is rarely indicated today, replaced instead by many well-designed braces and corsets. When considering a brace, remember that most of these patients will be better in a few days, and a brace is not indicated.

The treatment program previously described has been officially blessed by the Agency for Health Care Policy and Research (7), an arm of the American Government (US Department of Health and Human Services). The agency has, with great fanfare including media exposure, recommended a few days of bed rest, nonsteroidal anti-inflammatory drugs

(NSAIDs), a brace for return to work, physical therapy and manipulation for acute low back pain of less than 3 months' duration. They did not recommend acupuncture, transcutaneous electrical stimualation, trigger point injections, epidural injections, or traction. When "Big Brother" speaks, you just have to know it is right!

Prevention of Further Episodes

Regardless of how you treat these patients, they will get better. Your value as a health care professional is to attempt to prevent further attacks. Exercise in moderation on a regular basis is the most important step (see Chapter 13). It is prudent to discuss life-style factors that are detrimental to overall good health such as smoking and obesity.

Return to Function

Within a few days to a week most of these patients are back to work, within or outside of home. Hopefully you have them on a path of exercise and a healthier life-style to lessen the chance of further episodes.

Recurrent Aggravating Backache

This is probably the most common manifestation of disc degeneration and is the phase leading from dysfunction to instability. Rowe (79, 80), studying the incidence of low back pain in workers at the Kodak Company, found that 85% of the patients with backache had intermittent attacks of disabling pain every 3 months to 3 years, each attack lasting 3 days to 3 weeks. Between the attacks, the patients were relatively free from backache. The posterior joints are vulnerable to extension strains because degenerative changes in one or more discs may give rise to segmental hyperextension or persistent posterior joint subluxation. The facets of the involved segment or segments in these conditions are held at the extreme limit of extension; they have no safety factor of movement. A simply analogy can be drawn with the wrist. If a moderate blow is applied to the palm of the hand with the wrist in the neutral position, no pain results because the force of the blow is absorbed by the movement that occurs. If, however, the hand is hit with the same force, with the wrist in full extension, then this is painful because there is no safety factor of movement and the full brunt of the injury is transmitted to the capsule of the wrist (Fig. 14.21).

The same mechanical principle applies to the spine. In the neutral position moderate extension strains are not painful; but if a segment is held in hyperextension, there is no safety factor in movement and the extension strains of everyday living give rise to painful capsular lesions. The significance of extension strains is noted both in the history and examination of the patient.

Working with the hands above the head, such as in hanging up laundry, reaching, and so on, applies extension strains to the back and is painful. When the forward stooped position is maintained, the sacrospinales have to contract to hold the spine. With an unstable lumbar disc segment, in this position, the sacrospinales act as a bowstring producing hyperextension at the involved segment (Fig. 14.22). These patients complain of pain on stooping over the wash basin in the morning and when maintaining the bent forward position, as when making beds, and so on.

Sitting in a soft chair will allow the lumbar spine to become concertina-like and sag into hyperlordosis. These patients find it more comfortable to sit on a hard seat. Sitting in

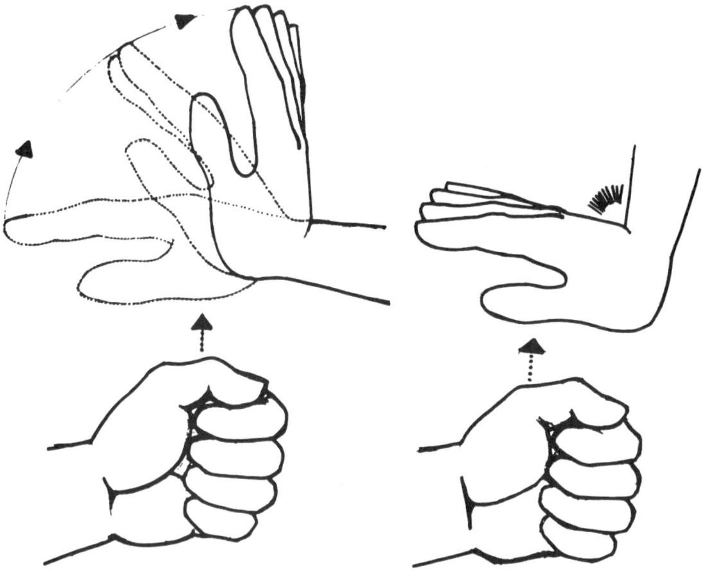

Figure 14.21 *The safety factor of movement. When a blow is applied to a wrist in the neutral position, the force of the blow is absorbed by the movement that occurs. When the same force is applied to the wrist in dorsiflexion, pain results because there is no safety factor of movement, and the full force of the blow is felt by the capsule of the wrist joint.*

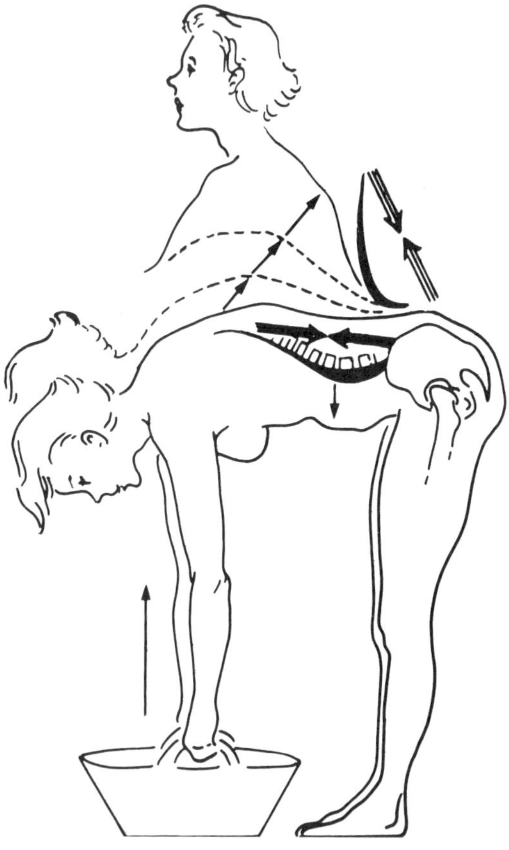

Figure 14.22 *When a patient bends forward with the knees straight and then tries to lift, the sacrospinales, when contracting, act as a bowstring and hyperextend the lumbar spine.*

a theater with the knees out straight and the floor sloping away will apply a significant extension strain to the spine, and the patients tend to irritate the patrons in the row in front by putting their feet on the back of their seat in order to keep knees and hips flexed. Similarly, sitting in a car with the knees held straight hyperextends the spine and makes prolonged driving uncomfortable.

When these patients stand for long periods of time, the lumbar spine sags into extension, and the patients automatically try to flatten the lumbar spine by flexing one hip and knee, as in the act of putting one foot on the seat of a chair or on a bar rail. Emotional tensions and frustrations will make the patient adopt the fight position, tightening up the sacrospinales. This posture will aggravate the pain, and the patient's increase in pain will aggravate his/her frustrations.

The pain experienced is commonly localized to the lumbosacral junction radiating out to one or both sacroiliac joints. If the pain intensifies it may radiate down one or both posterior thighs as far as the knee which may be confused with sciatica. On occasion, the pain may radiate into the groin and can be mistaken for hip disease.

On examination, the patients may demonstrate an increase in the normal lumbar lordosis, but more commonly they do not demonstrate any postural spinal abnormalities. They may, however, show many mechanical features that tend to aggravate hyperextension of the lumbar spine:

Weak Abdominal Muscles

These patients have difficulty in doing situps with their hips and knees bent and the palms of the hands clasped behind their heads. Because of the weakness of the abdominal muscles, when they lift both legs off the couch (bilateral straight leg raising) the weight of the legs tends to rotate the pelvis, hyperextending the spine and producing pain in the back (Fig. 14.23). Back pain reproduced by bilateral active straight leg raising is probably the best demonstration of the instability phase of lumbar disc degeneration aggravated by weak abdominal muscles.

Obesity

Excessive weight loading hyperextends the lumbar spine. This is particular)y apparent in the patient who has a "politician's pouch" (a protuberant fat abdomen). With the center of gravity anterior to the spine, the patient has to hyperextend his back to stand erect.

Tensor Fascia Femoris Contracture

Some patients, especially those with a mesomorphic build, have a tight tensor fascia femoris that tilts the pelvis forward (Fig. 14.24). With the pelvis fixed in this position, the lumbar spine must hyperextend to allow the spinal column to remain erect. When these patients stand against the wall with the back of the head, chest, buttocks, and heels touching the wall, they cannot flatten their lumbar spine. The only way they can flatten their backs against a wall is to step forward and bend their hips and knees, thereby relaxing the tensor fascia femoris and allowing the pelvis to rotate. On examination, adduction of the hip is markedly limited when the hip is internally rotated and extended at the same time.

Special note, then, is made of these aggravating factors: abdominal weakness, weight, and tightness of the tensor fascia femoris.

The physical findings in this stage of chronic degenerative disc disease are not very dramatic. If the patient is seen after the acute attack has subsided, movements of the lumbar spine may not be significantly limited. If muscle spasm is still present there may be maintenance of lumbar lordosis on forward flexion. On extending from the forward flexed position, however, the patient generally shows reversal of normal spinal rhythm. After starting to extend their backs, they will bend their knees and hips to tuck their pelvis under the spine in order to regain the erect position (Fig. 14.25). Extension in the erect position usually is limited and painful. If the examiner places his fingers on the anterior and posterior superior spines of the pelvis and then asks the patient to bend backward, the pelvis can be felt to rotate after approximately 20 degrees extension, and any further extension is painful.

Reversal of spinal rhythm on extending from the forward flexed position, pain on extension from the erect position, and pain on bilateral straight leg raising are common and, indeed, characteristic findings in chronic symptomatic degenerative disc disease. The demonstration of tenderness is not of significant diagnostic value and its distribution may be confusing. The injection of an irritating solution into the supraspinous ligament of L5

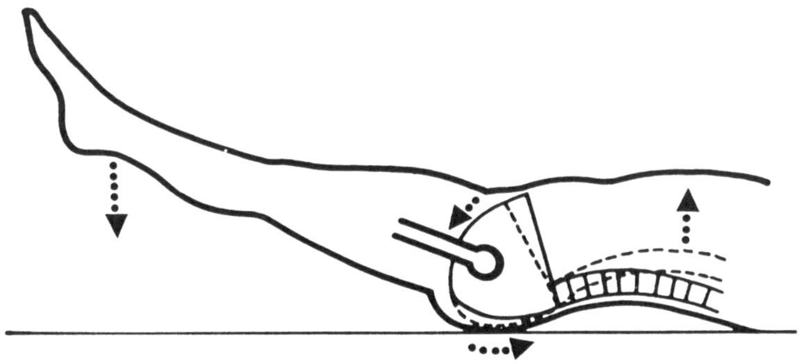

Figure 14.23 *When the patient carries out bilateral active straight leg raising, the weight of the leg causes the pelvis to rotate and thereby hyperextends the lumbar spine. Hyperextension of the lumbar spine in the presence of disc degeneration gives rise to pain. This is probably the most useful test to demonstrate the presence of painful segmental instability.*

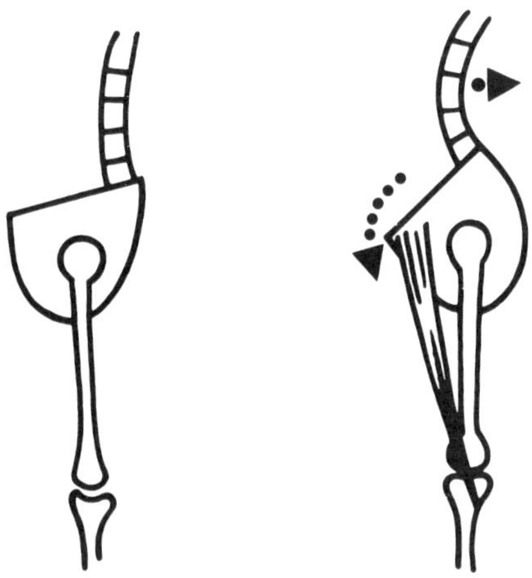

Figure 14.24 *A tight tensor fascia femoris, by rotating the pelvis anteriorly, produces hyperextension of the lumbar spine.*

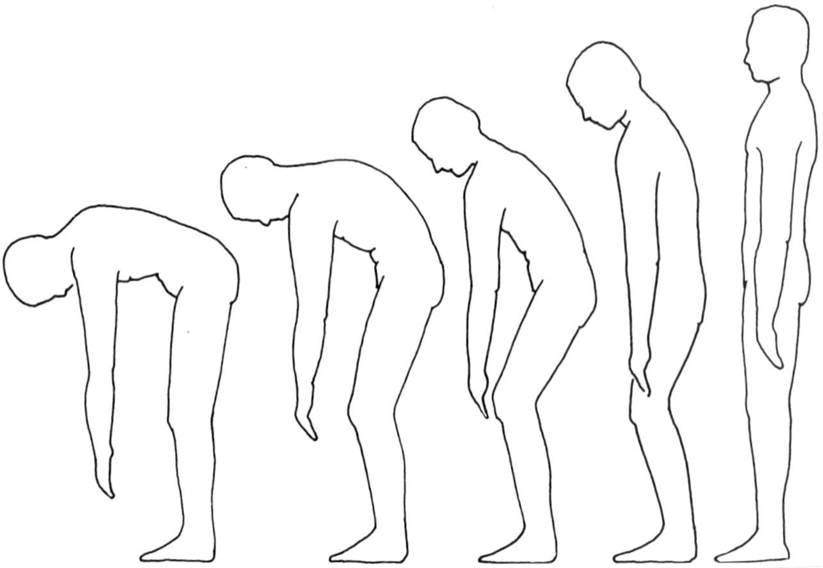

Figure 14.25 *With segmental instability, the patient will present reversal of normal spinal rhythm on extending from the forward flexed position.*

and S1 may give rise to local pain and also to pain referred to the sacroiliac joints and the buttocks or down the back of the thigh. Not only is pain referred in this distribution, but there may also be "referred tenderness." The upper outer quadrant of the buttock is normally tender on deep pressure. After the injection of hypertonic saline into the supraspinous ligament between L5 and S1, the upper outer quadrant of buttock becomes extremely tender and this form of "central irritation" may produce tenderness over the sacroiliac joints and tenderness on pressure over the back of the thigh. The physician must not allow himself to be led to believe that the demonstration of a point of tenderness indicates that the pathology lies deep to this area. It was because of this common zone of tenderness over the sacroiliac joints associated with degenerative disc disease that the diagnosis of sacroiliac joint lesions became so popular about a half century ago.

Treatment of the Instability Phase

In the treatment of recurrent aggravating discogenic back pain, the same general principles are employed as in the management of the acute incapacitating backache during its convalescent phase. Greater emphasis, of course, must be placed on the flexion exercise program and on general physical training.

With recurrent episodes of back pain of an aggravating rather than incapacitating nature, a sense of frustration on the part of the physician may result in the patient being thrown into the garbage dump of undirected physical therapy. If you are going to employ the services of a physical therapist, you must do so with reason and purpose. Physical therapy should never be employed as a form of entertainment until such time as nature cures the symptoms. Heat by itself and in whatever modality employed, although making the patient feel better temporarily, does little to speed the resolution of the symptoms. To request massage is no more than using the physical therapy department as a medically approved body rub parlor.

Physical therapists can be sensibly and usefully employed to teach patients how to carry out an exercise program and supervise their initial progress. Some patients are musculoskeletal morons. When trying to follow instructions on kickup exercises, these patients look like a butterfly having an epileptic fit. These patients need help and direction. Rotation exercises may place undue stress on the discs and the posterior joints and should only be undertaken by the very physically fit. Diverse corporal contortions may be inflicted on your patient and, although splendid in their place, such exercises should be kept in their place and reserved for the time when the patient has been symptom free for many months.

Discuss the exercise program you want with your physical therapist, so that, for better or for worse, you will know what exercises your patients are doing. Some patients need instruction in muscular relaxation far more than they need instruction in muscular contraction. Probably one of the most useful roles of the physical therapist is to teach the patient the technique of voluntary muscular relaxation. Probably the most important instructions the patient will receive from the therapist will be advice on how to pursue activities of daily living without reaggravating symptoms.

Your job is to emphasize the role of exercise in controlling symptoms and the negative impact smoking and obesity have on recurrent episodes of back pain. This is not a group of patients where you want to introduce the "crutch of bracing" and it is very important that you avoid long-term use of narcotics and mood altering drugs.

Chronic Persistent Backache

The bête noire of orthopedic surgeons is the syndrome of chronic, persistent discogenic low back pain, easily made intolerable by modest activity. These patients are in the midst of chronic spinal instability and have yet to advance into Kirkaldy-Willis's third phase of spontaneous stabilization.

Patients with a chronic persistent daily backache generally report a history of having been plagued by intermittent episodes of back pain for several years. Eventually, they reach the stage when the back pain never really leaves them. By pushing themselves, they may get through the average day with barely tolerable nagging discomfort in their back. They are very vulnerable to the traumatic insults of everyday life and, on minimal provocation, may get a "flare-up" of back pain. They have to be careful about everything they do and gradually, almost imperceptibly, their activities grind to a halt. They become the subjects of spinal rule, with their spine acting as a malevolent dictator, determining what they can do and what they cannot do. These patients then report the history of a back pain that seriously interferes with their ability to do their work and their capacity to enjoy themselves in their leisure hours.

When assessing such patients, it must be remembered that, although a chronic back pain may make the patient's life very miserable, persistent incapacitating back pain is most unusual. For example, if a woman presents with these complaints, the first question that the physician has to ask is "Why is this patient so disabled by the back pain she experiences?" It must be remembered that pain and disability are not synonymous. "The pain in my back is so severe I can't stoop to make the beds." This seems to be a perfectly reasonable complaint, but, nevertheless, it must be remembered that the patient is not describing the pain: she is describing her own reaction to the pain. Her next door neighbor with the same degree of pain may be out playing tennis. In chronic depressive states when the patient's emotional state is affected, the patient may describe an obviously unreasonable decrease of activities: "For the last 2 years the pain has been so bad that I have had to use two canes to get around the house, and I haven't slept for more than 1 or 2 hours any night," "I got a sudden severe attack of pain in the middle of the symphony concert and they had to carry me out on a stretcher." This grossly exaggerated degree of disability is obviously divorced from reality. Discogenic back pain never gives rise to this degree of physical impairment for this length of time. The magnification of the disability may be less bizarre. "I spend at least half the day lying down." "I can't walk a block."

Emotional problems commonly play a significant role in the disability resulting from chronic persistent low back pain. A patient with an hysterical personality tends to react hysterically to any pain, including a backache, but the histrionics generally subside as the pain abates. When the disability represents just one small facet of a general emotional breakdown, the symptoms will be intensified and perpetuated if too much attention is paid to them and too little attention is paid to the patient as a whole.

In the management of these patients, then, the important questions to answer are: "Why is this patient so disabled by the pain he/she experiences?" "Where has the breakdown occurred: in the patient, or in the spine, or in both?"

Examination of the spine will reveal the features described in patients suffering from recurrent back pain due to segmental instability: pain on extension of the spine, reversal of normal spinal rhythm, pain on bilateral active straight leg raising, and tenderness on palpation and manipulation of the lower lumbar spinous processes. It is frequently observed that the lower lumbar spine moves very little on forward flexion, a fact that can be measured by noting that the spinous processes do not separate very much on forward flexion. There are no signs of root tension, root irritation, or root compression.

Other factors contributing to the persistence of the pain may be noted: excessive weight, flabby abdominal muscles, a tight tensor fascia femoris. Radiographs will show the stigmata of degenerative disc disease at one or more segments (Fig. 14.26).

Treatment

No form of therapy will alter the degenerative changes that have occurred. Manipulation of the spine may result in a short-lived amelioration of symptoms but rarely, if ever, gives rise to permanent relief. Manipulation is most useful to break the pain cycle and allow a patient to pursue an appropriate exercise program.

In trying to outline a rational form of management of these patients, the following points must be remembered: (1) the natural tendency of the disease is eventually toward subsidence of symptoms and, occasionally, recovery; (2) no specific treatment alters the changes in the disc; and (3) treatment perforce must be directed at making the patient comfortable while nature effects the control of symptoms by stabilizing the painful motion segment.

When considering the means to make the patient comfortable, it must be remembered that (1) the pain is relieved by lying down, by unloading the spine; and (2) any activity that puts an extension strain on the spine increases the pain. Bearing these two points in mind, patients can be managed by unloading the spine in the following manner:

1. Losing weight, where indicated.
2. Wearing a corset with a strong abdominal binder to increase intra-abdominal pressure and bring the center of gravity nearer the spine. This should be seen by the doctor and the patient as a temporary step.

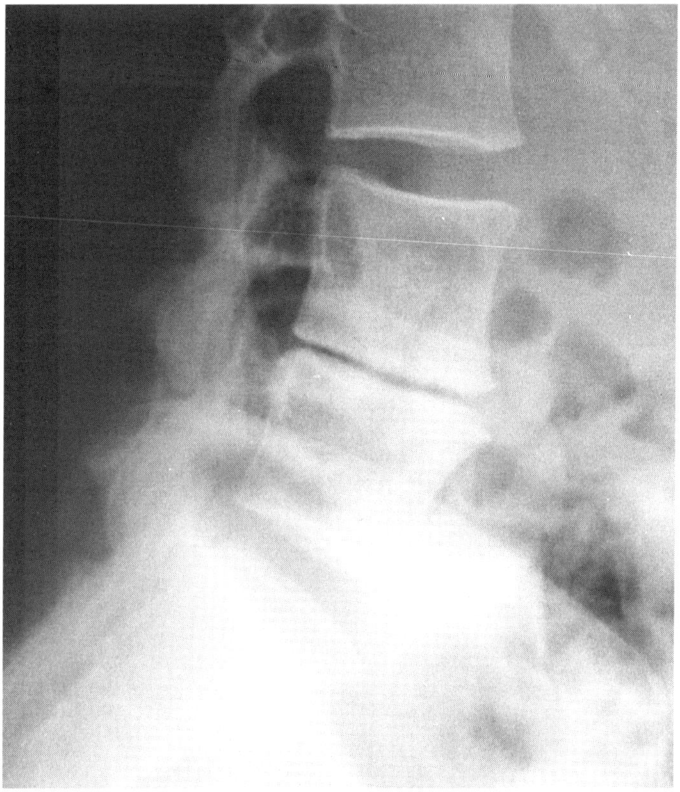

Figure 14.26 *A plain radiograph showing severe degenerative disc disease at L4–L5. You will meet this type of degenerative disc disease later in the chapter. Read on!*

3. Changing occupation. This course of action, although undesirable, may on occasion be the only realistic form of treatment. It most certainly must be considered before a spinal fusion for all workers engaged in heavy work.
4. Teaching the patient to guard his/her spine against the extension strains of everyday living. The symptom of chronic persistent discogenic low back pain is almost invariably associated with fixed hyperextension of the zygapophysial joints resulting either from segmental hyperextension or from disc narrowing with posterior subluxation. The posterior joints are maintained at the limit of extension and any further attempt at extension is painful.

Extension strains are common: reaching, pushing, sitting with the legs out straight, prolonged standing, walking with big strides, and so on. In the act of lifting with the knees straight, the sacrospinales act as a bowstring and extend the spine (Fig. 14.22).

The patients must be taught to modify activities and assume postures that maintain the lumbar spine in the neutral position. They must be given written instructions in this regard (Table 14.3).

Extension strains are more liable to occur if the trunk flexors are weak, and a prolonged program to build up the trunk flexors is an essential part of treatment. The kickup exercise-manipulation program is the simplest to learn and the one most readily accomplished and persevered with by the patient.

Table 14.3. Instructions for Patients on Flexion Routine

General Observations

Whenever possible, sit down. Sit with the knees higher than the hips. The best way of doing this is to sit with the feet on a foot stool. If no foot stool is available, cross the legs. Never sit with the legs out straight.

- Do not reach.
- Do not lift weights above the head or out in front of you.
- Do not stoop.
- Do not move furniture by pulling it in front of you.
- Do not push windows up.
- Do not put on weight.
- Do not get overtired.
- Do not maintain any one position for a prolonged period.

Sleeping

The mattress should be firm. If the mattress is soft, a board should be placed underneath it. Sleep on your side with your hips and knees bent.

Sitting

When driving a car, the seat should be as close to the steering wheel as possible, thereby flexing the knees and hips. When riding in a car, you should put a pillow behind your back so that you sit forward in the seat, again flexing the knees and hips. Whenever possible throughout the day, you should sit down with your knees higher than your hips in the "lazy boy" position.

Getting up from sitting

It is important not to arch the back on the act of getting up from sitting. Move to the front of the chair and stand up, keeping your back straight. Use your hands to help you if necessary.

Standing

The best way to stand is to adopt the posture commonly seen in a hotel bar: one foot on the ground and one foot on the brass rail. When the brass rail is not available, get one foot on any raised object: the bottom of a desk or the seat of a chair. NEVER maintain a stooped forward position when standing.

Lifting

Ideally, you should not lift anything heavier than 15 lb while your back is sore, and ideally you should not lift anything heavier than 50 lb for 6 months. When lifting something off the floor, bend the hips and knees, keeping the spine straight.

- NEVER bend over to lift something off the ground with the knees straight.
- NEVER hold anything weighing more than 15 lb more than 1 ft from the body.
- NEVER lift anything over 20 lb above the shoulder level.

Housework

Equipment. All equipment should have long handles so that you do not have to stoop too much.

Vacuuming. The vacuum should be pushed with short sweeps rather than long lunges. Do not try to vacuum the whole house at once.

Kitchen. Never reach for objects from high shelves. Rearrange your kitchen so that articles in daily use are on the first shelf above counter level. When you have to stand for any length of time (ironing or at the kitchen sink), stand with one foot on a box 9 inches high. Use the box as a step to reach for articles above shoulder level. When getting articles from cupboards underneath the counter level, bend your hips and knees, and squat down, keeping your back straight. Never bend forward with the knees straight to reach for anything from these low cupboards.

Laundry. When carrying laundry, it is best to carry the clothes in a small basket held against one side. Never carry a heavy laundry basket in front of you. It is better to make several trips than to stagger once under an enormous load.

Stairs. Avoid, as far as possible, going up and down stairs. Do all the housework you have to do upstairs and then leave the rest of the housework upstairs for the day.

Bedmaking. You have to bend forward when tucking in sheets, and this will aggravate your back pain. When your back pain is severe, if you cannot persuade some other member of the family to do this chore, the only way you can tuck in the sheets in comfort is to get on your hands and knees.

A corset should not be prescribed early in treatment. Flexion exercises and the flexion routine should be tried first and, as long as the patient shows some measure of improvement, they should be continued. If the patient reaches a plateau in recovery and is still plagued by back pain, a corset should be ordered (Fig. 14.27).

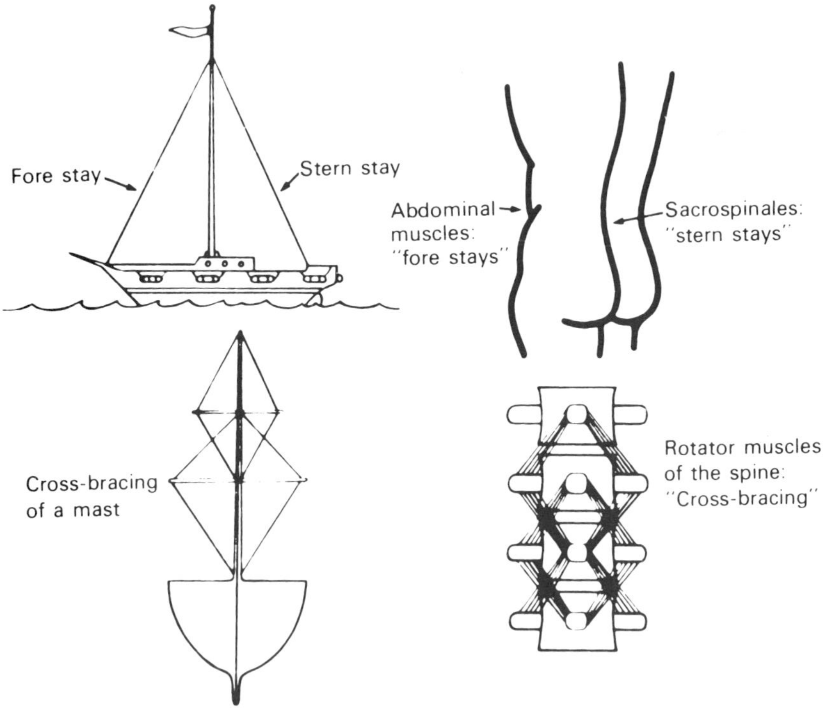

Figure 14.27 *It is interesting to note the similarity between the bracing used to support the mast of a ship and the muscular bracing of the human spine.*

As mentioned previously, patients derive the most benefit from a corset with a strong abdominal binder worn tightly, but a simple canvas corset cannot produce significant compression of the abdomen in thin patients, especially if they have a prominent rib cage. The most that can be done for these patients is to try to restrict movement to some extent with a high thoracolumbar brace.(TLSO)(2) The upper part of the brace must grasp the patient firmly around the lower rib cage and the pelvic band must fit snugly just below the iliac crest. Side and posterior steel supports will protect the patient, to some extent, against sudden jolts and jars. The posterior steel supports should not be curved in but should run in a straight line. The abdominal binder should be padded so that some pressure can be exerted against the abdominal wall (Fig. 14.28).

Once the back pain is under some control an increase in daily physical activities is an essential part of treatment.

We encourage our patients to join a health club and work out on a regular (3 to 4 times per week) basis. We instruct our patients to avoid impact/contact and lifting. The impact sports that should be avoided are running, skipping, stair-stepper, and volleyball. Basketball is a particularly poor choice for these patients because of both contact and impact. Our instructions on lifting are: never use two legs in the same moment of activity (Fig. 14.29). To be really effective, the progress of the patient must be checked regularly by the physician or by the physical therapist for a year. The treatment of a chronic, grumbling persistent back pain is like the treatment of a chronic alcoholic: nothing can be achieved during a single 15-minute consultation. If you are willing to follow through with these patients, or get a team to do this, in the well-motivated patient the result will be worth the effort.

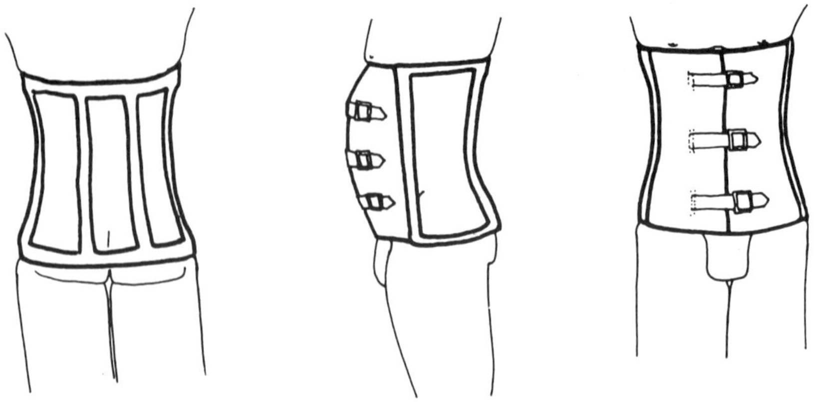

Figure 14.28 *A rigid spinal brace with posterior and side steels and a firm abdominal binder.*

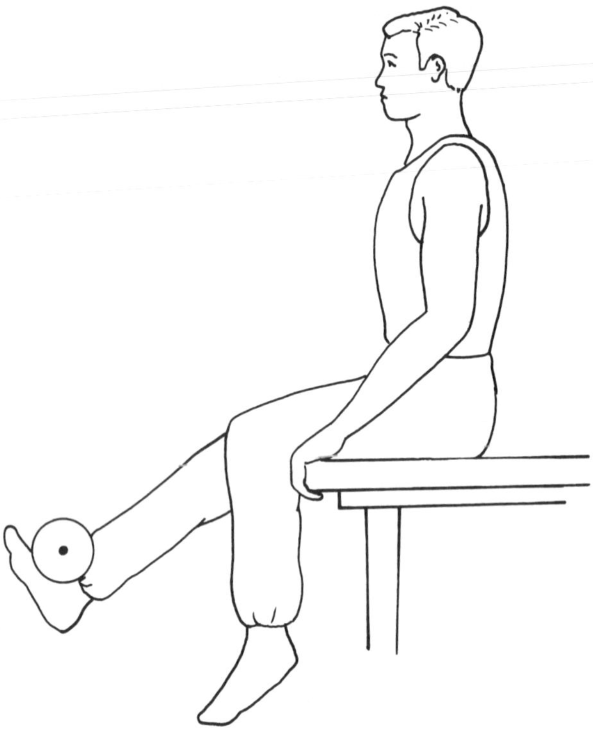

Figure 14.29 *Always use one leg at a time when working with a back pain patient. The use of two legs at the same time for weight lifting will immediately transfer forces to the back.*

Exercises: Flexion Versus Extension

Much of human low back pain is ascribed to the fact that we walk upright instead of on all fours, which in turn causes lumbar lordosis and extension strains. Over the years, much of our treatment has been directed at reducing the natural lordotic curve with Williams' flexion exercises.(101) More recently, McKenzie (62) has popularized the extension school and others have taken the best of both programs, combined with isokinetic theories of exercise, and spawned the exercise cult that is sweeping America with posh clubs containing expensive Cybex and Nautilus equipment. Some therapists believe that relaxation and stretching exercises are equally as important as flexion, extension, and/or isokinetic exercises. As a fifth option, most patients will choose the laissez-faire approach of exercising when they want and how they want: "walk a little, swim a little, and so on."

The basis of encouraging patients to consider exercises is: (1) Numerous studies have shown that a fit patient is less likely to end up with low back pain as a consequence of occupation.(14) (2) A fit person recovers faster and stays better longer after an episode of low back pain (6, 65).

Which exercise is best to help rehabilitate the patient is unknown. What is important is that the doctor recognize the patient who will respond to exercise therapy and the therapist, familiar with all theories and techniques, knows "when" to intervene with "what" technique. If the response desired is not being achieved, then the patient, therapist, and doctor should each be prepared to accept the limitations of exercise and either discontinue the exercise or change its nature. Continually flogging one particular exercise program because an individual believes fervently in its benefits is poor medicine.

Other Conservative Treatment Options

The most important treatment you offer a patient with mechanical low back pain is the passage of time, during which most disabilities will resolve.(5) Next in its effectiveness is the use of various forms of rest (bed, corset, weight loss, job modification) and the use of anti-inflammatory and/or analgesic medication. Short of these measures, there is very little else one can do to positively affect the natural course of the disease. We have discussed other treatments in other chapters, such as medications, braces, and exercises, and allow that they each have their own limitations.

Other Modalities

Heat, Ice, Short-Wave Diathermy, Ultrasound There is no scientific proof that the use of these modalities by themselves affect the natural course of low back disability.

Manipulation The self-administered manipulative exercises previously described may be of some benefit to the patient. Even better, is short term chiropractic manipulation. However, the institution of long-term treatment and preventative manipulation programs have no scientific basis for support.(31)

Education Patient education is an important aspect of treatment in many diseases. Providing a patient is receptive to this approach, attendance at back school (99) will help the patient understand "what went wrong" and hopefully encourage habits that will lower the incidence of recurrence of the disability. The school, generally directed by a therapist, will involve the patient in treatment and place the responsibility for improvement on the patient.(36)

Injections There is no scientific support for anything beyond placebo effect for injections into muscle, ligaments, trigger points, or facet joints. To some patients and some doctors, the occasional use of this placebo effect is beneficial. To make extensive use of these injections, although beneficial to the remunerative aspects of doctoring, is frustrating to the advancement of the science of low back pain.

Traction Many of us recall the days when patient after patient would be admitted to the hospital for traction. Fortunately, the cost of such treatment and the lack of a scientific basis (59) have largely put an end to such a useless endeavor. Now, we have evidence that bed rest beyond a few days, with or without traction, is detrimental to patients' muscle and bone mass, let alone their emotional well-being. To hang them up in traction has to be a form of cruel and unusual punishment.(59)

Miscellaneous Efforts The use of transcutaneous nerve stimulation, behavior modification, biofeedback, and psychotherapy are treatment efforts used in the management of chronic pain syndromes. Their indications and non-indications were discussed in Chapter 13 in the section on conservative treatment.

Degenerative Disc Disease with Special Status

There are five separate conditions we can lump in this group, including:

1. Isolated disc resorption.
2. Degenerative scoliosis.
3. The facet joint syndrome.
4. Internal disc disruption.
5. Cervicolumbar syndrome.

Isolated Disc Resorption

This is the easiest of the five special status conditions to deal with because it is easily recognized and easily treated. To "cut to the quick" of the subject, the patients are usually women; they have backache that totally dominates their life; they have the radiographic studies shown in Figure 14.30; they never get better with conservative treatment once they become symptomatic; and they all should have surgery. You might find this position a little dogmatic, so let us explore further.

In 1970, this condition was first described by Crock (20, 21, 93), who stressed three features.

1. The dominance of back pain (we agree).
2. The presence of bilateral leg pain due to nerve root encroachment in the foramen (we disagree) (see Figure 14.31).
3. The condition is more common than the ruptured disc (we disagree).

By definition, the term "isolated disc resorption" means the condition is isolated to one disc, whereas adjacent discs are normal. The usual involvement is L5–S1, although a few patients have L4–L5 involvement (Fig. 14.26). Only when the disc is completely resorbed (Figs. 14.30 and 14.31) has the definition of isolated disc resorption been fulfilled. Some degree of disc degeneration affecting multiple segments is simply degenerative disc disease and does not qualify for special status.

The patients are usually women, who have borne children and who may or may not recall a significant back injury many years earlier. They start with the usual history of intermittent episodes of back pain, and within 1 or 2 years, their disc space collapses, and they end up with constant back pain that totally dominates their life. They are unable to do

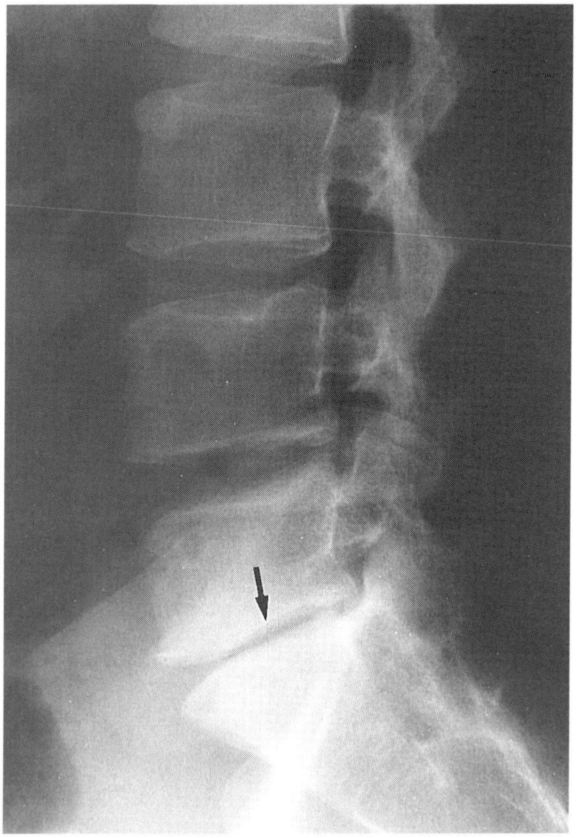

Figure 14.30 *Plain radiograph showing isolated disc resorption at L5–S1. Look back at figure 14.26.*

any activity other than rest in bed or stand and walk upright. As soon as they try to bend or lift, they develop significant back pain that takes hours of bed rest to settle. This is a combined picture of instability and inflammation. They are unstable in that the slightest level of activity triggers their back pain, yet on flexion-extension radiographs there is no instability demonstrated. The disc inflammation component is manifested by the persistent pain despite bed rest and the erosions in the endplate seen on plain radiographs (Figs. 14.26 and 14.30). The radiographic appearance is so unsettling that many of these patients undergo extensive investigation, including a CT-guided biopsy, despite the fact that there is no systemic or laboratory evidence of infection.

After months of failed, yet excellent conservative care, these patients presentwith the dominant symptom of back pain. Aside from some minor referred leg pain, there is no historical or physical evidence of radicular involvement. Crock originally stressed foraminal nerve root compression, but MRI (Fig. 14.31) shows that this is not present. The patients have a very stiff back and fail to reverse lumbar lordosis on forward flexion, yet often can reach the floor with their fingertips because of hip flexion.

Investigation is straightforward. The patients are usually young to middle-aged women in whom associated debilitating diseases, (eg, diabetes or immunocompromise) are not suspect. All you have to do is show that there is no fever and the white blood cell count and erythrocyte sedimentation rate (ESR) are normal; no other investigation is needed. Forget the ordering of bone scans, gadolinium enhanced MRIs, disc space biop-

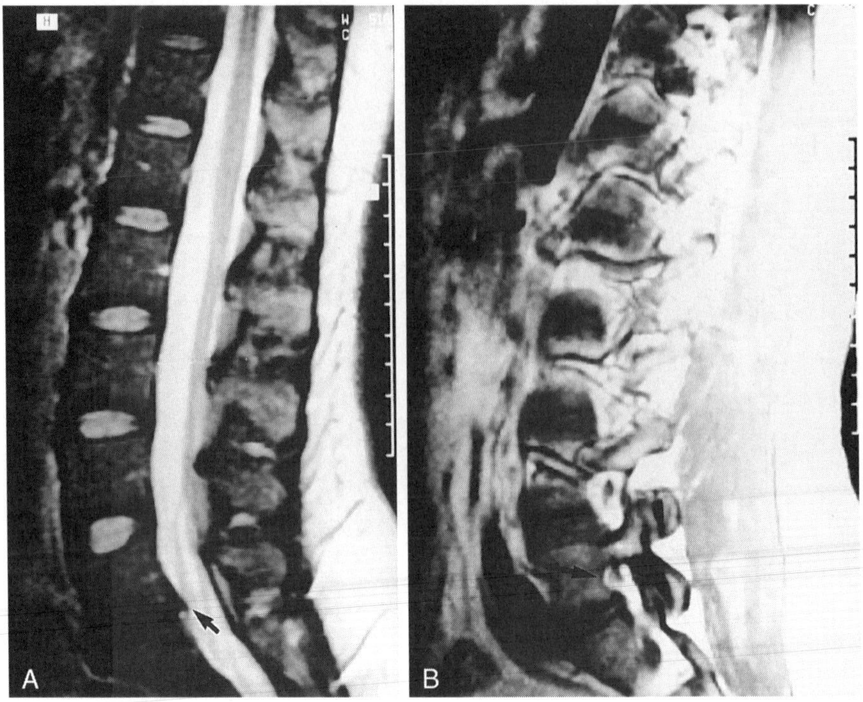

Figure 14.31 **A.** *Sagittal MRI (T2 weighted) showing isolated disc resorption at L5–S1 (the black disc, arrow). The rest of the discs have a high water content (bright signal).* **B.** *Parasagittal cuts showing the foramen at L5 to be wide open (arrow).*

sies, and EMGs. These tests will yield nothing. It is necessary to do an MRI with T2 sagittals (Fig. 14.32) to verify that the disc involvement is isolated, the adjacent discs are normal, and the foramen are open.

The pathology of this lesion is not understood. The condition is not unlike spondylodiscitis seen in ankylosing spondylitis and rheumatoid arthritis. Crock (21) has biopsied these discs at the time of surgery and has concluded the cause is a very active chemical process leading to degradation of the nuclear and annular portions of the intervertebral disc. The last phase of disc destruction is necrosis of the cartilaginous endplate, which leaves behind the worrisome cortical erosions seen on radiograph.

Treatment These patients almost always fail conservative treatment efforts and do very well with a limited (uninstrumented) lumbar fusion (Fig. 14.33).

Degenerative (Adult Onset) Scoliosis

Scoliosis (a frontal/coronal plain curve) is to be distinguished from a sagittal plain (kyphosis) malalignment (Fig. 14.34). It is reasonably common in adolescents (2–4% of the population) and may carry forward into adult years as an untreated condition. These patients present before the age of 40 with a painful deformity and very little in the way of neurological symptoms.

Adult onset scoliosis is a completely different problem and is not simply an extension of scoliosis from a young age.(51, 77, 86) It occurs in the older patient (over 50 years of

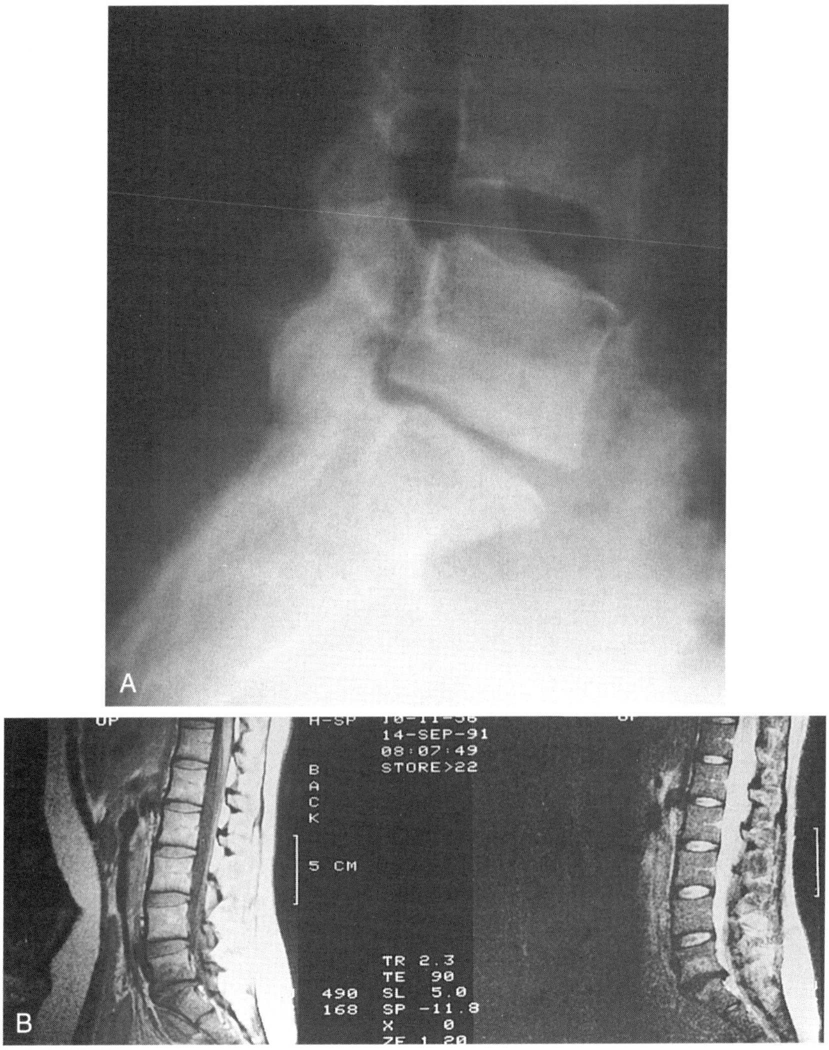

Figure 14.32 **A.** *plain radiograph showing isolated disc resorption at L5–S1.* **B.** *Sagittal MRI. Left: T1 weighted. Right: T2 weighted showing the black disc.*

age) and is secondary to degenerative disc and/or facet joint disease. It is present in 5% of patients over 50 years of age and is most often symptomatic in the female osteoporotic patient (female-male ratio = at least 2:1).

Etiology Degenerative facet and disc disease is universal. Degenerative scoliosis as a variety of degenerative disc disease develops because one facet joint wears and subluxes more than its mate (Fig. 14.35), which leads to a lateral subluxation and the subsequent development of the scoliosis.(76) Asymmetric disc space narrowing is also present (Fig. 14.35), either as a cause or a result. Osteoporosis is a constant feature in women who, in turn, usually have worse curves and more pain than men. A history of previous laminectomy, especially with loss of a facet joint, will accelerate the scoliosis.

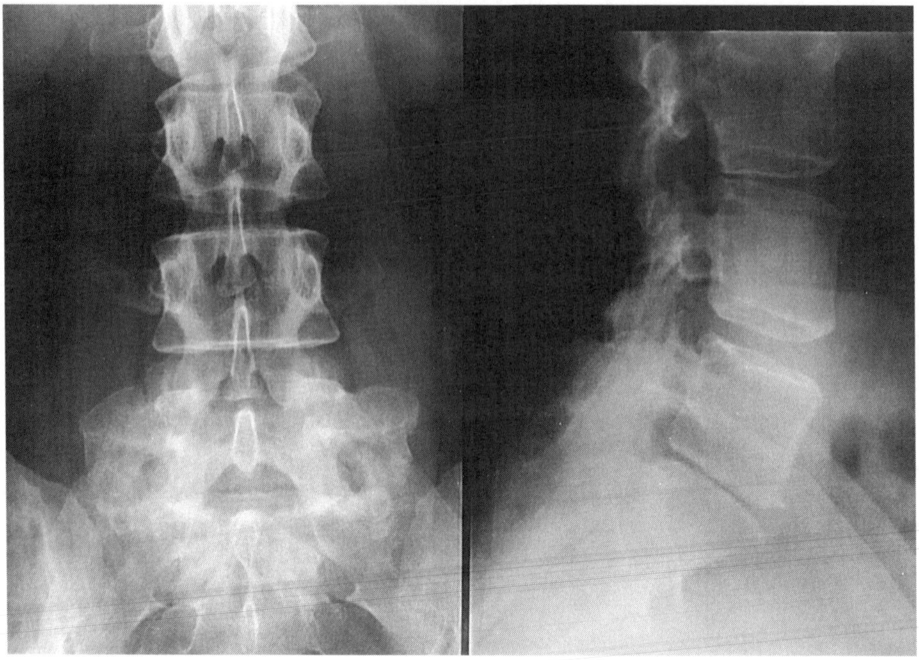

Figure 14.33 *A "limited" exposure for an L5–S1 uninstrumented fusion (left) for isolated disc resorption (right).*

Clinical Presentation The most common presentation is low back pain.(34) At least 50% of the patients will have neurological involvement, either in the form of monoradicular pain or claudicant leg pain due to spinal canal stenosis.

These patients all present with a long history of back pain, increasing in severity as the curve progresses. Curve progression may be up to 3 degrees per year and is more apt to occur in:

Women.
Individuals with osteoporosis.
Individuals with right-sided curves.
Individuals with shorter-segment curves.
Individuals with high Cobb angles (more than 30 degrees) on presentation.
Individuals with a rotation of Grade 2 or more (Fig. 14.36).
Individuals with a high L5–S1 junction (Fig. 14.37).
Individuals with significant lateral subluxation (Fig. 14.38)

On examination, patients will have an obvious lumbar curve. They usually stand in a forward flexed position with a loss of lumbar lordosis (the flat back). At least half of the patients will have decompensation (Fig. 14.39). Neurological examination will determine mono- or multiradicular involvement.

There may be a monoradicular complaint affecting either the lumbar or the sacral plexus, and it is important to distinguish between the two. Obviously, any anterior thigh pain with a depressed knee reflex and/or weakness of knee extension implicates the third or fourth lumbar nerve root and will routinely be due to compression on the concave side of the curve.

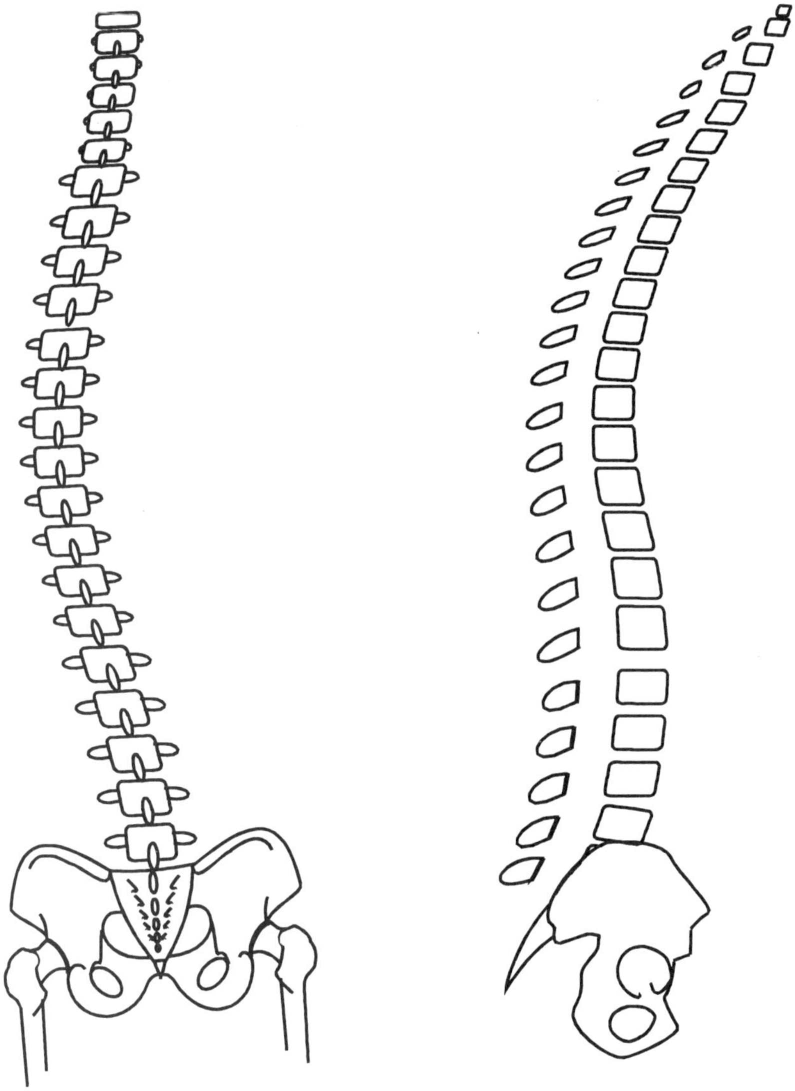

Figure 14.34 *Scoliosis, convex left, on the left; kyphosis on the right.*

Fifth lumbar or first sacral root involvement can be on either side of the curve. Generalized encroachment on the common dural sac is most pronounced at the apex of the curve (Fig. 14.40) and will cause a bilateral chronic radicular syndrome (spinal canal stenosis).

Curve Characteristics The curvature of adult onset scoliosis is most typically lumbar, which is another feature that distinguishes this condition from that of children (Table 14.4). Right-sided curves are equally as common as left, and usually no more than 6 vertebrae (average 4) are included in the curve (Fig. 14.35). Curves with a Cobb angle greater than 60 degrees are unusual, with most of these curves lying between 20 degrees and 30 degreees on patient presentation.

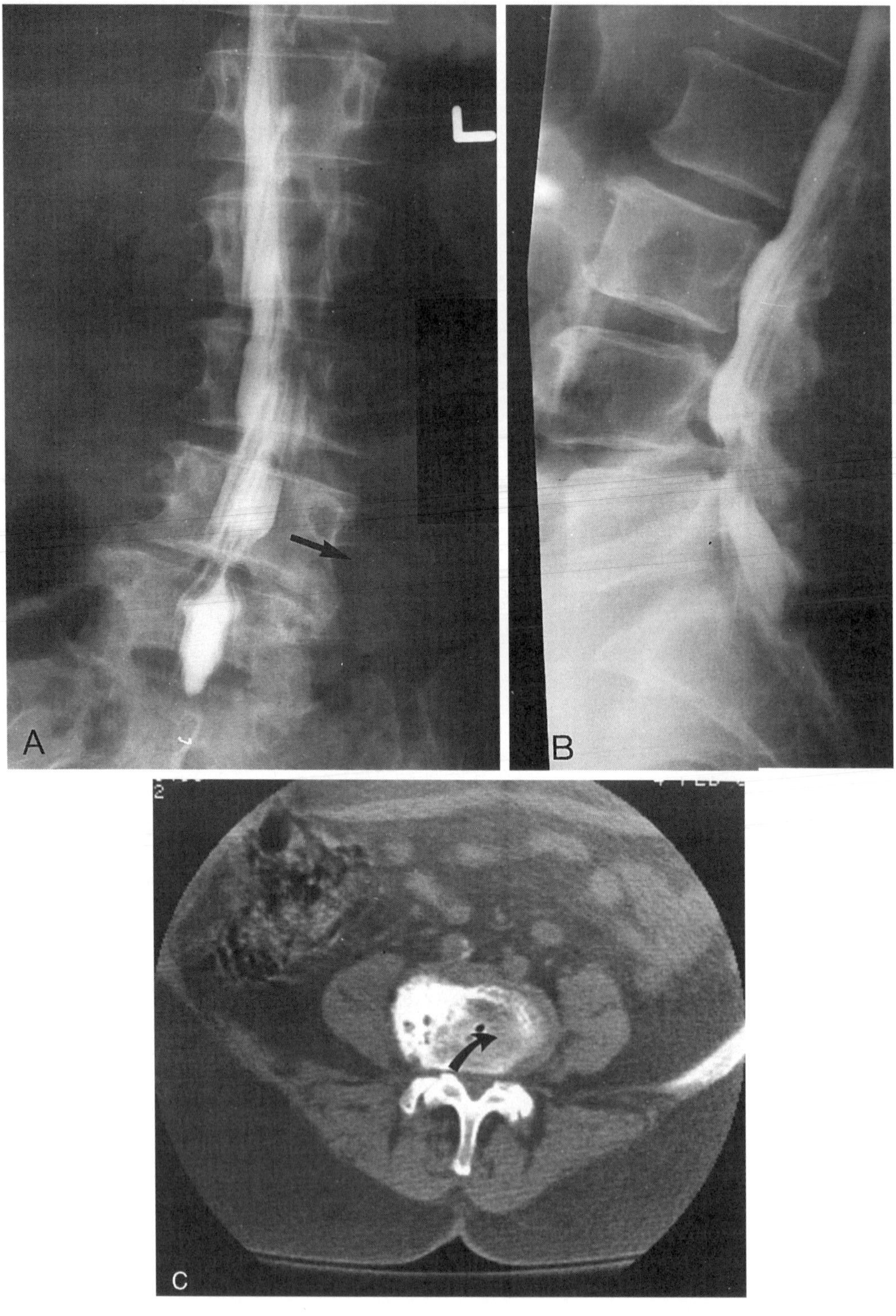

Figure 14.35 **A.** *A left lumbar degenerative scoliosis; the lateral spondylolisthesis of L4 on L5 (arrow).* **B.** *There is also a forward slip of L4 on L5.* **C.** *Note the facet joint subluxation, more on the right (arrow) than the left.*

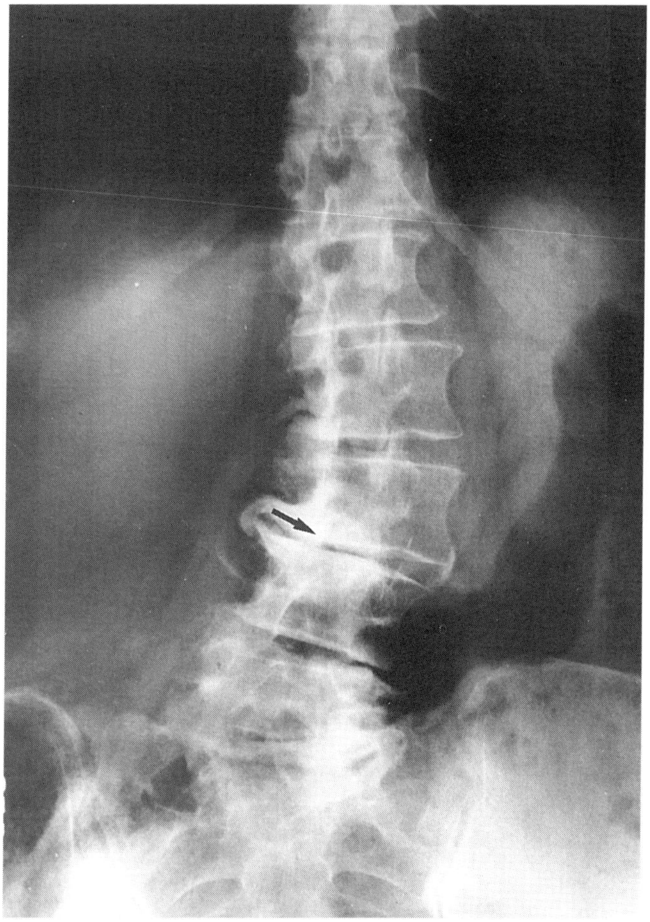

Figure 14.36 *Degenerative scoliosis showing significant rotation of spinous process (arrow).*

The apex of the curve is most often at L3. An apex at L2 will shift the curve into the low thoracic region and often be associated with a secondary curve just above the pelvis (Fig. 14.40).

Treatment These patients are incredibly difficult to treat because of many factors:

They are older (more concurrent medical problems).
They are osteoporotic.
They have often had previous surgery.
They all have significant back pain.

The universality of back pain mandates that any surgical procedure include a fusion. This in itself increases the level of difficulty in treatment because these patients have somewhat impaired wound healing potential simply because of their age. Add to that the requirement for a decompression of neurological structures and the requirement for multiple segments to be fused, and you have a setup for failure.

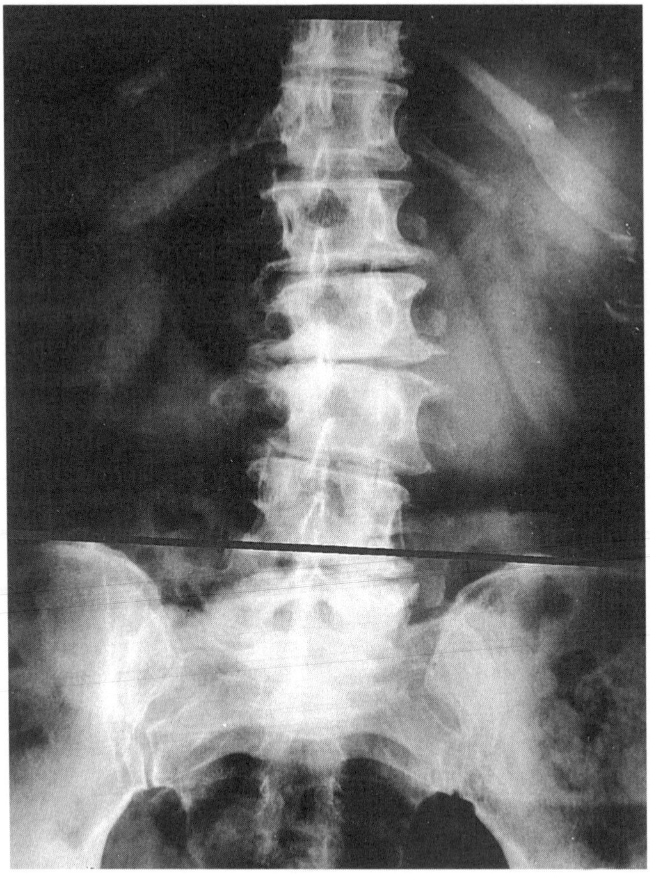

Figure 14.37 *Degenerative scoliosis with the intercrestal line through the L4–L5 disc space, which is considered to be a higher than normal lumbosacral junction.*

This has led most surgeons to the use of instrumentation to correct and stabilize the curve (Fig. 14.41), which seems to be a fine concept except that a segment of the spine is rigidly immobilized, stressing the segments above (Fig. 14.42). Over time, these unfused segments are likely to deteriorate.

Obviously, there is a message in this dismal discussion of surgical outcomes: do everything you can to treat these patients conservatively. Use physical therapy, bracing, epidural cortisone, and any other placebo-inducing treatment you can come up with. Above all, be open and honest with the patients when proposing surgery.

Surgery for Adult Degenerative Scoliosis The aim of surgery is to relieve neurological compression, fuse to relieve back pain, and obtain some (50%) curve correction. This is impossible without instrumentation. Because lamina have to be removed to accomplish the neurological decompression, the only viable instrumentation system is pedicle fixation.(58) Attempts should be made to avoid fusing to the sacrum; remember to build in some lumbar lordosis.

Surgery for monoradicular pain can be a limited microdecompression for L5 or S1 root involvement. For higher lumbar root involvement causing a monoradicular syndrome, a limited microdecompression will not work without a wide decompression and curve correction.

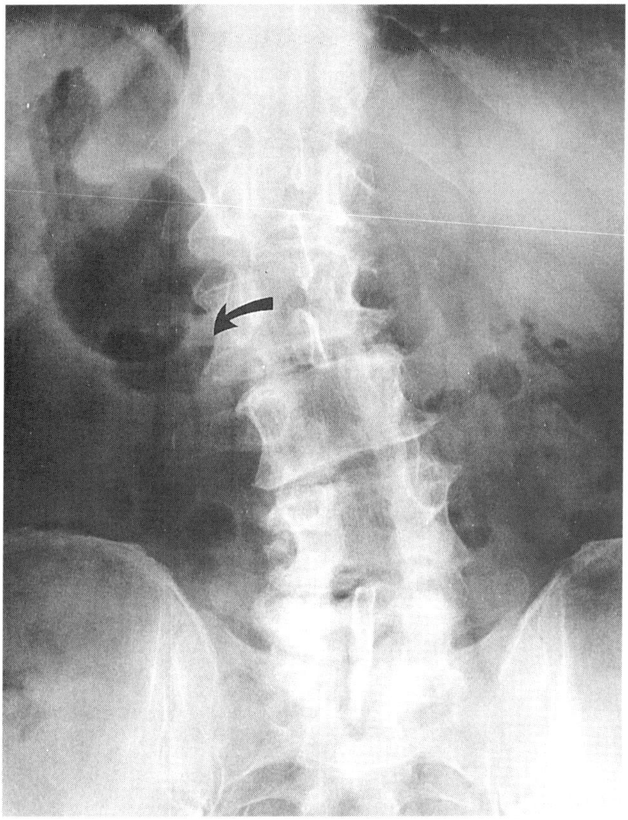

Figure 14.38 *Degenerative scoliosis with lateral subluxation of L2 (arrow, above a midline decompression at L3 and L4).*

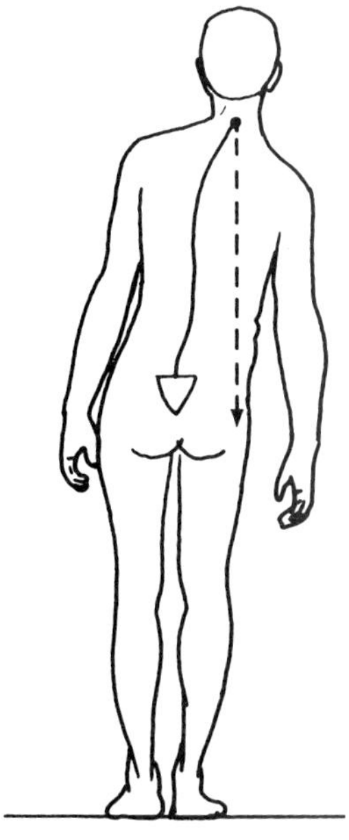

Figure 14.39 *Degenerative scoliosis with decompensation, that is, the upper torso is not centered on the sacrum.*

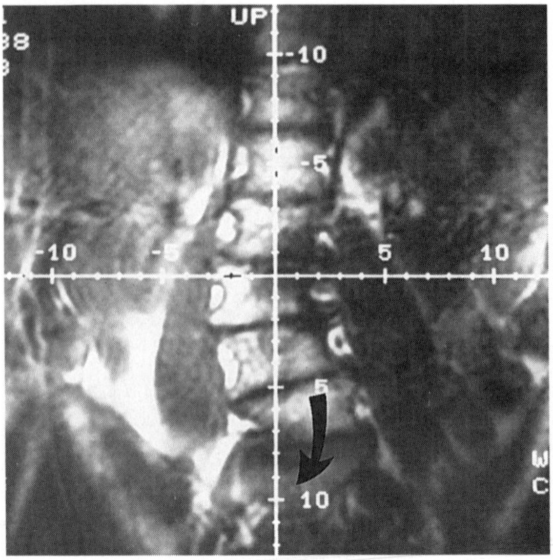

Figure 14.40 *A degenerative scoliosis on the MRI scout film. The root encroachment will be most severe in the "cross hairs" of the grid. Note the secondary curve heading toward the pelvis (arrow).*

Table 14.4. Characteristics of Scoliosis in the Young and Old

	Idiopathic Adolescent Scoliosis	Adult Onset Degenerative Scoliosis
Age	< 20 y	> 50 y
Sex	F > M	F > M
Location	Thoracic or thoracolumbar	Lumbar
Side	L > R	L = R
Length	Longer curves	Avg 4 vertebral segments in curve
Severity	Can be more than 60°	Rarely more than 60°
Vertebral deformity	Common (vertebral wedging and laminar changes)	Uncommon (degenerative changes on concavity)
Presentation	Deformity ± pain	Pain
Neurological involvement	Rare	Common

The Facet Joint Syndrome

In 1933, Ghormley (29) introduced the possibility that lumbar facet joints were a source of low back pain. A year later, his study was eclipsed by the report of Mixter and Barr (66) of the ruptured disc. Sixty-three years later, we still do not know what the facet joint syndrome is!

It is easy to postulate that the facet joints are a source of pain:

1. They are synovial joints, paired at each level, lined by hyaline cartilage, and encased in a capsule: they are a miniaturized version of a knee joint.
2. They are innervated by the medial branch of the posterior primary ramus (Fig. 14.43).
3. They degenerate in concert with the disc space (Fig. 14.44).

Yet numerous, recent, well-controlled studies suggest that directing treatment (facet joint blocks) at the facet joints is largely a waste of time.(44, 46)

Let us explore further.

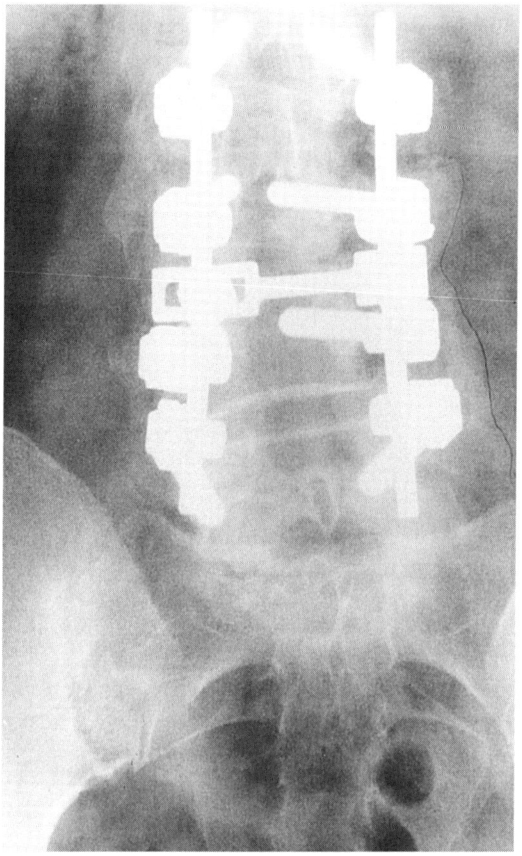

Figure 14.41 *Instrumentation for degenerative scoliosis.*

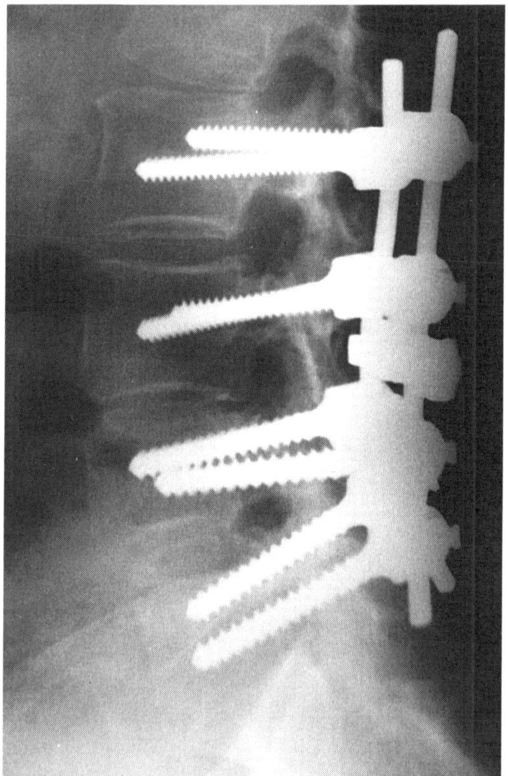

Figure 14.42 *The segment above the instrumented fusion is developing degenerative changes.*

Figure 14.43 *The innervation of the facet joints is from branches from the posterior primary ramus (arrow in the pedicle at L5).*

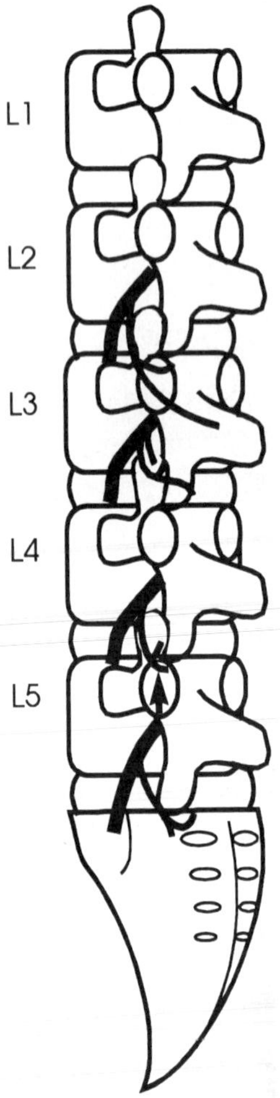

Biomechanically, the facet joints share the load in each spinal motion segment. Their primary function is to protect the disc space from shear and rotational (torsion) forces. Their secondary role is to share a low portion of the axial load when a person is standing (they share 0% of the axial load on the spine when you are sitting). When degenerative changes develop in the disc space, the facet joints share even more of the load.

There is no question that facet joints degenerate, just like knee joints degenerate. The work of Fairbank et al (24) and Mooney and Robertson (68) showed that the facet joints can be painful when appropriate stimulation is applied to the joint. Pathology, in the form of typical osteoarthritic changes, has been demonstrated in facet joints removed at surgery.(4)

So with the stress and strains on the facet joints, with the anatomy and innervation described, and with the degenerative changes that develop, why should not the facet joints be a source of low back pain, just as Ghormley proposed 63 years ago?

The patient with facet joint pain has been described by many authors, but each one has a different approach. Let us offer our description. The facet joint syndrome is really misnamed; it should be labeled painful osteoarthritic degeneration of the facet joint. That means that before you propose that someone's low back pain is arising from the facet joint, you should see some radiographic change of degeneration in the facet joint (Fig. 14.45). We do not wish to imply that all patients with facet joint degeneration on radio-

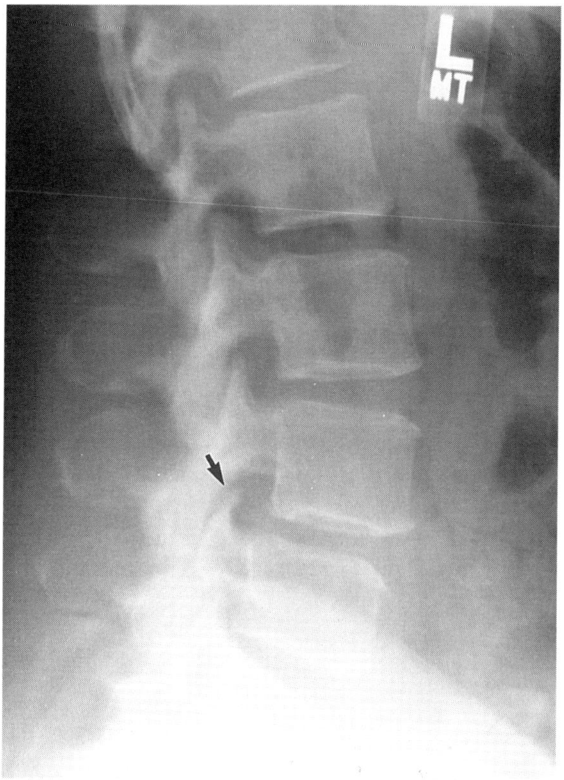

Figure 14.44 *A lateral plain film showing degenerative disc disease at L4–L5, with a degenerative spondylolisthesis. Note the associated facet joint changes, including the characteristic lipping of the tip of the superior facet (arrow).*

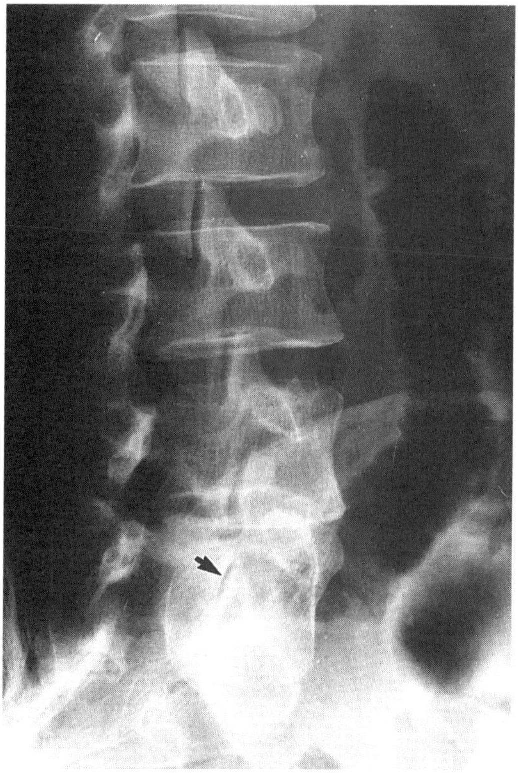

Figure 14.45 *An oblique view with early facet degeneration at L4–L5 and significant facet joint degeneration at L5–S1 (arrow).*

graph have pain, just as all patients with degenerative disc disease on radiograph do not necessarily have pain.

This concept of facet degeneration implies a number of clinical features:

The "syndrome" takes years to develop, which means it is a problem of older, not younger patients.
Although early osteoarthritic changes are subtle on radiographic examination and may be associated with intermittent back pain, once the facet joint syndrome reaches a bothersome level, it is a fairly constant mechanical back pain to the patient.
Because facet joints are paired at each level, it is hard to imagine that you can degenerate a facet joint on one side and not the other.
Thus, facet joint pain is almost always bilateral.

Other features of the facet joint degenerative syndrome include pain that is off the midline, that is, pure central back pain (Fig. 14.46) that is not arising from facet joints. Facet joint pain is referred to the proximal area of the sacroiliac joint and rarely is referred lower into the thighs. The patient complains of increased pain with extension activities that include standing, working overhead, using the sweeper, pulling, and so on. The pain is not

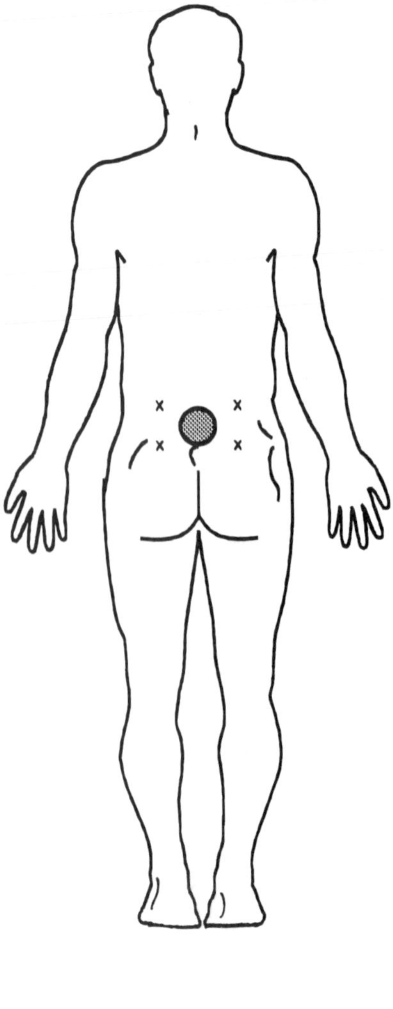

Figure 14.46 *Lumbar degenerative disc disease is a more central pain (cross-hatched area), whereas facet joint pain is off to the side (Xs) and is unilateral or bilateral.*

aggravated by and / or is relieved by sitting, walking, and lying down. Often, there will be a stiffness in the back on arising in the morning.

On physical examination, there is some stiffness to flexion and often increased pain on extension, especially into the lateral position (Fig. 14.47). Obviously, there will be no signs of root tension, irritation, or compression on examination of the lower extremities.

If this is an accepted description of the facet (joint) degenerative syndrome, then all of the published studies that suggest that the facet joint syndrome does not exist and injections of the facet joint are not worthwhile are contaminated with the following factors:

Patients too young.
Patients with a short history of back pain.(15)
Patients with no evidence of facet joint degeneration on radiograph.
Patients involved with workmen's compensation or motor vehicle accident claims (84).
Patients who have had previous surgery.

Fairbank et al (24) and Mooney and Robertson (68) have shown that pain can be reproduced and then diminished with facet joint injections of local anesthetics. The addition of steroids follows the same principles as injection of a knee joint for degenerative changes.

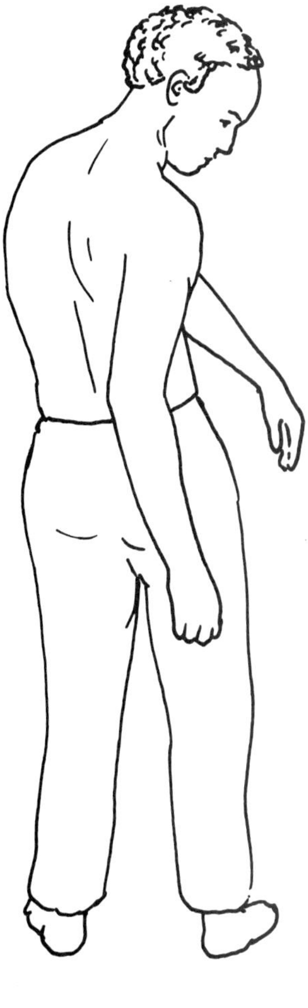

Figure 14.47 *Extension and lateral flexion will often increase pain arising from the facet joint.*

The procedure is known as a facet joint block and should be done bilaterally. Because facet joint degenerative disease advances in concert with the aging changes in the lumbar spine, it affects multiple levels, and thus multilevel facet joint injections (usually L3–L4, L4–L5, and L5–S1) are required. This is another problem with many of the published studies: too many single-level and single-sided facet joint injections.

Obviously, the facet (degenerative) syndrome is not resolved. All of the negative published studies have started with the premise—knowing the nature of the facet joints—that they must be a source of pain. But by including the wrong patient population in studying the efficacy of facet joint blocks with local anesthetic and steroids, these studies have concluded that the syndrome does not exist. Recognizing the weakness of the studies, the authors usually conclude their articles with the admonition that "this problem needs further study." Obviously!

Treatment of the Facet Degenerative Syndrome If you suspect the facet joints as the source of pain, a useful treatment modality is the multilevel, bilateral facet joint block (Fig. 14.48). A significant number of patients will be relieved of their symptoms in the long term, but a number will experience recurrent symptoms in a few days to a few months of injection. For all of these patients, a general fitness program of flexion-type exercises is indicated. For these patients, a facet joint rhyzolysis (Fig. 14.49) can be considered, but like all denervation procedures for arthritic joints, it is of limited usefulness. It is unusual that the facet joint syndrome would be severe enough to merit a decision to fuse the involved motion segments.

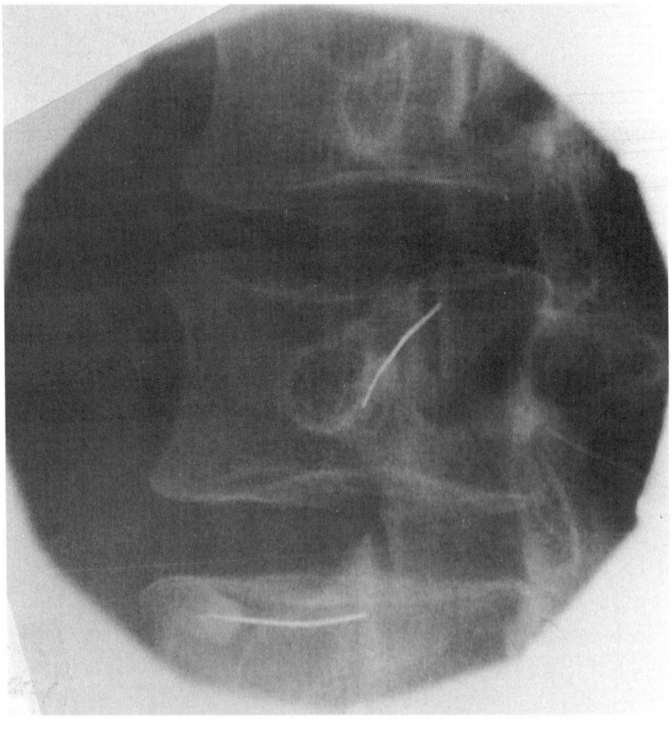

Figure 14.48 *Fine needles in the facet joints for the purpose of a block.*

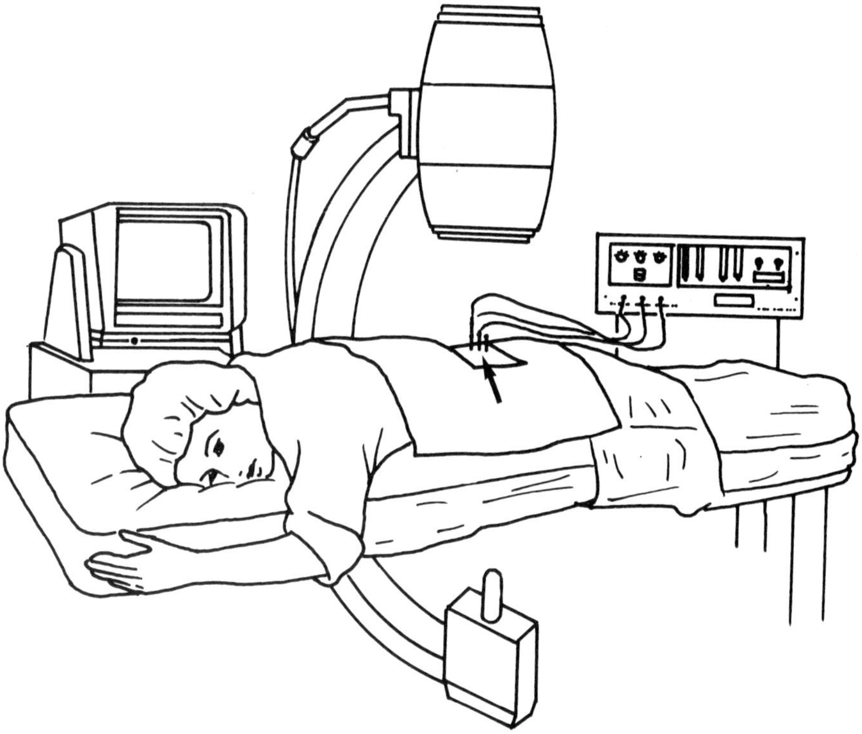

Figure 14.49 *A facet joint rhyzolysis, with the patient prone and image intensifier control to guide placement of the probes (arrow). The radiofrequency generator is in the background on the right.*

Internal Disc Disruption

Of those degenerative conditions with special status, isolated disc resorption and degenerative scoliosis are clearly established clinical problems; the facet joint syndrome is questionable. Internal disc disruption is a fancy description of Kirkaldy-Willis's first stage of degenerative disc disease. It presents as back pain with minor radiographic changes. Unfortunately, it has become the focus of discographers seeking the "pain generator" and surgeons looking for a reason, rather than the rationale, for surgery; this sometimes results in the performance of a 360-degree fusion for the "discogram discovered" lesion (Fig. 14.50). Unfortunately, there is not one controlled scientific study to support this course of action.

The term "internal disc disruption," like "isolated disc resorption," was also introduced by Crock. Although we agree with many of his concepts regarding isolated disc resorption, we think internal disc disruption is simply an early stage of disc degeneration and does not require special status. Crock coined the term to describe spinal and limb pains made worse by physical activity that stresses the "abnormal" disc. Profound loss of energy occurs, sometimes associated with significant reduction in body weight. A range of psychological disturbances often occurs. All this with normal looking plain radiographs!

Discography has become the simple test to prove the existence of this complex physical and psychological disability. More recently, Crock has opined that "MRI has become the

Figure 14.50 *A schematic of a 360-degree fusion (1) anterior interbody and (2) posterior rods and screws with bone graft (XX) in the intertransverse interval.*

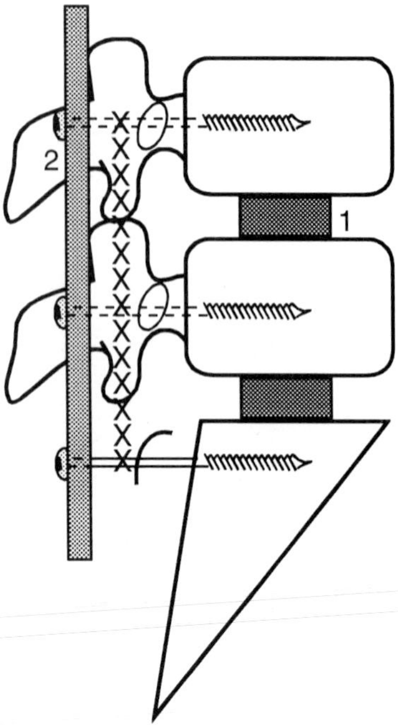

most important diagnostic test for internal disc disruption, largely replacing discography." "Nevertheless," he further opines "the significance of many of the findings referred to in MRI reports is still not clearly understood." This sounds like "a confession of inadequate radiographic diagnosis" for this condition.

Despite this tenuous means of diagnosis, Crock believes that very few of these patients get better with conservative care, and most require an anterior lumbar discectomy and fusion, single or multiple level, to remove "the pain generator."

We do not believe that this condition deserves the special status it seems to have acquired in some spinal centers. We also believe that internal disc disruption is simply Kirkaldy-Willis's first phase of disc dysfunction, from which most patients recover with the passage of time and appropriately prescribed nonoperative treatment measures.

Cervicolumbar Syndrome

Symptomatic degenerative disc changes are most commonly seen in the lower lumbar spine. Often, the changes are multisegmental and involve the whole lumbar spine, and on occasion the changes are multifocal, involving both the lumbar and cervical spine. It is to this latter group that the term "cervicocolumbar syndrome" has been applied. Commonly, the degenerative changes in the cervical spine are not symptomatic at the time that the patient is seen about low back pain, or else the symptoms are relatively minor, and the patient does not believe them worthy of mention. As part of conservative treatment, the patient may be given situp or kickup exercises. Situp exercises can place a severe extension strain on the neck, and in kickup exercises the patient may injure the neck by straining or overflexing (Fig. 14.51). As a result of the exercise program, the previously asymptomatic disc changes in the neck may become painful and may indeed constitute a significant continuing disability.

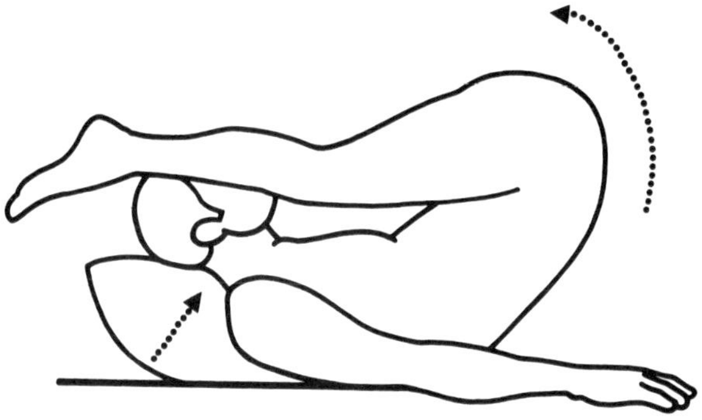

Figure 14.51 *With kickup exercises, the patient may put a severe flexion strain on the neck, particularly if the neck is not supported by a pillow.*

If a lumbosacral fusion is undertaken in such a patient, the hyperextended, rotated position of the neck adopted during the course of surgery may leave the patient with intractable cervicobrachial pain.

If, when the patient is first seen, symptoms are derived from the degenerative changes in both the cervical and lumbar spines, the patient presents the almost unbelievable picture of "total body pain," pain in the neck radiating to the occiput, to both shoulders, and maybe down the arms. In addition, these patients may have pain radiating to the chest. The lumbar disc changes result in low back pain frequently associated with referred pain to one or both legs (Fig. 14.52). It is little wonder, when confronted with such a picture, that the physician is defeated, and examination and treatment tend to be perfunctory.

An awareness of this syndrome is important to the physician. Before suggesting situp or kickup exercises for the treatment of low back pain, the patient should be specifically asked if he/she has any pain in the neck, shoulders, or arms. The neck should be examined carefully, with particular attention being paid to the first sign of symptomatic cervical disc degeneration, namely, painful limitation of extension of the neck. If there is any suggestion of cervical disc degenerative changes in such patients, the exercise program should be conducted with the patient's neck protected in a cervical collar.

When the patient complains of what appears to be total body pain, the possibility of a cervicolumbar syndrome should be considered, and its probability should be assessed by careful examination of both the cervical and lumbar spines. Admittedly, many of these patients are emotionally disturbed, but the emotional disturbance may be secondary to this irksome burden of pain. It is often wise to put the patient on a short course of adequate analgesia with mild sedation for a week, allow the discomfort to subside, and then re-examine the patient's clinical picture. There is no reason why simultaneous treatment for both the cervical and lumbar disc changes should not be performed.

Treatment of Symptomatic Lumbar Degenerative Disc Disease

We hope that you have the message by now! Most patients with axial (midline back) pain will respond to conservative care and the passage of time. Because these conditions are chronic, we advise against the use of narcotics and other mood altering drugs. The treatment should be confined to physical measures.

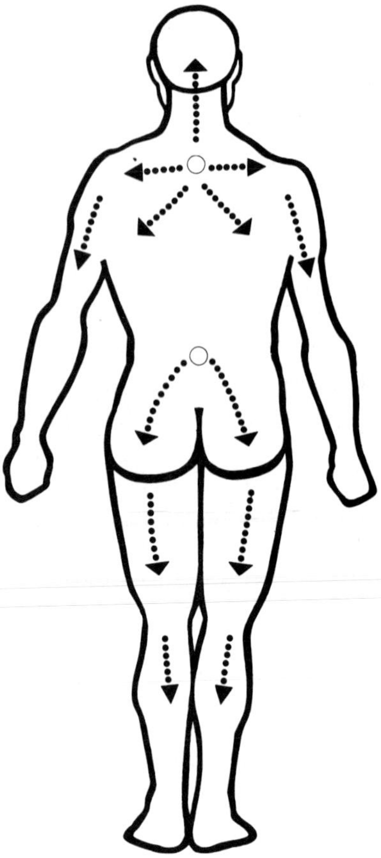

Figure 14.52 *Diagram to show the distribution of pain when symptoms are derived from degenerative disc disease in the cervical spine and the lumbar spine simultaneously. This gives rise to the unbelievable picture of total body pain.*

The choices are:

1. Rest.
2. Mobilization/exercise.

Rest

Certainly, bed rest has little role to play in the treatment of chronic low back pain. Occasionally, an acute episode will be so severe that a few days of bed rest is required. Most often bed rest is detrimental to these patients, reinforcing the idea that they have a serious problem and adversely affecting bone and muscle mass as well as disc and cartilage nutrition. We have the same feelings about a brace except in: (1) severe pain in a patient who must be ambulating, and (2) an older patient who cannot be treated in any other way because of co-morbid medical problems.

There are other forms of rest such as job or activity modification and weight loss that are worthwhile efforts. These were discussed in detail in Chapter 13.

Mobilization/Exercise

The management of chronic (axial) low back pain centers around the concepts of mobilization and exercise. The aim of this approach is to improve functional capacity, all the while encouraging the patient to take an active role and begin to cope with the pain. Letting the patient use the back pain as a barometer for activity will fail. Rather, set down a mobilization/exercise program and encourage the patient to follow that plan, regardless of the pain. These methods were discussed in Chapter 13.

Operative Treatment

It seems only reasonable to conclude that if mechanical low back pain is related to instability of a lumbar spine segment, stabilization (fusion) of that segment(s) will rid the patient of the wretched complaint. (53) Spine fusion as treatment of low back pain is rarely indicated. Nearly every back pain due to degenerative disc disease will settle to a tolerable level if the stress is taken off the spine by weight loss, strengthening of the abdominal muscles, the occasional use of temporary spinal support, and modification of activities that sometimes necessitates a change of employment.

A spinal fusion may be considered in those instances in which an emotionally stable patient is unable, or unwilling, to restrict work and pleasure activities or, despite doing so, is still disabled by recurrent episodes or persistence of incapacitating low back pain. The word "considered" is used advisedly. Before admission to the hospital, two things must be assessed in greater detail: first, the patient who has the backache and, second, the backache the patient has.

In the natural history of degenerative disc disease, the L5–S1 disc is usually the first to be involved, followed subsequently by changes in the L4–L5 disc. Clinical experience has shown that the degenerative changes in the lumbosacral disc are self-limiting and rarely give rise to prolonged symptoms. The L4–L5 disc is the "backache disc," and a single segment L4–L5 fusion is rarely indicated, except for isolated disc resorption. This means that most patients are faced with the requirement of at least a two-level fusion. That makes sense because the aging process is universal. As we get older, we wrinkle our skin, gray our hair, and wear out our discs. Doing a two-level fusion (L4 to sacrum) does not stop the aging process at L3–L4, especially if it is established at the time of the fusion. Let us repeat: Spine fusion as a treatment of low back pain is rarely indicated.

Surgical Options

Let us assume that you have that rare indication for a primary fusion for the treatment of discogenic low back pain. What are your options?

Surgical Approach

Primary fusions may be done posteriorly, anteriorly, or combined (the so-called 360-degree fusion). Except in some traumatic conditions (fractures) and tumors, we feel that there is no indication for a 360-degree fusion in the treatment of degenerative spines, so we will not discuss it further.

Technique of Spine Fusion

Operative techniques are the concern of the individual surgeon and are not dealt with here in any detail. Certain principles, however, are briefly discussed.

The modifications of the technique for spinal fusion initially described by Albee (1) and Hibbs (39) are legion. Initially, they consisted of corticocancellous grafts wired to or wedged between the spinous processes, reinforced with or replaced by multiple bone chips, sometimes additionally stabilized with a temporary fixation afforded by interspinous plates. Subsequent attempts to improve stability have resulted in the use of interlaminar rods and/or sublaminar wires, facet screws, and, most recently, pedicle screws. Internal fixation, however, only affords temporary stability; the bone graft must be incorporated to produce stabilization.

In the 1950s, with increasing surgical skills due largely to improved techniques of anesthesia, many surgeons, with thoughtless boldness, engaged in frontal assaults on the lumbar spine for degenerative disc disease. However, the initial wave of enthusiasm for anterior lumbar fusion has now largely receded for several reasons. Apart from the operative hazard of damage to major vessels and the nervi erigentes, unless a massive autogenous graft is employed to replace all of the excised disc, a pseudarthrosis is likely to occur. This is because it is easier for fibrous tissue derived from the remnants of the disc to invade the graft than it is for bone to grow from one vertebral body to the other. Cortical grafts inhibit the invasion of fibrous tissue, and thus fibular strut grafts are well suited for interbody fusion. To ensure solid bony fusion, a massive amount of donor bone must be employed, with the attendant problems of "donor site pain." Anterior spinal fusion is probably best used as a salvage procedure.

Posterior Lumbar Fusion

Para-articular or intertransverse fusions present several advantages:

1. There is a continuous bed to which the graft may be applied (Fig. 14.53).
2. The technique permits intra-articular fusion or facet fusion. It has long been established that the achievement of facet fusion is mandatory for the success of the extensive fusions performed for adolescent scoliosis. We believe that facet fusion is just as important in fusions for degenerative spine conditions.
3. The fusion mass lies nearer the axis of movement.
4. The graft does not extend medial to the facets, and the danger of an iatrogenic spinal stenosis, seen on occasion with routine posterior fusions, is thereby obviated.

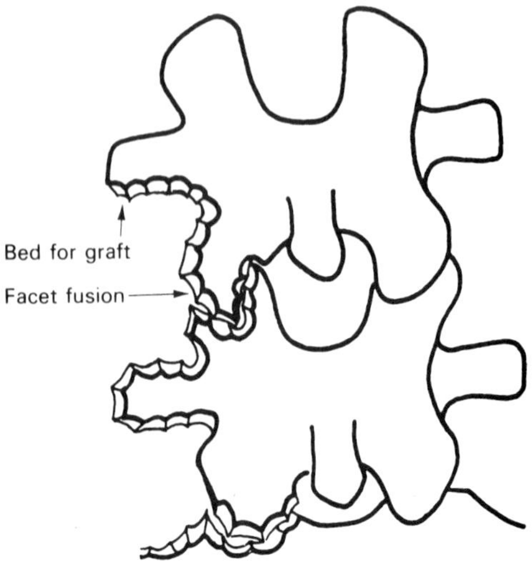

Figure 14.53 *When an intertransverse fusion is performed, there is a continuous bed of cancellous bone to which the bone graft can be applied. In addition to this, the intertransverse fusion can be combined with a facet fusion.*

Bone Graft Choices: Basic Considerations

The aim of bone grafting in lumbar degenerative disc disease is to get osteogenesis to occur. To achieve this, one needs to attend to two basic factors.

1. Stimulus. There must be a stimulus to the body to want to form bone, and that stimulus is in the form of the operative injury with the placement of the appropriate cells to form bone.
2. Environment. The host environment has to be inducive to the formation of new bone.

Each of these basic considerations will be covered in this chapter.

Alternatives in Bone Grafting

Various options are open when selecting material for a bone graft. At one time or another, the following choices need to be considered:

1. Genetic: autograft, allograft, xenograft.
2. Composition: cancellous, cortical.
3. Anatomic: size, shape, origin.
4. Method: vascularized, nonvascularized.
5. Preservation.
   a. Physical alteration: fresh, frozen, freeze-dried, irradiated, autoclaved.
   b. Chemical alteration: ethylene oxide, deproteinization, decalcification.
6. Substitutes.
   a. Cellular: marrow.
   b. Scaffolding: coral hydroxyapatite, hydroxyapatite, tricalcium phosphate (TCP), collagen fiber, biodegradable polymers. (polyglycolic acid)
7. Stimulation: electrical.

Ideal Bone Graft

The ideal bone graft material is:

1. Readily available.
2. Biologically inert and/or biodegradable.
3. Of the shape and size required.
4. In enough quantity.
5. Has a large enough surface (porosity) to be replaced by host bone.

Factors

When trying to understand bone grafting and arrive at the appropriate choice of materials, three factors have to be considered.

1. Biology,
2. Immunology, and
3. Biomechanics.

Biology

When a bone graft is placed in the lumbar spine, it is incorporated through healing by regeneration and not by scar. Any insult in tissues can heal by scar, and there is nothing the surgeon can do about this phenomenon. However, to get bone tissue to heal by regeneration takes much in the way of extra effort. Despite this extra effort, a number of bone grafts necrose, which accounts for the high nonunion rate in fusions for lumbar disc disease, especially intradiscal fusions. To prevent this, it is essential to understand the biological healing of a bone graft so that the surgeon can take steps to optimize the conditions for bone graft incorporation and achieve a solid fusion.

The standard for bone grafting in degenerative disc disease, is fresh, cancellous, autogenous bone, in enough quantity, laid in a good vascular bed with no extenuating circumstances such as nutritional depletion of the patient or scarring of the bed (Table 14.5). Any condition less than this optimal situation is going to increase the rate of nonunion/pseudarthrosis. Almost all of the following discussion centers on the fresh cancellous autogenous bone graft as being the only logical choice for grafting in lumbar degenerative disc disease.

Stages of Incorporation The five stages of incorporation of a fresh cancellous nonvascularized autograft are described in the following sections.

Stage I: Clot and Inflammation Within minutes to hours of the wound and the placement of the bone graft, hemorrhage occurs, which then is followed by the standard stages of inflammation, including clot and exudation (invasion of the area by inflammatory cells). The initial inflammatory cellular invasion is comprised of acute inflammatory cells (neutrophils), followed by chronic inflammatory cells (lymphocytes and macrophages).

Stage II: Revascularization or Osteoprogenitor Stage Within days of the wound, granulation tissue appears. The fibrous granulation tissue, in the form of blood vessels on a scaffolding, invades the graft as the inflammatory cellular exudate decreases. Along with blood vessels, the following appear:

Table 14.5. Technical Factors Contributing to a High Rate of Fusion

Donor Factors
The best bone is:
Autogenous
Freshly harvested
Cancellous
Great quantities
Recipient (Bed) Factors
A nutritionally intact patient (no excessive alcohol or smoking)
A bed with a good blood supply (no scarring)
A bed free of contamination (no tumor or infection)
A firm bed (no excessive tissue dissection)

1. Osteoblasts to clean up the bone debris;
2. Macrophages to clean up the cellular debris; and
3. Osteoprogenitor cells (mesenchymal cells): the source of the mesenchymal cell is the host, and these cells will only appear if an appropriate bed has been laid for the bone graft.

If cancellous bone has been the grafting material, then this stage of revascularization is completed within 2 weeks.(13) Cortical bone takes much longer for this stage to be completed because the cortical bone has to be resorbed through osteoclastic activity before any vascular invasion can occur. Up to this stage, there is not much difference between an autograft and an allograft. However, in the next stage the body's immune system will be stimulated if the grafting material is foreign to the body.

Stage III: Osteoinductive Stage This is the most vital stage with regard to bone graft incorporation. (13). The mesenchymal cells differentiate into osteogenic cells (osteoblasts). This is the most important source of osteogenic cells, although there are, in all, four sources of osteogenic cells:

1. Cells of the graft. A fresh cancellous bone graft will contain osteoblasts that will survive.
2. Cells from the host:
   a. The cambrial layer of the periosteum is a source of osteoblasts, especially in children.
   b. Cortical elements are probably the least important source of osteoblasts.
   c. The endosteum and marrow are the most important source of mesenchymal cells, with equal contribution from each one. It is these mesenchymal cells that ultimately contribute the most to new bone formation in the adult patient undergoing a fusion for lumbar degenerative disc disease.

There are two theories to explain why osteoinduction occurs.

1. The first theory states that the formation of bone is entirely due to the cells in the area stimulated by the injury of muscle dissection and decortication. It is simply the presence of osteogenic cells in the area that results in the formation of bone.
2. A more complicated theory is based on bone morphogenic protein (BMP). It is thought that BMP exists in the bone matrix and leads to the enhancement or the redirection of mesenchymal cells to form bone.(91) It is also thought to be the basis of ectopic and excessive bone formation in myositis ossificans around total hip revision, in paraplegia, and in ankylosing spondylitis.

This osteogenic or osteoinductive phase is well established within 1 month, and the majority of a cancellous bone graft is replaced within 3 months. Because of this timing, it is important to support a patient's back postoperatively with some form of bracing, waiting for this first stage of osteogenesis to occur. Sometime between 1 and 3 months, when osteogenesis is well established and the majority of the bone graft is replaced, it is important to stimulate the wound so that further new bone formation occurs on the basis of Wolff's law. (25)

As previously mentioned, it is at the stage of osteogenesis or osteoinduction that the antigen antibodies will affect the ultimate outcome if the grafting material is recognized as foreign.(27)

Stage IV: Osteoconductive Stage This stage is closely entwined with the osteoinductive stage, occurring over the same period of weeks to months. It is based on the fact that the grafting material serves as a passive template for the ingrowth of vascular and cellular activity. If a template is not present, then the osteoinductive stage cannot spread its wings, and a large enough fusion mass cannot occur. It is essential to this stage that the grafting material is in close contact with, as well as almost under compression with, the host bed. The one thing that will stop the osteoconductive phase is the formation of fibrous tissue, or the presence of fibrous tissue, between the graft and host bed. For this reason, it is futile to lay a bone graft in a scarred field because of the resultant inability of the host to bridge the gap between the scar tissue and the passive template of the bone graft.

Stage V: Incorporation and Remodeling If the stages just described have followed their normal course of events, and if enough bone has been formed, the body will remodel the graft to perform the mechanical function demanded of the graft. It is during this stage that stabilization of the motion segment is achieved, and backache decreases. This is facilitated by an increased activity program at approximately 2 or 3 months, which stimulates further new bone formation and remodeling on the basis of Wolff's law.(25) The final stage in remodeling is the accumulation of hemopoietic cells within the transplanted bone to form a marrow cavity. In an intertransverse graft, this is minimal, and in intradiscal and posterior grafts, it is almost nonexistent.

Dynamics of the Stages It is important to recognize that these stages of bone graft incorporation are not sequential but are, instead, closely entwined. There is a delicate balance between each of the stages, just as there is for a great classical music piece. Just because the violins start to play does not mean that the trumpets cease to be involved in the score. This delicate balance between osteoinduction and osteoconduction can be easily upset. Perhaps the most important thing that upsets this delicate balance is the body's immunological reaction to anything that is recognized as foreign.(27) This reaction results in slowing down of the osteoinductive stage, which, in turn, results in the breakdown of the scaffolding for osteoconduction. This accounts for the high failure rate in anything but fresh autogenous cancellous bone.

Creeping Substitution A cancellous bone graft is replaced by creeping substitution. New tissue invades along the channels made by the invading blood vessels or along preexisting channels in the cancellous transplanted bone. Leading this invasion are the osteoblasts, which lay down viable new bone on top of the necrotic old bone. The old bone is subsequently resorbed, and more new bone is laid down. The phenomenon of osteoblasts laying new bone on old bone, accompanied by the subsequent resorption of the old bone, is known as creeping substitution.

Cortical bone requires the reverse of creeping substitution for incorporation. First, cortical bone is in need of osteoclastic resorption of the bone before new bone can be laid down by osteoblasts. The phenomenon of creeping substitution is one of the major advantages of cancellous bone for grafting material. In addition, cancellous bone is revascularized in a broader and quicker fashion than cortical bone, which allows for an early and wide distribution to the phenomenon of creeping substitution. Finally, all cancellous bone is eventually replaced by new bone, which does not occur with cortical bone grafting. In cortical bone grafting, there is always some cortical bone that is never incorporated. It is unusual for much in the way of cortical bone to be used in bone grafting in lumbar degenerative disc disease, which is fortunate. Unfortunately, most of the bone removed at the time of a decompression for lumbar degenerative disc disease is cortical in nature, and this explains the very poor success rate when the bone removed at the time of surgery is used in an attempt to accomplish the fusion.

Failure of the Bone Graft

There are many fusions in lumbar degenerative disc disease that are not successful. The reasons are given in the following sections.

Local Causes of Failure

The Bed

1. If the bed is poorly vascularized through previous insult, such as surgery or radiotherapy, then there is no hope for the bone graft to be incorporated. Next to "fresh cancellous autogenous bone in great quantities," this is the most significant factor in successful bone grafting.
2. Site: In an intertransverse fusion, it is very important to save the intertransverse ligament and the decorticated transverse processes so that there is a firm bed for the bone-grafting material. Breaking off the transverse processes or destroying the intertransverse ligament takes away the foundation (bed) for the bone graft and introduces a degree of mobility that is bad for the bone graft.
3. Infection: Obviously, infection will interfere with incorporation of a bone graft.
4. Foreign objects (eg, bone cement) will interfere with bone graft incorporation.
5. Local bone disorders such as tumors will also interfere with bone graft incorporation.

Graft Material

1. Volume: If a less-than-optimum volume of bone grafting material is placed in the wound, then a strong fusion will not be achieved. The basic rule is that you can never have too much bone packed into the intertransverse or the intradiscal interval to achieve solid grafting.
2. Local disorders within the graft. Not unlike the bed, it is important that grafting material be uninfected and/or free of tumor cells.

General Conditions Poor general patient conditions (such as infection and nutritional deprivation) and the use of drugs (such as steroids and antimetabolites) will interfere with incorporation of the bone graft. The most significant general factor in bone graft incorporation is immunity. If the graft is recognized by the body as "non-self," the immunological reaction will be provoked, with detrimental effects on incorporation of the graft.

Failure If failure is to occur, there results a nonunion and resorption of the bone graft. It is a most frustrating experience when the patients return for their postoperative visits and are still complaining of pain a number of months after the fusion while radiographs show a poor fusion mass with pseudarthrosis.

Immunology

Problems with Autografting Although the best source of grafting material is the fresh cancellous autograft, it does introduce problems. The autograft requires a second incision with its associated time restraints. It introduces a second set of complications in the donor site, such as infection and pain. If a large mass of bone is required, then enough bone often cannot be obtained from the donor site. These problems have led to attempts to circumvent the use of autograft bone, largely in the form of allografting. This introduces a high risk of failure to the bone graft and, to this day, is not a suitable option for intertransverse or intradiscal fusions.

The two directions of circumvention are as follows:

1. Allografting bone. Today, this is the most frequent direction the surgeon takes to avoid the problems of autografting. There are renewed attempts to improve allografting by altering the allograft, histocompatibility matching, suppression of the immune response,(32) and vascularization of the graft immediately on placement.
2. Bone substitutes or composite grafts.(67)

Allografting (The Immunology of Bone Grafting) The greatest concern with allografting is the immunological reaction that interferes with satisfactory incorporation of the graft. In today's world, the transmission of disease, such as hepatitis and acquired immunodeficiency syndrome, is offering even further barriers to the use of allografting material. This aspect of disease transmission will not be discussed in this section; that is not to say that it is unimportant, but it is beyond the scope of this discussion.

Allograft and xenograft bone are recognized as nonself. This provokes the immunological reaction and results in rejection of the graft.

Antigenic (Non-Self) Components of Bone The antigenic components of bone are:

1. Cells. The cells of bone are the most significant source of antigens. Any cell, such as an osteogenic cell, a fibrous cell, or a cartilaginous cell, will contain proteins or glycoproteins on its cell surface that are noncompatible with the host.
2. Matrix. The proteoglycans of the matrix have antigenic characteristics that can invoke the immunological reaction.
3. Collagen. This is the least important source of antigens, but it is still a source of antigenic protein that can be recognized as non-self.

Histology of Rejection By the end of the second week, the immune response has started, and mononuclear cells invade the graft. This is at the end of the osteoprogenitor stage and at the beginning of the osteoinductive stage. It is the osteoinductive stage that is delayed by the appearance of immune cells.

The rejection histology is as follows: The inflammatory process soon includes lymphocytes. There is disruption of the vessels of the granulation tissue that are invading the graft. Eventually, the graft itself is encapsulated with a fibrous-like material, and the peripheral portion of the graft is resorbed. This breaks down the callus bridging between the host and the graft and ultimately results in failure of the graft with nonunion.

Through the work of many investigators, attempts have been made to reduce this rejection phenomenon. They are as follows:

1. Altering the allograft. The most effective method of altering the allograft appears to be freeze-drying of the grafting material. Other alterations that are less effective are freezing, decalcification, and deproteinization.
2. Histocompatibility matching.
3. Immunosuppression.(32)
4. Immediate vascularization.

Despite these efforts to reduce the rejection phenomenon, it is still the general experience that at least 25% of allograft material fails to incorporate.(27) This is a guaranteed failure rate that is too high to be acceptable for grafting in intertransverse and intradiscal fusions. For this reason, we do not recommend the use of allograft material.

Xenografts are mentioned only to be condemned. They provoke an even more profound immunological reaction than allografts, and eventually all xenograft material ends up as a sequestered fibrous-enveloped dead piece of bone. The immunological reaction occurs early in the osteoprogenitor stage. The more porous the implant, the more profound the inflammatory response. This is a strong position to take, but we think it is time for everyone to seriously look at the fusion rate in xenograft material and admit that there is an extremely high failure rate.

The only xenograft material used today is kiel bone (Surgibone). This is partly deproteinized bone from freshly killed calves. Immediately after death of the calf, the bone is harvested, washed in water, and then bathed in hydrogen peroxide. It is then passed through a fat solvent stage and subsequently dried with acetone. Sterilization is accomplished in the United States by use of ethylene dioxide and in Europe by use of gamma radiation.

Numerous other attempts at xenografts in the form of Boplant bone, which is freeze-dried calf bone, Oswestry bone, and Kobe bone, have been attempted. All of these xenograft materials provoke a significant immunological reaction and are associated with a very high pseudarthrosis rate. In the author's practice, they are unacceptable materials.

Biomechanics

In lumbar degenerative disc disease surgery, the biomechanical properties of the bone graft initially are not that important. In the end, one is trying to achieve a solid fusion and stabilization of a motion segment, and thus, biomechanics becomes more significant. Some surgeons feel that immediate stabilization is important, which is why they use rigid internal fixation with pedicle screws, plates, rods, and other devices. It is important in grafting for lumbar degenerative disc disease that one initiates the appropriate osteoprogenitor, osteoinductive, and osteoconductive stages. The earliest these phenomena are well established is sometime around 2 months. Before 2 months, it is imperative that the patient's back is protected (rest, corset support, and activity limitations). After that, you can mobilize the patient in a hope of invoking Wolff's law and stimulating the biomechanical aspects of the fusion mass.

Bone Substitutes

Because of the problems with allograft bone, attempts have been made to find bone substitutes.(41) The earliest attempt was the sprinkling of inorganic calcium in the area. It was initially thought that the excess of the calcium ion would stimulate mineral deposition. This was a failure.

Ceramics (Calcium Phosphate Ceramics) (37) Calcium phosphate biomaterials can be fused at high temperatures to form ceramics. These can be composed of hydroxyapatite or tricalcium phosphate (TCP). These products have a high degree of biocompatibility. Although both products are biocompatible, only TCP is biodegradable. These products can be used in the form of granular particles, porous intact implants, or dense intact implants. They must have an appropriate pore size between 100 and 400 μ, and, as such, they serve only as an osteoconductive mechanism.

There are drawbacks to the use of these ceramics, including their very brittle nature and the fact that they easily fracture. Sometimes the matrices do not get oriented in the correct direction and thus, retard remodeling. The use of ceramics requires a very stable interface between the living tissue and the biodegradable graft. If this does not occur, then a fibrous tissue membrane forms between the host and the graft and interferes with incorporation.

The Future It would appear that substitution for autogenous bone grafting will be directed away from allografting and toward composite grafting. A proposed composite graft would be as follows:

1. Marrow cells to introduce the osteogenic requirements.
2. BMP to introduce the osteoinductive requirements.(91)
3. Hydroxyapatite to introduce the osteoconductive requirements.

Obviously, this combination or composite graft will have to be laid in a good bed with (1) a good blood supply, (2) appropriate decortication, (3) appropriate immobilization, and (4) the absence of any soft tissue interposition. In addition, these materials will need to be placed in a patient that has the general conditions to incorporate the graft: good nutrition, the absence of steroid or antimetabolite drugs, the absence of excessive alcohol ingestion, and the absence of disease processes such as diabetes.

Conclusion If allografting is so unacceptable, then why does allografting work well in cervical fusions? A number of investigators are suggesting that you do not need any bone in an anterior cervical disc excision to obtain a fusion. Perhaps this accounts for the high fusion rate with allografting; that is, no grafting is necessary to achieve a solid cervical fusion.

If allografting is so poor for intertransverse fusions, then why does it work so well in scoliosis surgery? There are a number of reasons for this. Most scoliosis surgery, where allografting is being used, occurs in the younger patient population who have great healing potential. The allografting material is often mixed with autograft and laid on a very large bed of decorticated interlaminar bone. This solid bed is a great source of mesenchymal cells. Finally, there is usually rigid internal fixation placed at the time of scoliosis surgery. Thus, there are many factors present in scoliosis surgery that are conducive to allograft bone incorporation that are not present when doing intradiscal or intertransverse surgery. It is a mistake to transfer the concepts of allograft bone in scoliosis surgery to any use in intertransverse/intradiscal surgery. Stick with sufficient volume of fresh cancellous autograft to obtain your best results. In the future, look to composite grafting, not allografting, to resolve the problems in bone grafting.

Harvesting Autogenous Bone Graft

By way of introduction, let us state that the requirement for a separate incision to harvest autogenous bone will be unnecessary once bone substitutes are available. Although osteoconductive material such as coral (hydroxyapatite) is available, it is missing the osteogenic (cells) and osteoinductive components necessary for a viable solid fusion. Osteoinductive chemicals such as BMP have been successfully used in animals and are just starting into clinical trials. There is reason to believe that by the time the next edition of this book is written, we can drop this section on the harvesting of autogenous bone graft because of the usefulness of bone substitutes.

Technique Because the patient is usually in a prone (kneeling) position for posterior lumbar surgery, the posterior iliac crest (Fig. 14.54) is the natural choice for donor bone. We routinely use the right iliac crest and take the bone graft while standing on the opposite side of the operating table. An incision approximately 4 to 5cm long is started at the posterior superior iliac spine (Fig. 14.55). Do not extend the incision more than one hand's breadth away from the midline because you will cut the cluneal nerves, leading to an immediate postoperative numb buttock and later a neuroma.

Expose the outer aspect of the iliac crest subperiosteally, and place a bone graft retractor.

Save the entire thickness of the pelvic cortex, and start by taking slices of cortical cancellous bone from the outer table. Your first cut with the osteotome should be the distal cut; this is designed to avoid the sciatic notch (Figs. 14.55 and 14.56). Entering the sciatic notch with an osteotome may sever the superior gluteal artery and cause the loss of a

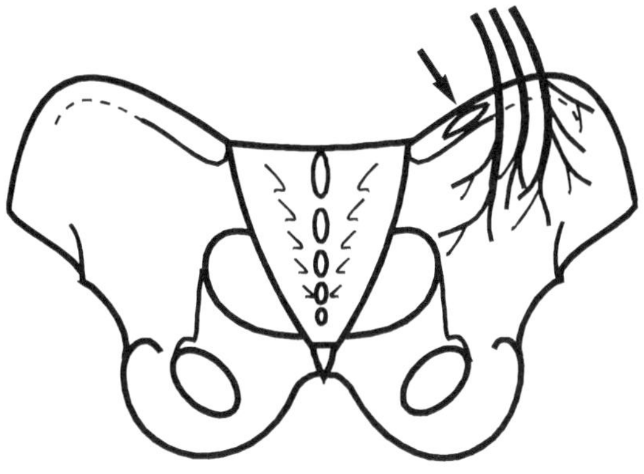

Figure 14.54 *The pelvis from behind showing the incision for a bone graft (arrow): keep it small, and keep it medial to the cluneal nerves.*

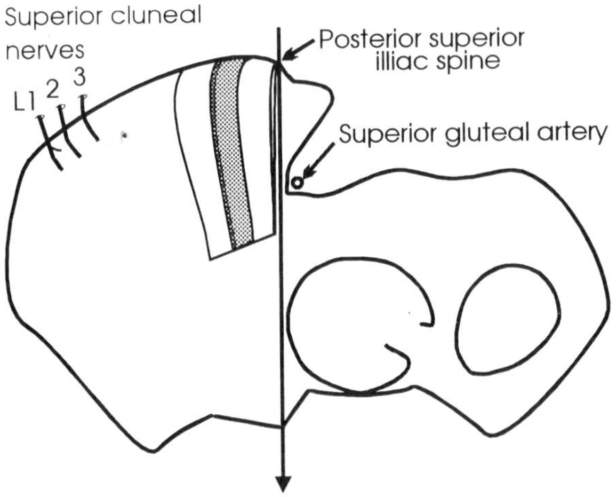

Figure 14.55 *The patient's hemipelvis as it appears on the operating room table. The cortex has been cut with an osteotome to allow for three cortical slabs of bone. As much cancellous bone as possible is removed deep to these cuts.*

considerable amount of blood. The sciatic nerve is also in the notch, and damage to it will be noticeable as soon as the patient awakens.

It is very important not to cross the inner cortex and damage the sacroiliac joint (Fig. 14.57). Harvest as much bone as you can, and remember the two admonitions about bone grafting:

You never have too much bone.
When you think you have enough bone, take a little more.

Closure is after you are satisfied the bleeding cancellous surfaces are controlled; this is accomplished with a tight closure.

Complications of Posterior Iliac Crest Harvest Complications of this procedure should be rare. The intraoperative complications of entering the sciatic notch and damaging the sacroiliac joint have already been mentioned. The minor but very annoying complication of cluneal nerve damage is easily avoided (Fig. 14.55).

In the immediate postoperative course, hematoma formation and/or infection are to be watched for. Each is an avoidable complication.

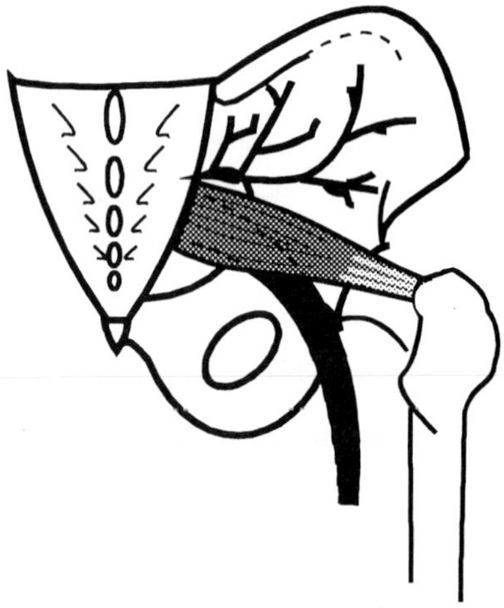

Figure 14.56 *The sciatic notch contains the gluteal arteries (above the piriformis) and the sciatic nerve inferior to the piriformis.*

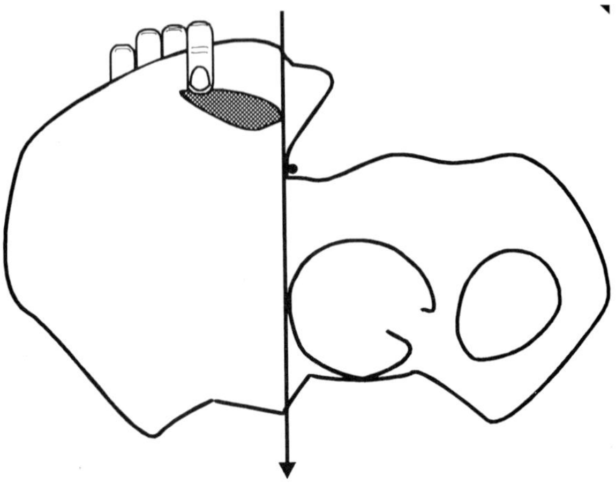

Figure 14.57 *Missing the sacroiliac joint: identify it by insertion of your fingertip to the proximal interphalangeal joint at a level just anterior to the posterior superior iliac spine.*

Donor Site Pain This is the most common complication of autogenous bone grafting and is very common in anterior iliac crest sites. It is less common, but troubling in posterior iliac crest sites and is prevented by the following:

1. The short incision.
2. Reserving the posterior cortex.
3. Avoiding the cluneal nerves.
4. Avoiding a postoperative hematoma or infection.

The Placement of the Posterior Bone Graft

To obtain a fusion, posterior bone grafting can be done in the midline or in the intertransverse interval (Fig. 14.58) or as an interbody fusion (Fig. 14.58). Almost no one does a midline posterior fusion today. Most surgeons prefer the intertransverse position, and some surgeons prefer the interbody position. Today, almost all posterior interbody fusions are combined with instrumentation and an intertransverse fusion. Except in revision surgery, we would not recommend this approach. For a primary single-level posterior fusion, we recommend the intertransverse fusion (Fig. 14.59). This is done through a limited posterior subperiosteal soft tissue envelope (Fig. 14.60).

The Limited Soft Tissue Envelope

Fracture surgeons have long recognized that extensive soft tissue damage interferes with fracture healing. It makes eminent sense that extensive soft tissue dissection in the intertransverse interval devitalizes the area and can lead to a poor fusion rate. It is on the basis of this fracture healing observation that we recommend the limited soft tissue envelope (Fig. 14.60) as the preparation for the bone graft.

This limited soft tissue dissection has the added benefit of more rigidly immobilizing the bone graft and enhancing healing (Fig. 14.60).

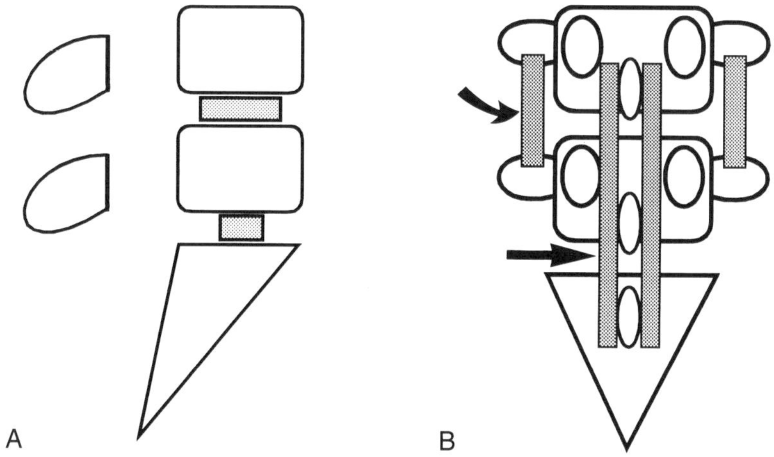

Figure 14.58 *Bone graft can be placed in* **(B)** *the midline (arrow), intertransverse interval (curved arrow), or* **(A)** *interbody. A small graft, not completely filling the intradiscal space, is shown at L5–S1; this is a bone graft that is likely to fail. The graft size at L4–L5 is more conducive to a solid interbody fusion.*

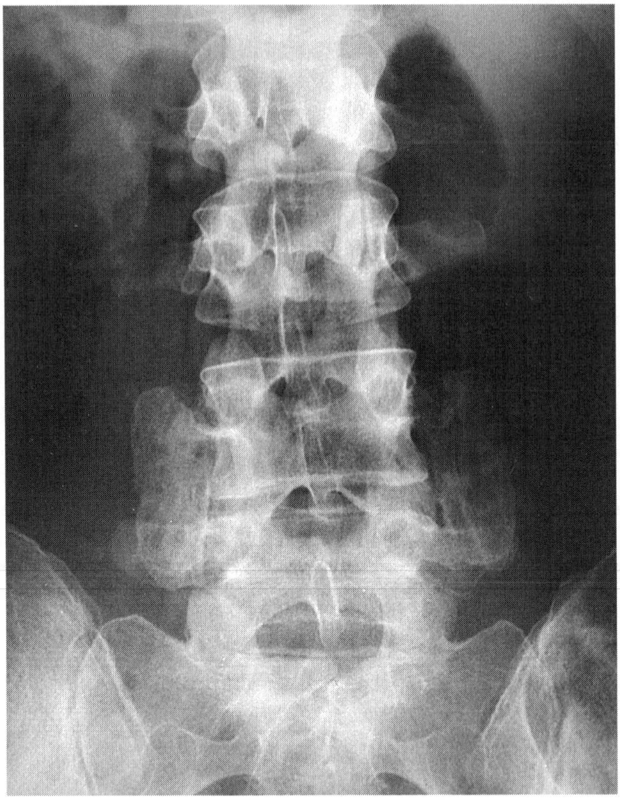

Figure 14.59 *A "floating" L4–L5 fusion for degenerative disc disease..*

To Instrument or Not to Instrument?

In the 1970s, European spine surgeons introduced pedicle fixation to the surgeon's armamentarium (Fig. 14.61). For 10 years after that, North American surgeons stuck with Harrington instrumentation, which was useful for treating spinal deformities but of little use in other spine problems. By the mid 1980s, North American spine surgeons had discovered the pedicle fixation systems, and their use grew exponentially. No one would disagree that pedicle instrumentation systems have been extended to treat degenerative disc disease of the lumbar spine, with some major problems presenting. The result has been intervention by the US Food and Drug Administration (FDA), leading to much confusion and consternation on the part of spine surgeons, considering the use of these systems in degenerative conditions of the spine.

Complications of Pedicle Screw Instrumentation Systems

Perhaps the best way to appreciate the resistance to pedicle screw systems is to look at the complications associated with their use (23):

Screw Malpositioning Placing a screw down the center of the pedicle is technically demanding. The screw may exit the pedicle and cause nerve root damage (Fig. 14.62) that can be permanent. This problem gets more serious the higher in the lumbar spine that screws are inserted. Screws may also break the pedicle and in turn damage nerve roots.

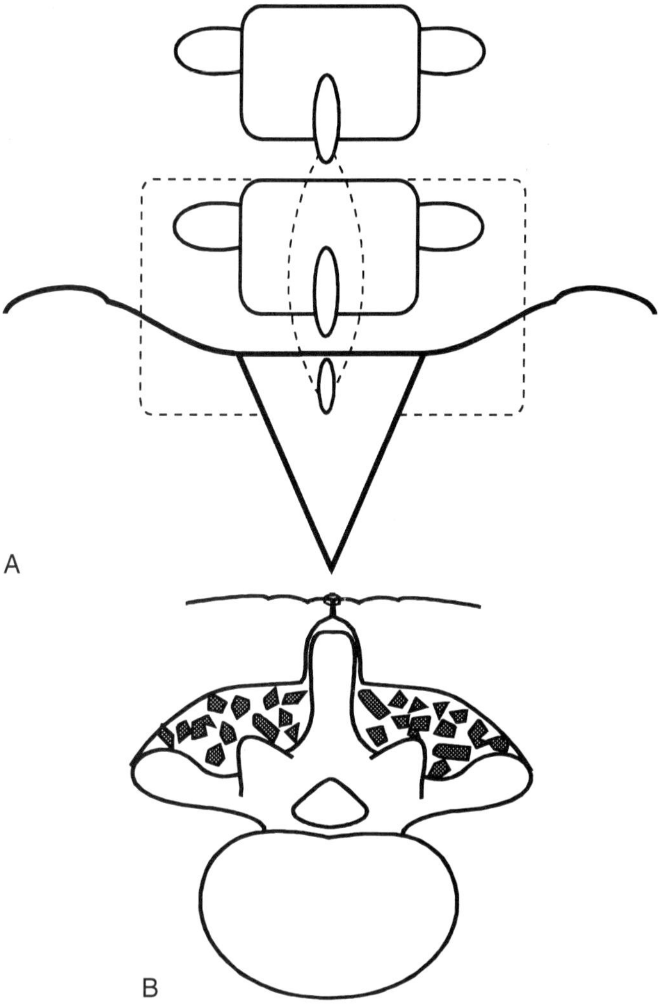

Figure 14.60 **A.** *The limited soft tissue envelope at L5–S1 is depicted as separate fascial incisions (dotted lines) for each side and limited soft tissue elevation as shown within the rectangular dotted line.* **B.** *An axial view of the limited soft tissue envelope, wherein the muscle serves as a firm cover for the bone graft.*

Implant Failure Screws break (Fig. 14.63), and the screw–rod-plate-rod junction can separate (Fig. 14.64). In osteoporotic bone the rigid nature of the construct may lead to screw pull out or the "windshield washer" phenomenon of screw loosening (Fig. 14.65).

Infection Pedicle screw instrumentation and fusion are long, tough cases. They require many members of the staff to assist (cell saver technician, radiographic technologist, spinal cord monitoring personnel, and so on). Because of the wide dissection needed to insert the instrumentation, more dead space and hematoma are left behind on closure. It is only reasonable to conclude that the postoperative infection rate will be high (up to 10% in some series).

The potential for infection may be further enhanced by the fact that you are often dealing with an older patient who has: somewhat impaired wound healing and a foreign (avascular) mass of instrumentation and bone graft (that can easily die instead of heal). Obviously, these infections are difficult (and expensive) to treat.

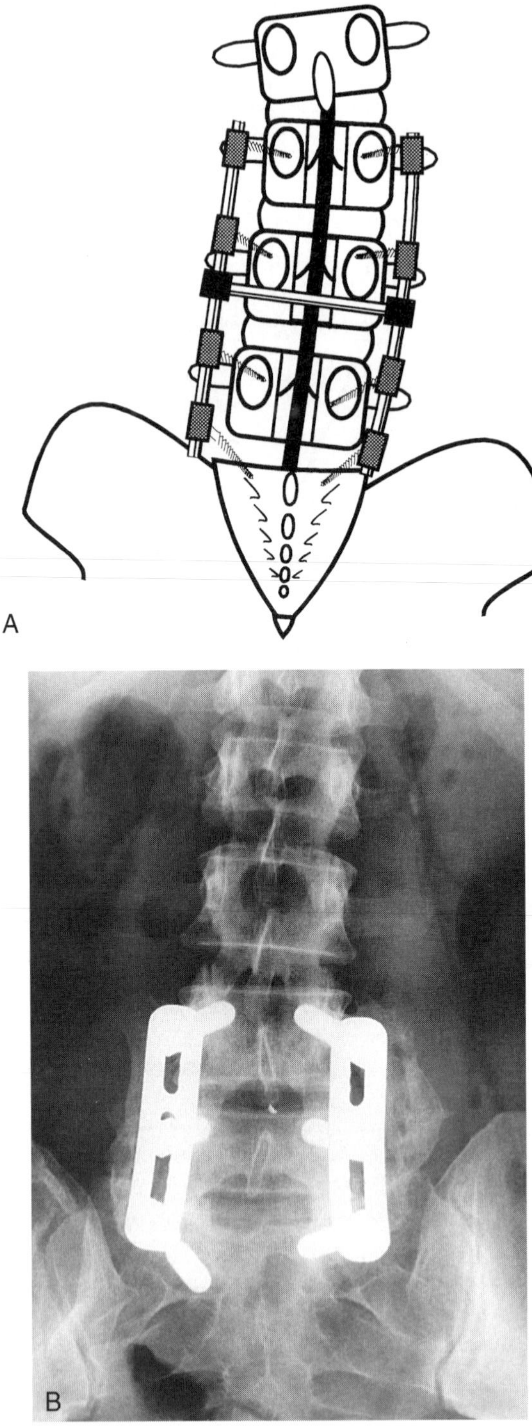

Figure 14.61 **A.** *A schematic of pedicle screw fixation of L3 to the sacrum.* **B.** *A two-level Steffee plate with pedicle screws.*

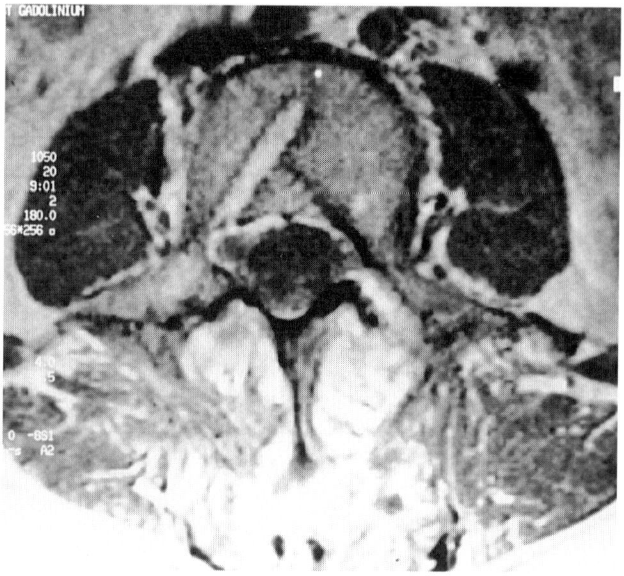

Figure 14.62 *An MRI (after pedicle screw removal) showing that the path of the screw was close to nerve roots on both sides.*

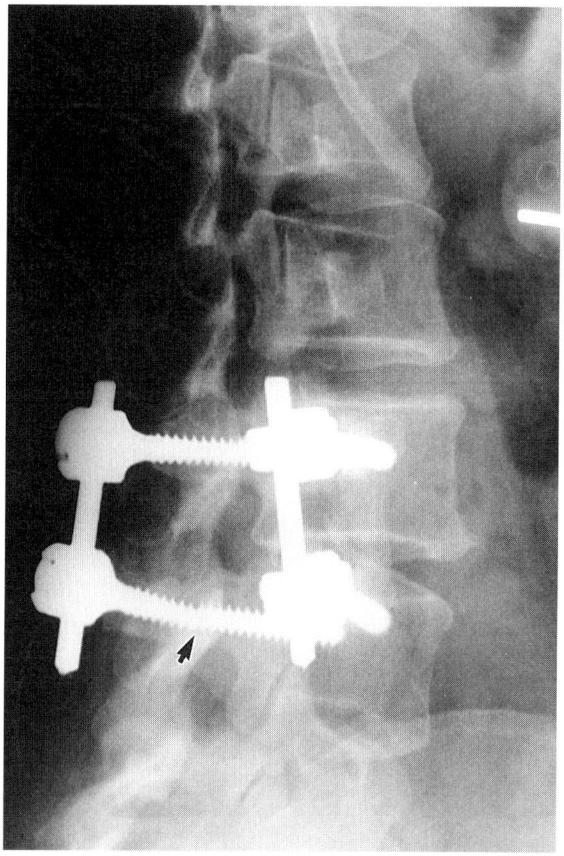

Figure 14.63 *Screw breakage (arrow).*

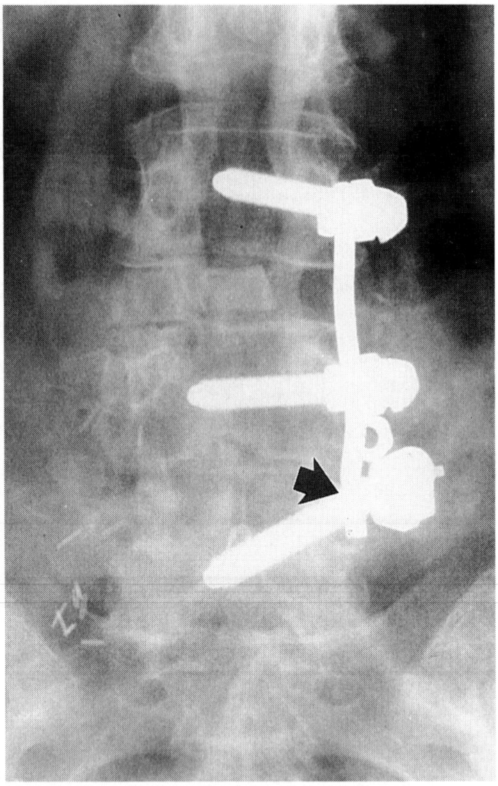

Figure 14.64 *Screw-rod separation (arrow).*

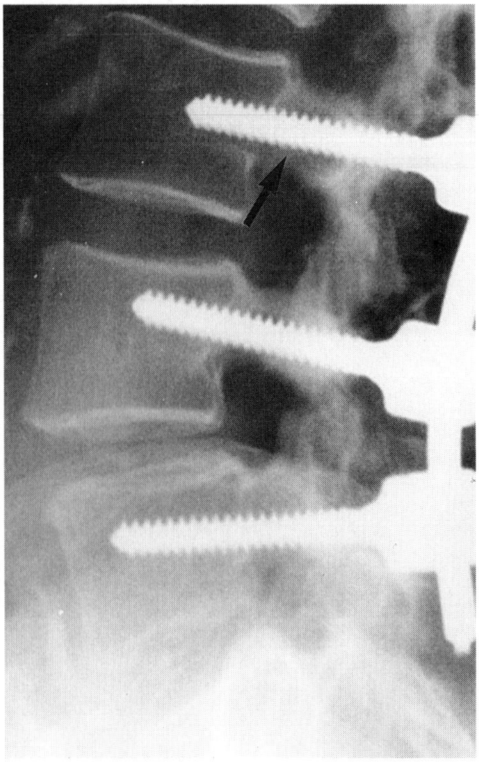

Figure 14.65 *The "windshield washer" phenomenon of screw loosening (arrow).*

Pseudarthrosis with Instrumentation The instrumentation systems have enjoyed wide support among spine surgeons because they decrease the pseudarthrosis rate.(57) It is still possible to end up with a pseudarthrosis in an instrumented fusion, which may be very hard to demonstrate on investigation and requires re-exploration of the fusion mass. When you combine a pseudarthrosis with one of the complications previously mentioned, you have a very difficult clinical problem, which often results in permanent long-term problems that are difficult to treat even with repeat surgery. Because of this possibility, a number of spine surgeons use these systems sparingly, or not at all (included among them is the senior author [JM]).

Painful Hardware In some patients, an apparently solid fusion may continue to be painful. In approximately 50% of these patients, removal of the hardware will result in relief of a significant amount of pain.

Degenerative Changes at the Motion Segment Above the Fusion The instrumentation systems' greatest advantage is the rigid immobilization of the instrumented segments and the higher successful fusion rates.(57) At the same time, this presents a disadvantage to the motion segment above the instrumentation, which becomes more mobile. This is apt to lead to degenerative changes that may become very symptomatic.

Miscellaneous Complications There are a number of miscellaneous complications such as screw perforation of a vessel anteriorly (Fig. 14.66) and damage to adjacent facet joints. These should not occur in skilled hands, but nevertheless they are complications associated with pedicle instrumentation, and not the uninstrumented intertransverse fusion. An allergy to the metal implant, although rare, has been reported.

General Complications Long, tough surgeries, with prolonged patient positioning on the operating table, are associated with higher complication rates (23) (Table 14.6).

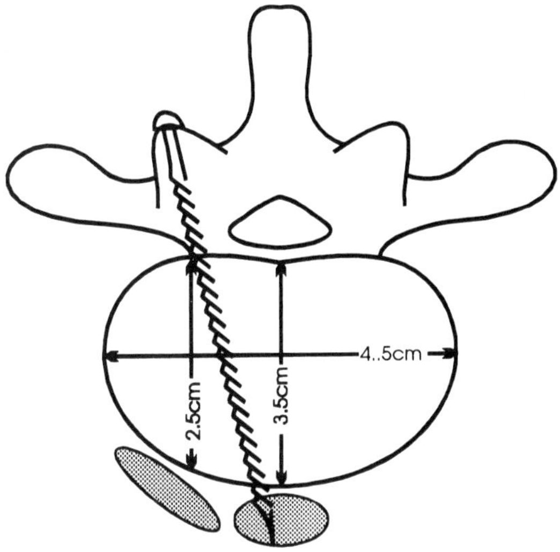

Figure 14.66 *Screw penetration of a vessel (aorta) anteriorly.*

The Biomechanical Principle of Stress Risers

Raising stress on spinal motion segments has the potential for increasing degeneration in those FSUs. Instrumented fusions are rigid constructs that raise stresses on adjacent motion segments (Fig. 14.67). The transfer of forces is most pronounced at the adjacent higher levels, and over the long haul, this transfer can lead to degeneration and symptoms at these unfused levels. This takes time (years) to develop, but it is our prediction that this will become the single biggest problem attendant on the use of spinal instrumentation for degenerative spinal conditions.

The Advantages of Pedicle Fixation

We have not painted a very nice picture for instrumented spinal fusions for degenerative spine problems. There is no question that the pedicle fixation systems have vastly im-

Table 14.6. Complications of Prolonged Operating Table Positioning

Pressure complications (eyes, ulnar and other peripheral nerves, and so on)
Phlebitis and pulmonary embolism
Atelectasis ± pneumonia
Urinary tract infection

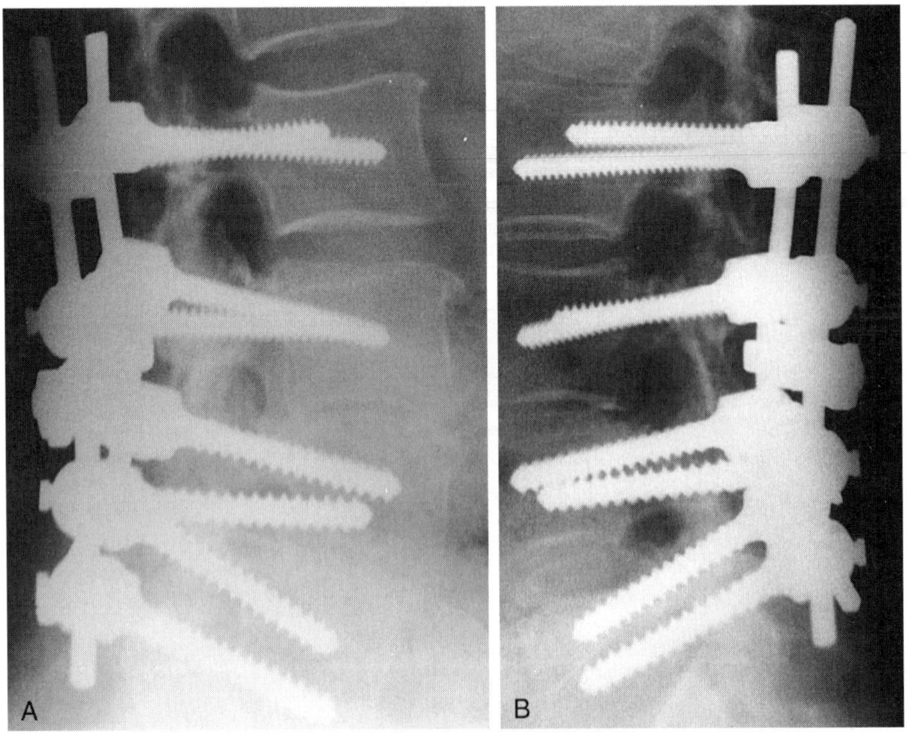

Figure 14.67 *The stress riser above a fusion:* **A.** *A normal L1–L2 disc above a three-level instrumented fusion.* **B.** *Degenerative changes have started to develop at L1–L2.*

proved the management of spinal fractures and deformity. There are serious questions being raised about their use in degenerative disc disease. Competent scientists have published good work on the advantages of instrumentation in degenerative spine problems, and their conclusions are that instrumentation will improve outcomes in degenerative spondylolisthesis, degenerative scoliosis, and salvage surgery. Instrumentation is of questionable value in single-level fusions, although Lorenz and co-workers (57) and Zdeblick(104) have published excellent studies in support of instrumentation. We believe that when compared with the limited lumbar fusion concept, there will be little advantage to instrumentation for a single-level fusion.

The problem is the role of instrumentation in multilevel lumbar fusions for degenerative disc disease. There is no question that the pseudarthrosis rate is high in uninstrumented multilevel lumbar fusions (up to 50%), which increases the failure rate. Also, there is no question that instrumentation decreases the pseudarthrosis rate, which has allowed surgeons to extend their indications for fusion in multilevel degenerative disc disease. But this has come with a higher price of complications, revision surgery, and long-term failure due to degenerative changes in adjacent motion segments. We agree with the study of Turner and colleagues, (89) which calls to question the merits of all lumbar fusions, but especially instrumented fusions.

Pedicle Screws: The Politics

It is a shame to have to introduce this aspect of pedicle screws, but it is important to see how political and bureaucratic steps affect the delivery of medical care in the United States. The center of this storm is the US Food and Drug Agency (FDA), which has had the power to regulate the marketing and sales of medical devices since 1976. In 1990 to 1991, the FDA became concerned with the fact that pedicle screw systems were being marketed and used without FDA approval, which threatened to limit the use of these systems by surgeons. To most surgeons, the FDA threat was an "Alice in Wonderland" move, because pedicle screws had revolutionized the treatment of spine fractures, and published studies showed their effectiveness in the management of spondylolisthesis.

Two efforts were launched. The first was an effort by manufacturers to prove that pedicle screws were used before the 1976 Medical Device Amendments. This has recently resulted in the FDA agreeing that pedicle screw systems could be used for the treatment of severe spondylolisthesis at the L5 level. The FDA did not mention or perhaps did not understand that some patients only have four lumbar vertebrae! Of course, the package insert must describe this use as "a pre-amendment, unclassified device system." The package insert must also carry a number of other warnings to surgeons that are too numerous to mention here. This decision came on the heels of a 4-year effort and untold hundreds of thousands of dollars spent by a manufacturer. Never mind, just add it to the already high cost of these implants!

The second effort was a major study sponsored by the North American Spine Society and directed by Yuan and co-workers.(103) These researchers presented results from thousands of cases studied showing that pedicle screws were very beneficial in the management of degenerative spondylolisthesis and spinal fractures. An FDA advisory panel has received this information, and in the summer of 1994 recommended that pedicle screw systems be down classified from Class III to Class II devices for the indications just mentioned. It will take months for this recommendation to move from one floor of the FDA building to another, but so goes the pace of the US government.

Things were so ridiculous in the United States that in 1993 and 1994, entire educational workshops were forced to delete the teaching of anything remotely connected with pedicle screw systems. Academic freedoms and freedom of speech were on temporary hold while the FDA pondered its navel! At the time of this writing, the FDA has not sanctioned pedicle screw insertion for anything other than severe (Grades 3 and 4) spondylolisthesis at L5–S1. Who knows what the future will bring? One thing for certain is that those bureaucrats who are deciding this issue are collecting a good paycheck and building a nice pension plan!

The Use of Electrical Stimulation to Augment Fusion

It has been long established by research in fracture healing that stresses in the area of active bone formation produce electrically negative signals. Less active areas of bone turnover were also noted to be electropositive. By the mid 1950s, researchers noted increased bone formation around the negative lead (cathode) in long bone healing. Although most of the investigation on electrical stimulation has centered around long bone healing, there have been published studies suggesting electrical stimulation may enhance the fusion rate in lumbar spine surgery. The fact that we are 40 years down the research road on electrical stimulation of spinal bone grafts without clear evidence of clinical efficacy should tell you how tenuous the claims are for improved lumbar fusion rates using electrical stimulation.

The theoretical foundation for electrical stimulation is based on good scientific evidence. A negatively charged electrode in an area of bone healing will consume oxygen and increase the pH, which is beneficial to bone formation. There may also be a direct stimulation of cells to increase their osteogenic activity. Kahanovitz (48) has shown that direct current stimulation of facet joint fusions in adult mongrel dogs increases the fusion rate to 100%. The problem has been to extend these excellent basic science works into the clinical realm to show efficacy. To date, there are as many clinical studies showing usefulness and uselessness.

Technique

There are two methods of applying electrical stimulation to lumbar fusions.

1. Implantable electrodes that apply direct current to the fusion site (Fig. 14.68).
2. Pulsed electromagnetic fields, worn in a brace (Fig. 14.68, B), that apply indirect current to the area of fusion.

Both mechanisms are safe. The direct current stimulation applies 5 to 20 microamperes constantly to the field, over a minimum of 20 weeks, through 2 to 4 electrodes. After 6 months, the subcutaneous battery pack is surgically removed, and the electrodes are left in place. To date, there have been no reports of adverse affects from this approach. The external electrical stimulator is inserted in a brace, and patients are instructed to wear the cumbersome apparatus 8 to 10 hours per day. The hope is that they will wear their stimulator at least 4 hours per day, but patient compliance has been a major problem in all research studies.

The authors' opinion is that properly selected patients, undergoing single-level fusions, and living up to the criteria outlined in Table 14.5, do not need electrical stimula-

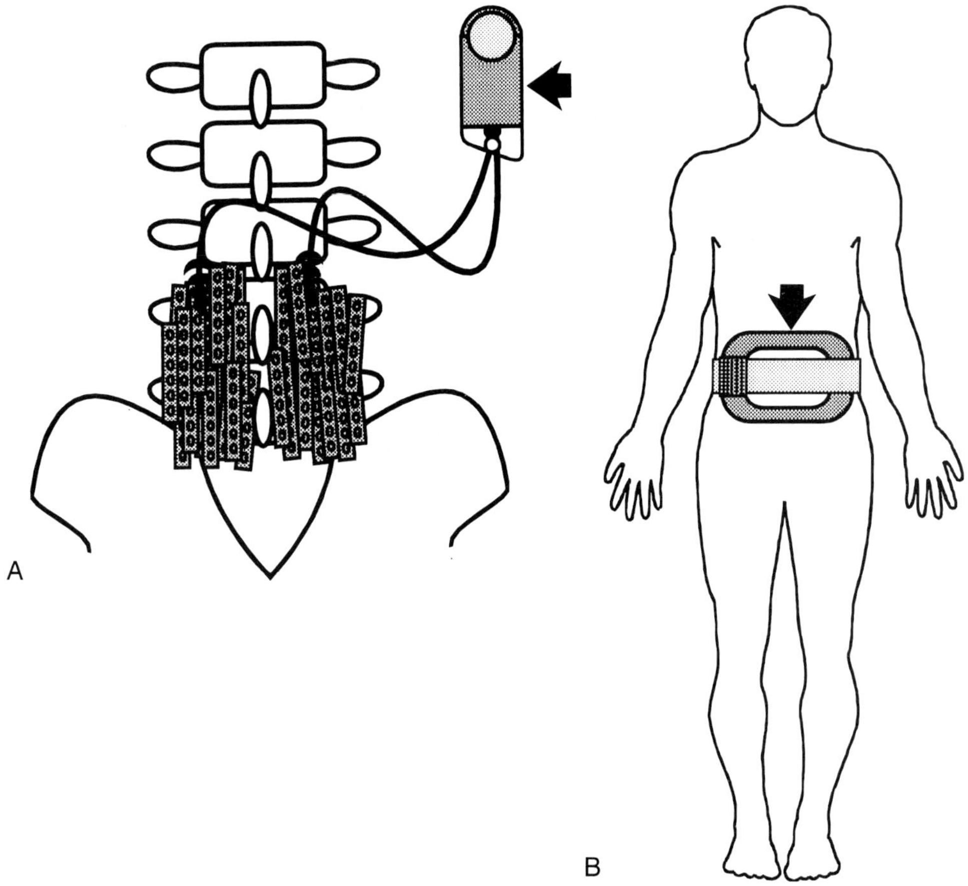

Figure 14.68 **A.** *Electrical stimulation: internal battery pack (arrow) implanted in muscle.* **B.** *Electrical stimulation: external brace (arrow) creating pulsed electromagnetic fields.*

tion to achieve a solid fusion. Using the limited soft tissue envelope to create the primary fusion bed is the most important of these principles. The use of electrical stimulation has led surgeons to extend their indications for fusions to patients who are undergoing multiple-level fusions, patients who are undergoing revision of failed fusions, smokers, and the malnourished. Further studies in this group of patients will show the futility of even operating on these patients, let alone adding the expense of electrical stimulation.

Postoperative Care of the Fused Lumbar Spine

It is essential that, before any fusion, the patient be made fully aware of the prolonged nature of the convalescence. The graft is rarely fully incorporated in under 9 months. Sedentary workers and housewives may return to their duties with some persistent discomfort in 2 to 3 months. Patients whose jobs require prolonged standing, climbing stairs, walking, repetitive bending, and stooping rarely return to work in under 6 months. Patients engaged in heavy work will take 1 year to return to work. None will really experience the full benefit of the operative procedure until approximately 1 year to 18 months after surgery. Unless the patient is fully aware of the time involved and is prepared for it, the operation may lead to financial disaster. These points are particularly applicable when spinal fusion is considered for the injured work man.

It is our routine to brace all patients for a minimum of 6 to 8 weeks postoperatively. The choice of a brace is not important. We use a simple corset for single-level fusions simply to remind the patient to keep the trunk straight and not bent. We avoid multilevel fusions for degenerative disc disease and thus avoid the requirement for a more rigid corset. We do not use corsets or braces with external electrical stimulators because we have not seen any scientific studies to support their usefulness.

All patients are instructed to supplement their daily diet with 1500 mg of extra calcium per day, along with multivitamins with iron.

From Day 1 of surgery, we encourage our patients to walk. On their first postoperative visit, we would like them to be walking up to 2 to 3 miles per day. Obviously, they are in their brace for this exercise. No other exercises are prescribed until the fusion mass shows signs of maturation.

The first postoperative visit is 6 to 8 weeks after surgery. At this time, radiographs and the patient's symptoms determine the need for further bracing for another 6 to 8 weeks. Patients with continuing back pain requiring analgesia and/or patients with less-than-optimal fusion mass (Fig. 14.69) are kept in their braces. A patient who is withdrawn from analgesic medication because of a reasonable comfort level and who shows signs of a good fusion mass (Fig. 14.69) is weaned from the brace and stepped up in activity.

For at least 3 months, patients are not allowed to smoke, drink excessively, or use

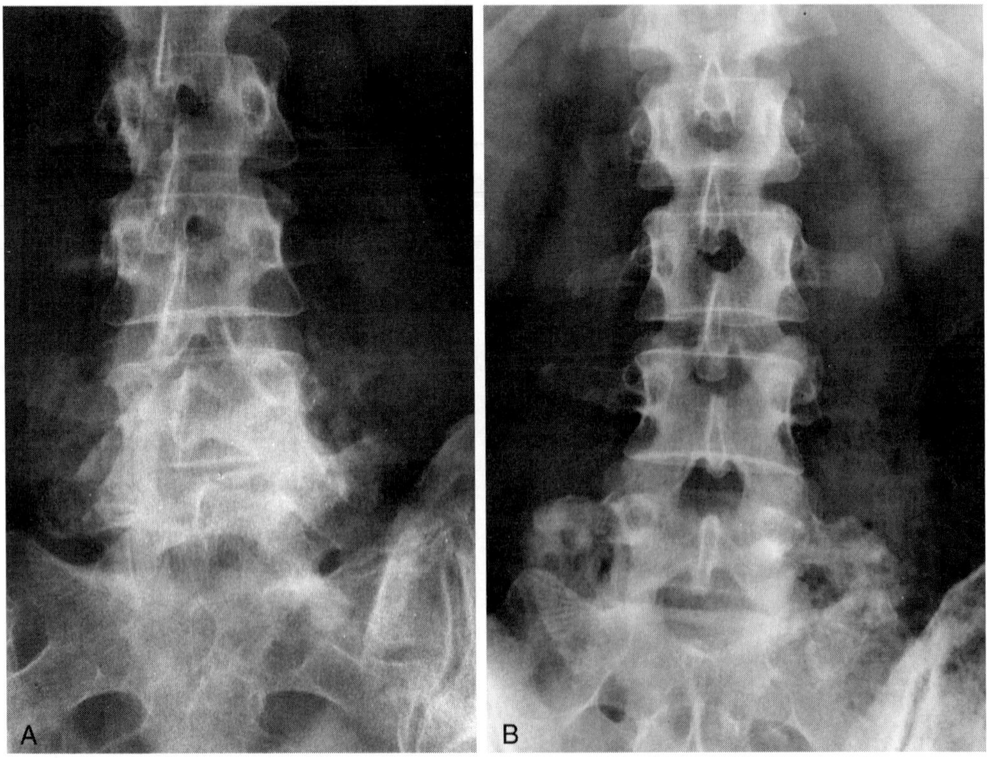

Figure 14.69 **A.** *A poor fusion mass (L4–L5, ie, last mobile level) at 6 weeks: the patient was kept in a brace and then went on to undergo a solid fusion.* **B.** *A good fusion mass (L5–S1) at 6 weeks.*

NSAIDs or aspirin-like products. They are asked to "treat themselves well," that is, lots of rest, limited sitting, and no work for at least 6 to 8 weeks.

Results of Lumbar Fusion

The results of lumbar fusion for degenerative disc disease are average at best. (3, 35, 89, 90) Expand the indications to multiple levels and add instrumentation, and the success rate may suffer even more.

It is very difficult to assess the failure or success of a procedure such as a spinal fusion. (73) If, in the reviews, subjective results are compared, many factors enter into the assessment of a patient. Even if radiographic results are compared, it is difficult to be sure whether a pseudarthrosis is present. However, in an attempt to assess the comparative success of fusion, our mentor (IM), many years ago, reviewed patients undergoing various fusions. The patients were those in whom a double segment fusion of L4 to the sacrum was carried out for degenerative disc disease. None of the patients had ever been subjected to any previous surgery, and the operations were never combined with laminectomy and discectomy. The operative procedure was performed in each instance by the same surgeon. Lateral stress films were studied 2 years after surgery. Although it is acknowledged that there are many sources of error in assessing the incidence of pseudarthrosis from lateral stress films, it was presumed that this error would be equally distributed throughout the whole series studied, and therefore, the series would indeed be comparable (Table 14.7). It can be seen from the analysis of this review that the results of intertransverse fusions compared very favorably with the results of other techniques.

The poor results of spinal fusion may be considered as stemming from three sources: the patient, the spine, and the surgeon.

The Patient Good results are rarely achieved in emotionally unstable patients with a low intelligence quotient (IQ), laborers engaged in heavy work who have no alternative mode of employment, the obese, and patients who are unable or unwilling to accept a temporary change in life-style. Every attempt should be made to avoid spinal fusion in the fat, flabby, fussed, and fearful. Every attempt should be made to avoid fusion in patients who are not capable of developing a solid fusion mass. This includes patients who are heavy smokers and drinkers, and any other nutritionally compromised individual.

The Spine It is dangerous to operate on a spine without irrefutable evidence of the involved segments. Carrying out a spinal fusion in persons whose spines shows multicentric disc degeneration is just patching an old coat, and good results cannot honestly be anticipated.

Concluding that a spine is not fused (pseudarthrosis) can be very difficult.(47) Plain and other radiographs (CT) are not sure methods, especially if instrumentation is in place (Fig. 14.70). The only sure way to determine if a spine is solidly fused is to re-explore, an expensive proposition in all patients with continuing pain following lumbar fusion.

Table 14.7. Results of a Series of Patients Undergoing Double-Segment Fusion[a]

Type of Operation	No. of Cases	Pseudarthrosis	Percentage
Anterior interbody fusion	54	16	30
Posterior fusion	174	30	17
Intertransverse fusion	138	10	7

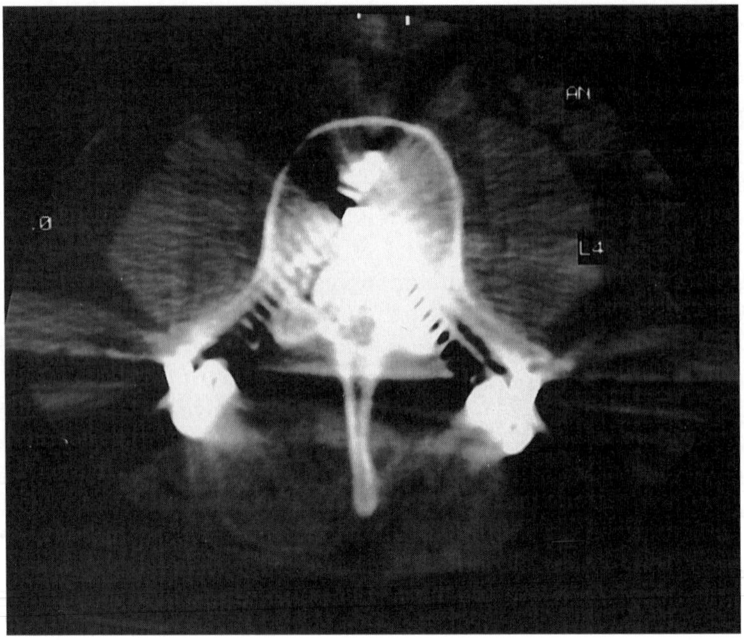

Figure 14.70 *A CT/myelogram with pedicle screws in place. The "scatter" from the screws makes it very difficult to assess the fusion mass.*

The Surgeon The surgeon may be responsible for a bad result not only because of poor technique but probably, what is more important and more common a cause is selection of the wrong patient. The results of spinal fusion are usually disappointing in the presence of financially supported back pain complaints or in those patients with a gross psychogenic magnification of symptoms, regardless of the underlying pathology.

The best results for spinal fusion are seen in the treatment of spondylolisthesis in the young, and in the emotionally stable, financially secure, and physically fit housewife, age approximately 40, who has degenerative disc disease involving one segment.

CONCLUSION

The classic disease model on which medicine is founded is known as the Sydenham model:

1. Signs and symptoms, when added together, suggest a pathology (etiology).
2. The diagnosis can be proved with appropriate tests.
3. There is a clearly prescribed treatment protocol that consistently alters the symptoms and signs (hopefully making them disappear, ie, cure).

The lumbar disc rupture, causing sciatica, fits this disease model. Lumbar degenerative disc disease does not.

In the mid 1800s, the building of the railroad was an important part of the industrial revolution. Laborers and passengers started to show up with low back pain. Legislation was enacted enshrining the concept that all back pain arose from injury and was due some sort of financial reward. Since the introduction of these laws, back pain has become as much a societal phenomenon as a medical problem.(71) It has become complicated by emotions, feelings about one's job or mate, financial reward, and so on. To step in with the simplistic concept of seeking the "pain generator" with both discography and the abolishing movement with an instrumented spinal fusion has caused considerable consternation for many health care professionals, insurers, and federal and state governments.

It is best to remember our admonitions throughout this chapter: Spinal fusion for disc degeneration is not commonly indicated. The emotionally stable, intelligent patient can usually keep this self-limiting condition under control with slight modification of daily activities, and the emotionally fragile are rarely helped by this surgical exercise.

REFERENCES

1. Albee FH. Transplantation of portion of tibia into spine for Pott's disease: a preliminary report. JAMA 1911;57:885–889.
2. Axelsson P, Johnsson R, Stromquist B. Effect of lumbar orthosis on intervertebral mobility. Spine 1992;17:678–681.
3. Axelsson P, Johnsson R, Stromquist B, Arvidsson M, Herrlin K. Posterolateral lumbar fusion: outcome of 71 consecutive operations after 4 (2–7) years. Acta Orthop Scand 1994;65:309–314.
4. Beaman DN, Graziano GP, Glover RA, Wojtys EM, Chang V. Substance P innervation of lumbar spinal facets. Spine 1993;18:1044–1049.
5. Bell GR, Rothman RH. The conservative treatment of sciatica. Spine 1984;9:54–56.
6. Biering-Sorensen F. Physical measurements as risk indicators for low-back trouble over a one year period. Spine 1984;9:106–119.
7. Bigos S, Bowyer O, Braen G, et al. Acute low back problems in adults. Clinical Practice Guideline, Quick Reference Guide Number 14. Rockville, MD: US Department of Health and Human Services, Public Health Service, Agency for Health Care Policy and Research, AHCPR Pub No. 95-0643, December 1994.
8. Boden SD, Davis DO, et al. Abnormal magnetic resonance scans of the lumbar spine in asymptomatic patients. J Bone Joint Surg 1990;72A:403–408.
9. Brightbill TC, Pile N, et al. Normal magnetic resonance imaging and abnormal discography in lumbar disc disruption. Spine 1994;19:1075–1077.
10. Brock M, Mayer HM, Weigl K. The artificial disc. Berlin: Springer-Verlag; 1991.
11. Brodsky AE, Binder WF. Lumbar discography: Its value in diagnosis and treatment of lumbar disc lesion. Spine 1979;4:110–120.
12. Buirski G. Magnetic resonance signal patterns of lumbar discs in patients with low back pain. A prospective study with discographic correlation. Spine 1992;17:1199–1204.
13. Burwell RG. Studies in the transplantation of bone. J Bone Joint Surg 1966;48B:532–566.
14. Cady LD, Bischoff DP, O'Connell ER, et al. Strength and fitness and subsequent back injuries in firefighters. J Occup Med 1979;21:169–272.
15. Carette S, et al. A controlled trial of corticosteroid injections into facet joints for chronic low back pain. N Engl J Med 1991;325:1002–1007.
16. Castagnera L, Lavignolle B, et al. Test de tolerance discale et Intérêt diagnostique et pronostique avant chimionucléolyse. Acta Orthop Belg 1987;53:184–194.
17. Cloward RB, Buzaid LL. Discography: Technique, indications and evaluation of the normal and abnormal intervertebral disc. Am J Roentgenol 1952;68:552–564.
18. Colhoun E, McCall IW, Williams L, Cassar Pullicino VN. Provocation discography as a guide to planning operations on the spine. J Bone Joint Surg 1988;70B:267–271.

19. Collis JS Jr, Gardner WJ. Lumbar discography: An analysis of one thousand cases. J Neurosurg 1962;19:452–461.
20. Crock HV. Isolated lumbar disc resorption as a cause of nerve root canal stenosis. Clin Orthop 1976;115:109–115.
21. Crock HV. Isolated disc resorption. In: Frymoyer, JW, ed. The Adult Spine. New York: Raven Press, 1991.
22. Esses SI, Botsford DJ, Kostuik JP. The role of external spinal skeletal fixation in the assessment of low-back disorders. Spine 1989;14:594–601.
23. Esses SI, Sachs BL, Dreyzin V. Complications associated with the technique of pedicle screw fixation. A selected survey of ABS members. Spine 1993;18:2231–2239.
24. Fairbank JCT, Park WM, McCall IW, O'Brien JP. Apophyseal injection of local anesthetic as a diagnostic aid in primary low back pain syndromes. Spine 1981;6:598–605.
25. Forrester JC, Zederfeldt BH, Hayes TL, Hunt TK. Wolff's law in relation to the healing skin wound, J Trauma 1970;10:770–779.
26. Fraser RD, Osti OL, Vernon-Roberts B. Discitis after discography. J Bone Joint Surg 1987;69B: 26–35.
27. Friedlaender GE, Strong DM, Sell KW. Studies on the antigenicity of bone. J Bone Joint Surg 1984;66A:107–112.
28. Frymoyer JW, Cats-Baril WL. An overview of the incidences and costs of low back pain. Orthop Clin North Am 1991;22:263–271.
29. Ghormley RK. Low back pain with special reference to the articular facets, with presentation of an operative procedure. JAMA 1933;101:1773–1777.
30. Gibson MJ, Buckley J, Mawhinney R, et al. Magnetic resonance imaging and discography in the diagnosis of disc degeneration: A comparative study of 50 discs. J Bone Joint Surg 1986;68B: 369–373.
31. Godfrey CM, Morgan PP, Schatzker J. A randomized trial of manipulation for low-back pain in a medical setting. Spine 1984;9:301–304.
32. Goldberg VM, Bos GD, Heiple KG, Zika JM, Powell AE. Improved acceptance of frozen bone allograft in genetically mismatched dogs by immunosuppression. J Bone Joint Surg 1984;66A: 937–950.
33. Graf H. Instabilité vertebrale, traitement à l'aide d'un système souple. Rachis 1992;4: 107–112.
34. Grubb SA, Lipscomb HJ, Conrad RW. Degenerative adult onset scoliosis. Spine 1988;13: 241–245.
35. Hanley EN. Lumbar spine fusion: Matching expectations and outcomes. AAOS Bull, April 1993, pp 6–7.
36. Hazard RG, Fenwick JW, Kalisch SM, et al. Functional restoration with behavioral support: a one year prospective study of patients with chronic low back pain. Spine 1989;14:157–161.
37. Heiple KG, Chase SW, Herndon CH. A comparative study of the healing process following different types of bone transplantation. J Bone Joint Surg 1963;45A:1593–1616.
38. Hess WF, Jackson RP, et al. Pain response by discography as a predictor of clinical outcome of patients with solid posterior lateral lumbosacral fusion. Poster Exhibit. New Orleans: American Academy of Orthopedic Surgeons; February 1994.
39. Hibbs RA. An operation for progressive spinal deformities: A preliminary report of three cases from the service of the orthopedic hospital. NY J Med 1911;93:1013–1020.
40. Holm S. Pathophysiology of disc degeneration. Acta Orthop Scand 1993;64(suppl 251):13–15.
41. Holmes RE, Salyer KF. Bone regeneration in coralline hydroxyapatite implant. Surg Forum 1978;24:611–616.
42. Holt EP, Jr. The question of lumbar discography. J Bone Joint Surg 1966;50A:720–726.
43. Hudgins WR. Diagnostic accuracy of lumbar discography. Spine 1977;2:305–309.

44. Jackson RP. The facet syndrome: myth or reality? Clin Orthop 1992;279:110–121.
45. Jackson RP, Cain JE, et al. The neuroradiographic diagnosis of lumbar herniated nucleus pulposus. Spine 1989;14:1356–1361.
46. Jackson RP, Jacobs RR, Montesano PX. Facet joint injections in low-back pain. A prospective statistical study. Spine 1988;13:966–971.
47. Johnson RG, Macnab I. Localization of symptomatic lumbar pseudarthroses by use of discography. Clin Orthop 1985;197:164–170.
48. Kahanovitz N. Electricity in spinal fusion. Rothman RH, Simeone FA, eds. The Spine. Philadelphia: WB Saunders; 1992.
49. Kirkaldy-Willis WH, Farfan HF. Instability of the lumbar spine. Clin Orthop 1982;165:110–123.
50. Konberg M. Discography and magnetic resonance imaging in the diagnosis of lumbar disc disruption. Spine 1989;14:1368–1372.
51. Korovessis P, Piperos G, Sidiropoulos P, Dimas A. Adult idiopathic lumbar scoliosis. Spine 1994;19:1926–1932.
52. Kuslich SD, Ulstrom CL, Michael CJ. The tissue of origin of low back pain and sciatica: a report of pain response to tissue stimulation during operations on the lumbar spine using local anesthesia. Orthop Clin North Am 1991;22:181–187.
53. Lee CK, Langrana NA. Lumbosacral spinal fusion. A biomechanical study. Spine 1984;9: 574–581.
54. Lee CK, Langrana NA, Parsons JR, Zimmerman MC. Prosthetic intervertebral disc (ch 96). In: Frymoyer JW, ed. The Adult Spine. Principles and Practice. New York: Raven Press; 1991; pp 2007–2013.
55. Lindblom K. Diagnostic puncture of intervertebral disks in sciatica. Acta Orthop Scand 1948;17:231–239.
56. Linson MA, Crowe CH. Comparison of magnetic resonance imaging and lumbar discography in the diagnosis of disc degeneration. Clin Orthop 1990;250:160–163.
57. Lorenz M, et al. A comparison of single-level fusions with and without hardware. Spine 1991;16:S455–S458.
58. Marchesi DG, Aebi M. Pedicle fixation devices in the treatment of adult lumbar scoliosis. Spine 1992;17:S304–S309.
59. Mathews JA, Hickling J. Lumbar traction: a double-blind study for sciatica. Rheumat Rehab 1975;14:222–225.
60. McCulloch JA, Waddell G. Lateral lumbar discography. Br J Radiol 1978;51:498–502.
61. McCulloch JA. Chemonucleolysis and experience with 2000 cases. Clin Orthop 1980;146: 128–134.
62. McKenzie RA. The Lumbar Spine. Mechanical Diagnosis and Therapy. Waikanae,1 New Zealand: Spinal Publications, Limited; 1981.
63. Milette PC, Melanson D. A reappraisal of lumbar discography. J Can Assoc Radiol 1982;33: 176–182.
64. Milette PC, Raymond J, Fontaine S. Comparison of high-resolution computed tomography with discography in the evaluation of lumbar disc herniation. Spine 1990;15:525–533.
65. Mitchell RI, Carmen GM. Results of multicenter trial using an intensive active exercise program for the treatment of acute soft tissue and back injuries. Spine 1990;15:514–521.
66. Mixter WJ, Barr JS. Rupture of the intervertebral disc with involvement of the spinal canal. N Engl J Med 1934;211:210–215.
67. Mooney V, Derian C. Synthetic bone graft. In: White AH, Rothman RH, Ray CD, eds. Lumbar Spine Surgery. St. Louis, Mo: CV Mosby; 1987.
68. Mooney V, Robertson J. The facet syndrome. Clin Orthop 1976;115:149–156.
69. Nachemson AL. Newest knowledge of low back pain. Clin Orthop 1992;279:8–20.

70. Nachemson A. Lumbar discography—where are we today? Spine 1989;14:555–557.
71. Nachemson A. Work for all. For those with low back pain as well. Clin Orthop 1983;179:77–85.
72. North Am Spine Society. Position statement on discography. Spine 1988;13:1343.
73. O'Beirne J, O'Neill D, Gallagher J, Williams DH. Spinal fusion for back pain: a clinical and radiological review. J Spinal Disord 1992;5:32–38.
74. Ordeberg G, Enskog J, Sjostrom L. Diagnostic external fixation of the lumbar spine. Acta Orthop Scand (suppl 251). 1993;64:94–96.
75. Perennou D, Marcelli C, Herrisson C, Simon L. Adult lumbar scoliosis. Spine 1994;19:123–128.
76. Pope MH, Frymoyer JW, Krag MH. Diagnosing instability. Clin Orthop 1992;279:60–67.
77. Pritchett JQ, Bortel DT. Degenerative symptomatic lumbar scoliosis. Spine 1993;18:700–703.
78. Report of the Commission of the Evaluation of Pain. Social Security Bulletin. Vol 50, No. 1, January 1987.
79. Rowe ML. Preliminary statistical study of low back pain. J Occup Med 1963;5:336–341.
80. Rowe ML. Low back pain in industry. A position paper. J Occup Med 1969;11:161–169.
81. Rhyne AL, Smith S. Outcome of unoperated discogram positive low back pain. Orlando, Fla: American Academy of Orthopedic Surgeons. Paper No. 395; 1995.
82. Sachs BL, et al. CT / discography in low-back disorders. Spine 1987;12:287–294.
83. Schaffer WO, Spratt KF, Weinstein J, Lehmann TR, Goel V. The consistency and accuracy of roentgenograms for measuring sagittal translation in the lumbar vertebral motion segment: an experimental model. Spine 1990;15:741–750.
84. Schwarzer AC, Aprill CN, Derby R, Fortin J, Kine G, Bogduk N. Clinical features of patients with pain stemming from the lumbar zygapopysial joint: is the lumbar facet syndrome a clinical entity? Spine 1994;19:1132–1137.
85. Shinomiya K, Nakao K, et al. Evaluation of cervical discography in pain origin and provocation. J Spinal Disorders 1993;6:422–426.
86. Simmons ED, Simmons EH. Spinal stenosis with scoliosis. Spine 1992;17:S117–S120.
87. Simmons EH, Segil CM. An evaluation of discography in the localization of symptomatic levels in discogenic disease of the spine. Clin Orthop 1975;108:57–69.
88. Simmons JW, Emery S, et al. Awake discography. A comparison study with magnetic resonance imaging. Spine 1991;165:S216–S221.
89. Turner JA, Ersek M, Herron L. Patient outcomes after lumbar spinal fusions. JAMA 1992;268: 907–911.
90. Turner JA, Herron L, Deyo RA. Meta-analysis of the results of lumbar spine fusion. Acta Orthop Scand (suppl 251). 1993;64:120–122.
91. Urist MR, Dawson E. Intertransverse process fusion with the aid of chemosterilized autolyzed antigen-extracted allogenic (AAA) bone. Clin Orthop 1981;154:97–113.
92. Vanharanta H, et al.The relationship of pain provocation to lumbar disc deterioration as seen by CT / discography. Spine 1987;12:295–298.
93. Venner RM, Crock AU. Clinical studies of isolated disc resorption in the lumbar spine. J Bone Joint Surg 1981;63B:491–494.
94. Waddell G. Clinical assessment of lumbar impairment. Clin Orthop 1987;221:110–120.
95. Waddell G. Low back disability. A syndrome of Western civilization. Neurosurg Clin North Am 1991;2:719–738.
96. Walsh TR, Weinstein JN, Spratt KF, et al. Lumbar discography in normal subjects. J Bone Joint Surg 1990;72A:1081–1088.
97. Wetzel FT, LaRocca SH, et al. The treatment of lumbar spinal pain syndromes diagnosed by discography. Spine 1994;19:792–800.
98. White AH III, Panjabi MM. Clinical Biomechanics of the Spine. Philadelphia: JB Lippincott; 1978, p223.

99. White AH. Back School and Other Conservative Approaches to Low Back Pain. St. Louis, Mo: CV Mosby; 1983.
100. Wiley JJ, Macnab I, Wortzman G. Lumbar discography and its clinical applications. Can J Surg 1968;11:280–289.
101. Williams PC. Examination and conservative treatment for disc lesions of the lower lumbar spine. Clin Orthop 1955;5:28–35.
102. Yasuma T, Ohno R, Yamauchi Y. False-negative lumbar discograms. J Bone Joint Surg 1988;70: 1279–1290.
103. Yuan HA, Garfin SR, Dickman CA, Mardjetko SM. A historical cohort study of pedicle screw fixation in thoracic, lumbar and sacral spine fusions. Spine 1994;19:2279S–2296S.
104. Zdeblick TA. A prospective, randomized study of lumbar fusion. Spine 1993;18:983–991.
105. Zucherman J, Derby R, et al. Normal magnetic resonance imaging with abnormal discography. Spine 1988;13:1355–1359.

15

Disc Degeneration with Root Irritation: Disc Ruptures

"Thou cold sciatica, cripple our senators and make their limbs halt as lamely as their manners."

— W. Shakespeare

INTRODUCTION

A patient with a mechanical compression of a lumbar nerve root will present with the complaint of leg (radicular) pain with or without associated pain in the back. However, it cannot be too strongly emphasized that the mere complaint of pain in the leg does not indicate, by itself, root irritation or root compression. Any painful lesion on the lumbosacral region may give rise to pain referred down the leg in a sciatic distribution. Diabetes can affect peripheral nerves and mimic sciatica due to a disc rupture.(9, 27)

Referred or "reflex" pain has the same neurophysiological basis as the referred pain to the shoulder associated with gallbladder disease and the referred pain down the arm associated with myocardial infarcts.

Referred leg pain derived from mechanical insufficiency of the lumbar spine is rarely experienced below the knee: it is not associated with paresthesia, and there is no evidence of root tension, as reflected by limitation of straight leg raising (SLR) or the presence of a positive bowstring sign.

In Chapter 7, which deals with the pathogenesis of symptoms associated with degenerative disc disease, the pathological processes giving rise to root compression are described. The following discussion of the clinical features of lumbar root compression is confined to describing the symptoms and treatment of the three most common groups seen in clinical practice: disc ruptures (this chapter), lateral zone disc ruptures and bony root entrapments (Chapter 16), and spinal canal stenosis (Chapter 17).

DISC RUPTURES (HNP)

To understand the clinical syndrome of lumbar root irritation and compression due to a disc rupture is to take the most important step in understanding all of low back pain. Although there is tremendous variation in the presentation of a patient with a disc rupture causing sciatica, there is a common thread of historical and physical features that allows for a fairly accurate clinical diagnosis.

Clinical Picture

History

Onset It is fairly constant that a patient who has radicular pain due to a disc rupture has, or had, back pain in their history. The exception to this is the younger patient who may manifest only leg pain as a symptom of the disc rupture and at no time will have had back pain. However, most patients with a disc rupture will have experienced some degree of prodromal back pain for varying lengths of time (from minutes to years). It may be intermittent in its occurrence and extended over a considerable period of time, representing the instability phase that Kirkaldy-Willis has described (Chapter 14). It may be acute, followed soon after by the onset of leg pain.

Approximately half of the patients will attribute their back pain to various forms of traumatic experience. This is especially prevalent in the litigation and compensation population but, in fact, is retrograde rationalization on the part of many patients. Experimental studies and careful statistical analysis of case histories (44) do not support the concept that direct trauma or sudden weight loading of the spine are the causal agents of disc rupture, although they may aggravate a preexisting asymptomatic degenerative condition.

Either in a gradual or sudden fashion, the pain will lateralize to the hip or leg. This moment of lateralization heralds the contact of the ruptured disc with the nerve root and may or may not be precipitated by a simple traumatic event, such as bending over in the shower to pick up the soap.

Location of Pain Various combinations of back, hip, and leg pain present. When trying to understand sciatica, think of five different areas: the back, the buttock, the thigh, the leg, and the foot. There may be symptoms in all five areas, or only in a few of theses areas.

The Back Back pain is considered to be pain localized to the midline lumbosacral region. Any radiation of pain from this area should most likely be considered lateralization of discomfort, and except for the vague referred pain, possibly indicative of radicular involvement. This is a rather controversial statement, but we think that as one gains more experience with radicular involvement, this historical feature will become more evident. Radiation to such areas as the sacroiliac joint region, the high iliac crest region, and the coccygeal region is more indicative of dural irritation than the commonly believed notion that the pain radiation represents muscular splinting of the back with referred pain. This is especially true if this referral is associated with leg pain characteristics as follows:

The Buttock In essence, the buttock is the proximal part of the leg (Fig. 15.1). The younger the patient, the more likely sciatica will be limited to the buttock and more proximal lower extremity. The nature of the pain in the buttock is usually one of a deep-seated, cramping pain that is especially aggravated by sitting.

The Thigh Pain in this area tends to be the sharpest component of sciatica and sometimes is described as having an associated superficial "burning-sensitive" feeling. For both L5 and S1 root involvement, it is located in the posterolateral or posterior thigh, and not lateral thigh. For higher lumbar root involvement, the sharp pain will be the anterior thigh. Unless the patient has a very sensitive bowstring sign, pain is usually absent from the popliteal fossa.

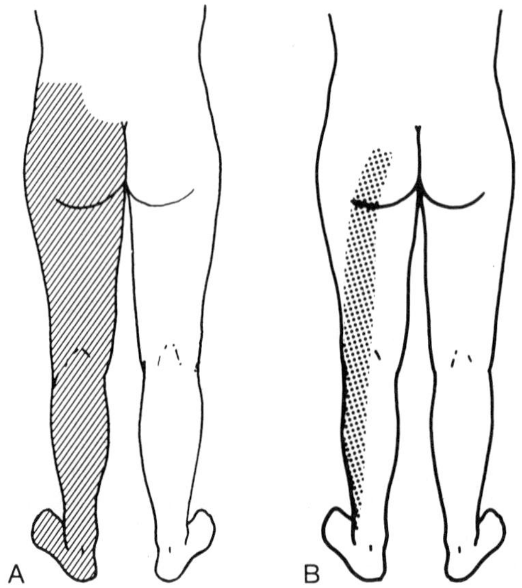

Figure 15.1 **A.** *The proximal part of the leg is the buttock. Pain in the buttock is considered leg pain.* **B.** *Radicular pain will be confined to a nerve root distribution in the leg.*

The Leg The sensation in this area can be mixed. For L5 to S1 root compression, the prevailing discomfort is a cramp and almost viselike feeling in the belly of the gastrocsoleus or peroneal muscles. In addition, the patient may report a paresthetic discomfort in the lateral calf (5th root) or back of the calf (1st root). Most, but not all adult patients with sciatica due to a herniated nucleus pulposus (HNP) will have pain below the knee. Again, the younger patient can be a trap, in that he/she may have pain only in the high iliac crest region, the proximal buttock, and/or thigh. Although rare, this does occur, and offers much confusion in the assessment of the young patient with a disc rupture.

Higher lumbar root lesions (L2, L3, L4) will have no pain below the knee. In L4 root involvement, the patient will often describe a paresthetic discomfort down the medial shin (below the knee), but not pain.

The Foot Unlike the calf, the most common symptom in the foot is paresthesia rather than pain. The lateral border of undersurface of the foot is often, but not always, involved with 1st sacral root compression, whereas the dorsum of the foot may be affected with 5th lumbar root involvement. It is unusual that the patient will complain of pain in the foot.

The term sciatica implies that the patient has leg pain. The younger the patient with a disc rupture, the more likely the sciatic pain will dominate the history. It is a good general rule that, regardless of age, if the radiating hip and leg pain is, at all times, less significant to the patient than the complaint of back pain, the sciatica is not likely due to a disc rupture.

In general, pain derived from the L5 to S1 root involvement courses down the posterior aspect of the leg, whereas lesions of the 2nd, 3rd, and 4th lumbar roots give rise to pain on the anterior part of the thigh.(64) It is routine for sciatic pain due to 5th and 1st root compression to radiate below the knee but, as often mentioned, the younger patient may not have this more distal radiation of discomfort. It is safe to teach that most sciatic pain due to root compression radiates below the knee, but there are exceptions to every generalization in medicine.

Paresthesia in the form of tingling, pins and needles, or numbness is of great value in localizing the level of root compression,(43) and the more distal its location, the more reliable it is in helping with root localization. If a patient can volunteer that the paresthetic discomfort is along the lateral border of the foot into the little toe or up the back of the calf, one can assume that the most likely nerve root involved is S1. Similarly, paresthetic discomfort over the dorsum of the foot or lateral calf implicates the 5th lumbar nerve root; paresthesia over the medial shin indicates 4th lumbar root involvement. Similarly, paresthetic discomfort centered around the knee indicates 3rd root involvement, and lateral thigh pins and needles indicates 2nd root involvement. If the paresthetic discomfort or numbness is vaguely described and has a stocking-and-glove-like distribution, it is not indicative of radicular involvement and is more suggestive of a neuropathy or psychogenic pain. Rarely, motor symptoms predominate and are more disabling to the patient. In such instances, the clinician has to beware of the presence of a spinal tumor or a peripheral neuropathy. When trying to determine the localization of leg pain, have the patient put his/her foot up on a chair and then draw the location of their symptoms (Fig. 15.2).

Aggravation Back and sciatic discomfort is spondylogenic in nature. That is to say, the pain is aggravated by general and specific activities and relieved by rest. Bending, stooping, lifting, coughing, sneezing, and straining at stool will intensify the pain. Which particular activity bothers a patient varies from patient to patient. Most patients with sciatica find difficulty in sitting, especially in a soft lounge chair, including most automobile seats. Standing and walking, although not comfortable, are usually more tolerable. Some patients may find other forms of activity aggravating, but a constant thread throughout the history of sciatica is the fact that some activity bothers the patient. The corollary is also true; if a patient with sciatica rests long enough, or gets into the proper position, some relief of the leg pain will ensue. Aggravation of sciatic discomfort by coughing and sneezing is one of the most commonly mentioned symptoms in textbooks. Although rather specific for radicular involvement, aggravation of pain due to coughing and sneezing is absent often enough from the history to be considered insensitive as a symptom.

Relief Most patients get some relief from lying in the hip-knee flexed position (Fig. 15.2, B). Sleeping is a more comfortable position for most patients when it is done with a pillow under the knees (Fig. 15.2, C) or on the asymptomatic side in the fetal position. Some patients have so much sciatic discomfort that there is no position of comfort. This is especially true for the high lumbar root lesions.

Unusual Referral Patterns of Pain On occasion, unusual referral patterns of pain may occur, such as perineal or testicular discomfort and lower abdominal discomfort. Waddell and Main (92, 93) have stated that referral of pain to the low sacrococcygeal region is suggestive of nonorganic involvement. We believe that just the opposite is true, in that patients with midline dural irritation will often refer discomfort to the lower sacrococcygeal region. Testicular pain is also common and somewhat confusing. Obviously, anyone with testicular pain needs to evaluated for a local testicular cause of their discomfort. In some cases, this referral to the testicular region, or perineum in women, is again due to irritation of the midline sacral nerve roots. On a rare

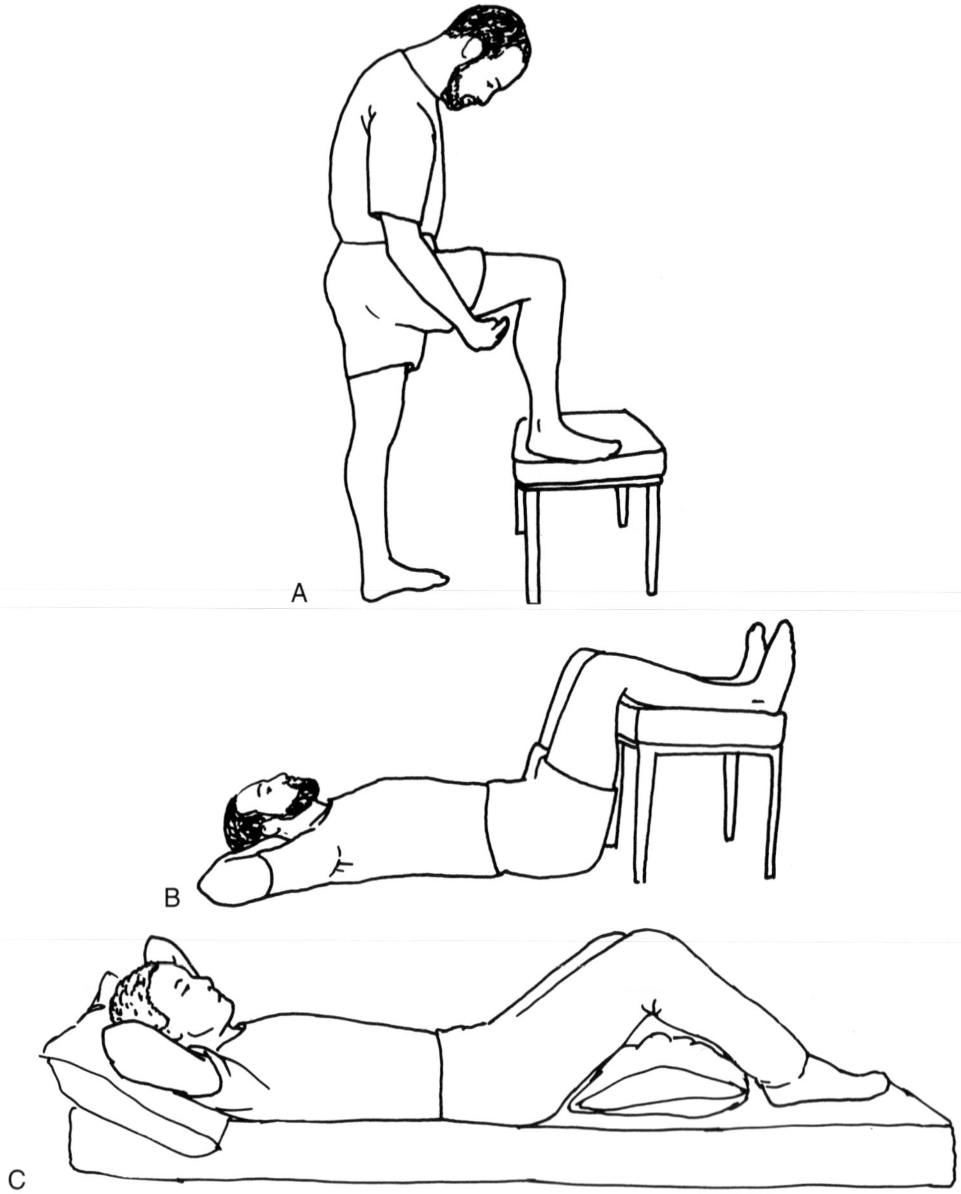

Figure 15.2 **A.** *Ask the patient to put their symptomatic foot up on a chair and draw the distribution of their leg pain. If they draw a line in a radicular distribution with one finger, you not only have the diagnosis of radicular syndrome, you can usually figure out which root is involved.* **B.** *Most patients with sciatica will have figured out that the fastest way to relief of some leg pain, when they get home from work, is to assume this position.* **C.** *The position of comfort when in bed (the semi-Fowler position).*

occasion, it is indicative of a higher lumbar disc lesion and represents the dermatomal radicular distribution of pain (L1 root).

Severe Sciatica On occasion, you will encounter a patient who has so much leg pain that he/she will not be able to localize the symptoms. These are the patients who say either, "fix my leg pain or amputate my leg." To persist in trying to get them to localize their leg pain or their paresthesias is fruitless. Get on with the examination and the diagnosis!

Physical Examination

The physical examination of a patient with sciatica due to a disc rupture is so variable as to be confusing. Some patients present with little in the way of back findings, with all of their findings confined to the lower extremities, whereas others present with incapacitating back spasm, sciatic scoliosis, and are significantly disabled. The common thread through this variable presentation is the fact that the majority of objective findings in a patient with sciatica due to a disc rupture will be in the lower extremity, rather than the back.

The Back

The posture is characteristic. The lumbar spine is flattened and slightly flexed. The patient often leans away from the side of pain, and this sciatic scoliosis become more obvious on bending forward. The patient is more comfortable standing with the affected hip and knee slightly flexed, a manner accentuated by asking the patient to flex forward (Fig. 15.3). In the very acute phase, these patients will walk in obvious discomfort, frequently holding their loins with the hands. The gait is slow and deliberate and is designed to avoid any unnecessary movement of the spine. With gross tension on the nerve root, the patient may not be able to put the heel to the floor and walks slowly and painfully on tiptoe. On rare occasion, this reaction may extend to needing crutches for ambulation.

Forward flexion may be permitted so the hands reach the knees by virtue of flexion of the hip joint. If the examiner keeps his/her fingertips on the spinous processes, it can be felt that the lumbar spine moves little because of splinting. Limitation of flexion in such instances is, therefore, the result of root tension and is due to the increase in leg pain. The degree of flexion should be recorded by measuring the distance between the fingertips and the floor.

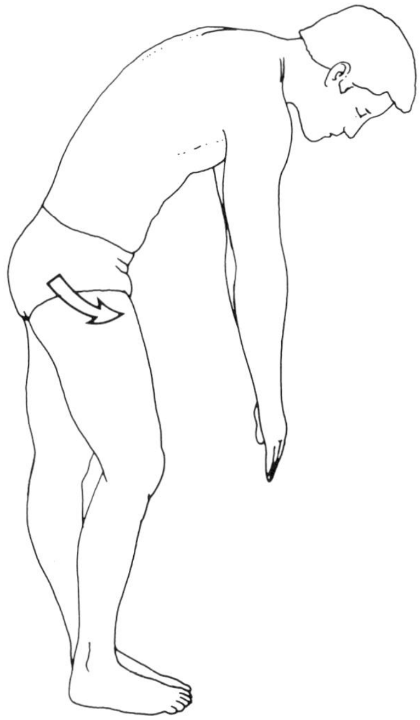

Figure 15.3 *The classic posture in sciatica on forward flexion; the knee of the affected leg flexes while the hip rotates forward (external rotation of hip to relax pyriformis).*

Extension is also limited, although to a lesser degree than flexion, and in most instances the pelvis starts to rotate as soon as the patient attempts to lean backward. The complaint on extension is usually back pain, but at times the patient may feel leg pain. It is our impression that the complaint of leg pain on extension is indicative of an extruded or sequestered disc.

Lateral flexion can be full and free to one side, but usually lateral flexion toward the concavity of the sciatic curve (side of sciatica) is limited. The phenomenon of sciatic scoliosis and the relief of aggravation of pain on lateral flexion have been attributed to the position of the protrusion in relation to the nerve root (Fig. 15.4). However, this may be a simplistic explanation in view of the fact that the sciatic scoliosis disappears on recumbency. This observation, the loss of lateral curvature of the lumbar spine on recumbency, differentiates the sciatic list from a fixed structural scoliosis.

Tenderness and Muscle Spasm

In the standing position, especially in the presence of scoliosis, muscle spasm can be observed. However, at rest, the spasm often subsides, and there is little tenderness to be found on examination. Selectively palpating and applying a lateral thrust to the spinous process may cause some back pain and, on the rare occasion, produce leg pain. The patient with sciatica due to a HNP, at complete rest in the prone position on the examining table, has little symptoms to be found in the back. The patient's major complaint is leg pain, and the majority of physical findings are in the extremity.

The Extremities

The cardinal signs of lumbar root compromise are root tension, root irritation, and root compression.

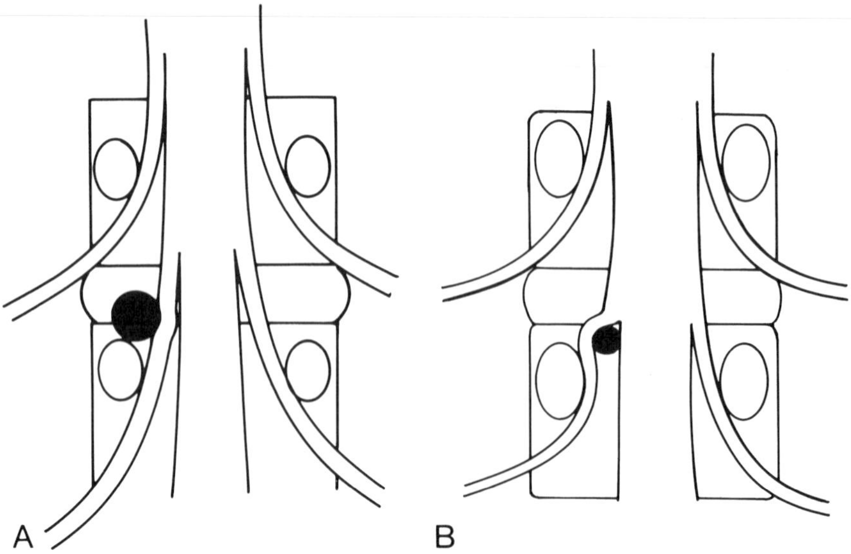

Figure 15.4 **A.** *A disc herniation lateral to the nerve root. Theoretically, lateral flexion to the same side would increase the pain.* **B.** *An axillary disc herniation. Theoretically, lateral flexion to the opposite side increases the pain.*

Root Tension and Irritation The term "root tension" denotes distortion of the emerging nerve root by an extradural lesion. The two most useful tests for the presence of root tension are limitation of SLR and the bowstring sign, the latter also arising in part from root irritation.

When testing straight leg raising, it is important not to hurt the patient. Never jerk the leg up in the air suddenly. The knee must be kept fully extended by firm pressure exerted by the examiner's hand, while the hip is slightly internally rotated and adducted. With the other hand under the heel, the examiner slowly raises the leg until leg pain is produced (Fig. 15.5). Two additional maneuvers are of vital importance to add significance to the finding of limitation of straight leg raising:

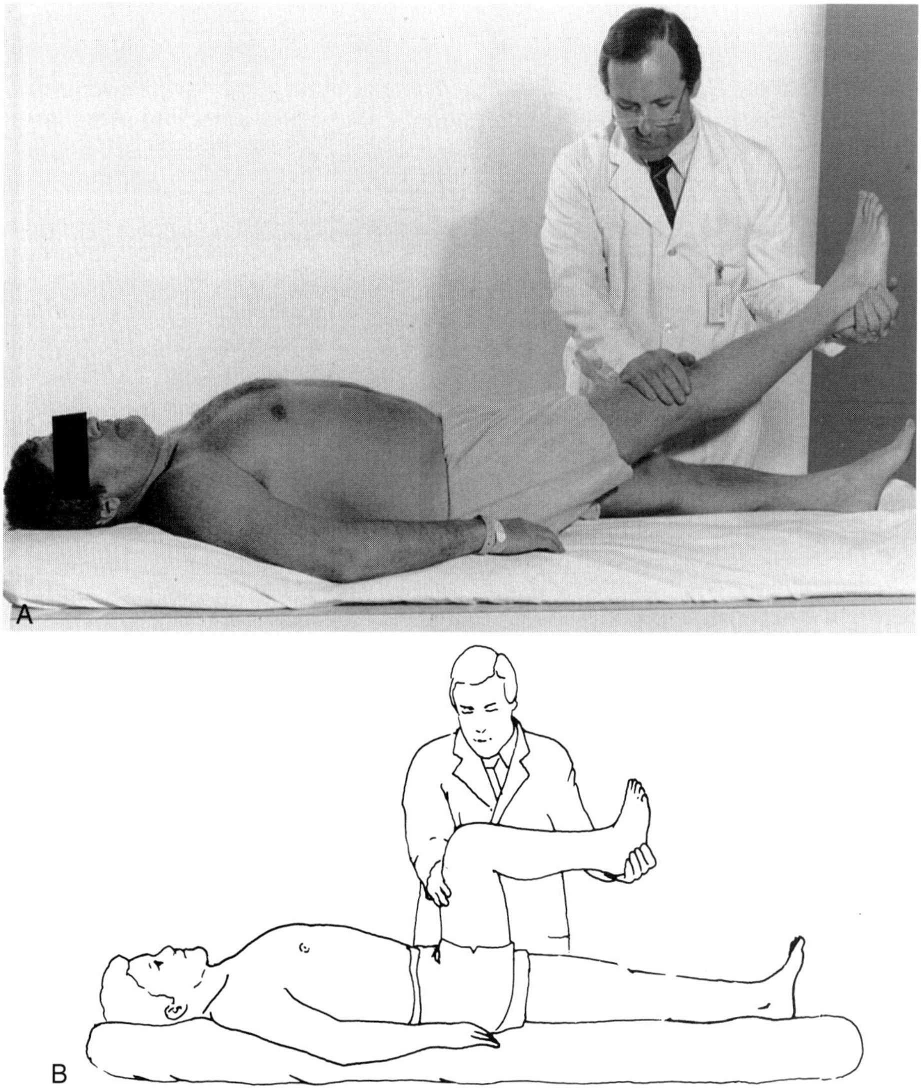

Figure 15.5 **A.** *The standard for the SLR test: knee straight, hip neutral or slight internal rotation, and slow lifting of the leg by the heel.* **B.** *Hip and knee flexion should relieve the pain of radicular origin.*

1. Aggravation of pain by forced dorsiflexion of the ankle at the limit of straight leg raising (A variation of Lasègue's sign).(83, 97)
2. Relief of pain by flexion of the knee and hip.

Physiogenic sciatic pain due to nerve root tension is always relieved by flexion of the knee and hip. Further flexion of the patient's hip with the knee bent does not reproduce and aggravate sciatic pain (Fig. 15.15). This phenomenon is only seen in the emotionally destroyed.

If SLR is permissible to 60 to 70 degrees before leg pain is produced, the finding is equivocal for an HNP. Below this level, the reproduction of pain on straight leg raising, aggravated by dorsiflexion of the ankle and relieved by flexion of the knee, is strongly suggestive of tension on the 5th lumbar or 1st sacral root. In patients in whom paresthesia in the foot is a predominant symptom, repetitive SLR, that is, "pumping of the leg," frequently intensifies the sensation of numbness.

Location of Pain on Straight Leg Raising The examiner is seeking to reproduce leg (buttock, thigh, and / or calf) pain when doing the SLR test. Reproduction of back pain, especially in the high ranges of SLR testing, is usually not indicative of root tension. However, there is one exception that is discussed later in this chapter under midline disc herniation.

False-Positive Straight Leg Raising Test Hamstring tightness may cloud the assessment of the SLR test. Patients with hamstring tightness have a generally tight body build (eg, inability to fully extend the elbow) and plenty of room between the wrist flexed, thumb abducted position, and the volar surface of the forearm (Fig. 15.6). Hamstring tightness should be bilateral, and the discomfort the patient witnesses is distal in the thigh, in the region of the hamstring tendons. Hamstring tightness does not radiate below the knee. Finally, other physical findings of root irritation and compression are absent in hamstring tightness.

False-Negative Straight Leg Raising Test On occasion, you will encounter a loose-jointed individual with sciatica due to an HNP. On SLR testing, you may not be im-

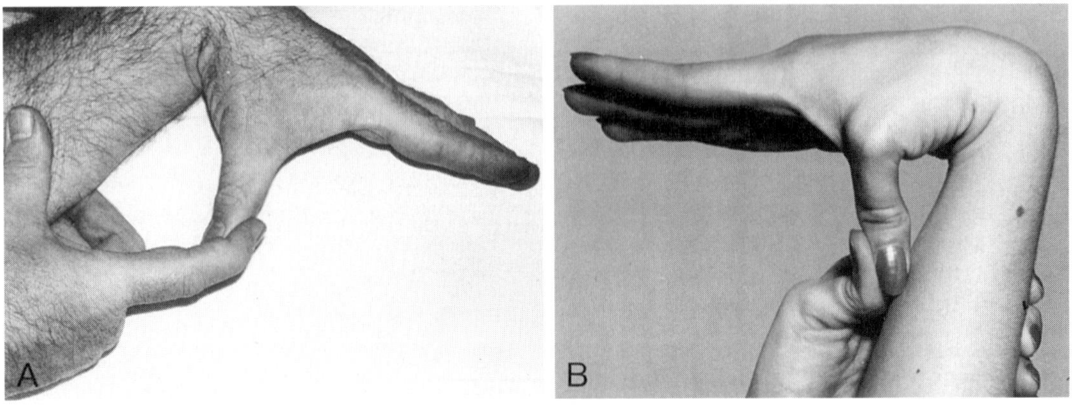

Figure 15.6 **A.** *A tight-jointed individual with limited abduction of thumb.* **B.** *A loose-jointed individual with much greater passive abduction ability.*

pressed with the degree of impaired SLR until you examine the unaffected leg and see the individual's ability to straight leg raise well beyond 90 degrees.

Bowstring Sign The bowstring sign (10) is an important indication of root tension or irritation. The examiner carries out SLR to the point at which the patient experiences some discomfort in the distribution of the sciatic nerve. At this level, the knee is allowed to flex, and the patient's foot is allowed to rest on the examiner's shoulder (Fig. 15.7). The test demands sudden, firm pressure applied to the popliteal nerve in the popliteal fossa. The action may startle the patient enough to make him jump, and this jump may hurt. To prevent this, first of all, tell the patient that you are just going to press firmly on the back of the knee and that it may hurt. Apply firm pressure to the hamstrings; this will not hurt. Then, move your thumbs over to the popliteal nerve. A positive bowstring test is reproduction of radiating leg discomfort. Most commonly, the radiating discomfort is pain felt proximally in the thigh and even into the back. Less commonly, radiating discomfort will travel distally, and this discomfort is more often paresthetic in nature than painful. If the test produces only local pain in the popliteal fossa, it is of no significance. This demonstration of root irritation is probably the single most important sign in the diagnosis of tension and irritation of a nerve root caused by a ruptured intervertebral disc.

Tests to Verify SLR Reduction When the patient sits with knees dangling over the side of the bed, the hip and knee are both flexed at 90 degrees. If the knee is now extended fully, the position assumed by the leg is equivalent to 90 degrees of straight leg raising (Fig. 15.8). If the patient is suffering from root compromise, this will cause sudden, severe pain, and the patient will throw his/her trunk backward to avoid tension on the nerve. This is commonly referred to as the "positive flip test." With the psychogenic regional pain syndrome, the patient will permit the examiner to extend the knee of the painful leg without showing any response at all.

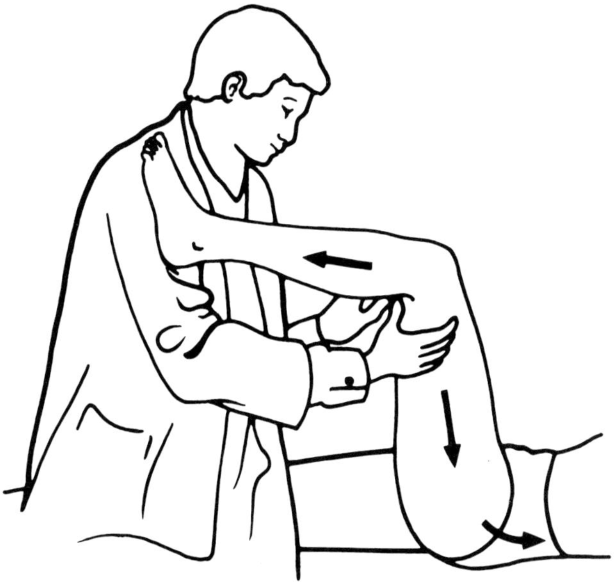

Figure 15.7 *The bowstring test.*

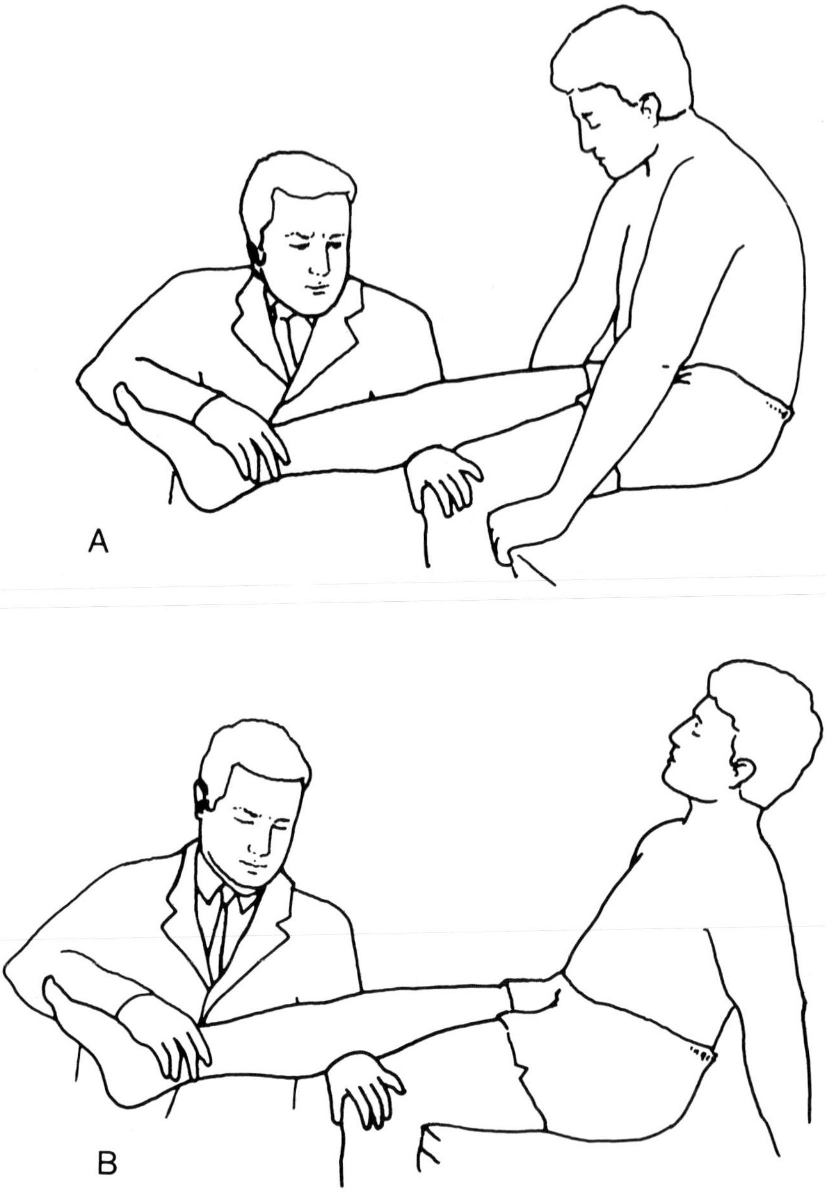

Figure 15.8 *The flip test (staged):* **A.** *Negative. No backward flip on 90 degrees of SLR because there is no root tension.* **B.** *Positive. Physical root tension (SLR test) causes patient to flip posteriorly when straight leg is raised.*

Crossover Pain (Well-Leg Raising Sign) There is some confusion as to what constitutes a positive crossed straight leg raising test.(102) Some have stated that a positive crossed SLR test occurs when you lift the symptomatic leg and produce pain in the asymptomatic leg. Historically, the original description of crossover pain was the reverse; that is, when lifting the well leg, pain crosses over into the symptomatic hip. Most people would agree that a positive crossed straight leg raising test occurs when the well leg is lifted and the opposite symptomatic side becomes more painful. This is indicative of a disc herniation lying medial to the nerve root, either in the axilla of the nerve root or in a midline position.

A variation in the crossover pain test is the sitting SLR test. If in the sitting position, SLR of the well leg crosses pain over to the symptomatic hip, this is pathognomonic of an HNP. This test is valuable in assessing a patient with combined organic and nonorganic features. It is of value in assessing patients with acute back conditions who have significant back pain in the supine position on straight leg raising tests. Some of them may be able to sit, and it is in this position that SLR testing can be done, with crossover pain being an early sign of an HNP, and the absence of SLR reduction or crossover pain indicating acute back muscle strain only.

Nonorganic Pain If the patient complains of severe sciatic pain when attempting to bend forward, and there is a suspicion that there may be a significant degree of functional overlay, the patient should be asked to kneel on a chair. This will relax the hamstrings and reduce the tension of the sciatic nerve. In this position, the patient is asked to bend forward. With a physiogenic source of pain, the patient will be able to bend the spine and let his/her fingertips go below the level of the seat. In the nonorganic pain phenomenon, even with the knees flexed and the patient kneeling on a chair, he/she will not allow the spine to bend (Fig. 15.9).

Nerve root pain is probably the result of a combination of pressure and an inflammatory response to the prolapsed disc material. This "inflammatory response," or "radiculitis," has been loosely termed "root irritation." Root irritation is an important factor in the demonstrated limitation of straight leg raising, and it would appear to be productive of peripheral muscle tenderness. Such tenderness is not always present, but, if demonstrable, it

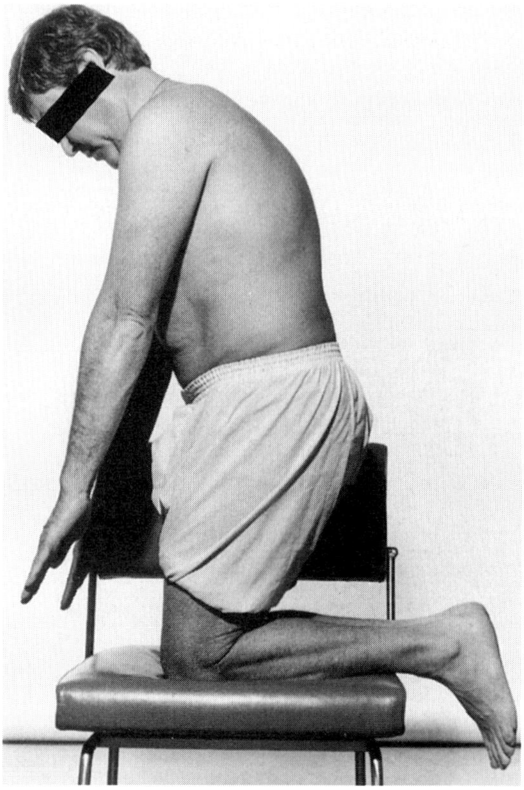

Figure 15.9 *Nonorganic reaction. The patient will not permit any flexion of spine in spite of relaxation of hamstrings.*

is of value in localizing the level of root involvement.(22, 87) Frequently, the calf is tender with S1 root lesions, the anterior tibial compartment is tender with L5 root involvement, and the quadriceps is tender when the 4th lumbar nerve root has been compromised.

The shin is the body image of the leg, and very marked tenderness on palpating the subcutaneous surface of the tibia should warn the clinician that the patient has a large emotional content in this total disability. In the psychogenic regional pain syndromes (Chapter 12), the patient frequently presents skin tenderness with pain on merely pinching the skin. Obviously, no meaningful statement can be made about the presence of deep muscle tenderness unless skin tenderness has been tested first. This is a trap for the unwary.

It should be noted that the upper quadrant of the buttock is a tender area in most people, with or without backache, and this area becomes increasingly tender in the presence of root irritation at any segment. The demonstration of this tenderness is of no localizing value. Patients with discogenic back pain with root irritation may also present tenderness over the sacroiliac joints and down the course of the sciatic nerve. This referred tenderness over the sacroiliac joint has given rise to confusion in the past, which results in the diagnosis of "sacroiliac strain" without any other clinical or radiological evidence of damage to the sacroiliac joint.

Femoral Nerve Stretch Figure 15.10 shows the femoral nerve stretch test. It is not nearly as satisfactory a test as is the SLR test, but is considered positive when unilateral thigh pain is produced and aggravated by knee flexion,(14) and it indicates tension on the 2nd, 3rd, or 4th lumbar roots. It is difficult to interpret in the presence of hip and/or knee pathology.

Impairment of Root Conduction (Root Compression) The diagnosis of disc rupture is in no way exclusively dependent on the demonstration of root impairment as reflected by signs of motor weakness, changes in sensory appreciation, or reflex activity. However, the presence of such changes reinforces the diagnosis.(29, 88) The common neurological changes are documented in Table 15.1.

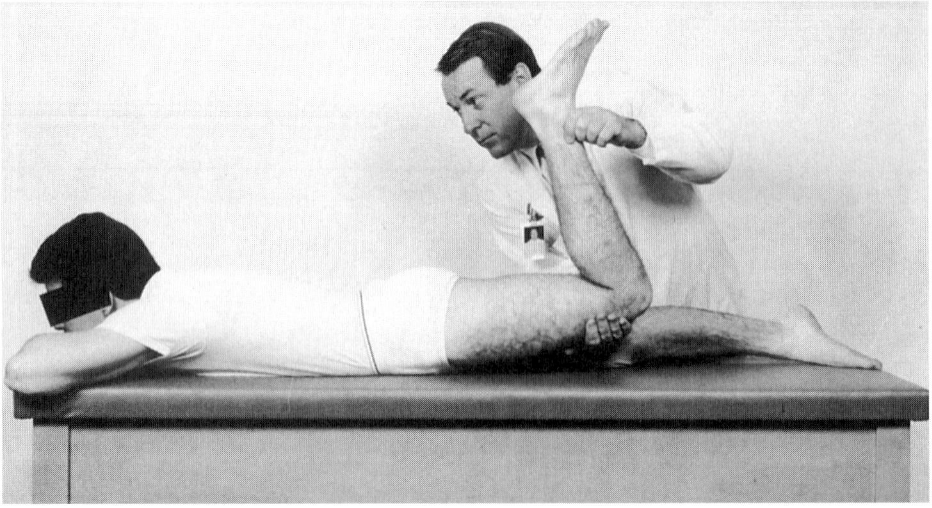

Figure 15.10 *The femoral nerve stretch test.*

Table 15.1. Common Neurological Changes in HNP

	Root		
	L4	L5	S1
Change			
Motor weakness	Knee extension, ankle dorsiflexion	Ankle[a] dorsiflexion EHL	Ankle plantar flexion FHL
Sensory loss	Medial shin below knee	Dorsum of foot and lateral calf	Lateral border of foot and posterior calf
Reflex depression	Knee	Tibialis posterior, lateral hamstrings	Ankle
Wasting	Thigh (no calf)	Calf (minimal thigh)	Calf (no thigh)

Key: EHL, extensor hallucis longus; FHL, flexor hallucis longus.
[a]To separate peroneal nerve palsy from L5 root, examine tibialis posterior (inversion/plantar flexion), which will be weak in latter and not in former.

Changes in Reflex Activity The ankle jerk may be diminished or absent with an S1 lesion. This is tested with the patient kneeling on a chair or sitting comfortably. If a patient's sciatica is so bad that he/she cannot sit with comfort, do not test any reflex in the sitting position, as the subconscious guarding and posturing required of the patient to become less uncomfortable will upset the assessment of reflexes. This guarding and posturing explains the occasional depression of a knee reflex seen in the presence of sciatica due to an L5–S1 disc protrusion. If the patient has suffered from a previous attack of sciatic pain with significant compression of the 1st sacral nerve to obliterate the ankle jerk, this may not return to normal. The absence of an ankle jerk, therefore, may merely be a stigma of a previous episode of disc rupture, and the present attack may be due to a disc rupture at another level. Scratching the sole of the foot, as in the plantar response, produces a reflex contraction of the tensor fascia femoris. This little known reflex is often lost with an S1 lesion.

With an L5 root compression, the tibialis posterior reflex (obtained by striking the tendon of the tibialis posterior near its point of insertion) may be absent. This is a pure L5 response. The clinician has to practice obtaining this reflex because it is not easy to elicit. Diminution of the lateral hamstring jerk is also seen on occasion with an L5 root compromise, but multiple innervation of this muscle group makes this an unreliable reflex. With L4 and L3 lesions, the knee jerk may be diminished.

Wasting Muscle wasting is rarely seen unless the symptoms have been present for more than 3 weeks. Very marked wasting is more suggestive of an extradural tumor than a disc rupture.

The girths of the thigh and calf should always be measured. This will act as a baseline, on occasion, to assess the progress of the lesion. It must be remembered that if there is gross weakness of the gastrocnemius, the main venous pump of the affected extremity is no longer working, and these patients may, indeed, show some measure of ankle edema. The combination of calf tenderness due to S1 root irritation and the observation of a swollen ankle may give rise to the erroneous diagnosis of a thrombophlebitis.

Motor Loss The weakness of the gastrocnemii is best demonstrated by getting the patient to rise on tiptoe five or six times (Fig. 15.11). The patient is asked if it requires more effort to rise on tiptoe on the affected extremity. If the quadriceps are weak, the physician must be wary of this before ascribing the difficulty of tiptoe rising to weakness of the calf muscles. If sciatic pain is severe, the test cannot be performed by the patient. Jumping on tiptoe may be painful, and it is not a good method of examination, although slight weakness may be assessed by asking the patient to walk backward and forward across the length of the examining room on tiptoes to find out whether the gastrocnemii tire more easily.

The power of ankle dorsiflexion is best tested by applying your full body weight to the dorsiflexed ankle (Fig 15.11). Testing the dorsiflexor by asking the patient to walk on his/her heels will only demonstrate marked weakness in this muscle group. Weakness of the flexor hallucis longus (S1) or weakness of the extensor hallucis longus (L5) is often the first evidence of motor involvement. The evertors of the foot may be weak with an L5 lesion. The gluteus maximus may become weak with lesions involving the 1st sacral nerve root, and this weakness may be demonstrated by the sagging of one buttock crease when the patient stands (Fig. 15.12). Weakness of the gluteus medius is seen with an L5 lesion and occasionally is marked enough to produce a Trendelenburg's lurch, particularly noticeable when the patient is tired. When the gluteus medius is involved, there is frequently marked tenderness on pressure over the muscle near its point of insertion, and this may be confused with a trochanteric bursitis or with gluteal tendinitis.

Quadriceps weakness is seen with an L4 and L3 lesion and can be assessed by the examiner placing his arm under the patient's knee and asking the patient to extend the knee against the resistance of the examiner's hand. However, this maneuver may produce pain, and a false impression of weakness is obtained. In such instances, it is better to have

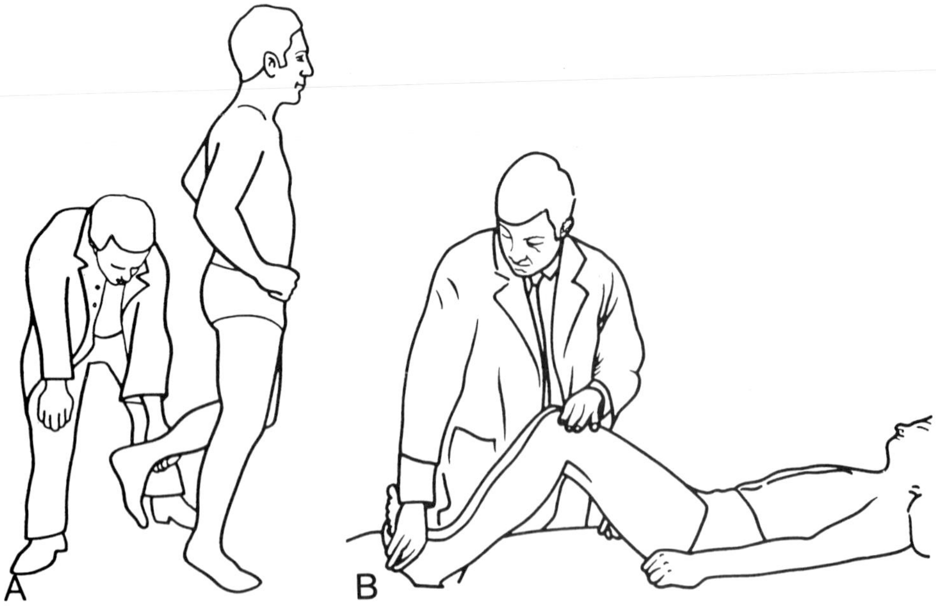

Figure 15.11 **A.** *It is important to recognize the fact that when trying to assess the strength of the gastrocnemius by asking the patient to rise on tiptoe, this action must be carried out repetitively and rapidly. The examiner is really attempting to assess fatigability of the muscle.* **B.** *Ankle dorsiflexion (L4 and L5 roots) is best tested in this position of comfort.*

the patient lying face downward and flexing his/her knees to 90 degrees and then assessing the power to fully extend the knee from this position (Fig. 15.13).

Sensory Impairment The regions of sensory loss are reasonably constant (Fig. 15.14). Within each dermatome, there appear to be areas more vulnerable to sensory loss that others. Loss of appreciation of pinprick is first noted in an S1 lesion below and behind the lateral malleolus and in an L5 lesion in the cleft between the first and second toes. Sensory appreciation is a subjective response and, as such, may at times be difficult to assess. Certain precautions must be followed. Sensibility varies in different parts of the limb. Identical areas in each limb must be tested consecutively. The examination must be carried out as expeditiously as compatible with accuracy, because the patient will soon tire of this form of examination, and answers may not be accurate. When the skin is pricked with a pin, the physiological principle of recruitment is present. The overall sensory appreciation is dependent then, not only on the action of the pinprick, but also on the number of pinpricks experienced.

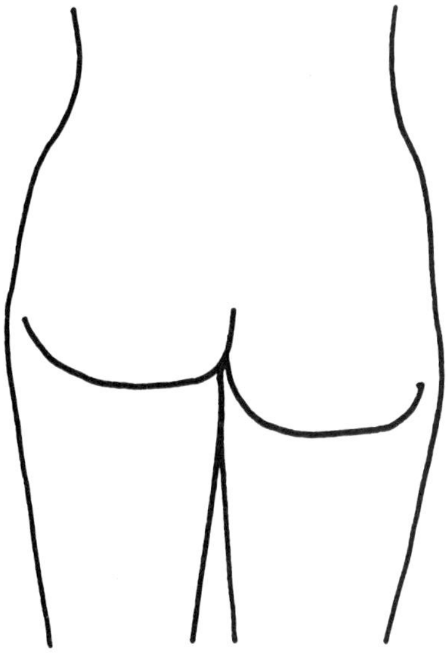

Figure 15.12 *The gluteus maximus is supplied mostly by S1. Lesions involving the first sacral root may cause weakness of the gluteus maximus, which is apparent on examination by the sagging of one buttock crease.*

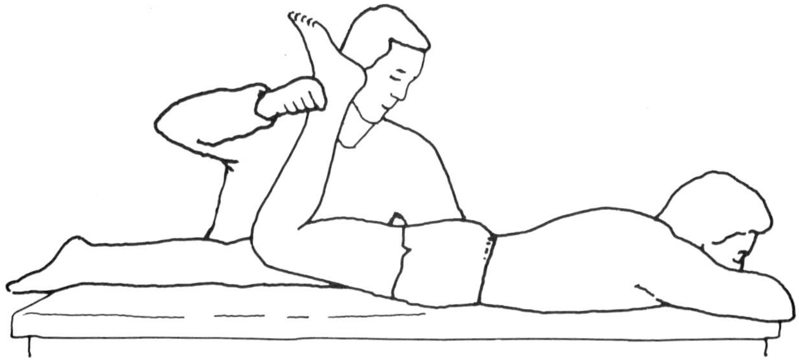

Figure 15.13 *Prone position for testing quadriceps strength.*

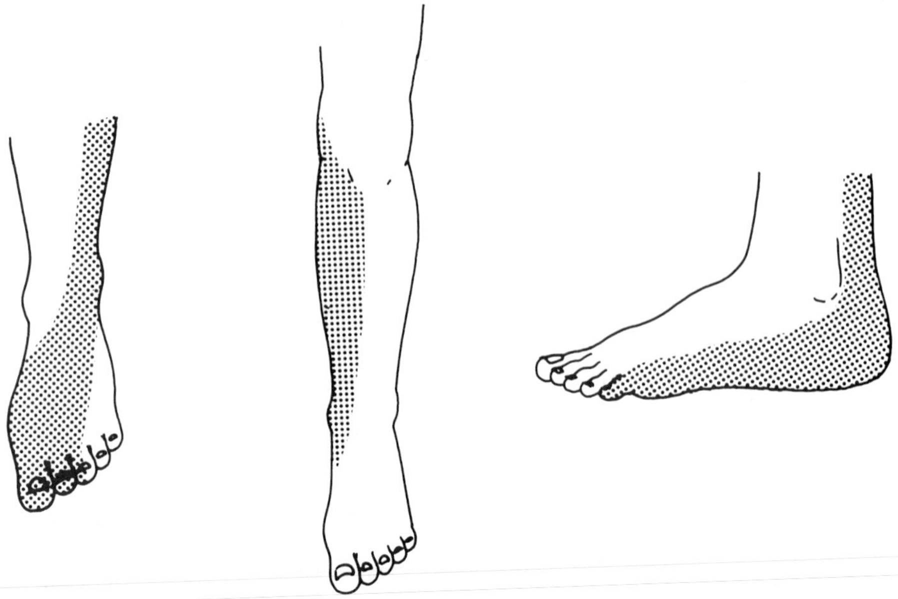

Figure 15.14 *The dermatomal areas supplied by each root where a sensory loss may be detected (left, L5; middle, L4; right, S1).*

A sensory examination is only interpreted as positive for a radicular lesion when the sensory loss approximates one dermatomal distribution, and the loss is not present in the adjacent ipsilateral dermatomes or the same contralateral dermatome.

Age Difference in the Presentation of a "Disc Rupture Causing the Acute Radicular Syndrome"

Throughout this discussion we have often referred to the different types of presentation for the acute radicular syndrome in young patients. In fact, the acute radicular syndrome from a disc rupture tends to have a characteristic presentation in the three age groups as outlined in Table 15.2.

High Lumbar Root Lesions

Higher lumbar root lesions (ie, L2, L3, L4) are a different breed (2, 24)! First lumbar root lesions also occur, but they are extremely rare. High lumbar root lesions are frequently missed, so let us try to prevent this by drawing all the historical and physical features together in point form.

1. High lumbar root lesions are almost always due to a disc herniation and rarely are caused by bony encroachment. Therefore, they present as an acute, rather than chronic, radicular syndrome.
2. They are difficult to diagnose because they are rare (5% of disc ruptures) and carry with them a significant differential diagnostic challenge. The most common condi-

tion confused with a high lumbar root lesion from a disc herniation is a diabetic femoral neuropathy.(9, 27)

3. These disc ruptures/root lesions usually occur in the older patient population (50 + years).
4. They are extremely painful, producing severe discomfort in the anterior thigh. The patients usually volunteer that they have so much pain that they are unable to sleep at night.
5. They almost all have a very positive femoral nerve stretch test (see Fig. 15.10).
6. They almost always have neurological changes (Table 15.3).
7. The best clinical clue as to the root involved usually comes from a very careful sensory history and sensory physical examination.
8. The lesions are very resistant to conservative care and are more likely to require surgical intervention.
9. At least 50% of high lumbar disc herniations occur in the foramen (51) and may be missed by the radiologist (Fig. 15.15).

Table 15.2. Clinical Picture of Sciatica in Different Age Groups

Symptom	Adolescent (<25 years)	Adult (30–50 years)	Senior Adult (55–80 years)
Pain	Typical radicular pattern, may not be below knee	Typical radicular pattern, almost always below knee	Typical radicular pattern, most severe below the knee
Paresthesia	50% chance of being present	Common	Most common
SLR reduction	Profound	Less than 50% of normal	Most often > 50% of normal
Neurological signs	> 50% chance of being absent	> 50% chance of being present	Most often present
Associated degenerative changes (spinal stenosis)	Rare	Occasional	Common
Response to conservative care	Recurrence rate of symptoms very high	Good response to conservative care	Limited tolerance for prolonged care
Protrusion/ extrusion	Protrusions very common	Protrusions less common	Protrusions rare

Table 15.3. Neurological Changes in High Lumbar Disc Ruptures

	L2	L3	L4
Motor weakness	Hip flexors[a]	Knee extensors[a]	Knee extensors[a]
Sensory loss	Lateral thigh	Patellar region	Medial shin
Reflex depression	0	Knee	Knee
Wasting	Thigh (minor)	Thigh	Thigh

[a]To separate pure femoral neuropathy (eg, diabetes) from root lesion, examine hip abductors, which are spared in the former and weakened in the latter.

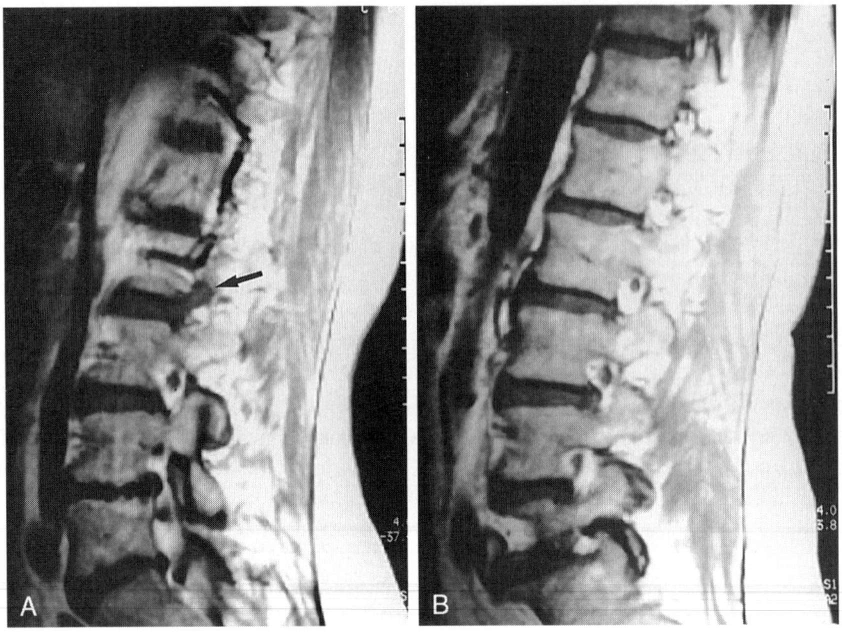

Figure 15.15 **A.** *An L2 foraminal disc (arrow) that would be easily missed on MRI. Compare the foramen on the opposite side* **(B).**

The Cauda Equina Syndrome

This is the third time that you have met the cauda equina syndrome (if you have been brave enough to read the book from the beginning!). The syndrome is a true spine surgical emergency that is often missed.(21, 59) The reason it is missed or there is a delay in diagnosis is that it is such a rare occurrence (less than four cases per year in a busy spine surgery practice), and the much more common presentation of a disc rupture causing sciatica is never an emergency. There is considerable evidence supporting immediate surgical intervention as the best way to relieve the syndrome. A delay in diagnosis with a poor outcome is often cause for a malpractice suit against everyone who missed the diagnosis.

The presentation is fairly classic. The patient usually has a prodromal stage of back pain and some leg symptoms. The leg symptoms are rarely severe in the prodrome, and it is rare that they have led to much in the way of treatment or even a magnetic resonance image (MRI). Without much in the way of intervening trauma, there is a dramatic increase in back pain and the occurrence of bilateral leg pain and perineal numbness. The numbness usually extends to the penis in men. The patient then notices an inability to void because of the paralysis of the S2, 3, and 4 roots in the cauda equina.

The condition is usually caused by a massive midline disc sequestration into the spinal canal, usually at L4–L5 but also at L5–S1 and L3–L4.(28) Higher disc ruptures are a rare cause of this syndrome.

If you are seeing the patient early in the presentation there will be marked reduction in SLR; numbness to pinprick in the perineal region (S2, 3, 4 dermatomes); and weakness corresponding to the level of the disc rupture. Reflexes will usually be depressed (eg, bilateral ankle reflex depression with either an L4–L5 or L5–S1 sequestered disc). The bladder will be full to palpation/percussion, and any passage of urine will be due to involuntary overflow incontinence. It is essential to do a rectal examination, at which time decreased tone in the external sphincter will be noted.

It is best to consider a cauda equina syndrome an all or nothing diagnosis, (ie, there is no such thing as a partial cauda equina syndrome that can wait until morning for reassessment). If there is any suspicion at all that bladder and bowel function are impaired, in a back pain patient, an immediate diagnostic study is indicated.(15, 69, 70) Our choice is for an emergency MRI (Fig. 15.16)

Double Root Involvement

Exclusive of the cauda equina syndrome, most patients you see with the acute radicular syndrome have single root involvement. The reason is obvious: most symptomatic disc herniations are single-level lesions. In fact, if you are reading an article on anything to do with disc ruptures, especially surgical treatment, and you see a high incidence of two level disc involvement (over 10%), you know the author has lost his/her way!

But double root involvement does occur in the occasional patient. Figure 15.17 shows how this occurs:

1. A disc rupture that migrates medially (usually L4–L5) so that L5 and S1 root impairment is evident on physical examination (see Fig. 15.17).
2. Any disc rupture that migrates cephalad and laterally. At the L5–S1 level, this would present as S1 and L5 root involvement, and an L4–L5 disc, migrating in this fashion, would present as L5 and L4 root involvement (Fig. 15.17).
3. A disc rupture that migrates cephalad and medially (Fig. 15.17).
4. A foraminal L4 disc rupture may present clinically as an apparent L4 and L5 root

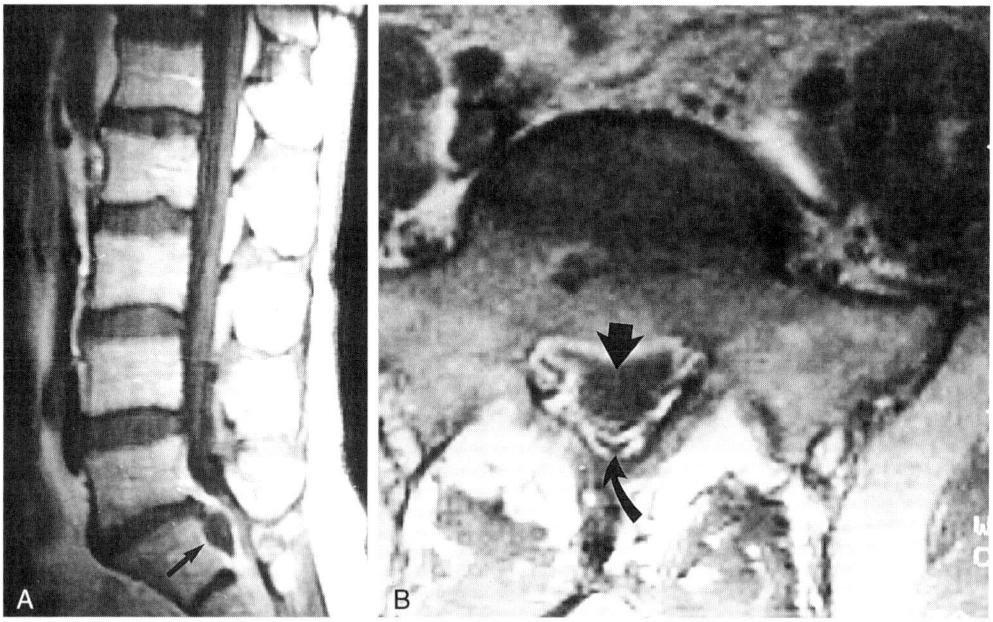

Figure 15.16 **A.** *Sagittal T_1 MRI with a large HNP at L5–S1 causing complete obliteration of thecal sac (arrow).* **B.** *Axial T_1 MRI showing the large HNP (big arrow) and the thinned residual of a common dural sac (curved arrow).*

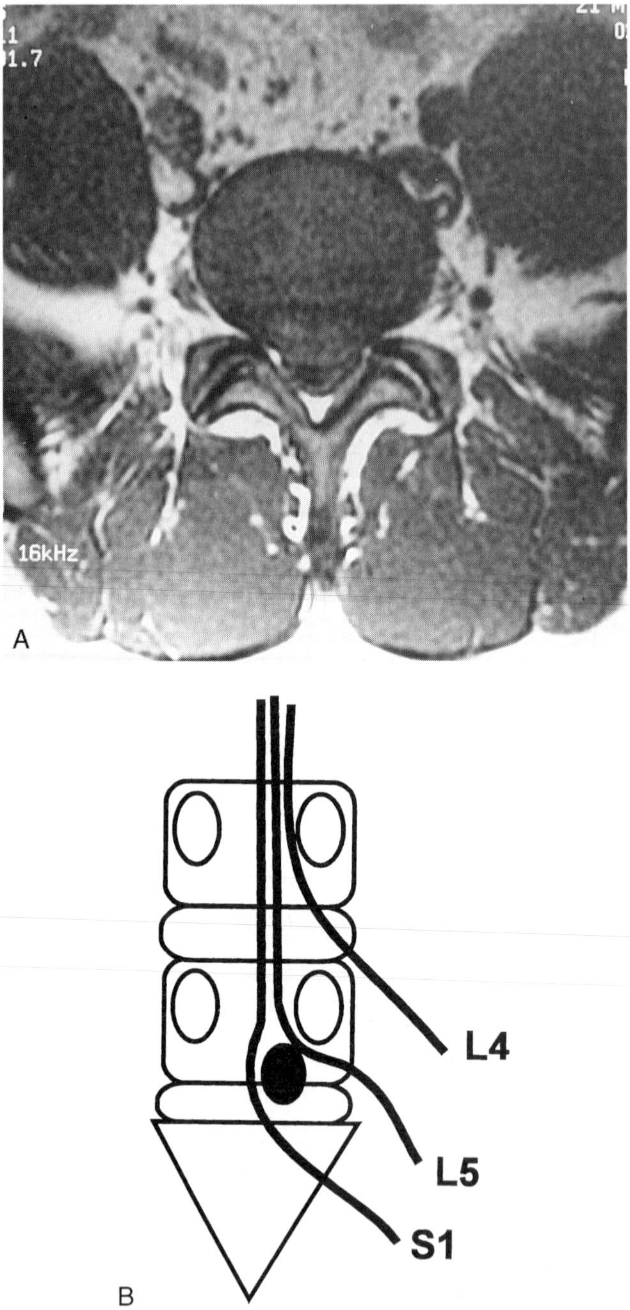

Figure 15.17 **A.** *Medial migration of a disc rupture at L4–L5; the patient had L5 and S1 root symptoms.* **B.** *Cephalad migration of an L5–S1 disc rupture on schematic impacting on the L5 and S1 roots.*

involvement because of the furcal nerve. This will be discussed in greater detail in the next chapter.

5. A rare double disc herniation.
6. A conjoined nerve root (Fig. 15.17) (62).

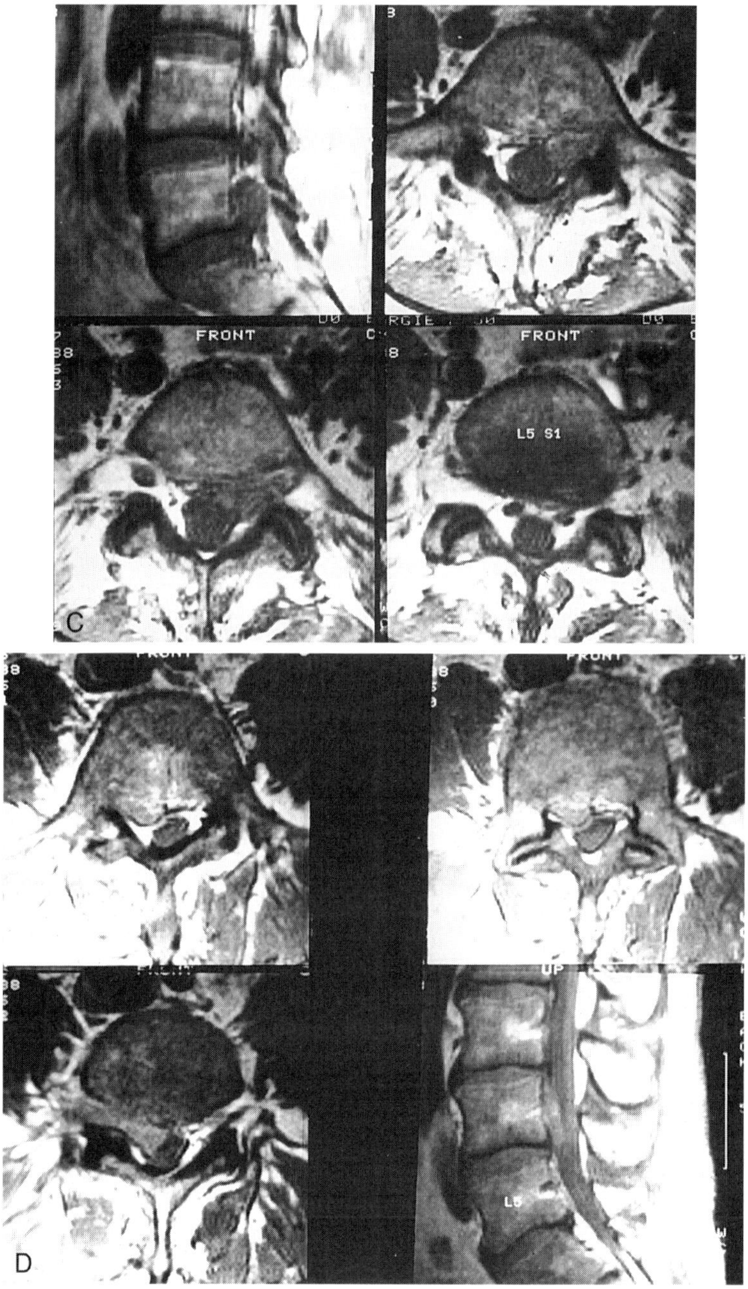

Figure 15.17 (continued) **C.** *An MRI of schematic in* **B. D.** *Cephalad and medial migration of a disc rupture at L4–L5 presenting as L4 and L5 root involvement.*

Remember one important rule about double root involvement: the densest neurological lesion determines the disc rupture level; for example, in Figure 15.17, the double root lesion was L5 and S1; the greater neurological lesion was S1 (the lesser, L5); thus, the HNP had to be L5–S1.

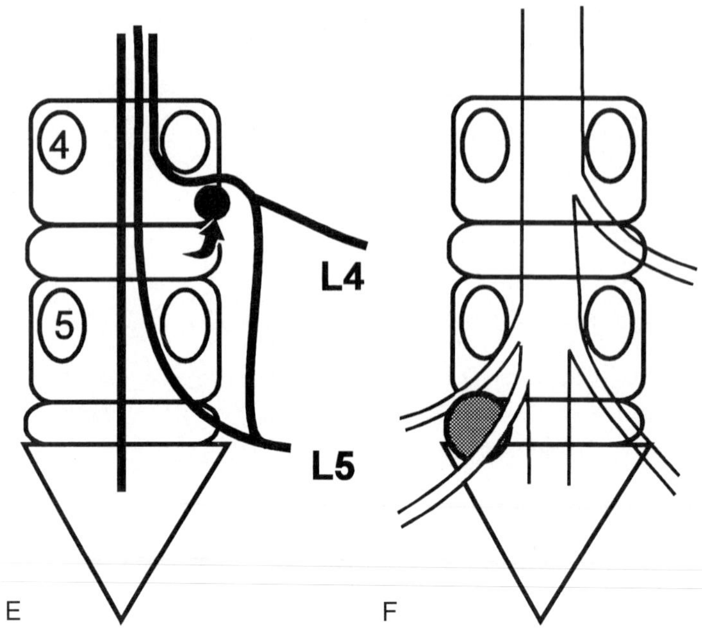

Figure 15.17 (continued) **E.** *A foraminal disc herniation impacts on the 4th root before the takeoff of the furcal nerve.* **F.** *A conjoint nerve root, when compressed, can present as a double root lesion, L5 and S1 in this schematic.*

Conclusion

There is nothing more constant in degenerative conditions of the lumbar spine than the many faces of presentation in a ruptured disc.(29) Although there is a multiplicity of clinical presentations, there is a common thread of: some degree of back pain, the dominance of leg pain, the significant root tension and irritation findings, and the variability in neurological findings. Recognizing these variations, and yet their constancy, allows one to be fairly accurate with a clinical diagnosis.(1) In fact, the patient with classical sciatica due to a disc rupture is one of the most obvious diagnoses in degenerative conditions of the lumbar spine and often can be made within a few moments of talking to the patient (Table 15.4). From an understanding of the patient with sciatica due to a disc rupture flows an understanding of patients with lateral zone stenosis, central canal stenosis, and the more elusive mechanical low back pain conditions with referred leg pain.

CONSERVATIVE TREATMENT

Once the clinical diagnosis of an acute radicular syndrome is made, a treatment regimen has to be designed to fit the patient's degree of disability and life-style. This can usually be done before extensive, expensive investigation, such as MRI or computed tomography (CT) scan. As mentioned in chapter 11 on Investigation, the acute radicular syndrome due to a disc rupture is a diagnosis based on history and physical examination. Only when conservative treatment has failed and surgery is being considered should an

Table 15.4. Criteria for the Diagnosis of the Acute Radicular Syndrome (Sciatica Due to an HNP)

1. Leg pain (including buttock) is the dominant complaint when compared with back pain.
2. Neurological symptoms that are specific (eg, paresthesia in a typical dermatomal distribution).
3. Significant SLR changes
   - SLR less than 50% of normal
   - Bowstring discomfort
   - Crossover pain

   } any one or a combination of these
4. Neurological signs: weakness, wasting, sensory loss, or reflex alteration (at least two of four).

[a]Three of four of these criteria must be present, the only exception being young patients who are very resistant to the effects of nerve root compression and thus may not have neurological symptoms (criteria 2) nor signs (criteria 4).

MRI be ordered. An MRI can also mislead you, showing multiple changes such as disc space narrowing and annular bulging at many levels that are all clinically insignificant.(4) A disc rupture causing sciatica is not a "blip" on MRI; it is a patient with lots of leg pain and positive physical findings.

Almost every episode of sciatica can be made better with conservative treatment.(46) At issue is:

1. How long will conservative care take relative to the demands of daily living?
2. What residual neurological deficit will be left (16)?
3. What if conservative treatment does not relieve the pain (3)?

Conservative treatment for an HNP is no different than for that for degenerative disc disease (DDD), the cornerstone being rest and time with appropriate medication support. The use of other treatment modalities are questionable in their effect. When conservative treatment fails, surgery is indicated.

Treatment obviously varies according to the severity of the root compression and can best be considered under the following clinical syndromes: aggravating leg pain and incapacitating leg pain.

Aggravating Leg Pain

These are patients, who after certain activities, develop a dull, nagging sciatic pain that slows them down. The patients learn to recognize that if they do certain things, their sciatica will flare up; they may have to give up playing golf or tennis, and they may markedly modify their work activities. Their pain is never sufficiently severe to stop them from getting on with their daily rounds, but it "bugs" them.

Theoretically, the best way to heal the underlying pathology would be to take all of the mechanical loading off the spine by putting the patient to bed for a number of days. However, the physician is treating a patient, not a spine, and, with the type of symptoms presented, it would be unreasonable to expect the patient to follow this sort of advice. The same principles, therefore, must be followed as in the treatment of chronic symptomatic degenerative disc disease.

Unloading the Spine

The following measures must be undertaken to take weight off the spine:

1. Loss of weight where indicated.
2. Modification of work and play activities: the flexion routine.
3. Increase of intra-abdominal pressure, temporarily by a corset, and permanently by building up the strength of the abdominal muscles. In thin patients, the corset will not be of much value unless it is padded well in front to add direct pressure on the abdomen. Some of these patients are better treated with a thoracopelvic brace to protect the spine against unexpected jars and strains.
4. Physical rest until the pain starts to abate. The patient should spend evenings in bed.

Anti-Inflammatory Drugs

The sciatic pain is due in part to a perineural inflammatory response to the protruded disc material. In many instances, this inflammatory change can be decreased by anti-inflammatory drugs, with aspirin being the best and cheapest.

Analgesics

As in all chronic pain problems, analgesics must be given on a time-dependent basis, not on demand.

Course

The majority of patients get better in approximately 6 weeks. In a few, however, the pain persists to a degree that demands further attention. Before considering surgical intervention, two alternative methods of treatment can be considered: infiltration of the nerve root sleeve under radiographic control with hydrocortisone, or enzymatic dissolution of the disc by the intradiscal injection of chymopapain (discussed later in this chapter).

Incapacitating Leg Pain

When the pain is incapacitating in severity, the patient must go to bed. The patient is allowed to move around in bed and assume whatever position is most comfortable. He/she may get up to use the toilet, using crutches if walking is difficult. After 48 hours of bed rest, many patients are relatively comfortable apart from sudden movements.

The patient should stay in bed until he/she has been relatively comfortable for 48 hours—except for the occasional journey to the toilet. How long should the physician persist with bed rest as a form of therapy? Many years ago, when the herniated disc was first described, physicians routinely demanded 6 weeks of complete bed rest. However, we must remember that 6 weeks in bed without any guarantee of recovery will be disastrous, not only to muscle mass and calcium balance, but also to the pocketbook. Most experts would agree that the maximal time in bed that a surgeon can demand from a patient who has shown no improvement whatsoever is 2 to 3 days.(46) If a patient has shown no improvement in both sciatic pain and SLR ability, it is unlikely that further bed rest will make a lasting difference. If a patient does not get better with time and conservative treatment, consideration must be given to operative intervention.

Exercise

Patients with the acute radicular syndromes should all go on the McKenzie exercise routine (see Fig. 13.7). This was discussed fully in Chapter 13 on conservative treatment.

Medication

Obviously, anti-inflammatory, analgesic, and, on some rare occasions, muscle relaxant medication, will help the patient comply with the prescription for bed rest.

Epidural Steroids

As discussed in Chapter 13 on conservative treatment, there has been no scientific support for the use of epidural steroids in the treatment of an acute disc rupture.(3) Occasionally, a situation presents where more aggressive treatment is indicated, but circumstances prohibit such a step. These include a pregnant woman with sciatica, a student heading into a few weeks of examinations, an elderly patient who wishes to avoid surgery, and a key athlete entering into a key game. In these situations, epidural cortisone injection might settle symptoms to a tolerable level. Except for pregnancy, epidural cortisone injection should probably be preceded by a 5-day course of oral steroids (eg, prednisone in a decreasing dose), provided there are no contraindications. It is likely that epidural injections of cortisone will offer short-term relief, with recurrence of symptoms probable, and a more definitive surgical decision will be required.

Miscellaneous Forms of Treatment

Traction Used as a method of holding the patient to the bed, traction is useful; used as a method to distract the disc, create negative pressure, and thus suck the ruptured disc back into place, it is useless.

Manipulation It is unwise to forcibly manipulate the spine of a patient with a disc rupture for fear of further disc displacement and more compromise of neurological tissue.

Investigation of the Patient with a Disc Rupture

Chapter 11 presented an in-depth discussion on investigation of patients with low back pain. Let us review some of the salient points relative to low back pain patients with a disc rupture.

1. Boden et al(4) have clearly established the fact that asymptomatic individuals can have MRI and CT scans showing abnormalities (including disc ruptures). To further confuse the issus, many authors have shown that patients with MRI/CT documented disc herniations causing sciatica, who lose their sciatic symptoms with conservative or surgical intervention, often have persistent defects shown on posttreatment scans that are little different from the pretreatment scans. Remember, what you see on MRI or CT scanning may not explain the patient's symptoms.
2. The diagnosis of a disc rupture causing sciatica is a clinical diagnosis. It is made after a history and physical examination and before expensive testing such as MR

imaging. Only when a patient fails to respond to conservative care or presents with severe neurological compromise is it time to start investigating.

3. The investigation of choice for any patient suspected of having a disc rupture and who has failed to respond to conservative care is an MRI. The advantages of MRI over myelography, CT/myelography, CT/discography, electromyelography, and thermography (Table 15.5) are so great that the discussion only flourishes in those jurisdictions that do not have MRI readily available (Fig. 15.18).
4. For an MRI to be interpreted as positive for a ruptured disc, it has to show a focal disc protrusion (see Fig. 15.18) and not a diffuse annular bulge. The focal disc protrusion must be at a level and side that fits the patient's neurology.
5. Remember the classification of disc ruptures—contained versus non-contained (Fig. 15.19).

Table 15.5. Advantages of MRI in the Investigation of a Patient with a Ruptured Disc

Tissue chemistry (with T1, T2 weighted images) is clearly demonstrated.
Two images, at right angles, are available (sagittal and axial).
The conus is viewed on sagittal cuts.
The foramina are more readily examined.
Greater tissue contrast sensitivity helps with the differential diagnosis of infection, tumor, and scarring.
Gadolinum enhancement adds a whole new dimension not available in other investigations.

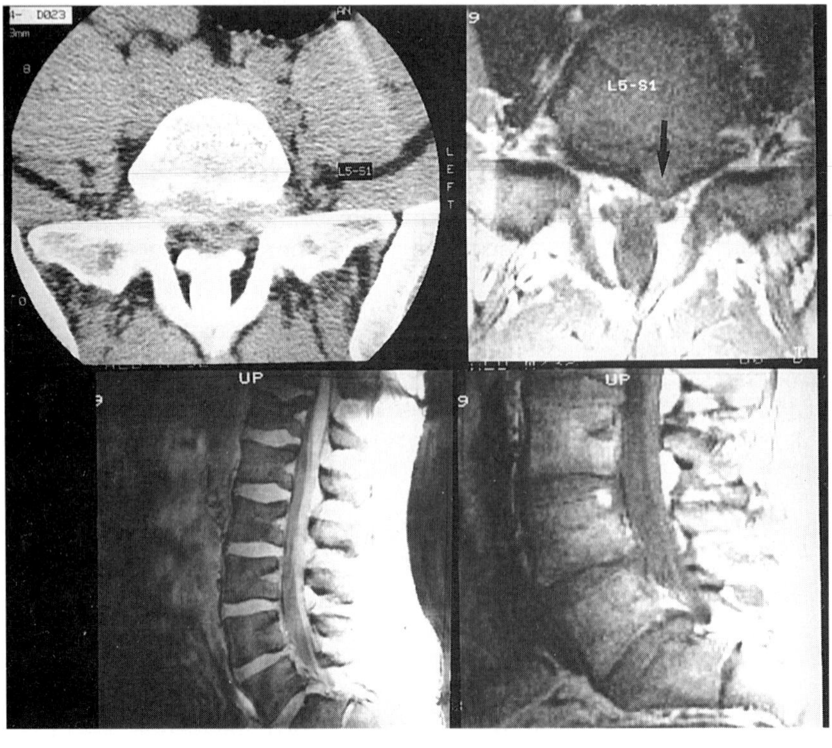

Figure 15.18 *A focal disc protrusion on MRI (T_1) arrow was present on CT (upper left) but was much more obvious on the sagittal (bottom) and axial MRI.*

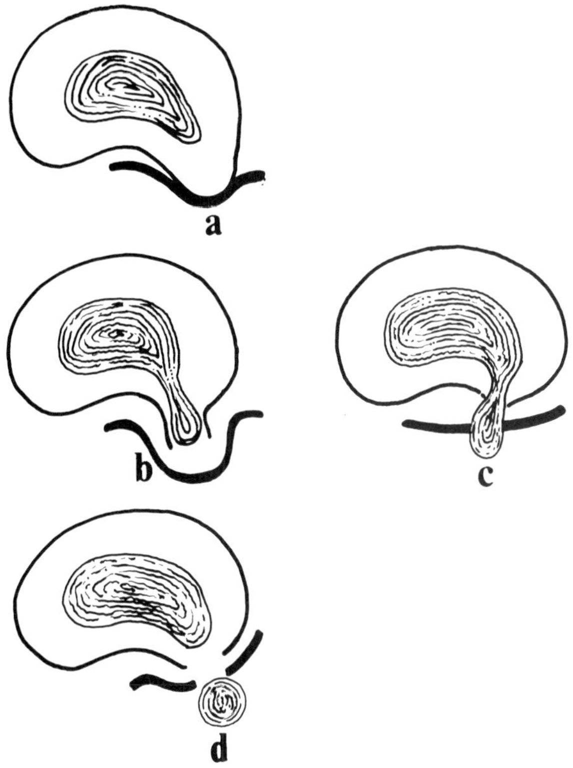

Figure 15.19 *Classification of disc ruptures: contained versus non-contained.* **(a)** *contained protrusion;* **(b)** *contained extrusion(subannular);* **(c)** *non-contained extrusion (transannular);* **(d)** *non-contained sequestration.*

6. Viewing of the sagittal cuts will give you a clue as to whether or not a disc is contained or non-contained (Fig. 15.20).
7. Remember that disc herniations can migrate (Fig. 15.21).
8. The differential diagnosis of a mass of material interfering with nerve root territory includes (Fig. 15.22):
   a. An HNP.
   b. An osteophyte (Fig. 15.22, A) (arrow) on CT, with an HNP.
   c. An epidural hematoma or abscess (Fig. 15.22, B).
   d. A neoplasm (neurofibroma) (Fig. 15.22, C).
   e. Meningocele / Tarlov cyst.
   f. Synovial cyst (Fig. 15.22, D)
   g. Scar.

Indications for Surgery

A General Statement

One only has to review the natural history of lumbar disc disease to realize that spinal surgeons play a palliative role in the management of this problem. The most outstanding study on the natural history of lumbar disc disease was done by Weber.(94) He randomly assigned large groups of patients with unequivocal signs of a disc herniation to surgical and nonsurgical groups. Table 15.6 summarizes his results. Weber has shown that, although

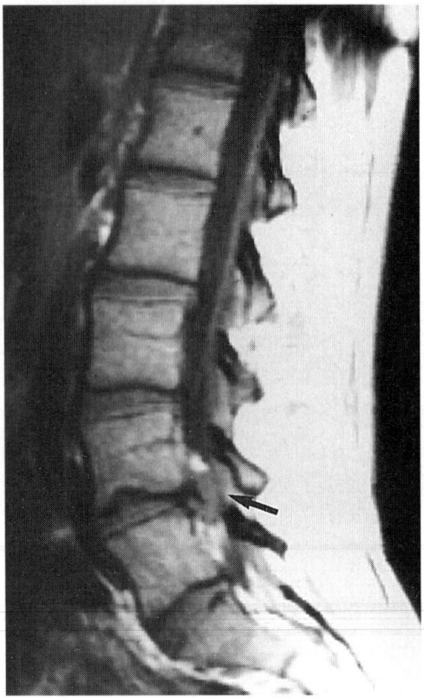

Figure 15.20 *A sagittal (T1) MRI with a fuzzy margin to the disc herniation (arrow) (likely non-contained).*

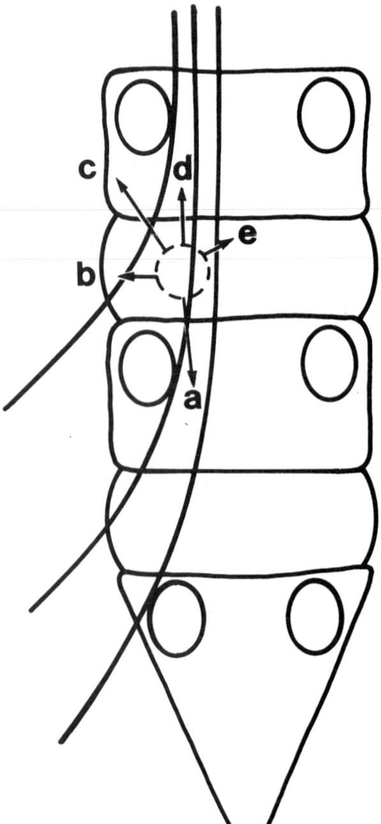

Figure 15.21 *Migratory patterns of disc ruptures.*

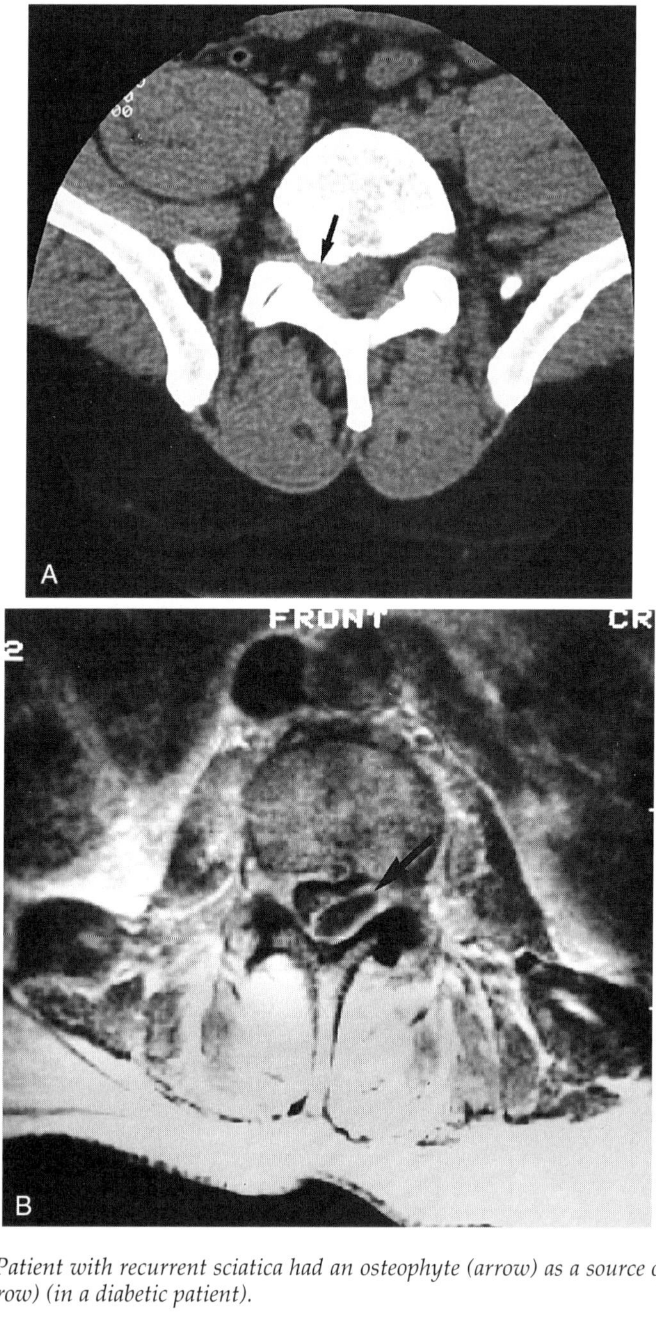

Figure 15.22 **A.** *Patient with recurrent sciatica had an osteophyte (arrow) as a source of symptoms.* **B.** *An epidural abscess (arrow) (in a diabetic patient).*

surgery initially increases the yields of good results, its advantages disappear on longer follow-up.

Hakelius (25) also completed a retrospective study of 583 patients with unilateral sciatica. His results were similar to Weber's in that the surgically treated patients initially had a better result, but by 6 months, there was no difference between the two groups of patients. He did show that on a 7-year follow-up, the conservatively treated group had somewhat more low back pain, more sciatic discomfort, more recurrences, and more lost time from work.

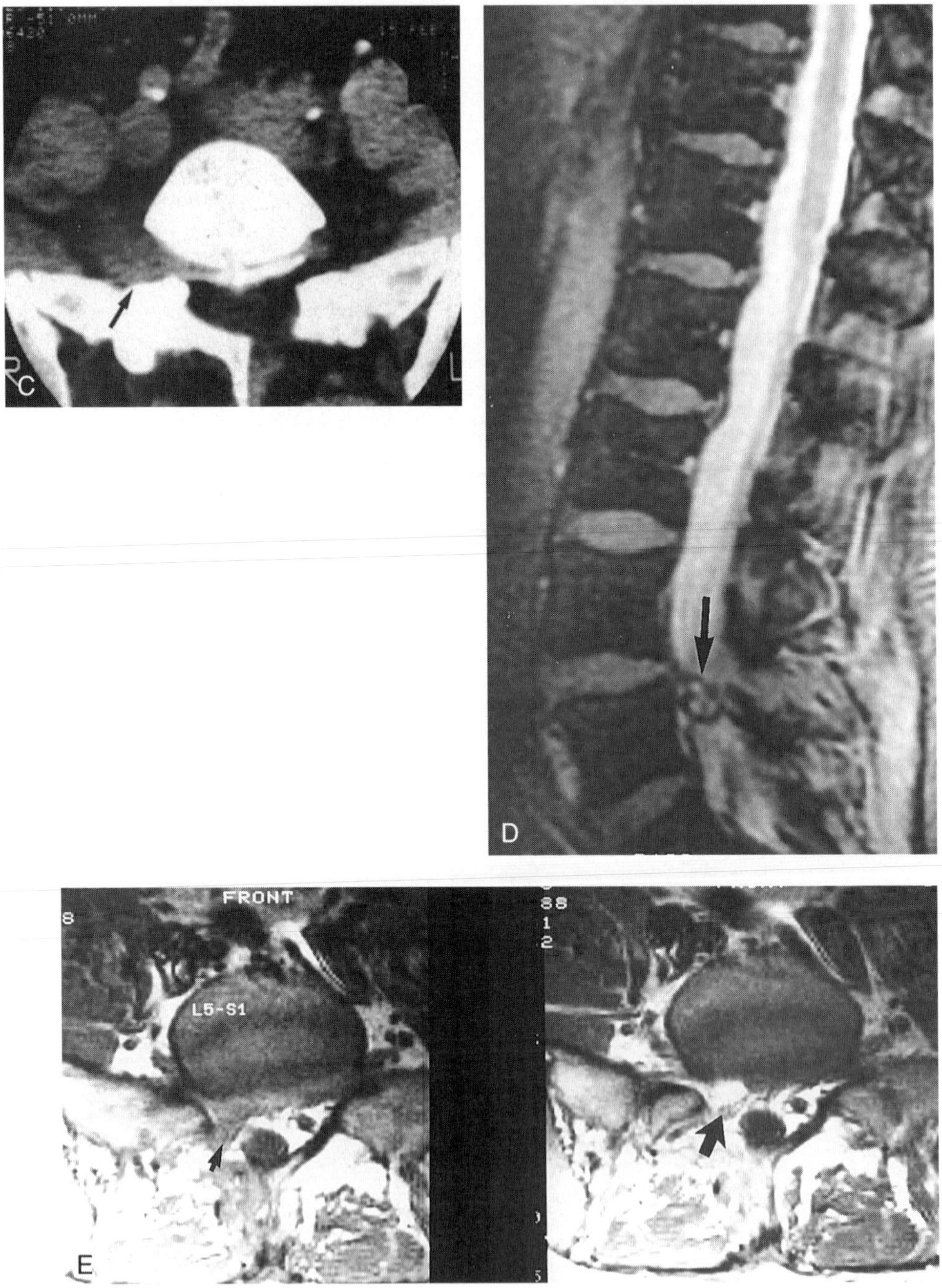

Figure 15.22 (continued) **C.** *Patient presented with right sciatica. The diagnosis: secondary carcinoma (primary lung). Note the bony erosions on the anterior aspect of the facet joint and ala of the sacrum (arrow).* **D.** *A synovial cyst (arrow).* **E.** *Scar on gadolinium-enhanced MRI: what looks like a recurrent disc herniation (left arrow) is all scar with injection of gadolinium (heavy right arrow).*

Table 15.6. Weber's Results of the Treatment of Lumbar Disc Herniation[a]

Year(s) (posttreatment)	Nonsurgical Results	Surgical Results
1	60% better	92% better
4	No statistical difference between the two groups	
10	No difference between 4-year and 10-year follow up	

[a]Data from Weber H. Lumbar disc herniation: a controlled prospective study with 10 years of observation. Spine 1983;8:131–140.

One can only conclude from these and other studies on the natural history of sciatica due to a disc herniation that it is a transient, self-limiting condition. Satisfactory resolution over time is likely to occur, regardless of the method of treatment intervention, be it surgery or conservative treatment. If one is proposing surgical intervention,(76) it becomes essential to prove that surgery carries with it a high rate of initial success with limited risk to the patient and at the least expense possible to the payers for the service.

The following is an enumeration of indications for surgery in HNP:

Absolute Indications

Bladder and Bowel Involvement: The Cauda Equina Syndrome The acute massive disc herniation that causes bladder and bowel paralysis is usually a sequestered disc that requires immediate surgical excision for the best prognosis.(28)

Increasing Neurological Deficit In the face of progressing weakness, it is wise to intervene early with surgical excision of the disc rupture.

Relative Indications

Failure of Conservative Treatment This is the most common reason for surgical intervention in the presence of a herniated nucleus pulposus. Ideal conservative treatment is treatment that occurs during at least 6 weeks and not more than 3 months and results in improvement in the patient's symptoms and signs. During that time, the amount of complete bed rest that should be prescribed is 2 to 3 days. Other conservative measure (3) such as medication (analgesic, anti-inflammatory, muscle relaxant); modalities (heat and cold); and exercises may be used. The key to measuring the success of conservative treatment is not only the patient's relief of pain but also the improvement in straight leg raising ability. If a patient goes to bed with appropriate medication for 2 to 3 days, and there is no improvement in sciatic discomfort or in straight leg raising ability, it is likely that the patient is going to follow a protracted conservative course, and surgical intervention is indicated. It is proposed that surgical intervention in the acute radicular syndrome occur before 3 months of symptoms to try and avoid the chronic pathological changes that can occur within a nerve root.

Recurrent Sciatica Conservative treatment can also fail in that the patient experiences recurrences of the sciatic syndrome. Table 15.7 outlines the use of "recurrences of sciatica" as an indication for surgical intervention.

Significant Neurological Deficit with Significant Straight Leg Raising Reduction This is a relative indication for surgical intervention for an HNP. Again, Weber (94) has shown that these patients eventually recovered just as well with nonsurgical intervention. These patients are in extreme pain and often cannot wait for the benefits of conservative care. On the rare occasion, these patients present with severe pain that has resolved as the neurological deficit has increased; they also should go to surgery when the MRI demonstrates a large HNP.

A Disc Rupture into a Stenotic Canal We are quick to intervene surgically when the neurological deficit is shown on MRI to be associated with a narrowed spinal canal such as acquired canal stenosis or subarticular stenosis or congenital stenosis.

Recurrent Neurological Deficit If a patient with sciatica and a neurological deficit has been successfully treated with conservative care, only to have a neurological deficit reappear with recurrent symptoms: operate.

Table 15.7. Recurring Sciatica[a]: Indications for Surgery

Episode of Sciatica	Prognosis
First	90% of patients will get better and stay better with conservative care.
Second	90% of patients will get better, but 50% of the patients will have a recurrence of symptoms. Consider surgery.
Third	90% of the patients will get better, but almost all will have recurrent episodes of sciatica. Propose surgery.

[a]This condition is to be distinguished from recurrent HNP (disc herniation recurring after previous surgery).

Table 15.8. Differential Diagnosis of Sciatica

- Intraspinal causes
  - Proximal to disc: conus and cauda equina lesions (eg, neurofibroma, ependymoma)
  - Disc level
    - Herniated nucleus pulposus
    - Stenosis (canal or recess)
    - Infection: osteomyelitis or discitis (with nerve root pressure)
    - Inflammation: arachnoiditis
    - Neoplasm: benign or malignant with nerve root pressure
- Extraspinal causes
  - Pelvis
    - Cardiovascular conditions (eg, peripheral vascular disease)
    - Gynecological conditions
    - Orthopedic conditions (eg, osteoarthritis of hip)
    - Sacroiliac joint disease
    - Neoplasms (invading or compressing lumbosacral plexus)
  - Peripheral nerve lesions
    - Neuropathy (diabetic, tumor, alcohol)
    - Local sciatic nerve conditions (trauma, tumor)
    - Inflammation (herpes zoster)

Contraindications to Surgical Intervention

Before intervening surgically for the acute radicular syndrome due to a lumbar disc herniation, it is essential to have an accurate clinical diagnosis of the cause of the sciatica (Table 15.8), an anatomical level of the lesion, and support for both clinical impressions by some form of investigation. If there is not a perfect marriage between the patient's clinical presentation, the anatomical level, and the structural lesion as demonstrated on myelography, CT scanning, or magnetic resonance imaging, the potential for a poor result increases dramatically.

Patients with a significant nonorganic component (Chapter 12) to their disability are usually a contraindication to surgical intervention. The presence of a nonorganic component to a disability does not immunize a patient from having a disc herniation. On the other hand, few patients with a significant nonorganic component to their disability do, indeed, have a disc rupture as part of their causative pathology.

Further contraindications to surgical intervention for a lumbar disc herniation are listed in Table 15.9.

TREATMENT OPTIONS

Before considering surgical intervention, remember: Successful surgical outcomes depend 90% on proper patient selection and 10% on surgical technique.

The principle of surgical intervention is to relieve neural compression without complications and, specifically, without creating instability. Surgery for a disc rupture is nerve root surgery, not disc surgery. Obviously, you need to remove offending disc material, but when you are finished, you must leave the nerve root free and mobile. The treatment choices include:

1. Chemonucleolysis.
2. Surgery.
    a. Posterior approaches
        - Standard laminectomy.
        - Microlaminectomy: posterior.
        - Microlaminectomy: lateral.
    b. Anterior approach.
    c. Percutaneous discectomy approach.

Table 15.9. Contraindications to Surgery for an HNP

- Wrong patient (poor potential for recovery, eg, workmen's compensation patient off work for more than 2 years)
- Wrong diagnosis, for example, other pathology causing the leg symptoms (see Table 15.8)
- Wrong level (see Chapter 19)
- A painless herniated nucleus pulposus (do not operate for primary complaint of weakness or paresthesia, in absence of pain)
- An inexperienced surgeon applying poor technical skills
- Lack of adequate instruments

Chemonucleolysis

Since it was first isolated by Jansen and Balls (36) in 1941, chymopapain has followed a checkered course to clinical acceptance. After 1964, when Smith (78) first reported its clinical use in the treatment of lumbar disc herniations, chymopapain was widely used in Canada, Great Britain, France, Germany, and the United States. However, a US double-blind study published in 1976 (75) led to the withdrawal of chymopapain from clinical use in the United States. Subsequent double-blind studies by Fraser;(18) Smith Laboratories(79, 80, 81, 82); and Travenol Laboratories (89) led the United States Food and Drug Administration (FDA) to reconsider chymopapain's position, and this agent was again released for general use in 1982. Surgeons accustomed to surgically excising space-occupying pathology were reluctant to embrace the concept of injecting a disc with chymopapain, a constituent of meat tenderizer. Further, 6 deaths and 37 serious neurological complications (79) had occurred in the United States in approximately 80,000 injections done during a time span of 18 months (ending time, 1984). Unfortunately, these events have served to undermine chymopapain as a clinical tool.

One manufacturer's claim that chymopapain was as good as surgery (92% success rate) (80) and unsupported claims of product superiority by competing firms fostered more credibility problems for this drug.

Despite the ongoing controversy that surrounds chymopapain, we continue to be convinced of its clinical efficacy as the last step in conservative care before surgery is considered.(90)

Pharmacology

Chymopapain is an extract of latex of the tropical fruit papaya.(36) Of the proteolytic enzymes in papaya, chymopapain is the most specific in its activity on the nucleus pulposus and the least antigenic. Despite the fact that it is less antigenic than papain, it is still a foreign protein to the human body and can precipitate allergic reactions.

Mechanism of Action

Tissue can be classified into two basic components, cells and noncellular matrix. The cartilage connective tissue of nucleus pulposus contains, obviously, cartilage cells; the matrix is made up of collagen, and proteoglycan-water complexes. This noncellular matrix of nucleus pulposus can be thought of as collagen-reinforcing bars laid in a viscoelastic base of proteoglycan and water. It is a very pliable structure designed to absorb force, but through the various effects of trauma and aging can be displaced, in whole or in part, from the disc space cavity into the spinal canal.

Chymopapain affects the proteoglycan-water aggregation of nuclear tissue. A proteoglycan aggregate is made up of many proteoglycan monomers (Fig. 15.23). A proteoglycan monomer is a protein core with glycosaminoglycan (mucopolysaccharide) side chains. Chondroitin sulfate and keratosulphate make up almost all of the glycosaminoglycan chains. A number of monomers then link to a central chain (hyaluronate) to form a proteoglycan aggregate. This proteoglycan aggregate imbibes water and cements itself among the collagen fibers to give the nucleus pulposus its viscoelastic structure. Proteoglycans are negatively charged. Because of the chemical makeup of proteoglycan and its fluid nature, it has the ability to absorb and dissipate water, thereby absorbing and dissipating forces across the disc space.

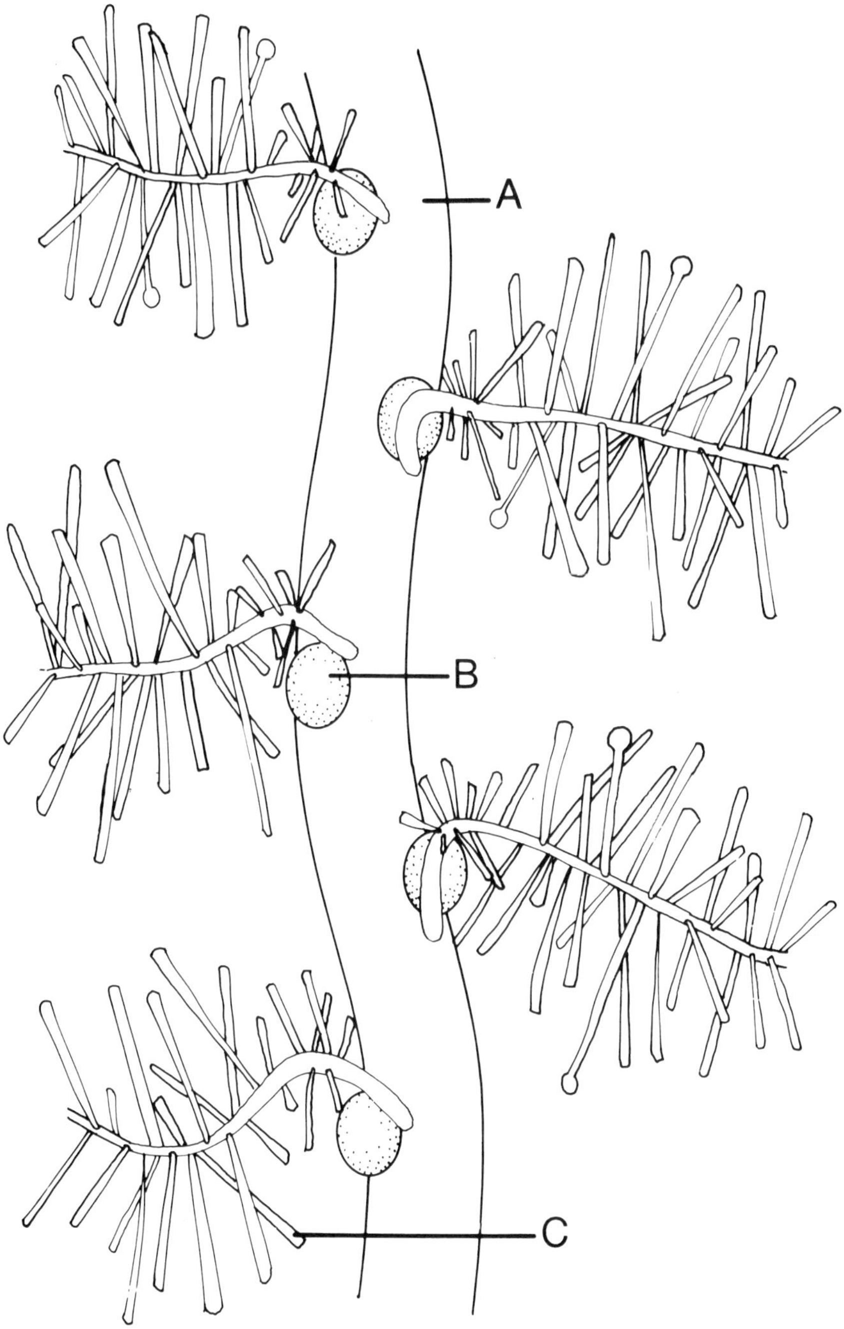

Figure 15.23 *The proteoglycan aggregate made up of* **(A)** *hyaluronate,* **(B)** *link protein, and* **(C)** *proteoglycan monomer.*

On displacement of nuclear material of a disc into the spinal canal, three local components can then contribute to the symptom of sciatica (Fig. 15.24). Chymopapain, positively charged, has a direct effect on the negatively charged proteoglycan aggregate by splitting off the glycosaminoglycan side chains, interfering with the ability of proteoglycan to hold water. This hydrolysis deflates the nuclear bulge and thus reduces pressure on the nerve root. Because collagen is not directly affected, there is still some mass of disc tissue present for weeks or months after chemonucleolysis (Fig. 15.25).

To understand the failure of the action of chymopapain in the extruded/sequestered disc, one must appreciate that in addition to the relatively inaccessible location of the disc fragment to chymopapain, the histological makeup of this mass of material lying in the spinal canal is almost uniformly collagenous and thus, unaffected by the enzyme. At the other end of the spectrum is an adolescent disc protrusion, which usually contains a considerable amount of proteoglycan, which will respond dramatically to the chymopapain.(48) One can appreciate that the combination of a displaced fragment and the collagenous nature of that fragment makes chymopapain injection for an extruded/sequestered disc a "fruitless endeavor."

Toxicology

Except for subarachnoid injection, chymopapain enjoys a wide margin of safety between the effective therapeutic dose and the toxic dose.(5, 6, 61) In animal experiments, there is a 100-fold margin of safety between the effective therapeutic dose and the toxic dose.(49, 61) Because chymopapain has no effect on collagenase structures such as bone, ligaments, muscle, nerve, and epidural tissue, it is very safe and has virtually no local complications when properly injected. Rydevik et al (72) reported adverse effects on nerve tissue in rabbit tibial nerves, but this has not been borne out with clinical work.(100)

Chymopapain is very dangerous when injected into the subarachnoid space.(49) It dissolves the basement membrane of the pia arachnoid vessels, resulting in subarachnoid hemorrhage. This hemorrhage can cause a local phenomenon such as arachnoiditis and cauda equina syndrome, or it can spread to the entire cerebrospinal fluid (CSF) space and

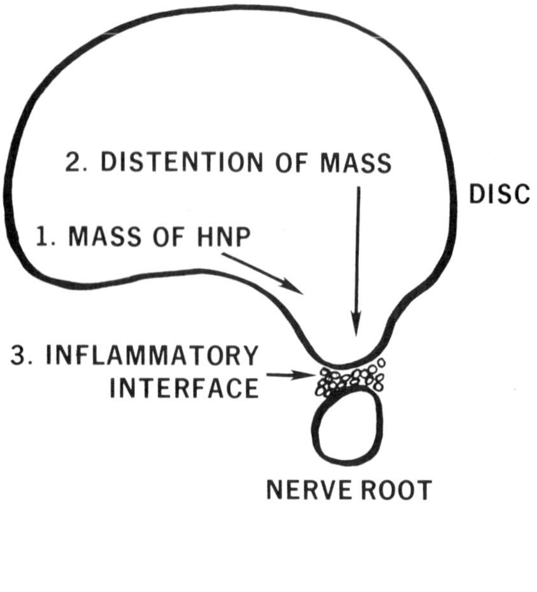

Figure 15.24 *The three local components that contribute to the pain of sciatica.*

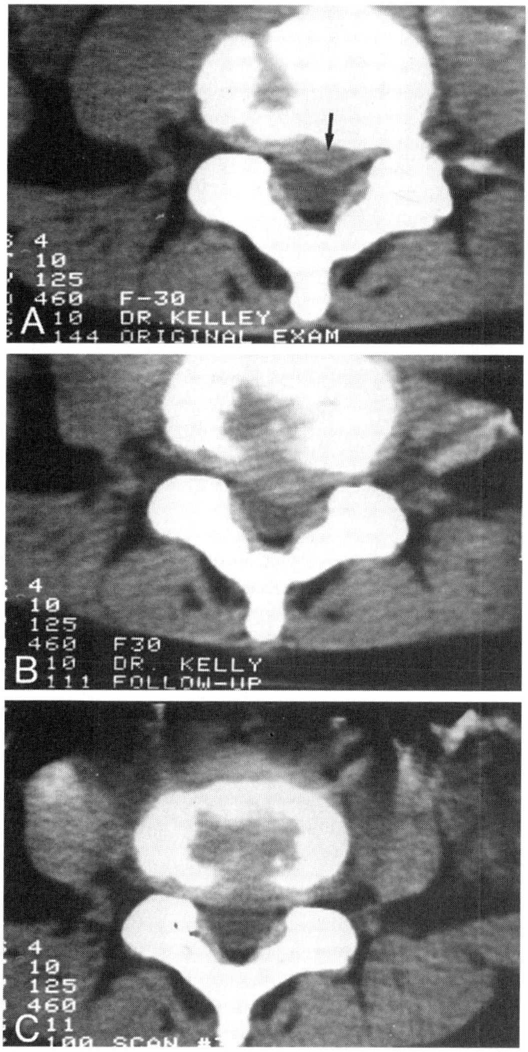

Figure 15.25 **A.** *Preoperative axial CT scan (arrow).* **B.** *One-month postchymopapain injection with relief of leg pain, yet persistence of "mass" on CT. The theory is that the hydrostatic distention has been "deflated" by the chymopapain, converting a hard "golf ball" mass to a soft "cotton ball" mass—the residual collagen.* **C.** *Six months later, no further treatment, the residual mass has disappeared, and the patient remains symptom free.*

cause the serious central nervous system neurological complications of subarachnoid hemorrhage.

In addition, there seems to be some sinister, albeit iatrogenic, delayed and possible hypersensitive effect of chymopapain in the subarachnoid space that has caused transverse myelitis in humans. These topics will be covered in the section on chymopapain complications.

As with any surgical procedure, it is difficult to obtain a good result to a treatment modality if one cannot recognize the patients that will respond to that treatment. There are very clear indications and contraindications to the use of chymopapain, and they are summarized as follows:

Indications

There is only one indication for chemonucleolysis with chymopapain: the herniated nucleus pulposus, causing sciatica, and unresponsive to conservative care. The diagnosis is based on the four criteria in Table 15.4.

Contraindication

Extruded/Sequestered Disc Within these four criteria there is the contraindication of an extruded/sequestered disc. This is a very difficult clinical diagnosis. We have reviewed 50 consecutive extruded/sequestered discs (documented at surgery), looking at all aspects of each patient's history and physical examination.(58) Age, sex, type of work, level of disc herniation, side of disc herniation, patient's smoking status, onset of symptoms, location of pain, nature of pain, aggravating factors, relieving factors, associated symptoms, progression of symptoms, nerve root tension findings, and neurological signs offered no clues as to whether the disc was contained or an extruded/sequestered fragment. With a few clinical exceptions, the diagnosis of an extruded/sequestered disc is best made on the basis of investigative studies. The following clinical findings point to an extruded/sequestered fragment, and discolysis is contraindicated: (1) cauda equina syndrome with bladder and bowel involvement, (2) large MRI or CT/myelography defect that is in association with a significant neurological deficit.

On investigation, the following findings are suggestive of either an extruded/sequestered disc or a chymopapain–nonresponsive disc herniation (Fig. 15.26): (1) a large HNP (filling more than 50% of the sagittal diameter on any one MRI or CT scan slice); (2) pedunculated shape to disc fragment (a disc fragment with a long sagittal dimension and a narrow stalk or coronal dimension); (3) a disc fragment that has migrated away from the disc space; (4) artifactual changes, such as calcification (osteophyte formation) or air in the fragment.

The following investigative findings suggest that a disc protrusion is present and chymopapain injection may be of benefit (Fig. 15.27): (1) a defect exactly opposite the disc space, (2) a shallow defect with more coronal breadth than sagittal depth.

Relative Contraindications

Spinal Stenosis Spinal stenosis affecting the canal or lateral zone will never respond to chemonucleolysis. Occasionally, these bony defects will be complicated by a disc herniation; it is highly unlikely that these combined conditions will be favorably altered by chemonucleolysis.

Previous Surgery Patients who have had previous surgery and suffer from recurrent disc herniations at the same level, same side, should not have chemonucleolysis. Patients who have had previous surgery and suffer from a disc herniation at a different level or opposite side (a rare occurrence) may benefit from chemonucleolysis.

Strong Contraindications

Degenerative Disc Disease and Facet Joint Disease Patients with back pain predominantly due to mechanical instability either within the disc space or within the facet joint will not respond to chymopapain injection.

Spinal Instability Patients with spondylolisthesis will not benefit from the injection of chymopapain at the slip level. In fact, the temporary instability that occurs at a disc space level after the injection of chymopapain (91) could result in an increase in the listhesis. This contraindication applies to both lytic and degenerative spondylolisthesis. There is always a possibility that a patient with spondylolisthesis has a symptomatic disc herniation at a level away from the slip, and that patient would qualify for a chymopapain injection, provided he/she fulfills the criteria for the diagnosis of a soft disc herniation causing sciatica.

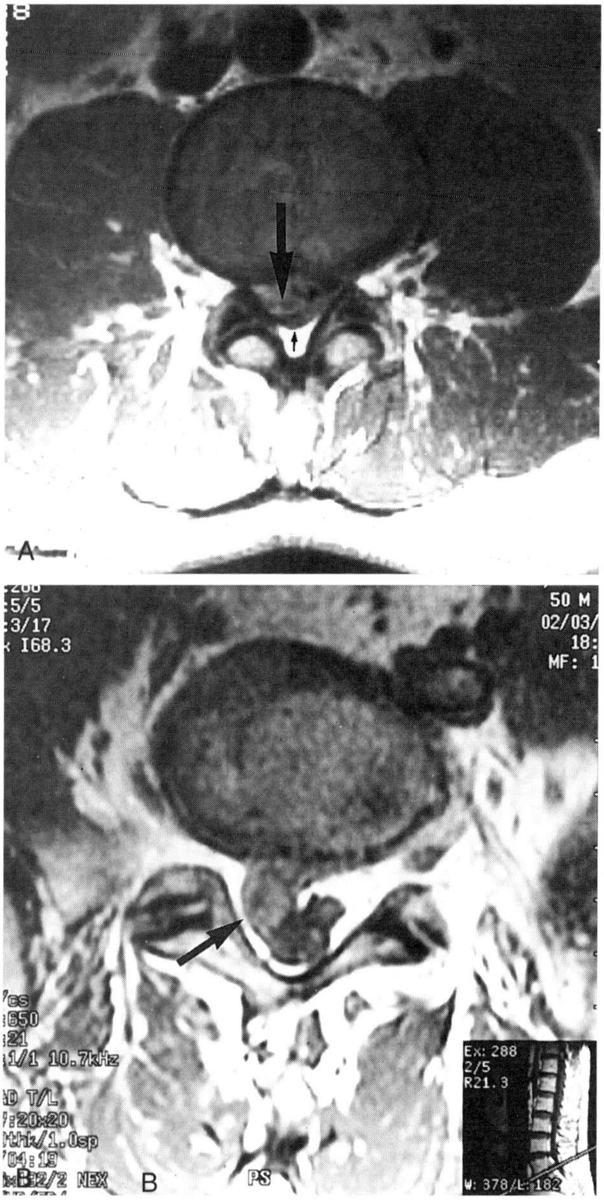

Figure 15.26 **A.** *A large HNP (arrow) almost obliterates the thecal sac (small arrow) in a congenitally small canal.* **B.** *A pedunculated HNP (arrow).*

Absolute Contraindications

Sensitivity to Chymopapain A patient may give a history of an allergy to the ingestion of meat tenderizer or foods containing chymopapain (beer, cheese, and some toothpastes). These patients are at risk for an allergic reaction and should not be considered for chymopapain injection. Obviously, injecting chymopapain into a patient who has a positive skin test (57) for chymopapain sensitivity is a contraindication. A patient who has

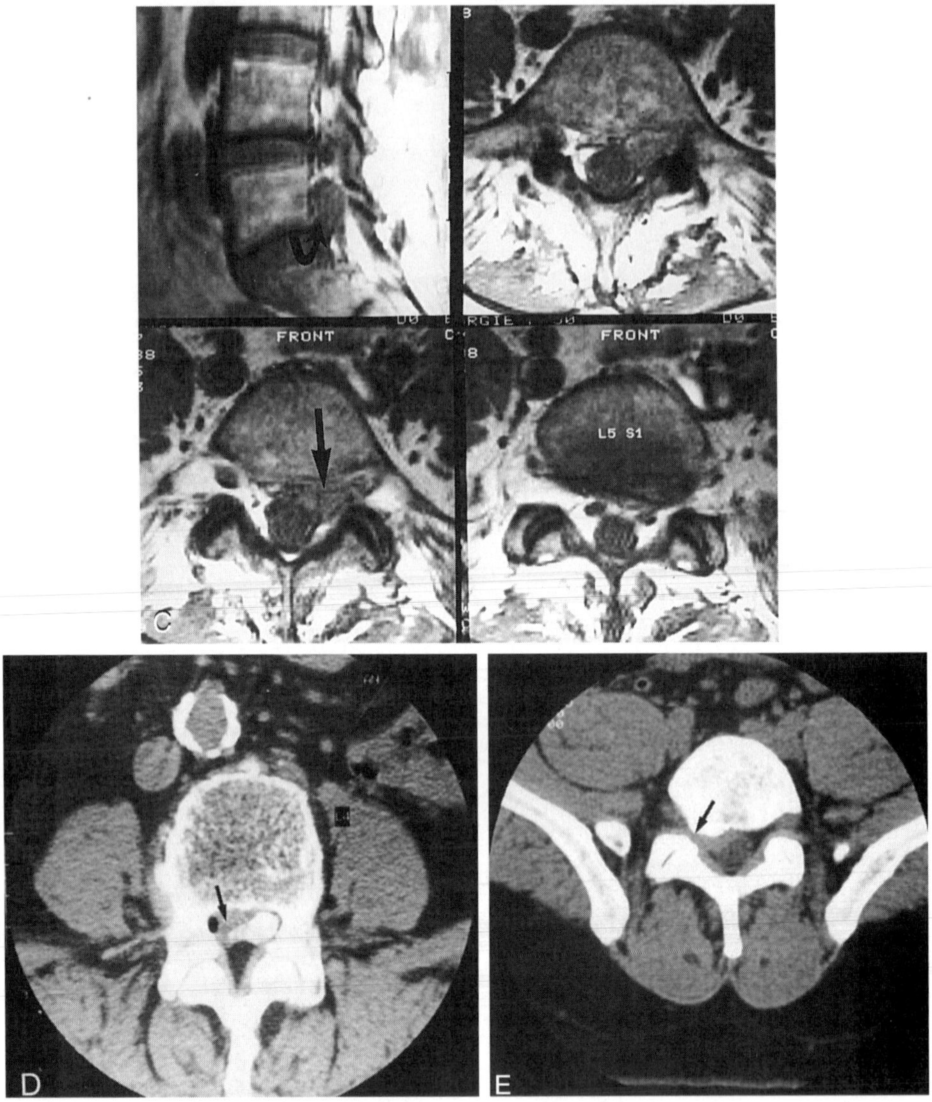

Figure 15.26 (continued) **C.** *A disc rupture that has migrated up into the second story of the anatomic segment (arrows). In fact, in the top right axial T1, the tip of the disc rupture is as high as the third story.* **D.** *Axial CT, artifact: gas in disc fragment, third story, L4, right (arrow).* **E.** *CT of L5–S1 HNP with osteophyte (arrow).*

had a previous chemonucleolysis may, after a long latent interval, develop another disc herniation at another level. Manufacturers are recommending against a second chymopapain injection. However, if that patient has a negative skin test, a repeated chemonucleolysis (different level) could be considered.(57)

Disc Herniations at Cord Levels To date, there is no recommendation for chymopapain to be injected into disc herniations at cord levels. The cord level that one might consider could be a thoracic or cervical disc. Unfortunately, most thoracic disc are calcified, and most cervical radicular syndromes are chronic, with an element of bony nerve root entrapment, and a chymopapain injection would be of no benefit. Presently, there is ongoing research on the use of

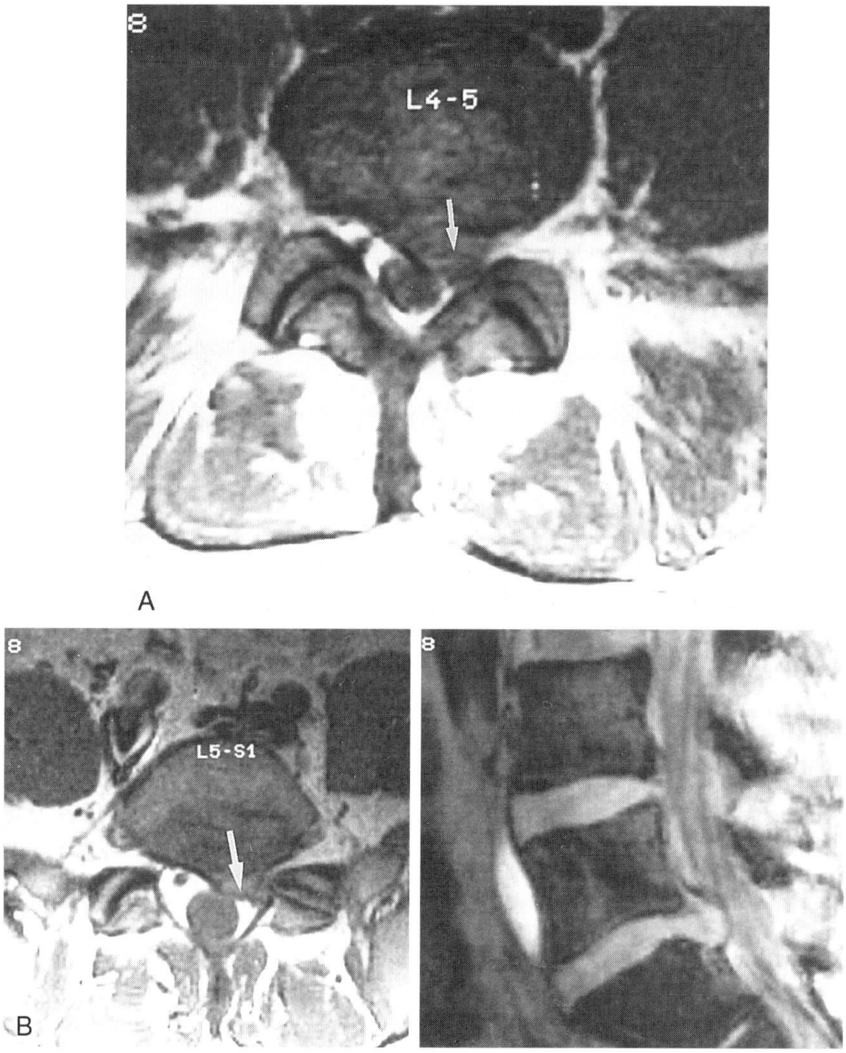

Figure 15.27 **A.** *A disc herniation in the 1st story (arrow).* **B.** *A disc herniation (L5–S1) that is "shallow in depth" compared with Figure 15.26, B (left, axial T1; right, sagittal gradient echo).*

chymopapain in the treatment of the infrequent recalcitrant soft cervical disc herniation, and a recommendation for or against injection into soft cervical or thoracic disc cannot be made.

Neurological Lesion of Unknown Etiology It is unreasonable to risk plant enzyme aggravation of a neurological problem of obscure etiology (eg, multiple sclerosis).

Pregnant Women Because the effect of chymopapain on the fetus is unknown, it is unreasonable to submit a pregnant woman and the fetus to the potential risks of a chymopapain injection.

Nonorganic Spinal Pain (See Chapter 12) Obviously, a chymopapain injection will not "dissolve away" nonorganic pain, the origin of which is far removed from the disc space.

Patient Age and Duration of Symptoms

Provided that the patient fulfills the criteria for the diagnosis of an HNP causing sciatica, patient age and duration of symptoms seem not to play a role in the response to chemonucleolysis. There is a tendency for the older patient or the patient with many years of symptoms to have a diagnosis such as spinal stenosis, and these patients in general do not fulfill the clinical criteria for the diagnosis of an HNP.

Preparation of Patient

Conservative Treatment All patients who are considered for chemonucleolysis must have failed to respond to excellent conservative therapy (including at least 2–3 days of complete bed rest). It is reasonable for a patient to spend 3 months attempting various forms of conservative care before opting for chymopapain injection. There are some patients with persistent sciatica that interferes significantly with their pattern of living or who have a pattern of living that does not allow for 3 months of conservative care. Early chemonucleolysis may be considered in this patient population. However, this represents a shortcutting of conservative care therapy and is really not consistent with our treatment philosophy.

Aim of Therapy

Because most disc ruptures occur at single levels, chemonucleolysis should be done only at single levels. Almost all of the patients who have failed chymopapain injection should go on to surgical intervention, because most of those patients will be found to have a sequestered or extruded disc.(54) Thus, in selecting patients for chymopapain injection, it is obvious that only those patients in whom you would expect a good surgical result are candidates for chymopapain injection. Chymopapain is not to be used as a catchall for those patients rejected for surgery.

Preoperative Chymopapain Sensitivity Testing

The best strategy for coping with chymopapain sensitivity and anaphylaxis is to identify beforehand the patients who are at risk and exclude them from the chymopapain injection. We have experimented with a sensitive and sufficiently specific skin test, the prick test.(57) Our more than 1500 consecutive patients now have had negative skin tests and have not had anaphylactic or other immediate hypersensitivity reactions.(56) We feel confident enough to recommend the chymopapain skin test to detect chymopapain sensitivity (see Appendix).

Serological tests for chymopapain antibody level (IgE) such as chymoFAST and radioallergosorbent test (RAST) are also available but are not considered as reliable as skin testing.

Technique of Chemonucleolysis

Considerable confusion arose when one manufacture (81) originally recommended the use of general anesthesia, premedication, a needle insertion site 8 cm from the midline, a 45-degree angle to approach the disc space, single-needle technique to get into the L5–S1 disc space, and the use of contrast material for discographic assessment for disc integrity. With the occurrence of the complications after the release of chymopapain in the United

States, a critical review suggested that a safer protocol was in order. For this reason, there have been some changes recommended in the technique of chemonucleolysis.(82) These are essentially the recommendations published by numerous authors (66) in the past and include the use of local neuroleptic anesthesia, the selection of a needle insertion site an adequate distance from the midline (10 cm average), the use of the double-needle technique at the L5–S1 disc space, and the avoidance of discography using contrast material.

Whether or not you choose to use contrast material, the basic technical rule is: You must know exactly where the needle tip lies before injecting chymopapain. If that requires the use of contrast material, you must use contrast material. The authors feel that, with proper needle insertion technique and good radiographic views at 90 degrees to each other, routine use of contrast material is not necessary to localize needle tip position.

Local Versus General Anesthesia Local anesthesia (augmented with neuroleptic agents) is the choice for the following reasons:

1. It is safer.
2. It is efficient: it shortens operating room (OR) time and the patient's length of stay in the hospital.
3. The patient avoids the complications of general anesthesia and intubation.
4. It allows for earlier intervention in the event of a complication, for example, anaphylaxis.
5. It preserves discometry or discography (with patient response), as a test.

In the face of a negative skin test, it is highly unlikely that a patient will experience a hypersensitivity reaction, and thus the main reason for suggesting general anesthesia is eliminated.

Premedication Test Dose Regimen The authors do not premedicate or test dose.(54) Rather than assume all patients are at risk and premedicate, the better approach is to try to identify reactors with an allergic history and skin test. Other tests, such as RAST or chymoFAST, are available.

The reasons for not premedicating are:

1. The incidence of anaphylaxis is low (0.35%) (26), and lower still with skin testing.
2. There is no scientific evidence that premedication lowers the incidence of anaphylaxis below the figure in our experience.
3. Any treatment regimen in medicine considered to be prophylactic in nature should contain the most effective agent: in anaphylaxis, this is epinephrine. Obviously, this agent cannot be included in a prophylactic program.
4. Patients who have been premedicated according to recommendations have experienced severe anaphylactic reactions.(81)
5. Patients who have received an intradiscal test dose (not skin test) of chymopapain have experienced severe anaphylactic reactions.(81)
6. Anaphylaxis requires aggressive treatment as follows:
    a. The doses of cortisone and antihistamines required to treat anaphylaxis are much greater than the recommended dose in the premedication regimen.
    b. The addition of epinephrine, which cannot be part of the premedication regimen.
7. The best defense against anaphylaxis is:
    a. Identification and exclusion of the hypersensitive patient (skin test).
    b. An alert, well-prepared team of assistants.

Operating Room or Radiology Department The OR has the greatest concentration of skilled personnel for managing the complications of discolysis. Generally speaking, life-threatening emergencies such as anaphylaxis severely stress a radiology department. On the other hand, if your operating room image intensifier capabilities are not good, you will have to consider the radiology department.

Position

The lateral position is the choice of most spine surgeons (Fig. 15.28). The prone position is acceptable, provided you do not get too far laterally with your puncture site. Theoretically, the bowel has not fallen away from the lateral abdominal gutter in the prone position. In the lateral position, the bowel falls away from the lateral gutter, and a 10-cm insertion site is very safe.

The principles of the lateral approach are:

1. Maintain the proper position of the patient. If you are doing the procedure in the lateral position, there is a tendency for the awake patient to roll out of the perfect lateral position. This is the most common mistake made by the beginner trying to get a needle into a disc space.
2. Select the correct disc. It is very important to see the front of the sacrum before selecting the disc space for injection. One can inadvertently put a needle into the L3–L4 disc space, believing it to be at the L4–L5 level. View the front of the sacrum before counting levels. Four or six lumbar vertebrae, or other congenital lumbosacral anomalies, may confuse the selection of the disc space to be punctured.

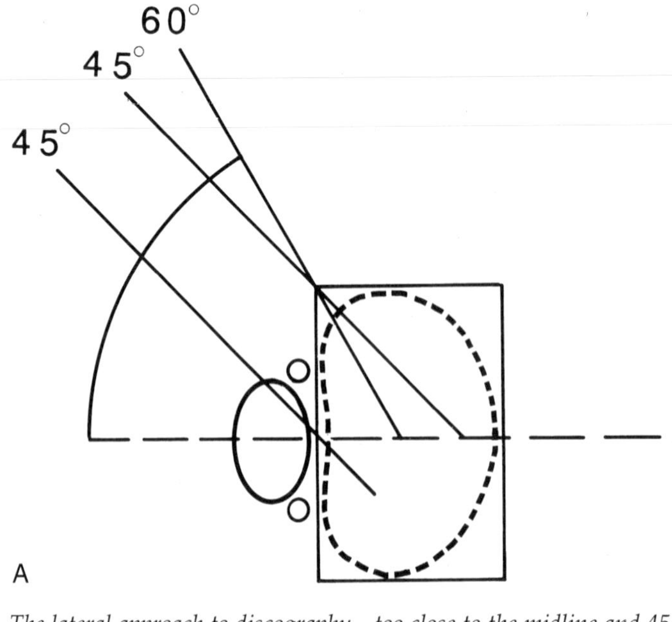

Figure 15.28 **A.** *The lateral approach to discography—too close to the midline and 45-degree angulation will direct the needle through the common dural sac. Too far from the midline and 45-degree angulation will direct the needle tip to the front of the disc space.*

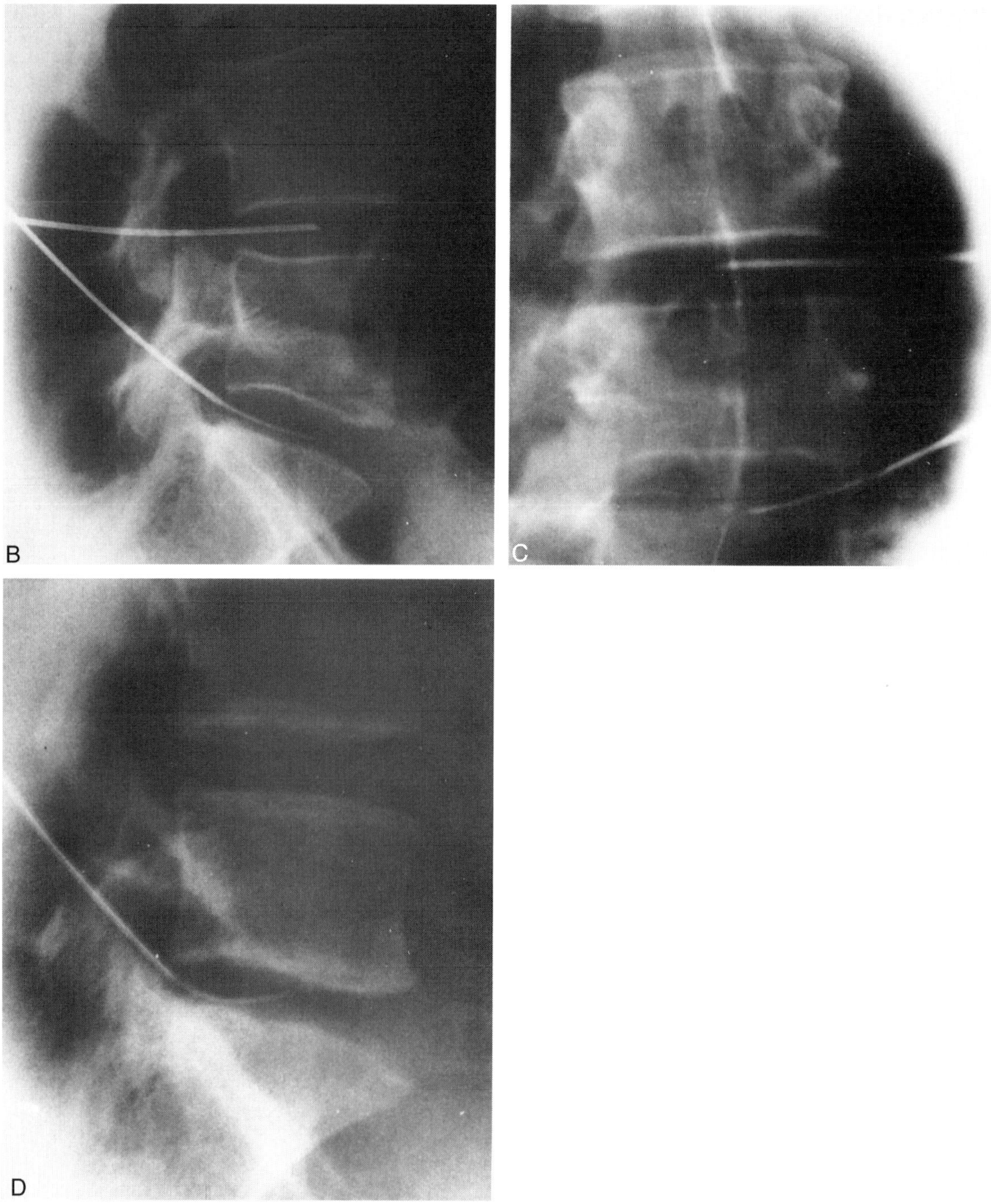

Figure 15.28 (continued) **B.** *Perfect positioning of needle tips on lateral.* **C.** *Perfect positioning of needle tips on AP. Just because needle positioning in both L4–L5 and L5–S1 is shown, it is not meant to suggest that two-level injections should be done.* **D.** *The bend sometimes required to get into the L5–S1 disc.*

3. Select the correct insertion site. It is important to get far enough from the midline. For the average patient, 10 cm from the midline, adjacent to the iliac crest, is the correct insertion site. For a larger patient, you sometimes have to go further than 10 cm from the midline, and for a small patient you would select a needle insertion site closer to the midline.
4. Approach the disc at the proper angle (see Fig. 15.28). The angle of approach to the disc space is closer to 60 degrees than 45 degrees. However, at all times it is important to remember that the needle must not penetrate the foramen and enter the spinal canal to puncture the subarachnoid space. (It is advisable to leave the stylet out of the needle as an additional precaution. Inadvertent puncture of the subarachnoid space is then heralded by the immediate backflow of CSF, which signals abortion of the procedure and rescheduling in 2 to 3 weeks.)
5. Position the needle tip in the center of the disc. The center of the disc space is defined as the middle third of the disc space on lateral radiograph and superimposed on the spinous process on anteroposterior (AP) radiograph (see Fig. 15.28).
6. Appreciate all of the intricacies of discometry (discography) (see Chapter 14).
7. Inject the proper amount of active chymopapain into a clean disc space. The dose of chymopapain ranges from .75 to 1.0 mL (2000 units Chymodiactin) (Boots Pharmaceuticals, Inc, 300 Tri-State International Center, Suite 200, Lincolnshire, Ill).

If more than three passes of the needle have occurred without entry to the disc space being achieved, abort the procedure. Similarly, if you penetrate the nerve root (ie, cause severe leg pain), abort the procedure. The authors recommend that after puncturing the skin, remove the stylet from the needle and advance the needle toward the disc space with an open lumen. If you inadvertently cross the subarachnoid space on advancing the needle, the immediate backflow of CSF will be ample notification to abort the procedure. Never abandon the lateral approach for the midline transdural approach.

Postoperative Care

The most important thing to recognize about postoperative management of the patient is the tremendous variation in patient response to the procedure and recovery from the chemical disc excision. Approximately 20% of the patients will have significant back pain (back spasms) immediately after the procedure. This is best managed with an intravenous or intramuscular dose of steroids. This back spasm usually settles within a few hours to a few days after the procedure. The pain is very severe and is usually more severe than pain the patients experience after surgical disc excision. However, 80% of the patients do NOT have excessive back pain, and their symptoms can be controlled by moderate doses of oral analgesics. Most patients benefit from a light canvas corset support to help them ambulate in the first few weeks after chymopapain injection.

Patients follow one of three courses with regard to postinjection leg pain. Often, there is very dramatic relief of leg pain, but most patients destined for a good result will notice a gradual reduction in their leg pain. Leg cramping and paresthetic discomfort in the leg are the last to disappear. The latter paresthetic discomfort often takes many weeks to go away. Rarely, a patient will notice a dramatic increase in leg pain immediately after injection. This patient requires swift surgical intervention (within a day or two of the procedure) to remove the extruded or sequestered fragment of disc material.

RESULTS

Results vary all the way from "no good" to 90 to 95% good. The authors have experienced approximately a 70% good result rate (49, 54, 55, 90, 95), slightly higher for younger patients, and slightly better at the L5–S1 level in all age groups.

The most common cause of failure is the sequestered or extruded fragment of disc material that has not been dissolved by chymopapain. Because the nuclear contents of the disc space have been dissolved by the chymopapain, very little work needs to be done within the disc space itself during surgery. In fact, microsurgery dealing solely with the spinal canal pathology is the treatment of choice in these patients.(45) Chemonucleolysis has not compromised surgical intervention in more than 350 cases in our practices.

It is obvious that the 70% good result rate is going to be improved upon only by correctly identifying the patient with an extruded/sequestered disc and using surgical excision in these patients.

Complications

The overall complication rate of chemonucleolysis is low.(61) Nordby (63), in a review of complications reported to the United States FDA from 1982 to 1991, described no serious complications since 1988. In 1987 and 1988, there was one serious complication per year, with the overall serious complication rate from 1982 to 1991 being 121 patients in 135,000 injections (0.09%). Bouillet (5, 6), in a survey of 43,662 injections in Europe, reported a rate of 0.44% for serious complications such as anaphylaxis, cerebral hemorrhage, cauda equina syndrome, and discitis. These two series have formally documented a much lower complication rate to chemonucleolysis versus surgery. Still, the unfavorable malpractice climate in the US drastically limits the use of chymopapain. Table 15.10 summarizes the complication rates.

Anaphylaxis Anaphylaxis occurs in 0.35% of patients who have not been prescreened. It is manifest by a profound drop in blood pressure and requires very vigorous immediate resuscitation to save the patient's life.(26) The cornerstone of treatment for anaphylaxis is appropriate doses of epinephrine, large volumes of intravenous fluids, steroids, and antihistamines.

With the use of skin testing, anaphylaxis is becoming a less frequent problem. The senior author (JM) has experience with 1500 cases of chymopapain injection preceded by

Table 15.10. Comparison of Surgical and Chemonucleolysis Complications

Complication	Surgery	Chemonucleolysis	
	(%)	United States (%)	Europe (%)
Mortality	0.3 (53)	0.02 (63)	0.0 (5,6)
Morbidity			
Serious	0.02 (59,67,83)	0.05 (63)	0.04 (5,6)
Anaphylaxis	0.00	0.05 (63)	0.06 (5,6)
Less serious	2.0 (59,87,63)	0.03 (63)	0.80 (5,6)
General	2–3	Extremely low	Extremely low

skin testing for chymopapain sensitivity. To date, there has not been an anaphylactic reaction in a patient who has had a negative skin test. This represents unpublished data from a combined study in Berlin, Germany, and Akron, Ohio.(56) Thus, the management of anaphylaxis has moved into the best medical realm, that of prophylaxis. Any patient with a positive skin test is eliminated from treatment with chymopapain.

Neurological Complications Chymopapain, with or without contrast material, when injected into the subarachnoid space, is almost certain to cause a disaster. Thus, it is extremely important that the needle tip does not cross the subarachnoid space on insertion into the nuclear cavity. If there is any question about the needle tip crossing the subarachnoid space at the time of needle insertion, the procedure should be aborted.

The possibility of a connection between the disc space and the subarachnoid space is the one drawback to not using contrast material at the time of needle placement. It is obvious, on injecting contrast material into the disc, that when it appears in the subarachnoid space (Fig. 15.29), there is a connection between the disc cavity and the subarachnoid space. The most common cause of this connection is crossing the subarachnoid space on needle insertion. It is the authors' opinion that whenever there is any degree of resistance of injection of test material into the nuclear cavity, it is highly unlikely that there is a connection between the disc space and the subarachnoid space. For this reason, it is possible to use a water acceptance test rather than contrast material at the time of chymopapain injection.

Injection of chymopapain (with or without contrast material) into the subarachnoid space may cause subarachnoid hemorrhage with cerebral complications, a cauda equina syndrome, or a delayed transverse myelitis. Recent preliminary experimental work (81) suggests that it is not chymopapain alone but rather the combination of chymopapain and contrast material in the subarachnoid space that is causing the serious neurological complications. Other research (95) would suggest that chymopapain alone is capable of causing subarachnoid hemorrhage and serious neurological complications.

The complication that has struck fear into most users has been transverse myelitis.(63) Six cases were reported following chemonucleolysis in 1983 and 1984. All were of delayed onset (many days to a few weeks) and caused total paralysis due to a high to mid-thoracic cord lesion. Three points are important:

1. There is some doubt that any of these cases are a direct result of the chymopapain injection.
2. There have been no cases of transverse myelitis following chemonucleolysis since 1984.
3. Fraser and Gogan (20) reported one case of transverse myelitis in his placebo group (no chymopapain injected) on 10 year follow-up.

One can only conclude that transverse myelitis as a complication of chemonucleolysis is rare.

Miscellaneous Complications Two miscellaneous complications require consideration. The first is root damage from penetration of the nerve root at the time of needle insertion. This usually occurs under general anesthesia when the spine surgeon is attempting to get the needle into the L5–S1 disc space.(101) Under local neuroleptic anesthesia, this is a very rare complication. Root penetration has led to some permanent causalgic syndromes.

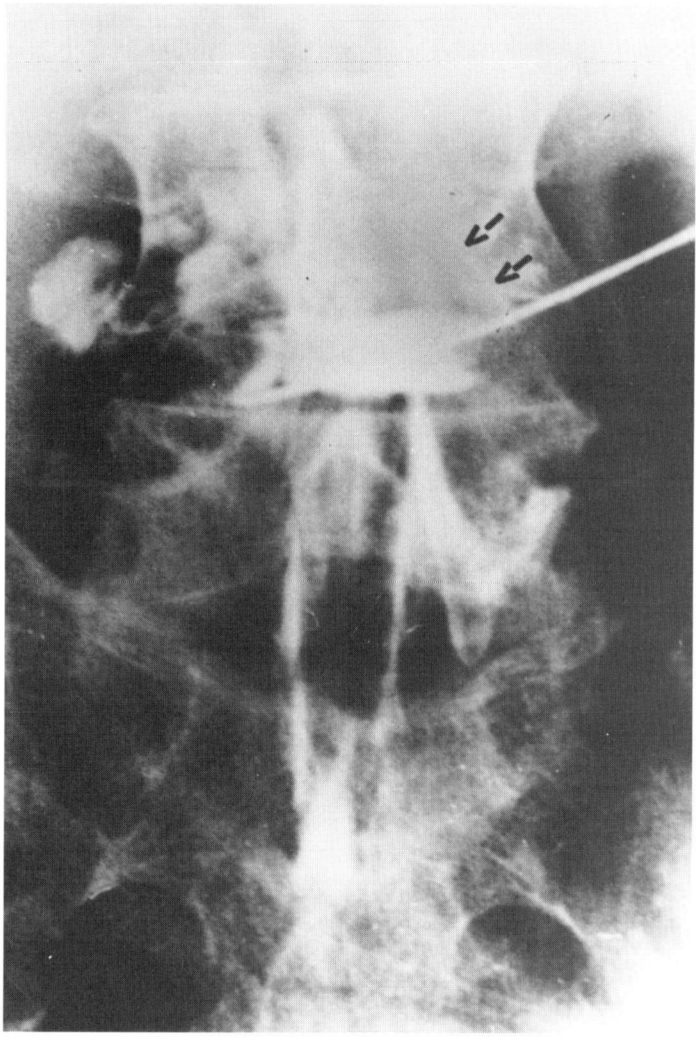

Figure 15.29 *AP of discogram, (arrows) superimposed on which is a myelogram, signifying a connection between the disc space and the subarachnoid space.*

A second complication is discitis. This is either a low-grade infective discitis or a chemical discitis that results in a prolongation of the patient's back pain and a typical radiographic picture (Fig. 15.30) (see Chapter 4). It is infrequent that one has to deal with a fulminating septic discitis with systemic manifestations. When this does occur, the basic principles of management of any infective discitis applies.

Postoperative Care

After chymopapain injection, patients are usually discharged from the hospital the same day or within 1 to 2 days. Analgesic medication is usually required for 1 to 2 weeks after discharge. The patient who is self-employed may feel compelled to return to work

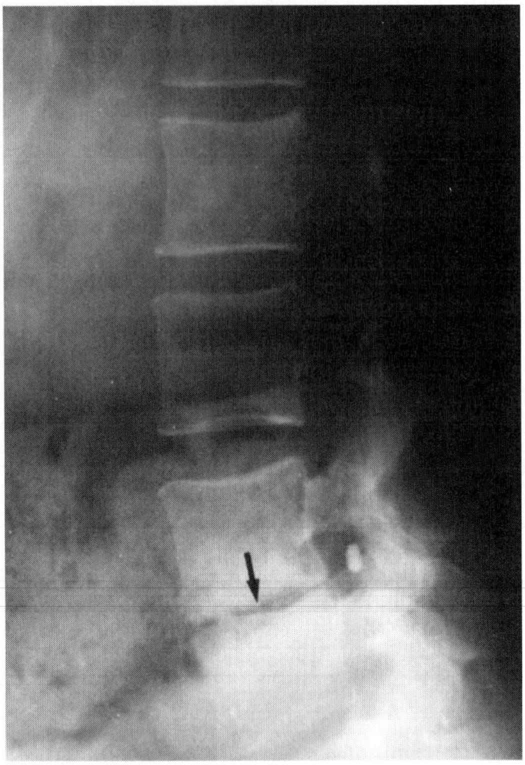

Figure 15.30 *Postchemonucleolysis discitis, L4–L5 (arrow).*

within the first week after injection. However, it is prudent for the patient with light occupational demands to wait 2 to 4 weeks before considering a return to work. Patients who have heavier work demands should convalesce for the same period as a patient who undergoes the standard laminectomy/discectomy. The return to leisure activity varies according to its form. The first leisure activity usually available to patients is swimming, which can be started 2 to 4 weeks after injection.

It is advisable to see the patient at 1 month for assessment, including a radiograph. Those patients who have lost most of their leg pain, have improved in SLR ability, and show disc space narrowing on a plain lateral radiograph, are destined for an excellent result. Patients with some improvements in leg discomfort and some improvement in SLR may be observed for a further 1 to 2 months before a decision about future treatment intervention is made. However, those patients who persist with unaltered leg pain 1 month after the procedure usually have persistent SLR reduction and can be considered to be a treatment failure. These patients need immediate surgical intervention. As mentioned earlier, most of these patients have an extruded or sequestered disc and will benefit from microsurgical (45) intervention. If you have been careful in selecting your patients and have had the assistance of a CT scan or MRI, most patients with lateral recess stenosis will have been promptly and correctly diagnosed, and thus eliminated from consideration for chemonucleolysis.

Failures

It is possible with any surgical therapy to select a patient with a nonphysical disability, to make the wrong diagnosis, or to do the wrong operation and end up with a poor result.

This has happened, and continues to happen, with selection of patients for chymopapain injection. Assuming a very infrequent complication rate that causes failure, it becomes obvious that true failures to chymopapain injection should almost always be due to pathology within the spinal canal, and almost always this pathology is an extruded or sequestered disc ± subarticular stenosis.

It should be possible to determine that a patient has failed to respond to chemonucleolysis at 4 to 6 weeks after injection. Subsequent surgery is not compromised by chemonucleolysis. In fact, there is a discolysis advantage because within a number of weeks of injection of chymopapain into the disc space, the disc space narrowing offers some degree of stability. Further, there is no nuclear material left within the disc space, and thus no extensive disc space dissection is needed. Finally, the absence of nuclear material within the disc space and the surgical removal of nuclear material within the spinal canal should result in an extremely low recurrence rate.(45)

Conclusions

Chemonucleolysis with chymopapain represents the least invasive, lowest risk, lowest cost surgical intervention for a patient with a herniated nucleus pulposus causing sciatica. Despite the recent serious complications and deaths, there is still a wide margin of safety between chemonucleolysis and surgical intervention for disc disease (see Table 15.10). In the properly selected patient, there is at least a 70% chance of a successful result.

In the authors' hands, chemonucleolysis with chymopapain has been a safe, simple, and effective treatment modality. The patient does not end up with an incision on his/her back. The patient is in hospital for a shorter time and, in some cases, a faster return to work is possible. Four long-term studies (48, 54, 66, 90) suggest that the long-term results are excellent, and the recurrence rate is extremely low. Finally, a failure to respond to chymopapain injection does not compromise any future surgical consideration.

SURGICAL TECHNIQUE

Introduction

The authors confine chemonucleolysis use to the younger patient (below ages 25–30).(48) Over the ages of 30 to 35, most patients will have a requirement for surgical intervention because of the high incidence of extruded/sequestered discs that tend not to respond to chymopapain treatment.

Posterior Approach

Most lumbar disc herniations requiring surgery will be approached posteriorly. The surgery can be done under general, spinal, or local anesthesia. The most expedient anesthetic is general, although there are surgeons who believe that the procedure is best accomplished under either spinal or local anesthesia.

Most surgeons agree that the kneeling position (Fig. 15.31) is the best for the surgeon and patient. It allows for a free abdomen, removing pressure from the inferior vena cava, and decreasing venous flow through Batson's plexus, which in turn reduces bleeding from epidural veins during surgery. In the kneeling position, one has to be mindful of a number of pitfalls, which are outlined in Table 15.11.

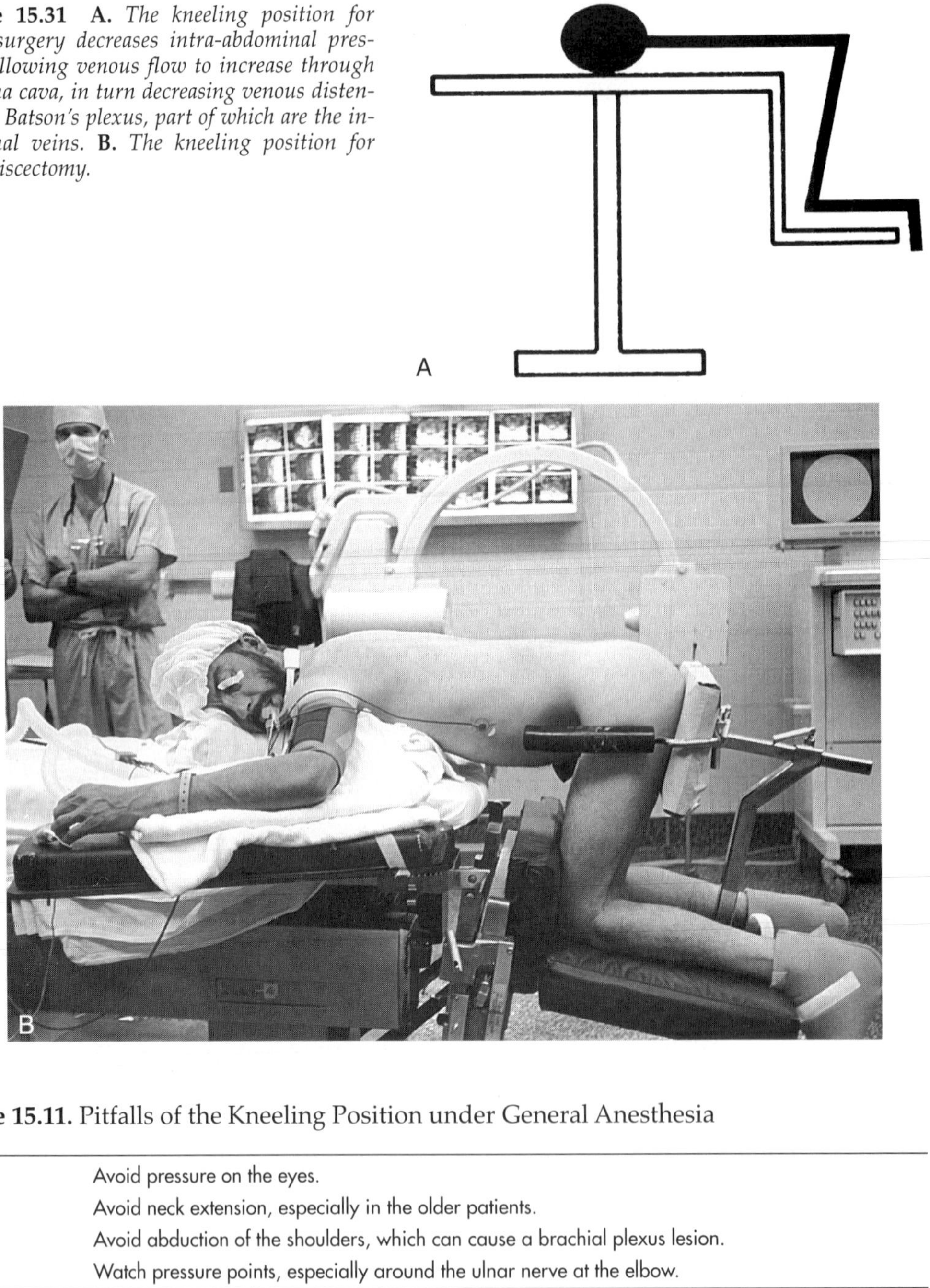

Figure 15.31 **A.** *The kneeling position for spine surgery decreases intra-abdominal pressure, allowing venous flow to increase through the vena cava, in turn decreasing venous distention in Batson's plexus, part of which are the intraspinal veins.* **B.** *The kneeling position for microdiscectomy.*

Table 15.11. Pitfalls of the Kneeling Position under General Anesthesia

Avoid pressure on the eyes.
Avoid neck extension, especially in the older patients.
Avoid abduction of the shoulders, which can cause a brachial plexus lesion.
Watch pressure points, especially around the ulnar nerve at the elbow.

Whether one should use no magnification or magnification (loupes or microscope) to accomplish the disc excision is unresolved. As long as the root is decompressed and the patient is relieved of symptoms, the mission has been accomplished. The microsurgeons believe this can be better accomplished with the assistance of the magnification and illumination of the microscope.(98) Critics of this approach cite inability to see everything and the possibility of leaving behind nerve root encroachment pathology (eg, lateral zone stenosis and retained disc fragments).(71) Supporters of microsurgery would reply that the eyes of a microsurgeon are the sophisticated images of MRI and an intimate knowledge of anatomy, which combine to tell you, before you make the limited skin incision, exactly what the root encroachment pathology is and where in the "anatomical house" it will be found. The road map in lumbar disc surgery is the MRI, not a long incision, wide exposure, and seek-and-find surgery.

The standard surgical approach for a laminectomy or a microdiscectomy has been outlined in many articles.(76, 85) Briefly, it is important to open the correct interlaminar space. Once within the laminar opening, the next exercise is to find the lateral border of the nerve root and reflect the nerve root and cauda equina sheath medially to expose the pathology. It is necessary to remove enough bone to see the lateral border of the nerve root. This may require removal of the medial edge of the superior facet of the anatomical segment below (Fig. 15.32). In trying to find the lateral border of the lumbar nerve root, there are a few pitfalls. The first problem is a nerve root that is displaced laterally by an axillary disc herniation. A second pitfall is the posterior displacement of a nerve root that occurs because of the location of the disc herniation, which places the nerve root at jeopardy when opening the ligamentum flavum (Fig. 15.33). It is important to remove all of the offending pathology, not miss any extruded/migrated disc fragments, and not leave behind bony nerve root encroachment. (See later section on "Complications of Microsurgery for Lumbar HNP.")

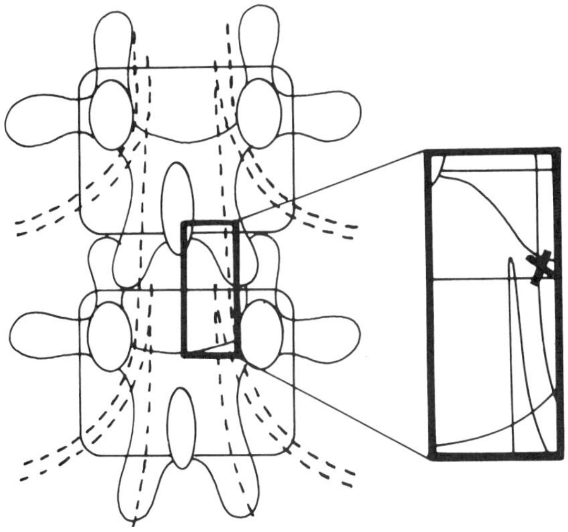

Figure 15.32 *To see the lateral border of the nerve root (x) through an interlaminar exposure, it is sometimes necessary to remove the medial edge of the superior facet.*

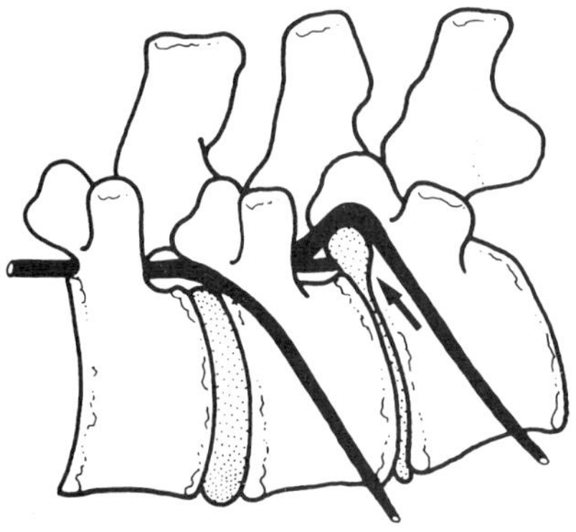

Figure 15.33 *A disc herniation at the inferior disc space (right) may displace the nerve root posteriorly (arrow), making it vulnerable to injury when the ligamentum flavum is opened.*

Ninety-five percent of surgery for lumbar disc herniations will occur at either L4–L5 or L5–S1, with the former tending to be the older patient and the latter tending to be the younger. Five percent of surgical interventions will occur at higher lumbar levels, such as L3–L4 and L2–L3.

It is important to be aware of root anomalies (62) that by their nature reduce nerve root mobility. Very small disc herniations can cause major sciatica symptoms in a patient with root anomalies. At the time of surgery, root anomalies lead to a very immobile nerve root, which leads to difficulty in getting at the more anterior pathology.

There is no uniform agreement on how much disc to remove. Williams (98) has proposed that only the ruptured portion of the disc be removed; Spengler (85) and Hudgins (34) have suggested a limited disc removal; the classic teaching is to remove all of the ruptured disc and as much intradiscal material as possible, including curettage of the endplates. We prefer the middle road of Spengler and Hudgins.

Most surgeons are now using prophylactic antibiotics at the time of and immediately after lumbar disc surgery. This is a carryover from implant surgery in orthopedics, and to date there are no statistically valid studies in the literature to support the use of prophylactic antibiotics at the time of lumbar disc surgery.

The aim of all surgical intervention is to reduce scar formation to a minimum. To this end, proposals have been made for the use of Gelfoam,(47) fat graft, and other materials.(103) The authors do not use any of these materials but rather rely on very limited microsurgical exposure and early mobilization to reduce scar tissue formation (Fig. 15.34).

Results of Posterior Microdiscectomy A study of 257 patients undergoing microsurgery for lumbar disc disease (17) (Table 15.12) revealed an 84% success rate and a 95% return to work rate in patients undergoing surgery for virgin lumbar disc herniations. Less successful but acceptable results were obtained in patients with compensation claims who had herniated nucleus pulposus and patients with previous spine surgery procedure (Table 15.13). Analysis of a complication rate of 10% (Table 15.14) revealed relative minor problems that did not affect outcomes, and a decreasing incidence of complications as experience with the procedure grew. The short-term success rate in this series compared favorably with standard laminectomy-discectomy. Along with the reduction of hospital stay (average, 2.3 days in this series), microsurgery delivered acceptable results in patients with lumbar disc herniation. With increasing confidence in the procedure, a majority of microdiscectomies are now done on an outpatient basis.

Complications of Microsurgery for Lumbar HNP There is more to learn from complications than from successes. Although there are many surgeons using microsurgical intervention for lumbar disc disease, there are many critics who believe that microsurgery is associated with several disadvantages and many additional risks. A major criticism is that inherent in the procedure are inadequate exposure of the nerve root and incomplete decompression of the encroachment pathology. Table 15.14 lists the complications experienced in the 257 microsurgical procedures done by the senior author (JM).

A general review of the literature reveals complications associated with any spine invasive procedure, as listed in Table 15.15.

There are some complications that are specific to microsurgical intervention:

Wrong Level Anyone doing any volume of microsurgery will admit that at one time or another, they have exposed the wrong level. This complication and its prevention are discussed in detail in Chapter 19.

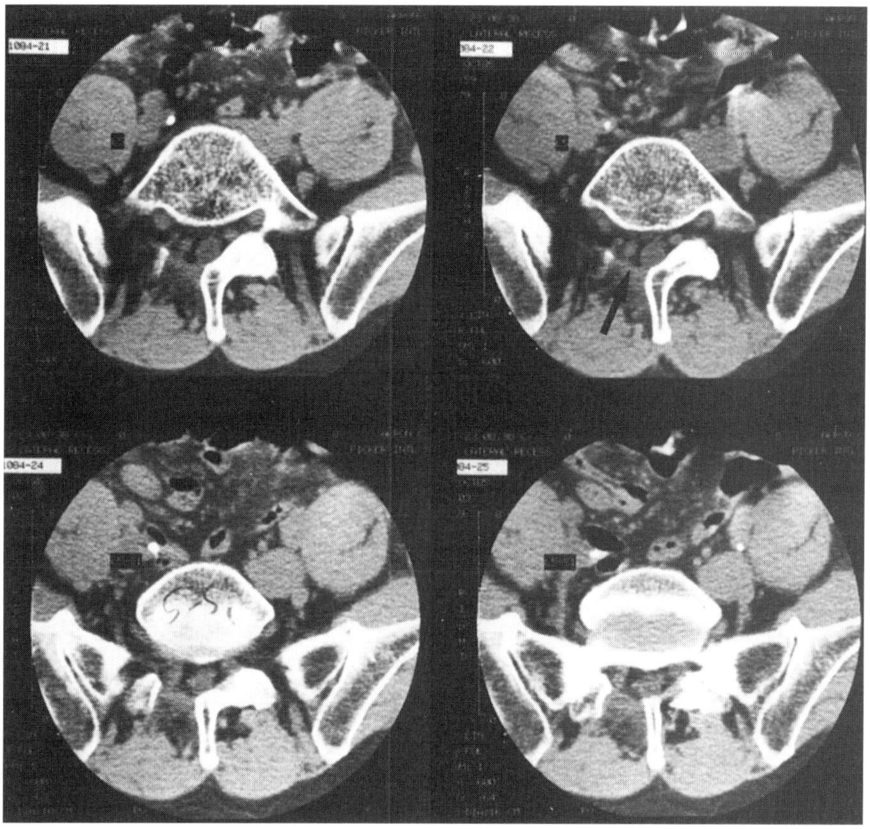

Figure 15.34 *The laminectomy membrane, L5–S1, right (arrow). No Gelfoam, no fat, just limited surgical exposure and early mobilization.*

Table 15.12. Follow-up of Patients Undergoing Microsurgery for Lumbar Disc Disease[a]

Number of patients operated on		257
Average length to follow-up		19 months
Number of patients followed up		249 (97%)
Case distribution		
Virgin HNP	119	
Lateral zone stenosis	24	
Previous procedure		
Chymopapain	70	
Laminectomy	10	
Fusion added to microdiscectomy	26	
	249	

[a]Personal series of senior author (JM).

Missed Pathology Many critics of microsurgery state that because of the limited operative field, it is easy to miss a fragment of disc material that has migrated away from the disc space, or miss bony encroachment.(71) Microsurgery for lumbar disc disease is not seek-and-find surgery; rather, by careful examination of the preoperative investigation, including the MRI or CT scan, the surgeon will know exactly what pathology is causing the symptoms and where the pathology is located.

Table 15.13. Results in Compensation Patients and Patients with Previous Surgery

		Compensation	Previous Surgery[a]
Satisfactory		66% (27)	69.7% (46)
Unsatisfactory		34% (14)	30.3% (20)
	Total	(100%) 41	(100%) 66

[a]Excluding those patients with lateral zone stenosis.

Table 15.14. Complications of Microsurgery for Lumbar HNP[a]

Condition	No. of Patients (%)	Results
Dural tear (minor)	6 (2.70)	Only 1 required repair, no problems
Wrong level exploration	6 (2.70)	Recognized and corrected at time of surgery
Hemorrhage requiring transfusion	3 (1.35)	Poor patient positioning and technique
Superficial wound infection	2 (0.90)	Resolved on antibiotics
Disc space infection	2 (0.90)	Resolved on antibiotics
Increased neurodeficit	2 (0.90)	Recovered quickly
Hematoma	1 (0.45)	Resolved spontaneously
Gastritis	1 (0.45)	Resolved
Urinary retention	1 (0.45)	Resolved
Total	24 (10.8)	

[a]Senior author's (JM) first 257 microdiscectomy procedures.

Table 15.15. Complications of Lumbar Spine Surgery [53]

Neurological damage with increased neurological deficit
Wound infection
Superficial
Deep
CSF fistula
Hematoma with or without cauda equina compression
Fatalities
Pulmonary embolus
Great vessel injury
Late complications
Spinal stenosis
Instability resulting in vertebral body translation
Scarring, with or without arachnoiditis

Reprinted with permission from Mayfield FH. Complications of laminectomy. Clin Neurosurg 1976;23: 435–439.

Intraoperative Bleeding Because of the very small incision and the limited operative field, a small amount of bleeding under the microscope appears as a major hemorrhage. It is important to take steps to prevent excessive bleeding during microsurgery, such as withdrawing patients from anti-inflammatory medications before surgery, positioning the patient properly on the table so there is no abdominal compression, and using hypotensive anesthesia. During the surgical exercise, all bleeders should be stopped the moment they occur; regular cautery should be used outside the spinal canal and bipolar cautery within the spinal canal. Since this initial experience with microsurgery (Table 15.14), the senior author (JM) has not transfused another patient.

Dural Injury The inexperienced surgeon with poor equipment is the one who causes neurological damage during microsurgical intervention. It is essential to train oneself in the technique and to have the proper instrumentation available to reduce dural injury to a minimum. In fact, under the microscope, the nerve root can be seen so well that an experienced microsurgeon is going to have less of a neurological complication rate than someone using a standard laminectomy approach without magnification.

Disc Space Infection Wilson and Harbaugh (99) have reported an increased incidence of disc space infection after microsurgery. These researchers proposed that manipulation of the microscope over the wound was the source of this increased infection rate. This occurred despite surgical draping of the microscope, which leaves exposed eyepieces that are not sterile. This has led to the use of prophylactic antibiotics and the proposal that manipulation of the microscope over the open wound should be kept to a minimum. Unrecognized disc space infections can quickly lead to disasters. (32)

Laminectomy Almost all of this section on surgical intervention has been about microsurgical intervention. There are still many surgeons who prefer the standard laminectomy/discectomy exposure, with or without loupe magnification. It really does not matter what technique you use to decompress the nerve root; if you fail to fully decompress the nerve root or introduce a complication to the equation, you have failed to serve the patient.

Special Situation with an HNP Disc herniations do not always occur in simple, uncompromised situations. Following are some unique situations relative to an HNP causing sciatica.

Herniated Nucleus Pulposus with Spondylolisthesis Patients with a spondylolisthesis may suffer from a disc rupture, which causes an acute radicular syndrome. Most of these will occur at the level above the spondylolisthesis (Fig. 15.35). A disc herniation at the same level of the slip usually occurs into the foramen (Fig. 15.35). For the former situation, simple disc excision or chemonucleolysis is all that is required; for the latter (disc excision at the slip level), discectomy should be accompanied by a stabilization procedure.

Herniated Nucleus Pulposus in Spinal Stenosis Spinal stenosis can occur in the central canal or lateral zones. It can be an asymptomatic or a mildly symptomatic condition that can suddenly convert to a significant disability when a disc herniation occurs. Investigation in these patients is somewhat inconclusive because the stenosis does not allow for a clear depiction of the disc rupture. It is only when the presenting symptoms are analyzed and the dominance of the leg pain is ascertained that one will suspect a small disc herniation in the presence of a stenotic canal or lateral zone stenosis. Simple microscopic removal of the disc herniation along with a local decompression of the stenotic segment is the proposed method of treatment. If, on history, the stenotic component was significantly symptomatic before the occurrence of the HNP, a wider decompression is needed to treat both the stenosis and the HNP.

Herniated Nucleus Pulposus in Instability Patients with a long history of back pain and significant degenerative disc disease revealed on plain radiograph may suffer from a disc herniation at the degenerative level. Whether or not this instability should be treated at the time of the disc excision is a difficult question to answer. We feel that if

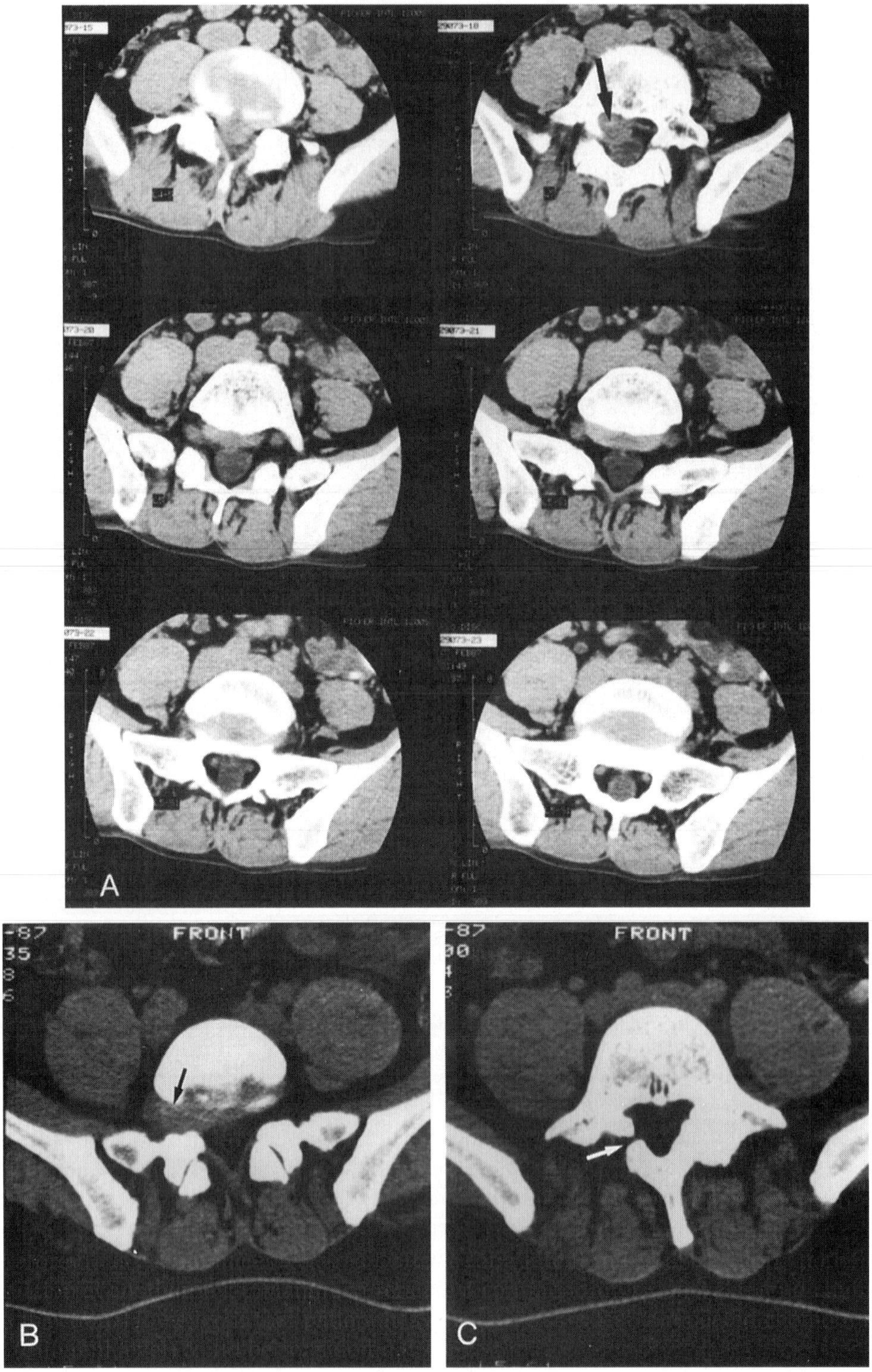

Figure 15.35 *Lytic spondylolisthesis with HNP on axial cut.* **A.** *HNP above spondylolysis at L4–L5, right (arrow).* **B.** *HNP (at slip level), that is, below lysis, L5–S1, right (arrow).* **C.** *The spondylolysis, L5, of patient in* **A.** *(arrow).*

the disc degeneration and HNP are confined to one level (see Chapter 14), it is reasonable to consider fusion. If the disc degeneration is present at multiple levels, either on plain radiograph, discography, or MRI, simple disc excision is the best choice.

Herniated Nucleus Pulposus in the Adolescent Patient The younger patient with a disc herniation is a special problem. As outlined in DeOrio and Bianco's series (13) from the Mayo Clinic, a number of these patients go on to repeat surgical procedures after their initial surgical intervention. Because of the high incidence of protrusions rather than disc extrusions, it is proposed that in this age group the optimal treatment is chemonucleolysis rather than surgical intervention.(48)

Recurrent HNP (After Discectomy) Reherniation of discal material occurs in approximately 2 to 5% of patients. The recurrence may occur at any interval after surgery (days to years) and is most often at the same level/same side. If the recurrence is at the same level/opposite side or another level, it can be considered a virgin HNP, and the principles discussed earlier in this chapter apply.

Unfortunately, most recurrences are same level/same side, and scar tissue from the previous surgery introduces a whole new element to diagnosis and treatment.

Summary

- Scarring "tacks" down the dura to the back of the disc space so that a smaller amount of herniated nuclear material is capable of producing a significant amount of pain and neurological deficit.
- Because of the immobility of the scarred dura, transdural ruptures, although rare, can occur.(33)
- Determining the anatomical level by clinical assessment can be difficult because:
- Some neurological changes are residual from the prior HNP.
- The dura may not only be immobilized, it may be distorted from the scar tissue, which leads to lower root involvement than usual for the level of the HNP (eg, a recurrent L4–L5 HNP may affect a number of sacral roots.)
- Investigation can be difficult to interpret because of the scar tissue. To a large extent, this reduces the reliability of myelography and has led to the use of intravenous Conray-enhanced CT and IV gadolinium diethylenetriamine penta-acetic acid–enhanced MRI (Fig. 15.36).
- Not only are the clinical assessment and investigation difficult, the surgery is also difficult and prone to complications such as missed pathology, dural tears, and neurological damage. A basic principle in repeated surgery is to gain as wide an exposure as possible to deal with the recurrent pathology. The microsurgeons are flying in the face of this principle, but with accurate localization of the recurrent pathology by preoperative investigation, microsurgical intervention presents some advantages.(19)

Anterior Approach

The anterior (through the abdomen) approach is mentioned only to state that the authors believe the needle, percutaneous, and microsurgical approaches are superior. The anterior discectomy (and fusion) technique should be reserved for the patient in need of salvage surgery, and it is too major an operative procedure for primary intervention for an HNP.

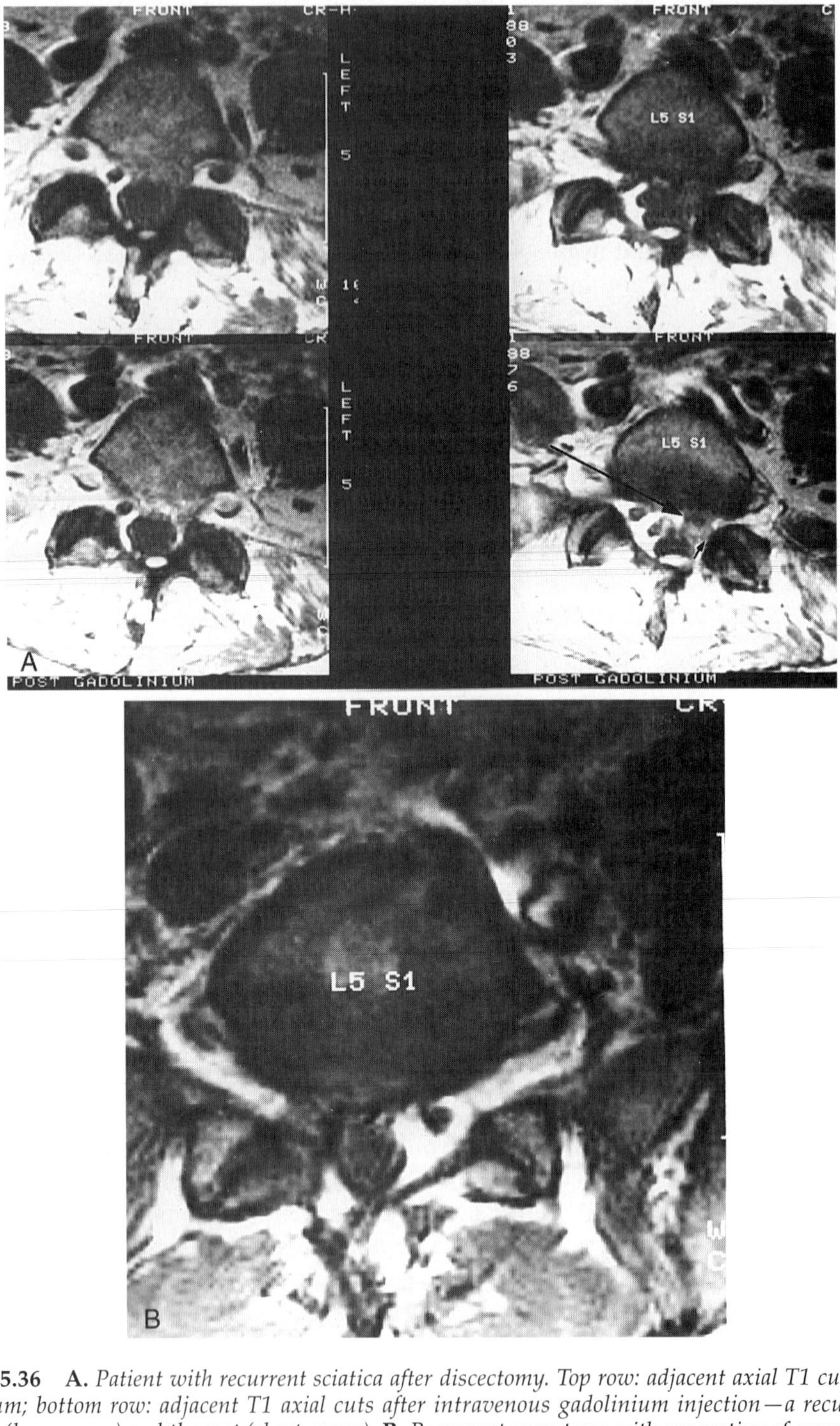

Figure 15.36 **A.** *Patient with recurrent sciatica after discectomy. Top row: adjacent axial T1 cuts without gadolinium; bottom row: adjacent T1 axial cuts after intravenous gadolinium injection—a recurrent disc fragment (long arrow) and the root (short arrow).* **B.** *Recurrent symptoms with suggestion of recurrent HNP until gadolinium was administered (arrow,* **C***).*

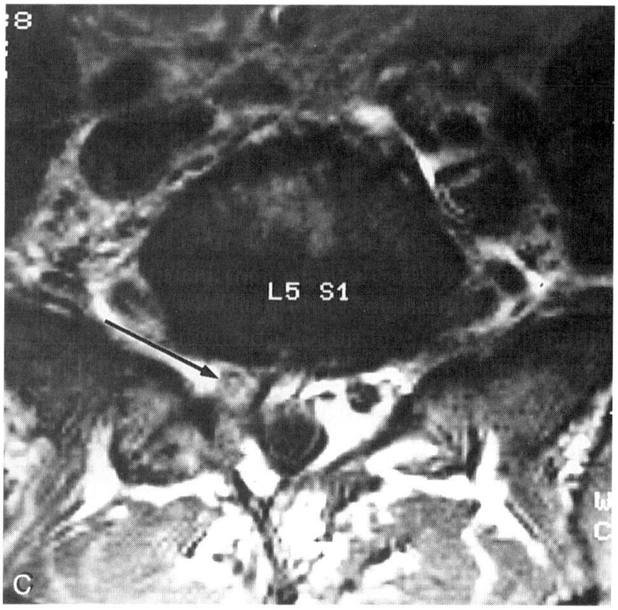

Figure 15.36 (continued)

Percutaneous Lumbar Disc Surgery

There is no question that surgery in general is moving toward least invasive/same day surgery procedures. For lumbar disc herniation, chemonucleolysis was one of those procedures. But as chymopapain complications mounted, other researchers developed yet more least invasive disc procedures, the second of which was percutaneous manual discectomy (30, 31). Subsequently, Kambin (39, 40, 41, 42) and Onik (50, 65) weighed in with their particular brand of percutaneous discectomy so that today we have as options the following:

1. Automated percutaneous lumbar discectomy (APLD) (Fig. 15.37).
2. Manual percutaneous lumbar discectomy (MPLD) with:
   a. Uniportal or biportal assist.
   b. Laser assist
   c. Working channel endoscope
   d. Laparoscopic and thoracoscopic approaches.

There are a number of poorly controlled anecdotal studies in the literature to show that percutaneous discectomy is effective in up to 85% of patients so treated.(39, 40, 41, 42) Two well-controlled studies by the Revel (68) and Findlay groups (8) have shown a success rate for APLD of 44% and 27%, respectively. These studies have seriously questioned the effectiveness of percutaneous discectomy procedures. Studies by Kahanovitz et al(38), Mathews et al(52), and Delamarter et al(12) have seriously questioned not only the efficacy of laser discectomy but the risks.(11) The authors would conclude from these studies that APLD and laser-assisted percutaneous discectomy should be abandoned.(11)

This leaves the manual percutaneous discectomy techniques to consider. One of the initial theories advanced in support of MPLD was the fact that the fenestration made laterally in the disc reduced the pressure within the disc herniation and lessened the sciatica.(35)

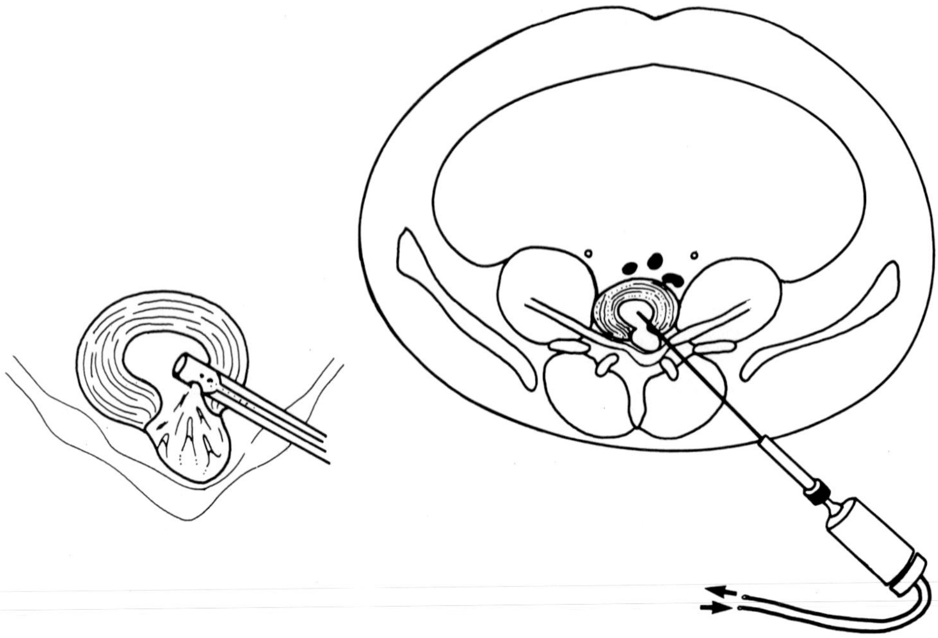

Figure 15.37 *The approach to percutaneous discectomy. The small diagram (left) represents the probe tip in the disc space, which sucks out the nuclear material.*

Some even went so far as to suggest that the reduced pressure would allow the protruded disc material to fall back into the disc space,(40,41) a concept never proved on any imaging study. The concept of an indirect MPLD violated many basic surgical principles:

1. Before a surgeon can effectively eliminate pathology, he/she must have direct view of that pathology.
2. Surgery for sciatica is really nerve root surgery, not disc surgery.(7, 23, 67, 96) The pinched nerve is causing the sciatica; it is necessary to unpinch it to relieve sciatica. The fact that additional pathology beyond a disc herniation (eg, bone spur, ligament hypertrophy, adhesions) can interfere with root function demonstrates the necessity of a direct view of the root pathology. MPLD takes the opposite approach; it attacks the disc first in an attempt to get to the nerve root.
3. More surgeons subscribe to the view that less is better within the disc space. Obviously, the root encroachment pathology has to be addressed, but no one has shown that an aggressive intradiscal excision improves the outcome of microdiscectomy. MPLD takes the reverse position of excising intradiscal material to get at the ruptured fragment.
4. Some percutaneous surgeons have suggested that their procedure is no different than knee arthroscopy when in fact there is a vast difference. Knee arthroscopy improved visualization of parts of the knee (eg, posteriorly) that were not well seen in open arthrotomy; knee arthroscopy is done through a low soft-tissue-to-portal ratio (Fig. 15.38), which is the reverse of MPLD (see Fig. 15.38); the visualization aids in knee arthroscopy are superior to those used in MPLD. Finally, the irrigation and cutting procedures are alot more favorable in the cavity of the knee than in the syndesmosis (non-cavity) of the intervertebral disc.

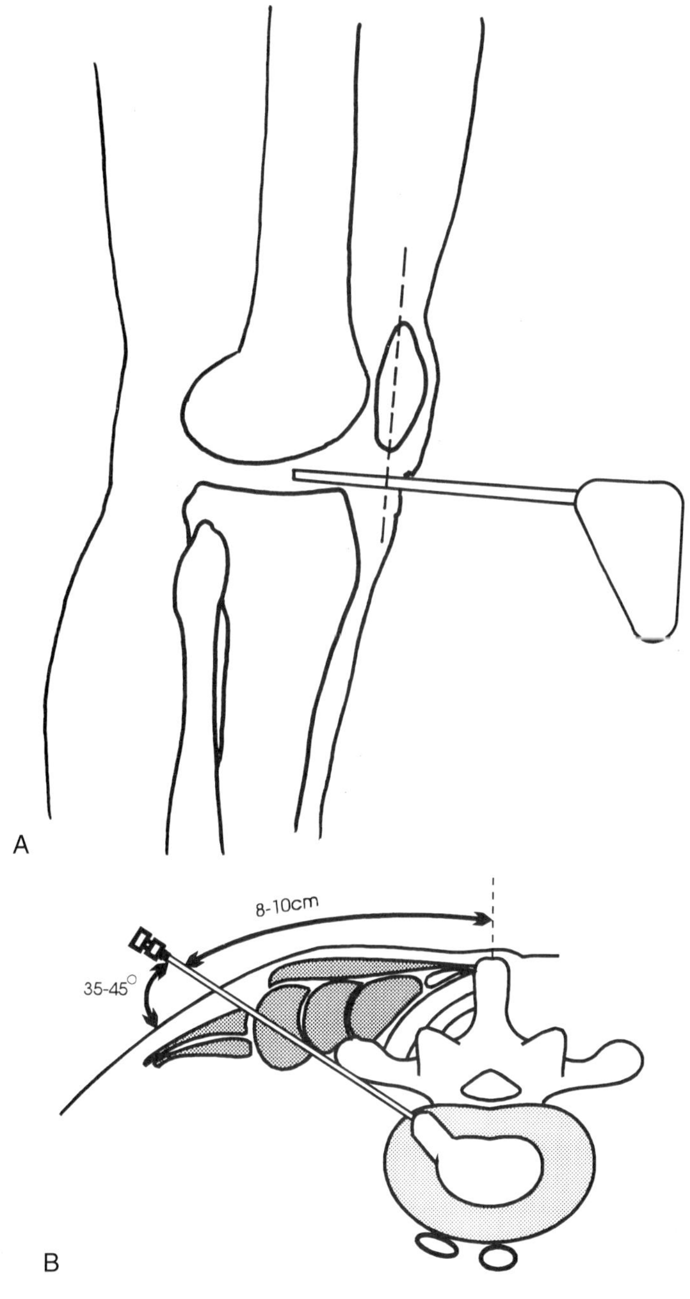

Figure 15.38 **A.** *Knee arthroscopy: soft tissue-to-cavity ratio is much less than that in B (please excuse the spine surgeon's version of an arthroscope!).* **B.** *Percutaneous discectomy: soft tissue-to-cavity ratio is much greater than that in knee arthroscopy, which makes scope manipulation more difficult.*

These facts have moved the percutaneous disc surgeons to emphasize the importance of seeing the back of the disc space with scopes that look posteriorly and instruments that turn the corner. Obviously, rapid technical changes are occurring as the percutaneous surgeons accept the importance of a direct view of the pathology. It remains to be seen if they can produce scientifically validated studies to show that they are on the right tract. For now, the authors consider all of the percutaneous disc procedures experimental, which is a view contrary to that of Schreiber's group.(74)

Unfortunately, the field is being patient and commercially driven, that is, "I want the probe surgery," "I want the profits." This opens the field to abuse that arises out of sweet talking vendors seeking a living and surgeons seeking a public identity. But we should all remember that the answers to patients should be different than those to shareholders in a company selling these tools, and that it is essential to produce scientific studies to support the cause of MPLD. To date, these studies are not available.(86)

Conclusion

Since Mixter and Barr introduced us to the disc rupture causing sciatica,(60) the acute radicular syndrome has become an easy condition to diagnose, most often responds to conservative treatment, and when that fails, it yields good results after surgery. For spine practitioners, and especially surgeons, this condition is a winner, gratifying to both the patient and the doctor.

The bony root entrapment syndromes and lateral zone disc herniations discussed in the next chapter are more difficult to diagnose and treat and thus have the potential for delivering less than satisfactory results to treatment intervention.

APPENDIX

Ingredients and Instructions for Mixing Skin Test Solution

Ingredients and Equipment

Buffer: Albany buffered saline and phenol diluent for allergenic extract: 4.5-mL vials.
Glycerol: 99.5%—any local pharmacy should have this.
Chymodiactin: Manufactured by Boots Pharmaceuticals, Inc. Obtain through your hospital pharmacy.
Dropper Bottles: Two small (1-oz) sterile dropper bottles.

Skin Test

Do not mix Chymodiactin with sterile water as indicated by the package insert. This is only for disc injection purposes. For the skin test, use 1 mL of buffer to mix Chymodiactin and withdraw from the vial and put into one dropper bottle. Add 1 mL of glycerol and shake. This skin test solution should set at room temperature for the first 24 hours so that the active enzymatic component is spent.

Control Solution

In the second dropper bottle, combine 1 mL of glycerol and 1 mL of buffer. You now have your control solution. Both of these solutions should be refrigerated when not in use.

Test

The standard prick test involves one drop of each solution on the skin that is then pricked. Read in 15 minutes. A positive test is a wheal of 5 mm or more, with a surrounding flare of 10 mm or more at the Chymodiactin test site that is much greater than that of the control site.

REFERENCES

1. Armstrong JR. Lumbar disc lesions. Pathogenesis and treatment of low back pain and sciatica. Baltimore: Williams & Wilkins; 1965.
2. Aronson HA, Dunsmore RH. Herniated upper lumbar discs. J Bone Joint Surg 1963;45A:311–317.
3. Bell GR, Rothman RH. The conservative treatment of sciatica. Spine 1984;9:54–56.
4. Boden SD, Davis DO, Dina TS, et al. Abnormal magnetic resonance scans of the lumbar spine in asymptomatic subjects. J Bone Joint Surg 1990;72:403–408.
5. Bouillet R. Complications of discal hernia therapy. Comparative study regarding surgical therapy and nucleolysis by chymopapain. Acta Ortho Belg 1983;suppl I:49-48.
6. Bouillet R. Treatment of sciatica. A comparative survey of complications of surgical treatment and nucleolysis with chymopapain. Clin Orthop 1990;251:144–152.
7. Brown HA, Pont MR. Disease of lumbar discs. Ten years of surgical treatment. J Neurosurg 1963;20:410–417.
8. Chatterjee S, Foy PM, Findlay GF. Report of a controlled clinical trial comparing automated percutaneous lumbar discectomy and microdiscectomy in the treatment of contained lumbar disc herniation. Spine 1995;20:734–738.
9. Chokroverty S, Reyers MG, Rubino FA, et al. The syndrome of diabetic amyotrophy. Ann Neurol 1977;2:181–194.
10. Cram RH. A sign of nerve root pressure. J Bone Joint Surg 1953;35B:192–195.
11. Delamarter RB. Personal communication; 1994.
12. Delamarter RB, Howard MW, Goldstein T, Deutsch AL, Mink JH, Dawson EG. Percutaneous lumbar discectomy: preoperative and postoperative magnetic resonance imaging. J Bone Joint Surg 1995;77:578–584.
13. DeOrio JK, Bianco AJ. Lumbar disc excision in children and adolescents. J Bone Joint Surg 1982;64A:991–996.
14. Dyck P. The femoral nerve traction test with lumbar disc protrusions. Surg Neurol 1976;6: 163–166.
15. Emmett JL, Love JG. Urinary retention in women caused by asymptomatic protruded lumbar disk: report of 5 cases. J Urol 1968;99:597–606.
16. Fager CA. Observations on spontaneous recovery from intervertebral disc herniation. Surg Neurol 1994;42:282–286.
17. Feldman R, McCulloch JA. Microsurgery for lumbar disc disease. In: McCulloch JA, ed. Principles of Microsurgery for Lumbar Disc Disease. New York: Raven Press; 1989.
18. Fraser RD. Chymopapain for the treatment of intervertebral disc herniation. Spine 1982;7:608.
19. Goald HJ. A new microsurgical reoperation for failed lumbar disc surgery. J Microsurgery 1986; 7:63–66.
20. Gogan WJ, Fraser RD. Chymopapain: a 10 year double blind study. Spine 1992;17:388–394.
21. Graf CJ, Hamby WB. Paraplegia in lumbar intervertebral disk protrusion, with remarks on high lumbar disk protrusion. NY Med J 1953;53:2346–2348.

22. Gunn CC, Chir B, Milbrand WE. Tenderness at motor points; a diagnostic and prognostic aid to low back injury. J Bone Joint Surg 1976;58A:815–825.
23. Gurdjian ES, Webster JE, Ostrowski AZ, et al. Herniated lumbar intervertebral discs—an analysis of 1176 operated cases. J Trauma 1961;1:158–176.
24. Gutterman P, Shenkin JA. Syndromes associated with protrusion of upper lumbar intervertebral disc. J Neurosurg 1973;38:499–503.
25. Hakelius A. Prognosis in sciatica: a clinical follow-up of surgical and non-surgical treatment. Acta Orthop Scand 1970;129(suppl):1–76.
26. Hall BB, McCulloch JA. Anaphylactic reactions following the intradiscal injection of chymopapain under local anesthesia. J Bone Joint Surg 1983;65A:1215.
27. Harati Y. Diabetic peripheral neuropathies. Ann Intern Med 1987;107:546–559.
28. Hardy RW Jr, David HR Jr. Extradural spinal cord and nerve root compression from benign lesions of the lumbar area. In: Youmans JR, ed. Neurological Surgery. Philadelphia: WB Saunders; 1990.
29. Hardy RW Jr, Plank NM. Clinical diagnosis of herniated lumbar disc. In: Hardy RW Jr, ed. Lumbar Disc Disease. New York: Raven Press; 1982, pp 17–28.
30. Hijikata S. Percutaneous nucleotomy. A new concept technique and 12 years' experience. Clin Orthop 1989;238:9–23.
31. Hijikata A, Yamagishi M, Nakayama T, et al. Percutaneous nucleotomy: a new treatment method for lumbar disc herniation. J Toden Hosp 1975;5:39.
32. Hlavin ML, Kaminski HL, Ross JS, et al. Spinal epidural abscess: a ten year perspective. Neurosurgery 1990;27:177–184.
33. Hodge CJ, Binet EF, Keiffer SA. Intradural herniation of lumbar intravertebra disc. Spine 1979;3:346–350.
34. Hudgins WR. The role of microdiscectomy. Orthop Clin North Am 1983;14:589–603.
35. Hult L. Retroperitoneal disc fenestration in lower back pain and sciatica. A preliminary report. Acta Orthop Scand 1950;20:342–348.
36. Jansen EF, Balls AK. Chymopapain: new crystalline proteinase from papaya latex. J Biol Chem 1941;137:459–460.
37. Javid JJ, et al. Safety and efficacy of chymopapain (chymodiactin) in herniated nucleus pulposus with sciatica. JAMA 1983;249:2489–2494.
38. Kahanovitz N, Viola K, Goldstein T, Dawson E. A multicenter analysis of percutaneous discectomy. Spine 1990;15:713–717.
39. Kambin P, Brager MD. Percutaneous posterolateral discectomy. Anatomy and mechanism. Clin Orthop 1987;223:145–154.
40. Kambin P, Gellman H. Percutaneous lateral discectomy of the lumbar spine —a preliminary report. Clin Orthop 1983;174:127–132.
41. Kambin P, Sampson S. Posterolateral percutaneous suction-excision of herniated lumbar intervertebral discs. Report of interim results. Clin Orthop 1986;207:37–43.
42. Kambin P, Schaffer JL. Percutaneous lumbar discectomy. Review of 100 patients and current practice. Clin Orthop 1989;238:24–34.
43. Keegan J. Dermatome hypalgesia associated with herniation of intervertebral disk. Arch Neurol Psychiatry 1943;50:67–83.
44. Kelsey JL. An epidemiological study of acute herniated lumbar intervertebral disc. Rheumatol Rehabil 1975;14:144–159.
45. Kitaoka H, McCulloch JA. Microdiscectomy for failed chemonucleolysis. Neuro-orthopedics 1988;5:45–51.
46. Lahad A, Malter AD, Berg AO, Deyo RA. The effectiveness of four interventions for the prevention of low back pain. JAMA 1994;272:1286–1291.
47. LaRocca A, Macnab I. The laminectomy membrane. J Bone Joint Surg 1974;56B:545–550.

48. Lorenz M, McCulloch JA. Chemonucleolysis for herniated nucleus pulposus in adolescents. J Bone Joint Surg 1985;67A:1402–1404.
49. Macnab I, McCulloch JA, Wiener DS, et al. Chemonucleolysis. Can J Surg 1971;14:280–284.
50. Maroon JC, Onik G. Percutaneous automated discectomy: a new method for lumbar disc removal. Technical note. J Neurosurg 1987;66:143–146.
51. Maroon JC, Schulhof LA, Kopitnik TA. Diagnosis and microsurgical approach to far lateral disc herniation in the lumbar spine. J Neurosurg 1990;72:382–387.
52. Mathews HH, Kyles MK, Fiore SM, Long BH. Laser disc decompression with KTP532 wavelength: a two year follow-up. AAOS presentation paper No. 292. Orlando, Fla; February 1994.
53. Mayfield FH. Complications of laminectomy. Clin Neurosurg 1976;23:435–439.
54. McCulloch JA. Chemonucleolysis for relief of sciatica due to a herniated intervertebral disc. Can Med Assoc J 1981;124:880–883.
55. McCulloch JA. Outpatient discolysis with chymopapain. Orthopedics 1983;6:1624–1628.
56. McCulloch JA, Brock M. Unpublished data,1985.
57. McCulloch JA, Dolovich G, Canham W. Skin testing for chymopapain allergy: a preliminary report. Ann Allergy 1985;55:609–611.
58. McCulloch JA, Lambe D. Unpublished data,1987.
59. McLaren AC, Bailey SI. Cauda equina syndrome: a complication of lumbar discectomy. Clin Orthop 1986;204:143–149.
60. Mixter WJ, Barr JS. Rupture of the intervertebral disc with involvement of the spinal canal. N Engl J Med 1934;211:210–215.
61. Morris J. Complications of chemonucleolysis. Presented at Spine Update, San Francisco; 1984.
62. Neidre AN, Macnab I. Anomalies of the lumbosacral nerve roots. Review of 16 cases and classification. Spine 1983;8:294–299.
63. Nordby EJ. Chemonucleolysis. In: Frymoyer JW, ed. The Adult Spine. New York: Raven Press; 1991, p 1744.
64. Norlen G. On the value of neurological symptoms in sciatica for localization of a lumbar disc herniation. Acta Chir Scand 1944;95(suppl):7–95.
65. Onik G, Helms CA, Ginsburg L, Hoaglund FT, Morris J. Percutaneous lumbar diskectomy using a new aspiration probe. AJR 1985;144:1137–1140.
66. Parkinson D, Shields C. Treatment of protruded lumbar intervertebral discs with chymopapain. J Neurosurg 1973;39:203.
67. Raaf J. Some observations regarding 905 patients operated upon for protruded lumbar intervertebral disc. Am J Surg 1959;97:388–397.
68. Revel M, Payan C, Vallee C, et al. Automated percutaneous discectomy versus chemonucleolysis in the treatment of sciatica. Spine 1993;1:1–7.
69. Rosomoff HL, Johnston JDH, Gallo AE, et al. Cystometry as an adjunct in the evaluation of lumbar disc syndromes. J Neurosurg 1970;33:67–74.
70. Ross JC, Jameson RM. Vesical dysfunction due to prolapsed disc. Br Med J 1971;3:752–754.
71. Rothman RH, Simeone FA, Bernini PM. Lumbar disc disease. In: Rothman RH, Simeone FA, eds. The Spine. Philadelphia: WB Saunders; 1982:508–645.
72. Rydevik B, et al. Effects of chymopapain on nerve tissue. Spine 1976;2:237.
73. Schreiber A, Suezawa Y. Transdiscoscopic percutaneous nucleotomy in disk herniation. Orthop Rev 1986;15:75–78.
74. Schreiber A, Suezawa Y, Leu H. Does percutaneous nucleotomy with discoscopy replace conventional discectomy? Eight years of experience and results in treatment of herniated lumbar disc. Clin Orthop 1989;238:35–42.
75. Schwetschenau PR, Ramirez A, Johnston J, et al. Double-blind evaluations of intradiscal chymopapain for herniated lumbar discs. Early results. J Neurosurg 1976;45:622.

76. Scoville WB, Corkilig G. Lumbar disc surgery: technique of radical removal and early mobilization. J Neurosurg 1973;39:265–269.
77. Shepperd JA, James SE, Leach AB. Percutaneous disc surgery. Clin Orthop 1989;238:43–49.
78. Smith L. Enzyme dissolution of nucleus pulposus in humans. JAMA 1964;187:137.
79. Smith Laboratories, Inc, Northbrook, Ill. Data from post-marketing surveillance, 1985.
80. Smith Laboratories, Inc, Northbrook, Ill.Product brochure.3
81. Smith Laboratories, Inc, Northbrook, Ill. Product brochure.4
82. Smith Laboratories, Inc, Northbrook, Ill. Product information letter, July 1984.
83. Spangfort EV. The lumbar disc herniation. A computer-aided analysis of 2,504 operations. Acta Orthop Scand 1972;142(suppl):1–95.
84. Spangfort E Lasègue's sign in patients with lumbar disc herniation. Acta Orthop Scand 1971;42:459–460.
85. Spengler DM. Lumbar discectomy: results with limited disc excision and selective foraminotomy. Spine 1982;7:604–607.
86. Spengler DM. Percutaneous Discectomy: Where's the beef? (editorial). J Spinal Disord 1990;3:383.
87. Smyth MJ, Wright V. Sciatica and the intervertebral disc. An experimental study. J Bone Joint Surg 1958;40A:1401–1418.
88. Spurling RG, Grantham EG. Neurologic picture of herniations of the nucleus pulposus in the lower part of the lumbar region. Arch Surg 1940;40:375–388.
89. Travenol Laboratories, Inc. New Drug Application 18–625. (Submitted to United States Food and Drug Administration on April 24, 1981.)
90. Tregoning GD, Transfeldt EE, McCulloch JA, Macnab I, Nachemson A. Chymopapain versus conventional surgery for lumbar disc herniation. J Bone Joint Surg 1991;73B:481–486.
91. Wakano K, Kasman R, Chao EY, Bradford DS, Oegema TR Jr. Biochemical analysis of canine intervertebral disc after chymopapain injection: a preliminary report. Spine 1983;8:59.
92. Waddell G, Main C. Assessment of severity in low-back disorders. Spine 1984;9:204–208.
93. Waddell G, Main CJ, Morris EW, et al. Chronic low back pain, psychological distress and illness behavior. Spine 1984;9:209–213.
94. Weber H. Lumbar disc herniation: a controlled prospective study with ten years of observation. Spine 1983;8:131–140.
95. Weiner DS, Macnab I. The use of chymopapain in degenerative disc disease: a preliminary report. Can Med Asoc J 1970;102:1252.
96. Weir BKA. Prospective study of 100 lumbosacral discectomies. J Neurosurg 1979;50:283–289.
97. Wilkins RH, Brody IA. Lasègue's sign. Arch Neurol 1969;21:219–221.
98. Williams R. Microlumbar discectomy: a conservative surgical approach to the virgin herniated lumbar disc. Spine 1978;3:175–182.
99. Wilson D, Harbaugh R. Microsurgical and standard removal of protruded lumbar disc. A comparative study. Neurosurgery 1981;8:422–427.
100. Wiltse LL. Chymopapain chemonucleolysis in lumbar disc disease. JAMA 1975:233:1164.
101. Wiltse LL, Widell EH, Hansen AY. Chymopapain chemonucleolysis in lumbar disc disease. JAMA 1975;231:474–479.
102. Woodhall B, Hayes GJ. The well-leg raising test of Fajersztajn in the diagnosis of ruptured lumbar intervertebral disc. J Bone Joint Surg 1950;32A:786–792.
103. Yong-Hing K, Reilly J, DeKorompay V, Kirkaldy-Willis WH. Prevention of nerve root adhesions after laminectomy. Spine 1980;5:59–64.

16

Disc Degeneration with Root Irritation–The Lateral Zone: Disc Ruptures and Bony Root Entrapment Syndromes

"Physicians think they do a lot for a patient when they give his disease a name."

— Immanuel Kant (1800)

INTRODUCTION

No better description of the lateral lumbar zone has been given than in Macnab's well-read and often quoted article on "Negative Disc Exploration,"(18) in which he introduced the term "hidden zone" (Fig. 16.1). Since that time, spinal surgeons have struggled to decompress that zone without removing the inferior facet to cause spinal instability. All too often, in the orthopedic community, the facet has been saved to the detriment of an adequate decompression of the foramen, whereas in the neurosurgical community, an adequate decompression has been completed at the expense of the facet joint, which has possibly led to subsequent instability. A recent study has shown that the single most detrimental event that precludes a good result to discectomy is the loss of a facet joint at surgery.

Two things have happened in the last 10 years to renew focus on the lateral zone: (1) The computed tomography (CT) scan and magnetic resonance image (MRI) have shown us just how much pathology can be located in the lateral zone. (2) The microscope has opened avenues for new approaches to this hidden zone.

The lateral zone is divided into three sections (regions) based on the relationship with the pedicle above. The first region, or entrance zone (Fig. 16.2), is designated the subarticular region because it lies immediately anterior to the medial edge of the superior facet. The second region, or midzone, is designated the foraminal region and lies inferior to the pedicle. The third and most lateral region of the lateral zone is known as the extraforaminal region or exit zone.

Subarticular Zone

The subarticular zone (Fig. 16.3) extends from the tip of the superior facet to the base of the superior facet. It has, as its anterior wall, the first story of the segment above and the

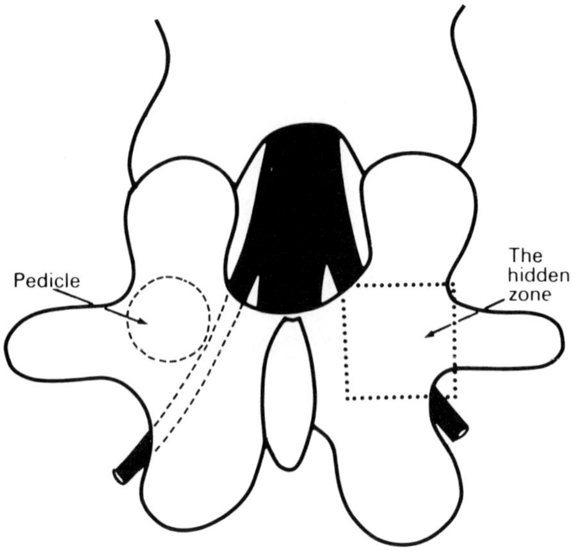

Figure 16.1 *The hidden zone.*

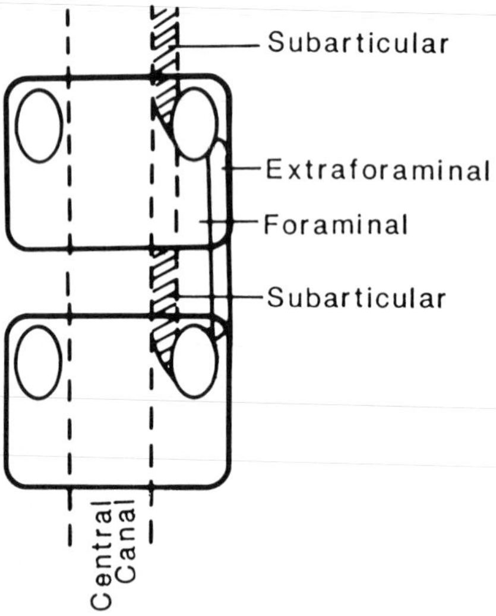

Figure 16.2 *The three sections to the lateral zone.*

third story of its own segment (Fig. 16.4). This zone has been designated the entrance zone by Lee et al (16), and contains the nerve root (Fig. 16.4).

Foraminal Zone (Foramen, Nerve Root Canal)

This middle zone has, as its upper and lower boundaries, the two adjacent pedicles (Fig. 16.5). The most important aspect of this zone is shown in Figure 16.6: the foramen or nerve root canal has no bony roof or posterior bony covering except at the L5 level, and there only its medial portion has a bony roof. The posterior cover or boundary of the foramen is the intertransverse ligament, an easy structure to cross to gain entry into the foramen. This zone is the midzone in Lee's classification and contains the dorsal root ganglion (Fig. 16.4).

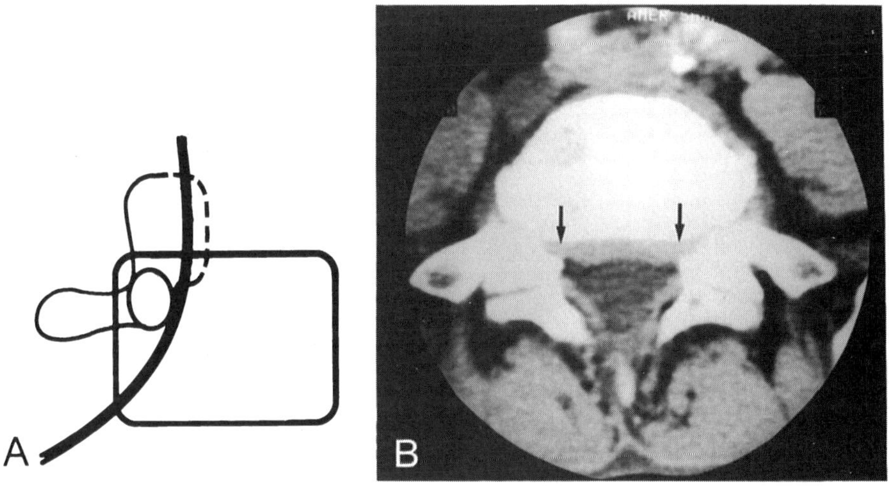

Figure 16.3 **A.** *Schematic of the subarticular zone: under the dotted "hypertrophied" medial edge of the superior facet.* **B.** *Hypertrophy of the medial edge of the superior facet (degenerative arthritis of the facet joint forming a "facet spur") creates the subarticular zone (bilateral L5–S1 in this axial CT [arrows]).*

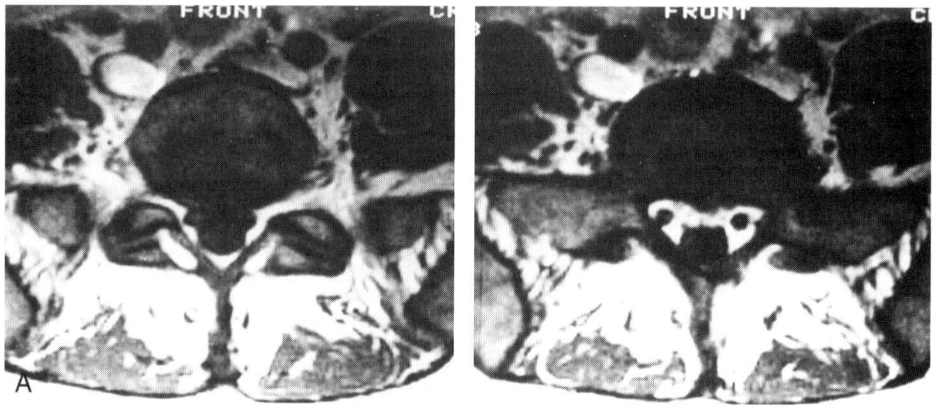

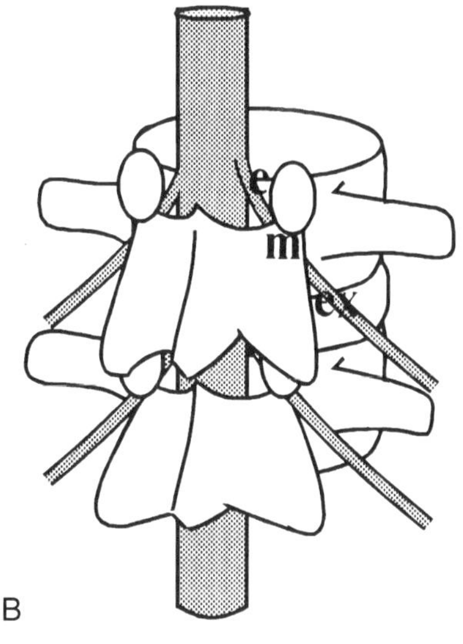

Figure 16.4 **A.** *The normal subarticular zone for the S1 root. Left, the cephalad portion, immediately adjacent to the medial edge of the superior facet, located in the first story of L5. Right, the caudal portion, again immediately adjacent to the medial edge of the superior facet, located in the third story of S1.* **B.** *The entrance (e), mid (m), and exit (ex) zones.*

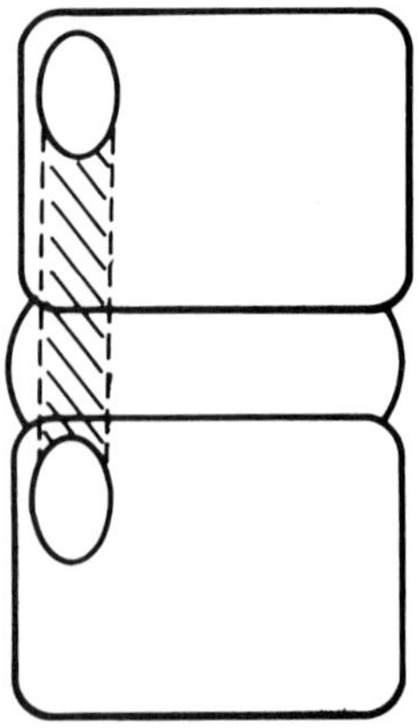

Figure 16.5 *The boundaries of the foraminal zone.*

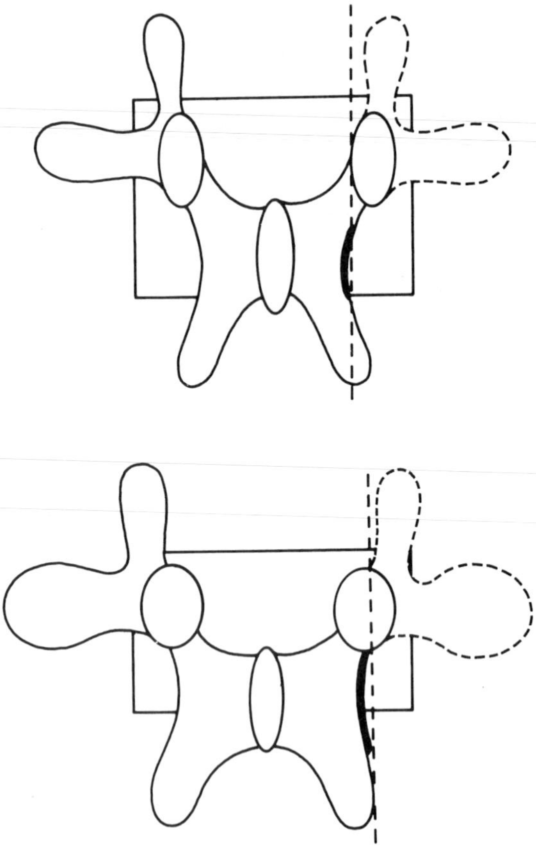

Figure 16.6 *Top, the lateral border of the pars is on the same sagittal plane as the medial border of the pedicle at all levels except L5 (bottom). The foramen, in other words, has no bony root.*

Extraforaminal Zone (Far Out Zone of Wiltse)

This zone (29) is the most lateral of the three subsections to the lateral zone (Fig. 16.7), and in Lee's classification is designated as the exit zone. It contains the peripheral nerve.

CLASSIFICATION OF DISORDERS

There are two lateral zone conditions that interfere with the smooth exit of a nerve root from the spinal canal:

1. Disc ruptures.
2. Degenerative disc disease with osteophytes.

Disc Ruptures

Macnab (18) was the first to describe the two disc ruptures that occur in the lateral zone (Fig. 16.8):

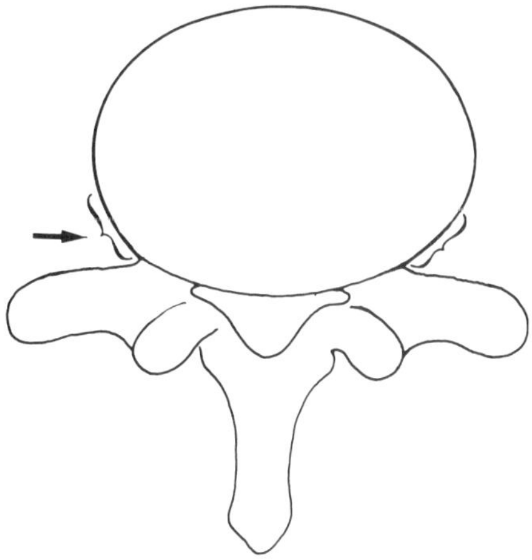

Figure 16.7 *The extraforaminal zone (braces and arrow on each side of vertebral body, adjacent to pedicles).*

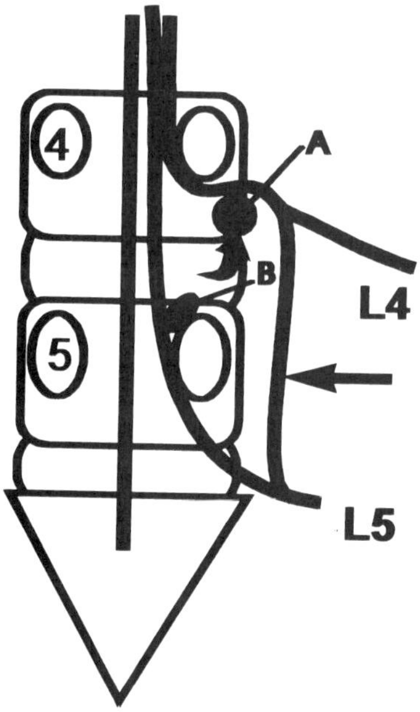

Figure 16.8 *The two disc ruptures into the lateral zone:* **A.** *A true foraminal rupture.* **B.** *Into "no man's land." The furcal nerve (arrow) is an important branch connecting the lumbar and sacral plexi, and is outside the spinal canal.*

1. The foraminal disc rupture (superior and lateral migration from the disc space below).
2. A disc rupture into "no man's land" (inferior and medial migration from the disc space above), so named because patients present with an obvious acute radicular syndrome, yet no lesion is seen on MRI and the subannular disc rupture can be easily overlooked in surgery.

The Foraminal Disc Rupture

Definition

There is considerable confusion of terminology when describing the foraminal herniated nucleus pulposus (HNP). What one author describes as a foraminal HNP,(2) another describes as extraforaminal,(21) whereas a different author includes annular bulging of segmental instability in the "catchall" category of a foraminal HNP.(7) For the purpose of this

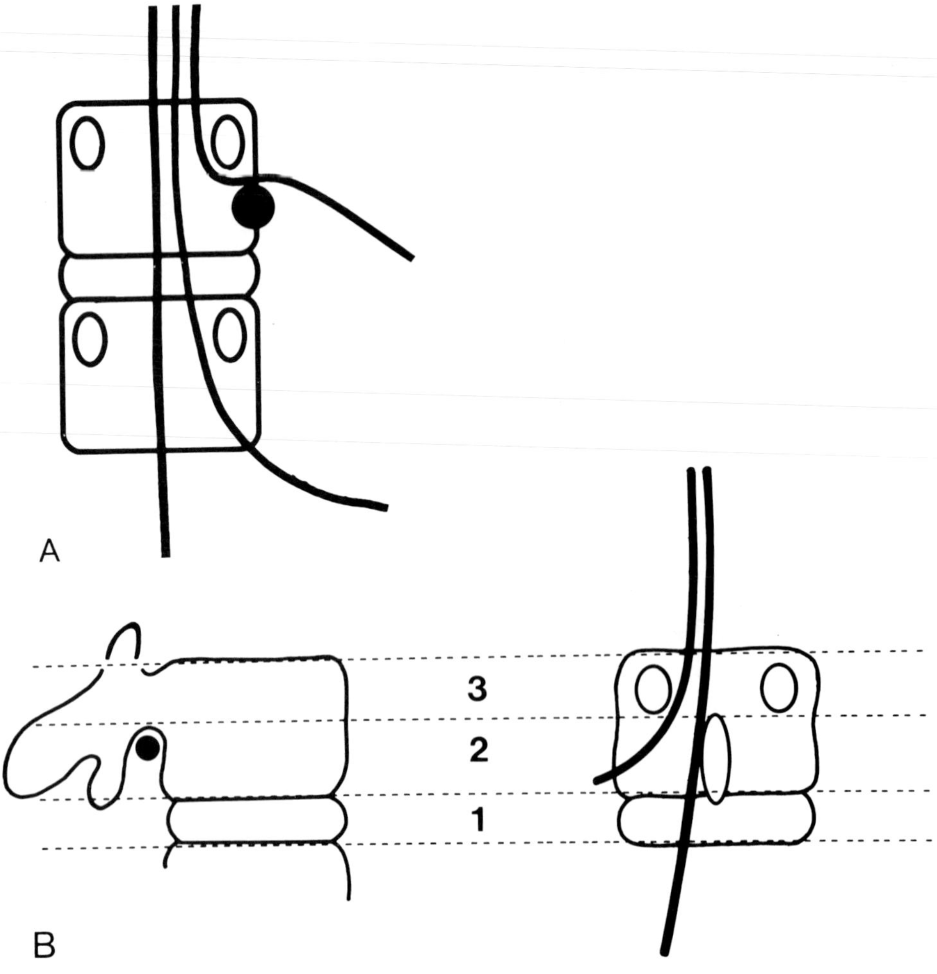

Figure 16.9 **A.** *A foraminal disc herniation on schematic.* **B.** *A foraminal disc herniation lies in the second story after migrating cephalad from the first story. It compresses the exiting nerve root rather than the traversing root.*

discussion, a foraminal disc herniation is described as a disc rupture that compresses the exiting, rather than the traversing, nerve root (Fig. 16.9), and causes a dominant radicular syndrome (ie, more leg pain than back pain). Anything else, (eg, annular bulging, patients with mostly back pain) is excluded from our discussion of the foraminal disc rupture.

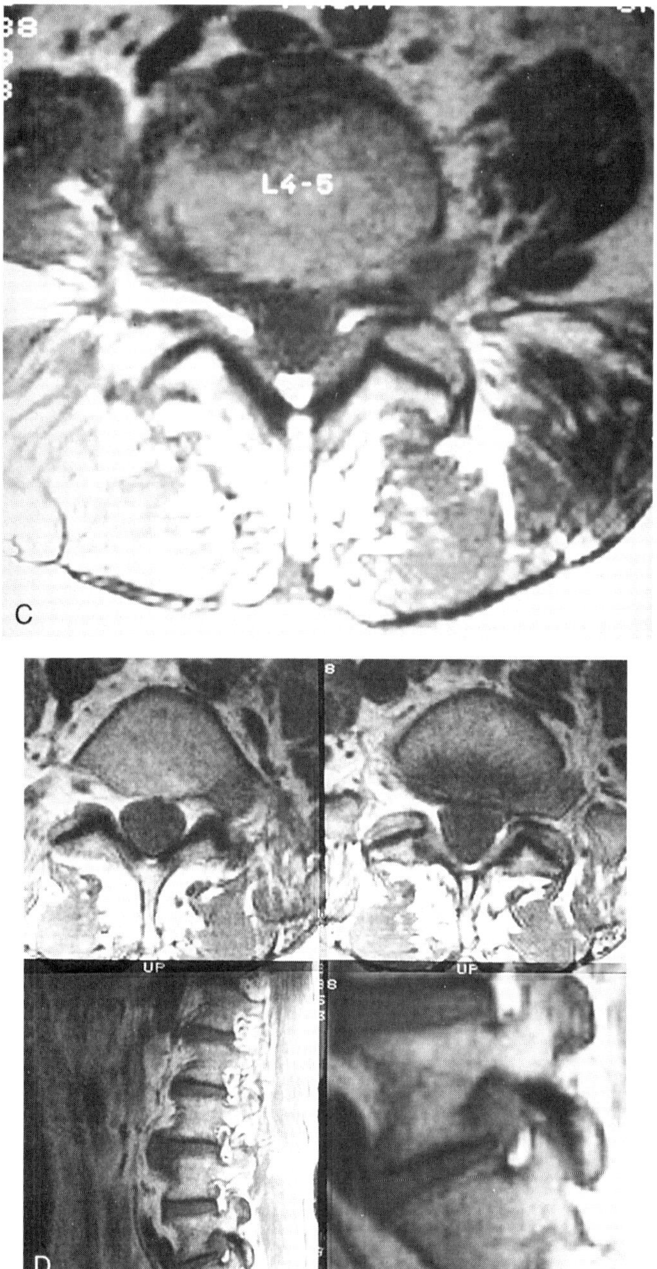

Figure 16.9 (continued) **C.** *A left foraminal disc herniation L4–L5 (T1 axial MRI).* **D.** *A foraminal disc herniation L5–S1 on MRI. This is an unusual location for a foraminal disc rupture, and 50% of foraminal disc herniations at this level will have an associated spondylolysis.*

The symptomatic HNP usually presents as an acute radicular syndrome. As described in the previous chapter, the classic posterolateral HNP is usually associated with more leg and buttock pain (than back pain), neurological symptoms and/or signs, and marked reduction of straight leg raising (SLR). The foraminal HNP also presents with dominant leg pain. Recent reports on foraminal HNP have brought the clinical and radiological description of this phenomenon to our attention.(1, 6, 13, 15, 17, 19) Because myelography was frequently nonconclusive for this type of disc herniation,(9, 22) the condition usually went undiagnosed in the past. However, with the advent of CT scanning and MRI as diagnostic modalities, the occurrence of foraminal disc herniations has turned out to be quite frequent.(11, 32)

Nature of the HNP

Figure 16.9 depicts an important aspect of the foraminal HNP. Disc ruptures are usually in the posterolateral portion of the disc space interval, that is, the first story. However, disc ruptures may migrate (Fig. 16.10), and the most common migratory pattern for a disc herniation is caudad, to lie beside the pedicle of the vertebral level below. This disc herniation has left the first story of one segment to enter the third story of the level below (Fig. 16.11). Less common is a laterally directed disc herniation as depicted in Figure 16.12. Note that this disc herniation is opposite the disc space and appears contiguous with the discal cavity. This direct lateral protrusion of disc material still lies within the first story of

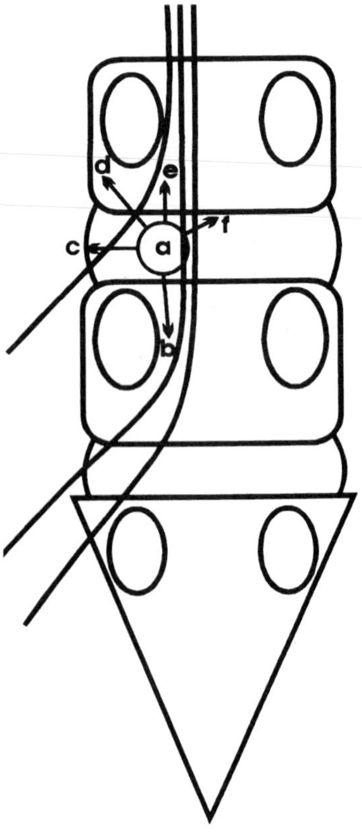

Figure 16.10 *(a) Circle represents the usual posterolateral location of an HNP. Migratory patterns of disc ruptures are: b, pedicle (third story); c, lateral (first story); d, foraminal (second story); e, behind vertebral body (second story); f, midline (first story).*

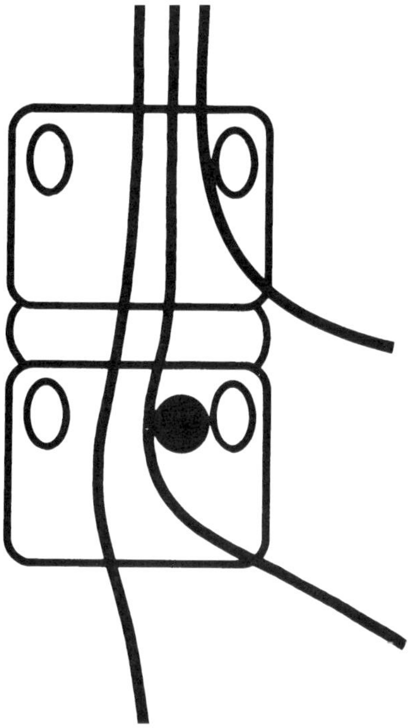

A

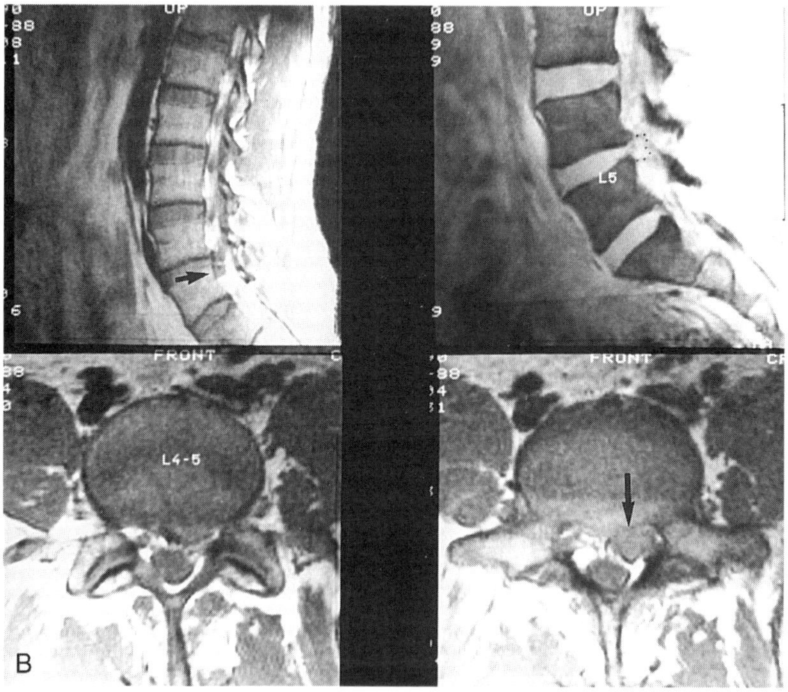

B

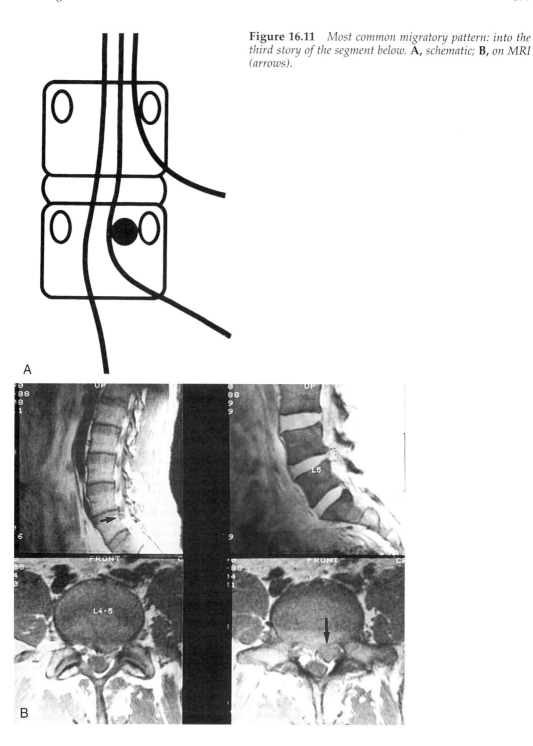

Figure 16.11 *Most common migratory pattern: into the third story of the segment below.* **A,** *schematic;* **B,** *on MRI (arrows).*

the anatomical segment. If a disc herniation migrates, not only laterally but also cephalad into the second story as depicted in Figure 16.9, it is likely to be an extruded or sequestered fragment of disc material. It is important to distinguish these two types of disc herniations because a lateral disc herniation is likely to be a simple protrusion, opposite

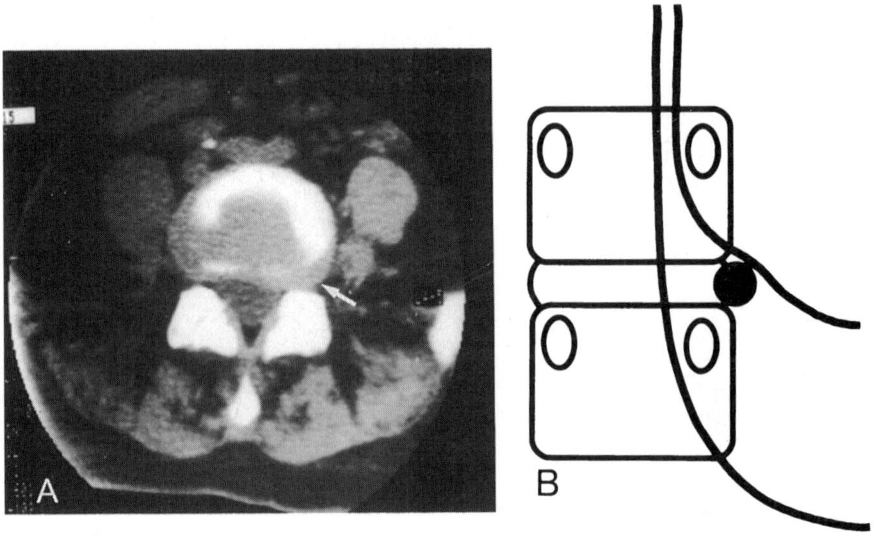

Figure 16.12 **A.** *A lateral disc bulge, (arrow), still in the first story. This most often is a manifestation of annular bulging and a stage of instability.* **B.** *Schematic of the location of a lateral disc bulge or herniation. Note its location in the first story versus the second story location of a foraminal HNP in schematic and Figure 16.9 A and C.*

and directly connected with the disc space, whereas the foraminal disc herniation, because it has left the first story to enter the second story, is no longer opposite the disc space and is almost certainly a disc extrusion or sequestration. This last type of disc herniation occurs in 1.7% to 4.4% (1, 9, 15, 22) of patients with a disc rupture and is the subject of this section.

Clinical Presentation of the Foraminal HNP

1. This is a disc herniation of the older population. The average age of a patient with a canal disc herniation is 40±2 years; the average age of a patient with a foraminal disc herniation is 60±2 years. (Women = Men, and Left = Right).
2. The radicular pain caused by this disc rupture is frightfully severe. More often than not, the patients arrive in wheelchairs, with a story of not having slept many a night because of the severity of pain. It is only natural to think of some catastrophic illness as the explanation. The radicular pain of this disc herniation is thought to be severe because the disc herniation lies against the ganglion (Fig. 16.13).
3. Almost all the disc ruptures will occur at the L4–L5 level or cephalad levels (Table 16.1). It is a rare disc herniation at L5–S1 (Fig. 16.9). A disc herniation in the fourth anatomic segment (L4–L5) will irritate and compress the exiting fourth lumbar nerve root. If most of the rest of the foraminal disc herniations occur above L4–L5, then the root afflictions will all occur in the lumbar (not sacral) plexus and present as anterior thigh pain.
4. Because the nerve root involvement is the lumbar plexus (femoral and obturator nerves), the anterior thigh pain will be associated with a positive femoral stretch test (Fig. 16.14). This very positive stretch test explains why patients cannot sleep at night on their backs with their legs down flat. Most patients will report that their

only sleeping position of comfort is lying on their affected side with the legs drawn up in the fetal position or sitting in a recliner chair. Very few patients will demonstrate SLR reduction.

5. The neurology in the patients is almost always positive. In fact, if there is not a strong historical and physical neurology component, watch out, you likely do not have a foraminal HNP. Historically, concentrate on the paresthesia, which will tell you the root involved (Fig. 16.16). The findings on neurological examination are outlined in Table 16.2. Remember, if you do not find neurological changes on clinical assessment, you are unlikely to find a foraminal disc herniation on investigation.

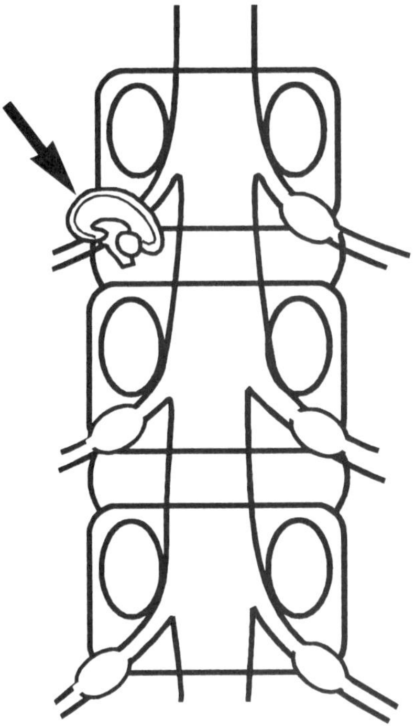

Figure 16.13 *The ganglion (arrow) is the brain of the motion segment and is extremely painful when compressed. (Adapted from Weinstein JN. Anatomy and neurophysiologic mechanisms of spinal pain. In: Frymoyer JW, ed. The Adult Spine. New York: Raven Press; 1991, p 597.)*

Table 16.1. Levels of Foraminal Disc Herniations

Foramen	% of Foraminal Disc Ruptures	As % of All Acute Radicular Syndromes[a]
L4 (from L4–L5)	50	1.5 (1.5/100 patients)
L3 (from L3–L4)	30	0.9 (1/100 patients)
L2 (from L2–L3)	12	0.4 (4/1000 patients)
L1 (from L1–L2)	2	0.06 (6/10,000 patients)
L5 (from L5–S1)	6	0.2 (2/1000 patients)

[a]Approximately 3% of all disc ruptures causing the acute radicular syndrome will occur in the foramen. From this column it is obvious that one needs to see alot of disc ruptures to see even a few foraminal disc herniations.

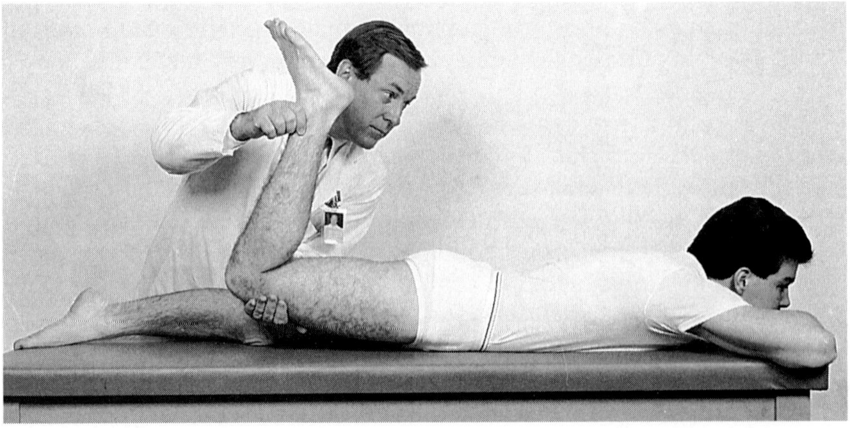

Figure 16.14 *The femoral stretch test.*

Figure 16.15 *The furcal nerve is a large extraforaminal branch carrying motor fibers for ankle dorsiflexion but not for extensor hallucis longus function.*

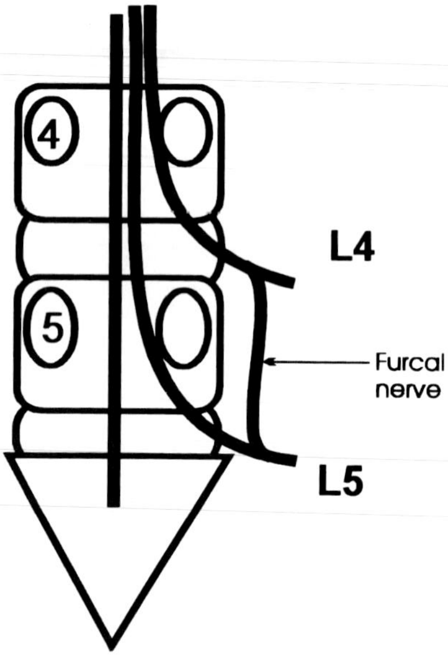

6. Concentrate on the sensory symptoms and signs to determine the root level. The difference between an L4 root lesion and an L3 root lesion is the fact that the sensory symptom and sign extend below the knee in L4 and concentrate around the knee in L3. Both root lesions will be associated with a depressed knee reflex and weak quadriceps.

The difference between an L2 and an L3 root lesion is even more subtle, except there is less tendency for the knee reflex to be depressed in an L2 root lesion.

7. Fifty percent of these disc ruptures occur at L4–L5 and appear to cause a double root lesion (Backache, Second Edition, p 342). The apparent double root lesion (L4 and L5 roots) is in fact a single root lesion that affects the furcal nerve (Fig. 16.15) and causes

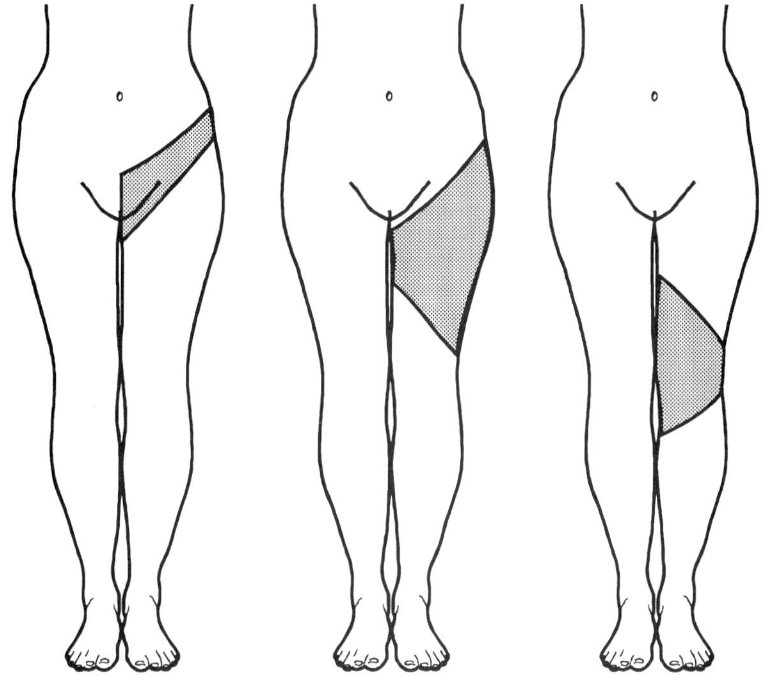

Figure 16.16 *The sensory distribution of the high lumbar roots (left to right, L1, L2, L3).*

Table 16.2. The Neurology of Foraminal Disc Ruptures

Foramen	Motor (Weakness)	Sensory (Loss)	Reflex (Depression)
L4	Knee extensors Ankle dorsiflexors	Medial shin	Knee
L3	Knee extensors	Patellar region	Knee
L2	Hip flexor Hip adductor	Lateral thigh	None
L1	Hip flexor	Groin	None
L5	Extensor hallucis longus	Dorsum of foot	None

weakness of the knee extensors and ankle dorsiflexors but spares the extensor hallucis longus.(14)

8. Obviously plain radiographs will not make the diagnosis but do reveal as yet an unexplained phenomenon: Why do almost all of these disc herniations rupture out of relatively normal (wide) disc spaces?
9. The diagnosis of a foraminal disc rupture has only been routinely made in the past decade because of CT scanning and MRI. Myelography alone will miss most foraminal disc ruptures (Fig. 16.17). The MRI is a better choice for diagnosis than the CT scan because:
   a. It depicts soft tissue changes better than CT (Fig. 16.18).
   b. It gives parasagittal views of the foramen (Fig. 16.19).

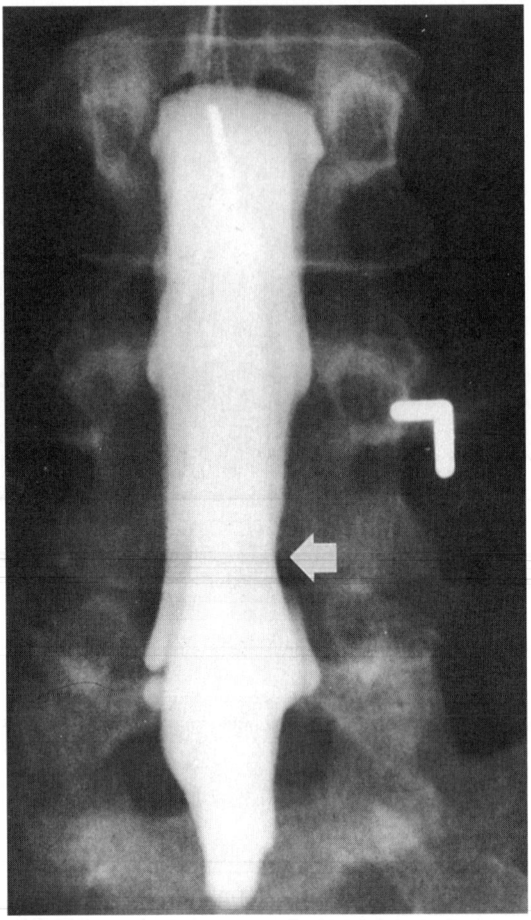

Figure 16.17 *AP myelogram in a foraminal HNP, L4, left. Note the slight defect in the dye column just above the L4–L5 disc space, left (arrow).*

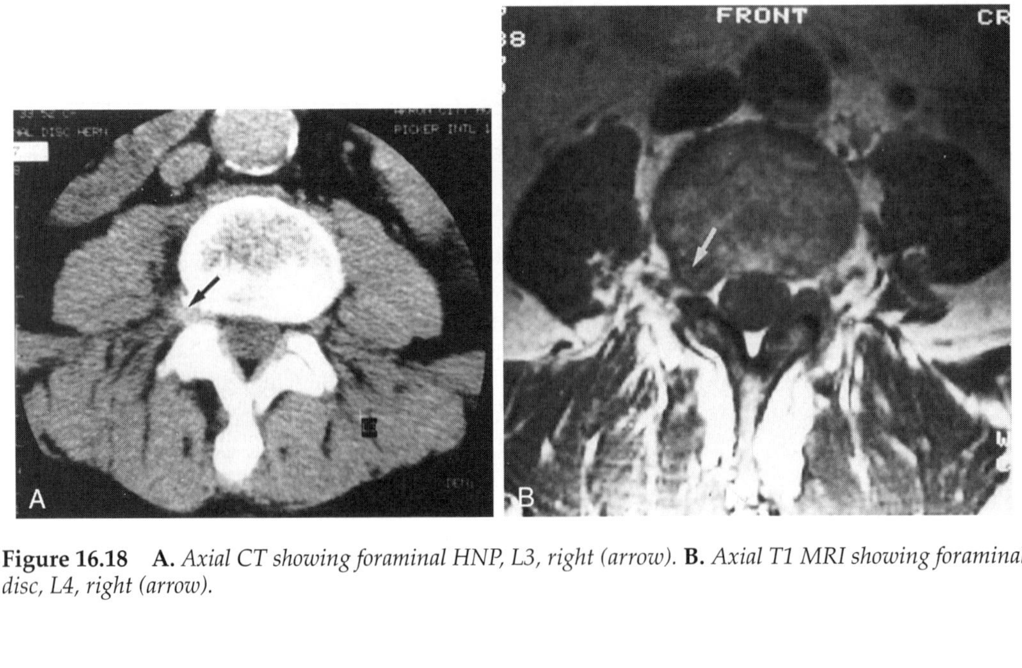

Figure 16.18 **A.** *Axial CT showing foraminal HNP, L3, right (arrow).* **B.** *Axial T1 MRI showing foraminal disc, L4, right (arrow).*

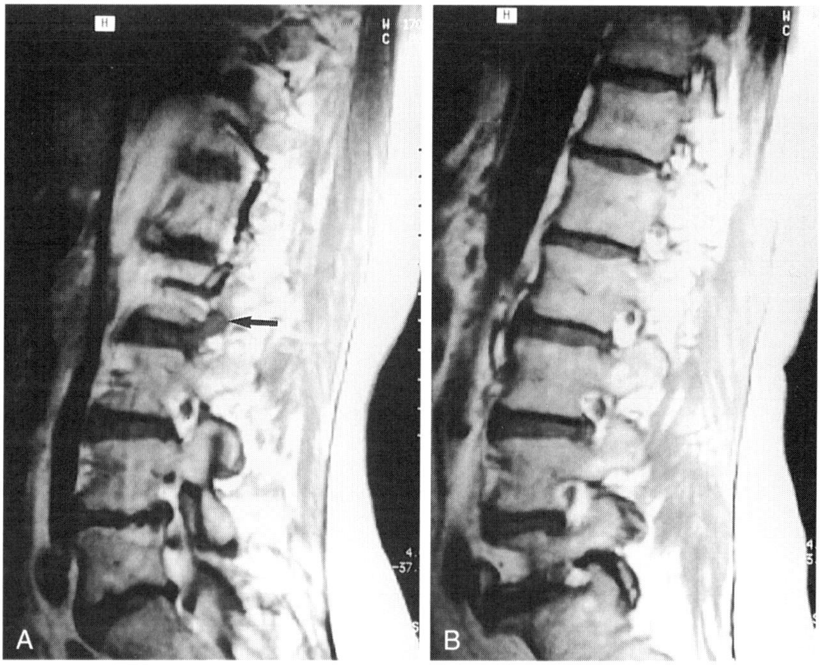

Figure 16.19 **A.** *A sagittal (T1) view of a foraminal disc L2 (arrow) and the open opposite foramen (right)* **(B).**

The Differential Diagnosis of a Foraminal Disc Herniation

There are obviously a few conditions that should not be confused with a foraminal HNP (23, 24) (Fig. 16.20). There is one condition that can easily be confused with the lumbar foraminal disc: diabetic mononeuropathy.

There are three neuropathic conditions that can occur in diabetes. We are all aware of the diabetic peripheral sensory neuropathy that presents as a bilateral stocking and glove sensory loss. Obviously, this condition would not be confused. The problem is diabetic mononeuropathy or plexus neuropathy that presents as a sudden onset of radicular pain. The usual affliction is to the femoral nerve, and the presentation is not unlike a foraminal disc rupture. The clinical clues that you may be dealing with a diabetic plexus neuropathy are the absence of back pain; the absence of any mechanical aggravation of the radicular pain (eg, coughing and sneezing); and the fact that more than one root is involved (eg, L3 and L4). Diagnosis is usually made when the MRI is negative, and a neurologist gets to look at the patient.

A less common condition that is missed is a retroperitoneal problem such as a renal cell carcinoma or any other infective or tumorous lesion that invades the femoral plexus.

Something that should not be missed is an osteoarthritic hip that causes groin pain and limp and interferes with a patient's ability to get a sock on (Fig. 16.21).

Treatment

All disc ruptures merit a trial of conservative care. But conservative care in this particular disc rupture should be limited because:

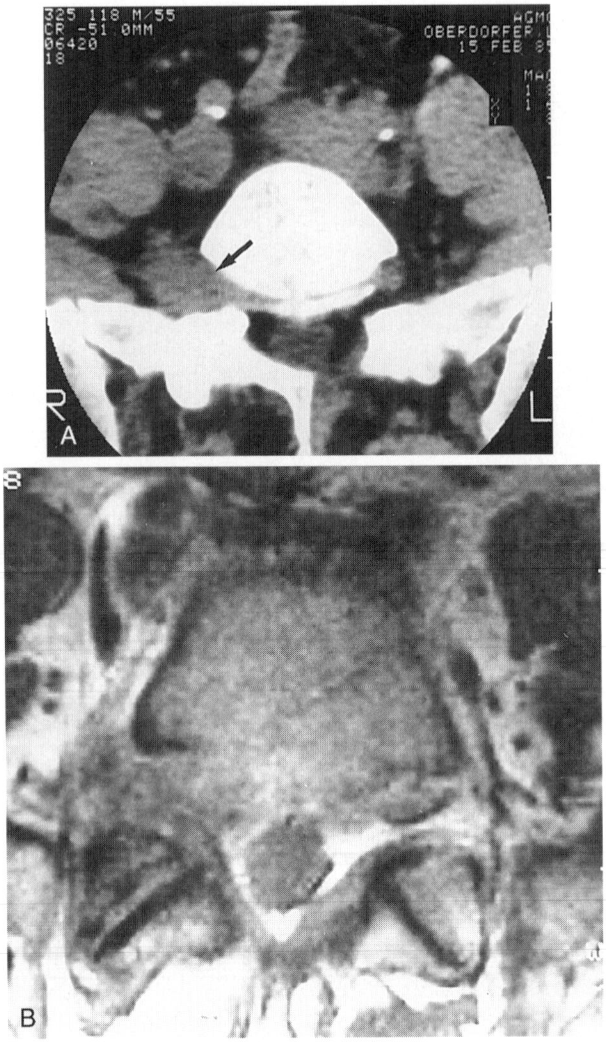

Figure 16.20 *Differential diagnosis of a foraminal disc:* **A.** *A tumor (arrow): a patient with a metastatic carcinoma of the lung who presented with an acute L5 radicular syndrome (CT scan).* **B.** *A synovial cyst wrapped around the 5th lumbar nerve root right (T1 axial MRI).*

1. The older patient should not be restricted to bed for a term longer than a few days.
2. The pain is so severe that nonsurgical care beyond 2 weeks is inhumane.
3. The neurological lesion is usually profound, that is, marked weakness of knee extensors, which is a major handicap to a lot of activities (eg, stairs, squatting, rough ground). The potential for neurological recovery is less in the older patient compared with the young patient; neurological compression should be relieved within 2 to 3 weeks if there is no sign of recovery.

Recommended Nonsurgical Care

1. Rest in the position of comfort, which is usually sitting (Fig. 16.22).

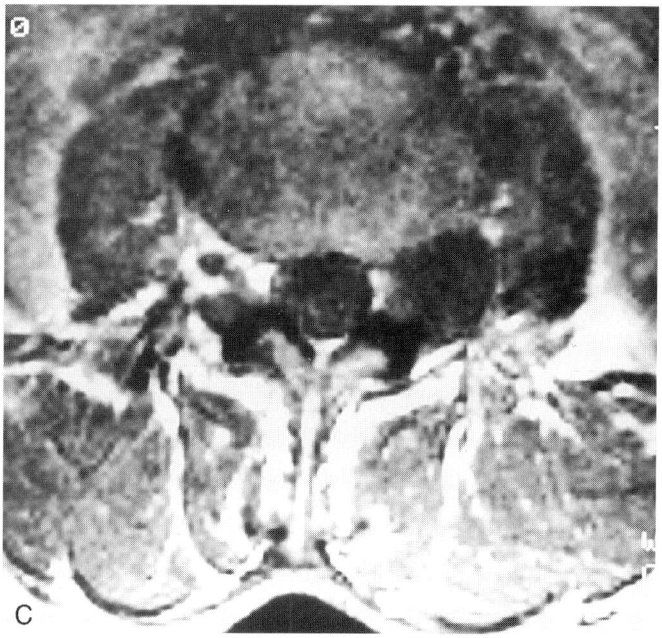

Figure 16.20 (continued) C. *A schwannoma L4 left (T1 axial MRI).*

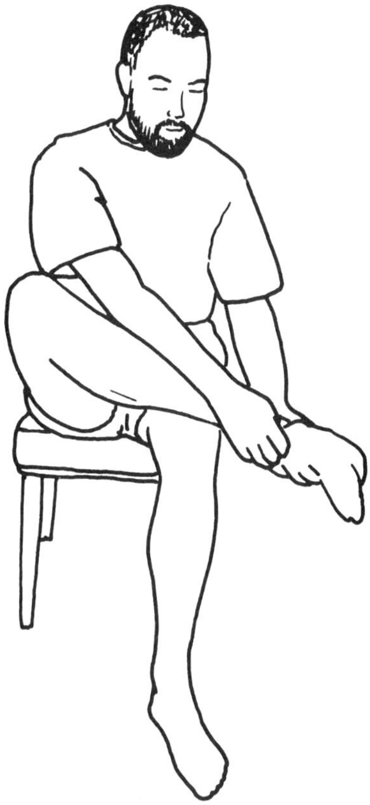

Figure 16.21 *A patient with osteoarthritis of the hip has trouble putting on a sock because of lost range of motion in the hip joint. A patient with a foraminal disc affecting the L1, L2, L3, and L4 roots can sit to put a sock on. A patient with an acute radicular syndrome affecting the L5 or S1 root cannot even sit to try and put a sock on.*

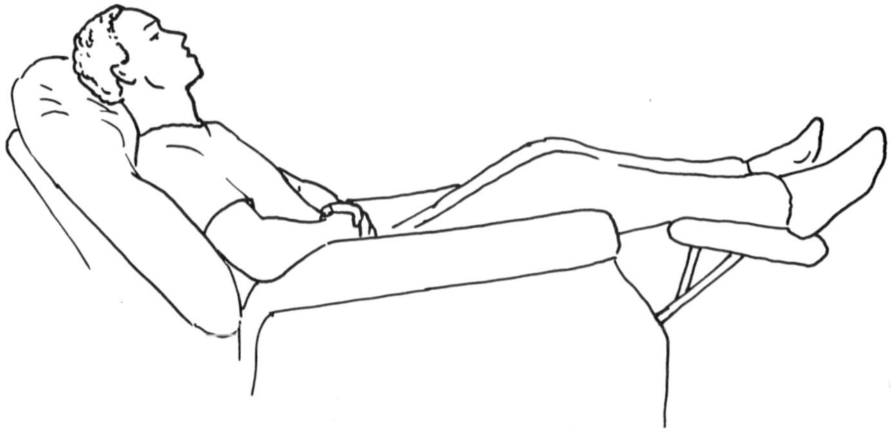

Figure 16.22 *Most patients with a femoral (and obturator) nerve root lesion find it difficult to lie in bed and learn quickly that the position of comfort is sitting.*

2. Use strong analgesics (oxycodone, fentanyl, or meperidine).
3. Use a brief course of oral steroids providing the patient is not diabetic, does not have a history of gastrointestinal ulcers, or does not have some other medical condition that precludes their use.
4. Use any other form of treatment (muscle relaxants, sleeping pills, heat, ice, and so on) that helps the patient cope.

Usual Course of Events with Nonsurgical Care

The authors have seen a few patients get better with conservative care. Those that do so will declare their course within 1 to 2 weeks. If there continues to be severe pain or worsening of the neurological lesion, do not procrastinate, operate.

The Approach to a Foraminal HNP (Excluding L5–S1)

The senior author (JM) stumbled along the learning curve with this disc herniation. Using a foraminal disc at L3–L4 as the example, the following surgical experience occurred. The initial approach was through the L3–L4 interspace, attempting to enter the foramen. On a few occasions, this resulted in fracturing the pars and losing the inferior facet (10) (Fig. 16.23). This obviously gave a good view of the foramen but did little for the stability of the segment. Next, switching to an L4–L5 foraminal disc, an attempt was made to come from the level above, that is, through the 3 to 4 interspace into the foramen of L4. This approach was used because of the particular arrangement of the lamina relative to the second, or foraminal, story of the vertebral segment (Fig. 16.24). This was equally unsuccessful with loss of some inferior facets. Presently, the approach taken is lateral to the pars (20, 26, 29, 31) using the anatomy depicted in Figures 16.25 and 16.26. This is most successful at the L4–L5 level and all levels cephalad. It is not advised for the rare L5 foraminal disc, which can be readily retrieved through a canal approach.

The approach to the L4, L3, L2, and L1 foramina is an easy approach made easier with the aid of the microscope. It is proposed only for disc herniations exclusively in the foramen

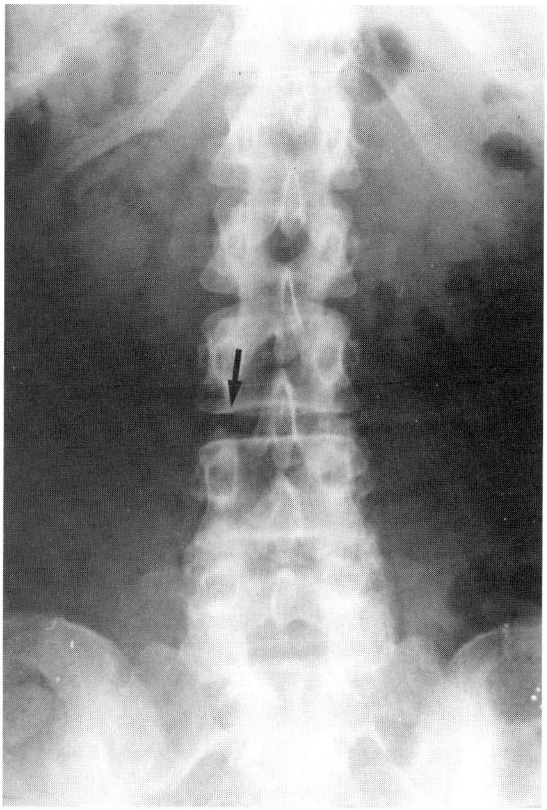

Figure 16.23 *AP radiograph showing the missing inferior facet, L3, right (arrow), inadvertently removed while trying to excise a foraminal disc through the interlaminar approach.*

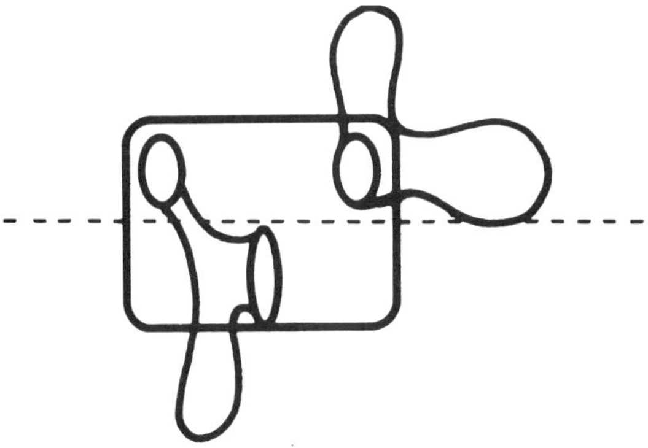

Figure 16.24 *The top edge of the lamina lies close to the bottom border of the pedicle, that is, at the junction between the second and third stories.*

(Fig. 16.27), because it is a single-level, non-expansile exposure. The sole purpose of this approach is to obtain a direct view of the disc rupture without sacrificing the facet joint.

The key to the microsurgical paraspinal approach is the pars interarticularis. It is the center of your surgical field beneath, which will lie the disc fragment. Using, as an example, an L4 foraminal disc rupture from an L4–L5 disc space, the microsurgical approach would be as follows:

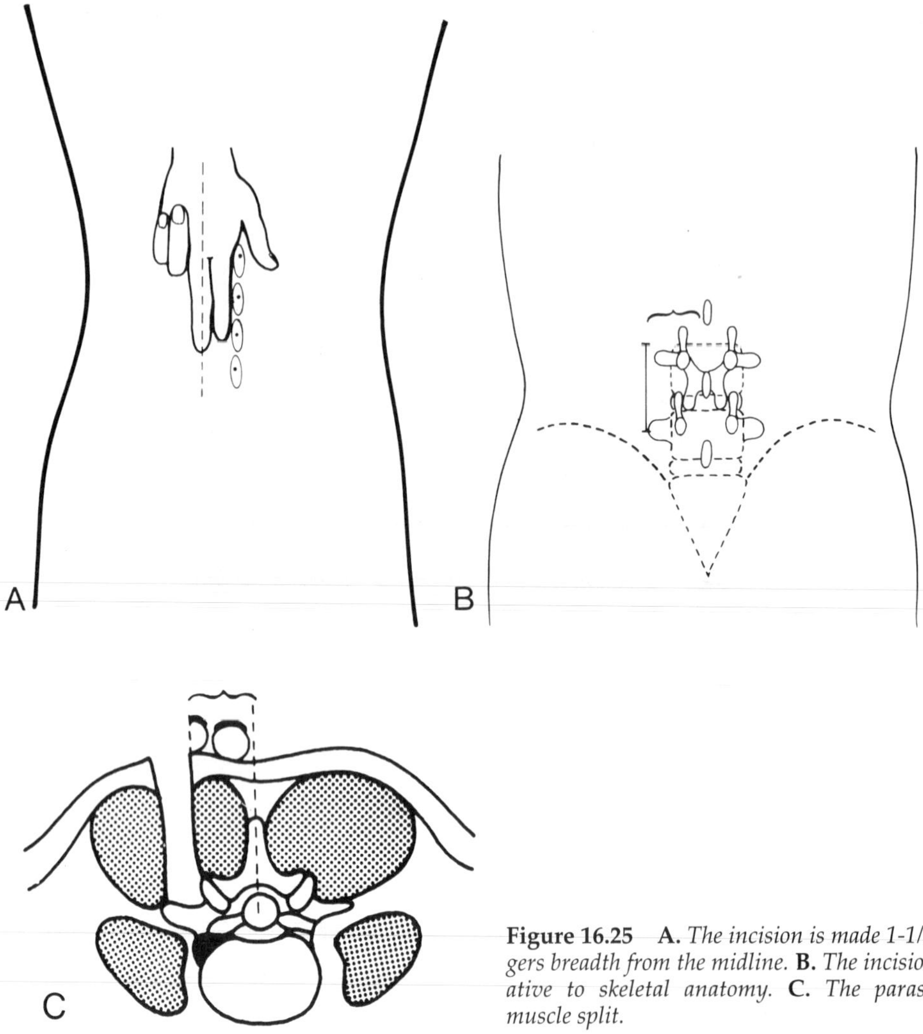

Figure 16.25 **A.** *The incision is made 1-1/2 fingers breadth from the midline.* **B.** *The incision relative to skeletal anatomy.* **C.** *The paraspinal muscle split.*

1. Mark the disc space above and below the disc rupture (ie, L3–L4 and L4–L5) (see Fig. 16.26). The pars you expose must fall between these two lines.
2. Split the paraspinals just lateral to the facet joints (see Fig. 16.25). This is usually a finger and a half's breadth off the midline.
3. Keep your eye and your dissecting finger on the pars. Position the double-bladed frame retractor so the medial blade is centered over the pars and the pars is clearly visible. If you start the intertransverse ligament exposure without a clear view of the pars, you will get too far laterally with your dissection.
4. Take the intertransverse ligament down as shown in Figure 16.27.
5. There are three things to remember about locating the nerve root:
   a. The exiting root will be just deep (anterior) to the pars and more often than not will be shoved up into the pars by the disc rupture.
   b. As with canal exposures, if you wish to find a root, find the medial border of the pedicle.

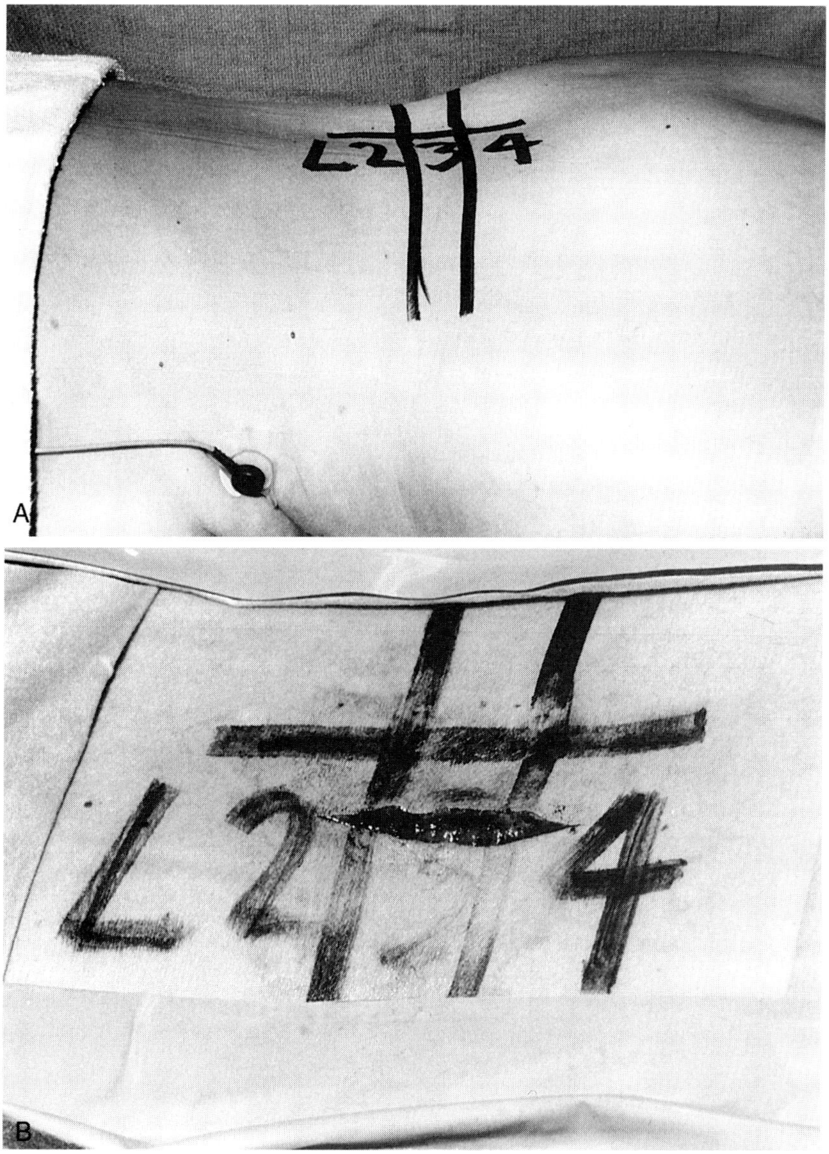

Figure 16.26 **A.** *Mark the disc space above and below the foramen to be approached (in this example, L2–L3 and L3–L4): the pars to be exposed lies between these lines.* **B.** *The skin incision centered over the pars to be exposed.*

c. The nerve root will be surrounded by a perineural mass of fat that needs to be gently removed to find the root.

6. Most foraminal disc ruptures are subligamentous extrusions that are found along the medial border of the root (Fig. 16.28). Occasionally, a free sequestered fragment will be found lateral to the root.
7. Remove not only the ruptured disc fragment but also follow its tract down into the disc space and remove any loose fragment from the intradiscal cavity.

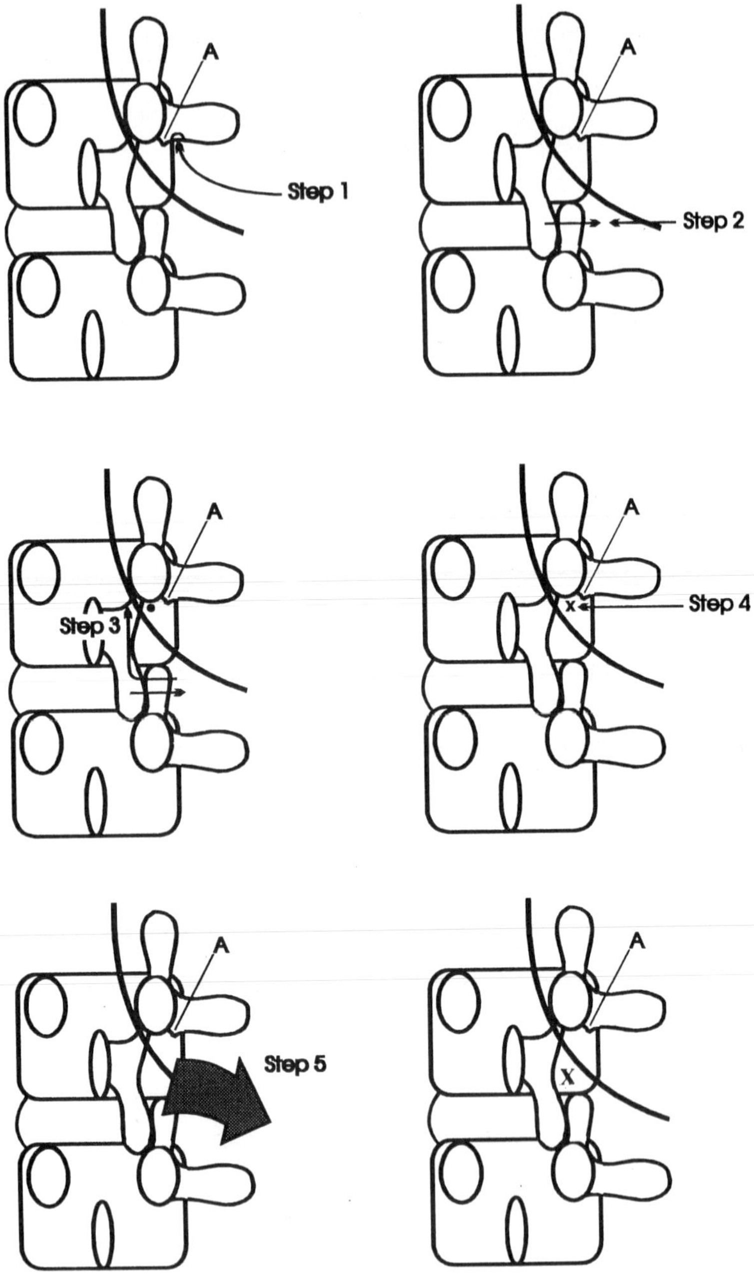

Figure 16.27 *The intertransverse approach, once the paraspinal exposure has been completed. Step 1: identify the accessory process and open the intertransverse ligament just lateral to the accessory process; this establishes depth perception for the nerve root. Step 2: open the capsule of the facet joint. Step 3: separate the medial extent of the intertransverse ligament from the ligamentum flavum by cutting up the lateral border of the pars interarticularis with a 2-mm rongeur. Step 4: join step 3 and step 1; you will be crossing over the top (posterior) of the nerve root at this point. Because of Step 1, you know the depth of the root. Step 5: reflect laterally the intertransverse ligament as a flap (heavy arrow). Step 6: find the nerve root by gently stroking the fat in the direction of the root. Most often, the disc herniation lies medial to the root (X), but be prepared for anything.*

Foraminal Disc Herniations at L5–S1 (Fig. 16.29)

Although rare, foraminal disc ruptures do occur at L5–S1. Because of the narrowed intertransverse window, the more lateral location of the pars, the broad transverse process of L5, and the shape of the ala of the sacrum, this disc rupture is best excised through a midline interlaminar exposure.

Complications

As mentioned, these disc herniations were approached initially in the standard interlaminar fashion, that is, an L4–L5 exposure for an L4 foraminal disc herniation. In three patients, the inferior facet was inadvertently sacrificed during exposure.

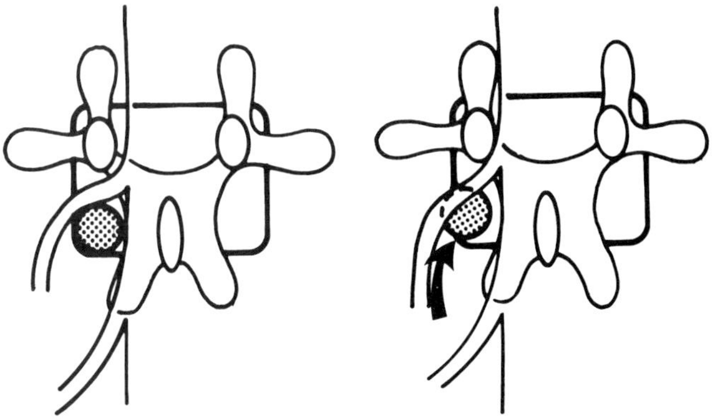

Figure 16.28 *Most foraminal disc herniations will be found along the axillary (medial) border of the nerve root (arrow).*

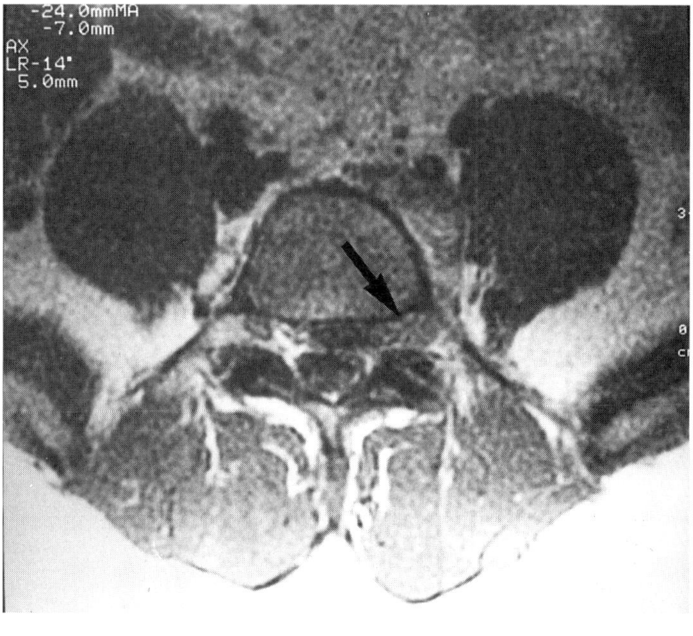

Figure 16.29 *A foraminal disc L5–S1 left on axial T1 MRI (arrow).*

In an early series,(8) one patient had a unilateral fusion to compensate and shows excellent results. The other two patients did not have a fusion, and although they have good results, they have vague sensations of weakness in their backs, which were only evident when they were called back for assessment. Two other patients had fusions at the time of surgery for an L5–S1 spondylolisthesis with a foraminal disc herniation. One had a unilateral intertransverse fusion under the microscope; the other had bilateral intertransverse fusion with a muscle-splitting paraspinal approach. Both patients have excellent results.

There was one serious complication in the 15 procedures (12 microdiscectomies and 3 chemonucleolyses in 13 patients). This was a disc space infection in a microsurgical patient. Staphylococcus aureus was cultured from his disc space through a percutaneous biopsy, and his disc space infection resolved with rest and appropriate antibiotic treatment.

Postoperative Course

A number of these patients do not follow a routine postoperative course following a foraminal disc excision. Because of irritation of the ganglion from the rupture or by the surgeon's manipulation of the root at surgery, and/or because of cautery of venules on the nerve root, the patients often linger with postoperative dysesthetic leg symptoms. Although relieved of their severe leg pain, they have a burning, uncomfortable feeling in their leg, which eventually disappears after a number of months. The senior author (JM) has seen three patients with a postoperative reflex sympathetic dystrophy that was very resistant to treatment.

Most patients will regain quadriceps strength, but few will regain their knee reflex. Management of these patients immediately postoperative and for a few months is not different than that described for the routine microdiscectomy.

Discussion

A foraminal HNP is a specific clinical entity. It is usually found in the older patient compared with the standard posterolateral disc herniation. Patients present with a story of sudden and intense leg pain with minimal back pain. The anterior thigh pain is severe enough that the sleep pattern is dramatically altered. On physical examination, the majority of patients present with a neurologic syndrome including motor, sensory, or reflex changes affecting one nerve root (usually L4). It is likely that the most common cause of fourth lumbar nerve root involvement from a ruptured disc occurs because of a foraminal herniated nucleus pulposus at the L4–L5 level rather than an L3–L4 disc herniation. The straight leg raising is only mildly decreased in this patient group, but the femoral stretch test is very positive if the fourth lumbar nerve root is affected.

The myelogram is usually nondiagnostic. The diagnosis is made with the CT scan (27, 28) or, better, with the MRI.(11) A number of CT scans in these patients were reported normal, because the original reviewing radiologist did not look at that area of the MRI or CT scan where a foraminal disc herniation occurs.

A foraminal disc herniation in this series was always a sequestered/extruded disc. Although conservative treatment should be tried, there is a growing pessimism that the patient will be able to tolerate the severe pain while waiting for conservative treatment to have its beneficial effect. In this older patient age group, with significant quadriceps weakness, there is a theoretical advantage to early decompression of the recently compressed fourth lumbar nerve root to assist in recovery of function. For some reason, the foraminal location of the ruptured fragment provokes more of an inflammatory response than usual, and, if patients are left too long with their symptoms, scarring around the fragment and the nerve root make dissection and removal more difficult.

The use of the microscope facilitated the surgical approach in these patients. It would appear that the best approach to a foraminal disc herniation is an approach lateral to the pars interarticularis (see Fig. 16.27).(26, 31) The lesson learned early in this experience was how easy it was to lose a facet joint when trying to enter the second story from the first story below (see Fig. 16.23).

A DISC RUPTURE INTO NO-MAN'S LAND

Definition

No man's land: "an unknown or unclaimed tract of usually barren land."

No man's land is depicted in Figure 16.8. It is a transitional area between the subarticular and foraminal regions. It is designated as no man's land because, as Macnab (18) pointed out, disc herniations can migrate here, causing significant root tension; yet this can be missed on investigation and at surgery.

The following rules govern no man's land:

1. Disc herniations do migrate into this area, especially in the older patient with degenerative narrowing of the disc space and/or subarticular stenosis.
2. The patient presents with dominant radicular pain often as severe as a foraminal disc.
3. The disc herniation will be missed on MRI for many reasons.
   a. The area is not well seen on MRI
   b. Degenerative changes such as subarticular stenosis obliterate any chance of seeing a disc rupture on MRI.
4. These disc ruptures are almost always subligamentous and, at surgery, Macnab's negative disc exploration is an easy task. You expose the interlaminar interval and note the nerve root is nonmobile. You palpate the disc and note little disc protrusion. Unless you open the annulus, you will miss the subligamentous disc extrusion (Fig. 16.30).

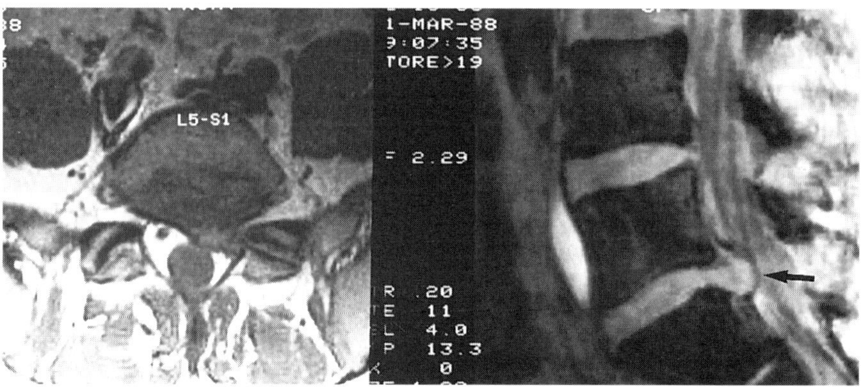

Figure 16.30 *Not a foraminal disc herniation on MRI, but a contained disc herniation that on the gradient echo sagittal is starting to migrate down behind the vertebral body of S1. Note the black line surrounding the disc herniation (arrow), which suggests containment.*

5. A very diligent search for the fragment of disc needs to be made because, in this age group, it is unusual to find one large contiguous fragment of herniated discal material. Rather, multiple fragments migrate into no man's land, and a careful search with blunt probes is necessary to prevent the leaving behind of any fragments.

NONDISCAL ENCROACHMENT IN THE LATERAL ZONE

Bony encroachment of nerve roots may occur in any of the three divisions of the lateral zone. The exact zonal location of the neurological compression is often difficult to pinpoint, which results in a high rate of failure to relieve symptoms with a limited microsurgical procedure.(8) To avoid this failure, it is necessary to review the details of the pathoanatomy.

There are four situations where nondiscal material can interfere with smooth root exit from the spinal canal: three of them bony, and one soft tissue:

1. Subarticular stenosis (Fig. 16.31).
2. Pedicular kinking in the foramen (Fig. 16.32).

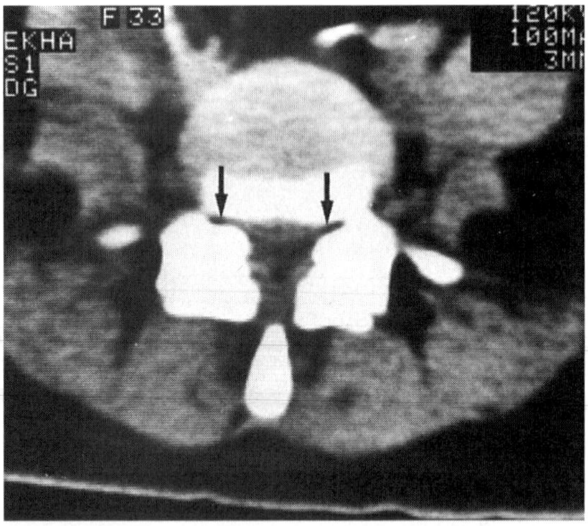

Figure 16.31 *Axial CT showing superior facet hypertrophy narrowing the subarticular zone (arrows), bilateral L4–L5 (compressing the fifth roots).*

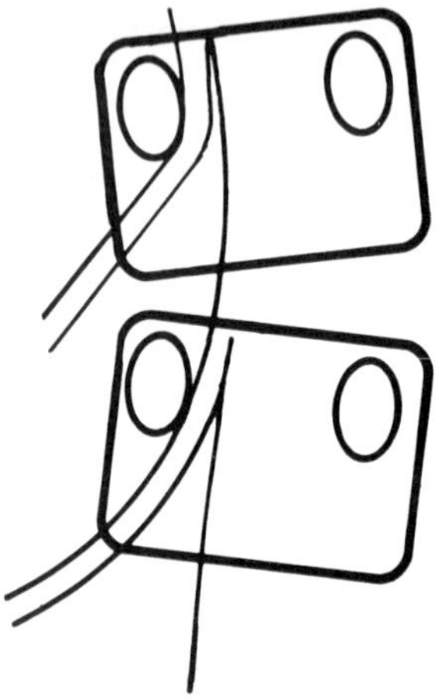

Figure 16.32 *Asymmetric disc space narrowing with pedicular kinking.*

3. Superior facet subluxation (Fig. 16.33).
4. Capsular hypertrophy (Fig. 16.34).

Before outlining these various scenarios, it is important to understand the double crush.

"Double Crush"

Figures 16.33 and 16.34 show how a facet joint, through bony hypertrophy or subluxation and/or capsular hypertrophy, may impinge on a nerve root. Using the superior facet of S1 as an example, medial edge hypertrophy encroaches on the first sacral nerve root in the subarticular zone, whereas capsular hypertrophy and osteophyte formation at its tip will impale the 5th lumbar nerve root in the foramen. If this occurs at the level above, (L4–L5),

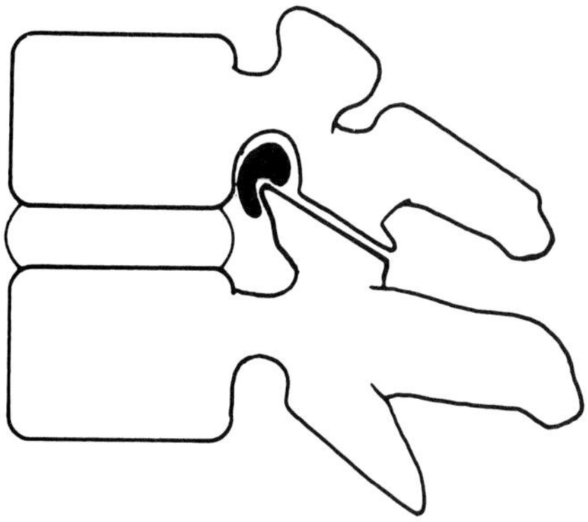

Figure 16.33 *Subluxation of a superior facet may compress the nerve root in its foramen.*

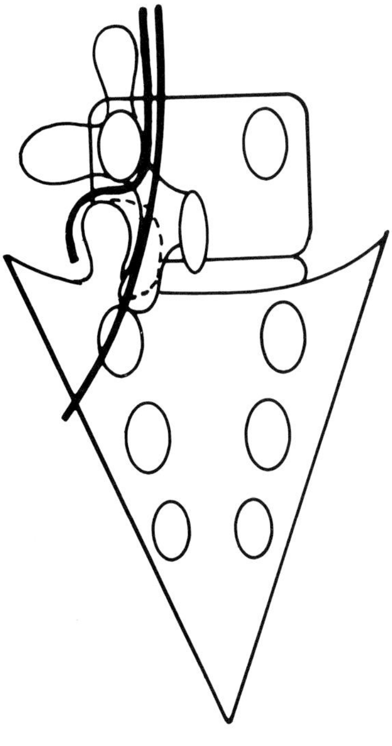

Figure 16.34 *The superior facet of S1 is capable of encroaching on two roots: the fifth lumbar root via the superior facet migration, and the first sacral root via medial facet hypertrophy.*

this is a reasonably easy clinical situation to sort out because one form of encroachment (subarticular) will cause radicular pain down the posterolateral aspect of the leg (L5 root), and the other syndrome (foraminal) will cause pain in the anterior thigh (L4 root).

Unfortunately, the double crush phenomenon occurs most commonly at the L5–S1 facet joint, where medial edge hypertrophy of the S1 facet will impale the first sacral nerve root, and superior tip pathology will encroach on the 5th lumbar nerve root. Both syndromes cause radiating posterolateral leg pain, one indistinguishable from the other. It is also possible for a single nerve root to be doubly crushed in a true sense. Figure 16.35 shows how this happens to the 5th lumbar nerve root.

Clinical Presentation

Most often, lateral zone bony encroachment is part of a more widespread canal stenosis.(3) So in reality, lateral zone stenosis should be lumped with the discussion on spinal canal stenosis. As with the chapter on spinal canal stenosis, we will split before we lump, that is, we will discuss the radicular syndrome associated with lateral zone stenosis because:

1. It may present as an isolated event affecting one nerve root (5)
2. If it is part of spinal canal stenosis, it is important to recognize the lateral zone stenosis so it can be dealt with at the time of surgery.

The clinical presentation of the chronic radicular syndrome was outlined in Chapter 7. Characteristic of this syndrome is the presence of claudicant radicular leg pain and the absence of hard neurological findings. It is this aspect that makes an L5 chronic radicular syndrome indistinguishable from an S1 chronic radicular syndrome. Other clinical characteristics of the chronic radicular syndrome incriminating chronic encroachment pathology in the lateral zone of the L5 or S1 root are:

Figure 16.35 *A true double crush: the fifth lumbar root by hypertrophy of the medial edge of the superior facet of L5, and in its foramen by the tip of the superior facet of S1.*

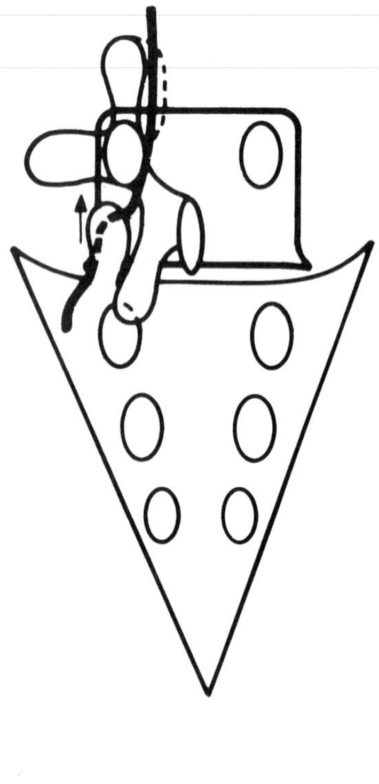

1. The older patient with a long history of back pain.
2. The back pain may be part of their complaint, but it is the chronic leg pain that brings them to you for an opinion.
3. The leg pain follows a very definite radicular distribution. (It is a more definite pain than the diffuse leg discomfort weakness and numbness seen in spinal canal stenosis).
4. The leg pain is aggravated by standing and walking and usually relieved by sitting (which is the reverse story to the radicular pain caused by a disc herniation).
5. The flexed position, such as leaning on a grocery cart, may relieve symptoms.
6. Leg symptoms take longer to go away with cessation of the aggravating activity than in vascular claudication.
7. SLR is not reduced to any great extent, although it will usually be reproductive of pain as compared with the asymptomatic side (Fig. 16.36).
8. Neurological symptoms (paresthesias) are often present, and neurological signs are subtle, that is, some extensor hallucis longus (EHL) weakness for 5th root but no drop foot.
9. On the rare occasion, a patient with bilateral bony encroachment causing a bilateral chronic radicular syndrome will present. This patient is very difficult to sort out until an MRI or CT scan is done, which demonstrates a relatively patent spinal canal with bilateral lateral zone encroachment (Fig. 16.31).
10. More commonly than that previously mentioned, a patient with double crush or a double nerve root lateral zone stenosis will present, causing considerable clinical consternation in sorting out the roots involved.
11. The clinical presentation of the unilateral chronic radicular syndrome is outlined in Table 16.3.

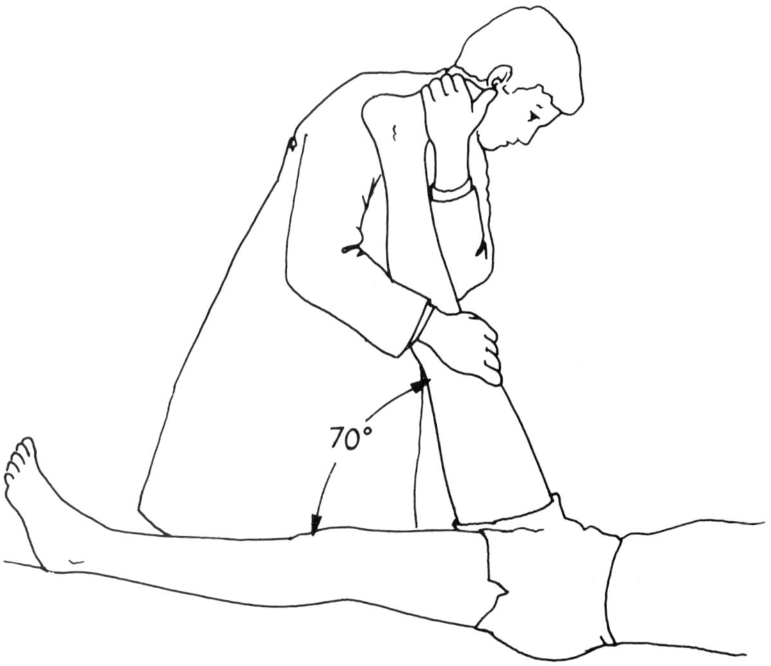

Figure 16.36 *Some, but not significant, SLR reduction occurs in the chronic radicular syndrome.*

Pathogenesis

Subarticular Stenosis

Hypertrophy of the medial edge of the superior facet narrows the subarticular zone from behind (Fig. 16.31). (3, 4, 5) From in front, an osteophyte from the inferior edge of the vertebral body or an HNP may further compromise the subarticular zone (Fig. 16.37). The critical dimensions for the subarticular zone should be determined at the top end of the third story (27) of the segment and are depicted in Figure 16.38.

The most significant form of medial edge hypertrophy occurs in degenerative spondylolisthesis (Fig. 16.39).

Foraminal Stenosis

There are many sources of nerve root encroachment in the foramen, exclusive of the HNP: (1) the uncinate spur (Fig. 16.40) (12);(2) the subluxed superior facet (Fig. 16.41); (3) capsular hypertrophy (Fig. 16.42); (4) disc space narrowing, especially if it is asymmetric (see Fig. 16.32) (18), causing pedicular kinking, that is, a longstanding lytic spondylolisthesis with foraminal encroachment of the 5th lumbar root. This condition was discussed in the chapter on spondylolisthesis.

Table 16.3. Unilateral Chronic Radicular Syndrome[a]

Older patient with long history of back pain.
Gradual drift of pain into buttock, thigh, and calf.
Eventual claudicant unilateral leg pain.
Distribution corresponds to root involvement (posterior leg for L5 and S1).
Often, but not always, proximal-to-distal spread.
Relief after many minutes in flexed position and, most often, with sitting.
Frequently, neurological symptoms (paresthesia).
Rarely, neurological signs.
Close to normal straight leg raising.

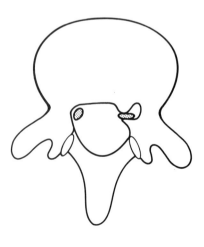

Figure 16.37 *The left nerve root as a "sandwich filler," an osteophyte from behind, and a disc bulge from in front.*

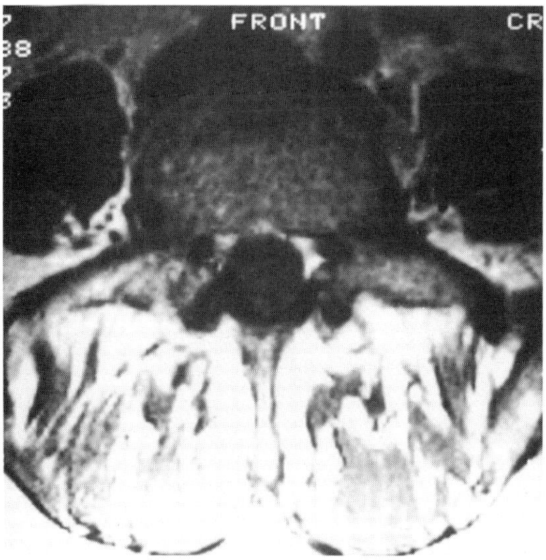

Figure 16.38 *The area to determine dimensions of the subarticular zone in the upper portion of the third story. This is a normal subarticular zone.*

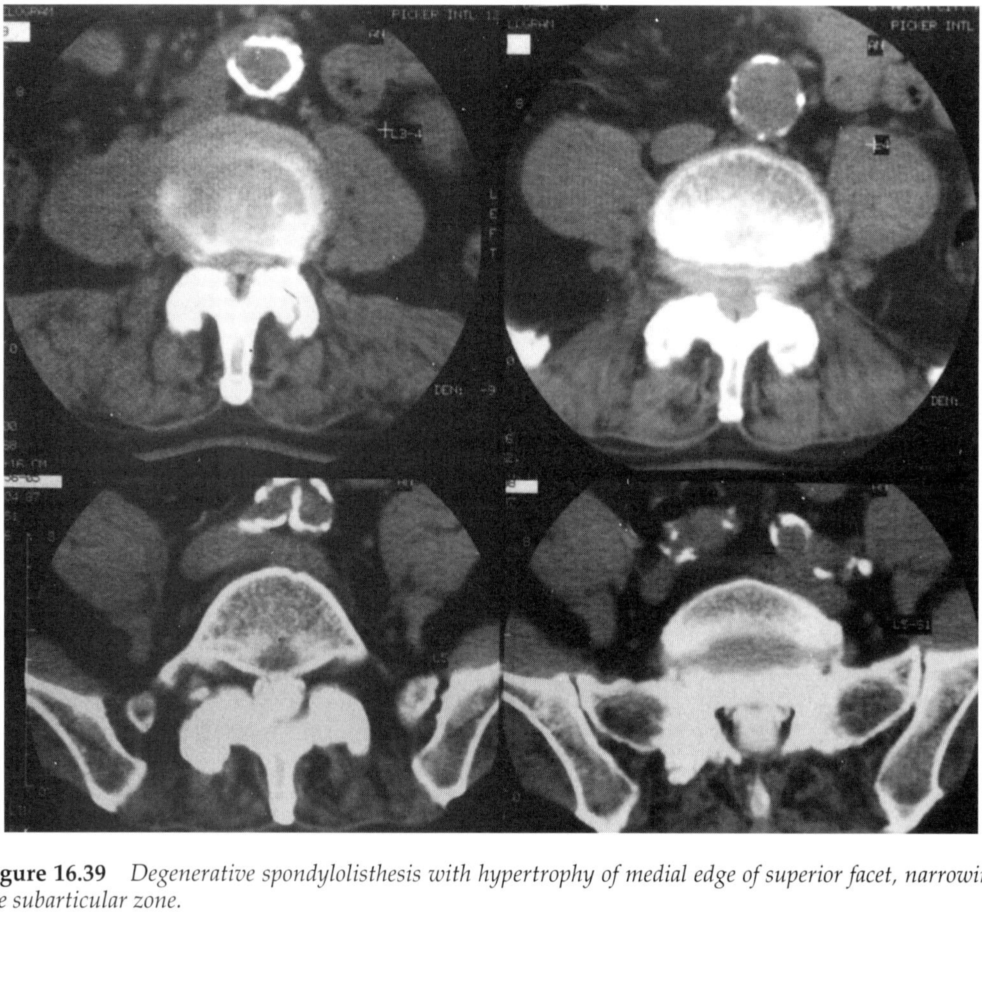

Figure 16.39 *Degenerative spondylolisthesis with hypertrophy of medial edge of superior facet, narrowing the subarticular zone.*

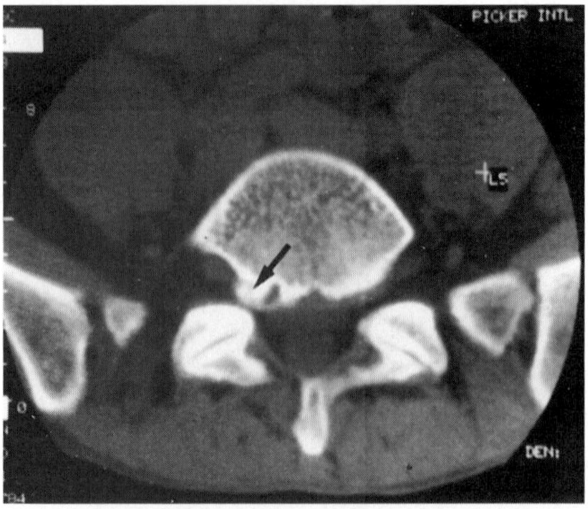

Figure 16.40 *The uncinate spur, right (arrow).*

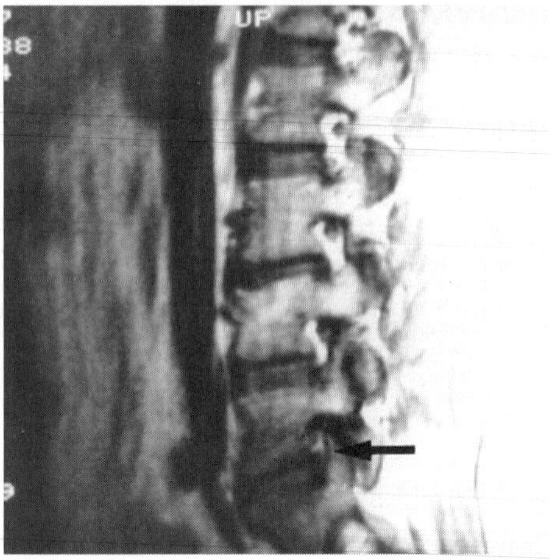

Figure 16.41 *A subluxed superior facet of S1, closing down the L5 foramen (arrow).*

Extraforaminal Stenosis

This condition has been described by Macnab (first edition of this book) and Wiltse (30) and is due to entrapment of the L5 nerve root between a deeply descending transverse process of L5 and the superior position of the medial sacral ala (Fig. 16.43).

Investigation

Plain radiography will always reveal degenerative changes with varying degrees of bony hypertrophy from the edges of the vertebral bodies and/or the facet joints. Myelography is occasionally useful but is so often false negative that it has been supplanted by CT and MRI.(12) If there is one place where sagittally reformatted CTs (27) are indicated, it is in the investigation of this patient (Fig. 16.44). Axial CT will readily show causes of subarticular stenosis, foraminal stenosis, and extraforaminal stenosis.

MRI will become increasingly useful to show pathology in the foramen (Fig. 16.45). At this particular stage of MRI development, CT scans are still superior for demonstration of the bony pathology in subarticular and foraminal stenosis.

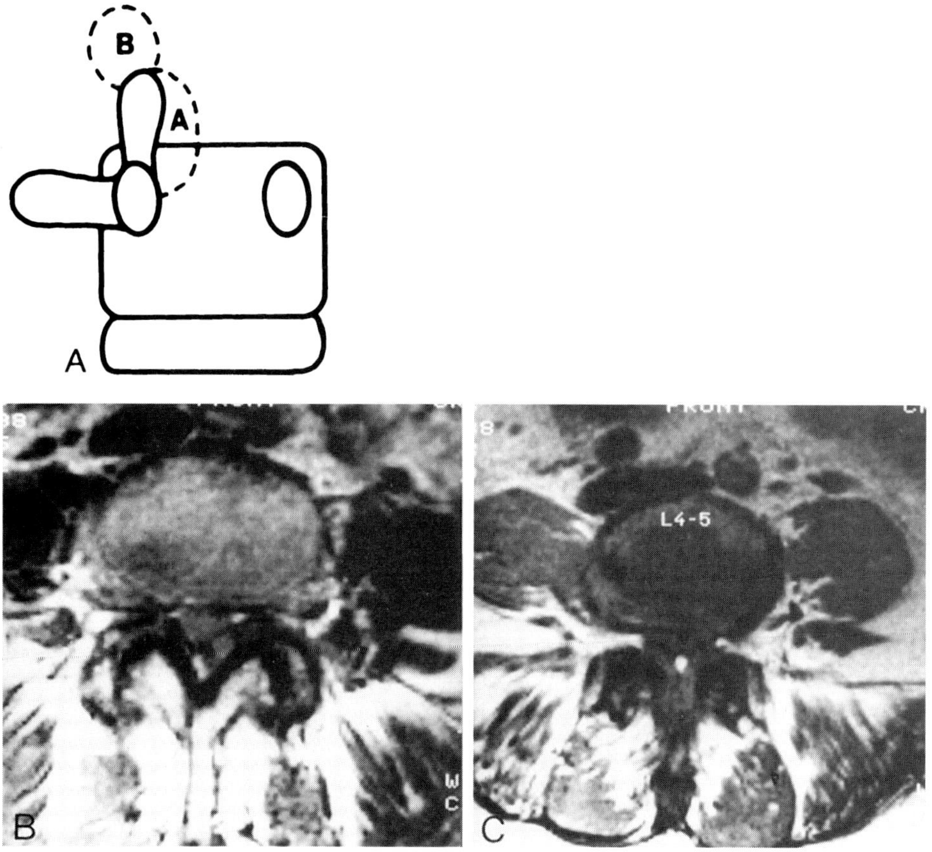

Figure 16.42 **A.** *Capsular hypertrophy* **(B)** *will compress the nerve root in the foramen above as shown on schematic.* **(A)**, *hypertrophy of the medial edge of the superior facet.* **B.** *MRI of both spinal canal and foraminal stenosis. The foraminal encroachment is from capsular hypertrophy. Compare this with* **C**, *spinal canal stenosis as well, but no capsular hypertrophy in the foramen.*

Determination of Root Involved

Because of the paucity of neurological findings, it is often difficult to tell whether symptoms are arising from the 5th lumbar or the first sacral root. Distinction between the two can be made in the following fashion:

1. On history, the patient may describe associated paresthesias that give a clue as to which root is being compromised.
2. On physical examination, there may be EHL (L5) weakness that is not present on the asymptomatic side. Rarely, if the S1 root is involved, will there be plantar flexion weakness.
3. An electromyograph (EMG) may show some changes that incriminate one particular nerve root. The limitations of EMG in this patient population and the false-negative examinations were covered in Chapter 11. These limitations are so common that the author does not feel that EMG offers very much to the investigation of a patient with chronic radicular pain.
4. Nerve root block (as described in Chapter 11) is probably the most important test for trying to decide which root is the source of the patient's chronic radicular syndrome.

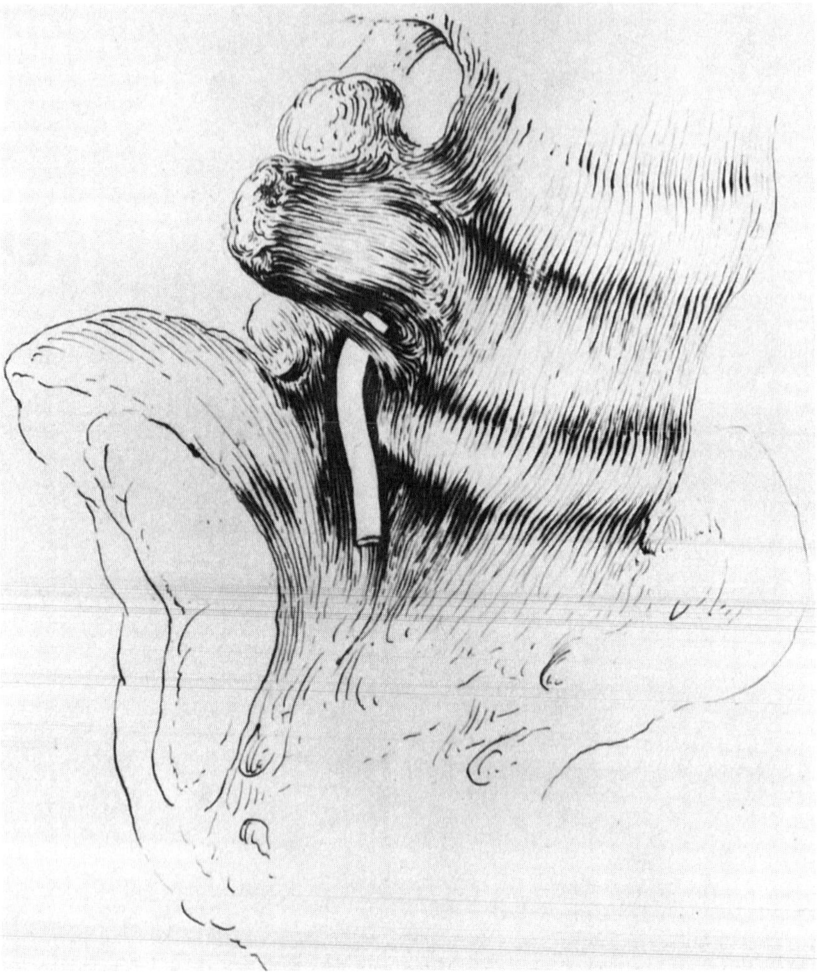

Figure 16.43 *There is a strong ligamentous band passing from the transverse process of L5 to the body of L5, which lies immediately cranial to the fifth lumbar nerve root as it courses over the ala of the sacrum. With marked narrowing of the lumbosacral disc, this ligament descends on the fifth lumbar nerve root like a guillotine and compresses it against the ala of the sacrum. Patients with this lesion will present with evidence of impairment of fifth lumbar nerve root function, but will not show any defect on myelographic examination.*

Nonsurgical Treatment

Once patients reach a state of disabling unilateral claudicant leg pain, it is unusual for them to respond to conservative treatment. Rarely, in their chronic unilateral radicular syndrome, they may temporize symptoms with various exercise routines and anti-inflammatory medications. It is usual that most of these patients will notice increasing symptoms and eventually require surgery. Enough patients with minor disability do improve with the passage of time and conservative treatment measures that surgical intervention should be reserved for the patient who is significantly disabled.(25) If they present in this state, there is little hope that conservative treatment will make a difference.

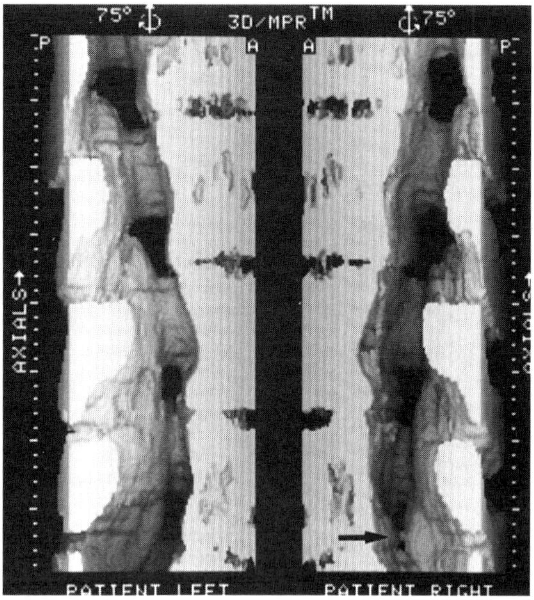

Figure 16.44 *A sagittal reconstruction of CT scan showing foraminal narrowing, L5, right (arrow).*

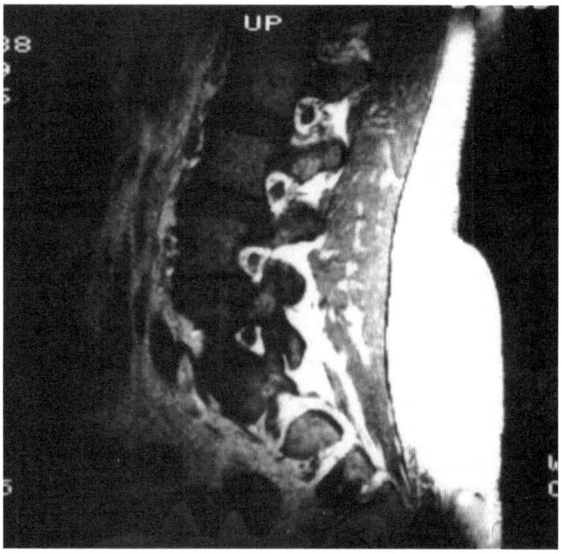

Figure 16.45 *T1 sagittal MRI, clearly showing normal foramen.*

Surgical Treatment

Entry into the spinal canal is usually more difficult in these patients because of the degenerative changes. Once inside the canal, it is probably easier to decompress a subarticular stenosis than it is to remove an HNP. There is only one caveat to obey: always identify the lateral edge of the nerve root as soon into the case as possible and before removing significant amounts of bone.

Surgical Decompression of Subarticular Stenosis

This is usually a simple exercise once you have gained entry to the spinal canal (Fig. 16.46).

Surgical Decompression of a Foraminal Stenosis

Not only is it difficult to recognize a foraminal stenosis location, it is also hard to decompress. The surest way to decompress a foraminal stenosis is to do a wide decompression, cutting across the pars and removing the inferior facet (Fig. 16.46). If there are alot of degenerative changes in the segment, with implied stability, this is the best approach. If there are minimal degenerative changes or an early degenerative spondylolisthesis, this is a disastrous approach, potentially producing postoperative instability requiring further treatment intervention. It is advisable to add an intertransverse fusion to this latter situation.

For the purpose of this chapter discussion, a method of accomplishing a foraminal decompression without destruction of the facet joint is presented. Two situations present:

1. The necessity to decompress the foramen alone, for example, capsular hypertrophy.
2. The necessity to decompress the foramen and the subarticular zone.

If the foraminal zone alone has to be decompressed, the lateral approach as described in the section on foraminal HNP is used. If a subarticular decompression is needed at the same time, the midline interlaminar approach is taken, extending the soft tissue exposure to the tips of the transverse processes so that an intertransverse interval decompression

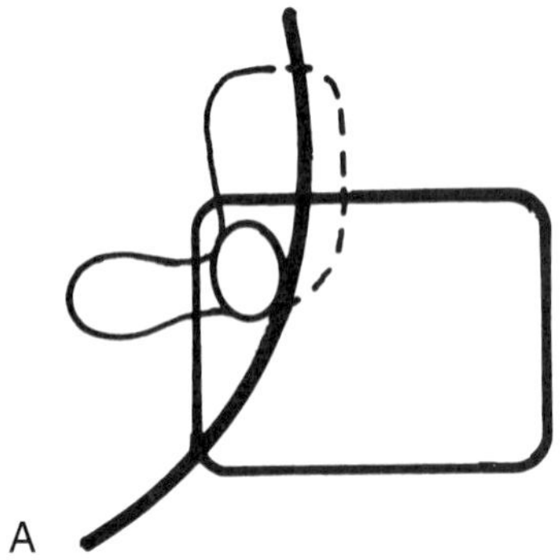

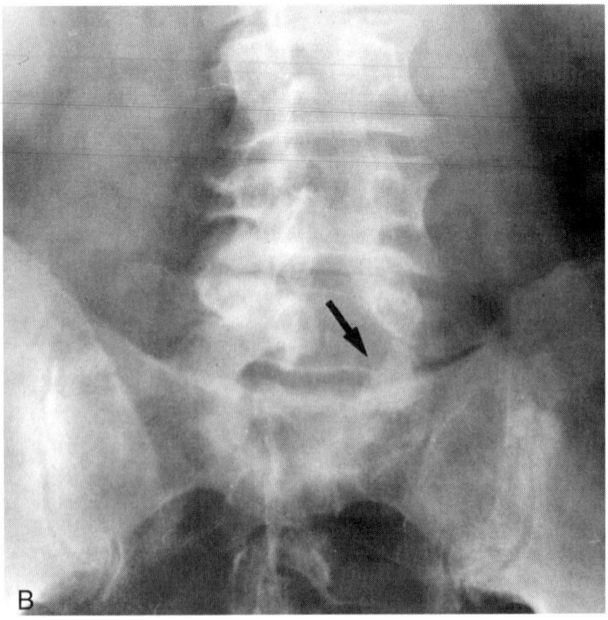

Figure 16.46 **A.** *Once inside the spinal canal, remove the medial edge of the superior facet so that it is flush with the medial border of the pedicle.* **B.** *To decompress the foraminal stenosis in Figure 16.44, the inferior facet of L5 and the tip of the S1 facet were removed (arrow).*

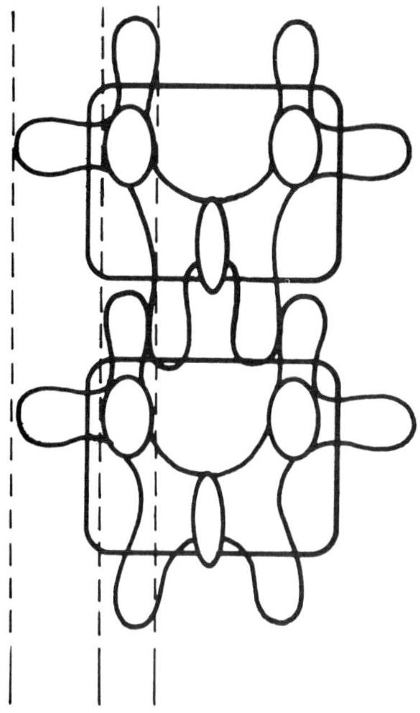

Figure 16.47 *By extending the standard midline exposure laterally (which means a longer incision), the pars and transverse processes can be viewed for a combined interlaminar and intertransverse exposure.*

can be added to the procedure (Fig. 16.47). Be sure to save as much of the superior lamina as possible so as not to weaken the pars.

Surgical Decompression in Pedicular Kinking

This condition is singled out to mention the high failure rate when attempting a single root decompression in degenerative scoliosis (Fig. 16.48). This has failed so often in the senior author's (JM) experience that it is obvious the only way these problems can be handled is with a more general approach to stabilize the curve at the time of a wide decompression.

Decompression of pedicular kinking of a nerve root in lytic spondylolisthesis was discussed in Chapter 5.

Prophylactic Decompression of the Asymptomatic Side

As is so often the case, degeneration of a lumbar vertebral segment causes bilateral changes; it is not unusual to see subarticular or foraminal stenosis as an asymptomatic condition on the opposite side (Fig. 16.49). Should you or should you not decompress the asymptomatic side? This is a discussion that quickly turns friends into acquaintances and neither opinion can support their position with any scientific fact. It is the authors' opinion that, at all times, the least possible "invasion" should be offered to a patient facing spinal surgery. In keeping with this philosophy, prophylactic decompression of the asymptomatic side is not considered. Those who would propose decompression of the asymptomatic side have problems when asked what to do about degenerative changes at other levels. The argument for prophylactic decompression can expose the patient to a multilevel major surgical exploration when a simple unilateral microsurgical decompression will relieve the leg pain that brought that patient to the surgeon for an opinion.

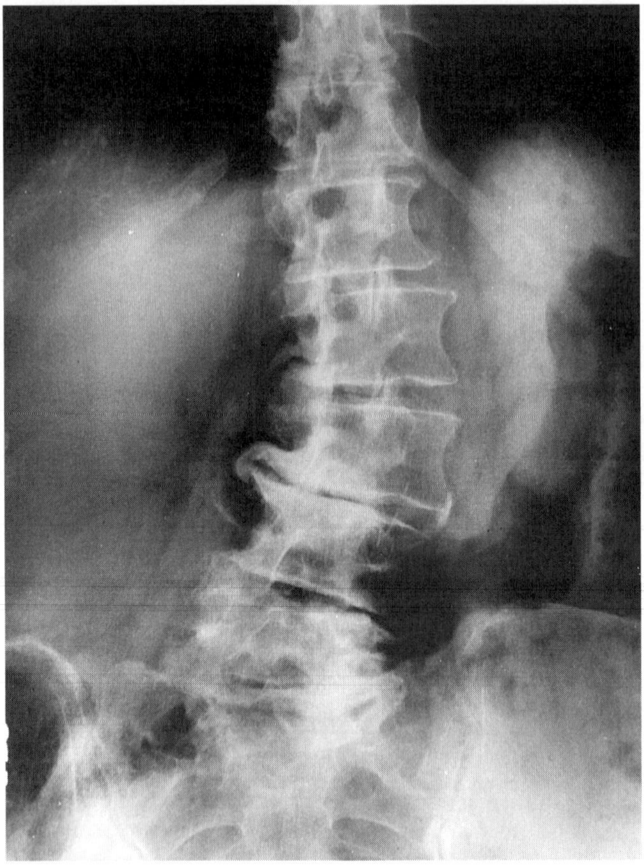

Figure 16.48 *Anteroposterior radiograph of degenerative scoliosis: a single root decompression at L4–L5 or above would be a waste of time.*

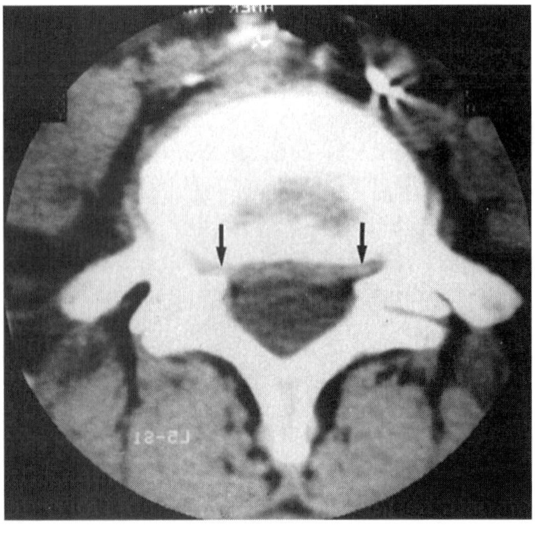

Figure 16.49 *Bilateral subarticular stenosis, L5–S1 (arrows), symptomatic on the left because of a disc herniation. Should the right subarticular stenosis be decompressed at the same time? We say no.*

Conclusion

The illumination and magnification available through the microscope have opened the lateral reaches of the spinal canal to decompression of the nerve root in the lateral zone. Be it an HNP or foraminal stenosis, the lateral approach to the lumbar nerve roots is a relatively easy procedure with the microscope as an aid. Decompression of a subarticular stenosis through the usual interlaminar exposure is also facilitated by the microscope.

REFERENCES

1. Abdullah AF, Ditto E, Byrd E, Williams R. Extreme lateral lumbar disc herniations. J Neurosurg 1974;41:229–234.
2. Broom MJ. Foraminal and extraforaminal lumbar disc herniations. Clin Orthop 1993;289:118–126.
3. Choudhury AR, Taylor JC. Occult lumbar spinal stenosis. J Neurol Neurosurg Psychiatr 1977; 40:506–510.
4. Ciric I, Mikhael MA, Tarkington JA, Vick NA. The lateral recess syndrome. J Neurosurg 1980; 53:433–443.
5. Epstein JA, Epstein BS, Senthal AD, Carras R, Lavine LS. Sciatica caused by nerve root entrapment in the lateral recess: the superior facet syndrome. J Neurosurg 1972;45:584–589.
6. Epstein NE. Far lateral lumbar disc herniation: diagnosis and surgical management. Neurol Orthop 1986;1:37–40.
7. Faust SE, Ducker TB, VanHassent JA. Lateral lumbar disc herniations. J Spinal Disorders 1992; 5:97–103.
8. Feldman R, McCulloch JA. Microdiscectomy for lumbar nerve root encroachment. In: McCulloch J, ed. Principles of Microsurgery for Lumbar Disc Disease. New York: Raven Press; 1989, pp 225–238.
9. Gado M, Patel J, Hodges FJ. Lateral disc herniation into the lumbar intervertebral foramen. AJNR 1983;4:598–600.
10. Garrido E, Connaughton PN. Unilateral facetectomy approach for lateral lumbar disc herniation. J Neurosurg 1991;74:754–756.
11. Grenier N, et al. MR Imaging of foraminal and extraforaminal lumbar disc herniations. J Comput Assist Tomogr 1990;14:243–249.
12. Heithoff KB, Ray CD, Schellhas KP, Fritts HM. CT and MRI of lateral entrapment syndromes. In: Genant HK, ed. Spine Update, 1987. Radiology Research and Education Foundation; San Francisco: University of California Printing Services; 1987.
13. Jackson RP, Glah JJ. Foraminal and extraforaminal lumbar disc herniation: diagnosis and treatment. Spine 1987;12:577–585.
14. Kikuchi S, Hasue M, Nishiyama K, Ito T. Anatomic and clinical studies of radicular symptoms. Spine 1984;9:23–30.
15. Kurobane Y, et al. Extraforaminal disc herniation. Spine 1986;11:260–268.
16. Lee CK, Rauschning W, Glenn W. Lateral lumbar spinal canal stenosis: classification, pathological anatomy and surgical decompression. Spine 1988;13:313–320.
17. Lejeune JP, Hladky JP, Cotten A, Vinchon M, Christiaens JL. Foraminal lumbar disc herniation. Spine 1994;19:1905–1908.
18. Macnab I. Negative disc exploration. J Bone Joint Surg 1971;53A:891–903.
19. Maroon JC, Kopitnik TA, Schulhof LA, Abla A, Wilberger JE. Diagnosis and microsurgical approach to far-lateral disc herniation in the lumbar spine. J Neurosurg 1990;72:378–382.

20. Melvill RL, Baxter BL. The intertransverse approach to extraforaminal disc protrusions in the lumbar spine. Spine 1994;19:2707–2714.
21. Novetsky GJ, Berlin L, Epstein A, Lobo N, Miller S. The extraforaminal herniated disc. AJNR 1982;3:653–655.
22. Osborne D, Heinz R, Bullard D, Friedman A. Role of computed tomography after negative myelography: foraminal neural entrapment. Neurosurg 1984;14:147–153.
23. Patrick BS. Extreme lateral ruptures of lumbar intervertebral discs. Surg Neurol 1975;3:301–304.
24. Postacchini F, Montanaro A. Extreme lateral herniations of lumbar discs. Clin Orthop 1979; 138:222–227.
25. Porter RW, Hibbert C, Evans C. The natural history of root entrapment syndrome. Spine 1984;9:418–421.
26. Ray CD. Far lateral decompression for stenosis: the paralateral approach to the lumbar spine. In: White AH, Rothman RH, Ray CD, eds. Lumbar Spine Surgery. St Louis: CV Mosby; 1987, pp 175–186.
27. Schubiger O, Valavanis A, Hollman J. Computed tomography of the intervertebral foramen. Neuroradiology 1984;26:439–444.
28. Williams AL, Haughton V, Daniels D, Thornton R. CT recognition of lateral lumbar disc herniation. AJNR 1982;3:211–213.
29. Wiltse LL, et al. The paraspinal sacrospinalis-splitting approach to the lumbar spine. J Bone Joint Surg 1968;50A:919–926.
30. Wiltse LL. Alar transverse process impingement of the L5 spinal nerve: the far-out syndrome. Spine 1984;9:31–38.
31. Wiltse LL, Spencer CW. New uses and refinements of the paraspinal approach to the lumbar spine. Spine 1988;13:696–706.
32. Zindrick MR, Wiltse LL, Rauschning W. Disc herniations lateral to the intervertebral foramen. In: White AH, Rothman RH, Ray CD, eds. Lumbar Spine Surgery. St. Louis: CV Mosby; 1987, pp 195–207.

17

Disc Degeneration with Root Irritation: Spinal Canal Stenosis

"The loss of youth is melancholy enough: but to enter into old age through the gate of infirmity, most disheartening."

— Horace Walpole, 1765

INTRODUCTION

Stenosis is defined as a narrowing or constriction of a passage or canal. When the term is applied to those changes that occur within the spinal canal, the additional connotations of irreversible and progressive narrowing of the canal are implied. Such irreversible narrowing is in contrast to the often waxing and waning symptoms of encroachment occurring with a herniated nucleus pulposus (HNP). Although both conditions are mechanical in nature, that is, aggravation with activity, relief with rest, there are often gaps of days to months in the history of patients with an HNP, during which time they function reasonably well. There are no gaps in the history of patients with spinal canal stenosis (SCS) except early in the disease. As the condition progresses, the patients separate into approximately two equal groups: one in which the symptoms relentlessly (and slowly) progress with no gaps of relief from leg pain, and a second group of patients with a nonprogressive collection of symptoms that wax and wane in severity.

Spinal stenosis occurs in mobile segments. Abnormal motion, usually secondary to degenerative disc disease, results in osteophyte formation, ligament infolding or hypertrophy, and annular bulging. The corollary is also true: Degenerative spinal stenosis does not occur at a nonmobile level.

The term claudication means "limp." Often, patients with spinal stenosis experience claudication or "limping," after walking. The lameness is thought to be caused by an upset in neurological function, thus, the term neurogenic claudication. Infrequently, patients with spinal stenosis do not have neurogenic claudication, but the symptom is prevalent enough that it forms the foundation of the definition of spinal canal stenosis: (1) claudicant limitation of leg(s) function, (2) clinical evidence of chronic nerve root compression with the presence of, (3) a stenotic spinal canal lesion on imaging and, (4) in the absence of vascular impairment to the lower extremities.

Neurogenic claudication is defined as posterior (or anterior thigh) and usually calf discomfort (pain, numbness, paresthesia, weakness, tiredness, heaviness), that is aggravated by both walking and standing and is relieved only after many minutes of resting in the flexed (sitting) lumbar spine position.

CLASSIFICATION

The standard classification of spinal canal stenosis is outlined in Table 17.1. (1) Although this classification and the term spinal stenosis is used by most authors to describe canal and "lateral recess" stenosis, we have arbitrarily divided stenosis into lateral zone stenosis (Chapter 16) and spinal canal stenosis. Although this division helps in understanding the two conditions, it is an artificial separation that often does not stand the test of clinical medicine, where the two conditions so often coexist.(8) The authors have decided that before "lumping" we will "split" and describe SCS.

The most common canal stenotic conditions are acquired: stenosis due to degenerative changes in the spinal canal or stenosis due to a degenerative spondylolisthesis. On occasion, these acquired conditions occur along with developmental conditions, such as a narrowed or abnormally shaped spinal canal. Purely congenital or developmental spinal stenosis is uncommon and will receive but brief mention in this chapter. This chapter will concern itself with the three most common forms of SCS.

1. Spinal canal stenosis with degenerative spondylolisthesis, the most common stenotic condition, occurs most often in women (female-to-male ratio = 6:1) (7, 9, 18) (Fig. 17.1) and predominantly in the first story of each anatomic segment.
2. Spinal canal stenosis without vertebral body translation is a condition equally distributed among men and women. (Fig. 17.2).
3. Spinal canal stenosis may be due to a combination of a congenitally (developmentally) small spinal canal, superimposed upon which are degenerative changes, further narrowing the spinal canal. This condition most commonly occurs in men of large stature (Fig. 17.3).

The latter condition (developmental/acquired) stenosis may appear before age 50, but most patients in the former two groups will present later in life, which introduces the potential for complication by other aging conditions, such as heart disease and hypertension. This necessitates special planning for steps such as surgical intervention. Spinal canal stenosis is one of the most challenging diagnostic and surgical exercises one encounters in degenerative spine conditions.(6)

Table 17.1. Classification of Spinal Canal Stenosis[a]

A. Congenital-developmental stenosis of the spinal canal
    1. Achondroplastic stenosis
    2. Normal patient with narrowed spinal canal
B. Acquired stenosis of the spinal canal
    1. Stenosis due to degenerative changes
    2. Stenosis due to degenerative spondylolisthesis
    3. Iatrogenic—postfusion stenosis
    4. Post-traumatic
    5. Miscellaneous skeletal diseases; eg, Paget's disease
C. Combined A and B

[a]Reprinted with permission from Arnoldi CC, Brodsky AE, Cauchoix J, et al. Lumbar spinal stenosis and nerve root entrapment syndromes: Definitions and classification. Clin Orthop 1976;115:4–5.

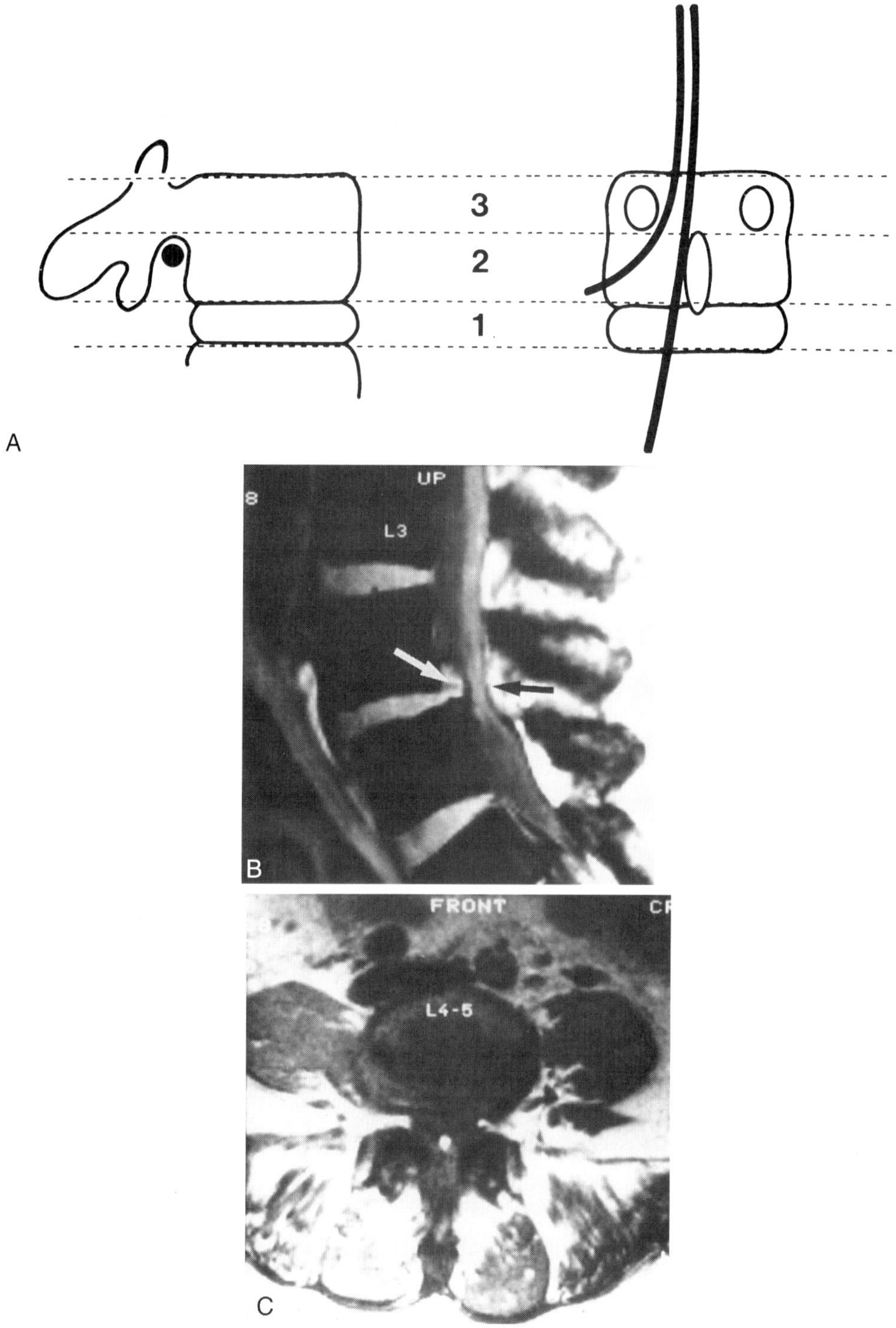

Figure 17.1 **A.** *The three stories of each anatomical segment. (How many times have you seen this schematic!)* **B.** *Sagittal MRI of degenerative spondylolisthesis and spinal stenosis showing annular bulging (white arrow) and ligamentum flavum hypertrophy (black arrow) causing stenosis in first story and upper portion of adjacent third story.* **C.** *Axial MRI in same patient showing ligamentum flavum hypertrophy, or folding, also contributing to stenosis.*

Figure 17.2 *Spinal canal stenosis without a slipped vertebrae:* **A.** *T1 sagittal—the stenosis does not appear that severe.* **B.** *T1 axial shows the true extent of the stenosis at L4–L5.*

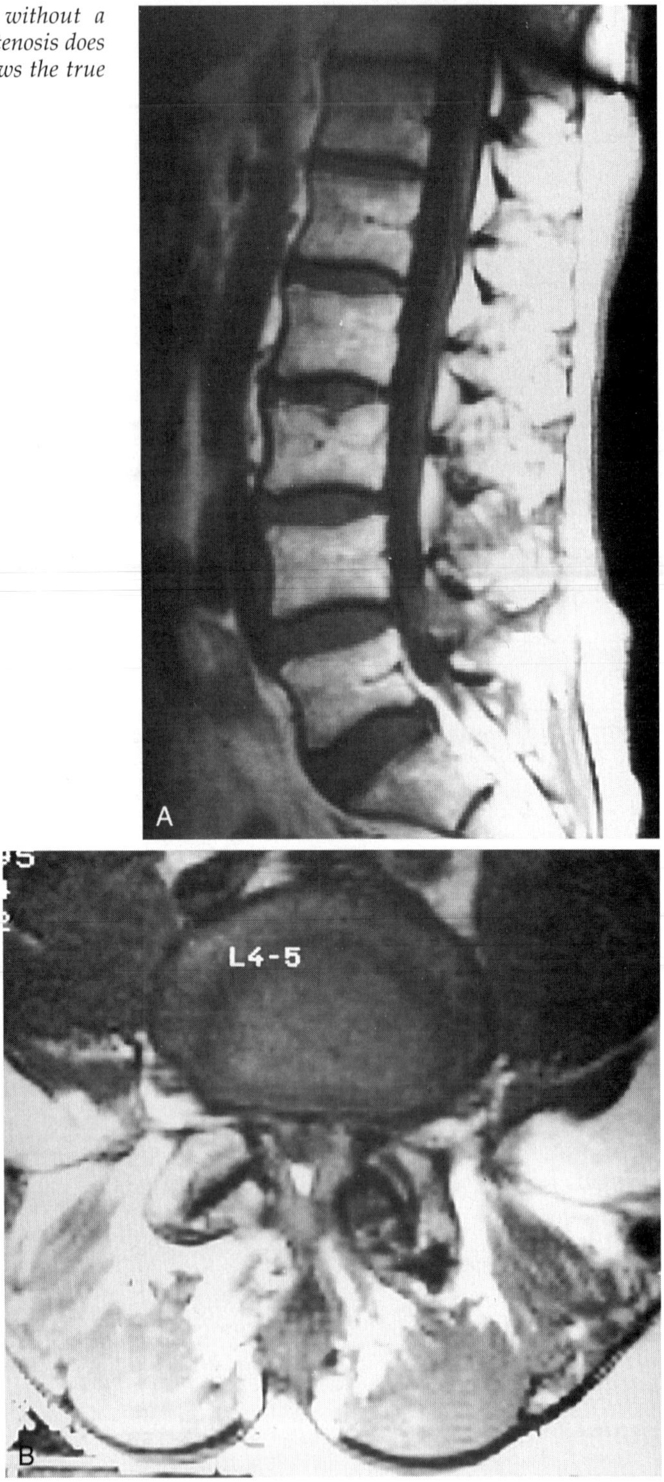

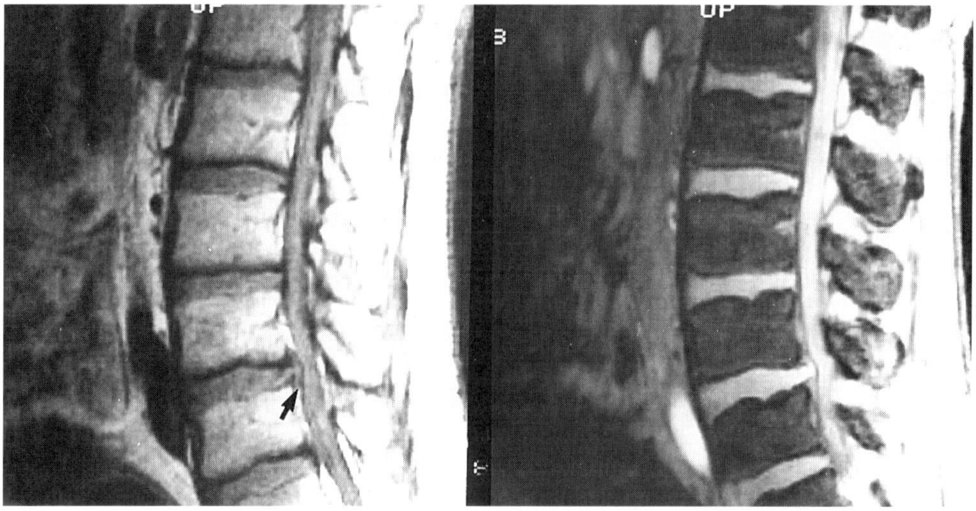

Figure 17.3 *Spinal canal stenosis without a slip but with a significant congenital narrowing of the spinal canal. Note the "global" nature of the pencil thin canal. This was a young patient tipped into symptoms by a disc herniation at L4–L5 (arrow).*

PATHOANATOMY: A SUMMARY

To understand the pathoanatomy of SCS, the reader is referred back to Chapter 1 on anatomy, paying specific attention to the first story of the anatomic segment (see Fig. 17.1), which is usually the greatest point of acquired stenosis (Fig. 17.4). Aside from the less frequent congenital narrowing of the spinal canal, the three structures that contribute to the canal stenosis are the ligamentum flavum, the facet joints, and the disc space. Notice in Figures 17.1 to 17.4 how this maximum effect is largely confined to the first story and upper reaches of the third story of the level below. This intrasegmental degenerative "napkin-ring" concept is the key to understanding the message of this chapter.

To take this concept further, consider the four factors, alone or in combination, that play a role in narrowing of the spinal canal:

1. Shape of the canal.
2. Degenerative changes reducing canal size.
3. Translation of one anatomic segment on the next.
4. Pre-existing congenital/developmental narrowing of the lumbar spinal canal.

Shape of the Canal

Figure 17.5. illustrates the three basic shapes of the lumbar spinal canal. The most common shapes are round and ovoid. Perhaps 15% of humans have a trefoil canal, and canals of trefoil shape are most vulnerable to the degenerative changes that decrease the space occupied by the neurological structures.

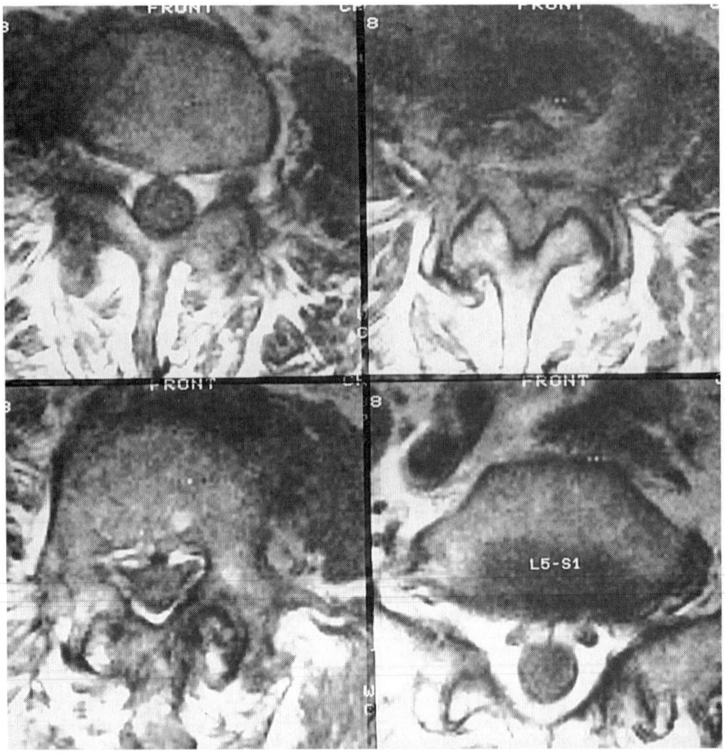

Figure 17.4 *Adjacent MRI T1 axial slices to show first story spinal canal stenosis (top right). Top left is second story of the fourth anatomic segment; bottom left is third story of fifth anatomic segment; and bottom right is first story of fifth anatomic segment (L5–S1 disc space).*

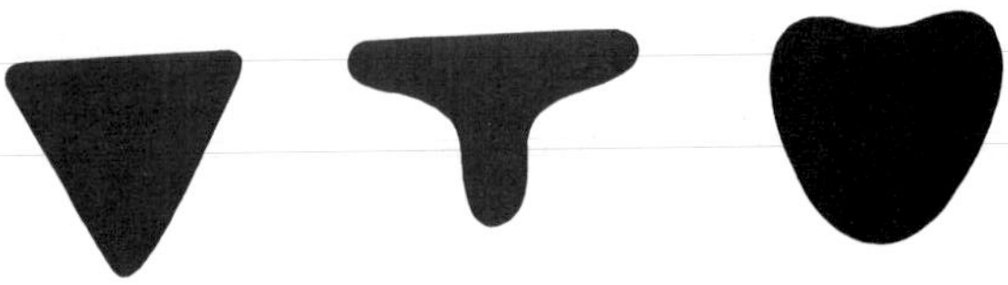

Figure 17.5 *The three shapes of the spinal canal as seen on CT scan or MRI: round (really triangular), trefoil, oval.*

Degenerative Changes

Degenerative changes can affect the disc interval, the soft-tissue supports, and the facet joints.(6, 13, 17, 21) Annular bulging, ligamentum flavum infolding or hypertrophy, and osteophyte formation encroach on the spinal canal to decrease the space available to the cauda equina.

The series of computed tomography (CT) scans and MR images (Fig. 17.6) again demonstrates that the degenerative spinal stenotic lesion is worst in the first story and upper portion of the third story of the segment below and least pronounced in the lower reaches of the third story and second story of the same segment.

Linking a series of segments together and being aware that canal stenosis is always most prominent in the first story, one can appreciate that the constriction of canal stenosis occurs between the takeoff of nerve roots (Fig. 17.7). Thus, canal stenosis at the disc space level of L4–L5 (first story of L4) is a constricting ring between the takeoff of the fourth root above and the fifth lumbar nerve root below.

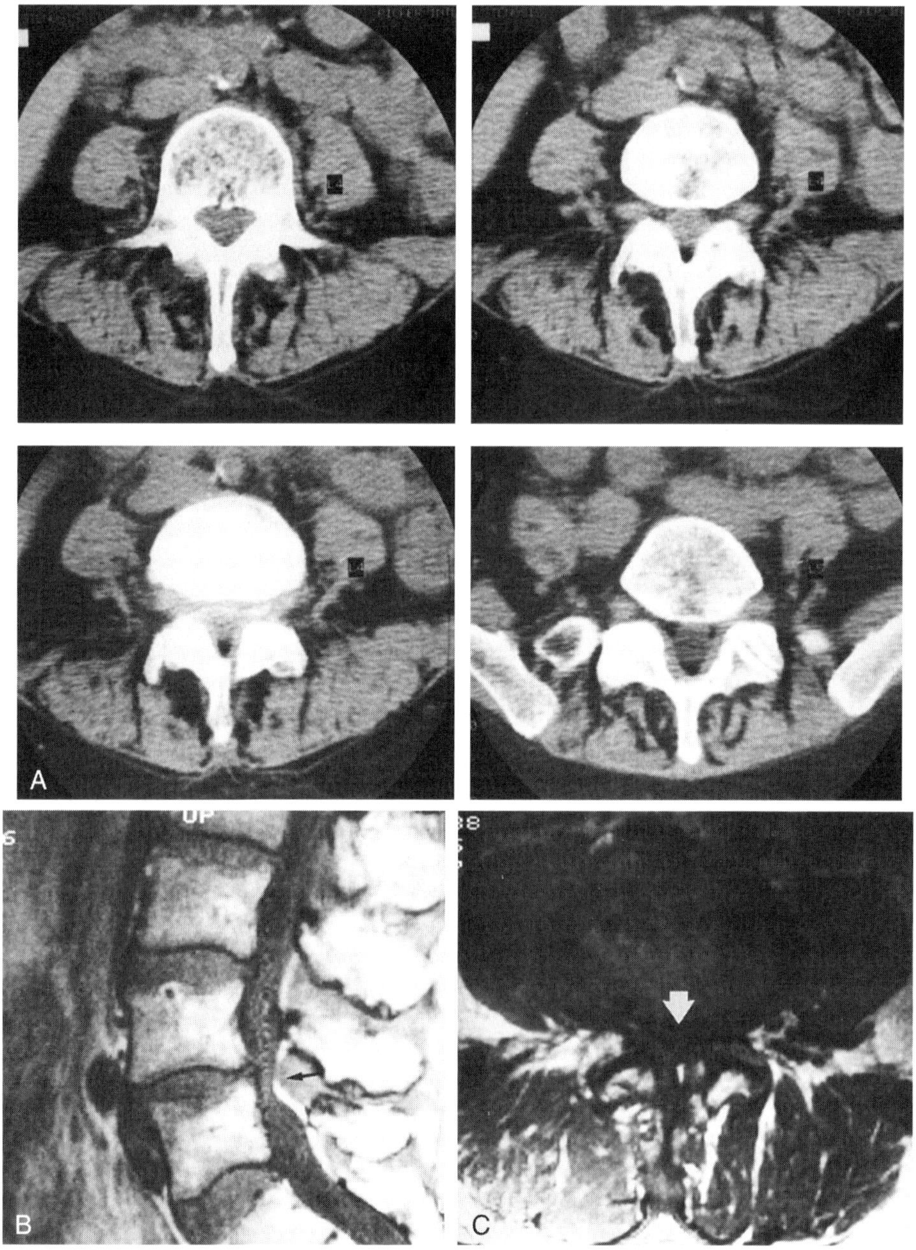

Figure 17.6 **A.** *CT of spinal canal stenosis. The stenotic lesion is greatest in first story of L4 (bottom left). The third and second story of L4 (top) and the second story of L5 (bottom, right) are relatively free of stenosis.* **B.** *Sagittal MRI showing a similar picture. Spinal canal stenosis is a lesion in the first and upper reaches of the adjacent third story, produced largely by the buckling of the ligamentum flavum from behind (arrow).* **C.** *Axial T1 MRI showing encroachmnet on space available for cauda equina (arrow) by hypertrophied ligamentum flavum and facet joints.*

Figure 17.7 *Schematic of the "napkin ring" stenotic lesion between the roots L4 and L5.*

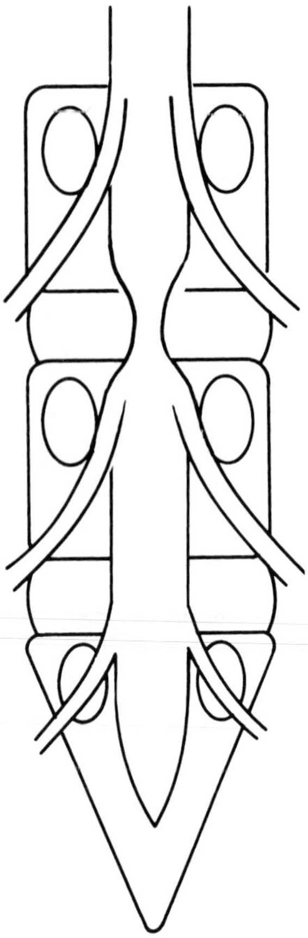

The hypertrophied ligamentum flavum enfolds to encroach posteriorly and is the major lesion in stenosis of the first story. Further first story canal encroachment occurs when the facet subluxation of a degenerative spondylolisthesis contributes inferior and superior facet bony masses to narrow the space available to the cauda equina (Fig. 17.8). Finally, annular bulging, with or without retrospondylolisthesis, contributes to anterior narrowing of the canal, the significance of which will be discussed in the section on surgical approaches.

In the second story, the anterior canal wall is formed by the inferior half of the vertebral body, which does not contribute to spinal stenosis. The one place in the second story where stenosis is said to occur is the very midline and posterior common meeting point of the superior edges of the lamina and spinous process (Fig. 17.9). This cortical edge can be likened to the wishbone of a chicken and is said to encroach on the midline of the dura at the junction of the second and third stories. But look at Figure 17.9, B. This is the second story of Figure 17.6, B and there is no stenosis.

The lateral portion of the second story is the foramen. As mentioned above, superior capsular hypertrophy, especially in degenerative spondylolisthesis, can protrude into this foraminal interval, producing radicular symptoms due to root encroachment in the lateral zone (Fig. 17.10).

Within the third story, there is virtually nothing that can cause acquired spinal stenosis. At the top end of the pedicle (third story) lies the bottom end of the superior facet. If it is hypertrophied, then lateral zone stenosis (subarticular form) can occur, but virtually nothing in the lower portion of the third story of an anatomical segment can contribute to central canal stenosis.

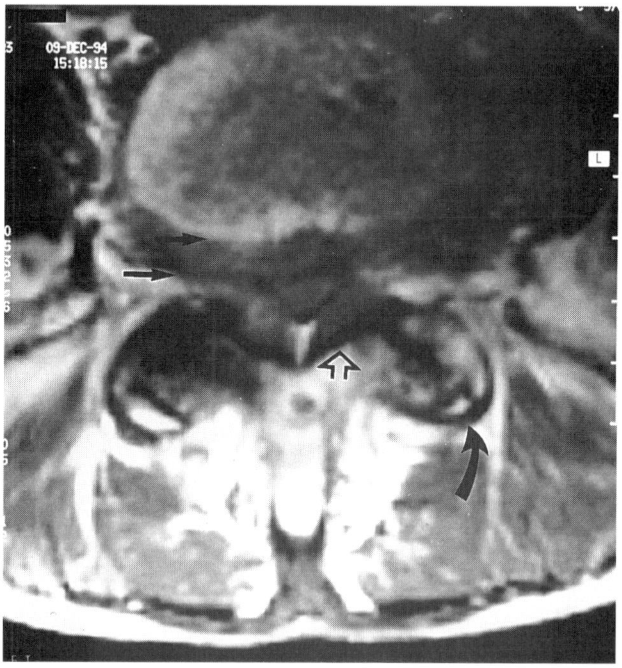

Figure 17.8 *Another example of spinal canal stenosis on T1 axial showing the two margins of the posterior vertebral body (arrows) of the "slip" and the ligamentum flavum hypertrophy (open arrow) and facet joint hypertrophy (curved arrow).*

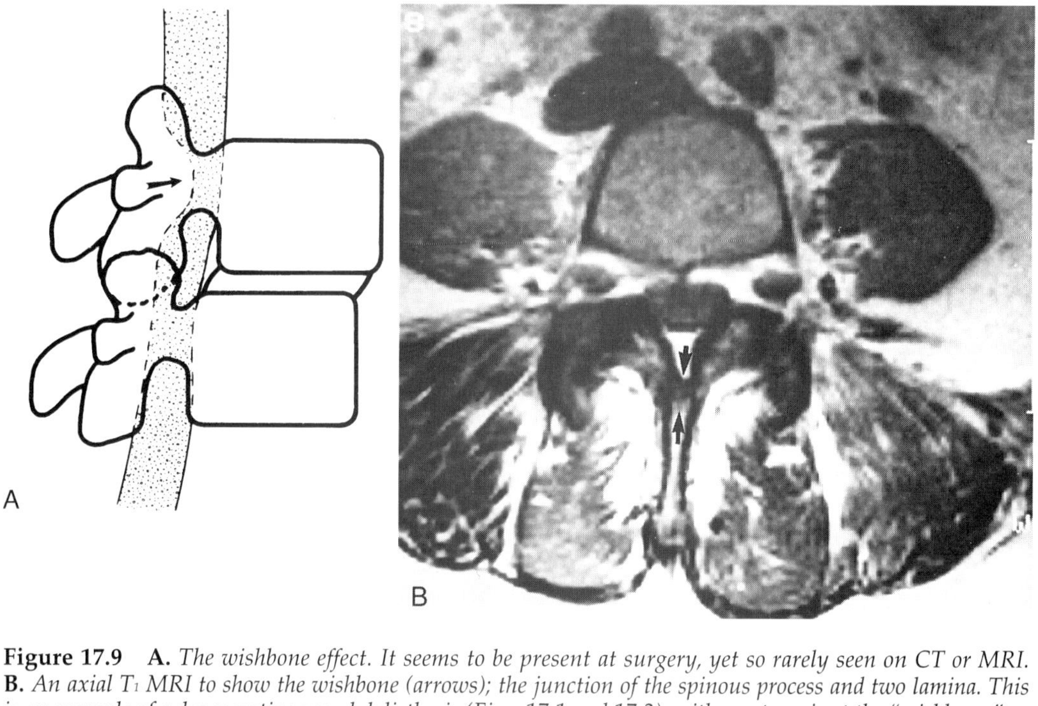

Figure 17.9 **A.** *The wishbone effect. It seems to be present at surgery, yet so rarely seen on CT or MRI.* **B.** *An axial T_1 MRI to show the wishbone (arrows); the junction of the spinous process and two lamina. This is an example of a degenerative spondylolisthesis (Figs. 17.1 and 17.2), with no stenosis at the "wishbone."*

Translation

When one anatomical segment translates on the next, a guillotining effect of the spinal canal occurs. The most common type of translation is degenerative spondylolisthesis, a forward or lateral slip of one anatomic segment on the next. Because of the intact neural arch, it has often been stated that the posterior elements of the cephalad segment impinge on the contents of the spinal canal (Fig. 17.11), when, in fact, the major lesion is still the ligamentum flavum and the facet joints. Lateral spondylolisthesis (Fig. 17.12) has the same effect on the space occupied by the cauda equina. Retrospondylolisthesis or posterior translation impinges least on the space occupied by the cauda equina except that it is usually part of the degenerative changes previously listed (Fig. 17.13.

CONGENITAL/DEVELOPMENTAL NARROWING OF THE LUMBAR SPINAL CANAL

The vertebral canal reaches its maximum size by 4 years of age. Thereafter, pedicles/vertebral bodies increase in size and the canal may change its shape, but the overall size of the canal changes little. Intrauterine factors such as drugs, alcohol, and smoking and environmental factors such as infectious diseases and malnutrition may potentially reduce canal size and result in a congenitally narrow canal. Because congenital/developmental stenosis is so prevalent among men of large stature (eg, the front line of football players), one has to wonder if spurts in vertical height before the age of four somehow reduce the cross-sectional area of the spinal canal. The analogy is a sausage tube held up by one hand maintains its maximal diameter, but when stretched fully by two hands (Fig. 17.14), quickly narrows in diameter. Whatever the insult, the spinal canal can be left in a

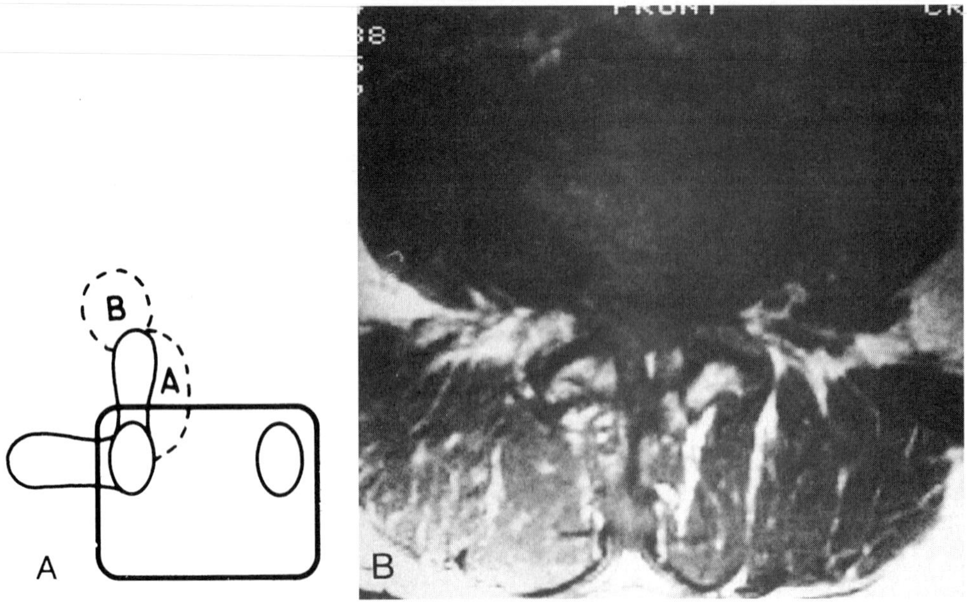

Figure 17.10 **A.** *Schematic showing effect of capsular encroachment on foraminal zone (B), and medial edge facet hypertrophy on the subarticular zone (A).* **B.** *MRI showing actual lesion.*

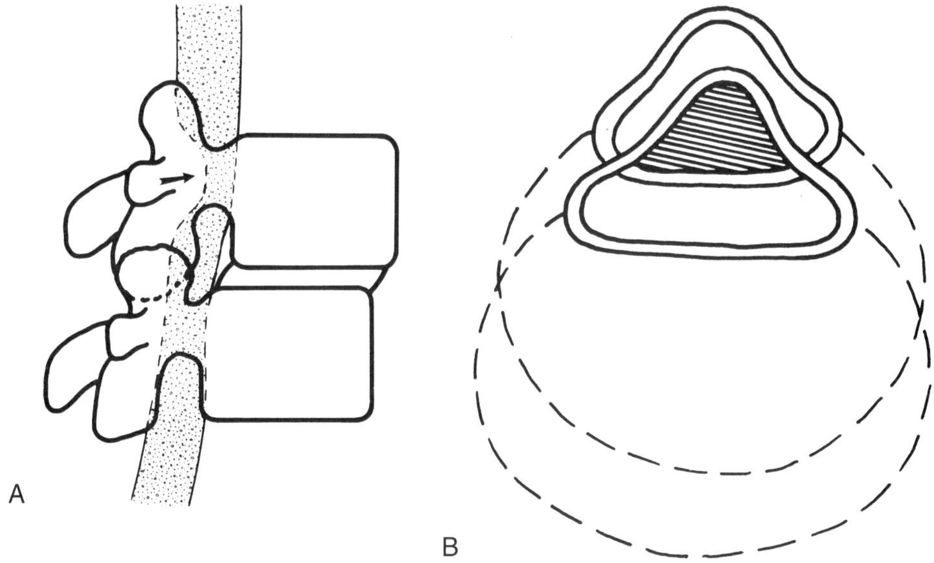

Figure 17.11 **A.** *The wishbone effect. It seems to be present at surgery, yet so rarely seen on CT or MRI.* **B.** *The so-called guillotining effect on the cauda equina of one posterior arch sliding over its mate. Hatched area is space left for cauda equina.*

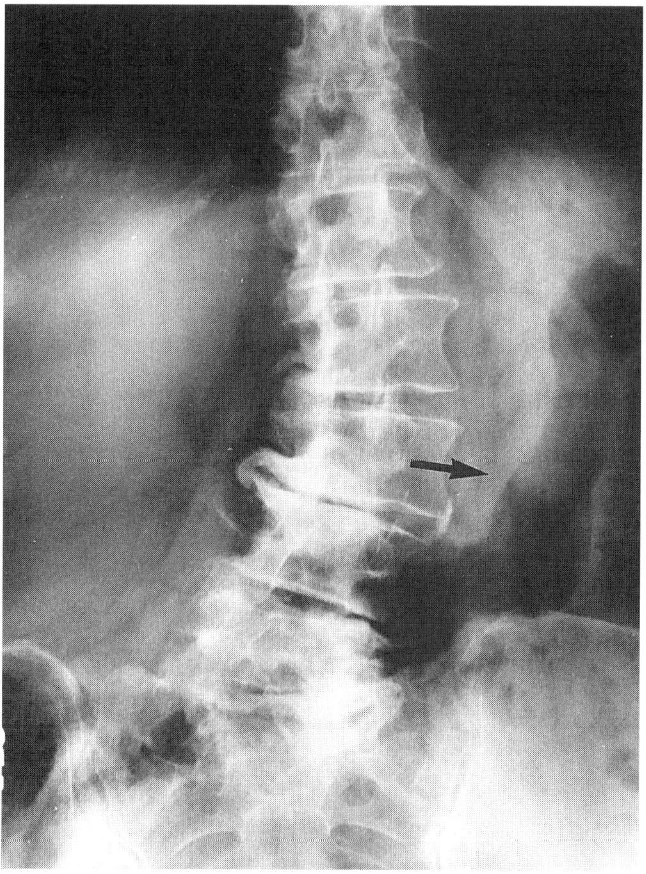

Figure 17.12 *Radiograph of a lateral spondylolisthesis (arrow) at the apex of a degenerative scoliosis.*

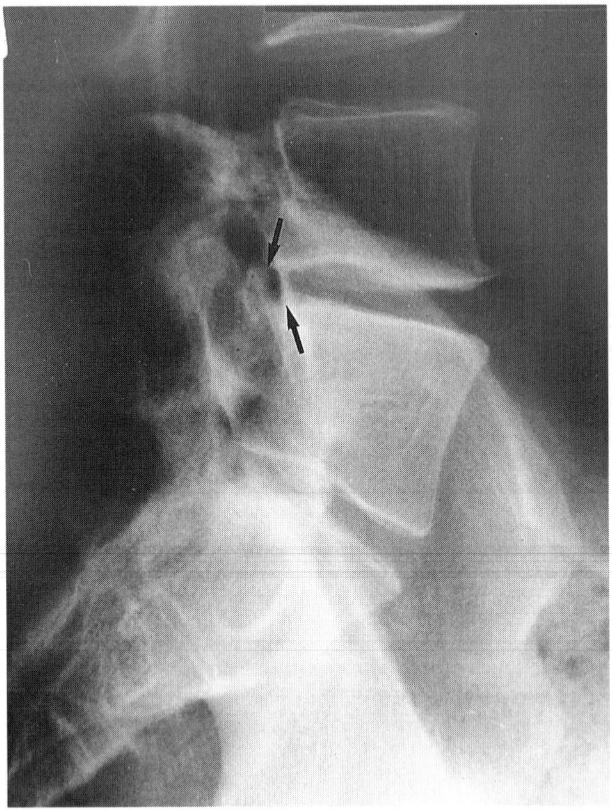

Figure 17.13 *A retrospondylolisthesis on plain radiograph at L4–L5 (arrows point to the respective corners of the vertebral bodies). Note how L4 is posterior to L5.*

narrowed state, vulnerable to isolated traumatic events or cumulative trauma causing degenerative changes, which leads to symptomatic spinal canal stenosis (Fig. 17.15).

Dimension of the Normal Spinal Canal

Porter (21) has done considerable work in measuring the normal lumbar spinal canal. The bony dimensions are fairly constant from L1 to L5 and are listed in Table 17.2.

MEASUREMENTS IN SPINAL CANAL STENOSIS

Verbiest (29) made a major contribution to our knowledge of how much the canal narrows in patients with spinal stenosis. Careful intraoperative measurements (at the level of the disc space, ie, first story) led him to identify three degrees of canal stenosis: no stenosis, relative stenosis, and absolute canal stenosis. Absolute SCS occurs when a sagittal diameter of less than 10 mm is noted. In a normal canal, the sagittal diameter is greater than 12 mm and may range up to 20 to 25 mm at L5–S1, normally the largest section of the spinal canal. The normal large diameters at L5–S1 contribute to the fact that SCS is rare at L5–S1 and is the reason why surgical decompression of the L5–S1 segment is so

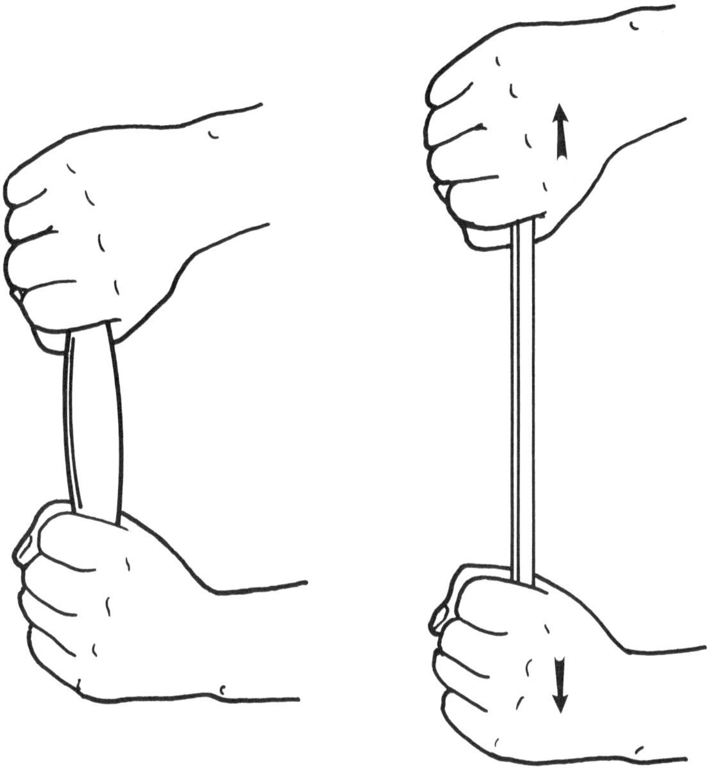

Figure 17.14 *In trying to understand congenital stenosis, think of the unstretched sausage tube (left) being stretched through sudden growth (right).*

Figure 17.15 *An example of congenital (global) spinal canal stenosis and an HNP (arrow) that precipitated the patient into a symptomatic state.*

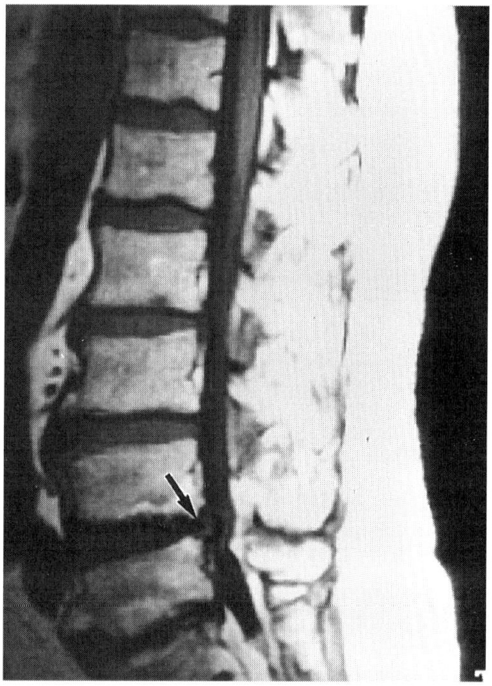

rarely indicated. Relative spinal stenosis occurs when the sagittal diameter is between 10 and 12 mm. Many attempts have been made to relate Verbiest's intraoperative measurements to plain radiographic films, all with limited success. Measurements applied to anteroposterior (AP) and lateral myelograms, axial CT scans and magnetic resonance image (MRI) are a better indication of the extent of stenosis.(20) Spengler's group (25), (in a CT scan study), took into account soft-tissue encroachment on the spinal canal, to conclude that the space available for the cauda equina should be measured as an area rather than a diameter. An area less than 100 mm (2) is considered to be indicative of relative spinal stenosis and a cross-sectional area of less than 65 to 70 mm (2) is indicative of absolute stenosis. As more MR images are studied, further understanding of the anthropometric aspects of SCS will follow. The use of CT and MRI to reveal both bony and soft tissue encroachment on the space available for the cauda equina have largely made spinal canal measurements obsolete.(28) To measure whether or not there is enough room for the cauda equina, use a simple "rule of the baby finger" (Fig. 17.16).

Table 17.2. Dimensions of the Spinal Canal (Midpedicle Level)

Midpedicle Level	Sagittal (mm)	Coronal (interpedicle) (mm)
L1	16	22
L2	15	22
L3	14	23
L4	13	23
L5	14	24

Figure 17.16 *The baby finger rule: in the top axial cut, the tip of the baby finger easily fits into the spinal canal—not so in the bottom axial cut (a stenotic level).*

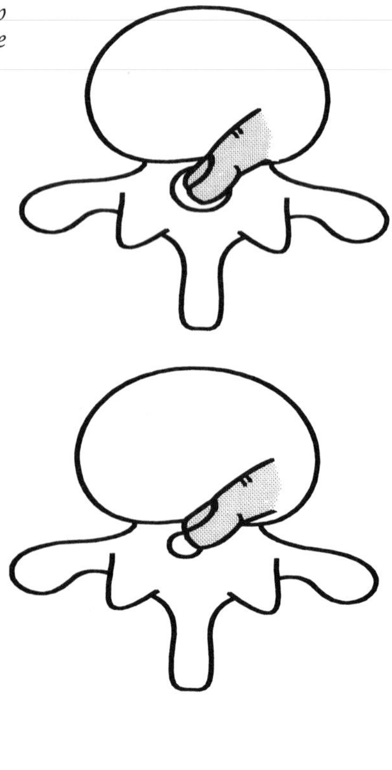

NEUROPATHOLOGY

A number of degenerative changes contribute to narrowing of the space available for the cauda equina. These include (Fig. 17.17) annular bulging or disc herniation anteriorly, facet hypertrophy or subluxation laterally and ligamentum flavum changes posterolaterally. The ligamentum flavum changes include loss of elastin fibers and hypertrophy of collagen fibers, fragmentation and infolding of the ligamentum (Fig. 17.17), edema, and substance deposit (Fig. 17.17).

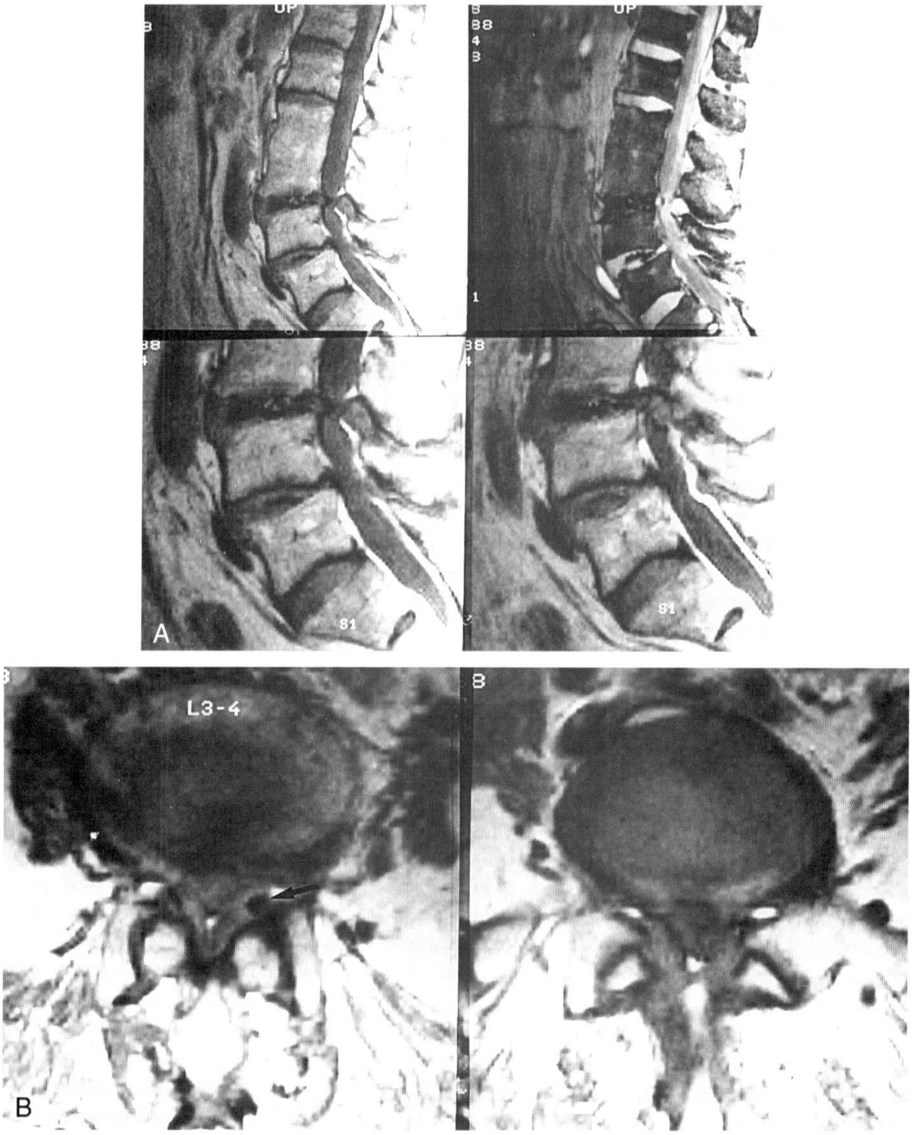

Figure 17.17 **A.** *Spinal canal stenosis on sagittal MRI showing a block vertebrae (L2–L3), annular bulging, and ligamentum flavum infolding at L3–L4 and a degenerative spondylolisthesis (slip) at L4–L5.* **B.** *Spinal canal stenosis on axial MRI showing ligamentum flavum hypertrophy and a "calcium" deposit (arrow) that is possibly part of a synovial cyst.*

Obviously, narrowing of the spinal canal constricts the dura and cauda equina nerves. The nerve roots themselves are constricted and often become adherent due to arachnoid changes. In a histological examination of the roots, Watanabe and Parke (30) found a reduction in the number of neurons, especially affecting large-caliber fibers. There were varying degrees of degeneration and demyelination with regeneration of nerve tissue. Morphological assessment of the vessels revealed that the arterioles were absent at the level of the constriction and more coiled on either side of the constriction. Venules were collapsed at the level of the lesion and engorged proximally, and there appeared to be more arterial venous shunts proximal to the stenotic lesion.

Synovial cysts are reasonably common in spinal canal stenosis (Fig. 17.18). They arise as outpouchings from the degenerative (synarthrodial) facet joint, and if they enlarge into the canal they may further compress a nerve root. They often become very adherent to the dura and can be difficult to excise because of this.

PATHOPHYSIOLOGY

SCS is a chronic rather than an acute compression of the nerve roots in the cauda equina. Although the cauda equina is often considered a peripheral nerve structure, its

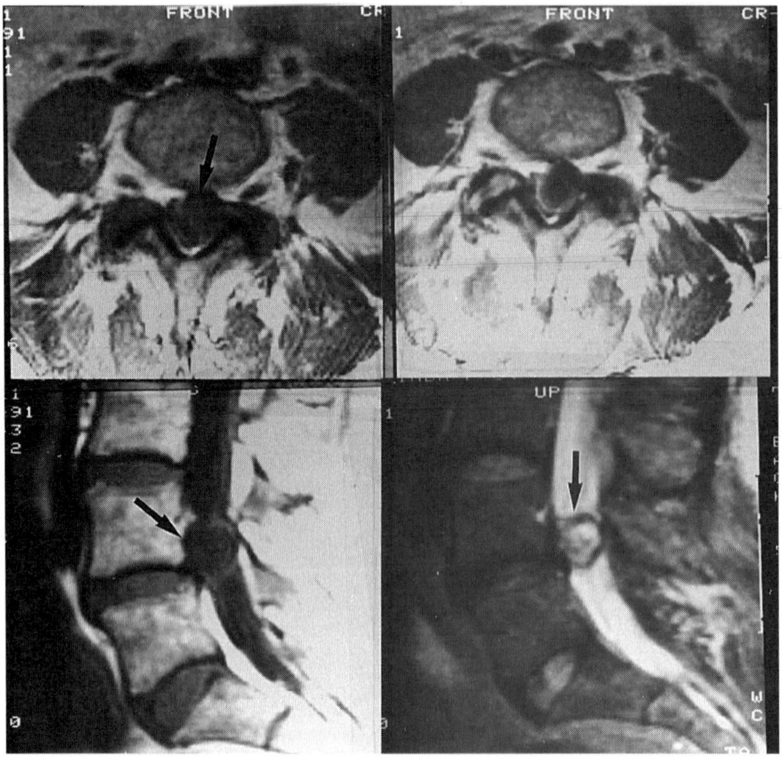

Figure 17.18 *A synovial cyst (arrow) at a very low grade "slip" L4–L5 contributing to some spinal canal stenosis. Gadolinium enhancement clearly outlines the cyst on axial T1 (top right). The bottom right is a T2 sagittal highlighting the "water" in the cyst.*

coverings and vascular anatomy are more like those of a central nervous system structure than those of a peripheral nerve, which makes them more susceptible to compression.

Obviously, compression of the cauda equina affects nerve conduction, resulting in the leg symptoms, with it likely that aging nerves are more susceptible to this compressive phenomenon. It is well known that the symptoms of spinal stenosis are exacerbated by activity, specifically involving extension of the back. Thus, any theory to explain the symptoms of spinal stenosis must account for this mechanical component. It is likely that symptoms are caused by a combination of mechanical and ischemic nutritional factors.(8, 21, 23)

The pathophysiology of spinal stenosis can be summarized as follows: The canal constriction or encroachment mechanically affects the cauda equina nerve bundle and the free flow of cerebrospinal fluid around this bundle. In turn, the nerve fiber is constricted and changes occur in the pia-arachnoid. When increased demands are placed on the cauda equina, such as when the patient walks, the body cannot satisfy the nutritional needs of the nerve roots because of the mechanical constriction and the associated ischemia. As well, the noxious by-products of metabolism build up in the constricted area and are not removed because of venous engorgement. Because of the mechanical compression shutting off the arterial blood flow to the constricted area of the cauda equina, arteriovenous shunts open on either side of the nerve root constriction, which in turn upset normal neurophysiological function. The result is ectopic nerve impulses that produce some of the painful paresthetic and cramping symptoms of spinal stenosis. It is obvious from clinical facts that this neurophysiological malfunctioning is more sensory than motor, which suggests that the large fiber sensory nerves are more susceptible to the compression than the motor fibers.

If the compression persists long enough, intraneural edema and fibrosis ensues. It is important to intervene surgically before symptoms progress to this stage, which is clinically evident as measurable weakness in the distal extremities.

Do not forget that the patient also experiences the mechanical symptoms of skeletal disease. These symptoms arise from degeneration within the disc spaces and the facet joints resulting in varying degrees of skeletal instability (backache).

CLINICAL PRESENTATION

Symptoms

Patients symptomatic with SCS may be categorized as (1) patients with only canal stenosis and (2) patients with both canal stenosis and lateral zone stenosis. The various combinations of canal and lateral zone stenosis are the reason for the rather confusing clinical picture presented by patients with SCS. For now, we have agreed to split and discuss the clinical presentation of canal stenosis.

Back Symptoms

Although back pain has been present for some years, almost all patients with spinal stenosis will present because leg symptoms have become disabling. They have put up with and adjusted to the back pain over the years, but the increasing limitation to walking due to leg "symptoms" is the "straw that broke the camel's back" and brought them to the doctor.

Leg Symptoms

The patient with canal stenosis has bilateral radicular symptoms. The bilateral leg symptoms are very diffusely localized and often described as a heaviness, general soreness, or weakness that occurs in both lower extremities, especially with walking. The reason for the diffuse vague leg symptoms rather than discrete radicular pain is due to compression of multiple roots rather than a single root, and an ischemic rather than an acute inflammatory origin of the radiculopathy. The distribution of the pain is most frequently to the buttocks, thighs, and calves because most stenotic lesions occur at L4–L5. If there is a higher level symptomatic stenotic lesion, anterior thigh discomfort will present. In addition, mild sensory symptoms in the form of paresthetic tingling or actual numbness are common. The patient may also describe night symptoms of restlessness in the legs or muscle cramps. The classic revelation by the patient is to volunteer that the symptoms are less aggravating in the grocery store, unbeknownst to them because they are leaning on the shopping cart in the flexed position (Fig. 17.19).

These symptoms are almost always of insidious onset, with the patient seldom presenting before 55 years of age. A sudden worsening of these symptoms is equated with a sudden increase in vertebral body translation or the occurrence of an HNP within the stenotic segment, an infrequent event. This latter condition usually occurs at a slip level and is usually accompanied by a dramatic increase in the radicular component of the symptoms.

Within the diffuse cauda equina syndrome may be a sharper radicular component. If it involves a single nerve root in the lateral zone the patient will describe a better defined

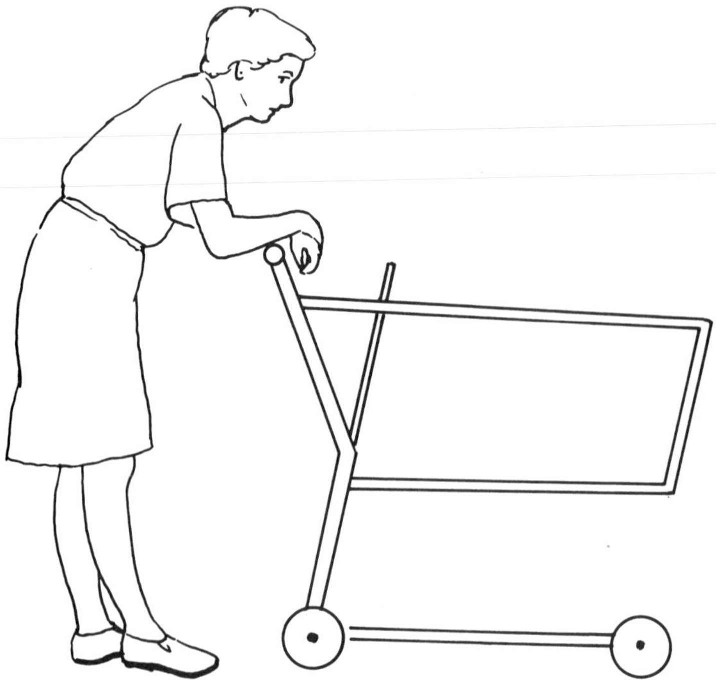

Figure 17.19 *The shopping cart sign: Most patients with spinal canal stenosis have noticed that they are able to walk further when leaning on a shopping cart (because they are flexing their stenotic canal and tensing (unfolding) the ligamentum flavum), which increases the space available for the cauda equina. It is such a common description in spinal canal stenosis that it is worth making it a specific question in your history.*

radicular distribution to the extremity pain, affecting one leg more than its mate. The radicular symptom of lateral zone stenosis described by the patient is more specific than the diffuse bilateral leg symptoms described by patients with SCS. However, the radicular component does not dominate the history, as with a disc herniation Both sets of symptoms are usually aggravated by walking and relieved by rest or standing in the forward flexed position.

Clinical symptoms of bladder and bowel upset are unusual in patients with SCS. However, many patient, with SCS have a subclinical upset in their bladder control, and other local causes of impaired bladder control.

At least 50% of stenotic patients will report an upset in balance or an unsteadiness of gait. On the rare occasion, a patient will present with symptoms of collapsing legs due to their weakness and will come to the spinal surgeon only after negative cardiac investigation. Finally, it is interesting to note that many patients have difficulty describing their symptoms and can do so only after surgical decompression of the spinal stenosis, has relieved the various feelings that they had in their legs. The reason for this is the fact that many patients have three or four different syndromes affecting their legs including neurogenic claudication, acute or chronic nerve root compression, low back pain and nonradicular lower extremity pain. Imagine trying to hear the strains of Beethoven rather than Chopin or Bach and hearing all three at the same time. It is no wonder that we do not understand the description of leg symptoms patients are offering up!

Both the backache and the leg symptoms of SCS are mechanical in nature. That is, they are aggravated by activity and often relieved significantly by rest. They are distinguished from vascular claudication in that the rest required for relief of neurogenic claudication is usually many minutes rather than a brief interruption in activities.

Signs

It is necessary to state clearly that often there is virtually nothing to find on physical examination,(7, 8, 10, 24) a fact that often relegates these patients to the scrap heap of a "functional illness." The diagnosis of SCS is made on history and verified on investigation. The main reason for doing a physical examination is to note that other conditions, such as vascular disorders, hip disease or neurological conditions, such as amyotrophic lateral sclerosis, are not present.

Examination of the back of a patient with SCS reveals three findings:

1. Loss of lumbar lordosis, with or without degenerative scoliosis.
2. Stiffness and loss of movement in the back.
3. A palpable step of a spondylolysthetic vertebral segment (Fig. 17.20), if vertebral translation is present.

Neurological examination of the extremities is often fruitless unless the stenotic condition has been present for a long time and is well advanced. In these infrequent cases, one sees a significant amount of weakness and sensory upset along with an absence of reflexes. However, patients with SCS are more usually seen early in the progression of symptoms, and one records little in the way of reduced straight leg raising. Although paresthetic discomfort is a common symptom in SCS, it is unusual to find a loss of sensation to pinprick testing, temperature, or light touch. Because of the age of patients, loss of distal vibratory sensation is frequent. Although many patients complain of weakness in their legs, a specific weakness is rarely noted unless the stenosis has been present for a

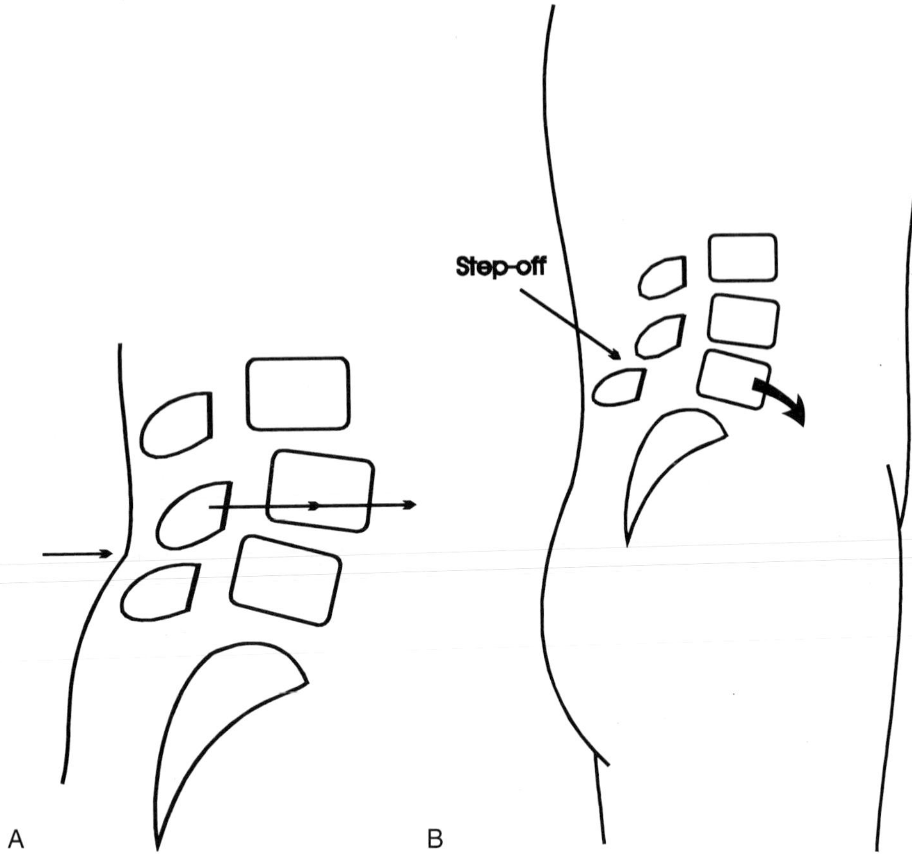

Figure 17.20 **A.** *Schematic of the palpable step in degenerative spondylolisthesis. The spinous process moves with the slipped vertebrae (double arrow). Compare the similar appearance to the skin crease step in lytic spondylolisthesis* **(B)**, *where the spinous process is left behind as the vertebrae (L5) slips forward (curved arrow).*

considerable time. It is usual to note that the ankle reflexes are much diminished over the knee reflexes (symmetric or asymmetric). However, that observation is frequent in many older patients without spinal stenosis. The observation of a discrepancy in reflexes gives us one useful rule: if a patient has brisk ankle reflexes they usually do not have spinal canal stenosis. (They may still have neurogenic claudication on the basis of bilateral subarticular stenosis of the 5th lumbar roots.) A femoral stretch test, if positive, suggests fourth root involvement either in the lateral zone or the cauda equina. There is a tendency for all signs to be more obvious immediately after the patient has been active.

The biggest problem with the history and physical examination of spinal stenotic patients is the fact they are in an age group where a host of other conditions may be in tandem with their spinal stenosis.

Tandem Stenosis

This is a term introduced by Epstein and co-workers (7) and Dagi et al (4) to describe a patient with both a lumbar canal stenotic lesion, and cervical spinal canal stenosis. It is reasonable to assume that the ravages of degenerative disc disease that narrow the lumbar spinal canal can also do the same thing to the cervical spinal canal. The cervical stenotic lesion causes cord compression or myelopathy (upper motor neuron lesion [UMNL]), whereas the lumbar stenosis causes nerve root compression (lower motor neuron lesion [LMNL]). This causes a mixed picture in the lower extremities. Patients will have hyper-reflexic knee jerks (UMNL), absent ankle jerks (LMNL), and equivocal or upgoing toes. The examiner focused on the lumbar canal stenosis will miss the cervical lesion, and an examiner similarly focused on the neck will miss the tandem lumbar stenosis.

Differential Diagnosis

The differential diagnosis of SCS (neurogenic claudication) versus vascular claudication is presented in Table 17.3. Although this table makes good script, and may even help you pass an examination, it is important to remember that spinal stenosis has many faces of presentation, some not clearly defined until the end of complete vascular and spinal investigation. Obviously, vascular claudication is the number one differential diagnosis. But other conditions that cause upset in walking also have to be included in the differential diagnosis. These include:

Table 17.3. Differential Diagnosis of Claudicant Leg Pain[a]

Findings	Vascular Claudication	Neurogenic Claudication (SCS)
Back Pain	Rare	Always in the past or present history
Leg Pain		
Type	Sharp, cramping	Vague and variously described as radicular, heaviness, cramping
Location	Exercised muscles (often calf, but may be buttock and thigh). May be one leg	Either typical radicular or extremely diffuse and almost always buttock, thigh, and calf in location. Always both legs in canal stenosis
Radiation	Rare after onset, but may be distal to proximal	Common after onset, usually proximal to distal
Aggravation	Walking, not standing	Usually aggravated by walking, but can be aggravated by standing
Walking uphill	Worse	Better (because back is flexed)
Walking downhill	Better (less muscular energy needed)	Worse (because back is extended)
Relief	Stopping muscular activity even in the standing position	Walking in forward, flexed position more comfortable; once pain occurs, relief comes only with lying down or sitting down
Time to relief	Quick (minutes)	Slow (many minutes)
Neurological symptoms	Not present	Commonly present
Straight leg raising tests	Negative	Mildly positive or negative
Neurological examination	Negative	Mildly positive or negative
Vascular examination	Absent pulses	Pulses present
Skin appearance	Atrophic changes	No changes

[a]Note that both conditions can coexist.

1. Bilateral hip joint disease.
2. Referred leg pain
3. Peripheral neuropathy.

Along with peripheral vascular disease, they form the "big four" in the differential diagnosis of SCS.

Bilateral Hip Joint Disease It is surprising the number of times this diagnosis is missed and patients are labeled as having SCS. Noting the groin pain along with the thigh pain (both aggravated by walking) will alert you to the possibility of hip joint disease. Inability to rotate the hip for daily tasks (eg, putting on one's socks and shoes) associated with a loss of hip range of motion on examination are the clues to radiograph the hips (Fig. 17.21).

Referred Leg Pain This concept was discussed in detail in Chapter 14. Referred pain is a diffuse discomfort in the legs not unlike that of spinal canal stenosis. It differs from the leg symptoms in SCS in that:

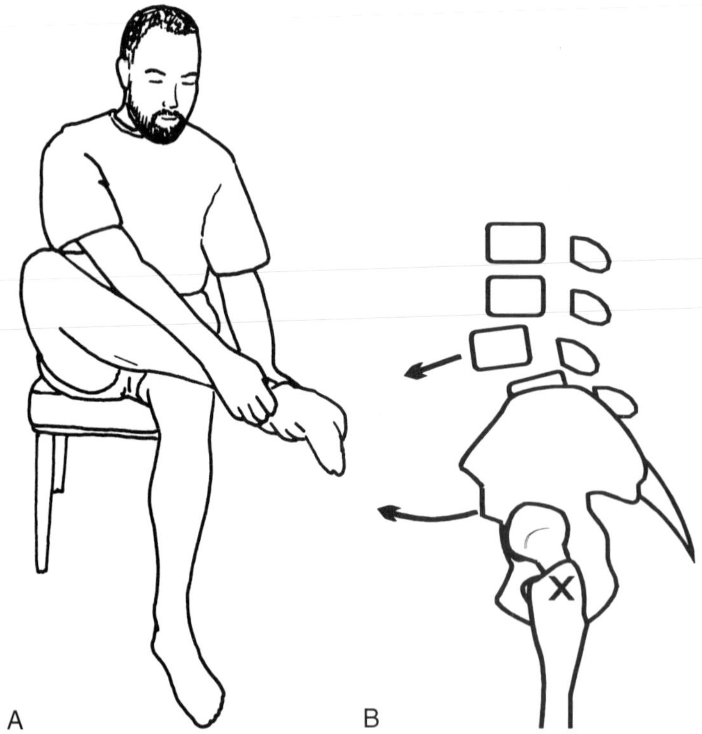

Figure 17.21 **A.** *A patient with an osteoarthritic hip has trouble externally rotating the hip to get a sock on: not a problem in spinal canal stenosis.* **B.** *The development of pain over the greater trochanter (X) is from a pelvic tilt (lower curved arrow) to compensate for the forward slip of the body (at L4–L5). The tensor fascia lata comes into play in an attempt to rotate (compensate) the pelvic balance. This causes pain over the greater trochanteric region. Another form of compensation is backward subluxation (retrospondylolisthesis) above, as shown in this schematic.*

1. Although it may occur with walking, it does not limit walking distance.
2. It rarely goes below the knees.
3. It is not associated with neurological symptoms (numbness, paresthesia).
4. The associated backache dominates the history.

Despite these clinical points it is still often difficult to distinguish between neurogenic claudication and referred leg pain even when testing with a facet joint block or doing an MRI.

Peripheral Neuropathy (PN) This is the toughest differential diagnosis of all and missing it has to be the most common reason for a failed outcome following spinal stenosis surgery. The two conditions (SCS and PN) may coexist in this age group. The clinical presentation of PN is dominated with neurological symptoms more so than pain and produces a more uniform distal stocking pattern of neurological deficits. These patients do not necessarily become aggravated by walking but they do experience unsteadiness that interferes with walking. Often, electrophysiologic testing is required to differentiate these conditions. Of course the absence of a stenotic lesion on MRI is a good reason to step back and consider the diagnosis of peripheral neuropathy.

A Word about Trochanteric Bursitis All too often spinal stenotic patients are given the diagnosis of trochanteric bursitis. This is followed by an injection of local anesthetic and steroid into the trochanteric area giving relief of symptoms due to a placebo effect. The relief is short-lived because the real condition is spinal stenotic alteration of the pelvic mechanics to accommodate changes in the lumbar spine (see Fig. 17.21).

INVESTIGATION

Investigation of a patient with SCS is often difficult to sort out. Because of the age group affected, it is important to rule out other conditions, such as infection, tumors, and other nonmechanical causes of back pain. A high percentage of these patients may also have vascular disease, and it is important to rule out symptomatic aortoiliac or femoral arterial insufficiency. Neurological symptoms require consideration of all possible causes, including generalized disorders unrelated to the spine.

Radiological Investigation

Plain radiographic films of most patients with low back pain are routinely ordered but yield little information about a patient with SCS except to show vertebral subluxations. Their greatest use is to rule out other conditions, such as tumors or infection. Radiographic films do reveal the degenerative changes within the disc space and the facet joints along with osteophytic formation. Subluxations are also obvious on plain radiographic films and bear on the surgical decision. Many investigators have attempted to define SCS by using radiographic measurements, but they have routinely failed. Perhaps the only plain radiographic observation suggestive of a stenotic spinal canal is a narrowing of the interlaminar space and/or short pedicles (Fig. 17.22).

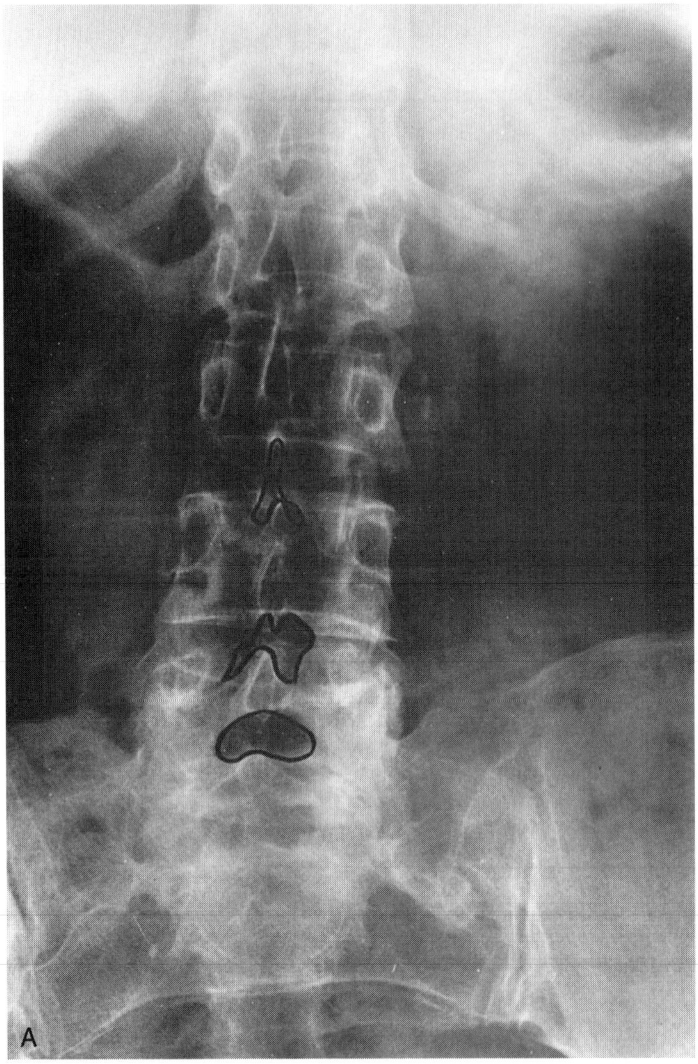

Figure 17.22 **A.** *Narrowing of interlaminar spaces L3–L4 and L4–L5 (normal at L5–S1) is suggestive of spinal stenosis.*

Some authors have advocated the use of standing films and flexion and extension films, but they yield little information that one cannot obtain with the preoperative investigation of MRI or CT/myelography.(25) Myelography has been the gold standard for the investigation of a patient with SCS. It is advisable to combine myelography with CT scanning while the contrast material is still present in the lumbar subarachnoid space.

Water-soluble, nonionic compounds are best used for myelographic examination of a patient suspected of having stenosis. They are better than oil myelographic compounds because they offer superior demonstration of the nerve roots. Another advantage of low-viscosity compound is its ability to slide by the block to show levels below the stenotic obstruction. This is most evident on CT/myelography (Fig. 17.23). In addition, redundant nerve roots are more readily demonstrated by water-soluble contrast material.(26)

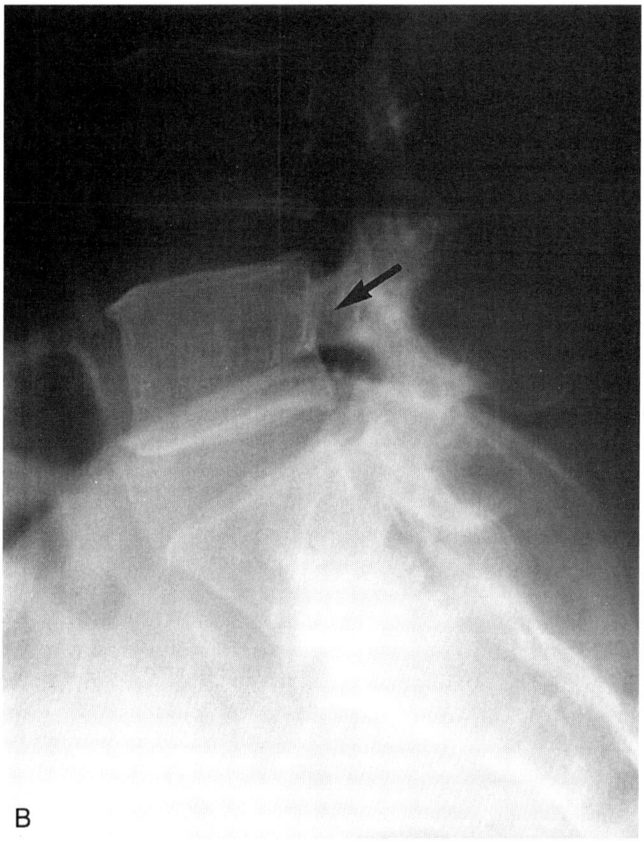

Figure 17.22 (continued) **B.** *Short pedicles at L5 (arrow), which suggest congenital spinal canal stenosis.*

The myelographic block of SCS is typical and described as either single level or multiple level. An incomplete obstruction is described as having an apple core appearance (Fig. 17.24) and a complete obstruction as having a paintbrush appearance (Fig. 17.25). These two changes are to be distinguished from the meniscal-like change that occurs with tumors of the spinal canal (Fig. 17.26).

A number of authors advocate functional myelography, which includes flexion and extension AP and lateral radiographic films during myelography. Again, the usefulness of this additional testing is low when compared with the benefits of CT scanning. Although myelography is considered the "gold standard" of investigation, CT/myelography has largely supplanted plain myelography in most centers. CT scanning is usually done from the midbody of L3 to the sacrum. Obviously, any disease above this level will not be demonstrated by CT scanning, making it essential for the clinician to predetermine the levels to be scanned. The added benefit of myelographic contrast material with CT will outline the true nature of the spinal canal below the level of the stenotic obstruction. CT/myelography allows detailed analysis of the first, second, and third stories of each segment (Fig. 17.23). In addition, myelography allows for screening of the higher lumbar levels to exclude unusual pathological conditions.

These imaging modalities are all preoperative tools that simply document a structural lesion that must marry perfectly with the clinical presentation.

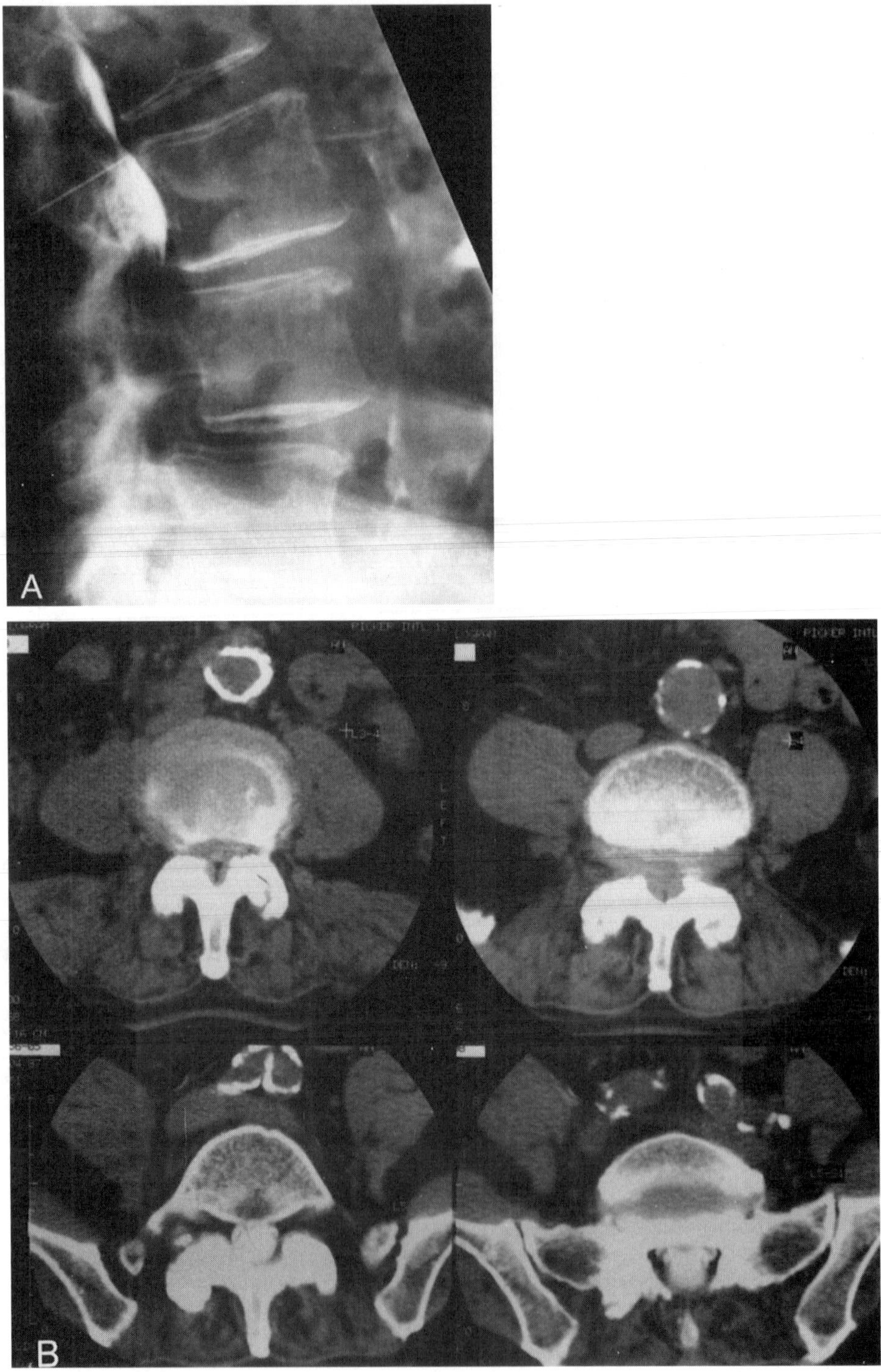

Figure 17.23 **A.** *Myelogram showing apparent complete block at stenotic site, L3, with no contrast at lower segments.* **B.** *Subsequent CT/myelogram showing flow of contrast past the obstruction at L4–L5 to L5–S1.*

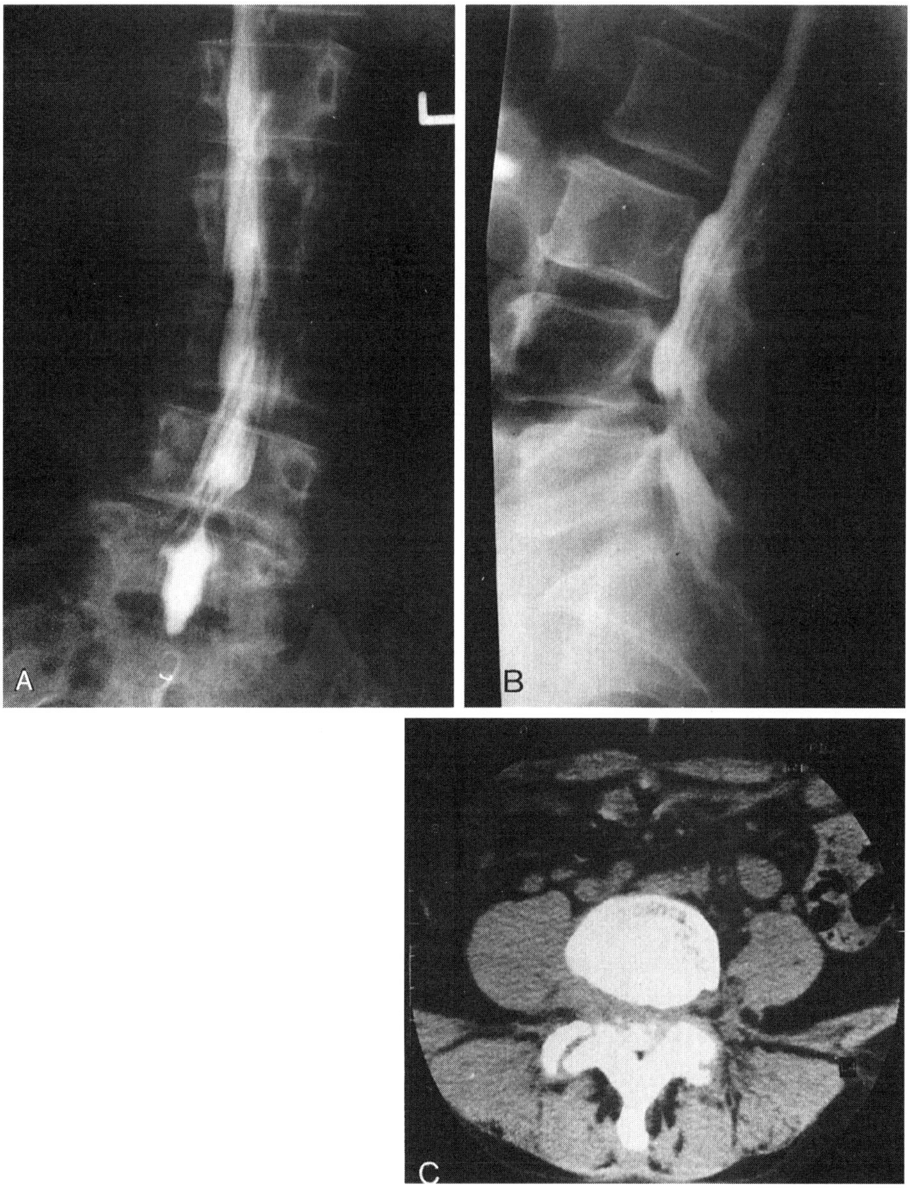

Figure 17.24 **A.** *AP myelogram showing lateral spondylolisthesis.* **B.** *Lateral myelogram, same patient, showing forward spondylolisthesis.* **C.** *CT myelogram, axial slice, showing resulting stenosis.*

Magnetic Resonance Imaging

MRI is used increasingly for imaging in SCS.(2) In fact, in most situations, except for a scoliotic patient with stenosis, it is superior to any other form of investigation (Fig. 17.1, 17.2, 17.3, 17.8). It is non-invasive, involves no radiation exposure, and provides two views at right angles to each other (sagittal and axial). Most important, the sagittal images are of all areas of the lumbar spine from the conus to S1.

MRI is notorious for underestimating the degree of canal stenosis.

Figure 17.25 *Complete obstruction producing paint-brush effect. Note the redundant nerve roots above the block.*

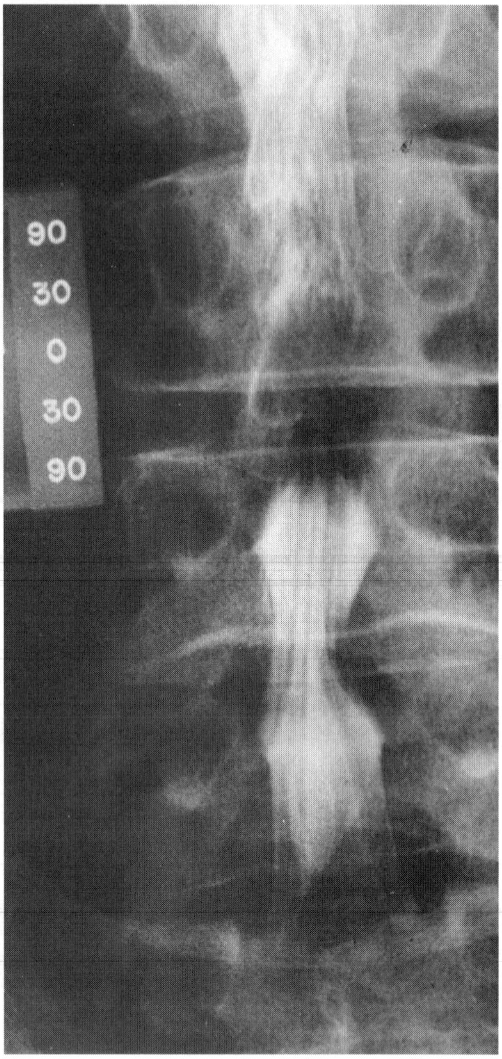

Miscellaneous Tests

Electromyograms and nerve conduction studies have not been useful in the assessment of a patient with SCS except to rule out other neurological disorders. Much work is presently proceeding on the use of somatosensory-evoked potentials to decide on the level of involvement in spinal stenosis.(5) To date, this work is not clinically applicable.

TREATMENT

Conservative Care

There is nothing fancy about conservative care in SCS. Rest in the form of corset support, weight loss and the use of a cane can be prescribed. Obviously, anti-inflammatory

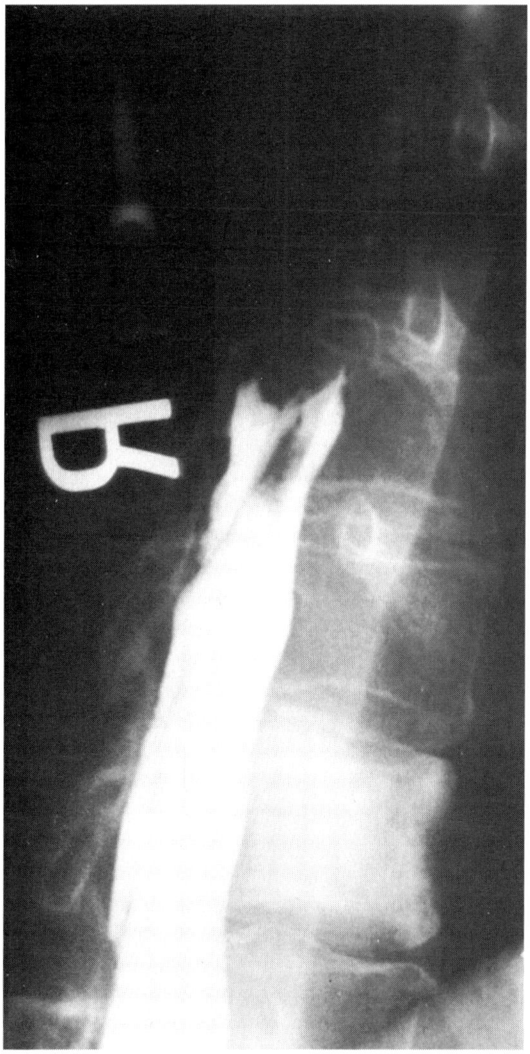

Figure 17.26 *Meniscal-like lesion of tumor obstruction to contrast flow.*

medication is useful, but be mindful of the side effects that are very prone to occur in this older age group. Heavy duty pain medication and muscle relaxants should be avoided because you are dealing with a chronic condition.

A Williams exercise program to reduce lumbar lordosis is very beneficial. Hyperextension exercises are to be avoided. Heat and/or ice, and modalities such as ultrasound are of limited benefit. It is unusual that manipulation affects leg symptoms, although it may be very beneficial for back pain.

Epidural cortisone is often prescribed for the treatment of SCS, yet there is not one article in the literature that supports the scientific basis for this treatment. In addition, successful installation of materials in the extradural space in older patients with the degenerative changes associated with stenosis can be very difficult. The final argument against steroid use in this patient population is the fact that the procedures are often done in a holding area in the operating room or radiology suite where sterile technique is below the standard of a surgical operating room. The authors have seen devastating consequences (infections), especially in a diabetic patient.

Calcitonin

Porter (22) has popularized the use of calcitonin in the treatment of neurogenic claudication. After it was noted that calcitonin had a beneficial effect on neurogenic claudication when used in Paget's disease, Porter proposed that it be used in spinal stenotic patients with Paget's disease. Its mechanism of action is unknown but it is thought to increase the blood supply to the cauda equina nerves and stabilize the neurotransmitting system. It has a widely recognized calming or placebo effect that may be its main mechanism of action. It has to be used intermittently, is expensive and has not been tested in controlled trials which may explain why it is not a popular form of treatment.

NATURAL HISTORY OF SPINAL STENOSIS

Although some patients with SCS experience temporary relief with conservative care,(13, 15) any patient with significant narrowing of the spinal canal and the disabling symptoms of SCS will ultimately need surgical intervention because of the progressive, relentless nature of SCS. Patients with a minimal to moderate lesion on MRI and moderate symptoms can often be helped by conservative care. Approximately 50% will not progress and may be managed conservatively, but 50% will experience increasing symptoms despite conservative care and eventually require surgery.

The following are indications for surgical intervention:

1. Failure of a patient with SCS to respond to standard conservative treatment measures.
2. Significant pain and disability in walking regardless of neurological findings and duration of symptoms.
3. Established weakness that is clinically measurable, regardless of duration of symptoms and conservative treatment.

TIMING OF SURGERY

Conservative care for this condition is associated with two drawbacks:

1. Benefit is often temporary unless the canal narrowing on CT is minor and the symptoms are minor.
2. Symptoms in the extremities usually occur after a long history of back symptoms, which at one time or another have been treated conservatively.

Patients become aware of this progression of symptoms despite bracing, therapy, and medication and are discouraged by the prospect of further conservative care. They are counting the years and often do not wish to expend them on previously tried conservative care. This may appear to be an aggressive surgical position; of course, all degenerative spinal conditions deserve a trial of conservative care, but, in particular, SCS deserves a good dose of common sense in making treatment decisions. Surgery is obviously elective and can be done when the patient is medically fit. Surgery should not be delayed many months or years, during which the patient may develop signs of weakness.

GENERAL MEDICAL CONSIDERATIONS

Spinal stenosis usually occurs in older patients, who often have associated medical problems. Often patients are wrongly denied surgery because of such conditions. Monitoring and fine-tuning of anesthetic agents in today's world are so good that only patients with severe general medical problems, for example, unstable angina, severe hypertension, or severe respiratory insufficiency, should be denied surgery. As long as the patient is aware of the risks, benefits, and alternatives, indicated surgery should proceed.

Many of our older patients are highly motivated and want to be active, and it is unfair to withhold surgery. Probably the most significant indicator of a good outcome of surgery is this high degree of motivation: "I would rather die than live the rest of my life immobile and restricted to the house."

One important point: older patients with SCS often have associated (symptomatic) vascular disease and osteoarthritis of the hip(s). It is best to deal with those conditions first, including surgery if indicated. In a significant number of these patients, symptoms thought to be due to spinal stenosis disappear when the vascular disease or hip disease is fixed. The opposite can happen as well. After the vascular disease or hip is fixed and the patients attempt to increase their activity, they may find limitations from the neurogenic claudication due to the spinal canal stenosis. As you can see, timing of surgery relative to other medical conditions becomes as much an art as science.

SURGERY

Although the primary goal is to relieve the patient's leg symptoms, one must not lose sight of the mechanical back pain that is present. It is important to explain to patients before surgical intervention that although relief of leg pain often occurs, it may not be complete and some back pain will almost certainly remain. But the residual symptoms should not restrict activities nearly to the extent of the preoperative symptoms.

Two surgical procedures, alone or in combination, are necessary to deal with SCS: (1) decompression of neurological structures, (2) stabilization of vertebral elements. Let us deal with each one of the three clinical presentations of SCS.

1. SCS without vertebral body translation.
   a. With a lot of back pain.
   b. With no back pain (mostly leg pain symptoms).
2. SCS with vertebral body translation (spondylolisthesis).
   a. With back pain.
   b. Without back pain (mostly leg pain symptoms).
3. SCS due to degenerative changes compromising a congenitally small canal.

SPINAL CANAL STENOSIS WITHOUT VERTEBRAL BODY TRANSLATION

Usually these patients have very little back pain and a fusion is not part of the game plan. If there is a reasonable component of back pain, it is usually due to multiple level degenerative changes and fusion is not a reasonable option. This latter situation is fortunately not common and the surgical decision centers around the nature and extent of the decompression.

Decompression

Length of Decompression

A number of general statements apply to decompression. Is it necessary to decompress every stenotic level seen on radiograph? Some decompress only those levels causing symptoms; others prefer to decompress every stenotic segment seen on radiograph. The tendency today is to do more levels, but limit the extent of the decompression at each level, an approach that will be commented upon later. Fortunately, in 50% of the SCS cases, the decompression can be confined to a single level, usually L4–L5, and usually the first story of L4 (Fig. 17.27). Decompression is usually not required in the first and second stories of L5, and thus stability of the lumbosacral junction can be maintained.

It is often stated that one should decompress to the level of a pulsating dura or to the level of epidural fat. Although this is a good goal, many times it is not achievable (7, 16). The clinical presentation and the structural defects as seen on investigation should guide the surgeon in assessing how far decompression should extend proximally and distally.

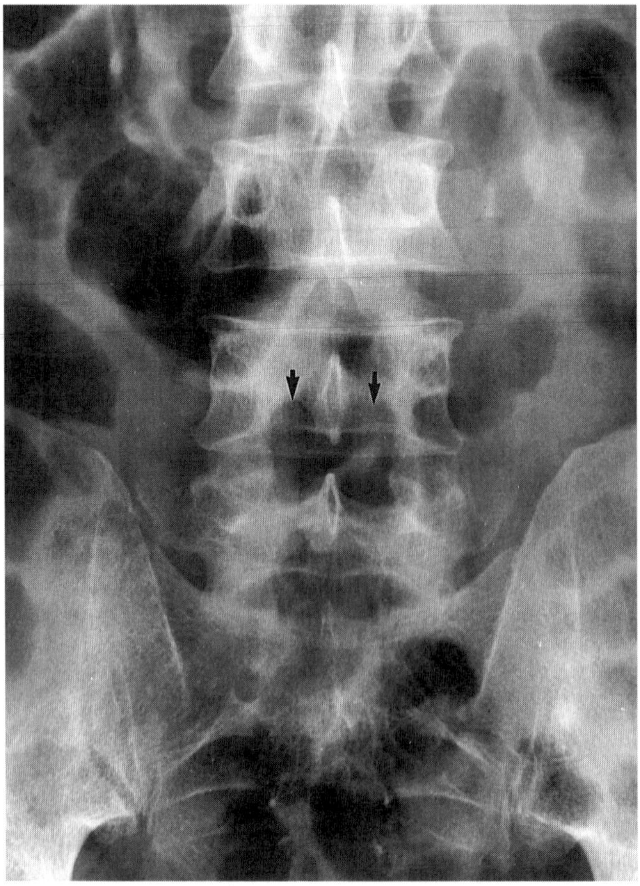

Figure 17.27 *AP radiograph of a single-level spinal canal stenosis decompression (laminoplasty) at L4–L5 (arrows at upper margin of laminar decompression).*

Width of Decompression

There are two choices in deciding how wide the decompression should be at each level.

1. Midline canal decompression saving the facet joints.
2. Midline canal decompression sacrificing one or both facet joints.

Suggested Guidelines for Length and Width of Decompression

1. Decompress all contiguous levels of canal stenosis (Fig. 17.28).
2. Ignore skip lesions (eg, L1–L2 when doing an L4–L5 decompression) unless the stenosis is severe and/or is producing specific symptoms.
3. Decompress both subarticular regions in each anatomic segment being decompressed (Fig. 17.29).
4. Read the foramen on MRI (Fig. 17.30) and decompress only those that are narrowed.
5. You may sacrifice a single facet joint in a patient with a narrowed disc space that has been stabilized by osteophytes.

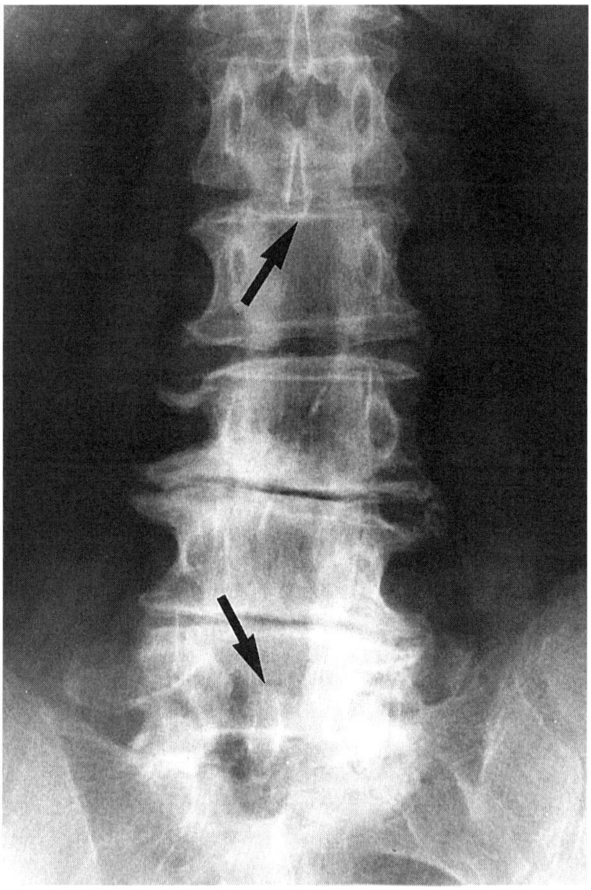

Figure 17.28 *A multilevel decompression for spinal canal stenosis extending from L1–L2 (top arrow) to L4–L5 (bottom arrow).*

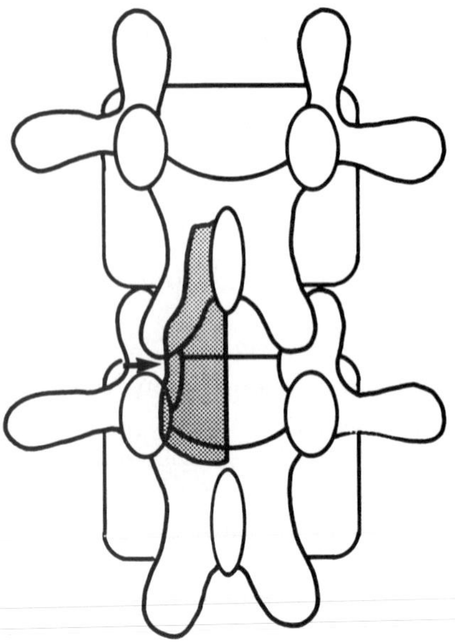

Figure 17.29 *The method of subarticular decompression by taking off the medial edge of the facet joint (arrow).*

6. Sacrificing a single facet joint in a younger patient with a wide disc space is likely to lead to future problems. Fortunately, this is a rare surgical problem because narrowed foramina tend not to occur at a nonslip level with a wide disc space.

Technique of Surgical Intervention

Positioning on the Operating Room Table

The kneeling position is preferred for patients having surgery for SCS (Fig. 17.31). The forced hip and knee flexion posture of the knee-chest position is probably unwise for these patients. Surgery for SCS usually lasts a few hours, and an older patient who stays in this position is at risk to lower extremity complications, such as thrombophlebitis. Before the patient is prepared and draped for surgery, an image intensifier needle identification of the surgical level is completed (Fig. 17.32). If the canal stenosis is confined to a single level, such as L4–L5, then the skin incision extends from the spinous process of L3 to the spinous process of L5. In the authors' experience, it is rarely necessary to decompress the first and second stories of the fifth segment, and thus a routine sacral exposure is not done.

Because the pathology is so confined to the first story and the upper reaches of the third story of the level below, it appears possible to relieve symptoms with an interlaminar decompression. If such a decompression were being carried out at the L4–L5 level, this can be accomplished by excising all the ligamentum flavum (L4–L5), the superior edge of the lamina of L5 bilaterally, the inferior one half of the lamina of L4 (which takes you up as high as the cephalad attachment of the ligamentum flavum), and the medial edges of the inferior and superior facets of L4 and L5, respectively. This is the so-called laminoplasty procedure (Figs. 17.33 and 17.34). This procedure can be done bilaterally through a unilateral portal (Fig. 17.35).

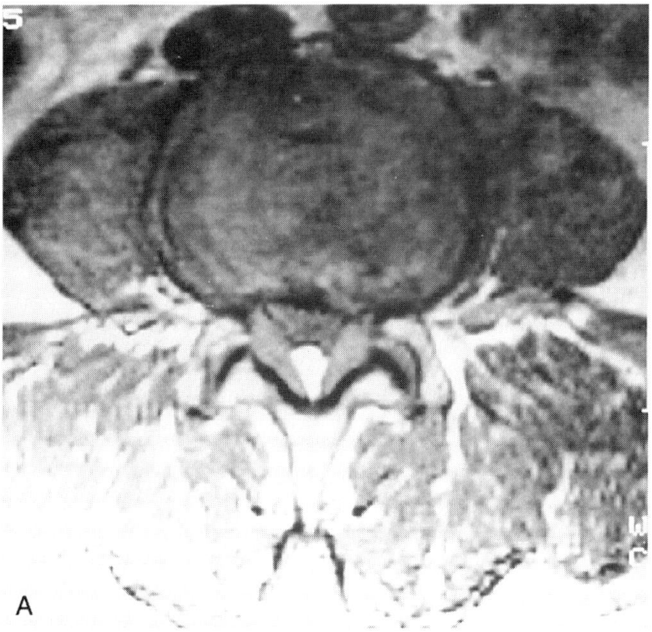

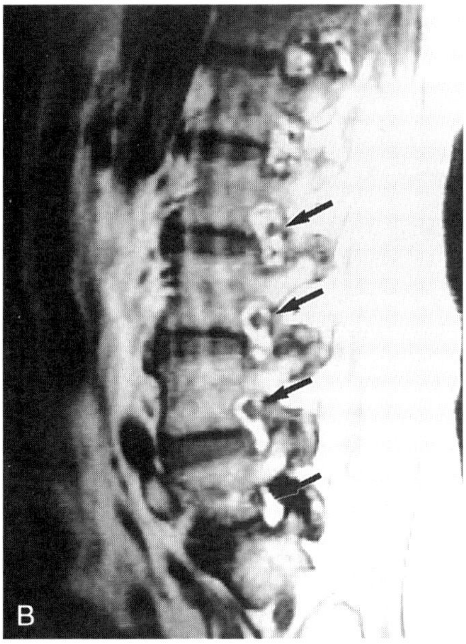

Figure 17.30 **A.** *A T1 axial MRI showing spinal canal stenosis.* **B.** *The foramina on T1 sagittal MRI are all wide open (arrows).*

Obviously, control of bleeding during surgery is important. Before surgical intervention, any medication, such as NSAIDs, which interfere with the clotting mechanism, must be discontinued. The kneeling position helps to keep pressure in Batson's plexus low, allowing for venous flow from the spinal epidural veins into the venacaval system. Although hypotensive anesthesia is very helpful in spinal surgery, it can be dangerous in these older patients. Finally, bipolar coagulation must be used around neurological structures. With these precautions, it is less likely that a patient would lose enough blood to require a blood transfusion.

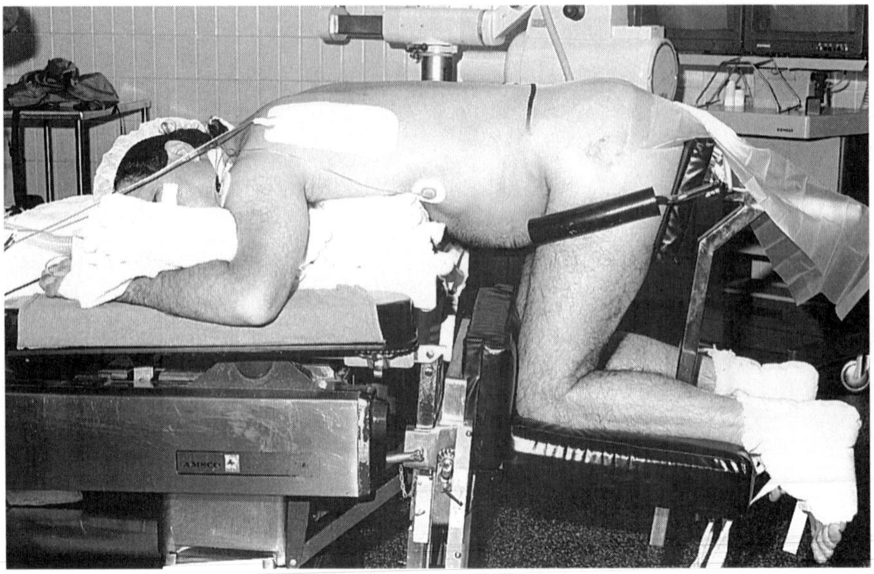

Figure 17.31 *The kneeling position for spinal canal stenosis surgery.*

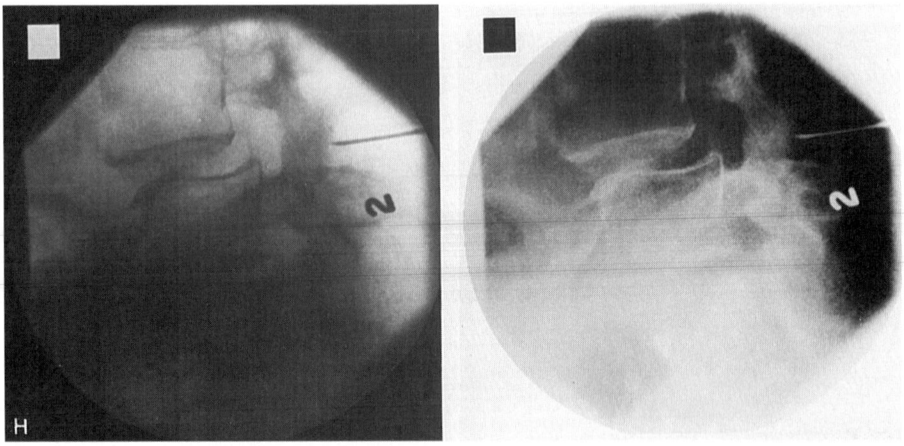

Figure 17.32 *Image intensifier identification of the slip level L4–L5 with a needle inserted at the inferior edge of the disc space.*

Method of Decompression

Probably the most important preparation for surgical intervention for SCS is to identify the segment involved and the number of stenotic stories within the segment. The most common set of circumstances is a significant spinal stenosis in the first story of the fourth segment (L4), and less significant stenosis in the second story of L4 and the third story of L5 below. In this situation, it is necessary to decompress the first and second stories of L4 and the third story of L5 (Figs. 17.27 and 17.36).

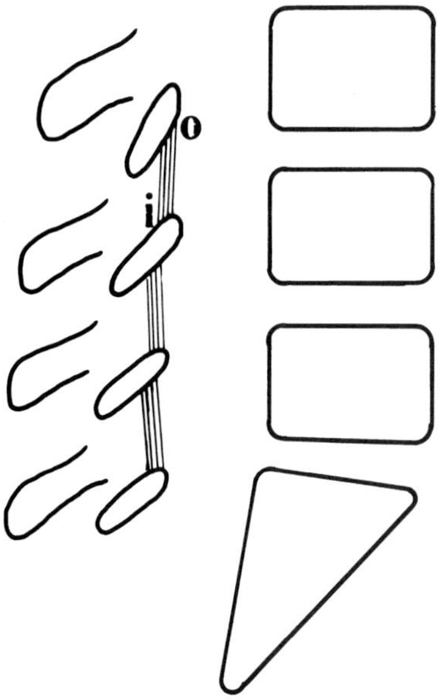

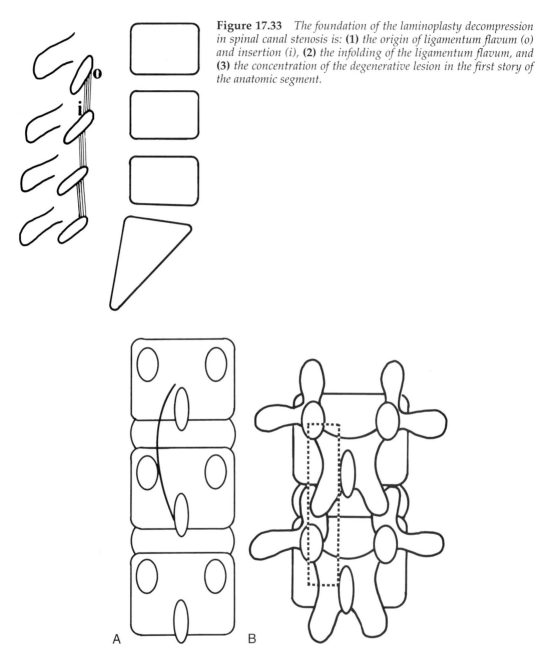

Figure 17.33 *The foundation of the laminoplasty decompression in spinal canal stenosis is:* **(1)** *the origin of ligamentum flavum (o) and insertion (i),* **(2)** *the infolding of the ligamentum flavum, and* **(3)** *the concentration of the degenerative lesion in the first story of the anatomic segment.*

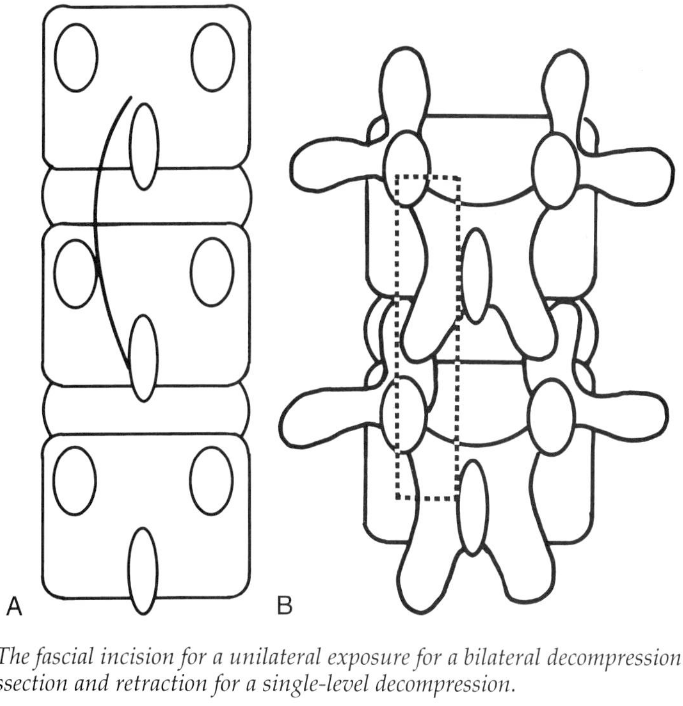

Figure 17.34 **A.** *The fascial incision for a unilateral exposure for a bilateral decompression.* **B.** *The extent of the submuscular dissection and retraction for a single-level decompression.*

Adhesions

It is often reported that adhesions are present between the dura and surrounding tissues, which make dissection difficult. In fact, adhesions "de novo" are rare; they do occur in the presence of a synovial cyst and, on occasion, in the concavity of a longstanding

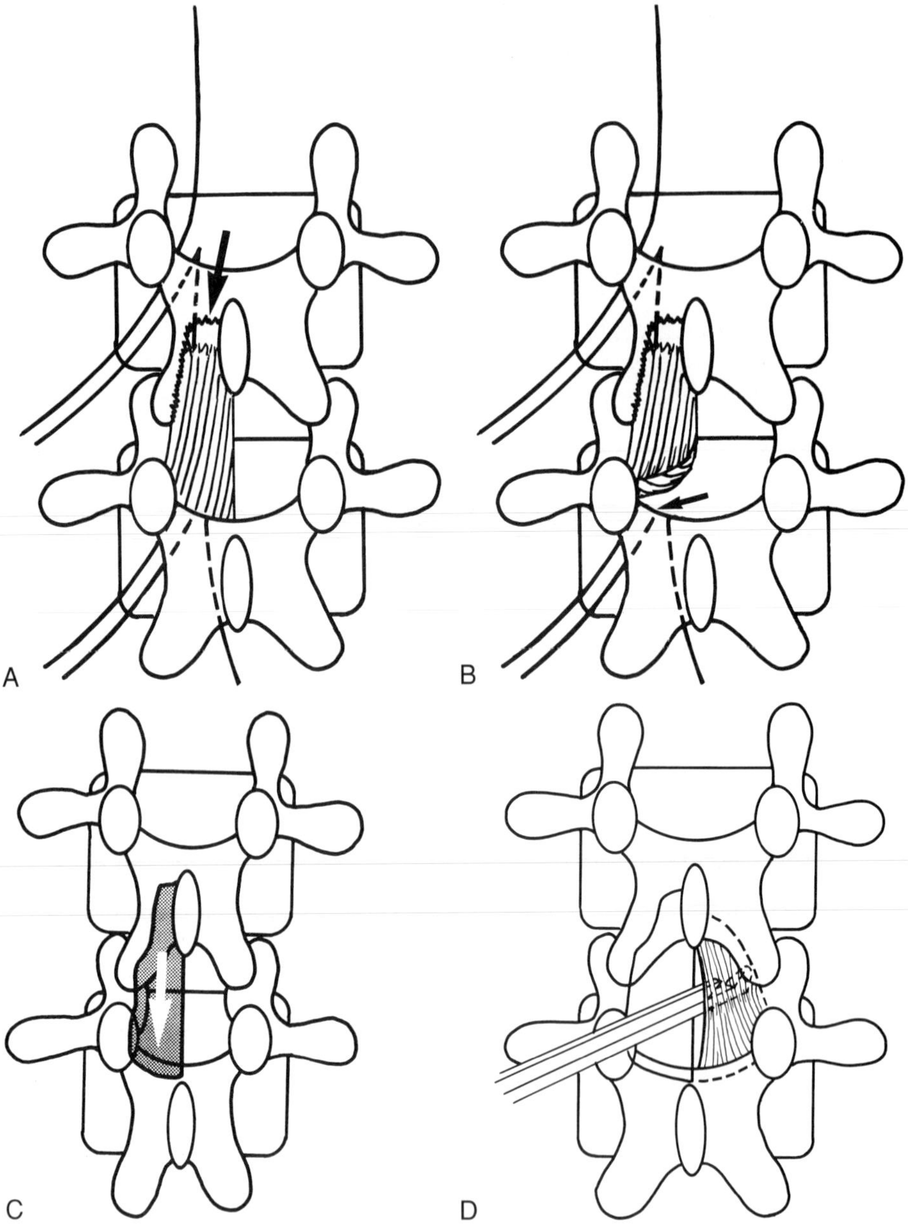

Figure 17.35 **A.** *The first step is to remove the inferior half of the cephalad lamina (arrow), to expose dura just cephalad to the origin of the ligamentum flavum.* **B.** *The second step is to remove the superior edge of the lamina below to detach the insertion of the ligamentum flavum (arrow).* **C.** *The third step is to remove the ligamentum flavum, along with the medial edge of the facet joint.* **D.** *After completion of the decompression on the ipsilateral side, the contralateral side can be decompressed. The surgeon uses the Kerrison rongeur to work under (anterior to) the intact interspinous/supraspinous ligament complex to remove the contralateral ligamentum flavum (along dotted lines).*

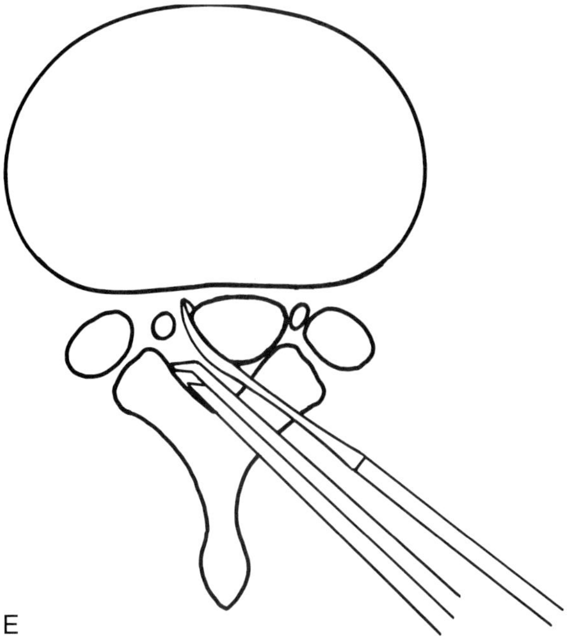

E

Figure 17.35 (continued) E. *An axial view of decompression of the contralateral side through the ipsilateral (unilateral) laminotomy defect.*

degenerative scoliosis. Aside from these two situations, adhesions are an uncommon limitation to decompression.

The Facet Joint

If no vertebral body translation is present, it is recommended that stability be preserved by saving each facet joint.

Disc

It is rare for discopathology to be a significant component of spinal stenosis (19) and thus, disc surgery is rarely needed at the time of a spinal stenosis decompression. It is prudent to avoid interfering with discal integrity because this increases postoperative instability. Be aware of the stenotic patient with dominant leg pain especially of sudden onset. They likely have a disc herniation hidden in their stenotic canal that will be impossible to see on MRI but easy enough to find at surgery only if you go looking for it!

Postoperative Care

Aside from the medical problems attendant on most of these patients, postoperative care for the decompression and fusion is very limited. The patients are ambulated as soon as possible (the day of surgery) in a light canvas corset. Discharge is usually 2 to 4 days after surgery with the activity level prescribed being a renewed commitment to walk.

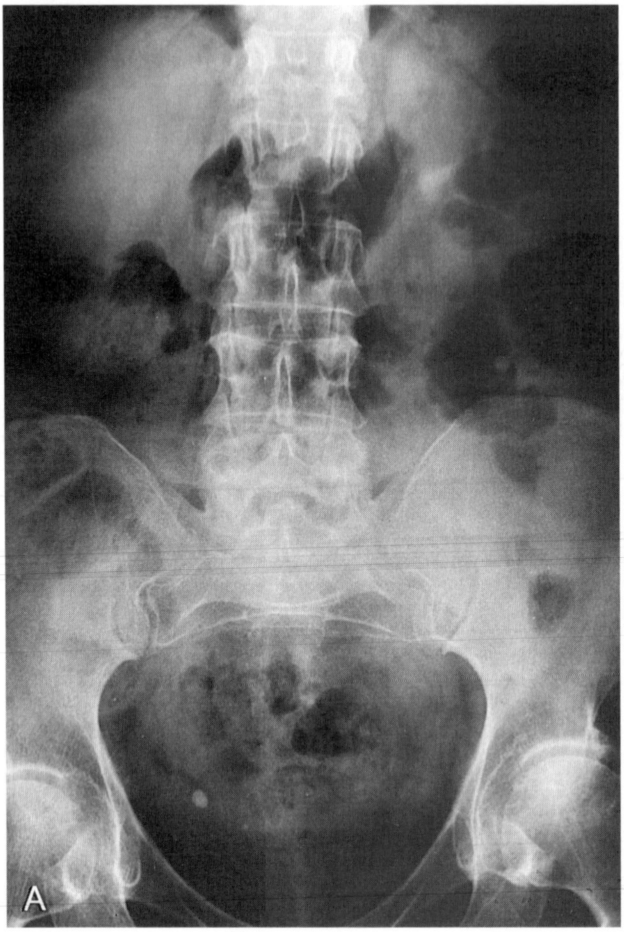

Figure 17.36 **A.** *A preoperative AP radiograph of spinal canal stenosis at L4–5.*

SPINAL CANAL STENOSIS WITH VERTEBRAL BODY TRANSLATION

Degenerative spondylolisthesis (Fig. 17.6, B) was first described by Macnab (18) as spondylolisthesis with an intact neural arch: the so-called pseudospondylolisthesis. It is the second most common form of spondylolisthesis in adults and affects the L4–L5 level most frequently. It may affect multiple levels (Fig. 17.37) and is at least five times more common in women. It is also more common when the last formed level is fixed to the pelvis (Fig. 17.38).

It is thought to be more common at L4–L5 because of the sagittal orientation of the facet joints at this level compared with the more coronally oriented facet joints at L5–S1. As well, L5–S1 is a more stable level because it is set down in the pelvis and anchored by the iliolumbar ligaments (Fig. 17.39).

The condition is aptly designated "degenerative" because it is thought to occur after long term instability (backache) due to degenerative changes in the posterior ligamentous

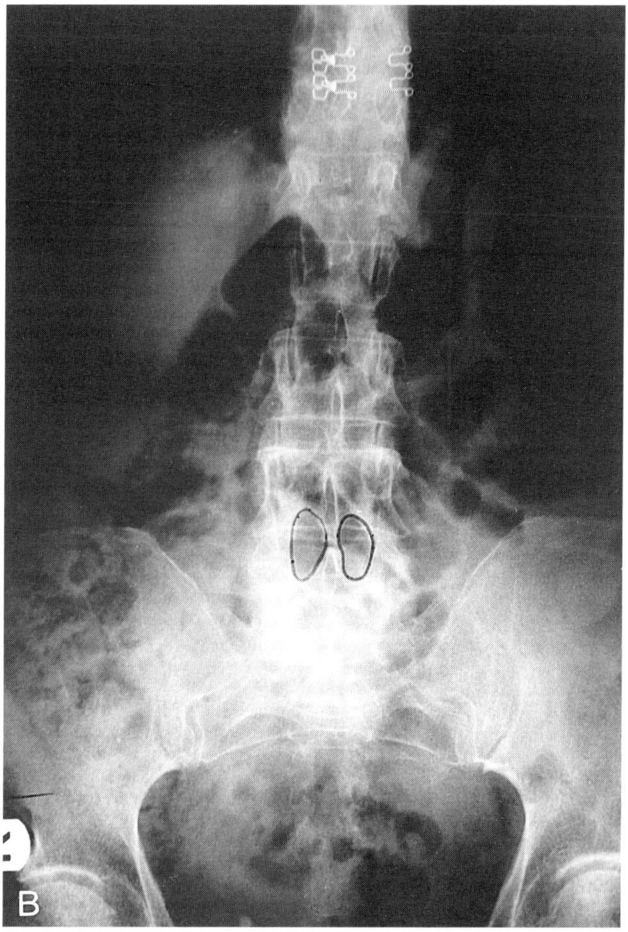

Figure 17.36 (continued) **B.** *A postoperative AP radiograph of spinal canal stenosis after a laminoplasty (outlined by black lines).*

structures, the disc space and especially the facet joints. All these changes allow for the forward slip of the cephalad vertebral body on its mate, not the reverse (Fig. 17.40).

When degenerative spondylolisthesis is associated with SCS, the patients can be divided into three groups.

Group One (Fig. 17.41)

A patient over 70 years of age.
Disc space narrowing at the slip level.
No increase in the extent of the slip on flexion films.
Little or no back pain (almost all leg pain complaints).

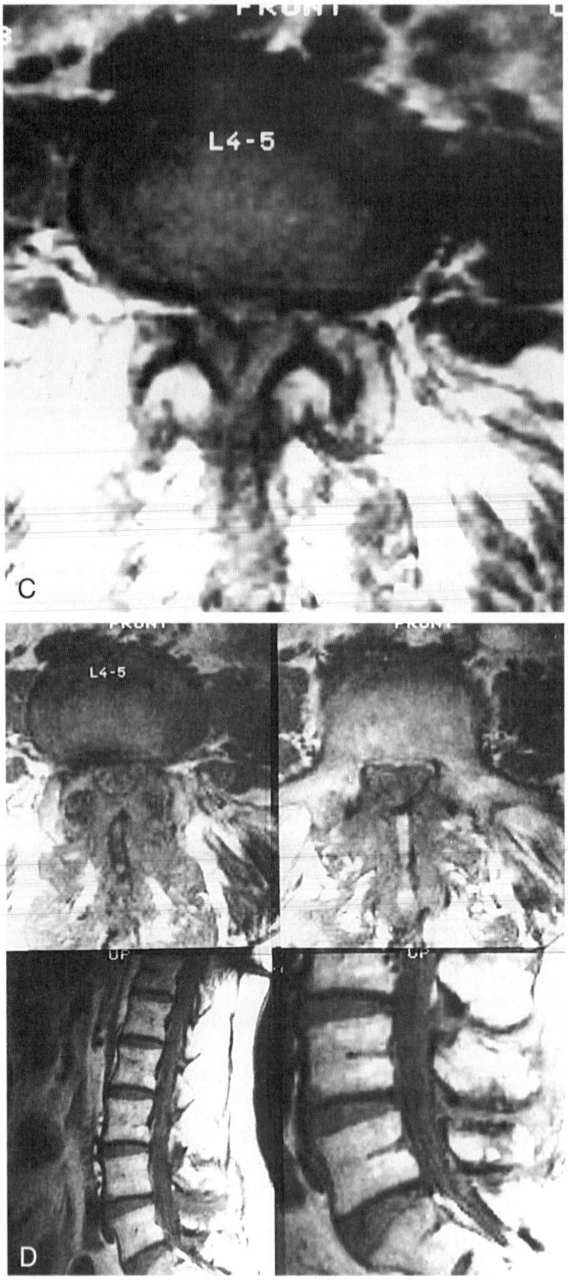

Figure 17.36 (continued) **C.** *A T1 axial MRI of L4–L5 before the laminoplasty.* **D.** *Axial and sagittal T1 MRIs after the microdecompression.*

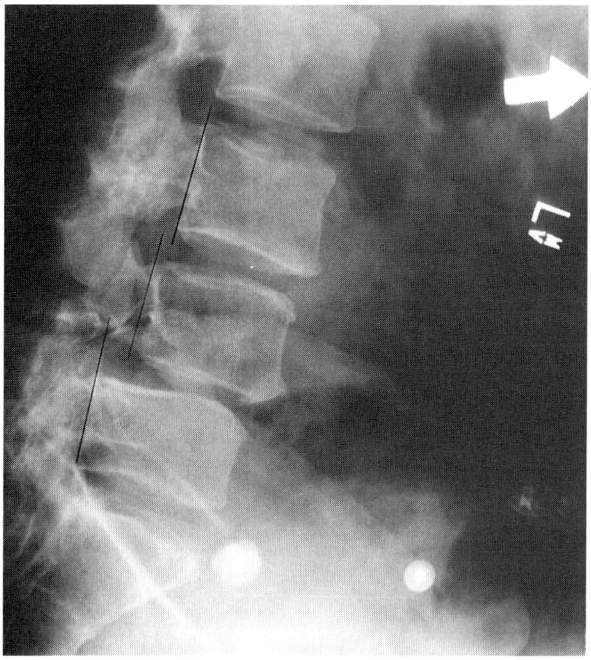

Figure 17.37 *A stair-step degenerative spondylolisthesis on flexion: L3 is slipped forward on L4, and L4 is slipped forward on L5.*

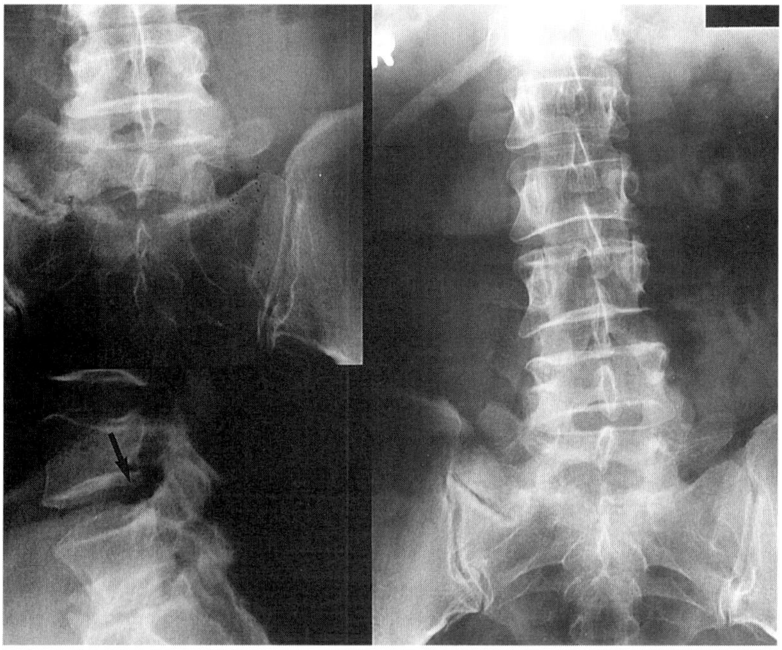

Figure 17.38 *Degenerative spondylolisthesis is more common when the last formed level is fixed to the pelvis. If you look closely at the bottom left lateral radiograph, you can see that the last mobile level (LML) is slightly forward on the last formed level (LFL) (arrow).*

Figure 17.39 *The iliolumbar ligaments.*

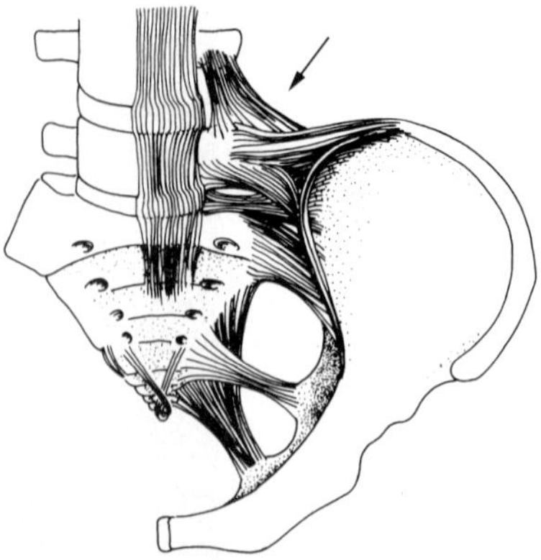

Figure 17.40 *A degenerative spondylolisthesis (top arrow) is shown and compared with a retrospondylolisthesis (curved arrow). The bottom arrow points to a fixed last formed level.*

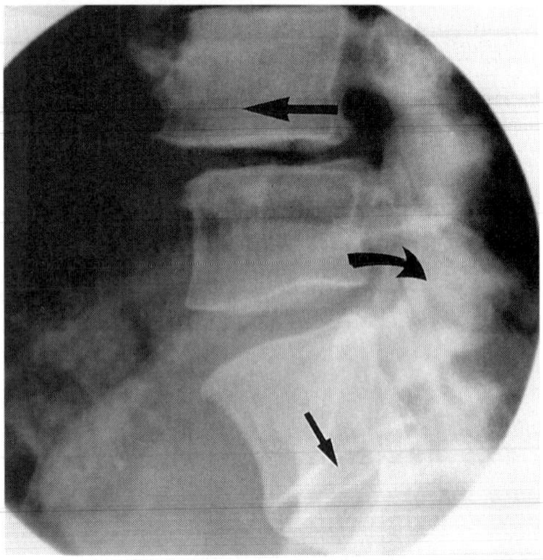

Group Two (Fig. 17.42)

A patient under 60 years of age.
A wide disc space at the slip level.
Evidence of instability on flexion/extension views.
A significant amount of back pain.

Group Three (Fig. 17.43)

Degenerative Scoliosis

This is a particularly difficult problem that will be discussed at the end of this section.

The division between group one and two is very artificial, with many patients falling into a large gray zone in between. However, to deal with the variations in the middle ground you have to understand the principles of management of the two groups at either end.

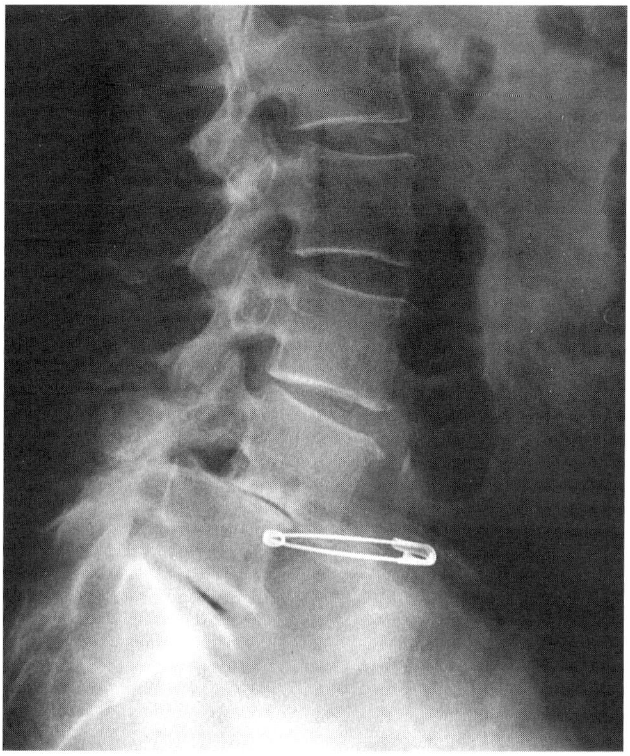

Figure 17.41 *The lateral plain film shows a degenerative spondylolisthesis with a narrowed disc space at the level of the slip: a fairly stable situation.*

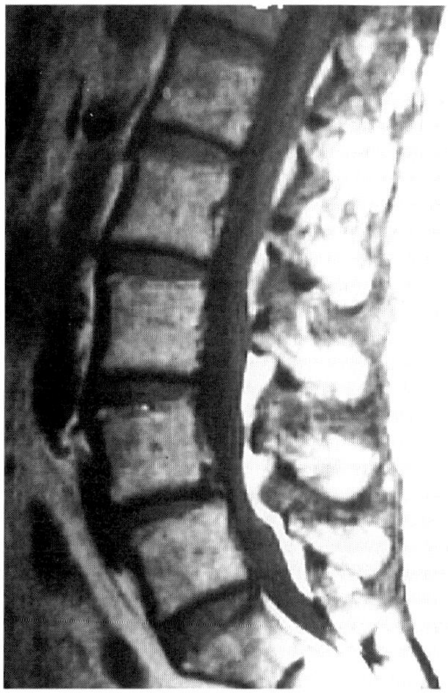

Figure 17.42 *The sagittal (T1) MRI shows a wide disc space (L4–L5) at the slip level: a relatively unstable situation.*

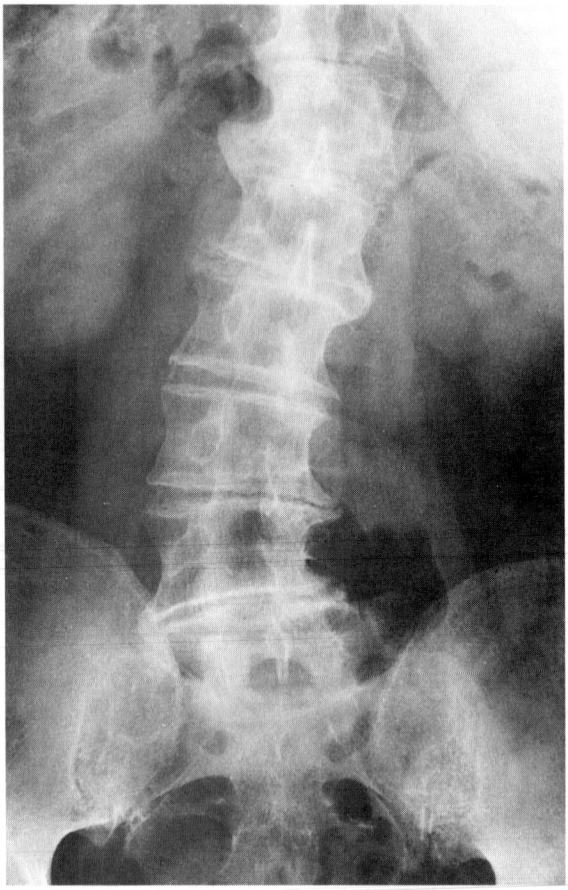

Figure 17.43 *A degenerative spondylolisthesis with scoliosis (AP radiograph).*

Group One

This group has reached the stabilization phase of Kirkaldy-Willis (see Chapter 7). The body, as natural defenses, through fibrosis of the disc and facet joint capsules and osteophyte formation, has stabilized the segment. These patients can be managed just like the spinal stenosis without slip – group, that is, decompression of the symptomatic segments without fusion.

Group Two

Obviously, patients in this group have unstable motion segments and require a fusion at the time of decompression.(11, 14) The addition of the fusion stabilizes the slip segment and prevents further postoperative increase in the slip, which may lead to a poor surgical outcome.(14) Having to remove a facet joint to decompress a foramen in this group makes a fusion a necessity.

Up for grabs is whether or not the fusion should be augmented with instrumentation.(3) These authors are split, with the senior author (JM) preferring no instrumentation (the minority position today) (Fig. 17.44), and the junior author (ET) preferring to stabilize the segment with instrumentation (Fig. 17.44). Note that both of these cases are floating fusions with no surgery (decompression/or fusion) being done at L5–S1.

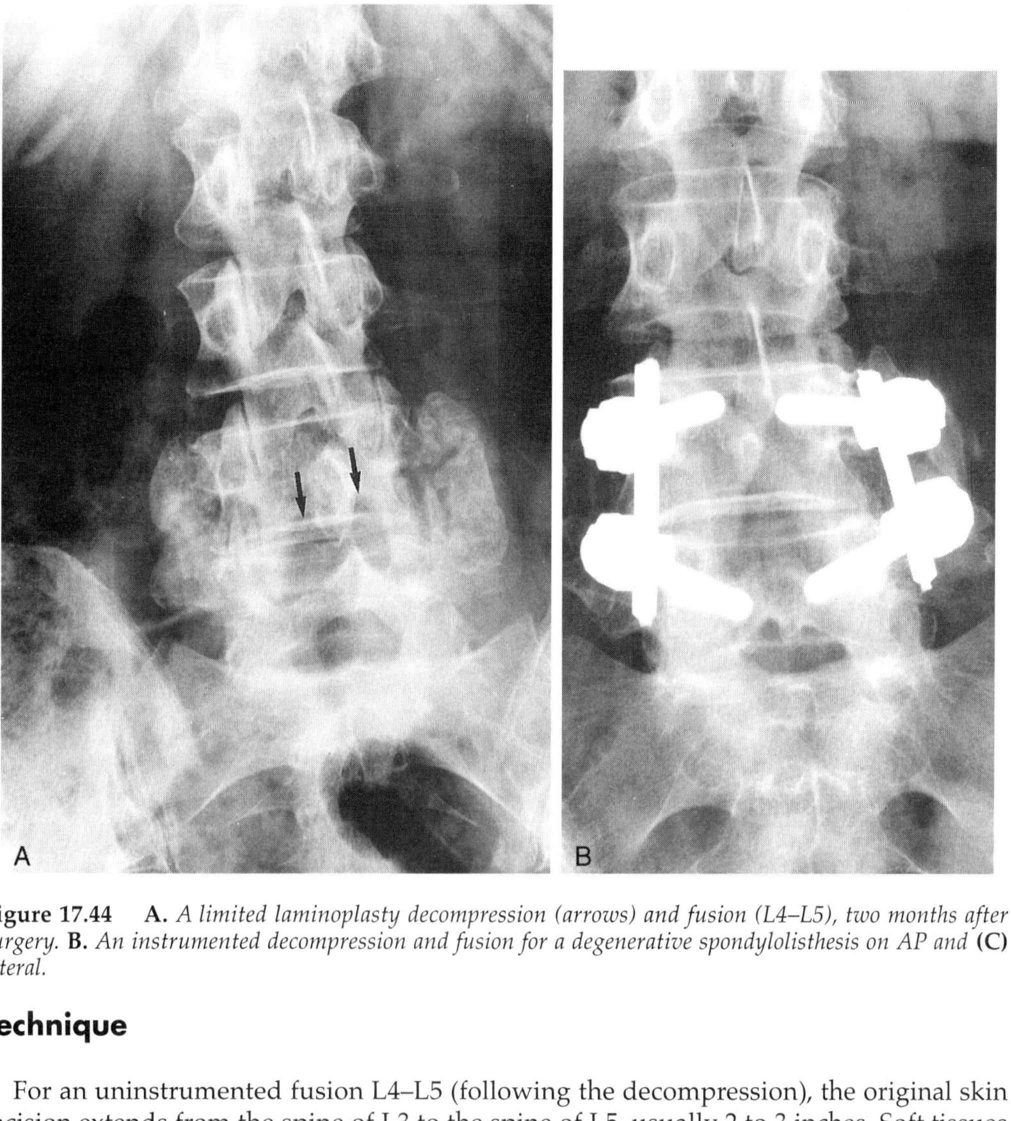

Figure 17.44 **A.** *A limited laminoplasty decompression (arrows) and fusion (L4–L5), two months after surgery.* **B.** *An instrumented decompression and fusion for a degenerative spondylolisthesis on AP and* **(C)** *lateral.*

Technique

For an uninstrumented fusion L4–L5 (following the decompression), the original skin incision extends from the spine of L3 to the spine of L5, usually 2 to 3 inches. Soft tissues are dissected off the spinous process and lamina of L3, L4, and L5. Inasmuch as the slip necessitates that a fusion is part of the procedure, the soft-tissue dissection must extend to the tips of the appropriate transverse processes; in this case, the transverse process of L4 and L5, bilaterally. This dissection can be accomplished through the 2-inch incision (Fig. 17.45).

The Decompression

Once the posterior elements are denuded of their soft-tissue attachments, one must make a basic decision as to where to start the decompression. The authors prefer to start the decompression in the most severely stenotic area. Many others recommend the reverse, but starting in the most severely constricted area poses less risk of injury to the bulging dura. In the standard case being described, the decompression starts medially at the inferior border of the lamina of L4. Figures 17.34 and 17.35 demonstrate the method of

Figure 17.44 (continued) C

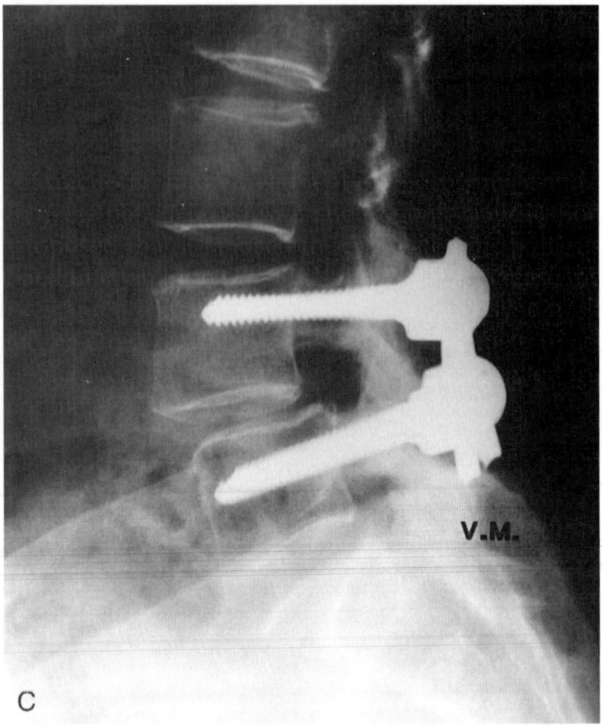

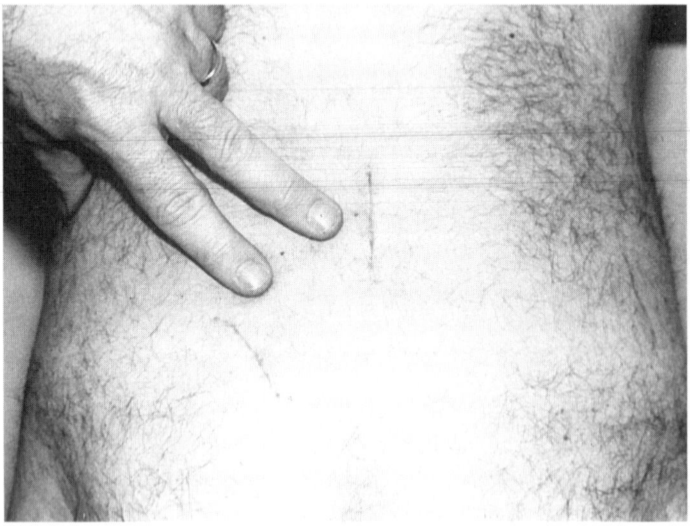

Figure 17.45 *The midline and donor incision for a single-level decompression and fusion without instrumentation.*

decompression of the fourth segment. The objective is to remove the lamina, and medial border of the facet of L4 along with the medial edge of the superior facet of L5. The ligamentum flavum, medial facet capsule, and superior facet capsule are carefully removed to complete the decompression.

Facet Joints

In the presence of a complete spinal canal obstruction with degenerative spondylolisthesis, there is a reasonable possibility of significant foraminal encroachment (see Fig. 17.30). This feature serves as the basis for those proposing an interbody fusion with instrumentation (Fig. 17.46). As mentioned in the previous chapter on lateral zone stenosis, there are three ways to deal with a tight foramen.

1. Directly open the foramen, which may mean removing the inferior facet (Fig. 17.47).
2. Restore disc space height with an interbody fusion (Fig. 17.46).
3. Immobilize the segment (Fig. 17.48).

The last of the three options is not often considered but is a viable consideration based on the fact that no matter how small the nerve root canal, if there is no movement, the nerve will not be a source of pain. The necessity for decompression of the foramen (second story) in slip levels comes from the fact that capsular hypertrophy is often present, impinging on the nerve root in the foramen (Fig. 17.49). Failure to decompress the foramen, in this patient, by removing the inferior facet and the capsule of the facet joint will leave the patient with residual leg symptoms.(12) In the case of an L4–L5 slip level, this would leave encroachment on the L4 roots, resulting in persisting postoperative anterior thigh discomfort.

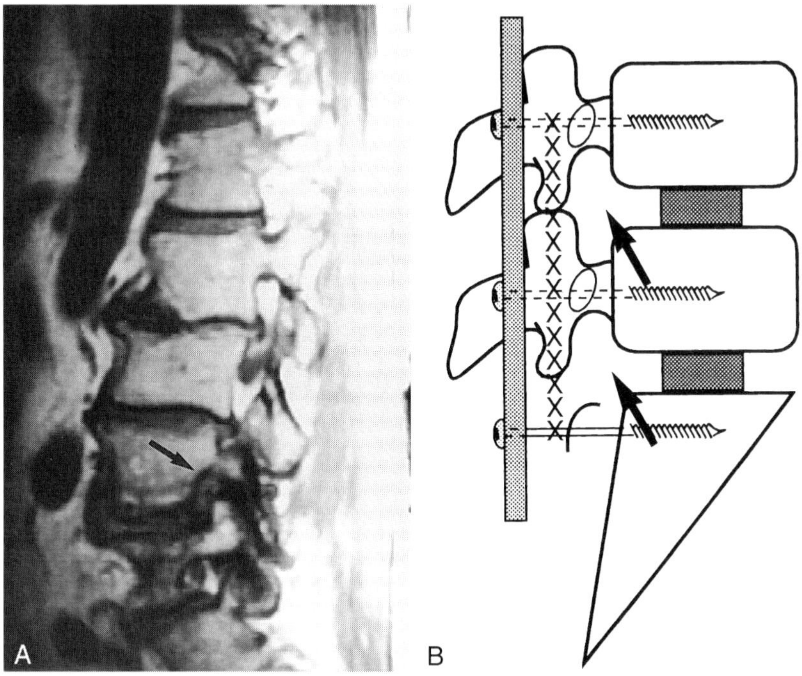

Figure 17.46 **A.** *A degenerative spondylolisthesis with foraminal encroachment at one level (arrow).* **B.** *The 360-degree fusion: interbody and posterolateral; the interbody fusion restores disc space height and reestablishes the patency of the foramen (arrows).*

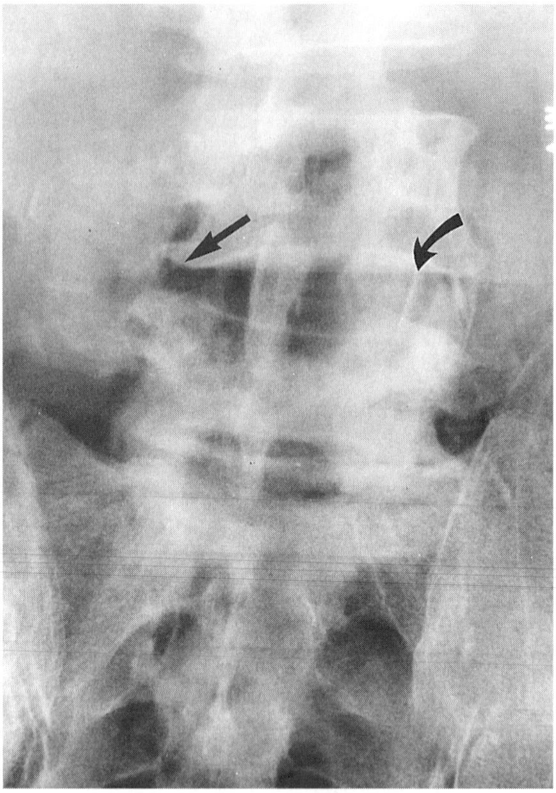

Figure 17.47 *To open the foramen on the left, the facet joint had to be removed (straight arrow), while on the right, the facet joint was left intact but fused after removing the cartilaginous surfaces (curved arrow).*

Fusion

Stabilization of Vertebral Elements

The controversy about stabilization or fusion of slip levels in spondylolisthesis, has been resolved by long-term results (11, 12, 13, 14). If a slip level is not fused at the time of decompression, there is a tendency toward a postoperative increase in the slip and a higher incidence of disabling back pain.(14) It is recommended that all slip levels, forward and lateral, be fused at the time of decompression, regardless of whether or not facet joints have been removed during the decompression. The recommended fusion is intertransverse (see Figs. 17.44, A, and 17.48).

SPINAL STENOSIS WITH DEGENERATIVE SPONDYLOLISTHESIS AND A DEGENERATIVE SCOLIOSIS

There is no more vexing problem in a degenerative spine than a lateral slip (spondylolisthesis) that leads to a degenerative scoliosis. Despite decompressions and fusions with or without instrumentation in this group, the results are universally poor. The management of this problem calls for a very sophisticated level of surgical expertise that is beyond the scope of this text.

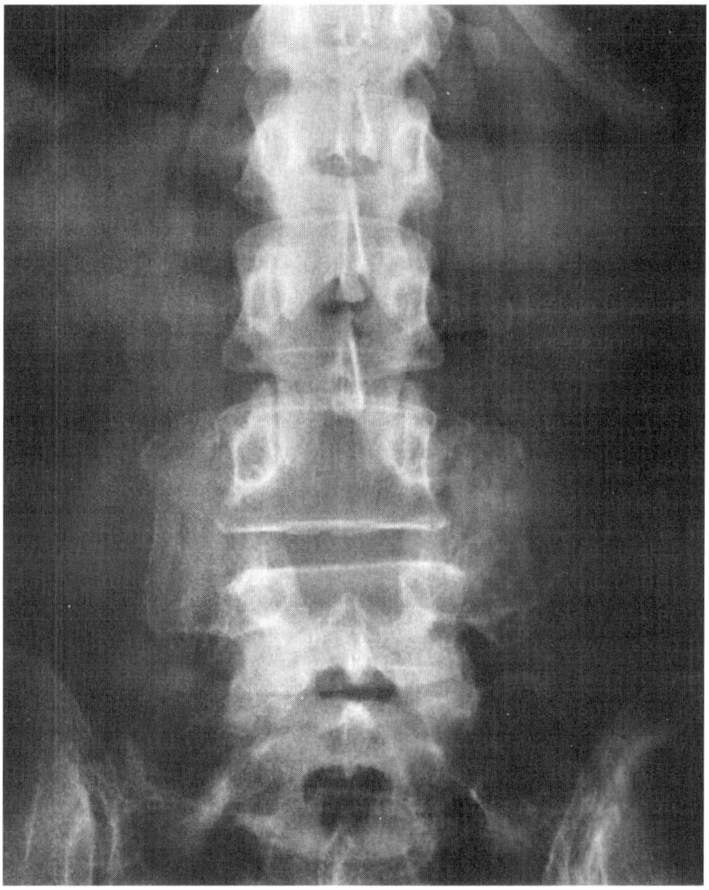

Figure 17.48 *Spinal canal stenosis. Another example of a single level decompression (L4) and a floating fusion, leaving L5–S1 untouched. (A fixed, formed level is below "L5–S1").*

CONGENITAL/DEVELOPMENTAL SPINAL CANAL STENOSIS

This condition is not at all uncommon, although it does not occur with the frequency of acquired SCS with and without degenerative spondylolisthesis. The mistake in this condition is to miss the global (congenital) stenosis (Fig. 17.49) and see this as a simple degenerative SCS meriting a laminoplasty type of decompression.

There are some basic rules to follow in understanding congenital SCS.

1. The condition usually occurs in men of large stature (male-female ratio = 10:1).
2. The patients present at a younger age and may present the classic picture of a disc herniation. It is only after an imaging study that the spinal canal stenosis is noted.
3. The stenosis affects all three stories of each anatomic segment (Fig. 17.50) (ie, global non-segmental) and is not intrasegmental as in degenerative SCS (Fig. 17.6, B).
4. It is unusual for a degenerative spondylolisthesis to be present. Therefore most operative decisions center around a decompression only (Figure 17.50 is the exception, not the rule!).

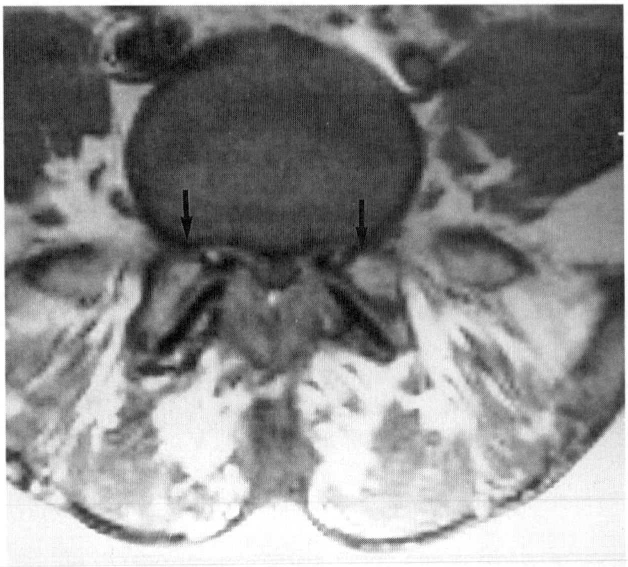

Figure 17.49 *An axial T1 MRI showing congenital stenosis with degenerative changes in the ligamentum flavum and capsule that increase the canal stenosis, and contribute to bilateral foraminal narrowing (arrows).*

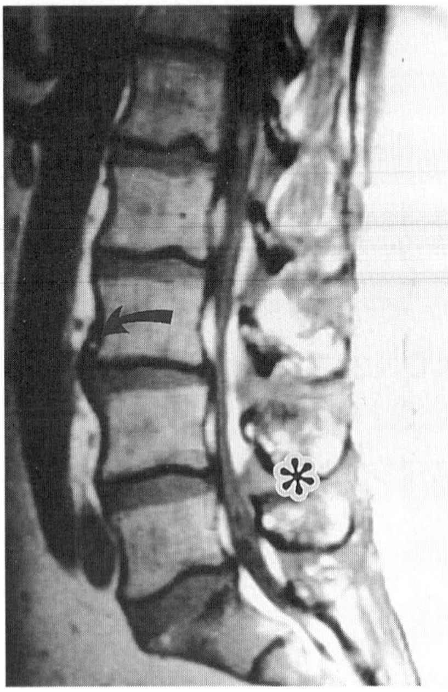

Figure 17.50 *A combined congenital and acquired spinal canal stenosis. Note the "pencil-thin" common dural sac from L1–L2 to L5–S1. This is the congenital "global" stenosis rather than an intrasegmental (first story) stenosis shown in the schematic in Figure 17.7. In addition, there is ligamentum flavum hypertrophy at L4–L5 (*), a slight forward slip (degenerative spondylolisthesis) at L4–L5, and an obvious forward slip at L3–L4 (arrow).*

5. It is unusual for foraminal stenosis to be present.
6. If neurological changes are present (eg, with an HNP) the neurological tissues are very sensitive to surgical retraction, and it is easy to increase a neurological deficit.
7. Most important, all three stories of each stenosed anatomic segment need to be decompressed. This usually means a multilevel decompression that most often extends from L2–L3 to L5–S1. Rarely is a fusion needed provided you save the facet joints.

8. Excessive retraction of nerve roots at the time of decompression, and especially if a disc herniation is present will result in an increased neurological deficit postoperatively.

Outcomes of Surgery

Surgery for SCS makes patients better, not normal.(27) Relief of leg pain is a reasonable expectation although chronic neurological changes (eg, weakness) will not be improved. Hopefully their progression will be arrested. Relief of back pain, even with a fusion is a little more tenuous with most patients ending up with some degree of residual backache. Fortunately, most patients are in an age group in which they do not wish to dig ditches and move furniture on a regular basis, and this lessened demand usually spares the back.

A poor initial result will not improve over time. If the patients initial result is less than optimal it usually means a missed diagnosis of an associated condition such as a peripheral neuropathy. Other causes of a poor result include decompression at the wrong level, an inadequate decompression at the right level or irreversible neurological changes.

Over time, approximately 20% of the patients will deteriorate in function. This is due to multiple factors including the continuous ravages of aging (the "rust" years), laminar regrowth and re-establishment of further stenosis.

Overall, two thirds of patients can anticipate a good, but not excellent, long-term result.

CONCLUSION

SCS is a relentlessly progressive narrowing of the lumbar spinal canal that insidiously decreases the space available for neurological structures. The resulting symptoms are quite disabling yet present little clinical evidence of nerve root involvement. The diagnosis is often elusive until the patient undergoes myelographic and/or CT investigation and/or MRI.

Surgery is the fate of at least 50% of patients with SCS. Symptoms can be temporarily relieved by conservative measures, but the degenerative changes of aging are relentless. The spinal canal may continue to narrow, and surgery may eventually be required.

The surgical procedures that are useful are a simple midline canal decompression, a wider decompression with removal of the facet joints, and stabilization procedures for slip levels. These three approaches have met with good results. Fortunately, because patients with SCS are older, they do not make great demands on the back postoperatively. If these patients required the ability to do heavy lifting, then backache postoperatively would be a limiting factor. In general, the results of surgical intervention for these patients are very gratifying.

REFERENCES

1. Arnoldi CC, Brodsky AE, Cauchoix J, et al. Lumbar spinal stenosis and nerve root entrapment syndromes: definitions and classification. Clin Orthop 1976;115:4–5.
2. Boden SD, Davis DO, Dina TS, Patronas NJ, Weisel SW. Abnormal magnetic resonance scans of the lumbar spine in asymptomatic subjects. A positive investigation. J Bone Joint Surg 1990; 72A:403–408.

3. Bridwell KH, Sedgewick TA, O'Brien MF, Lenke LG, Baldus C. The role of fusion and instrumentation in the treatment of degenerative spondylolisthesis with spinal stenosis. J Spinal Disord 1993;6:461–472.
4. Dagi TF, Tarkington MA, Leech JJ. Tandem lumbar and cervical spinal stenosis. J Neurosurg 1987;66:842–849.
5. Dvonch V, Scarff T, Bunch W. Dermatomal somatosensory-evoked potentials: their use in lumbar radiculopathy. Spine 1984;9:291–293.
6. Ehni G. Significance of the small lumbar spinal canal: cauda equina compression syndromes due to spondylolysis. J Neurosurg 1969;31:490–494.
7. Epstein NE, Epstein JA, Carras R, Lavine LS. Degenerative spondylolisthesis with an intact neural arch: a review of 60 cases with an analysis of clinical findings and the development of surgical management. Neurosurgery 1983;13:555–561.
8. Epstein JA, Epstein BS, Lavine LS. Nerve root compression associated with narrowing of the lumbar spinal canal. J Neurol Neurosurg Psychiatry 1962;25:165–176.
9. Epstein JA, Epstein BS, Lavine LS, Carras R, Rosenthal AD. Degenerative lumbar spondylolisthesis with an intact neural arch (pseudospondylolisthesis). J Neurosurg 1976;44:139–147.
10. Getty CJM. Lumbar spinal stenosis: the clinical spectrum and the results of operation. J Bone Joint Surg 1980;62B:481–485.
11. Herkowitz HN, Kurz LT. Degenerative lumbar spondylolisthesis with spinal stenosis. A prospective study comparing decompression and intertransverse process arthrodesis. J Bone Joint Surg 1991;73:802–808.
12. Herno A, Airaksinen O, Saari T. Long-term results of surgical treatment of lumbar spinal stenosis. Spine 1993;18:1471–1474.
13. Johnsson K. Lumbar spinal stenosis: a clinical, radiological and neuro-physiological investigation. Malmo, Sweden: Special publication of Department of Orthopaedics, Malmo General Hospital, Lund University; 1987.
14. Johnsson KE, Willner S, Johnsson K. Postoperative instability after decompression for lumbar spinal stenosis. Spine 1986;11:107–110.
15. Johnsson K, Rosen I, Uden A. The natural course of lumbar spinal stenosis. Acta Orthop Scand 1993;64(suppl 251):67–68.
16. Katz JN, Lispon SJ, Larson MG, et al. The outcome of decompressive laminectomy for degenerative lumbar spinal stenosis. J Bone Joint Surg 1991;73A:809–816.
17. Kirkaldy-Willis WH, Wedge JH, Yonk-Hing K, Reilly J. Pathology and pathogenesis of lumbar spondylosis and stenosis. Spine 1978;3:319–328.
18. Macnab I. Spondylolisthesis with an intact neural arch—the so-called pseudospondylolisthesis. J Bone Joint Surg 1950;32B:325–333.
19. Macnab I. Negative disc exploration. J Bone Joint Surg 1971;53A:891–903.
20. Management of Back Pain. In: Porter RW, ed. Edinburgh, Scotland: Churchill Livingstone; 1993, pp 59–72.
21. Porter RW. Central spinal stenosis: classification and pathogenesis. Acta Orthop Scand 1993; 251(suppl):64–66.
22. Porter RW. Neurogenic claudication and root claudication treated with calcitonin. Spine 1988;13:1062–1064.
23. Rydevik B. Neurophysiology of cauda equina compression. Acta Orthop Scand 1993;251(suppl): 52–55.
24. Schatzker J, Pennal GEF. Spinal stenosis, a cause of cauda equina compression. J Bone Joint Surg 1968;50B:606–618.
25. Schonstrom HSR, Bolender NF, Spengler DM. The pathomorphology of spinal stenosis as seen on CT scans of the lumbar spines. Spine 1985;10:806–811.

26. Tsuji H, Tamake T, Itoh T, et al. Redundant nerve roots in patients with degenerative lumbar spinal stenosis. Spine 1985;10:72–82.
27. Turner JA, Ersek M, Herron L, Deyo R. Surgery for lumbar spinal stenosis: an attempted meta-analysis of the literature. Spine 1992;17:1–8.
28. Ullrich CG, Binet EF, Sanecki MG, Kieffer SA. Quantitative assessment of the lumbar spinal canal by computed tomography. Radiology 1980;134:137–143.
29. Verbiest H. Pathomorphologic aspects of developmental lumbar stenosis. Orthop Clin North Am 1975;6:177–196.
30. Watanabe R, Parke W. Vascular and neural pathology of lumbosacral spinal stenosis. J Neurosurg 1986;64:64–70.

18

Differential Diagnosis of Low Back Pain

INTRODUCTION

This question is frequently asked by doctors at various stages of training and practice experience:

"How can I assess and treat a patient with back pain when the diagnosis is so elusive?" It is hard on the ego to assess a patient and fail to arrive at a concrete diagnosis on which to base a treatment program. The result often is a treatment program based more on hope than science. This should not be so. In today's medical world, our clinical skills and our investigative tools are such that we should be able to arrive at the correct diagnosis for most patients with "lumbago or sciatica." This chapter outlines the simple steps needed to assess a patient who presents with a complaint of low back pain.

ASSESSMENT METHOD

Do not initiate your assessment with a long list of time-consuming differential diagnoses on your menu. In family practice, this presents an overwhelming burden to the multitude of chief complaints heard during a day. Instead, adopt a simple, methodical approach. Your goal is to sort those patients who have mechanical or structural problems in the low back from those who have not. In a family practice setting, perhaps 20 to 25% of patients presenting with low back pain will have a source outside of the back as the cause of their symptoms. This fact presents many pitfalls for the unwary. For this reason, accurate evaluation requires a logical, step-by-step method. The foundation of this method is the clinical assessment / the good old-fashioned history and physical examination. Investigations such as computed tomography (CT) scanning and myelography should play a secondary role to clinical assessment. Today, our investigative tools are so sophisticated that one can find pathology on investigation in almost every patient whether or not the patient is sick.(1, 2) Moreover, minor insignificant pathology can become the red herring that causes you to miss the symptom producing lesion.

THE CLINICAL APPROACH

In assessing a patient with a low back complaint, ask yourself five questions:

1. Is this a true physical disability or is there a setting and a pattern on history and physical examination to suggest a non-physical or nonorganic problem?
2. Is this clinical presentation a diagnostic trap?
3. Is this a mechanical low back pain condition, and if so, what is the syndrome?
4. Are there clues to an anatomic level on history and physical examination?

5. After reviewing the results of investigation, what is the structural lesion and does it fit with the clinical syndrome?

Although these questions may not be answered sequentially during the history and physical examination, they ultimately must be answered sequentially before arriving at a diagnosis and prescribing a treatment program. That is to say, do not answer Question 5 and plan a treatment program until you have satisfactory answers to each preceding question. Probably the biggest pitfall is to answer Question 3 before you have satisfactorily answered Questions 1 and 2. The answers to Questions 1 and 2 should routinely be made outside the hospital, and before CT, myelography, magnetic resonance imaging (MRI), and other sophisticated investigative modalities are used. The classic trap is to ignore Questions 1 and 2 and admit a patient with a complaint of low back pain to the hospital, with sophisticated investigative tools, and then prescribe a treatment plan based on false-positive findings.

Question 1

Is this a true physical disability, or is there a setting and a pattern on history and physical examination to suggest a non-physical or nonorganic problem? That medicine should concern itself with the whole person is often stated but frequently ignored. The hallmark of a good clinician is the ability not only to diagnose disease but also to assess the "whole patient." No test of the art of medicine is more demanding than the identification of the patient with a nonorganic or emotional component to a back disability.

Remember the disability equation presented in Chapter 12:

Disability = A + B + C
where:
A = the physical component (disease).
B = the patient's emotional reaction.
C = the situation the patient is in at the time of disability
(eg, compensation claim, motor vehicle accident).

Each patient presenting with a back disability may have some component of each of these entities entwined in their disability. For example, a patient presenting a collection of symptoms, with no physical disability evident on examination, should lead one to think of the other aspects of the equation and look for emotional disability or situational reactions.

A classification of nonorganic spinal pain is presented again in Table 18.1. The term nonorganic has been chosen over other terms such as nonphysical, functional, emotional, and psychogenic. At this time reread Chapter 12. The conditions classified in Table 18.1 are such a common part of practice you cannot remind yourself enough to consider them in your differential diagnosis.

Commit Table 18.2 to memory. If you are puzzled by a patient with a complaint of low back pain, revisit Question 1: Is this a true physical disability? Specifically look for some or all of these symptoms and/or signs. If they are present, stop! Do not order expensive tests and treatment but rather seek help from someone more skilled in the evaluation of these non-organic syndromes.

Table 18.1. Classification of Nonorganic Spinal Pain

Psychosomatic spinal pain
Tension syndrome (fibrositis)
Pure Psychogenic spinal pain
Psychogenic spinal pain
Psychogenic modification of organic spinal pain
Situational spinal pain
Litigation reaction
Exaggeration reaction

Table 18.2. Symptoms and Signs Suggesting a Nonorganic Component to Disability

Symptoms	
	Pain is multifocal in distribution and nonmechanical (present at rest).
	Entire extremity is painful, numb, and/or weak.
	Extremity gives way (as a result, the patient carries a cane).
	Treatment response:
	A. No response.
	B. "Allergic" to treatment.
	C. Not receiving treatment.
	Multiple crises, multiple hospital admissions/investigations, and multiple visits to doctors.
Signs	
	Tenderness is superficial (skin) or nonanatomic (eg, over body of sacrum).
	Simulated movement tests positive.
	Distraction tests positive.
	Whole leg weak or numb.
	Academy Award performance.

It is important to stress that one swallow does not make a spring! The fact that a patient has one of these findings does not mean the patient should be classified as a exaggerator or litigant reactor. It is important to stress that a collection of symptoms and signs should be present with the appropriate clinical setting to make the diagnosis of exaggeration behavior. Waddell et al (3) have documented the significant symptoms and signs that, when collected together, suggest that a nonorganic component to a disability is present. These symptoms and signs have been scientifically documented as valid and reproducible. As a screening mechanism they are an excellent substitute for pain drawings and psychological testing.

Every human attends the school of survival. Sometimes the lessons lead patients to modify or magnify a physical disability at a conscious or unconscious level. Another word of caution: the presence of one of these nonorganic reactions does not preclude an organic condition such as a herniated nucleus pulposus. The art of medicine is truly tested by a patient with a physical low back pain who modifies the disability with a nonorganic reaction of tension, hysteria, depression, or emotional factors.

Question 2

Is this clinical presentation a diagnostic trap? It is too easy, when trying to arrive at a mechanical diagnosis, to fall into the many traps in the differential diagnosis of low back pain. An example is the young man in the early stages of ankylosing spondylitis who presents with vague sacroiliac joint pain and mild buttock and thigh discomfort who is thought to have a disc herniation. The patient with a retroperitoneal tumor invading the sacrum or sacral plexus may present with classic sciatica and also be diagnosed as having a disc herniation. It is not uncommon that patients with pathology within the peritoneal cavity will refer pain to the back. To avoid missing these various diagnostic pitfalls, always ask yourself the second question: Is this clinical presentation a trap?

Two broad categories of disease are included in this question:

1. Back pain referred from outside the spine may come from within the peritoneal cavity (eg, gastrointestinal tumors or ulcers) or from the retroperitoneal space (genitourinary conditions, abdominal aortic conditions, or primary or secondary tumors of the retroperitoneal space). These patients can be recognized clinically on the basis of two historic points. First, the pain is often nonmechanical in nature and troubles the patient just as much at rest as it does with activity. Second, the pain in the back often has the characteristics of the pain associated with the primary pathology, that is, if the primary pain is colicky, the back pain will be colicky.
2. Painful, non-degenerative conditions arising from within the spinal column, including its neurologic content. This group is subdivided into:
    a. The differential diagnosis of low back pain or lumbago (Table 18.3)
    b. The differential diagnosis of radicular pain or sciatica (Table 18.4).

Table 18.3. Differential Diagnosis of Nonmechanical Low Back Pain

Referred pain (eg, from the abdomen or retroperitoneal space)
Infection: bone, disk, epidural space
Neoplasm
Primary (multiple myeloma, osteoid osteoma, and so forth.)
Secondary
Inflammation
Miscellaneous metabolic and vascular disorders such as osteopenias and Paget's disease

Table 18.4. Differential Diagnosis of Sciatica

Intraspinal causes
Proximal to disk: conus and cauda equina lesions (eg, neurofibroma, ependymoma)
Disk level
Herniated nucleus pulposus
Stenosis (canal or recess)
Infection: osteomyelitis or diskitis (with nerve root pressure)
Inflammation: arachnoiditis
Neoplasm: benign or malignant with nerve root pressure
Extraspinal causes
Pelvis
Cardiovascular conditions (eg, peripheral vascular disease)
Gynecologic conditions
Orthopedic conditions (eg, osteoarthritis of hip)
Sacroiliac joint disease
Neoplasms
Peripheral nerve lesions
Neuropathy (diabetic, tumor, alcohol)
Local sciatic nerve conditions (trauma, tumor)
Inflammation (herpes zoster)

These patients have nonmechanical back pain or a pain characteristic for the primary pathology. Radiating extremity pain is not common unless neurologic territory has been invaded by the disease process, which usually occurs late in the disease. Unfortunately, many of these conditions are not obvious on history and physical examination and are often missed on reviewing plain radiographs. The following diagnostic tests are useful as a screening mechanism:

1. Hemoglobin, hematocrit, white blood cell count, differential, and erythrocyte sedimentation rate (ESR).
2. Serum chemistries, especially calcium, acid and alkaline phosphatase, and serum protein electrophoresis.
3. Bone scan. These three screening tests can be completed outside of the hospital and almost routinely identify these conditions. MRI will start to play a bigger role in the diagnosis of these various nonmechanical conditions.

Although the most common cause of leg pain in a radicular distribution is a structural lesion in the lumbosacral region, there are many other causes of radiating leg discomfort that must be considered. Missing these conditions is probably the most common error made in a spine surgical practice. For example, the high sensitivity of today's investigative modalities is capable of showing a minor and insignificant herniated nucleus pulposus when, in fact, the patient has a conus tumor higher in the spinal canal (Figure 18.1). This situation is being abetted by the tendency to perform a computed tomography (CT) scan and skip myelography in an attempt to arrive at a structural diagnosis for mechanical low back pain. This may seem a good idea to avoid the complications of myelography, but it will present problems unless you adhere to the following rule: An equivocal CT scan requires completion of myelography. As more MRI is done, the issue is going to be resolved. Soon, all patients with low back pain who do not respond to usual conservative treatment measures will be mandated by government or an insurance clerk to have an

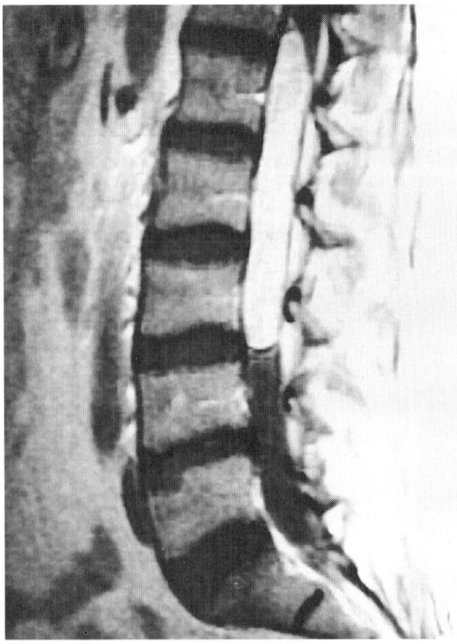

Figure 18.1 *Gadolinium-enhanced sagittal MRI of high lumbar schwannoma that was not seen on initial unenhanced MRI.*

outpatient hematologic and serum screen, a bone scan, a CT scan, or MRI. (Is it far down the road that one day robots will deal with the structural lesion?)

Etiology of Radiating Leg Pain

Space does not permit discussion of all the differential diagnoses of radiating leg pain, but three common conditions must be recognized:

1. Cardiovascular conditions (peripheral vascular disease).
2. Hip pathology.
3. Neuropathies.

Cardiovascular Conditions Cardiovascular disorders in the form of peripheral vascular disease can cause leg discomfort that is easily confused with nerve root compression. Because these conditions tend to occur in the older patient population, they may coexist. Table 18.5 separates vascular claudication from neurogenic claudication.

Hip Pathology Usually, it is easy to diagnose conditions of the hip because they so commonly cause pain around the hip and specifically pain in the groin. An early clue to hip pathology is the patient's statement that he/she cannot comfortably put on his/her socks (external rotation) (Fig. 18.2).In addition, walking causes a limp, and physical examination reveals a loss of internal rotation early in the disease. Occasionally, however, a patient with hip pathology will have no pain around the hip and will have only referred pain in the distal thigh. In these patients, it is easy to miss hip pathology unless one specifically examines the hip for loss of internal rotation. If there is any doubt, an radiograph of the hips must be taken, and if still in doubt a bone scan will be required.

Table 18.5. Differential Diagnosis of Claudicant Leg Pain[a]

Findings	Vascular Claudication	Neurogenic Claudication
Pain		
Type	Sharp, cramping	Vague and variously described as radicular, heaviness, cramping
Location	Exercised muscles (usually calf and rarely includes buttock, almost always excludes thigh)	Either typical radicular or extremely diffuse (usually including buttock)
Radiation	Rare after onset	Common after onset, usually proximal to distal
Aggravation	Walking, especially uphill	Not only aggravated by walking, but also by standing
Relief	Stopping muscular activity even in the standing position	Walking in the forward flexed position more comfortable; once pain occurs, relief comes only with lying or sitting down
Time to relief	Quick (seconds to minutes)	Slow (many minutes)
Neurologic symptoms (Paresthesia)	Usually not present	Commonly present
Straight leg raising tests	Negative	Mildly positive or negative
Neurologic examination	Negative	Mildly positive or negative
Vascular examination	Absent pulses	Pulses present

[a]Be wary of the patient in whom both conditions coexist.

Figure 18.2 *A patient with hip disease has trouble getting his/her leg into position (hip externally rotated) to put on socks. A patient with an acute disc herniation cannot get socks on because he/she cannot even sit to try and get the leg into this position!*

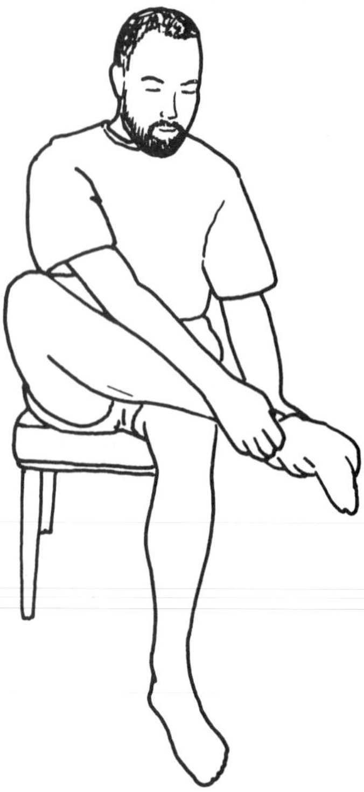

Neurological Disorders Someone who sees a lot of patients with low back pain will quickly realize that they must be a good neurologist. This is a major advantage of a neurosurgically trained spine surgeon over an orthopedically trained spine surgeon. But all is not lost if one takes a simple step by step approach to the patient who presents with weakness, sensory upset, pain and instability in the lower extremities. If pain is the predominant lower extremity symptom and follows a typical radicular distribution, there is a reasonable chance you are dealing with nerve root encroachment from a disc or osteophyte. But if weakness, sensory upset and / or instability is / are the dominant symptom(s), watch out: there is a good chance you are dealing with a primary neurological disorder. How do you approach such a patient?

Weakness as a Symptom

Weakness comes in many forms. For the poor historian it is one of the first words they reach for to describe almost any problem with the legs. It is used to describe generalized fatigue regardless of cause, for example, anemia. A true motor weakness will affect one or both limbs or a muscle group and will originate in the motor unit or the proximal motor pathways in the spinal cord, brain stem and cortex. Table 18.6 outlines the clinical aspects of weakness to help distinguish central from peripheral lesions. The next step in evaluating weakness is to separate the myopathies form the neuropathies. A good general rule is that the more proximal and symmetric the weakness the more likely you are dealing with a myopathy. The more distal lesions, symmetric or asymmetric are more likely polyneuropathies.

Table 18.7 classifies extremity weakness and sensory upset. Look back at Table 18.4 and recognize it as a table outlining the differential diagnosis of radiating leg pain. When you

Table 18.6. Symptoms and Signs of Central vs Peripheral Weakness

	CENTRAL	PERIPHERAL
Symptom	Diffuse weakness, associated stiffness	Localized to specific muscle group
Distribution	Proximal > distal	Proximal or distal
Tone	Increased (spastic)	Decreased (flaccid)
Reflexes	Increased	Decreased or absent
Path Reflexes	Upgoing toes	None
Rapid Alternating Movement	Poor	Slight impairment unless gross weakness
Atrophy	Limited	Limited to significant
Fasciculation	Absent	Present

Table 18.7. Classification of Extremity Weakness/Sensory Deficit

- Etiological classification
  - Congenital
  - Acquired
    - Trauma
    - Infection
    - Neoplasm
    - Degeneration
    - Metabolic
- Anatomical Level
  - Spinal cord
  - Anterior horn
  - Dorsal root ganglion
  - Peripheral nerve
  - Myoneural junction
  - Muscle
- Symptoms
  - Weakness
  - Sensory
  - Combined motor/sensory
  - Associated symptoms (eg, pain)

look at Table 18.7 you are looking at a different set of symptoms, that is, weakness and sensory deficit.

As depicted in Table 18.7, these neurological disorders can be classified according to etiology, anatomical level, and symptoms. Because the nerve fiber tracts involved lie so close to each other in the spinal cord and brain stem, it is often the case that the symptom complex for these deficits will be mixed.

Table 18.8 shows the working classification used in this section. Lesions will be discussed according to their anatomical level, that is, spinal cord, anterior horn, peripheral nerve, myoneural junction, and muscle. This is a simple classification but is not always correct in that some of the disorders discussed will affect more than one anatomical location. Also, etiological factors are considered in a simplistic fashion and sometimes are not clear-cut etiological factors. Even the subclassification of neurological presentation is simplistic in its concept but complicated in its application. If this were not the case, there would be no need for the specialty of neurology! Finally, many of these conditions bear little resemblance to differential diagnostic factors in sciatica. They are mentioned for completeness.

Trauma (Table 18.9)

Spinal Cord Shock Spinal cord shock is a stage of areflexia and flaccid paralysis that may occur immediately after a significant injury to the spinal cord. It lasts a varying length of time but usually reverses itself in a few hours to a few days. During the stage of spinal shock, there is virtually no physiological function present below the level of the lesion. The end of spinal cord shock is the time when any reflex arc reappears. The reflexes most often assessed in orthopedics is the bulbocavernosus reflex and the anal wink. After the return of these reflex functions, it is then time to assess the extent to the neurological lesion. If there is no motor or sensory function detected below the level of the spinal injury, then the spinal cord lesion can be considered total. If there is any sparing (such as sacral sparing) or a flicker of motor function, then the spinal cord lesion can be considered incomplete with some functional return to be anticipated. After spinal shock passes, the neurological state below the level of the lesion is one of spasticity. In addition, there may be excessive responses, such as the primitive withdrawal reflex or the mass reflex.

Brown-Séquard's Lesion (Fig. 18.3) Brown-Séquard's lesion is a hemisection of the spinal cord. The sensory loss, including pain and temperature loss, is in the contralateral extremity. The motor weakness is in the ipsilateral extremity below the level of Brown-Séquard's lesion. There is also posterior column loss of position and vibration sense.

Central Cord Syndrome This is the most common of the incomplete spinal cord lesions. It is a lesion similar to syringomyelia and is the result of interruption of the decussating pain and temperature fibers as well as the motor tracts at the level of the cord lesion. Because more distal motor tracts already present in the cord are displaced laterally by entering fibers, the motor lesion is more profound in the distal upper extremities than it is in the lower extremities. Figure 18.4 explains the anatomical basis for this phenomenon. The

Table 18.8. Workable Classification

Anatomical Level
Etiological classification
Neurological presentation

Table 18.9. Anatomical Level: Spinal Cord

Trauma
Transection
Brown-Séquard's
Central cord
Anterior cord
Posterior cord
Degeneration of tracts
Multiple sclerosis
Friedreich's ataxia
Subacute combined degeneration
Degeneration of sections of the spinal cord
Cervical disc disease with myelopathy
Syringomyelia

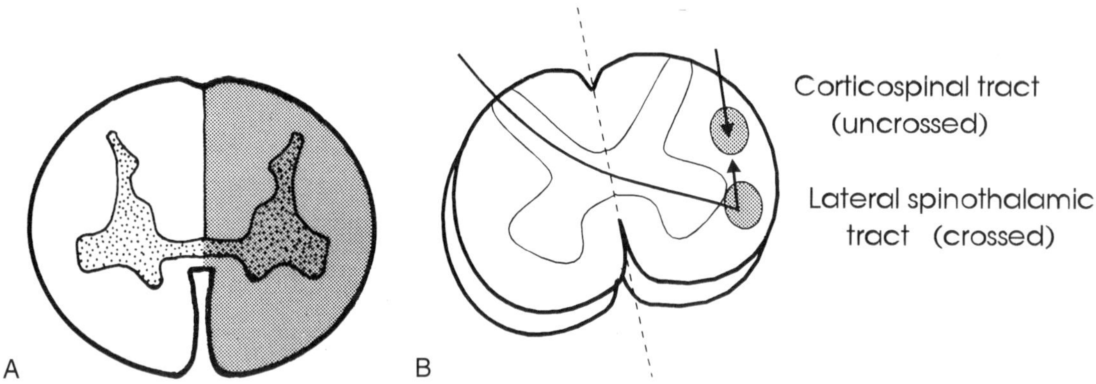

Figure 18.3 **A.** *A Brown-Séquard's cord lesion (shaded area). These lesions are rarely this symmetrical.* **B.** *The hemitransection of the cord (dashed line) of the right half of the spinal cord would produce motor paralysis on the same side (the corticospinal tract [anteriorly]) and sensory loss (the crossed lateral spinal thalamic tract [posteriorly]).*

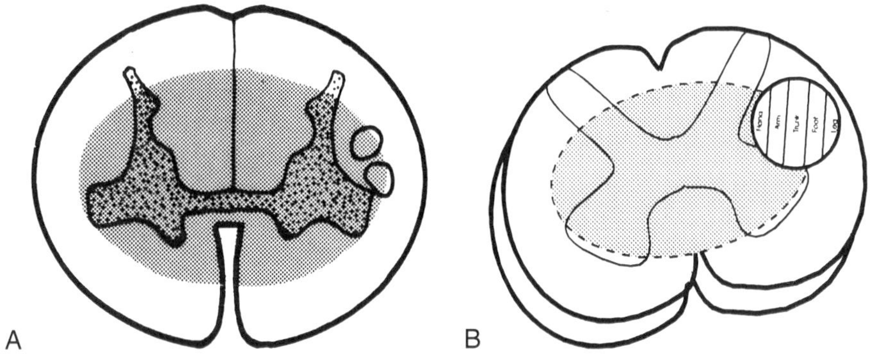

Figure 18.4 **A.** *Central cord syndrome: damage has occurred in the central shaded area that more affects the medial tracts (hands) than the lateral tracts (legs)* **(B).**

injury is usually secondary to a hyperextension injury of the cervical spine, especially in a patient who has a compromised spinal canal, either through birth or through degenerative changes. The pathogenesis of the lesion is thought to be interruption of the vascular supply to the central part of the cord, resulting in ischemic necrosis.

The disproportionate weakness in the arms and legs is manifest by greater weakness in the arms than in the legs and a more significant weakness in the hands than in the proximal upper extremity. The sensory symptoms are in the form of a burning dysesthetic discomfort in the arms as a result of damage to the spinothalamic fibers as they cross anteriorly.

Posterior Column This is a rare spinal cord lesion. In the days of syphilis and tabes dorsalis, we had an example of a nontraumatic form of posterior column disease. This resulted in sensory ataxia and varying degrees of radiating lower extremity pain and sensory loss. When it is the result of spinal cord injury, it is almost always part of corticospinal tract damage.

Anterior Cord Syndrome This is also a rare traumatic phenomenon. It is an upset in pain and temperature appreciation. There are occasions when there will be an infarct of the anterior portion of the cord, and this is usually a more extensive lesion involving the anterior two thirds of the cord, leaving only posterior column function intact (Fig. 18.5).

Degeneration of Tracts (Table 18.9)

Multiple Sclerosis Multiple sclerosis is a reasonably common affliction of young adults, occurring in 40 to 60 people per 100,000 population. The early symptoms depend on the location and the number of plaques of degeneration in the spinal cord. Early symptoms usually involve visual disturbances, paresthetic discomfort, gait disturbances, and brain-stem syndromes.

The visual disturbances are in the form of photophobia, pain on eye movements, and sudden unilateral blindness.

Sensory symptoms include paresthesia, dysesthesia, and Lhermitte's sign with a positive Romberg's test. These symptoms are the result of posterior column demyelination, and it is this collection of symptoms that occasionally offers some diagnostic difficulty to the spinal surgeon.

The gait disturbances are in the form of unsteadiness of gait with a positive Romberg test (unsteadiness on feet with the eyes closed).

The brain-stem syndromes involve multiple cranial nerves with appropriate symptoms indicating the cranial nerve involvement. If the degenerative plaques are specific for the corticospinal tracts, then the patient will experience muscle fatigue, stiffness, weakness, and spasticity. Occasionally MS will present with lower extremity pain that mimics sciatica.

Friedreich's Ataxia Friedreich's ataxia is an autosomal recessive inherited neurological disorder. The main symptom is ataxia, which has its onset between 4 and 20 years of age. The most usual clumping of patients is around the age of puberty. There is ataxia with a lower extremity motor and sensory component. There is an early loss of proprioceptive sensation. The effect on the corticospinal tracts results in weakness and pes cavus formation. In the cranial nerves, nystagmus will occur early; optic atrophy and blindness will occur late in the disease. Reflexes are lost early in Friedreich's ataxia, and the Babinski's extensor response is usually positive.

Patient's with Friedreich's ataxia usually go on to an early demise between the ages of 25 and 30. From the onset of the first symptoms to a wheelchair existence and death is approximately 5 years.

Figure 18.5 *Anterior cord lesion (shaded area).*

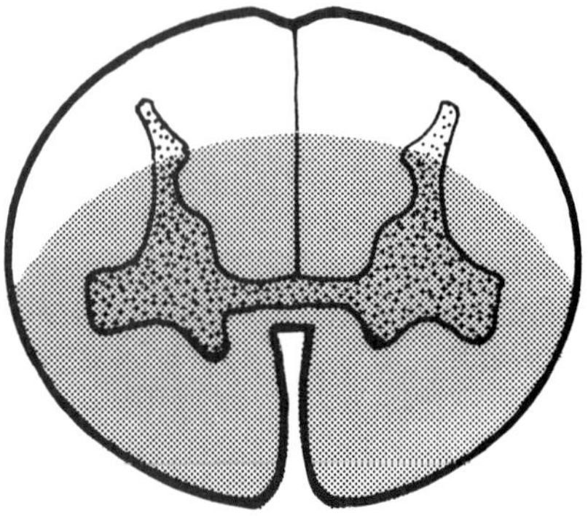

The lesion in Friedreich's ataxia involves (1) degeneration in the posterior columns, thereby upsetting position and vibration senses, (2) degeneration in the lateral corticospinal tract, resulting in loss of motor power, and (3) degeneration in the posterior and anterior spinal cerebellar tracts, resulting in ataxia.

Subacute Combined Degeneration of the Spinal Cord This condition occurs secondary to vitamin B12 deficiency. There is swelling of the myelin and subsequent demyelination in the lower cervical and thoracic posterior columns.

The general symptoms of anemia, including fatigue and weight loss, are present. Neurologically, the patients will present with a tingling, burning type of dysesthetic discomfort in the distal extremities. It may occur first in the feet and may be unilateral, thereby confusing the spinal surgeon evaluating lower extremity symptoms.

Later in the disease, the lateral columns and the spinocerebellar tracts will be involved, leading to stiffness and spasticity. If not detected early, vitamin B12 deficiency will lead to severe degeneration in the spinal cord, resulting in spasticity, bladder and bowel upset, mental disturbances, and sensory loss.

Degeneration of Sections of the Spinal Cord (Table 18.9)

Cervical Disc Disease with Myelopathy Degenerative cervical disc disease may result in the formation of ridgelike prominence across the back of the disc space that encroaches on the spinal cord. It is likely that this results in a compression ischemia of the tracts of the spinal cord, resulting in degeneration and the clinical picture of myelopathy. The onset of myelopathic symptoms is insidious. On occasion, trauma will result in a fairly rapid change in the presentation of the myelopathy. The usual presentation is one of slow onset paresis and spasticity as a result of damage to the corticospinal tracts. This may result in paresthesia and clumsiness of the hands but more likely will present as instability of gait. There is a striking absence of pain in the lower extremities with cervical myelopathy; this should lead the spinal surgeon to look outside of the lumbar spine for the source of the lower extremity symptoms. There presence of bilateral diffuse lower extremity weakness with hyper-reflexia and a positive Babinski's response should point to the cord levels as the source of the pathology. These levels are above L2, and the most common location for such pathology is the cervical spine. The presence of Lhermitte's sign—namely, tingling in all four limbs or electric shocklike feelings down the back, produced by neck flexion—further suggests the neck as the source of the patient's disability.

Tandem Stenosis It makes sense to conclude that if one part of the spinal canal narrows to constrict neurological tissue, another part of the spinal canal can do likewise. When this simultaneously involves the cervical and lumbar canals it is known as "tandem stenosis." The cervical canal narrowing produces myelopathy (a upper motor neuron lesion), and the lumbar stenosis produces a partial lower motor neuron lesion of the cauda equina. This can be quite confusing when examining the lower extremities, with the usual picture being brisk knee reflexes, suppressed ankle reflexes and equivocal Babinski's responses. Weakness is detectable proximal and distal and a sensory loss is usually not apparent.

Syringomyelia Syringomyelia is a condition of cavitation or syrinx formation in the central area of the spinal cord. As time passes, the size of the lesion gradually expands. This expansion produces neuronal and tract damage. The usual location of a syrinx is in the cervical and upper thoracic segments.

Initially, the lesion destroys the pain and temperature fibers crossing the central gray matter. This is depicted in Figure 18.6 and results in a capelike distribution to the loss of pain and temperature function in the upper extremities. Later in the disease process, the pyramidal tracts and posterior columns are compressed, resulting in symptoms usually appearing first in the hands.

The onset of the disease is late in the second decade through the 5th decade, with the average age of onset being 30. There is a variable progression in the disease, with 50% of the patients ending up in a wheelchair in 20 years. The classic sign of syringomyelia is a disassociated sensory loss with a capelike loss of pain and temperature in the presence of preservation of touch and position.

Anatomical Level: Anterior Horn Level (Table 18.10)

Motor Neuron Disease This is a general term used to designate a progressive disorder of motor neurons resulting from degeneration in the spinal cord, brain stem, and motor

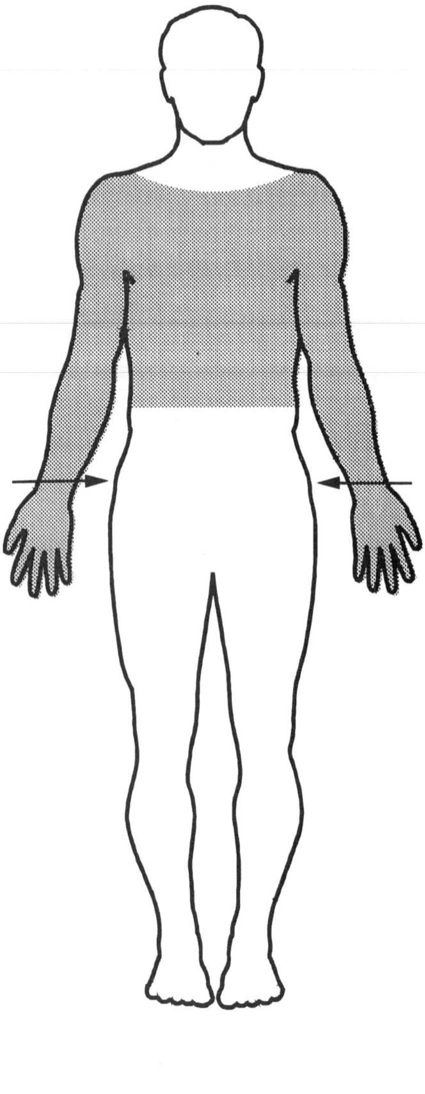

Figure 18.6 *Syringomyelia: the capelike area of impaired sensation to pain and temperature (touch, position, and vibration are spared). As the lesion expands in the spinal cord, a flaccid paralysis (anterior horn) develops in the distal upper extremity (distal to arrows).*

Table 18.10. Anterior Horn Disorders

Motor neuron disease
Amyotrophic lateral sclerosis
Progressive muscular atrophy
Primary bulbar palsy
Spinal muscular atrophy
Poliomyelitis
Tetanus

cortex. It occurs most commonly in middle-aged men and is manifest clinically by muscular weakness, atrophy and corticospinal tract signs in varying combinations. It usually ends in death in 2 to 6 years.

Amyotrophic Lateral Sclerosis This is the most common motor system disorder with amyotrophy and hyperreflexia combined. It most often starts in the hand, with awkwardness of fine movements and stiffness in the fingers. It may also start in the neck and trunk, and on the rare occasion its initial manifestations will be in the lower extremities. Eventually, the trait of atrophic weakness of hands and forearms, slight spasticity of the legs, and generalized hyperreflexia is present in the absence of any sensory or sphincter upset. Later, the disease spreads to involves the neck, tongue, pharynx, and laryngeal muscles. The confusion for the spinal surgeon comes about when the initial symptom of this disorder is a dropped foot, but on careful examination, the patient will be noted to have a diffuse lower extremity weakness and spasticity with hyper-reflexia.

Progressive Muscle Atrophy This is a symmetrical wasting and weakness of the intrinsic hand muscles. It slowly progresses to involve the rest of the arm. It is a variant of amyotrophic lateral sclerosis and is usually symmetrical.

Progressive Bulbar Palsy The first manifestation of bulbar palsy is an affliction of the muscles of the jaw, face, tongue, and pharynx. Its earliest manifestation is difficulty in articulating. It eventually spreads to respiratory muscles. It is not usually a differential diagnostic problem for the spinal surgeon.

Heredofamilial Forms of Progressive Muscular Atrophy (Spinal Muscular Atrophy) This condition is represented by the floppy baby syndrome, which is the infantile form of spinal muscular atrophy known as Werdnig-Hoffmann atrophy. It can have a later onset between the ages of 3 and 18, and this proximal spinal muscle atrophy results in a significant scoliosis.

Poliomyelitis Poliomyelitis is a familiar condition of an acute febrile systemic illness that results in a lower motor neuron lesion of muscles. It is due to a viral invasion of the anterior horn cells. It can affect higher centers in the form of a bulbar palsy, but the most common form is an affliction of the extremities.

Tetanus Three bacterial toxins affect humans. Tetanus affects the motor neuron; diphtheria affects the peripheral nerve; botulism affects the neuromuscular junction. Tetanus toxin attaches to the motor neuron cell and causes tetanic spasms, which first affect the jaw, face, and swallowing, and subsequently spread to involve the entire body. Tetanus is never a differential diagnostic problem to the spinal surgeon.

Dorsal Root Ganglion Herpes zoster is the viral infection that affects the dorsal root ganglion. The virus migrates up the peripheral nerve to the dorsal root, a migratory pattern that may occur early in life, leaving the virus dormant for years. It is then excited as an etiological agent and causes acute inflammatory reaction in the dorsal root ganglion. The initial manifestation is pain in a nerve root distribution followed by a skin rash in the same distribution. It can also spread to the anterior horn and cause a polio-like illness.

Clinically, usually only one root is affected. Although it is primarily in the lower thoracic region, it can occur in the lumbar region and present confusion to the spinal surgeon because of the radicular distribution of the pain. Eventually, a chickenpox-like rash appears in the same radicular distribution to establish the diagnosis. The pain may be present prior to the appearance of the rash by a few days, but eventually the rash will appear and disappear in 1 to 4 weeks. There are occasions, especially in the debilitated patient, where the syndrome persists as a painful rash.

Peripheral Nerve Polyneuropathies

Table 18.11 classifies the polyneuropathies. Polyneuropathies are slowly developing afflictions of multiple peripheral nerves. They may start primarily in one nerve (mononeuritis) and spread to involve multiple nerves (polyneuritis), a spread that is usually slow. Some may remain as mononeuropathies. Polyneuropathies are most often sensory in their onset, distal in their location, and lower extremity in their affliction. They are most characteristically asymmetrical. Subsequently, they will include weakness as part of their presentation. On physical examination, there is loss of reflexes. Electromyogram (EMG) assessment will demonstrate loss of innervation in the form of fibrillation potentials. The pathology in neuropathies and other degenerative neuropathies. In the hereditary and toxic neuropathies, the pathological lesion is in the axon.

Table 18.11. Polyneuropathies

Genetically determined
Hereditary motor and sensory neuropathies
Peroneal muscular atrophy (Charcot-Marie-Tooth)
Neuronal type of peroneal muscular atrophy
Hypertrophic neuropathy (Dejerine-Sottas)
Polyneuropathy or porphyria
Metabolic
Diabetic
Symmetrical distal diabetic neuropathy
Asymmetrical proximal diabetic neuropathy
Amyotrophy or myelopathy in diabetes
Hypothyroidism
Nutritional (undernourished)
Infectious diseases
Guillain-Barré syndrome
Leprosy
Collagenoses
Periarteritis nodosa
Toxic
Lead and alcohol
Miscellaneous
Neoplastic
Ischemic

Genetically Determined Polyneuropathies

Peroneal Muscular Atrophy (Charcot-Marie-Tooth) There is a relationship between Charcot-Marie-Tooth atrophy and Friedreich's ataxia. A pure Charcot-Marie-Tooth disorder is considered an inherited peripheral neuropathy affecting particularly the distal reaches of the peroneal nerve, manifested by pes cavus in childhood. It is associated with absence of ankle jerks. It can occur in this pure form, but often there are additional degenerative changes in the pyramidal tracts and the posterior columns, putting it into the same family as Friedreich's ataxia.

The neurological manifestations are weakness and wasting in the distal peroneal nerve distribution. This may be manifest as a drop foot with overpull of the gastrocnemius and posterior tibial muscle to give an equinovarus deformity with a caval foot and claw toes. In the more severe forms, there is an affliction of the upper extremities. These is rarely a sensory component to this neurological disorder, although there may be impairment of vibration sense distally.

Neuronal Type of Charcot-Marie-Tooth Atrophy This is a neurological disorder that appears later in life and affects predominantly the peripheral nerves of the lower extremities. The lesion is actually in the anterior horn cell, and this condition should be classified as an anterior horn cell disorder.

Hypertrophic Neuritis (Dejerine-Sottas disease) This is a polyneuropathy not unlike Charcot-Marie-Tooth atrophy. It begins early in childhood and is manifest by a motor involvement much more severe than Charcot-Marie-Tooth atrophy.

Porphyria Porphyria usually presents with acute abdominal symptoms in the form of colic, constipation, and vomiting. In addition, there is a generalized polyneuropathy that can be severe to the point of flaccid tetraplegia.

Metabolic Peripheral Neuropathies The most common peripheral neuropathy that a spinal surgeon will face as a differential diagnostic problem is diabetic neuropathy. This is a disease of the Schwann cell. The Schwann cell needs insulin to make myelin; when this cell is deprived of insulin, there will be myelin degeneration. Ischemia also plays a role in these disorders. There are various forms of diabetic peripheral neuropathy listed in Table 18.12.

Symmetrical Distal Diabetic Neuropathy This is predominantly a sensory neuropathy that occurs in the elderly mild diabetics. They complain of restlessness, pain, and inability to sleep at night because of the distal lower extremity symptoms. They can have extraordinary complaints, yet they have virtually nothing in the way of physical finding. If present long enough as a pathological entity, the patients will display a stocking and glove type of sensory loss. By the time the polyneuropathy extends up to the level of the thighs, there will be a similar phenomenon occurring in the hands.

Table 18.12. Diabetic Peripheral Neuropathy

Symmetrical distal
Asymmetrical proximal mononeuropathies and cranial neuropathies
Diabetic amyotrophy

There is a motor form of symmetrical distal diabetic neuropathy that occurs in upper extremities in men. It is a rare phenomenon, occurring in 1 of 200 sensory neuropathies seen.

Asymmetrical Proximal Mononeuropathy (Single Root or Local Involvement of Two or More Nerves [Multiplex]) This condition results from a stroke of the vasa nervorum of the peripheral nerve. It is manifest by radicular pain of sudden onset, almost identical to a herniated nucleus pulposus. However, the pain is more commonly in the femoral nerve distribution, most common in the older patient; the pain is nonmechanical in nature in that it bothers the patient day and night. The vital point on historical examination is the absence of back pain. The vital observation on physical examination is the unusual absence of root tension signs such as straight leg raising (SLR) reduction. Although the sensory symptoms predominate, it is the authors' experience that mononeuropathy affecting the formal of the lumbosacral roots had a more significant motor and reflex component on examination. The diagnosis is supported by abnormal blood sugars and electrical studies showing slowed nerve conduction velocities and the presence of fibrillation potentials, positive waves at rest, and a decrease in the number of motor unit potentials on EMG. As time passes, this condition tends to improve. Symptoms of asymmetrical proximal diabetic neuropathy can be precipitated by a minor disc herniation that may point the treating surgeon to operative intervention, only to result in a poor outcome because of the undetected diabetic neuropathy.

Diabetic Amyotrophy This is a particular problem of the adult-onset, obese, mild diabetic. It is a generalized condition of rapid onset manifested by weight loss and proximal weakness, especially in the psoas, gluteal, and quadriceps muscles. There is often a mild associated prodromal state. Over the course of a few weeks, the patient is unable to walk because of the severe weakness. These patients may have had a preexisting symmetrical distal sensory neuropathy and then experienced the onset of their proximal pain and severe weakness with wasting. Bladder and bowel function is always spared. From a differential diagnoses aspect, there is no back pain in diabetic amyotrophy and the neurological manifestations are of significant proximal weakness and less in the way of pain. In addition, the severe neurological involvement, symmetrical in nature, in the absence of bladder and bowel involvement, is a clue to the diagnosis.

Infectious Diseases

Guillain-Barré Syndrome The Guillain-Barré syndrome occurs following viral infection and is predominantly motor (and minimally sensory) in its manifestations. It occurs in young or middle-aged adults, more commonly men than women. It begins as a paresthetic sensation in the hands and/or the feet. It is at this moment that it can be seen by a spinal surgeon. Quickly, it spreads to become severe weakness of the extremities, especially in the proximal girdle muscles. This weakness may be accompanied by a general feeling of soreness. Cranial nerves can be involved. Again, bladder and bowel functions are spared, and there are minimal sensory findings. The patient is areflexic.

The concern with Guillain-Barré syndrome is the severe respiratory problems that can ensue.

Collagen Disorder

Polyarteritis Nodosa with Mononeuropathy Multiplex This is another peripheral neuropathy in which there is an upset in the vascular supply to a nerve. It has a presentation typical to a disc herniation, with radicular pain and paresthesia. Very quickly, a significant paralysis ensues and spreads to multiple nerves. Usually, the patient will experience the systemic manifestations of the collagen disorder, such as painful joints. Hypertrophic superficial cutaneous nerves, secondary to collagen deposition, may be palpated.

Disease of the Neuromuscular Junction

Myasthenia Gravis This is an acquired autoimmune disease in which antibodies are formed that bind to the acetylcholine receptors at the myoneural junction, resulting in interference with the transmission of nerve impulses. The condition occurs in young adults, more commonly in women than men (3:1). In the generalized form, there are varying degrees of severity. It often starts in the bulbar nerves, especially those nerves controlling the eyes. It then spreads to the neck, arms, and legs, and is ultimately manifest by significant weakness. Symptoms fluctuate during the day's activities, with the patient usually better in the morning and worse by the end of the day.

Muscular Lesions

Polymyositis This is an inflammatory myopathy in the category of autoimmune disease. It is frequently of insidious onset and occasionally of acute onset. Symptoms are progressive weakness of the limb girdle, trunk, and neck flexor muscles. Muscle pain may be associated with the condition, and if the changes are more pronounced around the neck and shoulders, the condition is easily confused with cervical disc disease having bilateral referred shoulder pain. Some patients have the typical skin changes of dermatomyositis.

Clinically detectable weakness distinguishes this condition from polymyalgia rheumatica. The diagnosis can be confirmed by muscle biopsy (showing muscle necrosis and repair), increased serum levels of muscle enzymes, and EMG changes (increased insertional activity and fibrillation potentials).

Polymyalgia Rheumatica This disease of elderly patients who have symptoms of malaise, weight loss, and an increased ESR as part of a myalgic picture. The pain may be confined to the shoulder girdle region, but is more often diffuse.

The absence of weakness, with normal creatine phosphokinase enzymes and normal EMG examination, distinguish this problem from polymyositis.

Conclusion

Although there are many other causes of extremity symptoms not listed in this table (Table 18.11), it is important to recognize that the table includes most causes of lower extremity pain. Extremity symptoms such as numbness and weakness, in the absence of pain, should suggest very strongly that a primary neurologic disorder is possible rather than a mechanical low back condition.

Question 3

Is this a mechanical low back pain condition, and if so, what is the syndrome? The two important words are "mechanical" and "syndrome." Mechanical pain is pain aggravated by activity such as bending and lifting, and relieved by rest. There may be specific complaints relative to household chores or specific work efforts. These mechanical pains are usually relieved by rest. Although these statements seem straight forward, clinical assessment is not always easy. A poor historian may not be able to relate a history of mechanical aggravation or relief. In addition, if significant leg pain is present, implying a significant inflammatory response around the nerve root, then much rest will be needed before the patient describes a relief of leg pain. Significant mechanical back pain may sometimes be aggravated by simply rolling over in bed. To the unsophisticated historian, this may have the appearance of nonmechanical back pain. However, if one takes a careful history, and if a patient is a good historian it is possible to determine that mechanical back pain is pain aggravated by activity and relieved by rest.

The second important word is "syndrome." It is much safer to make a syndrome diagnosis for mechanical low back pain and then, after investigation, try matching a structural lesion with the clinical syndrome. There are two reasons for taking this approach:

Today's investigative techniques are so sophisticated that it is possible to find abnormalities whether a patient has symptoms or not. A patient may have an obvious structural lesion such as spondylolisthesis, yet may have an acute radicular syndrome due to a disc herniation at a level other than that of the spondylolisthesis. In fact, a patient with spondylolisthesis may have any one of the potential diagnoses discussed in this chapter. To focus on the structural lesion of spondylolisthesis shown on radiograph and ignore the history and physical examination will lead to errors in diagnosis and treatment.

There are basically two syndromes in mechanical low back pain (Table 18.13): (1) lumbago (back pain), and (2) sciatica (radicular leg pain syndrome). Before enlarging on these syndromes, it is well to take a moment to reflect on the concept of "referred pain." Many experts state that leg pain that does not go below the knee and is associated with good SLR ability is likely referred leg pain. This idea is further entrenched if there is an absence of neurologic symptoms or signs. The gate control theory of pain is one of the theories used to explain referred pain. The phenomenon is thought to occur when painful stimuli are reflexively shifted around at the cord level. This shunting results in pain being felt in a myotomal or dermatomal distribution (eg, legs) away from the origin of the pain. The concept is altogether too simplistic and needs to be reworked in light of new investigative techniques such as CT scanning and MRI. We predict that referred leg pain will be a lot less common than originally thought. It is more likely that patients labeled as having referred pain for their leg radiations have various degrees of radicular pain due to nerve root encroachment by either bone or chronic disc herniations.

The diagnosis of referred leg pain should be reserved for the patient who has the following clinical presentation:

Table 18.13. Syndromes in Mechanical Low Back Pain

Lumbago: mechanical instability
Sciatica: radicular pain
Unilateral acute radicular syndrome
Bilateral acute radicular syndrome
Unilateral chronic radicular syndrome
Bilateral chronic radicular syndrome

1. There is significant mechanical back pain present as the source of referral.
2. The leg pain affects both legs, is vague in its distribution, and has no radicular component.
3. The degree of referred leg discomfort varies directly with the back pain. When the back pain increases in severity, the referred leg pain occurs or increases in severity. Conversely, a decrease in back pain results in a decrease in the referral of pain. Referred pain is less likely to radiate below the knee.
4. There are no neurologic symptoms or signs in concert with the complaint of referred leg pain.

It is safer to assume that any patient with radiating leg pain, especially unilateral leg pain, has a radicular syndrome until proven otherwise.

Lumbago–Mechanical Instability

The lumbago–mechanical instability syndrome is easy to recognize. These patients present exclusively with lumbosacral backache aggravated by activities such as bending, lifting, and sitting. The pain may radiate toward either iliac crest, but does not radiate down into the buttock or legs. The pain is almost always relieved by various forms of rest, for example, reduced activity, weight reduction, corset support, or bed rest. Most patients have no trouble describing these relieving efforts.

Most importantly, there are no associated leg symptoms or signs. (See Chapter 14 for a complete discussion of these patients).

Radicular Syndromes

The radicular syndromes have been describes in Chapters 15, 16, and 17. If you have time, go back and browse!

Summary

Tables 18.14, 18.15, and 18.16 summarize some of the important historic and physical features on which to build the diagnosis of an acute radicular syndrome.

Bilateral Acute Radicular Syndrome (The Cauda Equina Syndrome) Fortunately, the bilateral acute radicular syndrome is rare. Unfortunately, there is frequent delay in diagnosis, jeopardizing long term function of the bladder and bowel. Although we have covered this topic in Chapter 15, let us review it again because it is such an important clinical setting. To start, recognize that the chronic cauda equina encroachment of spinal canal stenosis does not cause bladder and bowel impairment, even in the face of significant physical compression of the cauda equina roots. On the other hand a large sequestered disc rupture (acute) at L3–L4, L4–L5, or L5–S1 can seriously impair cauda equina function. Patients usually have a problem of back symptoms that suddenly worsen. The syndrome includes back pain, bilateral leg pain, saddle anesthesia, bilateral lower extremity weakness, bladder (urinary) retention, and lax rectal tone. This presentation requires urgent medical attention almost always including a CT/myelogram or MRI and surgical decompression within hours of first seeing the patient. It is usually due to a massive midline sequestered disc. The syndrome is manifest by the sudden onset of bilateral leg

Table 18.14. Criteria for the Diagnosis of Acute Radicular Syndrome[a]

Leg pain (including buttock) is the dominant complaint when compared with back pain

Neurologic symptoms that are specific (eg, paresthesia in a typical dermatomal distribution)

Significant SLR changes (any one or a combination of these)
  A. SLR less than 50% of normal
  B. Bowstring discomfort
  C. Crossover pain

Neurologic sign (see section on anatomic level)

[a]Three or four of these criteria must be present, the only exception being young patients who are very resistant to the effects of nerve root compression and thus may not have neurologic symptoms (Criterion 2) or signs (Criterion 4).

Table 18.15. The Difference in Presentation of the Acute Radicular Syndrome in Various Ages

	Young (<30 y)	Adult (35–55 y)	Older (60+ y)
Symptoms			
Leg pain	usually the only symptom	some BP, but LP dominates	usually BP, but LP still dominates
Paresthesia	often absent	usually present	almost always present
Signs			
SLR	very positive (often 10–20% of normal)	less than 50% of normal	occasionally good ability
Neurological signs	absent in at least 50% of patients	sometimes absent	almost always present

Key: BP = buttock pain; LP = leg pain.

Table 18.16. Common Neurologic Changes in Acute Radicular Syndrome

Change	L4	L5	S1
Motor weakness	Knee extension	Ankle dorsiflexion	Ankle plantar flexion
Sensory loss	Medial shin to knee	Dorsum of foot and lateral calf	Lateral border of foot and posterior calf
Reflex depression	Knee	Tibialis posterior	Ankle
Wasting	Thigh (no calf)	Calf (minimal thigh)	Calf (minimal thigh)

pain usually accompanied by bladder and bowel impairment. It is obviously an emergency and is a diagnosis that is rarely missed.

Unilateral Chronic Radicular Syndrome The difference between acuteness and chronicity in a radicular syndrome is often difficult to measure. The severity and the duration of the syndrome usually combine to distinguish acute from chronic radicular pain. Chronic unilateral radicular pain is usually a complaint for many months or more. It follows a typical radicular distribution, including pain below the knee, and is usually associated with much in the way of mechanical back pain. Both pains are usually aggravated by walking. Neurologic symptoms are less prevalent than in the acute radicular syndrome, and are sometimes extremely diffuse and nonlocalizing. SLR ability is usually much better than 50% of normal, and bowstring discomfort and crossover pain are not seen in this syndrome. Neurologic findings are very few and usually not helpful in localizing the degree of nerve root involvement. For a complete discussion of this syndrome, see Chapter 16.

Bilateral Chronic Radicular Syndrome The bilateral chronic radicular syndrome is known as neurogenic claudication and was discussed in Chapter 17. However, bilateral leg symptoms specifically aggravated by walking are present in only 50% of patients with chronic bilateral radicular syndrome. For this reason, the term chronic bilateral radicular syndrome is preferred. This syndrome differs from the unilateral radicular syndrome in two ways:

1. Both legs are affected rather than one leg.
2. The pain of the bilateral radicular syndrome may not be a typical radicular-type pain. Some patients describe typical claudicant leg pain in a radicular distribution. Other patients describe a diffuse type of claudicant leg discomfort that cannot be localized to a radicular distribution.

Many other symptoms are present in this syndrome including weakness, "heaviness," and "rubberiness" in the legs. Numbness is also prevalent in this syndrome and is often of no value in localizing which nerve roots are compromised. There is a typical march phenomenon with the chronic bilateral radicular syndrome. Symptoms get much worse with prolonged walking, radiate further down the leg, and ultimately interfere with the ability of the patient to ambulate. Some patients may report noticing that if they attach themselves to a shopping cart and walk in the flexed position, they can get more distance before their leg symptoms appear. Characteristically, physical examination in chronic bilateral radicular syndrome reveals little. SLR is usually very good, and if the syndrome is due entirely to canal narrowing rather than lateral recess narrowing, there are limited neurologic findings except for mild weakness in the roots distal to the lesion and bilateral ankle reflex suppression. Rarely does the syndrome progress to the point where the patient has significant weakness requiring a wheelchair.

Question 4

Are there clues to an anatomic level on history and physical examination? Is there an anatomic level clinically? This is an important intermediate question to consider between a syndrome diagnosis and a structural diagnosis. If it is possible to determine an anatomic level clinically, then any structural lesion has to be at the appropriate level. Otherwise, it cannot be considered a significant defect. A patient who has an anatomic level of S1 root involvement rarely should have a structural diagnosis localized to the L3–L4 interspace!

There are three ways to determine an anatomic level: distribution of leg pain, neurologic symptoms, and neurologic signs.

Distribution of Leg Pain

Pain in the posterior thigh and posterior calf distribution incriminates the 5th lumbar root or the first sacral root. Whether this pain is posterior or posterolateral in the thigh and calf is of little use in separating 5th lumbar root lesions from 1st sacral root lesions.

However, pain down the anterior thigh almost certainly incriminates the 4th lumbar nerve root or higher lumbar nerve roots, and excludes involvement of the 5th lumbar or 1st sacral roots.

Neurologic Symptoms

A paresthetic discomfort with a dermatomal distribution is the most helpful historic feature in localizing an anatomic level. Paresthetic discomfort along the lateral edge of the foot incriminates the 1st sacral nerve root, paresthetic discomfort over the dorsum of the foot and the lateral calf incriminates the 5th lumbar nerve root, and paresthetic discomfort down the medial shin incriminates the 4th lumbar nerve root.

Neurologic Signs

The diagnosis of acute radicular syndrome is in totally dependent on the demonstration of root impairment as reflected by signs of motor weakness or changes in sensory appreciation or reflex activity. However, the presence of such changes reinforces the diagnosis. The common neurologic changes are summarized in Table 18.16.

Question 5

After reviewing the results of investigation, what is the structural lesion and does it fit with the clinical syndrome? The potential structural lesion diagnoses are listed in Table 18.17. This table covers only degenerative conditions of the spine; it omits postoperative scarring of arachnoid or nerve roots and fractures and dislocations. It is important to stress here that it is possible to have multiple syndromes related to a single structural lesion. For example, a degenerative spondylolisthesis can cause both mechanical instability (back pain) and bilateral claudicant leg pain as a result of encroachment on the spinal canal. Table 18.18 links syndromes with structural lesions.

Conclusion

It is important to make a clear-cut syndrome diagnosis on the basis of a history and physical examination, and match it to a clear-cut bona fide structural lesion on investigation. Failure to do this leads to wrong diagnoses and futile treatment interventions.

Table 18.17. Structural Lesions in Mechanical Low Back Pain

Instability
Intrinsic to disc—degenerative disc disease
Extrinsic to disc
Facet joint disease
Spondylolisthesis
Soft tissue lesions—muscle spasm; ligamentous strain
Herniated nucleus pulposus (HNP)
Narrowing of spinal canal
Spinal canal stenosis (SCS)
Lateral zone stenosis (LZS)

Table 18.18. Relationship of Syndromes and Structural Lesions

Lumbago	DDD FJD Spondylolysis/spondylolisthesis Soft tissue
Unilateral acute radicular	HNP HNP + LRS
Unilateral chronic radicular	LRS HNP
Bilateral acute radicular	Central HNP
Bilateral chronic radicular	SCS

Key: DDD = degenerative disk disease; FJD = facet joint disease; HNP = herniated nucleus pulposus; LRS = lateral recess stenosis; SCS = spinal canal stenosis.

Methods Used to Document the Structural Lesion

Steps to document the presence of a structural lesion in mechanical low back pain should be taken only after a satisfactory answer has been obtained for Questions 1, 2, and 3. Seeking a structural lesion in a patient with an unrecognized nonorganic problem is usually a waste of time and money, and is a danger to the patient.

False-positive investigative findings are easy to come by with today's sophisticated techniques.(2) Before entertaining each of these possible investigative procedures, it is assumed that a thorough history, physical examination, and other necessary investigations have satisfactorily answered Questions 1 and 2. For a run through of the investigative procedures useful and useless, you are referred back to Chapter 11.

Conclusion

The assessment of a patient with a low back disability does not need to be difficult. By keeping a simple system in mind, it is possible to arrive at a good clinical impression by asking yourself the following five questions and committing yourself, eventually, to sequential answers.

1. Is this a true physical disability, or is there a setting and a pattern in the history and physical examination to suggest a nonphysical or nonorganic problem?
2. Is this clinical presentation a diagnostic trap?
3. Is this a mechanical low back pain condition, and if so, what is the syndrome?
4. Are there clues to an anatomic level on history and physical examination?
5. After reviewing the results of investigation, what is the structural lesion, and does it fit with the clinical syndrome?

Do not commit yourself to any major investigative step until Questions 1 and 2 have been adequately answered. Then, if you are satisfied that you have a mechanical low back pain problem, dissect it into a syndrome first, an anatomic level second, and a structural lesion third. The structural lesion diagnosis should fully support the clinical syndrome and the anatomic level. If not, take one step back and repeat the history and physical examination. Listening to the patient's story, doing a thorough physical examination, and supporting your diagnosis with investigation is the best way to avoid erroneous diagnoses and ill-fated surgery.

REFERENCE

1. Bell GR, et al. A study of computer-assisted tomography. Spine 1984;9:552–556.
2. Boden SD, Davis DO, Dina TS, et al. Abnormal magnetic resonance scans of the lumbar spine in asymptomatic subjects. J Bone Joint Surg 1990;72:403–408.
3. Waddell G, McCulloch JA, Kummel EG, et al. Non-organic physical signs in low back pain. Spine 1980;5:117–125.

19

Complications and Failures of Spinal Surgery

"There is not a fiercer hell than the failure in a great object."

— John Keats

INTRODUCTION

Although spine surgery covers a broad range of procedures for trauma, tumors and degenerative conditions, this chapter will limit the discussion to that of failures for degenerative conditions. Failures in spine surgery are a fact of life because of the multifactorial nature of the problem. But should it be that way? A spine surgeon presenting his success/failure rate to a meeting of total joint surgeons would be ridiculed for such an abysmal record compared to the outcomes for total joint. But how often do the total joint surgeons, when faced with a poor outcome, have to face the three generalized categories of failures in spine surgery:

Wrong patient.
Wrong diagnosis.
Wrong operation?

There are many factors to consider when dealing with a failure of spine surgery. We ask the same question again: should it be that way? By reading this chapter maybe we will all become more discrete in our choice of patients, our diagnosis and our surgical exercise

One of the most difficult problems in spinal surgery is the assessment and management of patients still seriously disabled by backache, despite one or more attempts at surgical correction of the underlying lesion. (35) Such failures are nearly always compounded by a variable and varying mixture of inadequate preoperative assessments, errors in operative technique, and emotional breakdown of the patient either antedating or following surgery.(13) It is convenient to consider these separately under the headings listed in Table 19.1.

Although surgeons take much of the blame (and deservedly so) for creating the monstrous problem of the failed back surgery syndrome (FBSS), it is important to remember that some aspects of conservative care are also capable of delivering patients into the failed back syndrome, vis-à-vis:

Table 19.1. Failures of Spine Surgery

Preoperative errors
Wrong patient
Wrong diagnosis
Intraoperative errors
Wrong level
Wrong operation
Wrong syndrome
Incomplete surgery
Complications (immediate/local)
Postoperative failure
Complications
Arachnoiditis
Change of symptoms or recurrence of symptoms

1. Although Weber (33) and Hakelius (8) have shown that long term there is little difference in outcome between surgical and nonsurgical treatment of sciatica, others, as well as Weber's study, have shown that prolonged nerve root compression may lead to intraneural fibrosis and permanent residual symptoms. Nachemson (18) has suggested that nerve root compression beyond 3 months has the potential of permanent sequelae and recommends that nerve root decompression occur before that time has slipped by with prolonged conservative care.(24)
2. It is now becoming apparent that prolonged bed rest has detrimental effects on muscle bulk and bone mass. Many years ago, it was routine for a practitioner to a request of a patient up to 6 weeks of bed rest. Later, the standard of conservative treatment became 2 weeks of bed rest, but even that duration can result in significant and irreparable loss of muscle and bone mass, especially in the older patient. It seems only reasonable to limit complete bed rest to 2 to 4 days and, if there is no appreciable change in symptoms or signs, to consider other avenues of treatment. It is our recommendation that if patients with significant sciatica do not notice relief of some leg pain and improvement in straight leg raising (SLR) ability after 2 to 4 days of bed rest, they are more likely to follow one of two courses: a requirement for prolonged conservative care before satisfactory relief of symptoms, and a higher likelihood of recurrence after initial success with conservative care.

If pain and SLR ability does not improve after 2 to 4 days of complete bed rest, there is a higher likelihood that surgical nerve root decompression will be required to effect permanent relief of the patient's symptoms.

3. Too often, the emotional and financial well-being of the patient suffers with prolonged conservative care. This has the potential for precipitating a nonorganic component to the disability equation, and even though this is a secondary phenomenon initially, it may become the primary reason for inability to achieve a good surgical result even when a clear structural lesion is present.

Although all patients deserve a reasonable trial of conservative treatment, it is prudent to consider early surgical intervention in the patients with a significant mechanical syndrome (eg, unilateral acute radicular pain) and unequivocal MRI evidence of a structural lesion (eg, HNP). To do less than that exposes the patient to the risk of joining the ranks of the chronic low back pain syndrome because of prolonged or poorly planned conservative care. On the other hand, to rush a patient to the operating room without the benefit of a trial of conservative care and/or without a clear structural lesion being demonstrated on investigation, will almost certainly contribute to the large group of individuals known as the FBSS patients

PREOPERATIVE ERRORS

Selection of the Wrong Patient for Surgery

It is a constant theme throughout this book that, when contemplating back surgery, one should look at the whole patient. To ignore obvious emotional and situation pressures deflecting the patient toward a larger or longer period of disability will result in failure of the surgical exercise. The reader is referred to Chapter 18 and reminded that the first question to be asked in the differential diagnosis of any low back disability is:

"Am I dealing with a true physical disability, or are there features on history or physical examination to suggest there is a nonorganic component to the patient's disability equation?"

All too often this question is only answered in the affirmative after failed surgery.

It is not infrequent that a surgeon is faced with a patient who has a protracted disability. The patient has been in and out of work; in and out of hospital; in and out of physical therapy departments; in and out of the offices of drugless practitioners. It is understandably tempting to regard this long period of disability as indicating severe pain. However, if this group of patients, suffering from low back pain only, cannot be retrained to undertake lighter jobs, then a desperation fusion will be unlikely to succeed.

In this regard, it must be emphasized that a patient cannot describe the pain; he/she can only describe the disability. Pain and disability are not synonymous and the disability complained of is not necessarily indicative of the degree of pain experienced.

In the simplest superficial analysis, disability has three components: the pain, the patient's reaction to the pain, and the situation prevailing at the time of the pain. A certain degree of what might be termed a functional reaction can be regarded as normal. When the functional response is gross, it becomes a major part of the disease process. This concept is best exemplified by describing three hypothetical workmen, three bricklayers who presented with the same degree of disability. They had pain in their backs; although they could walk around, they could not do their work. They could not climb ladders, nor carry bricks, nor stoop to lay the bricks. They were not able to describe the amount of pain they had; they could only describe their disability. They all had degenerative disc disease. The radiographs could not describe how much pain they were experiencing. All that was known was that the disability claimed by all three was the same: they could not work. In one patient (patient A), the disability was largely due to the anatomical basis of his pain. In another patient (patient C), there was little anatomical source of pain, but he was overcome by the functional reaction or the emotional response to his discomforts (Fig. 19.1).

Surgery meticulously performed might overcome 90% of the anatomical basis of the disability. The first patient (A) would be cured and would be able to return to work, but even with 90% of the organic basis of his disability removed, the third patient (C) would still be incapacitated (Fig. 19.2). In such instances, because of failure of treatment, the functional reaction will get worse, and the story of patient C is best exemplified by the letters that were written to the workmen's compensation board about him:

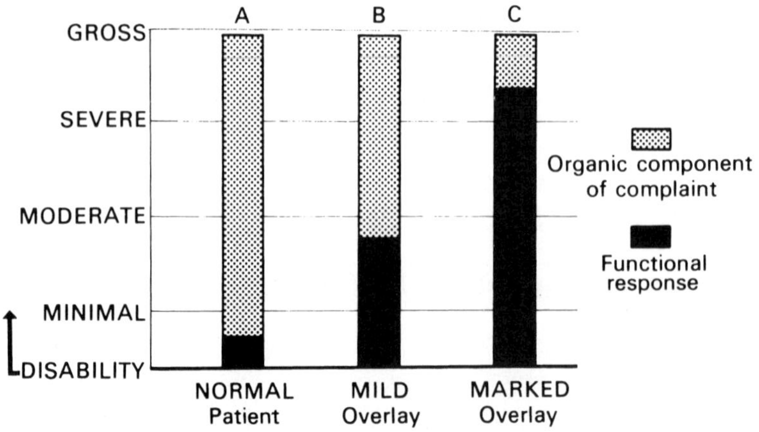

Figure 19.1 *Functional overlay. Three patients (A, B, and C) with apparently identical disability.*

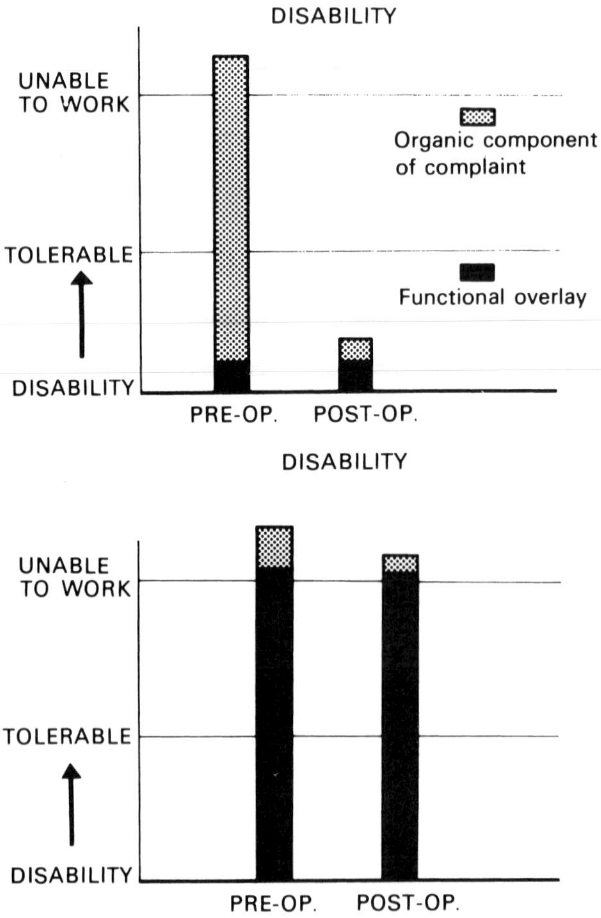

Figure 19.2 *Diagram to show that although removal of the organic basis of pain will produce a good result in the emotionally stable patient (top), the continuing emotional turmoils in the patient with significant functional overlay (bottom) result in perpetuation of the disability after operation.*

"Dear Sirs:

I saw this very pleasant claimant, George Smith, today, and the poor fellow has not responded to conservative therapy at all. He is totally unable to work. His radiographs show marked disc degeneration, and I plan to bring him into the hospital for a local fusion."

"Dear Sirs:

I operated on George today, and I am sure he will do well."

Dear Sirs:

I saw George Smith today, and I am a little disappointed with his progress to date."

"Dear Sirs:

Smith's radiographs show a solid fusion, but he shows surprisingly little motivation to return to work."

"Dear Sirs:

This dreadful fellow Smith."

"Dear Sirs:

Smith obviously needs psychiatric help" (Fig. 19.3).

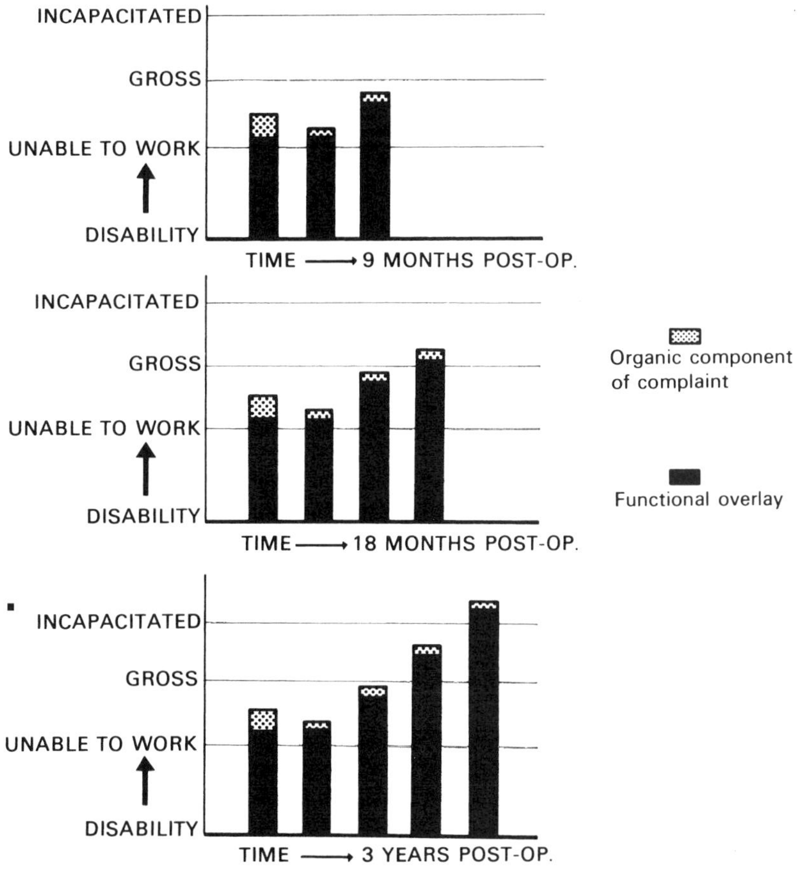

Figure 19.3 *Diagram shows how increasing emotional breakdown will produce increasing disability after surgical intervention.*

Patients A, B, and C all presented with the same disability. They were bricklayers who could not work. They had the same radiographic changes, but the constitution of their disability varied enormously, and, predictably, the results of operative treatment varied also (Fig. 19.4).

In patient C, the degenerative disc disease was not causing too much pain, and in better emotional health, the discomfort he experienced would not have taken him to a doctor. However, because of factors outside his spine, in fact, outside his soma, he was totally disabled by his discomfort; and this disability was later compounded, perpetuated, and exaggerated by the failure of surgical treatment.

Patients A and C do not really constitute much of a problem because the gross functional overlay of patient C is usually recognizable. These two groups of patients have been discussed in detail throughout this book to emphasize the fact that pain and disability are not synonymous. The middle group, patient B, typifies the most difficult problem. The surgeon who regards a functional overlay as a solid contraindication to operation will not help patient B even though he does have an organic basis of discomfort.

There are two important aspects in the management of patient B that must always be kept in mind: first, the recognition of the organic basis of pain, despite the clouding of the clinical picture by the functional elements; and second, an analysis of the constitution of the functional component of the disability.

The functional overlay is derived from a combination of many factors. A large part of the emotional overlay is due to the patient's personality; the patient may have no drive, no motivation, and may even be a psychopath. Whatever it is, it probably cannot be altered. It is important to recognize a gross personality defect because these patients will not do well with treatment directed solely at their spines.

Other factors must be considered, such as the patient's affect or mood, the significance of pain to the patient, and the patient's ability to adjust to his/her environment. The importance of financial security and work demands are obvious. Finally, the reaction of the patient to pain must be considered: the individual's pain tolerance and pain threshold. If the patient, because of inheritance or constitution, for example, tends to have an exaggerated reaction to any painful stimulus, it makes it very difficult to recognize the fact that the patient is suffering from an organic lesion.

For example, a patient may react violently at the limit of one phase of clinical examination: SLR. On experiencing discomfort, the patient may writhe, groan, shout, bang his/

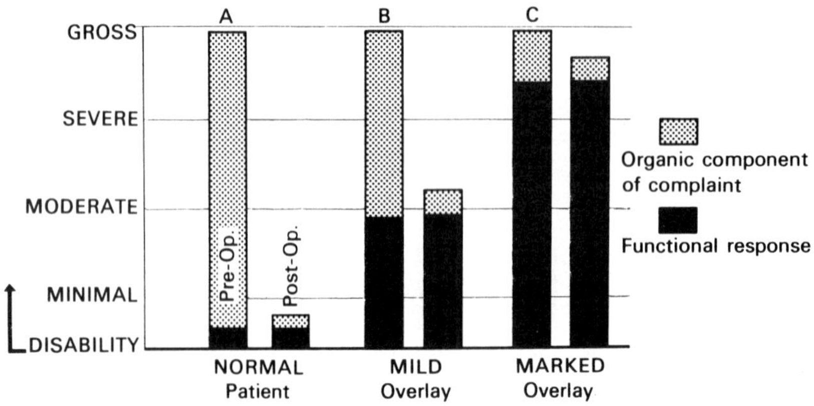

Figure 19.4 *Diagram to show the relationship between the functional overlay and the response to treatment in patients A, B, and C.*

her hands, and finally collapse, sobbing and weeping. Such patients react excessively to pain produced by an organic disability. However, when this excessive reaction is of a hysterical nature, it becomes extremely difficult to determine whether the problem is one of a hysterical patient with pain or a patient with hysterical pain. Suffice it to say, if these considerations are made preoperatively, it is less likely that the patient will fail to respond to surgical intervention because of nonorganic factors.

With the heightening criticism directed at spine surgeons for the all too frequent poor outcome, we are looking at the many factors that lead us into failure. It is becoming more apparent that the nutritionally compromised patient does not have the physical foundation for adequate wound healing.(7) The authors are becoming more convinced that the heavy smoker and/or drinker has also compromised wound healing, specifically graft incorporation, and is more likely to end up with a pseudarthrosis after attempted fusion.

Wrong Diagnosis

There are many pitfalls awaiting the unwary in evaluating and treating low back and leg pain. If an incorrect diagnosis was the basis of the surgical procedure, there is virtually no hope of a successful outcome. The "step back and take a long look" approach is then indicated. The second question to be answered satisfactorily is: Did I fall into a diagnostic trap and make an error in diagnosis (Tables 19.2 and 19.3)? (See Chapter 18.)

Table 19.2. Differential Diagnosis of Nonmechanical Low Back Pain

Causes of nonmechanical low back pain	
Referred pain (eg, from the abdomen or retroperitoneal space)	
Infection	—bone, disc, epidural space
Neoplasm	—primary (multiple myeloma, osteoid osteoma, and so forth)
	—metastatic
Inflammation	—arthritides such as ankylosing spondylitis
Miscellaneous metabolic and vascular disorders such as osteopenia and Paget's disease	

Table 19.3. Differential Diagnosis of Sciatica

Intraspinal causes
Proximal to disc: conus and cauda equina lesions (eg, neurofibroma, ependymoma)
Disc level
herniated nucleus pulposus
stenosis (canal or recess)
infection: osteomyelitis or discitis (with nerve root pressure)
inflammation: arachnoiditis
neoplasm: benign or malignant, with nerve root pressure
Extraspinal causes
Pelvis
Cardiovascular conditions (eg, peripheral vascular disease)
Gynecological conditions
Orthopedic conditions (eg, osteoarthritis of hip)
Sacroiliac joint disease
Neoplasms (invading or compressing lumbosacral plexus)
Peripheral nerve lesions
Neuropathy (diabetic, tumor, alcohol)
Local sciatic nerve conditions (trauma, tumor)
Inflammation (herpes zoster)

INTRAOPERATIVE ERRORS

Wrong Level

It seems rhetorical to state that even though you make the right diagnosis in the right patient, operating at the wrong level will fail to cure the disease. There is more "wrong level" surgery being done than we, as surgeons, have admitted. This occurs in two situations: (1) preoperative selection of the wrong level for surgery; (2) making the technical error of selecting the wrong level intraoperatively.

Wrong Level Diagnostic Error

This most often occurs in the chronic unilateral and bilateral radicular syndromes. Examples are shown in Figures 19.5 and 19.6.

Wrong Level Technical Error

It is not too difficult to intend to operate at the L4–L5 level, and mistakenly enter the L3–L4 level. Most often, this mistake is discovered intraoperatively and corrected. To discover it postoperatively when the patient's symptoms persist is most disheartening. The error occurs as the result of: congenital lumbosacral anomalies or poor judgment.

Congenital Lumbosacral Anomalies The reason congenital anomalies can lead to wrong level exploration is because our radiological colleagues speak a different language (Fig. 19.7) regarding these anomalies. Because of this lack of a common meeting ground, the radiologist reading the film may inadvertently number congenital lumbosacral anomalies differently than the clinician, which may contribute to a wrong level exploration. The reason for this is that orthopedic surgeons tend to read lumbar spine radiographs from the bottom up and radiologists tend to read lumbar spine radiographs from the top down (L1 to the sacrum) (Fig. 19.7).

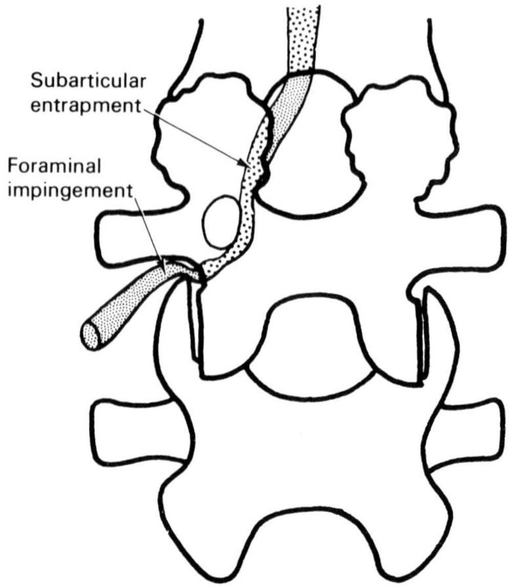

Figure 19.5 *The emerging nerve root may be compressed at more than one site. In this diagram, the nerve root is shown to be compressed as it passes through the subarticular gutter. It is also trapped in the foramen by the tip of the superior articular facet. The error in diagnosis occurs when one of the lesions is missed.*

Definitions When faced with congenital lumbosacral anomalies and the potential for numbering errors, the following definitions are offered. A formed lumbar segment is described as any anatomic segment that has an interlaminar space and a formed disc space (Fig. 19.8). A mobile lumbar segment is any lumbar vertebrae free of pelvic or rib attachment (Fig. 19.8). There is a tendency, which makes embryological sense, that the extent of formation of the disc space parallels the extent of formation of the interlaminar space; that is, the more rudimentary the disc space, the more rudimentary the interlaminar space

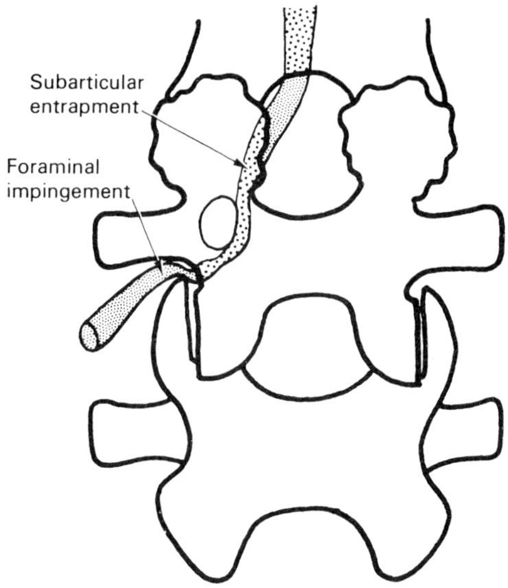

Figure 19.6 *Diagram showing apophyseal stenosis that results in the compression of two nerve roots. The diagnostic error occurs when only one root is thought to be causing symptoms.*

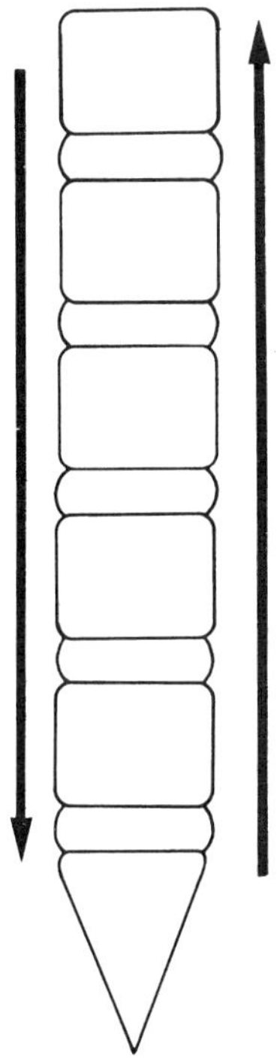

Figure 19.7 *Schematic showing scizophrenic approach to reading radiographs. The radiologists read and count from the top down; the spine surgeons read and count from the bottom up.*

Figure 19.8 **A.** *In a normal lumbar spine, there are five vertebrae, which are free of rib and pelvic bony attachment. The last interlaminar space is outlined.* **B.** *A schematic depicting the last mobile segment. (LML = last mobile level; LFL = last formed level.)*

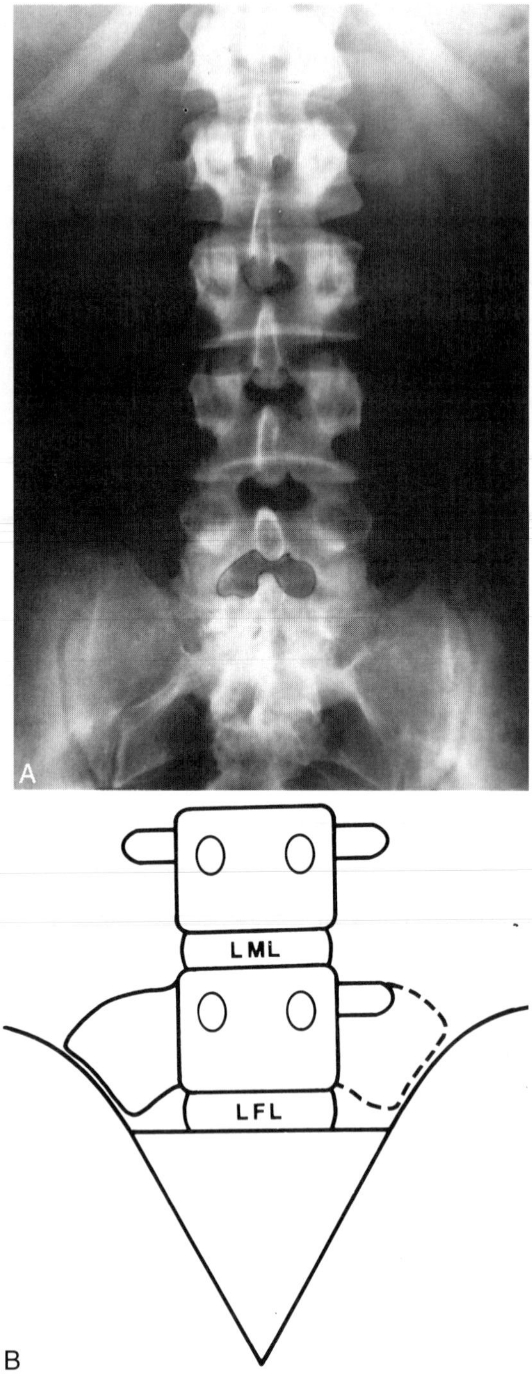

(Fig. 19.9). Even a rudimentary interlaminar space, exposed in a limited fashion, can appear as a normal interlaminar space. It represents entry into a nonmobile level that rarely harbors pathology, and a wrong level exposure. These congenital anomalies were fully discussed in Chapter 1.

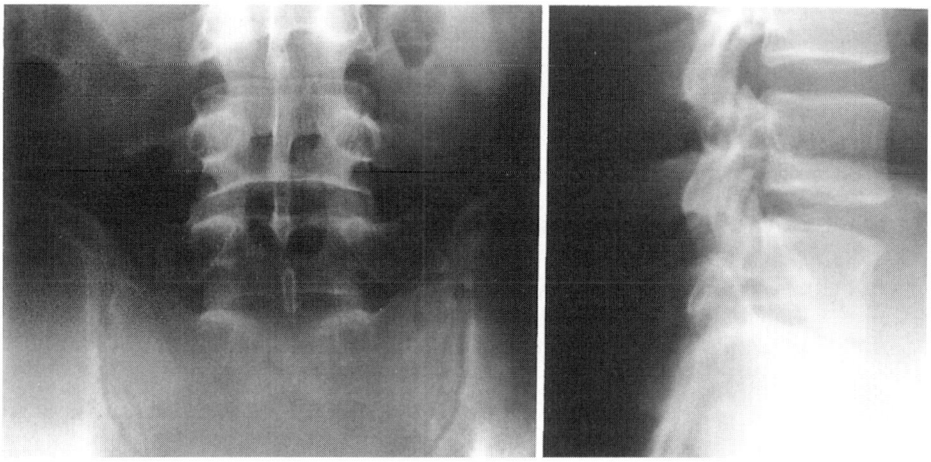

Figure 19.9 *A fixed last-formed lth its rudimentary disc on lateral.*

Poor Judgment Assuming the correct patient has been selected and the correct diagnosis has been made in regard to the nature and location of the pathology, how does a surgeon avoid the technical error of wrong level explorations? The standard method is to make a long incision, exposing the last mobile level (usually L5–S1) regardless of the level of planned surgical intervention. Despite this approach, wrong level exposures still occur, usually because of misinterpretation of the mobility of the last exposed level. Limit the surgical incision so that the last mobile level is not routinely exposed and the incidence of wrong level exploration can rise significantly.

Anyone doing any volume of spine surgery, especially microsurgery, will admit that at one time or another, they have been in at the wrong level. When embarking on a spine surgical career, admit immediately that wrong level exposure will be a constant problem and routinely plan the operative exposure to prevent the occurrence. All of the residents in our program are taught that the three most common errors in limited spine surgical exposures are:

1. Wrong level exploration.
2. Wrong Level Exploration!
3. WRONG LEVEL EXPLORATION!!

Once the resident and the surgeon have conquered this problem, they will be over a complication that occurs all too often in spine surgery, especially procedures attempted through limited exposure.

Despite an awareness of the problem of wrong level exposure, and despite careful preoperative marking (see Chapter 15), there are still occasions (guestimated at 1 in 50 procedures) when the authors expose the wrong interspace. To fail to recognize this at the time of surgery is unacceptable. The golden rules to prevent this combination of events are:

1. Know unequivocally what pathology you are going to find, and if it is not there, you are at the wrong level.
2. If there is any reason to suspect that you are at the wrong level, obtain an intraoperative radiograph (Fig. 19.10).

Wrong Operation, Wrong Syndrome

If you are satisfied that no error was made in the differential diagnosis of low back pain or sciatica, and the operation was done at the correct level, then was an error made in the third question? That is, is this a mechanical low back pain condition and, if so, what is the syndrome (Table 19.4)?

Surgery for degenerative conditions in the lumbar spine is of two basic types:

1. Encroachment surgery is for nerve root compromise by soft tissue (eg, disc, ligament) or bone (eg, osteophyte, vertebral body translation).
2. Stabilization surgery is for a painful motion segment.

There are many occasions when both surgeries (decompression and fusion) are indicated. However, if one type of surgery was carried out and the patient fails to improve,

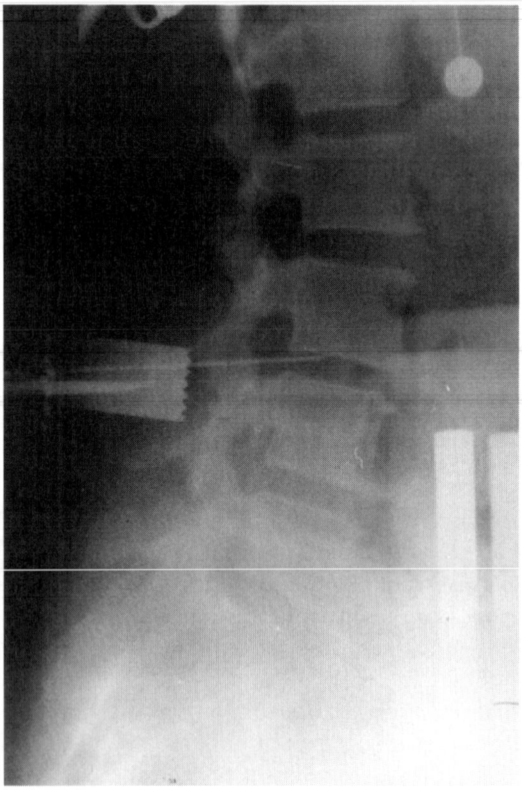

Figure 19.10 *The intent was to enter L4–L5 through a limited microsurgical incision. No pathology was found after the interlaminar exposure, and an intraoperative check radiograph revealed why no pathology was located!*

Table 19.4. Syndromes in Mechanical Low Back Disorders

Lumbago–Back Pain (Mechanical Instability)
Sciatica–Radicular Pain
Unilateral acute radicular syndrome
Bilateral acute radicular syndrome
Unilateral chronic radicular syndrome
Bilateral chronic radicular syndrome

was the wrong operation performed on the basis of an incorrect preoperative diagnosis? Was encroachment surgery done when stabilization surgery was indicated (14)? This is a common error and is most often due to referred leg pain being confused for radicular leg pain; removal of a "sucker disc" (Fig. 19.11) with the result being even more instability and more back pain.

Wrong Operation, Incomplete Surgery

An example might be failure after laminectomy for spinal stenosis due to incomplete apophyseal decompression. Incomplete decompression of the involved nerve roots is seen in the following circumstances: missed fragment of ruptured disc material. A reasonable criticism of microdiscectomy is the potential, because of a limited surgical field, to leave behind fragments of ruptured disc. This topic was discussed in Chapter 15. The two basic rules to prevent this are:

1. You are doing nerve root surgery, not disc surgery: be sure you are leaving behind a mobile root.
2. Know the size and location of your ruptured disc fragment. The MRI routinely underestimates the size of the fragment.

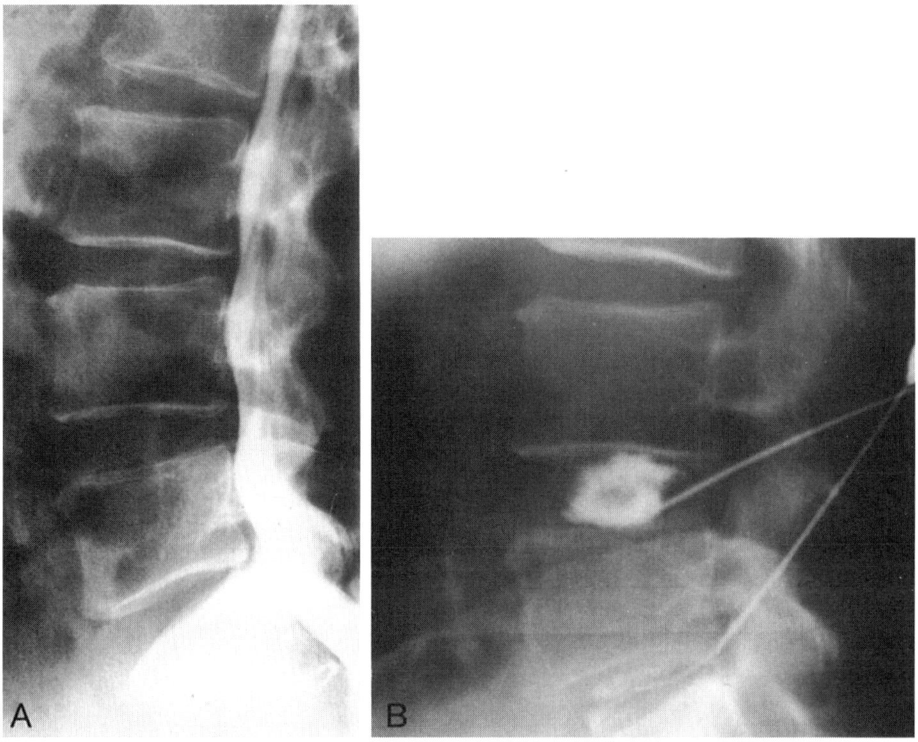

Figure 19.11 **A.** *A lateral myelogram, with a slight "bulge" at L4–L5.* **B.** *Subsequent normal discogram at L4–L5 and a degenerative disc at L5–S1.*

Entrapment of a Nerve Root at More Than One Site

This error will be avoided if the mobility of the root is assessed after the apparent source of compression is removed. It should be possible to displace a normal or completely decompressed nerve root at least 1 cm medially. The S1 root can normally be displaced to the midline (Fig. 19.12).

Involvement of More Than One Root

Incomplete decompression may result when more than one root is involved in an apparently unisegmental degenerative stenosis. This source of failure emphasizes the need for complete preoperative evaluation of the roots involved. The surgeon must know what roots to explore.

Overlooked Apophyseal Stenosis

A decompression laminectomy for spinal stenosis is always started by the removal of a portion or the whole of one or more laminae. If this is technically difficult because of shingling or overgrowth of the laminae, it is understandable that the surgeon confine his/her attention to a midline decompression. Even though a very complete midline decompression is performed, the patient will not be helped if, as is commonly the case, he/she is suffering from both canal stenosis and concomitant lateral zone stenosis giving rise to root compression. This error is more likely to occur if the lateral zone stenosis is at a different segment from the canal stenosis.

Here again, an accurate preoperative assessment followed by a preoperative design of the procedure required will avoid this only too frequent source of error.

Incomplete Midline Compression

Sometimes a midline decompression is incomplete. It must be remembered that this operation is most frequently performed on older patients with the surgeon being under-

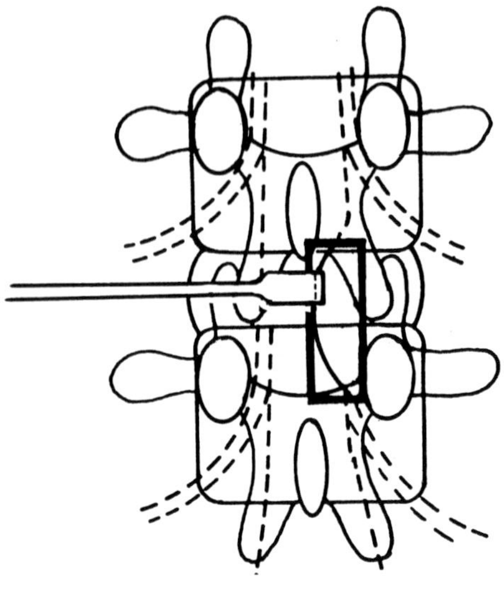

Figure 19.12 *The L5 root can often be retracted to the midline (providing there are no adhesions, no stenosis, and a normal takeoff of the root from the common dural sac). The S1 root can be easily retracted to the midline.*

standably reluctant to carry out extensive surgery. The operation is frequently tedious, hemorrhagic, time consuming, and apparently destructive. Despite the temptation to short-circuit the operative procedure, when the patient's symptoms superficially appear to stem from laminar compression at one or two segments only, decompression must occur at the appropriate levels.

Foraminal Disc

Macnab's landmark article on "Negative Disc Exploration" (14) described the foraminal disc. If you are in the canal looking for a foraminal disc there is a good chance you will miss it, and the patient will wake with identical leg pain. This topic was well covered in Chapter 16.

Conjoint Nerve Root

A small disc herniation compressing a conjoint root can not only produce a lot of sciatica, it can be a very difficult fragment to retrieve. This combination of events occurs most often at L5–S1 and requires a wide decompression, without sacrificing the facet joint, and removal of the fragment under the axilla of the root.

Complications Related to the Surgical Procedure

Classification

Complications to any surgical procedure can be classified into (1) general or local; (2) early (immediate) or late (delayed); and (3) specific or nonspecific (Table 19.5).

The topic of deformity surgery, including the implantation of internal fixation devices, has been mentioned on a few occasions in this book. The increasing popularity of these devices is introducing a whole new class of complications, including neurological damage and vertebral element fracture from the various hooks, screws, plates, and rods. We are in the early innings of a contest between the biological plasticity of the spine and the rigidity of the implants. Over the next decade, the indications and complications of use will become clear and be the basis of a separate textbook. For the purpose of this chapter, discussion of these particular complications will be omitted (see Chapter 14 for a limited discussion).

Complication Rate

Most surgeons rarely have complications! Better stated, most surgeons do not remember (or subconsciously forget) their complications until they complete a follow-up study. Their understanding of adverse effects is even clearer if that follow-up study is completed

Table 19.5. Generic Classification of Early (Immediate) Complications of Surgery

General
Local
Nonspecific
Specific to lumbar spine surgery

by an independent observer. Many studies (15, 21, 22, 27) have appeared in the literature describing complication rates; they are listed in Table 19.6.

Complications

Immediate general complications such as intraoperative anesthetic complications, hypotensive complications, and delayed general complications, such as postoperative thrombophlebitis, pulmonary embolism, atelectasis, and urinary retention are part of everyone's surgical practice. Readers are referred to other texts for a discussion of these general adverse events.

Early complications to lumbar disc surgery (excluding lumbar fusion) have been artificially divided into local specific and nonspecific complications:

Local Nonspecific Complications Local nonspecific complications are those that can occur in association with any lumbar disc operation. They include: (1) major vessel or visceral injury, (2) cauda equina injury, (3) foreign body retention, and (4) pressure complications secondary to positioning on table.

Local Specific Complications Local specific complications are those that can occur in association with any lumbar disc operation but are more likely to occur as a surgeon is learning the technique of microsurgery. They include: (1) wrong level exposure, (2) missed pathology, (3) intraoperative bleeding obscuring the visual field, (4) dural injury, (5) root injury, and (6) disc space infection.

Major Vessel or Visceral Injury(3, 4, 9, 10, 26) Major vessel or visceral injury occurs when an instrument penetrates the anterior annulus. Figure 19.13 demonstrates how this occurs. If you are a surgeon who believes that all of the discal material possible should be removed,(28) then this is a complication that must be prevented. The instrument that does the damage is usually a pituitary rongeur or curette, and the complication occurs when either instrument is inserted too deeply into the disc space.

If the complication is major vessel injury it is immediately apparent because of excessive hemorrhage and a fall in blood pressure. Once recognized, the lumbar wound must

Table 19.6. Complication Rates (%) from the Literature

Complication	Spangfort's (27) Literature Search	Spangfort's (27) Series (2504 operations)	Mayfield's (15) Series (1408 operations)	Ramirez and Thisted (21) Series (28,395 operations)
Mortality	0.3	0.1	0.4	0.06
Thrombophlebitis	N/S	1.0	N/S	N/S
Pulmonary embolus	1.7	1.0	0.2	0.2
Cauda equina syndrome	N/S	0.2	0.07	0.08
Wound infection	2.9	3.8	1.0	0.3
Root damage	N/S	0.5	0.1	0.2
Dural tear	N/S	1.6	0.7	0.1

Key: N/S = not stated.

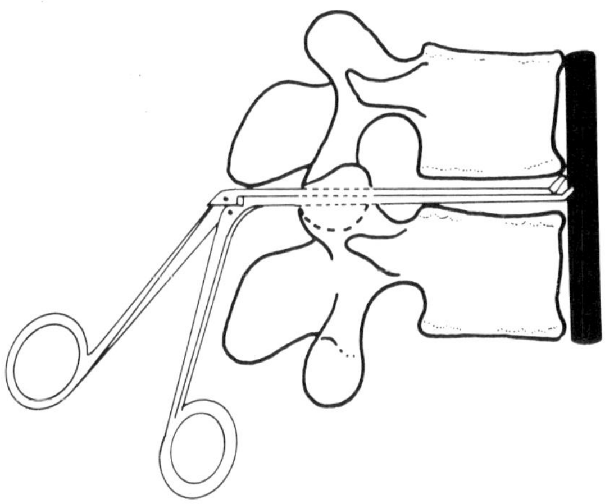

Figure 19.13 *Perforation of the anterior annulus with a sharp instrument may damage the aorta. Redrawn from Crock HV. A Short Practice of Spinal Surgery. New York: Springer-Verlag; 1993.*

be closed immediately and the patient rolled into the supine position for laparotomy and repair or ligation of the injured vessel. Less often, damage to the vessel will be limited to the outer layers of the vessel wall, leading to the delayed formation of an arteriovenous fistula. If the injury is to viscera (26) (ureter, small bowel, bladder) and is not accompanied by vascular injury as well, it more often goes undetected until the first few days postoperatively when systemic changes and abdominal symptoms signal intraabdominal pathology. On rare occasion, the astute surgeon will see bowel or ureter tissue when the forceps are removed from the disc space. If this fortunate observation of this unfortunate event occurs, immediate surgical repair is indicated.

Cauda Equina Injury The term cauda equina syndrome (CES) denotes the postoperative appearance of a compressive neuropathy involving multiple lumbar and sacral roots. The involvement of the roots from S2 caudally, with bladder and bowel dysfunction, is the hallmark of a cauda equina syndrome. Associated, usually, are varying degrees of motor and sensory deficits in the lower extremities. Compression of the cauda equina may have occurred during the surgery, from excessive retraction on the dural sheath, but more often is a delayed complication (hours or days) caused by a growing extradural hematoma.

Clinical Presentation

Most CES starts in the recovery room or soon after the patient arrives back on the floor. Less commonly they will evolve slowly over the first few postoperative days.(24)

The features are: (1) numbness in the perineum; (2) urinary retention or incontinence; (3) decreased rectal tone; (4) progressive motor weakness, starting in the feet and ankles; (5) decreased sensation starting in the perineum, sacral strips, and the feet; (6) progression of the motor and sensory dysfunction. Often enough, the postoperative presentation of the CES is absent leg pain, so do not get lulled into thinking the absence of leg pain post decompression, rules out the cauda equina syndrome.

McLaren and Bailey (16) have pointed out that this complication is more prone to occur when a limited laminectomy, through a standard incision, is done in the presence of a stenotic spinal canal. The cornerstones of treatment of this complication are early recognition and immediate evacuation of the hematoma with a wider decompression of any residual stenotic segments.

Foreign Body Retention Everyone is aware of a patient who, after persisting postoperative symptoms, was found at surgery (reoperation) to have a retained cottonoid or other foreign material pressuring the nerve root. Every surgeon can only insist on time-honored nursing protocols, at the time of closure, to prevent this complication.

Complications Secondary to Positioning on the Operating Room Table Most surgeons use a variation of the kneeling position for lumbar disc surgery. This is an interesting phenomenon because most reports on the lateral position report fewer complications from positioning on the OR table. Almost all of the complications from improper positioning of a patient, under general anesthesia, are related to prolonged pressure on neurological structures. These include (1) brachial plexus stretch, (2) radial nerve palsy, (3) ulnar nerve palsy, and (4) peroneal nerve palsy.

The most serious of all of these neurological complications is stretching of the brachial plexus, which is prone to occur in the heavy-set, muscular man with arthritic changes in the neck. In these patients in particular, and all patients in general, the neck should be place in a position of slight flexion (in particular: no extension). The shoulders are to be in no more than 90 degrees of abduction and should be in some flexion.

Other neurological structures prone to pressure palsies are the ulnar nerve, peroneal nerve, and radial nerve (listed in order of frequency). Careful padding of the relative pressure points will prevent injury to the nerves. Other areas that may be pressure damaged in the kneeling position are the eyes, breasts and chest cage, and the prepatellar region. Careful padding is necessary to prevent their occurrence.

Complications Specific to Lumbar Microsurgery

The previously described delineation of complications specific to microsurgery can occur in association with any lumbar disc operation but there are other specific complications that are more likely to occur in operations with limited exposure, that is, microsurgery. They are listed as follows:

1. Those critical of microsurgical techniques cite these specific complications (and rightfully so) (6).
2. Those microsurgeons who have traveled the learning curve (and are prepared to be honest about their experiences) agree that these complications are prone to occur.
3. Forewarned and/or experienced microsurgeons can reduce the incidence of these complications.
4. The advantages of microsurgery are enough to stimulate everyone to understand these pitfalls.(36, 37)
5. Once accepted as a group of complications prone to occur under the microscope, and once technically mastered, the use of the microscope will actually reduce the complication rate.

Wrong Level The complication of wrong level exposure has been discussed ad nauseum in the previous sections. There is a reason for this emphasis!

Missed Pathology If the wrong level is exposed and not recognized, then obviously pathology will be left behind. The error, however, is more likely to occur when the correct level is explored, disc is removed, and either more discal fragments are left behind or bony subarticular or foraminal stenosis is not decompressed. This issue was also discussed in the previous section.

The prevention of this complication is as much an attitude as a technique. Before the surgical exposure it is essential to know what pathology is present (disc and/or bone) and exactly where it is located in the various stories of the anatomical segment.

Successful use of limited surgical exposure for lumbar root encroachment is based on the attitude that spine surgery is no longer seek-and-find surgery and that aids such as loupes and the microscope do not perform the surgery; they merely facilitate the surgeon's efforts.

In the end, the mission must be completed: remove all pathology that is interfering with root function, be it bone or disc, without creating instability.(28)

Intraoperative Bleeding Obscuring the Visual Field If a limited surgical exposure is being used, a small amount of bleeding appears as a major hemorrhage under the microscope. Preparing for this potential complication is summarized in Table 19.7.

Dural Injury It is not possible to perform a large volume of spine surgery, especially through a limited surgical exposure, and not cause injury to the dura. Hopefully, it is infrequent! It is not necessary that this include injury to the nerve root but it may be an associated complication.

Causes of dural tears during lumbar spine surgery include:

- Inappropriate instrumentation.
- Overaggressive surgical technique.
- Pathology, such as a large HNP, displacing the dural sac or nerve root posteriorly, where it is more prone to damage during incision of the ligamentum flavum.
- A very thin ligamentum flavum, as occurs in congenital lumbosacral anomalies. These are more prone to occur at L5–S1. The surgeon, unaware of this lack of ligament substance, makes the standard incision in the ligament only to see cerebrospinal fluid (CSF). The senior author (JM) has watched in horror as a spine fellow pushed a narrow spooned Cobb through the interlaminar space in the same situation. Although the dura was lacerated by this error, fortunately, there was no damage to the cauda equina.
- Previous surgery with scarring of the dura.
- A necessary dural opening to deal with intradural pathology (rare in routine lumbar spine surgery).
- Secondary to spontaneous intradural extension of the pathology (eg, intradural HNP, also rare in lumbar spine surgery).

Table 19.7. Steps Necessary to Reduce Intraoperative Bleeding

Careful history regarding unusual bleeding during previous surgery
Coagulation studies where indicated
Remove patients from medications that interfere with coagulation (most important, discontinue all NSAIDs for at least 10 days)
Proper OR positioning of patient to remove pressure from abdominal vena cava

Intraoperative steps
  Limited surgical exposure
  Expeditious surgery
  Coagulate bleeders as they appear

Concern with Dural Tears Obviously, dural tears are not desired, but they do occur. They are of concern because:

1. They result in a loss of CSF that results in postoperative low pressure headaches.
2. They represent a potential entry route for infection.
3. They can lead to immediate postoperative leaks of CSF through a fistulous tract in the wound.
4. If undiscovered and unrepaired, they may form pseudocysts (pseudomeningocele) in the region of the nerve root, entrapping nerve roots or producing symptoms by mass effect.

The appearance of nonbloody (clear) fluid in the wound should alert the surgeon to the possibility of a dural tear being present. There are other possibilities for the appearance of this clear fluid including a CSF leak from yesterday's myelogram; synovial fluid from a synovial cyst; the scrub nurse handing you wet tools.

These three situations are self-limiting flows of fluid. In the case of the synovial cyst, the fluid has a yellowish tinge. The persistent flow of clear fluid, especially with respiratory inspiration is the signal that a dural tear is present and must be found. The principles of repair of dural tears are (5):

1. Recognize the tear, its extent, and the necessity for immediate repair. Under the microscope, dural leaks are being viewed with 5 to 10 times magnification. A small puncture, not much larger than a needle puncture rent in the dura, does not need to be repaired. Any dural injury that has length to it, that is, can be closed with one or more 6–0 to 7–0 sutures, must be repaired.
2. Assure that the exposure is wide enough and the field dry enough that an adequate repair can be accomplished. This may mean extending the microsurgical incision and bony decompression.
3. The author's preferred method of repair is direct suture, using a thin fat graft to assure a watertight repair (Fig. 19.14). Larger defects that cannot be closed in a direct fashion as in Figure 19.14 can be closed with a fascial graft.

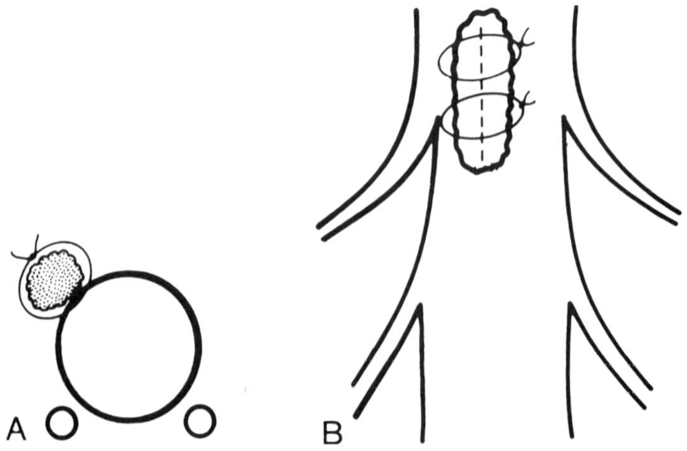

Figure 19.14 **A** *and* **B.** *Dural repair in two steps: direct repair of defect and oversewn fat graft.*

4. Once the repair is completed, the integrity of the repair should be tested with a Valsalva maneuver.

Probably, the most important step to prevent late complications is to suture the muscle tightly down on the laminar defect overlying the repair (Fig. 19.15) and complete a water tight closure at every level of suture.

Other methods of dural repair such as a Gelfoam patch, muscle patch, and gels have been tried without success. Newer products such as Gelfilm and fibrin glue are showing promise. Ignoring the dural rent (except for pin holes) and keeping the patient in bed postoperatively is also unlikely to be successful.

Postoperatively, the patient should be kept in bed for 2 to 7 days, 2 days to facilitate sealing of the repair and up to 7 days to deal for the low pressure headache.

Root Damage Root damage at the time of microsurgery is almost always associated with dural injury. It is difficult, but possible, to damage the root in the foramen and not have a dural tear. It is more likely that the root injury is proximal to the ganglion and that the appearance of clear CSF is the first indication of trouble. When searching for the source of the CSF, the appearance of severed rootlets is proof of the root damage. Root damage can also occur without a dural tear, as the result of excessive traction.

Factors leading to root damage are: (1) poor instrumentation; (2) aggressive surgical technique; (3) inadequate exposure before retraction of the root; (4) distortion of normal root location by the pathology; (5) excessive retraction, especially if adhesions are present or a very large axillary disc is present; (6) anomalous roots.

The instrument that does the damage is usually the Kerrison rongeur, used in an aggressive manner. The injury occurs close to the takeoff of the root (Fig. 19.16) and occurs because of failure to obey one cardinal rule of spine surgery: Before placing a sharp instrument in the spinal canal and before retracting the root, clearly define the lateral border of the nerve root.

Treatment There is nothing one can do to lacerated rootlets except to place them back within the dural sheath if possible. Repairing the laceration in the dural nerve root sheath is not only impossible but inadvisable because you will cause isolated root stenosis and

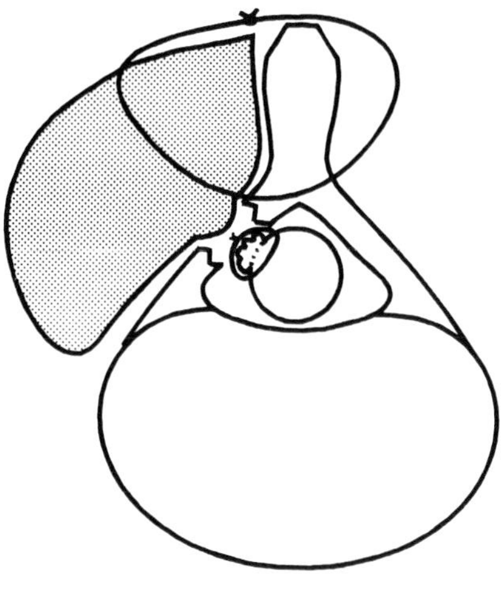

Figure 19.15 *After the dural tear has been repaired, use a couple of large sutures through the interspinous ligament to suture the paraspinal muscles down on the repair.*

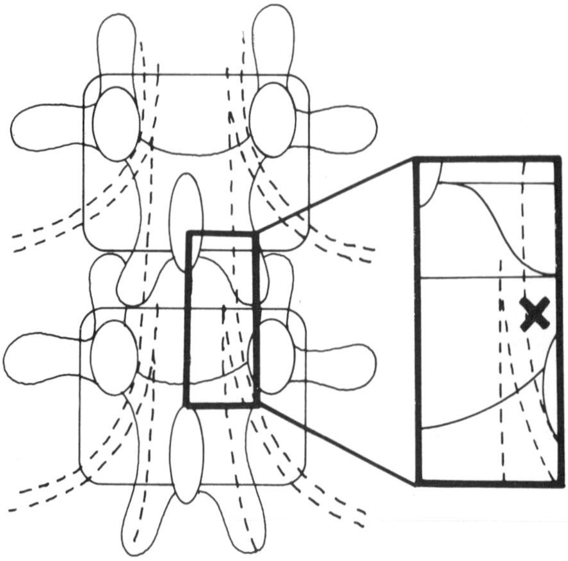

Figure 19.16 *X marks the spot where root damage occurs. The usual combination is an inadequate exposure of the lateral edge of the nerve root and discal displacement of the root in the area marked with X; for example, an axillary disc (see Fig. 12.26).*

recurrent postoperative leg pain symptoms. Fortunately, the damage of a few rootlets results in limited neurological dysfunction because of multiple sources of innervation for most lower extremity motor and sensory function.

Postoperative Failures

Disc Space Infection The incidence of disc space infection in microsurgery is approximately 1%. (11, 37) The incidence of disc space infection for standard laminectomy/discectomy is approximately 1/2% across the literature.(15, 20) It is thought that there is a higher incidence of disc space infection in microsurgery because the microscope is over top of the open wound, introducing the possibility of manipulating the exposed, unsterile eye pieces by the surgeon or an assistant.

To prevent this, make all microscope adjustments before draping the microscope and moving it over the patient. Also, position the microscope for the ligamentum flavum incision and then limit future manipulations of the microscope during the case. To adjust the focus on the microscope during the case, either raise or lower the OR table (and thus the patient) or raise and lower the microscope with a floor-operated control. In this fashion, one can avoid touching the microscope after it is placed in its correct position and thus reduce the possibility of contamination coming off the microscope and entering the surgical field.

Prophylactic Antibiotics Most surgeons would agree that surgery involving the use of implants (eg, total hip) requires the use of prophylactic antibiotics. Few surgeons would agree on the use of prophylactic antibiotics in a microsurgical spinal operation.(30) With an approximate rate of disc space infection of 0.5 to 1% it would require a prospective, multicentered trial of 2000 to 3000 patients to determine the effectiveness of prophylactic antibiotics. At this stage of writing, the use of prophylactic antibiotics in lumbar microsurgery is empirical and the surgeon's choice. The authors use one intravenous (IV) dose of an appropriate first generation cephalosporin at the beginning of the surgical procedure. If a foreign body is implanted (eg, instrumentation), a course of antibiotics is required immediately postoperatively.

When infection does occur postoperatively, it can range from a low virulent pathogen causing an indolent and easily missed disc space infection to an aggressive, resistant, hospital-based pathogen that infects disc and bone, forms abscess, causes septicemia, and threatens the patient's life. The wide variation in presentation often leads to delayed diagnosis and treatment. The principles of diagnosis and treatment of postoperative wound disc or bone infection are no different than those described for hematogenous spine infections described in Chapter 4.

Arachnoiditis (Spinal) Arachnoiditis, by definition, is an inflammation of the pia-arachnoid membrane, resulting in adhesions between nerve roots and between the pia mater and the arachnoid membrane.

There are two arachnoid membranes in the spinal canal (Fig. 19.17): the pia-arachnoid, a rich vascular membrane closely adherent to the spinal cord and cauda equina nerve roots; and the arachnoid membrane, an avascular membrane composed of fibrous and elastic tissue, more closely related geographically to the dura mater. Between the pia mater and the arachnoid membrane lies the subarachnoid space, where CSF normally flows.

Etiology

There does not appear to be one single cause of arachnoiditis. In any series of patients with arachnoiditis, there is a common thread of one or more of the following factors.

1. Prior lumbar spine surgery.
2. Prior myelogram with oil-based or ionic water-soluble contrast agents.
3. Prior spinal injury, usually an HNP or spinal stenosis and, on occasion, blunt spine trauma. Obviously, direct dural injury from penetrating traumas, such as a bullet wound, can cause dural and arachnoid scarring.

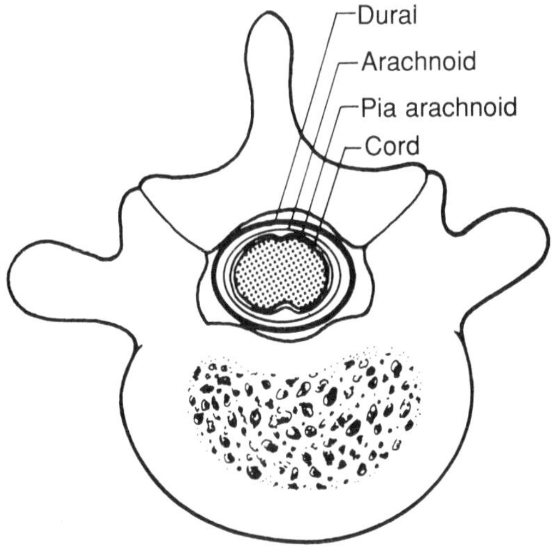

Figure 19.17 *The arachnoid membranes within the dural sheath.*

Postoperative epidural scar formation is a natural consequence of any spinal operation and, more often than not, is asymptomatic. It is not to be used interchangeably or confused with spinal (adhesive) arachnoiditis. On the other hand, most cases of spinal arachnoiditis are preceded by lumbar spine surgery. It has been difficult for many to accept myelography as an exclusive etiological agent for many reasons. One is that lumbar arachnoiditis is never (rarely) seen after cervical myelography. Another is that the lumbar arachnoiditic lesion is almost exclusively at the site of the pathology and/or the surgical exposure. Also, arachnoiditis is rarely seen in the caudal sac, where contrast agents such as Pantopaque (iophendylate, Lafayette Pharmaceutical, Lafayette, Ind) stay, sometimes for years.

With myelography being ordered less frequently as MRI assumes an increasing role in spinal diagnosis, the true effect of contrast materials on the arachnoid membranes will be determined. The authors predict that the incidence of arachnoiditis will remain unchanged because the major etiological factor is likely the combination of lumbar spinal pathology and surgery.

Other etiological agents causative of arachnoiditis include a subarachnoid hemorrhage, meningitis, spinal anesthesia, and intrathecal chymopapain injection. Recently, Nelson (19) has called attention to the obvious danger of intrathecal methylprednisolone acetate and the potential danger of epidural cortisone injections as a causative factor in arachnoiditis.

Clinical Presentation Arachnoiditis has a slow, insidious onset at varying intervals after the etiological insult. Initially, the patient may complain of leg pain in a single root distribution, but eventually there is a complaint of back pain (100%) and various degrees and types of bilateral leg symptoms (75%). The symptoms are strikingly aggravated by activity and, surprisingly, unrelieved by rest. Other symptoms may include nighttime leg cramps, paresthesia, dysesthesia, motor weakness, and sphincter dysfunction (25%). Most men are impotent as a result of arachnoiditis.

There is no typical picture of arachnoiditis, with some patients functioning very well with few symptoms (a rare occurrence) despite documented arachnoiditis on myelography; other patients may present with bizarre symptom complexes and physical signs, unfortunately resulting in the occasional erroneous diagnosis of psychogenic pain. A few patients with severe involvement reach a suicidal level of depression.

The characteristic physical findings, if any, are multiple root involvement on motor and sensory examination and mild SLR reduction.

Pathology Early in the disease, a fibrinous exudate, devoid of cells, envelops the pia-arachnoid and nerve roots. As the roots adhere to each other with this glue, more collagen is formed, which leads to the formation of more root adhesions. The end-stage scarring of arachnoiditis is no different than the pathology seen in other serous cavity inflammations, such as peritonitis, pericarditis, and pleuritic disease.

Stages of Arachnoiditis Staging of arachnoiditis has been developed on myelography (more recently on MRI) and at surgery:

Stage 1 Radicular stage, during which the pathology is confined to a single or a few roots. At this stage, the roots are obviously inflamed and swollen.

Stage 2 Arachnoiditis stage where roots clump together because of the fibrinous exudate but still occupy the central subarachnoid space.

Stage 3 Adhesive arachnoiditis where roots are densely adherent to the periphery of the spinal dural canal, leaving an empty central cauda equina canal. At this stage, the roots are atrophic and scarred.

Investigation Until recently, the standard of investigation for arachnoiditis has been myelography. Myelographic changes early in the disease include root sleeve cutoff and clumping of roots (Fig. 19.18) and homogeneous contrast pattern without root shadows. Later, the contrast column takes on the appearance of candle drippings and/or loss of fine root detail at multiple levels (Fig. 19.19), with varying degrees of filling defects and CSF or contrast filled cysts. These changes extend over a few to many lumbar spinal levels. Occasionally, they are confined to a single level in the form of a complete block, although many of these so-called "arachnoiditis" patients turn out to have spinal stenosis without arachnoiditis.

Ross (23) and co-workers have described the MRI appearance of arachnoiditis based on the examination of MRIs and myelograms in 12 confirmed patients (Fig. 19.19). They described three types of changes:

Type 1: Roots are adherent and clumped centrally.
Type 2: Roots are clumped peripherally and the meninges are thickened There is the appearance of the empty dural sac.
Type 3: No roots are seen because they are one amorphous mass with the dura and CSF. These patients have a complete block on myelography.

Treatment Unfortunately, there is little one can offer the patient with arachnoiditis. Various surgical procedures have been proposed, such as neurolysis, with or without the dura sewn open, with or without the intrathecal administration of lysing agents. None of these proposals have stood the test of timely follow-up of the patient.

The various conservative treatment measures used in chronic pain centers seem to be of limited use.

These are an unfortunate group of patients, hopefully reduced in numbers as MRI assumes a more dominant role in investigation and surgery becomes a more precise exercise conducted through a limited surgical exposure.

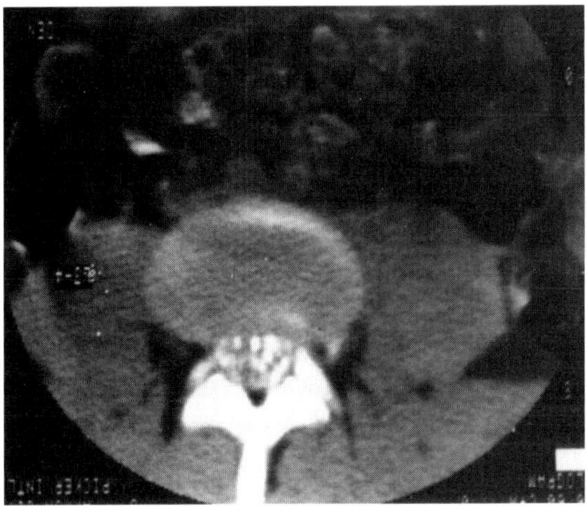

Figure 19.18 *Arachnoiditis: root clumping on CT.*

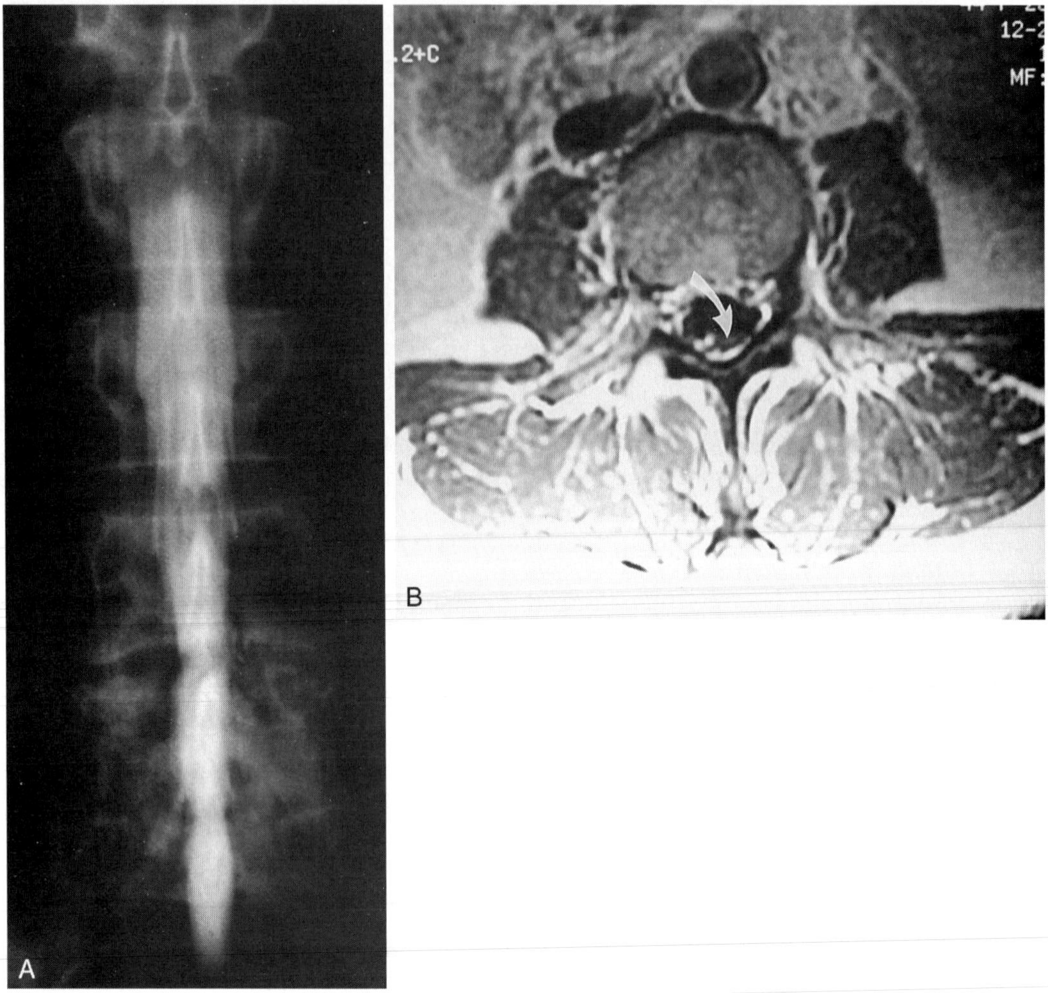

Figure 19.19 **A.** *Severe arachnoiditis: loss of root detail and root cutoff at multiple levels.* **B.** *An axial T1 MRI with arachnoiditis: note the irregular outline of the common dural sac, clumping of the roots (arrow), and increased signal from fatty degeneration in the roots.*

Change of Symptoms or Recurrence of Symptoms

It is almost impossible to separate "change" from "recurrence" of symptoms without an overlapping classification. To present a symptom-based approach to this group of failed spine surgical patients, we have divided the patients into two groups: those undergoing encroachment surgery and those undergoing stabilization surgery.

Obviously, a patient undergoing both encroachment and stabilization surgery could have failures from either group.

Failures After Encroachment Surgery

The reason for the original surgery in this group of patients obviously was based on the diagnosis of radicular pain from various causes. Failure of the surgery to cure the disease can arise from one of four scenarios.

1. The patient wakes with identical leg pain.
2. The patient reports relief of leg pain and notices increased back pain.
3. The patient notices a change in leg pain postoperatively.
4. The patient reports relief of leg pain for varying lengths of time and then notices recurrence of leg pain.

Patient Wakes with Identical Leg Pain

When the patient wakes with identical leg pain, a mistake has been made and cannot be wished away. The most common error is surgery being done at the wrong level or incomplete surgery being done at the right level! These problems have been discussed so many times in this book you are probably tired of reading it! Wait until it happens to you, as it does to everyone doing any volume of spine surgery!

Less often, the reason for persistent leg pain is an erroneous operating diagnosis, such as a missed conus tumor, extrapelvic conditions, or other diagnoses listed in Table 19.3.

Relief of Leg Pain/Increased Back Pain

The sciatic pain may be relieved, but the patient may be plagued by continuing back pain. In many of these patients, if you go back over their initial history you will find that their story was one of recurrent episodes of backache of increasing severity, duration, and frequency, culminating in an attack of incapacitating sciatic pain that necessitated operative intervention. These patients have been suffering for a long period of time from segmental instability giving rise to low back pain. The disc rupture, even though it precipitated the operative intervention, is only one part of the mechanical insufficiency of the spine. Removal of the disc alone in these patients will leave them with the same type of back pain of which they complained in the past. This is the group of patients who should be treated initially by combining disc with fusion, where this is feasible.

If the laminectomy involves destruction of the posterior joints, it may well lead to subsequent back pain, particularly if the involved segment is very mobile; indeed, if decompression requires a total excision of one or both posterior joints, then a segmental fusion is mandatory.

When operating upon a listhetic segment, be it a spondylolytic or degenerative spondylolisthesis, it is essential to avoid removing the disc at the slip level at all costs. Obviously, no symptom-producing pathology can be left behind, but all too often there is no real symptom-producing pathology present in the disc at the slip level, yet it is "decompressed" anyway. This removes one of the few soft-tissue stabilizers left and may result in an increased slip postoperatively. If a fusion was not done at the time of disc excision, increasing back pain postoperatively will make a fusion necessary in many of these patients.

Change in Leg Pain

When the patient notices a change of leg pain postoperatively, one of the problems that may arise after laminectomy is subsequent peridural and periradicular fibrosis.(15) This unfortunate sequel is much more likely to occur in the extensive laminectomy required for decompression of the cauda equina and the emerging nerve roots in a patient suffering from multisegmental spinal stenosis. Some surgeons prefer to use a thin fat graft, as an interposition membrane placed between the dura and the sacrospinales but there is no uniform agreement among spine surgeons regarding fat grafts.

The patient with root scarring notices some relief of leg pain postoperatively only to notice the gradual recurrence of leg pain in the same preoperative distribution. This time around, the pain is more constant in its presence and although aggravated by activity, it is not totally relieved by rest. The pain usually has a dysesthetic component to it.

Unfortunately, little can be done surgically for this complication, with palliative conservative measures offering some hope of control.

Recurrent Leg Pain

Compared with the patients with acute and chronic unilateral radicular syndromes, as described in Chapters 15 and 16, patients with a recurrent HNP or lateral zone stenosis differ in one major way—they have had previous surgery. Otherwise, they present with dominant radicular symptoms, clear evidence of nerve root tension (SLR reduction), and varying degrees of neurological involvement.

A recurrent HNP almost always occurs at the location of the previous surgical exercise (same level / same side).

Patients who have recurrent HNP do have a difference in neurological presentation. Because of the scar tissue tacking the dural sheath and its contents to the back of the disc space, a small disc herniation is capable of causing significant pain and neurological changes. Unusual neurological patterns may also occur and may include double root involvement that is more common than in a virgin HNP; for example, because of scar tissue fixing the dura to the L4–L5 disc space, a recurrent L4–L5 HNP, same level same side as the previous HNP, may cause both fifth and first root involvement.

There is apt to be more of a discrepancy between the root involved and the anatomical level of the HNP. We have seen a patient with a wide L4–L5 decompression suffer an HNP at L3–L4 and present with S1 neurological symptoms and signs. He had a wide and long L4–L5 decompression extending up to the L3–L4 disc space with an intertransverse fusion. Many years later, the recurrent HNP at L3–L4 came to lie against the scarred immobile dura in the midline and caused S1 neurological involvement.

Caution Just because a patient presents with recurrent sciatica, after previous surgery, does not guarantee that the symptom is due to recurrent lumbar spine pathology. All the respect paid to the differential diagnosis of sciatica is due these patients who, in fact, may have a conus tumor or diabetic neuropathy.

Nature and Site of Recurrent Pathology Recurrent HNP most often occurs at the same level / same side (80–90%). The next most frequent site of a recurrent HNP is a different level (10%), and a recurrent HNP, same level, opposite side, has an incidence of occurrence of 5% at most.

Recurrent pathology caused by lateral zone stenosis usually occurs at the same level as previous surgery and may occur on one or both sides. The pathology is usually facet subluxation into the foramen, due to developing instability after the prior surgical procedure. Discussion of lateral zone pathology is contained in Chapter 16. The patient with a recurrent HNP same level / opposite side or different level than previous surgery can be treated as a virgin HNP with no hesitation to plan a microsurgical procedure. Unfortunately, the bulk of patients with recurrent symptoms are in trouble with a recurrent HNP, same level / same side.(34) It is these patients who can be handled with a well-planned microsurgical procedure.

Investigation of the Patient with Recurrent Herniated Nucleus Pulposus (HNP) There is a tendency for clinicians and radiologists to get lost in the minutiae of investigating a patient with recurrent HNP. A patient who has had previously successful disc surgery and notices the sudden recurrence of leg pain, with significant SLR reduction, and renewed neurological symptoms and signs has a recurrent HNP. What else could it be? It then becomes necessary for the investigation to document the lesion. It is not a question of whether or not a recurrent HNP can be found on investigation but rather a question of what is the best test to document the location of the recurrent pathology. Too many patients with significant recurrent sciatica have been told that the investigation has revealed scar tissue and not a recurrent HNP and that they will have to live with their symptoms.

Tests that are of little value in documenting the structural lesion in recurrent pathology include myelography; myelogram/computed tomography (CT); plain CT; electromyography; and discography.

All of the previously listed tests lack both sensitivity and specificity in documenting the occurrence of a disc herniation at a previously operated level. Specifically, myelography,(1) with or without postinjection CT scan, cannot distinguish scar from a recurrent HNP. Teplick et al (31) have attempted to distinguish scar from recurrent HNP on plain CT scan by the shape of the defect, the deformity of the dural sac, and other parameters. Like myelography, these distinctions are not sensitive or specific enough to be used with any authority to document the presence or absence of a recurrent HNP.

Tests Useful in Documenting the Structural Lesion in Recurrent Pathology

Magnetic Resonance Imaging Because MRI is capable of showing biochemical changes as well as morphological characteristics of tissues, it has become the investigative procedure of choice for recurrent HNP.(2)

In the immediate postoperative period, the MRI changes, due to the hemorrhage and edema of wound healing, produce dramatic changes (see Fig. 19.20). These changes preclude a useful study until wound healing is completed and scar lissue begins to mature (6–12 weeks). Beyond this time, MRI changes of epidural scar versus recurrent HNP are viewed according to the following criteria: (1) location of the mass in the epidural space, (2) signal intensity, (3) mass effect, and (4) gadolinium enhancement (Fig. 19.21).

Tables 19.8 and 19.9 summarize the prevailing thought on MR images in recurrent HNP versus scar tissue. Sagittal and axial views are complementary in making the determination.

IV (Conray-60) Enhanced CT This test has been surpassed by gadolinium-enhanced MRI, but is still being used in some centers. A protruding disc in a patient who has not undergone operation is outlined by epidural fat (Fig. 19.22). In patients who have had previous surgery a recurrent HNP occurs into extensive epidural fibrosis and the distinction between disc and scar is not delineated by fat.

Schubiger and Valavanis (25) suggested the use of intravenous contrast material to distinguish between scar tissue and recurrent disc. The theoretical basis for this procedure is the vascularity of scar tissue and the avascular nature of disc.

The protocol is as follows:

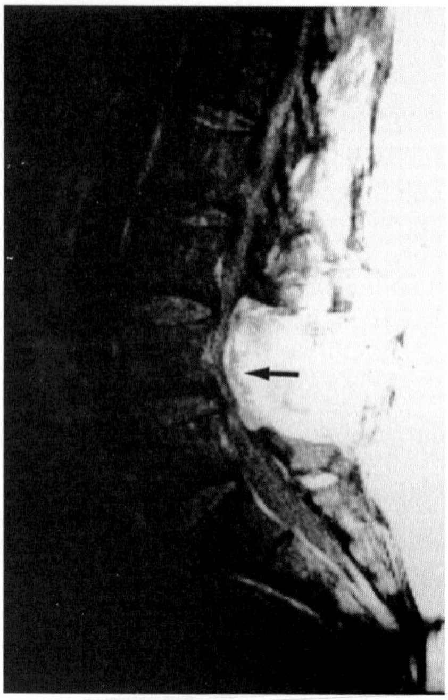

Figure 19.20 *A postoperative complication. A massive hematoma (arrow) (high-signal intensity) causing cauda equina compression (10 days postoperatively).*

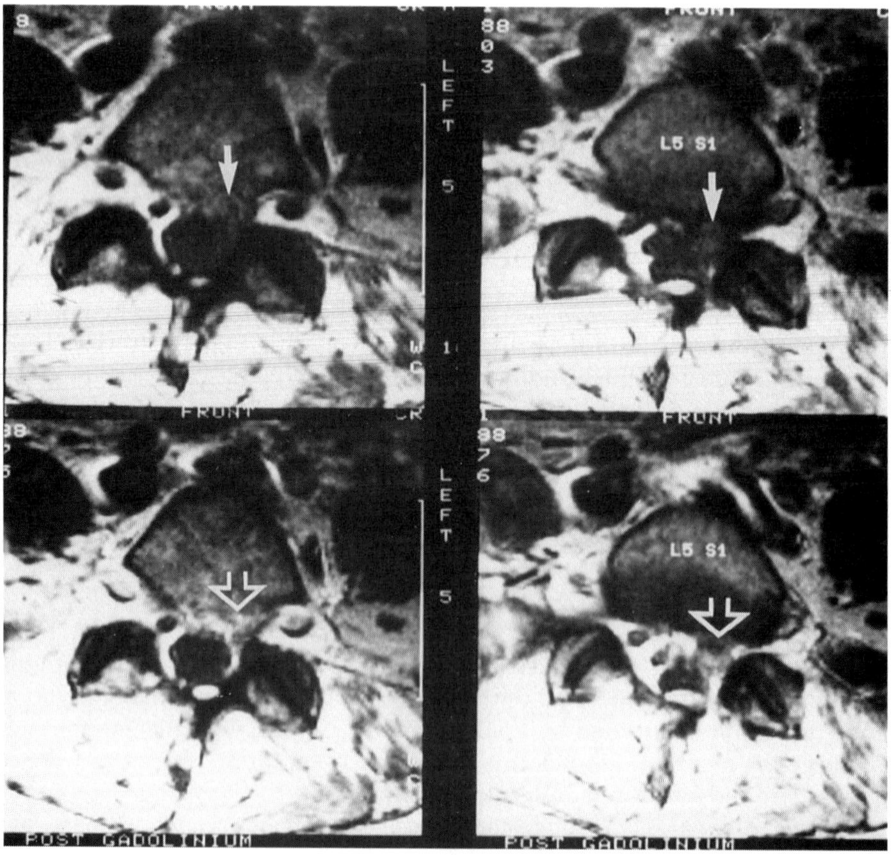

Figure 19.21 *Top row—a patient with recurrent left leg pain and a mass (T1 axial MRI) at a site of previous surgery. Bottom row—post-gadolinium injection shows no recurrent fragment (left bottom), but a very definite recurrent disc herniation in T1 axial MRI (bottom right [arrow]).*

Table 19.8. MRI in Scar vs Recurrent HNP, Axial Views

Factors	Scar	Recurrent HNP
Epidural location	Follows line of last surgical procedure	Opposite disc space
Mass	Conforms to space, retracts dura	Compresses (displaces) dura
Signal intensity (relative to annulus)	Hypo- or isointense on T1-weighted images	Hyperintense on T1-weighted images
Gadolinium	Enhances (Fig. 15.30)	Does not enhance

Table 19.9. MRI in Scar vs Recurrent HNP, Sagittal Views

Factors	Scar	Recurrent HNP
Epidural location	Axial better	Contiguity with disc space
Mass	Axial better	Axial better
Signal intensity (relative to annulus)	Same as axial, No difference on signal intensity on T2 weighted	Same as axial,
Gadolinium	Axial better	Axial better

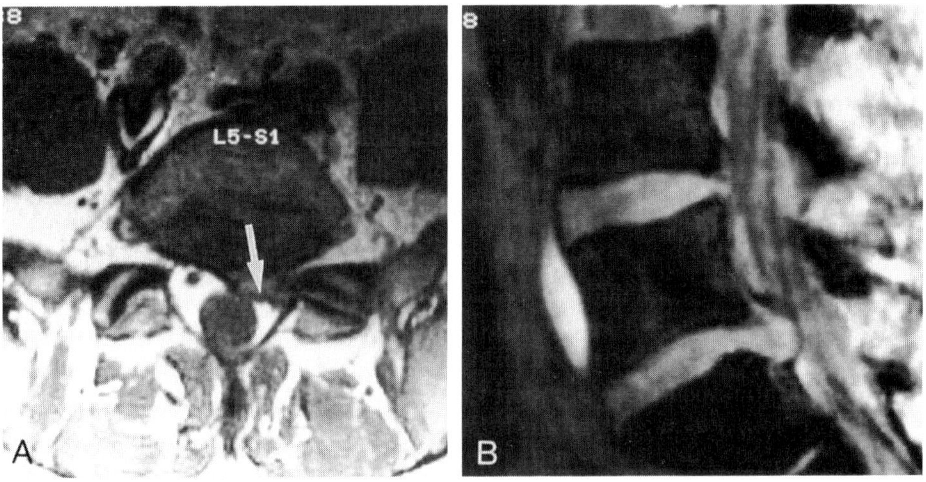

Figure 19.22 *A nonoperated HNP is outlined by high-signal intensity of fat (L5–S1, left).*

1. Before scanning, an IV line is started.
2. The patient has a regular CT scan according to a protocol that includes a nonangled gantry.
3. IV contrast is given first as a bolus of 150 mL of Conray-60 and secondly as a follow-on drip of 150 mL.
4. Scan cuts are immediately redone at the previously operated level, ensuring that the cuts for the enhanced scans were performed at the same levels and in the same planes as the unenhanced studies.

A focal unenhanced lucency, in a position where nerve root would not be expected, likely represents recurrent herniated nuclear fragments (Fig. 19.23).

The disadvantages of IV-enhanced CT are that the test is very operator dependent; there is an added dose of radiation; and the high iodine load usually limits examination to one disc space per session. For these reasons, many investigators continue to look to a plain CT for the differential diagnoses.

On a plain CT, without IV enhancement, the characteristics of scar tissue are that the scar conforms to the available epidural space and follows the direction of the previous surgery. That is, a wide laminectomy will have a wide scar; a scar will not appear deep to the intact lamina (Fig. 19.24); and a previous foraminotomy will result in scar formation into the foramen.

Another characteristic is that the scar can retract the dural tube. Note in Figure 19.24 how the dural sac is retracted by scar to the right-sided laminotomy defect. Recurrent HNP, on the other hand, has: (1) the effect of a mass (displacement of dural sac); (2) the mass is usually just opposite the disc space in a position contiguous with the annulus; (3) a different density within the scar tissue.

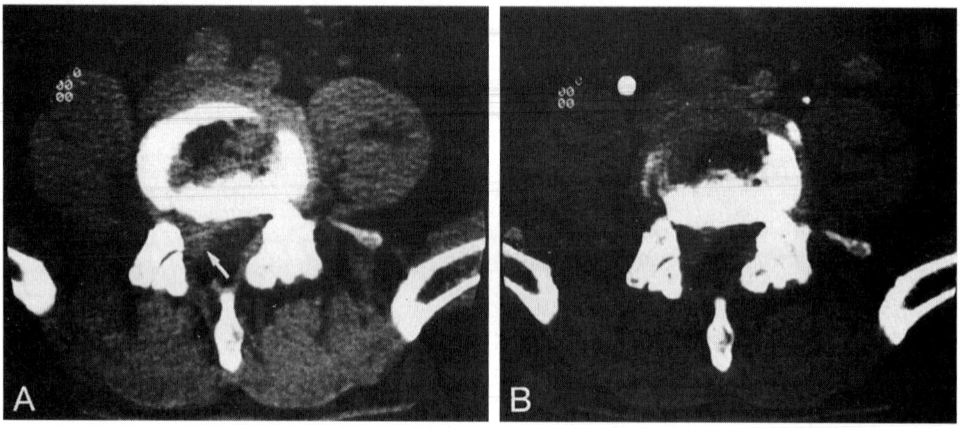

Figure 19.23 **A.** *Preinjection CT showing density, right (arrow).* **B.** *Post-Conray-60 injection. Scar tissue, which is vascular, takes up the contrast; disc, which is avascular, does not.*

Figure 19.24 *A mass of tissue (arrow) deep to lamina in a patient with recurrent sciatica is unlikely a scar and more likely a recurrent disc rupture.*

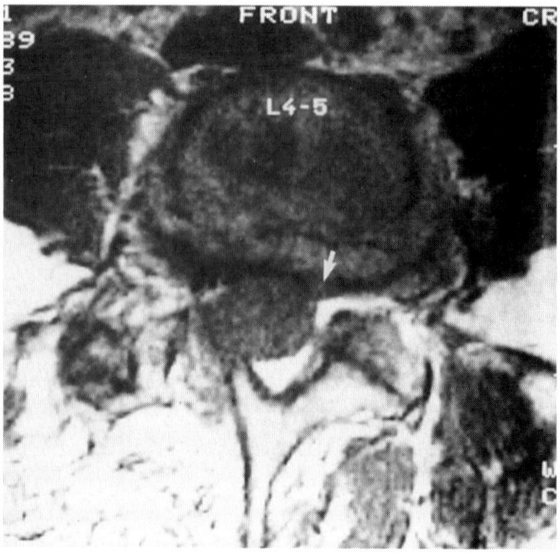

Despite these prescribed differences between scar and recurrent HNP, practical application is not universally fruitful. Because of this problem, other methods such as gadolinium-enhanced MRI are more rewarding

Treatment of Recurrent Herniated Nucleus Pulposus Although all patients with sciatica, recurrent or not, deserve a trial of conservative care, there is reasonable expectation that patients with a recurrent HNP will persist with their symptoms and require surgical intervention.(34) Conventional surgical dictum is that repeat surgery, anywhere in the body, is best done through a wide exposure. Those familiar with the use of the microscope disagree.(11, 36) If there is any indication for the use of the microscope in lumbar spine surgery: this is it. The illumination and magnification better show the difference between scar and neurological tissues, making it a safer operation.

Failures After Spinal Fusion

Failures after spinal fusion may be considered under the headings of (1) pain derived from the grafted area, (2) pain derived from the spine above the graft, and (3) donor site pain.

Pain Derived from the Fused Areas

When Dr. Macnab wrote the first edition of this book, spinal instrumentation was seldom used in lumbar spine fusion. Since the introduction of spinal (pedicle) instrumentation systems,(29) a large number of lumbar fusions are augmented by instrumentation. Needless to say this advance has been associated with a whole new set of complications.(12, 17) When you set out to achieve a fusion (for back pain) and fail to obtain a solid arthrodesis, you have the number one complication of spinal fusion.

Pseudarthrosis

Radiologically, a pseudarthrosis may be difficult to demonstrate. Moreover, a pseudarthrosis can be present without pain and the mere demonstration of the lesion does not necessarily mean that the source of the patient's continuing disability has been found.(38) Increasing work tolerance after infiltration of the pseudarthrosis with local anesthetic tends to indict the lesion as the source of pain, although it must be remembered that an injection of this nature is a powerful hypnotic suggestion. In order to arrive at any valid conclusion, it is necessary to assess the suggestibility of the patient first by observing the result of injection of normal saline. Discography may well prove to be the best diagnostic tool. Discography in the presence of a solid fusion, although demonstrating an irregular pattern, is generally painless. If there is a pseudarthrosis, discography is painful at the involved segment. Dr. Macnab opined that this technique carries with it an accuracy rate of about 80%; we have broad doubts about discography and limited experience in this specific problem.

Other investigative steps often used to try and demonstrate a pseudarthrosis are flexion/extension films and three-dimensional CT reconstruction. The problem with all of these investigations is the high level of false positive and false negative outcomes. This has lead to the opinion of many spine surgeons that the only consistent way to prove or disprove a pseudarthrosis is surgical reexploration of the fusion mass, looking for a pseudarthrosis and/or detecting movement of vertebral segments within the fusion mass .

In the surgical management of a pseudarthrosis, the failure rate of refusion has been alarmingly high. This probably arises from the fact that it is difficult to obtain, in the fusion area, a good vascular bed with a potent source of osteoblasts capable of revascularizing and reossifying the graft. It is best to reoperate on the spine in an area in which there has been no previous interference. If the previous fusion was midline, an intertransverse fusion is the best approach for repair. If the previous fusion was intertransverse, then the fusion bed should be along the spinous processes. If the previous fusion was a combination of an intertransverse and posterior fusion, the so-called "Cowl" fusion, then an anterior interbody fusion is the only feasible method of salvage. There are studies supporting the use of pedicle instrumentation for posterior revision surgery.(32)

Root Compression The patient may develop symptoms and signs of root compression that may be due to a rupture of an intervertebral disc underneath the fusion or it may be due to an iatrogenic spinal stenosis. A ruptured disc very rarely occurs under a solid spinal fusion; it is much more likely to occur in the presence of a pseudarthrosis. In those instances in which there is a ruptured disc under a fusion that is irrefutably solid, in all probability it was present at the time the fusion was performed.

Whereas the symptoms resulting from a recent disc rupture are fairly rapid in onset, the symptoms resulting from an iatrogenic spinal stenosis are slow in developing (Fig. 19.25). The clinical picture is clear-cut. A patient with a solid spinal fusion, usually intertransverse and incorporating the L4–L5 segment, which before operation had radiological evidence of interlaminar narrowing, slowly develops the claudicant type of sciatic pain

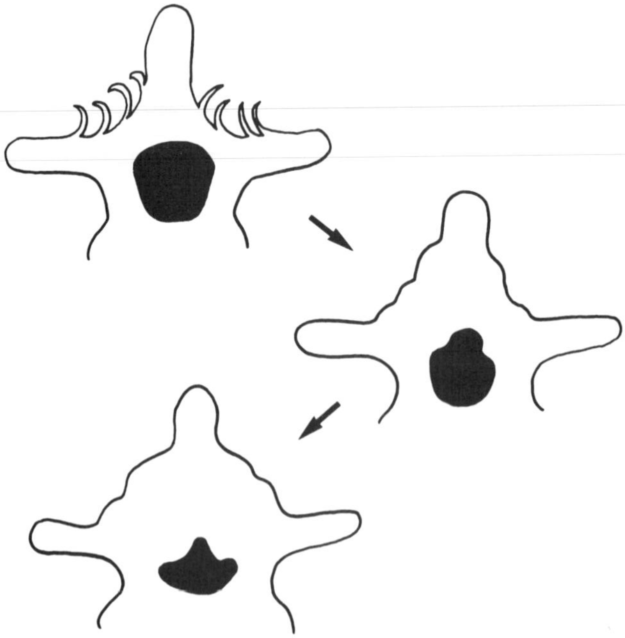

Figure 19.25 *Any operative procedure that involves discortication of the lamina may result subsequently in gross thickening of the lamina. If the spinal canal was narrow at the time of operation, further narrowing induced by the thickening of the lamina may precipitate the symptoms of spinal stenosis.*

that one associates with root compression secondary to spinal stenosis. On examination, these patients frequently present evidence of impairment of root conduction at more than one segment.

Pain Derived from the Spine above the Graft

Spondylolysis Acquisita A spondylolysis may develop at the segment above the spinal fusion. Spondylolysis acquisita is probably much more common than previously acknowledged because it may well be missed on a routine lateral view taken for the postoperative assessment of the stability of a spinal fusion. It is probably advisable in all patients who have undergone a spinal fusion and subsequently suffer from persisting discomfort to take oblique views of the spine to show the pars interarticularis of the segment above the lesion.

The exact etiology of the lesion is not known. It may be a stress fracture. The development of a stress fracture may be predisposed to by dissection of the muscle masses away from the lamina at the segment above a spinal fusion. A dissection such as this would interfere to a fairly marked degree with the venous drainage of the lamina, giving rise to partial death of bone in this area. If, subsequently, extra stresses are placed on such a bone by the placement of a graft below it, then the pars interarticularis may break and spondylolysis develop.

The lesion is not seen in patients in whom an intertransverse fusion has been carried out. Theoretically, spondylolysis acquisita should not occur with an intertransverse fusion because the site of the lesion is supported by the uppermost portion of the graft (Fig. 19.26).

Lumbodorsal Strain The significance of a chronic lumbodorsal strain after a lumbosacral fusion has not been sufficiently recognized. When the lumbosacral segment is fused, extra mechanical stresses are placed on the lumbodorsal junction and a previously asymptomatic degenerative change at this level may, after lumbosacral fusion, produce pain referred to both buttocks and down as low as the great trochanters.

Here again, treatment is prophylactic, recognizing the possibility and investigating the probability in every patient considered for spinal fusion. If the lesion does occur, there is no reason why a localized segmental fusion should not be undertaken.

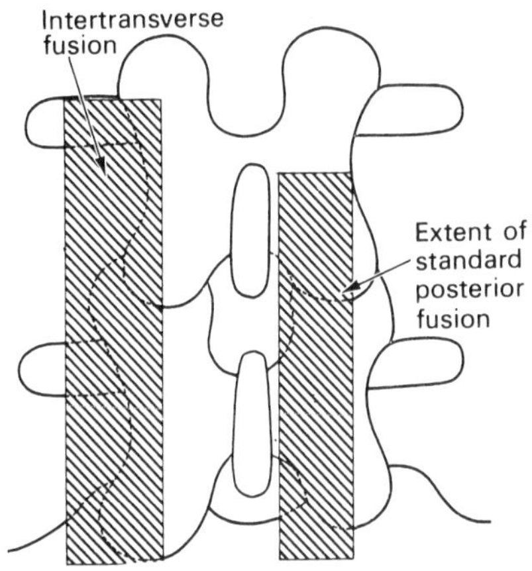

Figure 19.26 *An intertransverse fusion supports the pars interarticularis of the proximal vertebral segment in a spinal fusion. Because of this, spondylolysis acquisita is not seen with intertransverse fusions.*

Complications Related to Use of Instrumentation Systems

As discussed in the chapter on lumbar fusion (Chapter 14), there are two ways to try to immobilize a spine with instrumentation: (1) hold onto the pedicle; (2) hold onto the lamina. By far, the most popular of these methods are those systems that hold onto the pedicles. Complications attendant upon the use of these systems include (1) infection; (2) root irritation or injury; (3) screw/plate, rod breakage or disengagement; (4) degenerative changes at the motion segment above the fusion; and (5) painful hardware. These complications were described in detail in Chapter 14.

Pseudarthrosis with Instrumentation

The instrumentation systems have enjoyed wide support amongst spine surgeons because they decrease the pseudarthrosis rate.(29) It is still possible to end up with a pseudarthrosis in an instrumented fusion. It may be very hard to demonstrate on investigation and require reexploration of the fusion mass. When you combine a pseudarthrosis with one of the complications previously mentioned you have a very difficult clinical problem, that often results in permanent, long-term problems, difficult to treat even with repeat surgery. Because of this possibility, a number of spine surgeons use these systems sparingly or not at all (included amongst them is the senior author JM).

Donor Site Pain

Continuing pain may be derived from the donor site. The superficial gluteal nerve (cluneal nerves) crosses the iliac crest approximately the breadth of four fingers away from the midline (Fig. 19.27). If an incision over the iliac crest is used to obtain the graft,

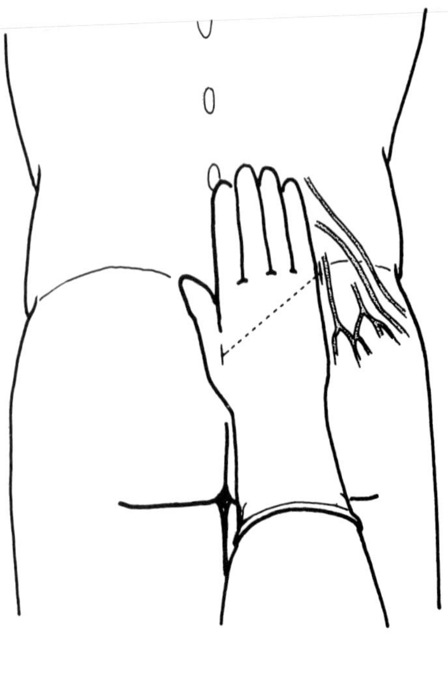

Figure 19.27 *The superficial gluteal nerve crosses the iliac crest approximately the breadth of four fingers away from the midline.*

the superficial gluteal nerve may be divided and trapped in the scar and become a source of pain. It is preferable to curve the lower end of the midline incision to expose the posterior superior iliac spine and obtain bone from this site.

The treatment of neuroma pain is very ungratifying and all efforts must be made to avoid cutting these nerves. If the patient had unilateral leg pain before surgery, it is wise to make the donor site incision on the opposite iliac crest so that residual postoperative symptoms due to root pathology are not confused by the potential for neuroma formation.

Sacroiliac Pain

Sacroiliac instability may occur if the donor site encroaches markedly on the sacroiliac joint, particularly if the iliolumbar ligament is divided. This is probably the most important of all the stabilizing ligaments of the sacroiliac joint. In cadavers, if this ligament is divided, the sacroiliac joint can be opened up easily, like the two halves of a book. Patients with sacroiliac instability will present with pain over the sacroiliac joint and the pain will radiate down the lateral aspect of the great trochanter onto the front of the thigh. Weightbearing on the involved extremity increases the pain, and the patients tend to limp with a combined Trendelenburg and antalgic gait. The pain is reproduced by straining the sacroiliac joints by resisted abduction of the hip and is temporarily relieved by infiltration of the involved sacroiliac joint with local anesthetic. With gross instability, movement at the symphysis pubis may be observed when the radiographs are taken with the patient standing first on one leg, then on the other (Fig. 19.28).

Some of these patients may even require a sacroiliac fusion to get rid of this troublesome, residual, significant disability.

Diagnoses of Questionable Significance

On occasion, failed low back pain patients reach an intolerable state symptomatically and, with the failure of accepted medical treatment, they reach for anything that offers hope. They fall into the hands of unscrupulous practitioners with legitimate and not so legitimate backgrounds; they are "awakened to new hope" with fancy-sounding diagnoses of questionable significance. Such diagnoses include fat nodule entrapment, neuroma formation, and various tendinitis and bursitis conditions. Before following this direction, these patients should be encouraged to attend the many fine chronic pain clinics or rehabilitation centers specializing in these problems. Readers are referred to Chapter 20 and Wilkinson's book (35) for further reading about this most difficult group of patients.

CONCLUSION

The intention of every surgeon is to make an accurate diagnosis as to the cause of symptoms and try, with a skillful surgical procedure, to relieve the symptoms. Surgeons are not perfect, and sometimes the outcome of surgery falls short of expectations of the patient and the surgeon. In today's legal climate in the United States, this failure of the surgeon to achieve a good result is called a complication and is grounds for a malpractice action. Surgeons, in this unchecked environment, are being forced into the role of guarantors, a godlike position many are finding difficult to sustain. Whether an unanticipated result to spine surgery is a complication, an adverse effect, iatrogenic, or act of God is not

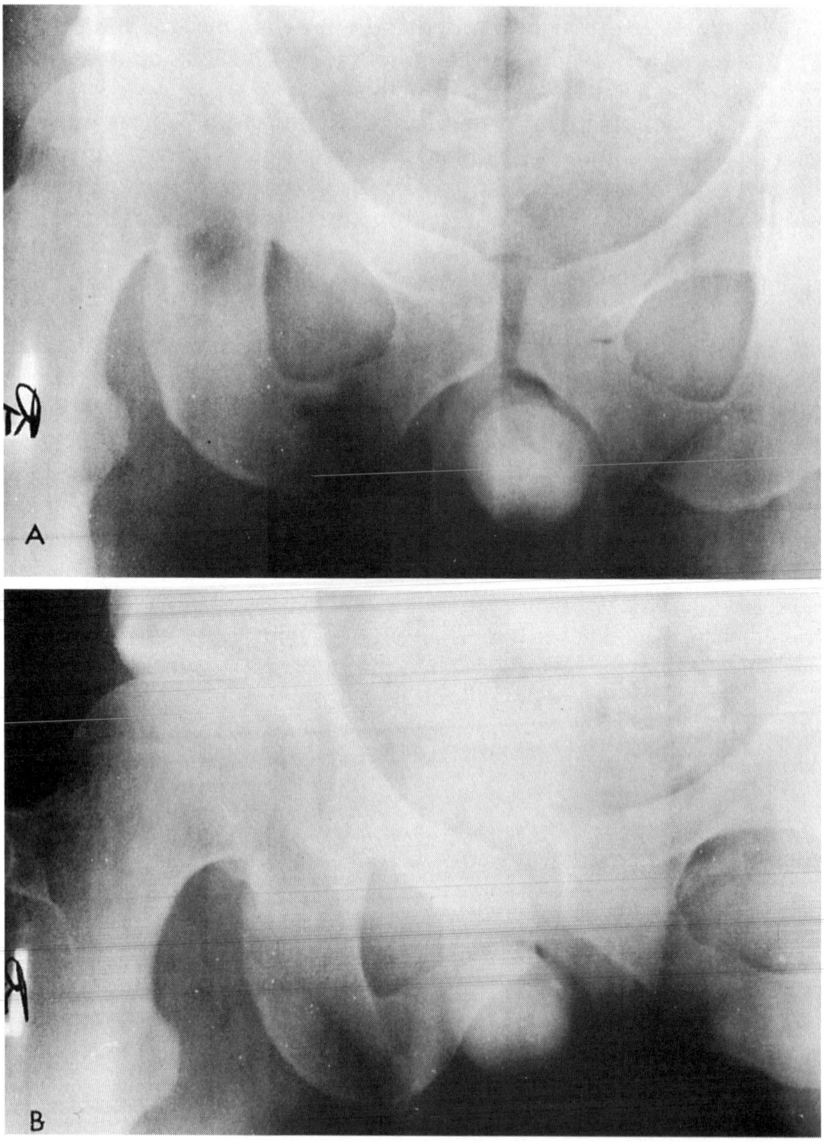

Figure 19.28 *Instability of the symphysis pubis associated with sacroiliac instability. This patient had instability of the left sacroiliac joint. In the first radiograph* **(A)**, *the patient is standing on his right leg, and in the second radiograph* **(B)**, *he is taking full weight on his left leg. Note the gross excursion of the symphysis pubis that is demonstrated when the patient takes his weight on the left leg.*

at issue in this chapter. The situations described represent occurrences that direct the result of surgery away from the goal the patient and the surgeon are trying to achieve. For centuries, surgeons have recognized these happenings as either complications, the results of their misadventures and technical errors, or acts of God, but all leading to a less-than-acceptable result of the surgical exercise. Less-than- acceptable results in surgery for lumbar disc disease do occur.

Unfortunately, these patients fall victim to the misconception that failed back surgery can only be cured by more surgery by the same surgeon. In the end, they appear in the clinics for patients with failed back surgery after multiple surgeries and multiple investigations. Most of these patients end up abusing narcotics and becoming psychologically destroyed. If there ever is a place for preventative medicine, this is it.

REFERENCES

1. Braun IF, Horfman MD, Davis PC, Landman JA, Tindall GT. Contrast enhancement in CT differentiation between recurrent disc herniation and postoperative scar: prospective study. AJNR 1985;6:607–612.
2. Bundschuh CV, Modic MT, Ross JS, Masaryk TJ, Bohlman H. Epidural fibrosis and recurrent disk herniation in the lumbar spine: MR imaging assessment. AJNR 1988;9:169–178.
3. Capana AH, Williams RW, Austin DC, Darmody WR, Thomas ML. Lumbar discectomy — Percentage of disc removal and detection of anterior annulus perforation. Spine 1981;6:610–614.
4. DeSaussure RL. Vascular injury coincident to disc surgery. J Neurosurg 1959;16:222–229.
5. Eismont FJ, Wiesel SW, Rothman RH. Treatment of dural tears associated with spinal surgery J Bone Joint Surg 1981;63A:1132–1136.
6. Fager CA. Progress, reason, and fallacy in today's world of neurosurgery. W James Gardner Lecture. Cleve Clin Quart 1987;54:261–270.
7. Greene K. Preoperative nutritional status of total joint patients: relationship to postoperative wound complications. Presented at American Academy of Orthopaedic Surgeons Annual Meeting. Las Vegas, Nevada; February 1989.
8. Hakelius A. Prognosis in sciatica: a clinical follow up of surgical and non-surgical treatment. Acta Orthop Scand 1970;129(suppl):1–76.
9. Harbison EC. Major vascular complications of intervertebral disc surgery. Ann Surg 1954; 140:342–348.
10. Holscher EC. Vascular and visceral injuries during lumbar disc surgery. J Bone Joint Surg 1968;50A:383–393.
11. Hudgins WR. The role of microdiscectomy. Orthop Clin North Am 1983;14:589–603.
12. Kostuik J. Surgical treatment of failures of laminectomy and spinal fusion. Lumbar Spinal Stenosis. St. Louis: Mosby YearBook; 1992; pp 425–470.
13. Long DM, Filtzer DL, BenDebba M, Hendler NH. Clinical features of the failed-back syndrome. J Neurosurg 1988;69:61–71.
14. Macnab I. Negative disc exploration. J Bone Joint Surg 1971;53A:891–903.
15. Mayfield FH. Complications of laminectomy. Clinical Neurosurg 1976;23:435–439.
16. McLaren AC, Bailey SI. Cauda equina syndrome: complication of lumbar discectomy. Clin Orthop 1986;204:143–149.
17. Mueller WM, Larson SJ. Complications of spinal instrumentation. In: Tarlov EC, ed. Complications of Spinal Surgery. Neurosurgical Topics. Park Ridge, Ill: American Association of Neurological Surgeons; 1991, pp 15–21.
18. Nachemson A. Advances in low-back pain. Clin Orthop 1985;200:266–278.
19. Nelson DA. Dangers from methylprednisolone acetate therapy by intraspinal injection. Arch Neurol 1988;45:804–806.
20. Pheasant HC. Sources of failure in laminectomies. Orthop Clin North Am 1975;6:319–329.
21. Ramirez LF, Thisted R. Complication and demographic characteristics of patients undergoing lumbar discectomy in community hospitals. Neurosurgery 1989;25:226–231.
22. Rish BL. A critique of the surgical management of lumbar disc disease in a private neurological practice. Spine 1984;9:500–504.
23. Ross JS, et al. MR imaging of lumbar arachnoiditis. AJR 1987;149:1025–1032.

24. Rydevik B, Brown MD, Lundborg G. The pathoanatomy and pathophysiology of nerve root compression. Spine 1984;9:7–15.
25. Schubiger O, Valavanis A. CT differentiation between disc herniation and postoperative scar formation. The value of contrast enhancement. Neuroradiology 1980;22:251–254.
26. Smith RA, Estridge MN. Bowel perforation following lumbar disc surgery. J Bone Joint Surg 1964;46A:826–828.
27. Spangfort EV. The lumbar disc herniation. A computer aided analysis of 2,504 operations. Acta Orthop Scand 1972;142(suppl):1–95.
28. Spengler DM. Lumbar discectomy: results with limited disc excision and selective foraminotomy. Spine 1982;7:604–607.
29. Steffee AD, Biscup RS, Sitkowski DJ. Segmental spine plates with pedicle screw fixation: a new internal fixation device for disorders of the lumbar and thoracolumbar spine. Clin Orthop 1986;203:45–53.
30. Tenney JH, Vlahov D, Salcman M, Ducker TB. Wide variation in risk of wound infection following clean neurosurgery. J Neurosurg 1985;62:243–247.
31. Teplick JG, Teplick SK, Haskin ME. The postoperative lumbar spine. In: Yost MJD, ed. Computed Tomography of the Spine. Baltimore: Williams & Wilkins; 1984.
32. Thalgott J, et al. Reconstruction of failed lumbar surgery with narrow A-O DCP plates for spinal arthrodesis. Spine 1991;16:5170–5175.
33. Weber H. Lumbar disc herniation: a controlled prospective study with 10 years of observation. Spine 1983;8:131–140.
34. Weir BKA, Jacobs GA. Reoperation rate following lumbar discectomy. An analysis of 662 lumbar discectomies. Spine 1980;5:366–370.1.
35. Wilkinson HA. The Failed Back Syndrome, Etiology and Therapy. Philadelphia: Harper & Row; 1983.
36. Williams RW. Microlumbardiscectomy: A l2-year statistical review. Spine 1986;11:851–852.
37. Wilson DH, Harbaugh R. Microsurgical and standard removal of the protruded lumbar disc: a comparative study. Neurosurgery 1981;8:422–427.
38. Zucherman J, Schofferman J. Pathology of failed back surgery syndrome. In White AH, ed. Failed Back Surgery Syndrome. Philadelphia: Hanley & Belfus. Vol 1, no 1, 1986, pp 1–12.

20

Management of Chronic Low Back Pain

"It's not so much the pain the man has, it is more the man who has the pain."

— Ian Macnab (1950s)

INTRODUCTION

If you are at all familiar with books or articles on low back pain, you will have noticed that sections on chronic pain and/or failures of surgery are at the end. They are not there because the topic is an afterthought; rather they are there in the hope that you will be tired of reading by the time you reach the section and will gloss over what has to be a major failure of society and professionals to resolve the problems of low back pain.

In the epidemiology chapter (Chapter 8), you read that 80% of the population will suffer from an episode of low back pain sometime in their life.(11) If this is so, the obvious question is, "why don't we have a nation of back cripples?" The answer is equally obvious: "because most back pain sufferers get better spontaneously." In most cases, it does not matter if the patient rubs peanut butter on their back or goes to a "specialist," they are likely to improve spontaneously!

So why is there a problem called chronic low back pain? There are two factors that lead patients to fall into this classification:

1. Society (politicians) has created some pretty juicy entitlement programs that pay 100% of wages (sometimes tax free) while you are off work.(26) If you have no motivation to work (you do not like your job or your boss), long-term back disability is an attractive option.
2. As the number of spine surgeons increases, the rate of back surgery increases exponentially (Table 20.1). Failures of spine surgery are all too common, occurring in 15 to 40% of surgeries (2, 4, 10). With 300,000 low back operations per year in the United States, there is added 45,000 to 120,000 patients with chronic low back pain on the basis of failed back surgery (FBS). The next year an equal number will be added, and on and on and on. Low back pain is an industry, and chronic low back pain is a cottage industry of doctors, lawyers therapists, counselors, insurance companies, and so forth that generates handsome profits.(26) Is there any wonder we have not solved the problem of low back pain!

Furthermore, new tests (magnetic resonance imaging [MRI]) and new spine procedures (pedicle instrumentation) have allowed those in the field to discover new diseases

Table 20.1. Spine Surgery in the United States

Year	Surgery Rates	Chronic Pain Patients	No, of Orthopedic and Neurosurgeons
1979	147,000/y	20,000+/y	4.6/100,000[a]
1990	179,000/y	40,000+/y	7.6/100,000

Data compiled from: Cherkin DC, et al. An international comparison of back surgery rates. Spine 1994; 19:1201–1206; Taylor VM, et al. Low back pain hospitalization: Recent United States trends and regional variations. Spine 1994 19: 1207–1213.
[a]Number after slash in fourth column represents the general population.

and assault the back with big operations that are loaded with complications leading to the FBS.

Finally, it is important for the doctor and the patient to accept the following:

1. Back pain is often part of the aging process, and there is no "cure" for aging.
2. Spine surgery, hopefully, makes patients better, but will never make a patient normal.

DEFINITION OF CHRONIC LOW BACK PAIN

Chronic low back pain describes a patient who is functionally disabled (for work or play) beyond a period of 6 months. The disability may arise out of failed conservative care or failed surgery.

THE APPROACH TO THE PATIENT WITH CHRONIC LOW BACK PAIN (CLBP)

Assessment of the patient with CLBP follows a series of questions.

Step 1: What is the Setting in which the Disability is Occurring?

Patients with CLBP are difficult diagnostic and treatment problems. They require extensive time and many specialists to diagnose and treat them. They are probably best handled in institutions who dedicate resources and personnel to the cause.(29)

On referral to these centers, patients are requested to bring all records and radiographs pertaining to their past care and surgeries. The four most important historical features to be decided on seeing such a patient are:

1. The role that litigation, compensation, and attorneys are playing in the disability.
2. The length of time off work.
3. The level of drug use.
4. The rate of recidivism, that is, how many times has the patient been through a treatment program, only to have the disability recur?

A patient deep into litigation, off work for more than a year, on daily narcotic or mood altering drugs cannot be successfully treated in any setting.(21, 31, 32, 33) Treating patients with these factors still in place more often than not leads to temporary improvement under the intense scrutiny of a pain center, but recurrence of the depth of disability as soon as medical supervision is removed. A patient who has been through a chronic pain center and has failed to improve or has recurrence of disability is unlikely to be improved by extensive and expensive repetition of care. There are always exceptions to every general statement, but they are few and far between in the patients with CLBP.

Step 2: What Has Been Missed?

Failures of care can have many causes but two constant themes recur:

1. Failure of the doctor to recognize psychosocial factors adversely affecting the patient (Question 1 in Chapter 18 and fully discussed in Chapter 12).
2. Failure to diagnose a condition that is not at the disc space level. (Question 2 in Chapter 18). The differential diagnosis of CLBP (see Table 18.3) and sciatica (see Table 18.4) includes an extensive list of conditions.

Step 3: Is this a Failed Back Surgery?

This topic was extensively covered in the preceding chapter (Chapter 19) on Complications and Failures of Spine Surgery. It is best to look at failed back surgery in terms of the following factors:

1. When did the failure occur?
   a. Did the patient wake up with the same symptoms?
   b. Did the patient have a pain-free interval between the index surgery and the recurrent symptoms?
2. What is the nature of the symptoms: back pain, leg pain, or both?

Table 20.2 summarizes this approach, and each condition has been discussed in Chapter 19. In reading this table, accept that we have ruled out psychosocial factors and the non-organic pain problems discussed in Chapter 12. This topic has been mentioned so many times during this book it is time to back off! We will also assume that no traps such as an aortic aneurysm, arthritis in the hip, etc., have been missed (ie, Question 2 in Chapter 18 has been satisfactorily answered). What is outlined in Table 20.2 are the local causes of the FBS. Macnab's landmark article on negative disc exploration (22) (Table 20.3) is also presented in Table 20.3.

Step 4: What is Significant on History and Physical Examination?

Obviously, patients with chronic low back pain need a careful history and physical examination. In fact, many will need multidisciplinary assessment, including psychological testing.(35)

The history and physical examination needs to be as detailed as that outlined in Chapters 9 and 10. Salient features relative to Tables 20.2 and 20.3 are:

Table 20.2. Failed Back Surgery

Timing of Failure Related to Surgery	Symptom Associated with Failure: Predominant Back Pain	Predominant Leg Pain
Immediate (Day 1)	Creation of acute instability (eg, sacrificing both facet joints) Wrong level fusion	Wrong level exploration Retained fragments of disc Missed pathology (see Table 20.3) Root injury Conjoint root Complication of root (eg, root penetration by pedicle screw) Root damaged by intraoperative cautery
Intermediate (Wk)	Infection discitis osteomyelitis epidural abscess Instability: failed instrumentation Paraspinal muscle insufficiency from denervation Fusion of too few levels Abutment of instrumentation Donor site pain	Infection Recurrent disc herniation The battered root Meningeal cyst Reflex sympathetic dystrophy Retained foreign body such as a cottonoid
Mid-term (Months) to Late-Term (Y)	Instability pseudarthrosis at segments adjacent to fusion failed instrumentation Fracture Painful hardware	Recurrent disc: disc herniation Scarring: epidural or arachnoiditis Stenosis above fusion at level of previous surgery lateral zone

Table 20.3. Causes of Negative Disc Exploration[a]

Pathology	Frequency (N)	Satisfactory Results (%)[b]
Foraminal migration	9	88
Pedicular kinking	12	91
Facet impingement	19	84
Spinal stenosis	8	87
Lateral herniation	2	100
Root adhesion	6	0
No abnormality detected	12	50

[a]Reprinted with permission from Macnab I. Negative disc exploration. An analysis of the causes of nerve-root involvement in 68 patients. J Bone Joint Surg 1971; 53A:891–903.
[b]Percentages are given only for emphasis; the numbers in each group are too small to indicate anything but trends.

1. Identical leg pain is almost certainly missed pathology (eg, wrong level).
2. New location of significant leg pain soon after surgery is usually an intraoperative lesion affecting the root (eg, a pedicle screw touching the root).
3. Less leg pain in the same preoperative location with increased neurological symp-

toms (paresthesia, weakness) is indicative of excessive intraoperative nerve root retraction.(1)

4. Non-mechanical night time pain of delayed onset should immediately raise the suspicion of infection.(7)
5. The sudden onset of significant radicular leg pain after a pain free interval is almost certainly a recurrent disc herniation (see Chapter 15). A major problem in sorting out these patients is to decide what neurological symptoms and signs are old and which are new. This is done largely on history, determining if new paresthesias or new weakness has developed.
6. The gradual onset of moderate radicular leg pain within weeks of surgery and after a pain-free interval is usually associated with root scarring or the formation of a meningocele.(25)
7. The gradual onset of diffuse bilateral leg pain that is non-claudicant in nature points to arachnoiditis.(13, 16, 27)
8. The gradual and delayed onset (months to years) of diffuse bilateral leg pain that is claudicant in nature is most often associated with spinal canal stenosis, that may be developing at the mobile level above a fusion.(12, 14, 18, 19)
9. The patient that persists with back pain after a fusion operation, who notices a gradual increase in back pain with activity has a pseudarthrosis of the fusion until proved otherwise.(12)

Step 5: What Constitutes Effective Investigation for the CLBP Patient?

The first thing to reach for in the CLBP patient is the plain radiograph.(5) It will quickly reveal most sources for back pain as a continuing cause of symptoms, for example, failed hardware, pseudarthrosis and wrong level surgery. A plain lateral radiograph will also give early clues to the presence of a disc space infection (Fig. 20.1).

If you suspect a postoperative infection, a fever, an elevated white blood cell count, and an extremely high erythrocyte sedimentation rate will support the diagnosis.(7) The indications for and types of bone scans useful to you in this situation are discussed in Chapter 11.

MRI is the most effective radiological modality to investigate scar and recurrent disc pathology.(3, 8, 28) The addition of gadolinium (8, 17) (Fig. 20.2) allows for quick resolution as to the cause of most persistent or recurrent radicular pain. Helical computed tomography (CT) is most useful for the evaluation of the patient with a suspected pseudarthrosis.

Tests that depend on patient response for evaluation have a limited role to play in CLBP. These procedures include the facet joint block, epidural injections and root blocks.

Electromyography is also of limited use in the evaluation of these patients (see Chapter 11).

Step 6: How Do You Treat the Patient with Chronic Low Back Pain and/or the Failed Back Syndrome?

First, accept that it is not easy. This is not a patient you see in your office for a few minutes; this is a patient that requires a considerable amount of assessment and treatment time by a multidisciplinary team.(29) Remember, when you are getting ready to do your first operation, you have the best chance to prevent the failed back surgery syndrome.(9,

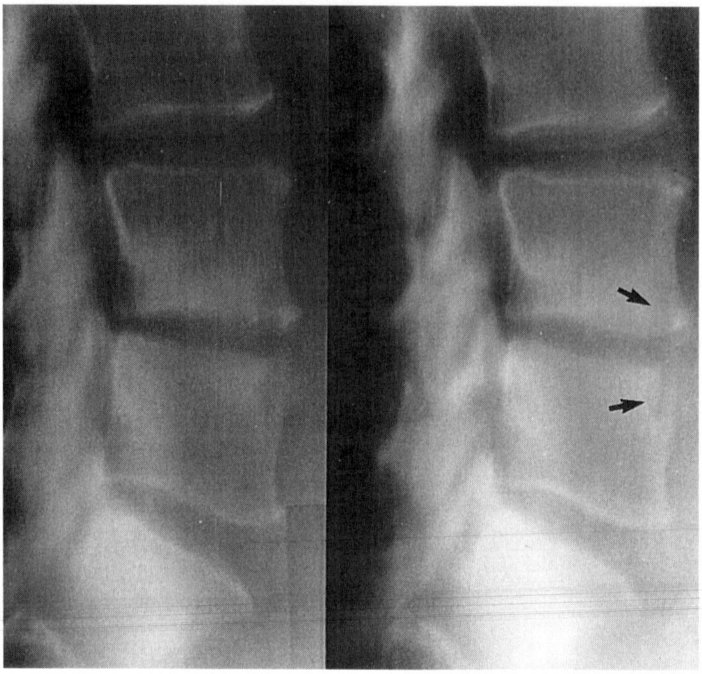

Figure 20.1 *Very early signs of a disc space infection: narrowing of the L4–L5 disc and erosions anteriorly (arrows). These are adjacent tomogram cuts.*

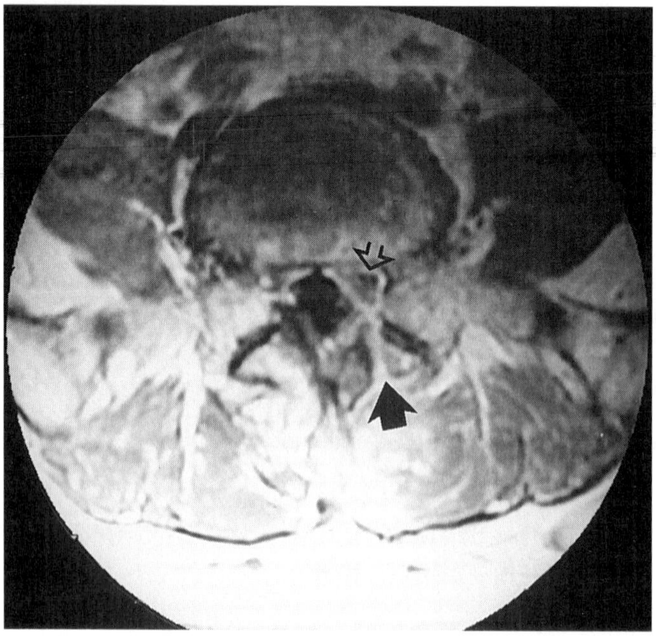

Figure 20.2 *A gadolinium-enhanced (T1) axial MRI showing a recurrent disc fragment surrounded by a high signal intensity arrow (open arrow). The heavy arrow points to the laminotomy defect made at surgery.*

34) Surgery done for soft indications in a poorly motivated patient has no chance for success. It is only natural for a surgeon to think that repeat surgery will help a FBS. There is little support for this position in the literature.(12, 34) In fact a second operation will make only 50% of the patients better and 20% worse. The third operation on a patient's back will make more patients worse rather than better.(34) There are very few indications for multiple back operations.

There are some conditions that are readily treated by further surgery:

1. Missed pathology and wrong level surgery.
2. A recurrent disc herniation.
3. The development of spinal canal stenosis at a previous discectomy level or above a fusion.
4. Postoperative conversion of a dominant radicular pain (disc excision) to a dominant back pain due to isolated disc resorption (6) (Fig. 20.3). If the disc degeneration is confined to one level, these patients can be helped by a lumbar fusion.
5. The occurrence of leg pain immediately after pedicle screw insertion with a CT scan showing the screw in the region of the nerve root.
6. Meningeal cyst causing leg pain.(25)

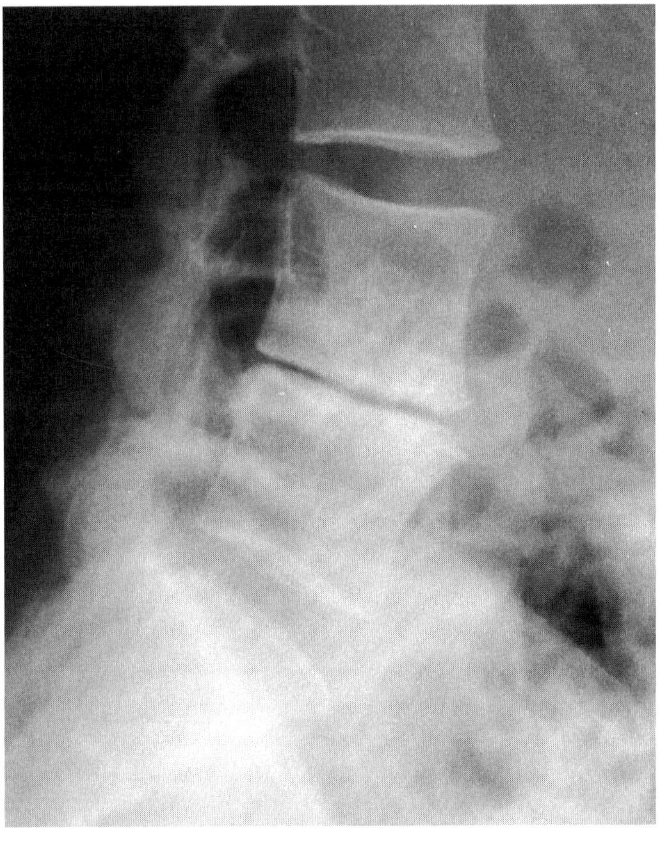

Figure 20.3 *An isolated disc resorption (postoperative) at L4–L5.*

There are some conditions that you cannot help with repeat surgery:

1. Scarring: either epidural or arachnoiditis.
2. Scarred root(s) from misplaced pedicle screws.
3. A pseudarthrosis that has had one attempt at revision surgery.

Above all, remember that a patient off work for more than one year is unlikely to return to work via a trip through the operating room. Accept when you encounter a patient with CLBP or FBS that the chronicity of the pain has changed many circuits in the neurological system. Simply concentrating on a suspected peripheral source to the pain is often not enough to relieve the patient's suffering.

Most patients with chronic low back pain and the failed spinal surgery syndrome are best treated conservatively.(15) Use of appropriate medications, transcutaneous electrical nerve stimulation units, spinal cord stimulation, trigger point injections, and so forth were discussed in Chapter 13. More sophisticated techniques of relaxation therapy and biofeedback regimens are often helpful and were also discussed in Chapter 13.

THE ROLE OF A CHRONIC PAIN CLINIC

Patients with CLBP and/or FBS are frustratingly difficult to treat. They are most often a mixture of physical and emotional disability with drug and vocational problems added. Few improve in any setting except a multidisciplinary pain diagnostic and management center.

The goals of such a clinic are to get the patient to take control of their problem. They have to understand through education that:

1. Their pain is not imagined and is real pain.
2. There is no cure, just relief from pain.
3. There is a difference between hurt and harm: the latter event is rare in its occurrence.
4. That increased physical activity will in turn improve the mental outlook and reduce the need for drugs.
5. Because their condition is chronic, there is a danger of drug dependency.
6. The goals of the program will not be met without family support. Equally important is a spouse who encourages self-reliance and is not over-supportive to the point of negating the advances of the team of therapists.
7. That personnel in the pain clinic will ignore pain behavior (eg, emergency calls for pain medication) and evidence by the patient of increasing self reliance will be rewarded.

THE ROLE OF LITIGATION IN CLBP

Anyone who doubts the ability of a continuing law suit or workmen's compensation claim to interfere with the goals of rehabilitation is not familiar with extensive literature in this field and is naive in an understanding of human nature. We all attend the "school of human survival" which conditions us to seek out means of support for ourselves and our families. If that support is potentially there through litigation or compensation, some patients will seek that survival route. Whether it is pursued at a conscious or subconscious level is unimportant. What will happen is the perseveration of symptoms and failure of treatment. All patients in these settings should be encouraged to seek an endpoint to litigation/compensation disputes. There are many barriers to patients earnestly and honestly seeking this course (Fig. 20.4).

FUNCTIONAL RESTORATION

A number of centers have developed a variant of the chronic pain center with Functional Restoration Programs. Mayer and co-workers (23, 24) have popularized this approach (Table 20.4), the basis of which is the significant level of deconditioning in most CLBP patients.

Their five-step program concentrates on accurately measuring the extent of deconditioning, followed by active exercises to recondition the patients. This exercise program is supervised by physical and occupational therapists and is designed to mobilize and strengthen the weakened back.(30) The final step in reconditioning is a work simulation effort ("whole body training") by the patient.

Equally important, and constituting 50% of the program time is an extensive effort to deal with the psychosocial aspects of the disability. The first step is detoxification of the patient heavily dependent on analgesics. These patients do need some medication support but this is closely supervised down to light analgesics and/or nonsteroidal anti-inflammatory drugs. Antidepressants are also useful as discussed in Chapter 13.

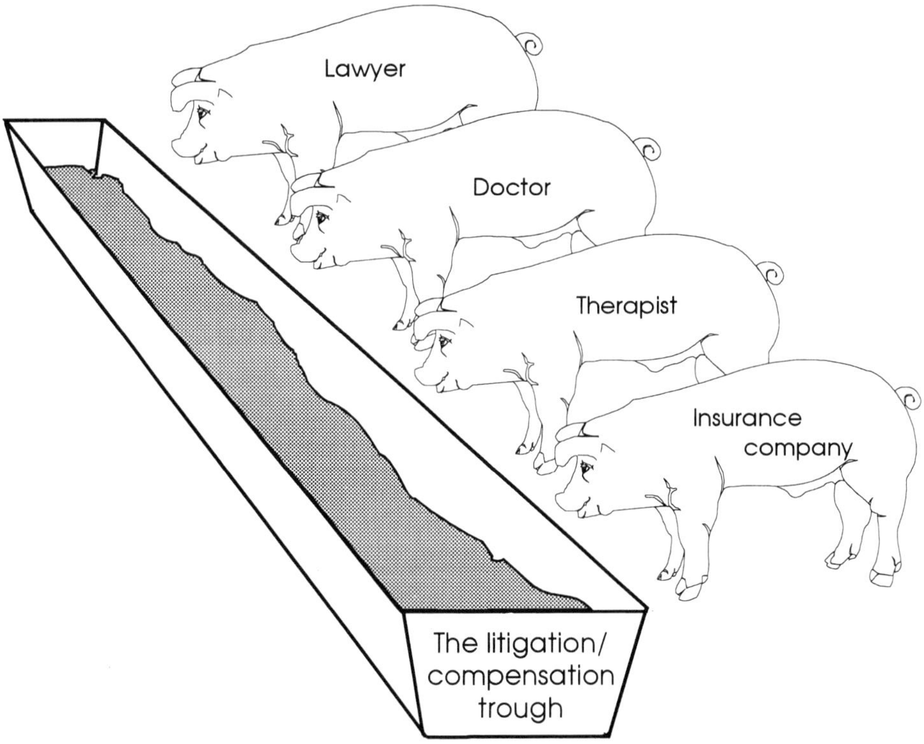

Figure 20.4 *The barriers to the termination of a claim are the many professionals who depend on keeping patients sick to maintain their professional income stream.*

Table 20.4. Critical Elements of a Functional Restoration Program[a]

Quantification of physical function and patient self-report
Physical reconditioning of the injured functional unit
Work simulation and whole-body retraining
Cognitive-behavioral multimodal disability management program
Ongoing outcome assessment using objective criteria

[a]Reprinted with permission from Mayer T, et al. Functional restoration. In: Hardy RW, ed. Lumbar Disc Disease. New York: Raven Press; 1993, pp 309–319.

The final step in functional restoration is vocational counseling and an active attempt to link the patient with suitable employment as the ultimate goal. With good outcome studies Mayer has shown a high level of success with this approach. Studies by Mayer (23) and Hazard (15) have shown an 80% maintenance of work effort 1 and 2 years after the completion of functional restoration.

Prevention of CLBP and FBS

The best approach to CLBP and FBS is simply not to let it happen. Prevention comes through early intervention of appropriate conservative care in the spine disabled patient. The best way to prevent failed spine surgery is not to operate. But if symptoms persist despite appropriate conservative care and the problem is clearly defined on MRI and confined to one spinal segment, surgery often delivers a good outcome. Multiple level surgical procedures for predominant back pain syndromes have a high rate of surgical failure and probably should be abandoned.

At all times the treating clinician needs a clear understanding of the psychosocial barriers to adequate treatment outcomes. Denying that litigation and workmen's compensation does not raise these barriers displays a lack of understanding of the weight of literature on the subject.

CONCLUSIONS

The best approach to the patient with CLBP is prevention. Early intervention in the spine injured patient with judicious conservative care and the avoidance of surgery, unless there is a clear-cut lesion on investigation to explain the patient's symptoms, are the foundation of this preventative efforts.

REFERENCES

1. Bertrand G. The "battered" root syndrome. Orthop Clin North Am 1975;6:305–310.
2. Boden SD, Wiesel SW. The multiple operated low back patient. In: Rothman RH, Simeone FA, eds. The Spine. WB Saunders; 1992, pp 1899–1905.
3. Bundschuh CV, Modic MT, Ross JS. Epidural fibrosis and recurrent disc herniations in the lumbar spine: MR imaging assessment. Am J Radiol 1988;150:923–932.

4. Burton CV, Kirkaldy-Willis WH, Yong-Hing K, Heithoff KB. Causes of failure of surgery on the lumbar spine. Clin Orthop 1981;157:191–199.
5. Byrd SE, Cohn ML, Biggers SL, et al. The radiographic evaluation of the symptomatic post-operative lumbar spine patient. Spine 1985;10:652–661.
6. Crock HV. Internal disc disruption: a challenge to disc prolapse fifty years on. Spine 1986; 11:650–653.
7. Dall BE, Rowe DE, Odette WG, Batts DH. Postoperative discitis: diagnosis and management. Clin Orthop 1987;224:138–148.
8. Delamarter RB, Ross JS, Marsaryk TJ, Modic MT, Bohlman HH. Diagnosis of lumbar arachnoiditis by magnetic resonance imaging. Spine 1990;15:304–310.
9. Finnegan WJ, Tenlin JM, Marvel JP, et al. Results of surgical intervention in the symptomatic multiply-operated back patient. J Bone Joint Surg 1979;61A:1077–1082.
10. Frymoyer JW. The role of spine fusion. Question 3. Spine 1981;6:284–290.
11. Frymoyer JW. Back pain and sciatica. N Engl J Med 1988;318:291–300.
12. Frymoyer JW, Matter RW, Hanley EN, Kuhlmann D, Howe J. Failed lumbar disc surgery requiring second operation: a long term follow-up study. Spine 1978;3:7–11.
13. Guyer DW, Wiltse LL, Eskay ML, Guyer BH. The long-range prognosis of arachnoiditis. Spine 1989;14:1332–1341.
14. Hanley EN Jr, Shapiro DE. The development of low-back pain after excision of a lumbar disc. J Bone Joint Surg 1989;71A:719–721.
15. Hazard RG, Fenwick JW, Kalisch SM, et al. Functional restoration with behavioral support: a one year prospective study of patients with chronic low-back pain. Spine 1989;14:157–161.
16. Hoyland JA, Freemont AJ, Denton J, Thomas AM, McMillan JJ, Jayson MIV. Retained surgical swab debris in post-laminectomy arachnoiditis and peridural fibrosis. J Bone Joint Surg 1988;70B:659–662.
17. Hueftle MG, Modic JM, Ross JS. Lumbar spine: post operative MR imaging with Gd-DTPA. Radiology 1988;167:817–824.
18. Johnsson KE, Redlund-Johnell I, Uden A, Willner S. Preoperative and postoperative instability in lumbar spinal stenosis. Spine 1989;14:591–593.
19. Johnsson KE, Willner S, Johnsson K. Postoperative instability after decompression for lumbar spinal stenosis. Spine 1986;11:107–110.
20. Langenskydd A, Kiviluoto O. Prevention of epidural scar formation after operations on the lumbar spine by means of free fat transplants. Clin Orthop 1976;115:92–95.
21. Long DM, Filtzer DL, BenDebba M, Hendler NH. Clinical features of the failed-back syndrome. J Neurosurg 1988;69:61–71.
22. Macnab I. Negative disc exploration: an analysis of the causes of nerve-root involvement in 68 patients. J Bone Joint Surg 1971;53A:891–903.
23. Mayer T, Gatchel R, Mayer H, et al. A prospective two-year study of functional restoration in industrial low back injury: an objective assessment procedure. JAMA 1987;258:1763–1767.
24. Mayer TG, et al. Objective assessment of spine function following industrial injury: a prospective study with comparison group and one-year follow-up. Spine 1985;10:482–493.
25. Miller PR, Elder FW, Jr. Meningeal pseudocysts (meningocele spurius) following laminectomy. J Bone Joint Surg 1968;50A:268–276.
26. Nachemson A. The lumbar spine, an orthopedic challenge. Spine 1976;1:59–71.
27. Quiles M, Marchisella PT, Tsairis P. Lumbar adhesive arachnoiditis: etiologic and pathologic aspects. Spine 1978;3:45–50.
28. Ross JS, Masaryk TJ, Modic MT, et al. Lumbar spine: postoperative assessment with surface-coil MR imaging. Radiology 1987;164:851–860.

29. Seres JL, Newman RI. Results of treatment of chronic low back pain at the Portland Pain Center. J Neurosurg 1976;45:32–36.
30. Sihvonen T, Herno A, Paljarvi L, Airaksinen O, Partanen J, Tapaninaho A. Local denervation atrophy of paraspinal muscles in postoperative failed back syndrome. Spine 1993;18:575–581.
31. Spengler DM, Freeman C, Westbrook R, Miller JW. Low-back pain following multiple lumbar spine procedures. Failure of initial selection. Spine 1980;5:356–360.
32. Spengler DM, Freeman DW. Patient selection for lumbar discectomy: an objective approach. Spine 1979;4:129–134.
33. Waddell G. Failures of disc surgery and repeat surgery. Acta Orthop Belg 1987;53:300–302.
34. Waddell G, Kummel EG, Lotto WN, Graham JD, Hall H, McCulloch JA. Failed lumbar disc surgery and repeat surgery following industrial injuries. J Bone Joint Surg 1979;61A:201–207.
35. Waddell G, McCulloch JA, Kummel E, Venner RM. Non-organic physical signs in low-back pain. Spine 1980;5:117–125.

21

Disability Assessment in Low Back Pain

"A physician is obligated to consider more than a diseased organ, more even than the whole man—he must view the man in his world."

— Harvey Cushing (1869–1939)

INTRODUCTION

As a practicing physician, you may be called on to participate in a disability assessment of a patient. Your involvement may come about because you are the treating doctor and require nothing more than to provide your office notes; other times you will be requested to submit a formal report on your patient, outlining your opinion as a diagnosis, the causation of the condition, treatment required, and the prognosis. Some doctors act as independent medical examiners (IME) with no responsibility for past or future treatment of the patient. As an "unbiased" observer they are asked to assess a patient, and file a report. Some doctors generate the majority of their income doing this work and all too often their "unbiased" position becomes compromised, and they become known as defense or insurance doctors; others develop biases in the opposite way and become known as plaintiff or claimant doctors. Some lawyers, representing the patient/client in this setting establish cozy relationships with these doctors, leading to many abuses in the system. The result is a wide variation in the opinion of the treating physician and the IME leading to adjudication, a make work project for all involved, and a drain on the limited financial resources. As a make-work project for many professionals, it more often than not leads to abuses to the patients/clients in workmen's compensation and motor vehicle accident claims.

In the United States, the systems that may require your input include the workmen's compensation system, private disability insurance, personal injury claims or the Social Security disability insurance. Other countries have variations of these systems, and in fact many of the social plans in America have been borrowed from European systems. Because we have limited knowledge of systems outside of the United States, we will confine our comments to the American scene.

Workmen's Compensation Claims

If a patient has suffered an injury on the job, he has a workmen's compensation claim. Covered under this claim will be costs for medical care, payment of some percentage of lost wages and awards for permanent disability. The workmen's compensation system varies from state to state in the United States, and from country to country in the world. Insurance premiums in the United States are determined by industry injury histories (the construction industry pays higher premiums per worker's wage than the less dangerous office workers' field). The premiums are paid by the employer to state agencies or private insurance carriers or, if the company is large enough they will be self-insured. The monies so collected are used to pay the workers' benefits and administer the system.

Private Disability Insurance

Many self-employed individuals will purchase disability insurance to cover any physical or emotional problem that prevents them from generating an income. Many companies provide this coverage for employees as part of their benefits package. To lessen the premium bite there is usually a long waiting period of 30, 60, 90, 120, or 365 days before the policy pays off. This is unlike workmen's compensation coverage, which kicks in immediately after injury and inability to work. It is rare that an IME is required for private disability insurance because the primary care doctor can usually provide the necessary medical intervention. In addition, the long-term medical problems that qualify for insurance, are usually clear diagnostic situations. The long waiting period between the onset of the disability and the payment of benefits serves as a significant deterrent to disability claims in this category.

Personal Injury Litigation

If an individual suffers an injury as the result of a motor vehicle accident or a slip and fall on someone else's property (the two most common settings), it is their right to sue the involved party for negligence. The two most common injuries are the neck injury suffered as the result of a rear-end motor vehicle collision, and a low back injury as the result of a slip and fall on a wet floor in a store. There is almost always a lawyer involved on behalf of the claimant/plaintiff, which more often than not, results in an opposing lawyer being hired by the defending insurance company. As the treating physician for the injuries suffered you may be asked for your office notes or a report. This is the most common setting for an IME by a so-called "unbiased" doctor.

Medical Malpractice

Medical malpractice is another form of personal injury litigation that is resolved in civil court. In this situation, a claimant is alleging that what a doctor did or did not provide in the way of diagnoses or treatment was incorrect and negligent, leading to harm to the patient and impairment of the patient's life-style.

Social Security Disability Insurance and Supplemental Security Income (SSI) Programs

These government programs pay individuals after a long period of absence from work and are designed as a social net for individuals not covered by any of the three previously mentioned insurance situations. Causation is not an issue in these assessments. What is needed is a clear diagnosis of the illness, and the likelihood that the illness is so severe that any substantial gainful employment will not be possible for at least 1 year. If the illness is likely to result in death, the claimant qualifies for SSI. All claimants in these systems must take a means test to demonstrate financial need, must have worked 5 years out of the past 10, and have been unemployed for 6 of the past 12 months. Payment for these disability awards is financed by payroll taxes. Claims against this system were rising rapidly in the mid to late eighties leading to a tightening of the criteria for awards. The result has been very few awards for patients disabled by low back pain, unless the patient has suffered a spine fracture with paraplegia, or has other medical problems associated, that add up to a significant long-term disability.

All of these situations are so different from the everyday practice of medicine. It takes a special kind of listening to a patient's collection of symptoms, a detailed physical examination and often extensive investigation to establish the diagnosis. Then there is the giving of a prognosis, the introduction of treatment and hopefully a resulting cure. For the common cold, a skiing injury or a myocardial infarct, these are fairly straightforward clinical situations, unencumbered by a patient trying to prove an illness for financial support. The added factor of insurance and secondary gain and the added players such as an insurance company, lawyer and / or workmen's compensation system can easily deflect an illness away from the Sydenham-established disease model of illness, that is, symptoms and signs that point to a diagnosis, which has attached to it a course of treatment, that hopefully will result in a cure. To prepare yourself for these disability assessments, you require a clear understanding of low back pain (Chapters 12 to 18), and be aware of the non-organic factors that can alter the patient's illness behavior (Chapter 12).

DEFINITIONS

Before going any further, it is essential that you understand some terms:

Impairment

Your involvement in the assessment of a patient for insurance claims purposes will require you to report only on physical impairment. What is the loss of physical function in quantifiable anatomic or physiologic terms? You will be further required to state if the impairment is temporary or permanent.

Disability

"Disability" is a legal and administrative term. With the doctor's impairment report, an administrative system and / or the courts will determine (rate) the overall disability. This system will consider a multitude of factors in addition to the physical impairment report including the emotional state of the claimant and other social factors such as training, education, job experience, and so forth. With this information, the administrative system will arrive at an estimate of the diminished capacity for everyday activities and work. This is the disability equation introduced in Chapter 12.

Whole Man

This term was coined many years ago before "political correctness" arrived on the scene. There was no attempt to exclude women from the process, but in today's world we best use the term "whole person."

A whole person is the sum of his/her anatomic parts. A lumbar spine is only part of a person and thus a low back disability can only be partial.

Acute vs Chronic Pain

Acute Pain

Acute pain rarely represents a dilemma in impairment ratings. Acutely painful conditions readily demonstrate a level of pain commensurate with the physical findings making impairment obvious. Usually an acutely painful condition will subside and not require an impairment rating.

Chronic Pain

If an acutely painful condition does not subside, obviously it becomes a chronic pain. The patient will participate in prolonged treatment and multiple assessments. If this occurs in a secondary gain situation, the patient will have to prove continuing pain and impairment, a difficult thing to do. How do you prove you have pain? How do you measure pain? There has been no scientifically valid method of measuring pain. Soon the chronic pain becomes a self-sustaining condition picking up the additional baggage of emotional distress, resentment toward the causation and other social implications. The condition becomes resistant to treatment, especially surgical intervention. With this background, you are asked to give a physical impairment rating!

Impairment Rating

A number of organizations have published manuals to assist in the standardization of impairment assessment. The most widely used of these is the American Medical Association Guides to the Evaluation of Permanent Impairment ("Guides"). Also, the American Academy of Orthopedic Surgeons publishes a manual for surgeons in evaluating permanent physical impairment. Other jurisdictions and organizations have produced additional guides, but despite of all these efforts, there is still a wide variation from doctor to doctor is assessing the percentage of impairment in the same patient. This raises serious questions about the process of impairment rating. This concern is further compounded by the administrative system that awards disability pensions based on these widely divergent impairment ratings, which they combine with other psychosocial and economic factors. Obviously, there is as much, if not more, politics and bias in the system as there is science. Scientists have tried to improve the system and have failed. Since this is the system you have to deal with, let us run through it and let us start with the simple task of the percentage impairment rating. Note that the "Guides" specifically exclude the rating of loss of function. That is the purpose of the adjudication system i.e. receive the impairment rating from the doctor and along with consideration of other psychosocial factors arrive at a (functional) disability rating which is converted to "dollars."

The Percentage Impairment Rating

The manual of the American Academy of Orthopedic Surgeons defines physical impairment as a purely medical condition. Permanent physical impairment is any anatomical or functional abnormality or loss after maximum medical rehabilitation has been achieved and which abnormality or loss the physician considers stable or non-progressive at the time the evaluation is made.

As a physician assessing a claimant, it is your job to provide a percentage rating of the permanent physical impairment and the loss of permanent physical function to help the administrators determine the depreciation of earning capacity and, in turn, the amount of the award.

In the end you are required to give your opinion of percentage impairment based on your own knowledge and experience. If you are using the American Medical Association guide, you will be considering the following four factors:

1. Range of motion of the lumbar spine.
2. Neurological impairment.
3. Diagnosis.
4. Psychological dysfunction.

Range of Motion (ROM)

Figures 21.1 to 21.4 show the recommended way of measuring lumbar ROM with an inclinometer. Note the use of the inclinometer for the quantification of straight leg raising (SLR). Table 21.1 shows how your measurements are applied to the lumbar spine so that you can arrive at a percentage impairment of that area.

Neurological Impairment

This is the most scientific of the impairment ratings because it is based on objective tests of reflex, sensory and motor loss. Table 21.2 shows the method of grading sensory loss.

The combination of a motor and a sensory loss to signify impairment of a single root are outlined in Table 21.3.

The next step is to evaluate the diagnosis, as shown in Table 21.4. This table shows a quick capsule summary of how a percent impairment of the whole person can be estimated and given a numerical value.

Unfortunately, the system is not as simple as we are leading you to believe. Assessing impairment is very complicated and beyond the scope of this book. For those interested in disability assessment you are referred to the "Guides" and other official organizations that have issued guidelines for impairment and disability rating. Grasping the system is very difficult and complex to the point that many doctors avoid getting involved at all in these assessments.

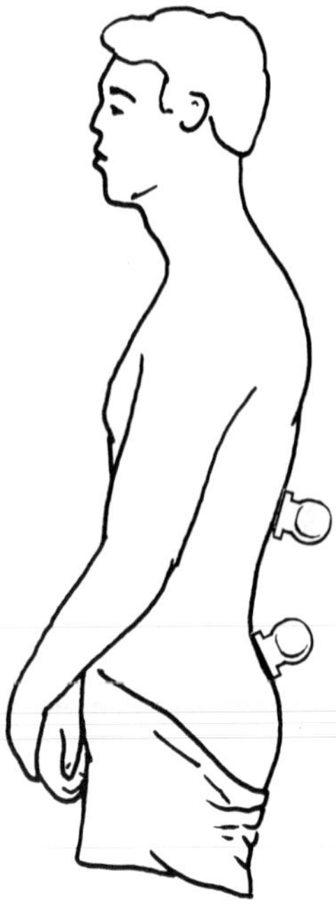

Figure 21.1 *In neutral, the inclinometer is set on both a T_{12} marking line and the sacrum: each time, the inclinometer is set at 0 degrees.*

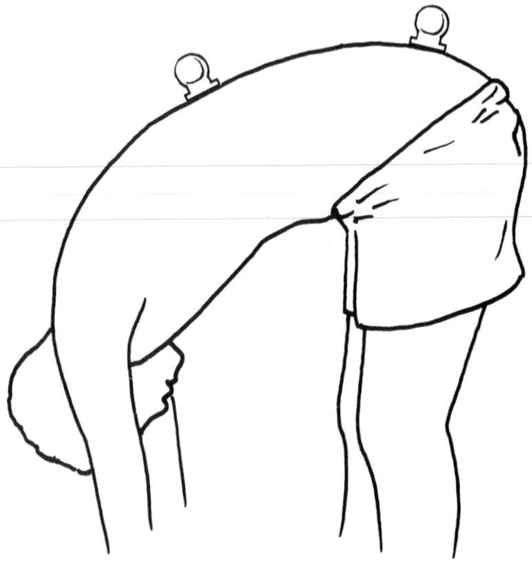

Figure 21.2 *After flexion, place the inclinometer again on the sacrum to record the flexion angle. Then, move the inclinometer to the T_{12} skin mark and record the lumbar flexion angle.*

The Workmen's Compensation System

In addition to impairment rating, there are other requirements of you when assessing a workers' compensation claimant. These include the following:

1. Determine causality.
2. Determine apportionment.
3. Decide if maximum medical improvement has occurred, that is, end of healing.
4. Decide if disability is temporary or permanent.
5. Provide a work capacity evaluation.

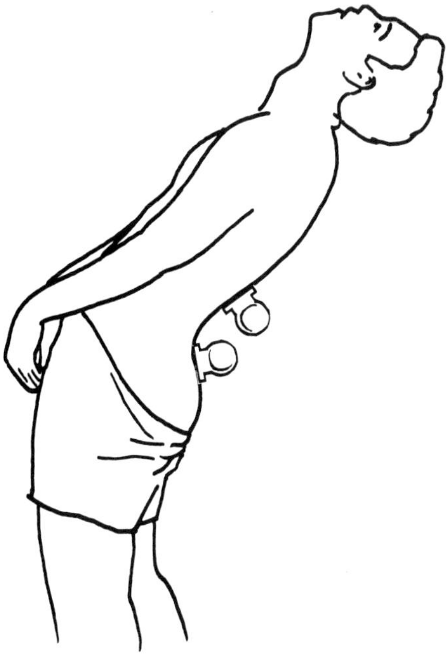

Figure 21.3 *After resetting the inclinometer, extension can be measured in the same fashion as flexion. It is prudent to repeat the measurements for flexion and extension a number of times to obtain valid measurement.*

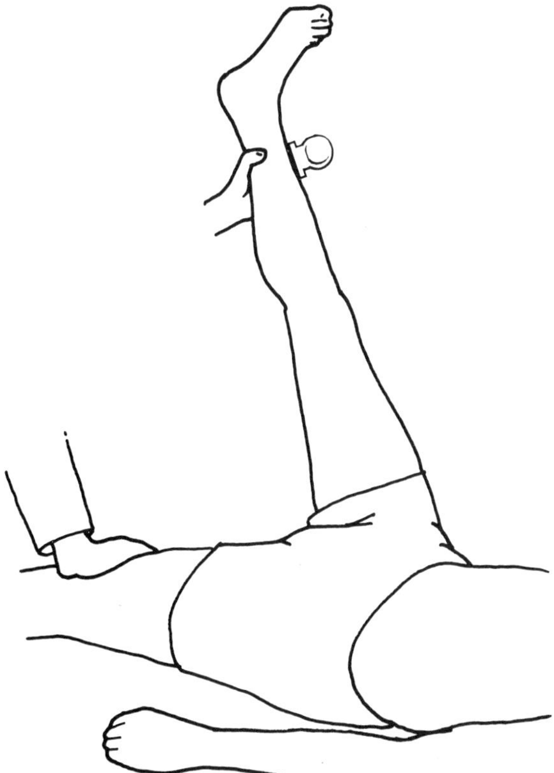

Figure 21.4 *The inclinometer can be used to measure straight leg raising.*

Table 21.1. Impairment Due to Abnormal Motion of the Lumbosacral Region: Flexion and Extension[ab]

Sacral (hip) flexion angle(°)	True lumbar spine flexion angle (°)		% Impairment of whole person
45°+	60°+		0
	45°		2
	30°		4
	15°		7
	0°		10
30–45	40+		4
	20		7
	0		10
0–29	30+		5
	15		8
	0		11
True lumbar spine extension from neutral position (0°) to:	**Degrees of lumbosacral spine motion**		
	Lost	**Retained**	
0°	25	0	7
10°	15	10	5
15°	10	15	3
20°	5	20	2
25°	0	25	0

[a]Use this table only if the sum of sacral (hip) flexion and sacral (hip) extension is within 15° of the straight leg raising test on the tighter side. From AMA Guides to the Evaluation of Permanent Impairment. Fourth Edition. The Musculoskeletal System. Chicago: American Medical Association. 1993; Chapter 3, p 128.
[b]The proportion of flexion and extension of total lumbosacral motion is 75%

Determine Causality

What is the relationship between the claimants condition and the work accident? For the young healthy claimant who has a sudden lifting incident at work that produces immediate back pain, the problem is simple. There is a direct relationship between the diagnosis and the accident. For the claimant who accumulates multiple small traumas and eventually fits in to allow back disability, the problem is much more difficult.

It is important to understand that workmen's compensation systems are "no-fault." Unless there is gross negligence on the part of the employer, the only determination of causality centers around the relationship of the medical condition to an incident or accident that occurred while working.

Determine Apportionment

This is a very difficult area of assessment that asks you to deal with pre-existing conditions versus current injury. The classic example is the young man, with an undiagnosed asymptomatic isthmic spondylolisthesis, discovered on radiograph, after he suffers a lifting injury at work that results in back pain.

The American Medical Association (3) has determined that the physician should have a substantive basis for apportionment and indicated it can be of five types:

Table 21.2. Sensory Loss in an Extremity Resulting from Spinal Disease or Injury: Grading Scheme and Procedure for Determination*

Grading Scheme

Description	Grade (%)
1. No loss of sensation, or no spontaneous abnormal sensations	0
2. Decreased sensation with or without pain, which is forgotten during activity	5–25
3. Decreased sensation with or without pain, which interferes with activity	30–60
4. Decreased sensation with or without pain, which may prevent activity (minor causalgia)	65–80
5. Decreased sensation with severe pain, which may use outcries as well as prevent activity (major causalgia)	85–95
6. Decreased sensation with pain, which may prevent all activity	100

Procedure

1. Identify the area of involvement, using the dermatome chart.
2. Identify the nerve(s) that innovate the area(s).
3. Find the value for maximum loss of function of the nerve(s) due to pain or loss of sensation or pain, using the appropriate table.
4. Grade the degree of decreased sensation or pain according to the preceding grading scheme.
5. Multiply the value of the nerve (from the appropriate table) by the degree of decreased sensation or pain.

Reprinted with permission from Engelberg AL, ed. Guides to the Evaluation of Permanent Impairment. Chicago: American Medical Association; 1993.

Table 21.3. Impaired Nerve Function of Lower Extremity Measured by Sensory and Motor Criteria[a]

Nerve root impaired	Maximum % loss of function due to sensory deficit, pain, or discomfort	Maximum % loss of function due to loss of strength	% impairment of lower extremity[b]
L3	5	20	0–24
L4	5	34	0–37
L5	5	37	0–40
S1	5	20	0–24

[a]Reprinted with permission from Engelberg AL, ed. Guides to the Evaluation of Permanent Impairment. Chicago: American Medical Association; 1993.
[b]Conversion tables (not shown) allow lower extremity impairment to be estimated for the whole person.

1. An occupational disorder aggravated by a supervening non-occupational disorder.
2. An occupational disorder aggravated by a supervening other occupational condition arising out of and in the course of employment by the same employer.
3. An occupational disorder aggravated by a supervening other industrial condition arising out of and in the course of employment by a different employer.
4. An occupational disorder aggravated by a pre-existing non-occupational condition.
5. An occupational disorder aggravating a pre-existing non-occupational condition.

Table 21.4. Diagnostic Related Estimates: Lumbosacral Spine Impairment Categories

DRE impairment category	Description	% impairment of the whole person
I	No complaints or symptoms	0
II	Minor impairment: clinical signs of lumbar injury are present without radiculopathy or loss of motion segment integrity	5
III	Radiculopathy: evidence of radiculopathy is present	10
IV	Loss of motion segment integrity; criteria for this condition are described in Section 3.3b, p 95 of Guides to the Evaluation of Permanent Impairment. Fourth Edition. American Medical Association; 1993.	20
V	Radiculopathy and loss of motion segment integrity	25
VI	Cauda equina-like syndrome *without* bowel or bladder impairment	40
VII	Cauda equina syndrome *with* bowel or bladder impairment	60
VIII	Paraplegia	75

Maximum Medical Treatment

To meet this requirement, you must look into the biological crystal ball and decide if the patient will improve further with time and/or treatment or whether the patient is on a plateau of recovery and will not improve further. If the latter is the case, the patient is deemed, by your opinion, to have reached maximum medical improvement (MMI).

Determine if Disability is Temporary or Permanent

Under most workmen's compensation statutes, disability is divided into three periods:

1. Temporary total disability: is that period in which the injured person is totally unable to work. During this time the patient is almost always on treatment and has not reached MMI.
2. Permanent partial disability: is that period after maximum medical improvement has been reached and the claimant may be considered for some kind of gainful occupation. A pension decision is also made at this time based on your impairment rating.
3. Permanent total disability: is that period after maximum medical improvement has been reached and the claimant cannot be expected to return to any gainful employment. These are extreme situations such as loss of sight in both eyes, amputation of both legs or both arms, or paraplegia/quadriplegia. Obviously, this becomes a time for a pension award.

Work Capacity Evaluation

If the patient has reached maximum medical improvement and is ready to return to work you will often be asked to fill out a functional capacities form (Table 21.5) You will see on this form examples of physical job requirements for which you are to provide two answers:

Table 21.5. Estimated Functional Capacities Form

Policy No. ________________Claim No. ________________

Please complete the following items based on your clinical evaluation of ________________________________.
Any item that you do not believe you can answer should be marked N/A.

In an 8-hour workday, the patient can: (Circle full capacity for each activity)

									Continuously	With Rests
Sit	1	2	3	4	5	6	7	8(h)	_______	_______
Stand	1	2	3	4	5	6	7	8(h)	_______	_______
Walk	1	2	3	4	5	6	7	8(h)	_______	_______

	Never	Occasionally 0 to 33%	Frequently 34 to 66%	Continuously 67 to 100%
Lift				
10 lb	_______	_______	_______	_______
11–20 lb	_______	_______	_______	_______
21–50 lb	_______	_______	_______	_______
51–100 lb	_______	_______	_______	_______
Carry				
10 lb	_______	_______	_______	_______
11–20 lb	_______	_______	_______	_______
21–50 lb	_______	_______	_______	_______
51–100 lb	_______	_______	_______	_______
Bend	_______	_______	_______	_______
Squat	_______	_______	_______	_______
Crawl	_______	_______	_______	_______
Climb	_______	_______	_______	_______
Reach above shoulder level	_______	_______	_______	_______

Patient can use hands for repetitive actions such as:

	Simple grasping	Pushing & Pulling	Fine Manipulating
Right	Yes______No______	Yes______No______	Yes______No______
Left	Yes______No______	Yes______No______	Yes______No______

Patient can use feet for repetitive movements, as in operating foot controls:

Right	Left	Both
Yes______No______	Yes______No______	Yes______No______

Restriction of activities involving:

	None	Mild	Moderate	Total
Unprotected heights	_______	_______	_______	_______
Being around moving machinery	_______	_______	_______	_______
Exposure to marked changes in temperature and humidity	_______	_______	_______	_______
Driving automotive equipment	_______	_______	_______	_______
Exposure to dust, fumes, & gases	_______	_______	_______	_______

Can patient now work? ________________________________

Part-time: (h/d) ________________________________

Full-time: (yes) ________________________________

Disability Rating________________%

Date________________Physician ________________________________

Please put additional comments on other side

1. Can the worker do this job?
2. If so, for what percent of a normal work day can the worker do that particular activity?

Because most physicians have little knowledge of a work setting, this exercise is arbitrary and potentially full of error.

In response, more sophisticated evaluation systems, such as muscle testing, have been developed. To date, there is no scientific evidence that these systems are any better than your guesswork on a work capacity evaluation.

YOUR LEGAL RESPONSIBILITY

Once you agree to look after an injured worker or provide an IME in a workmen's compensation or personal injury case, you are obligated to provide a report of your findings and your opinions. If there is substantial agreement between all medical examiners in the case, the administrative system is ready to draw a conclusion as to disability and award. This is known as settling out of court and is almost always the case in workmen's compensation claims and usually the case in personal injury claims. If there is not common ground between medical examiners (eg, one examiner finds no physical impairments, and another describes a significant disability), then the difference has to be resolved by adjudication. This adjudication system involves legal council to the parties involved (claimant/plaintiff vs insurance/defendant). This in turn may require you to testify as to your opinions and be cross-examined by opposing council. Your appearance may be by deposition (written or video) or an actual court appearance.

Deposition

At your convenience, the two lawyers involved in the case will request to sit down with you and, under oath, question you about your opinion. These meetings are usually at the end of a long office day, which makes you vulnerable to tough questions. Most orthopedic surgeons and neurosurgeons arrange to do this in their office; the setting may be an oral examination only or an oral examination recorded on videotape for future presentation if and when a trial occurs.

The advantage of this setting is that council can follow a set of written questions and if any surprises appear, council has time to prepare for rebuttal before trial. The advantage for you as a doctor is the convenience of arranging a time that disrupts your practice the least. The disadvantage of deposition testimony is that they are more easily arranged than court testimony, which lawyers may use against each other i.e. you become the foil. Another disadvantage is in the fact there is no judge present to rule on procedures and objections. Despite these problems, the majority of doctors who are required to participate in these disputes do so through depositions.

Court Appearance

You or legal council may decide that your testimony as to your opinion is best provided in a court room. For the uninitiated doctor this can present an unnerving experience. It should not be. Remember that the court considers you an expert witness who can testify as to fact as well as add your opinion regarding interpretation of facts. Very few witnesses are allowed that status, which makes you an important player in the administrative decision. The court will treat you courteously and with deference, provided you abide by the authority and rules of the court.

To best serve as an expert witness, the following recommendations are made:

1. You are an independent expert witness (not a factual witness) and can render an opinion based on your medical expertise (knowledge, experience, and judgment).
2. You are an independent professional and not an advocate for the defense or the plaintiff.
3. Do not lose your temper and/or argue with the lawyer asking questions.
4. Dress like a professional. Act like a professional (eg, stand still in the witness stand). Speak like a professional (slowly and audibly). Maintain eye contact with the judge and jury.
5. KISS (Keep It Simple, Stupid!) Avoid medical terms (jargon) that the court may not understand.
6. If you do not understand a question, ask that it be repeated. If you are asked to answer "yes" or "no" to a question and do not feel that you can do so, state the reason and ask permission to answer the question in the manner you deam appropriate.

In the end, the two opposing lawyers will have brought out all the evidence, for or against the claimant, so that a jury of six citizen peers can decide on whether or not a financial award is to be made, and what amount that award should be.

CONCLUSIONS

When you consider that 80% of the population will experience low back pain sometime in their life, that each year 2 to 5% of adults will seek treatment or lose time from work because of low back pain, you realize how significant an issue LBP is in our society. Some of these individuals will become disabled and require long-term support and/or a disability decision.

To cope with this, we have developed a specialty interest in the condition. We have spine surgeons and physicians; we have clinics dedicated to low back pain; we have therapists specializing in low back pain. Low back pain has become an industry unto itself in medicine. With all this high energy and intellect dedicated to the problem you would expect improved results. Just the opposite! As the number of specialists in the field has increased, so has the incidence of long-term low back disability. Why?

One reason for our failure is the fact that we are dealing with the symptom of pain. It is very subjective, and its report by the patient is not only influenced by the exciting pathology, but also the patient's emotions, beliefs, and attitudes. The assessment of this multivariate set of factors requires a skill seldom found in one individual.

Second, subjective low back pain is not always associated with objective physical findings. If some physical findings are present, such as a loss in ROM, which of the 19 joints within the lumbar spine is the source?

Third, what is the relationship between pain, physical impairment, and disability?

It is a hopelessly complex equation that requires the patient's input, the doctor's assessment, and the interpretation of the administrative/legal system. When we consider the high level of intellectual energy involved, we should be able to conclude that we have a fail-safe system. Instead, we have a failed system of disability assessment that is unscientific, loaded with special interests, generates wonderful fees for the participants, but more often than not dehumanizes and demoralizes the legitimate claimant and rewards the fraudulent claimant. If ever a situation calls out for reform, it is the American way of handling low back pain and the disabilities that may become associated with it.

REFERENCES

1. American Academy of Orthopaedic Surgeons Manual for Orthopaedic Surgeons in Evaluating Permanent Impairment. Chicago; 1966.
2. Disability Evaluation under Social Security. A Handbook for Physicians. Washington, DC: US Department of Health, Education and Welfare; 1979.
3. Engelberg AL, ed. Guides to the Evaluation of Permanent Impairment. Chicago: American Medical Association; 1993.

22

Low Back Pain in Special Situations: Pregnancy; Children; Sports Medicine

"Specialized knowledge will do a man no harm if he also has common sense, but if he lacks this, it can only make him more dangerous to his patients."

— Oliver Wendell Holmes (1809–1894)

LOW BACK PAIN IN PREGNANCY

Introduction

Pregnancy exacts its toll on the female body including the low back. It is estimated that 50% of women who are pregnant will experience low back pain at some time during the pregnancy.(28, 33) In Sweden, low back pain is the most common cause of sick leave during pregnancy with 70% of pregnant women averaging 9 weeks of sick leave.(30) The problem is more prevalent in Caucasians than Hispanics and is more common and more severe in multiparous women.(28) It does not appear to be more frequent in women who are overweight, who gain excessive weight during pregnancy or who carry heavy babies.

Mechanisms

There are two major factors that lead to the increased incidence of low back pain in pregnancy:

1. The presence of a fetus in the pelvis, anterior to the lumbar spine, increases lumbar lordosis, and decreases the support of the abdominal muscles.(23) Along with the weight of the baby, this increases the biomechanical stresses on the lumbar spine, increasing the discomfort.
2. The hormone relaxin,(22) decreases collagen stiffness in the pelvic support ligaments, allowing for increased mobility and, in the end, widening of the symphysis pubis and sacroiliac joints.

Clinical Presentation

There are three potential diagnostic groupings (13, 23) to consider when the pregnant patient presents with low back pain:

1. Low back pain from mechanical strain on the lumbar spine. This may be associated with referred leg pain (see Chapter 14). The problem rarely presents before 5 months and surprisingly often starts to improve toward the end of pregnancy.
2. Any pregnant woman can be afflicted with any of the hundreds of conditions mentioned in Chapter 18 on differential diagnosis. Pain of onset in the first trimester will fall into this classification. A disc rupture with sciatica is one of those diagnoses.(11, 20) Fortunately, it is rare in pregnancy.
3. Sacroiliac (SI) joint pain, which is located low and laterally over the SI joints. Sometimes, there is associated referred anterior thigh pain (Table 22.1). The pain is more severe and more disabling than the mechanical low back strain. Also, the pain will persist through the end of pregnancy. A few women will continue with severe disabling pain in the immediate postpartum period that may take a few months to go away.(29)

Examination of patients in the first two groups will be no different than that described in Chapter 10. Patients with SI joint insufficiency need special tests for SI joint function (Fig. 22.1).

INVESTIGATION

It is reasonable to carry out routine blood tests to be sure there is no sinister cause for the back pain. Radiographs should not be done in the first trimester and probably should not be ordered at any time during the pregnancy unless absolutely indicated. Although MRI is not recommended during pregnancy, there are a few reports in the literature that describe MRIs done during pregnancy with no adverse effects.(24, 37) No other investigations are indicated for mechanical low back pain or SI joint dysfunction. If you are dealing with a low back problem that has serious consequences for the mother, then no limitations should be placed on investigation. The authors cannot recall such a situation in many years of practice.

Table 22.1. SI Joint Dysfunction in Pregnancy

- A history of time- and weight-bearing–related pain in the posterior pelvis, deep in the gluteal area
- A pain drawing with well-defined markings of stabbing in the buttocks distal and lateral to the L5–S1 area, with or without radiation to the posterior thigh or knee, but not into the foot
- A positive "posterior pelvic pain provocation test"
- Free movements in the hips and spine and no nerve root syndrome
- Pain when turning in bed

Reprinted with permission from Östgaard HC, et al. Reduction of back and posterior pelvic pain in pregnancy. Spine 1994; 19:894–900.

TREATMENT

The mainstay of treatment includes the invocation of the various forms of rest, graded according to the severity of the pain. Severe low back pain obviously requires complete bed rest. Most often, the mechanical low back pain patient can be supported by a maternity corset, and patients with SI joint pain can be supported with a belt that cinches the pelvis rather than supports the abdomen.

A physical therapist is of particular help to these patients with regard to instructions for activities of daily living, that is, do not wear high heel shoes; avoid certain lifting positions; and ways to sit, stand, and rest (the semi-Fowler position, Fig. 22.2).

Medication should be used sparingly and only on the approval of the obstetrician.(3) For pain relief, use acetaminophen and avoid acetylsalicylic acid and nonsteroidal anti-inflammatory drugs (NSAIDs). Methocarbamol as a muscle relaxant appears to be safe.

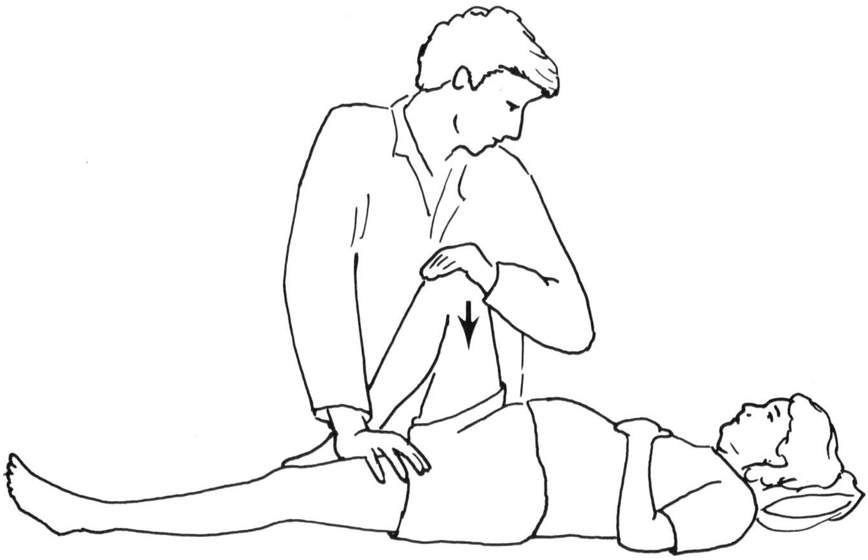

Figure 22.1 *With the hip flexed to 90 degrees, downward pressure (arrow) is applied to the femur. This stress on the sacroiliac joint will produce pain in an unstable sacroiliac joint.*

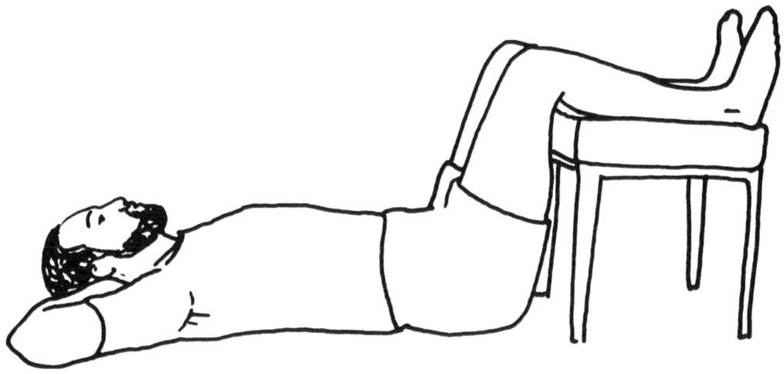

Figure 22.2 *This is a great way for a patient to assume the semi-Fowler position.*

Limited modalities can be used. There is no indication for manipulation of the pregnant woman's spine.

The appearance of low back pain in a pregnancy should rarely constitute an indication for abortion.

Patients with SI joint dysfunction have the most pain and are most resistant to treatment efforts. They require alot of support and not alot of aggressive therapy with admonitions to "do more." This latter course often leads to immense frustration on the part of the mother.

Occasionally, a patient will present with severe sciatica, unresponsive to prolonged periods of bed rest, or rarer still a pregnant patient may present with a cauda equina syndrome. It is possible to operate on these patients under local anesthetic with extensive patient and fetal monitoring to remove the offending disc rupture.

DELIVERY

We take the position that the method of delivery and the anesthetic used should not be affected by the low back problem, unless the patient has an obviously symptomatic disc rupture. In these very rare situations, pushing during delivery could worsen the disc rupture or severely increase the sciatica. In this case, a cesarean section is a good choice for delivery. It is extremely rare that this approach will result in any harm to the baby or to the mother's low back.

After delivery, it is best to wait 6 weeks before taking any steps to investigate or add aggressive treatment steps to the regimen. By this time, most mechanical low back problems will have settle spontaneously. Mothers who are breast feeding need to continue their limited use of medication.

PREVENTION

The lumbosacral mechanical syndromes can be lessened in severity with an exercise program instituted before pregnancy and into the first trimester.(30) Exercises can be continued into the second and third trimesters but become less effective in controlling symptoms.

There is little one can do to prevent SI joint dysfunction.

PROGNOSIS

Unfortunately, the occurrence of back pain during one pregnancy usually means the earlier onset of more severe back pain during subsequent pregnancies.(28) These are not episodes that are harmful to the patient and hopefully can be lessened by the treatment measures previously mentioned.

LOW BACK PAIN IN CHILDREN

Introduction

Low back pain in adults is second only to the common cold as a disabling symptom; more than 80% of adults, at some time in their lives, will have an episode of low back pain. Low back pain in children is a rare complaint (4, 14); it is as unusual a complaint in children as it is usual in adults. With its rarity as a complaint in children, it often is an elusive and delayed diagnosis.

Added to the problem is the fact that children play down their symptoms (so they can keep playing with their buddies), give a vague or no history (the very young), and are brought in by parents who may easily play down changes in posture and gait. It is easy to understand why the cause of low back pain in children has the potential for going undiagnosed for many months.

Differential Diagnosis

Children do not degenerate (physically!); the many degenerative conditions listed in Chapter 18, on the differential diagnosis of low back pain do not apply to children. The differential diagnosis of low back pain is best thought of in six broad categories (36) (Table 22.2) and two age groups, young and old (Table 22.3).

Table 22.2. Differential Diagnosis of Low Back Pain in Children

1. Mechanical Causes
   - Postural
   - Muscular
   - Overuse
   - Trauma
   - Herniated nucleus pulposus
2. Developmental
   - Spondylolysis/spondylolisthesis
   - Scheuermann's disease
   - Scoliosis (secondary)
3. Inflammatory
   - Discitis
   - Infection (osteomyelitis/discitis)
   - Collagen/vascular disorders (juvenile rheumatoid arthritis)
   - Inflammation (SI joints)
   - Disc calcification
4. Neoplasms
   - Spinal canal
   - Vertebral column
   - Retroperitoneal
5. Tethered Cord
6. Psychogenic

Table 22.3. Diagnosis by Age in Children

Less than 10 years of age
- Infection
- Tumor
- Psychogenic

More than 10 years of age
- Spondylolysis/spondylolisthesis
- Scheuermann's disease
- Overuse and postural
- Herniated nucleus pulposus
- Tumor/infection
- Neurological: spinal dysraphism

Mechanical Disorders

Postural/Muscular Disorders

Children do the most darned things and muscular strain of the low back may be the outcome. Simply putting in time with these children will allow for resolution of their symptoms: so they can continue to do the darnedest things!

Overuse Syndromes

Children, trying to improve performance, may push their backs to muscle fatigue. (2) The mild, diffuse backache is handled by taking the patient out of their sport for a few days of rest. The quick resolution of symptoms can then be followed by a gradual aerobic, muscle strengthening and sport specific rehabilitation program.(25)

Trauma

A child's spine is very flexible, which explains why fractures and associated injuries are rare. The two most common outcomes of trauma to a child's spine are:

1. Spondylolysis.
2. Slipped vertebral apophysis.

Spondylolysis This is the most common diagnosis made for the cause of back pain following trauma to the young spine. The topic was covered in Chapter 5.

Slipped Vertebral Apophysis: Posterior Vertebral Rim Fracture This is a variant of the disc rupture and occurs exclusively in the young spine (7, 9) (Fig. 22.3). The usual disc involved is L4–L5 (the inferior ring apophysis of L4) and the usual cause is a traumatic event that loads the disc to the point of fracturing the rim apophysis.

The ring epiphysis appears at 6 years, ossifies by the 13th year, and fuses to the vertebra body at approximately 17 years. Most of these patients will present between the ages of 13 to 17 years with a history of sudden injury in contact sports or activities such as weight lifting. Their clinical presentation will be no different than a disc rupture that causes sciatica. The diagnosis will become evident on computed tomography (CT) or magnetic resonance imaging (MRI). If their sciatica is very symptomatic, it is unlikely that conservative care will lead to resolution of symptoms, and more likely disc and ring apophysis excision will be needed.

Herniated Nucleus Pulposus

The young patient with a disc rupture is an unusual patient.(10, 19) It is usual for the majority of these patients to go undiagnosed for many months because of the absence of back pain. Their dominant buttock and thigh pain is often labeled "hamstring spasm."

There is little clue as to the cause of the disc rupture except the children are often very athletic and come from families with a high incidence of back troubles. The diagnosis is made on the basis of dominant extremity pain (Fig. 22.4) and usually significant straight leg raising reduction. There is often no neurological change detected on extremity examination.

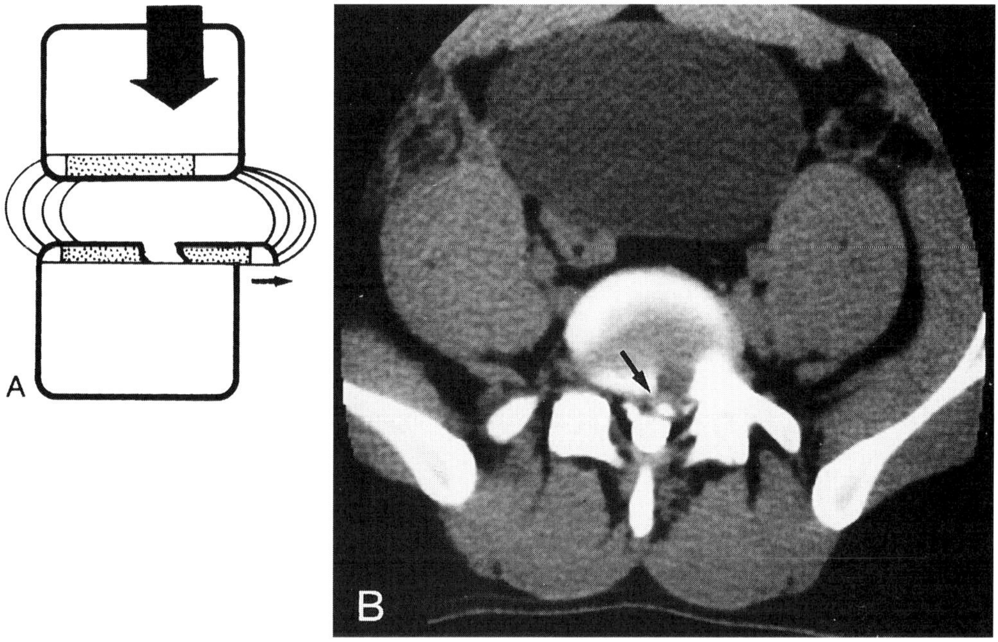

Figure 22.3 *An injury to the ring apophysis* **(A)** *will result in a cartilage component* **(B, arrow)** *to a disc rupture; this injury almost always is confined to the adolescent age group.*

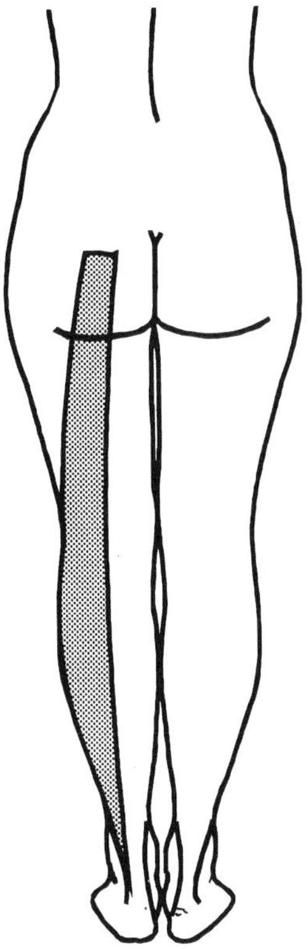

Figure 22.4 *Children rarely have back pain as part of their history: all their pain is located in the leg and more often than not does not radiate below the knee, that is, hamstring spasm.*

The diagnosis is made on MRI, which most often will show multiple levels of disc degeneration in addition to the single-level disc rupture (Fig. 22.5). As with apophyseal rim fracture, if the sciatica presents as a significant symptom (the usual presentation), conservative care is of limited value, and most children will require surgical intervention.(6, 8) We recommend chemonucleolysis (21) in the adolescent disc herniation for reasons that were discussed in Chapter 15.

Developmental

Spondylolysis/Spondylolisthesis

See Chapter 5 for a discussion of these related diagnoses.

Scheuermann's Disease

Although this condition may affect the lumbar spine (Fig. 22.6), it's effects are more likely to fall on the thoracic spine and cause kyphosis (4) (Fig. 22.7). Because of endplate growth disturbances, wedging of the vertebral bodies occurs, leading to the kyphosis. Associated changes include disc space narrowing and the formation of Schmorl's nodes. Three contiguous disc

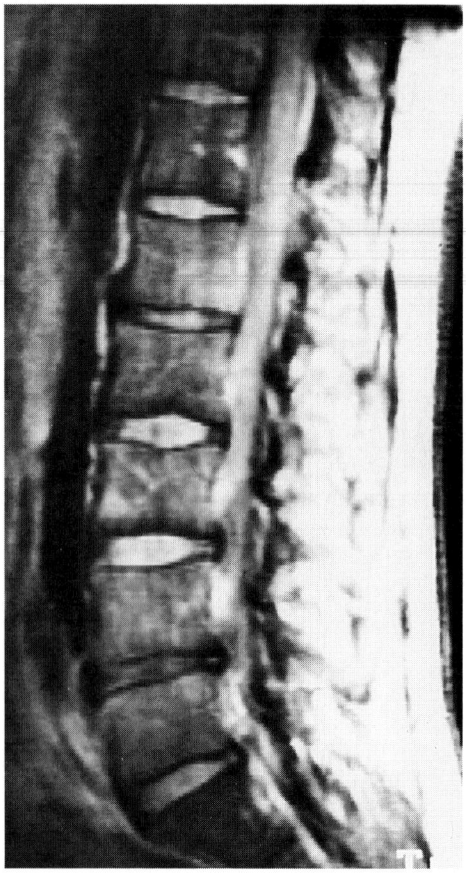

Figure 22.5 *T2 sagittal MRI in a young patient with a herniated nucleus pulposus at L4–L5 but degenerative changes at multiple levels.*

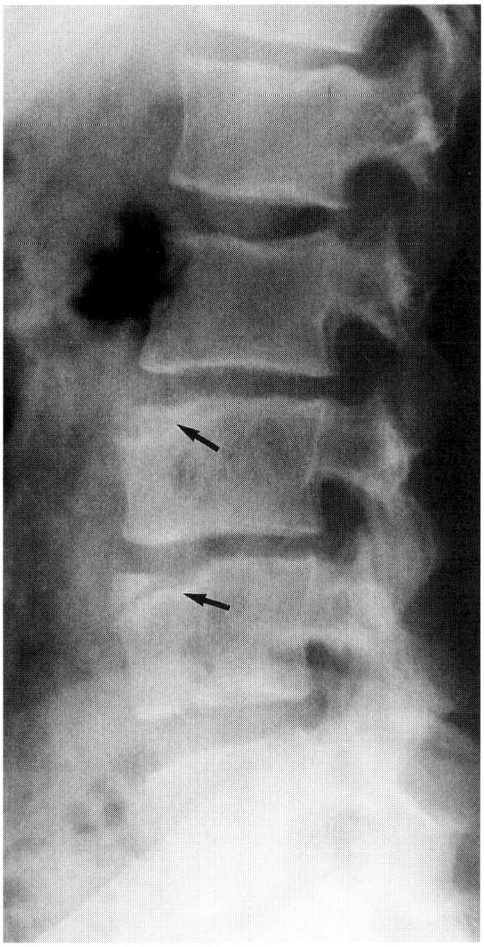

Figure 22.6 *A two-level epiphysitis (arrows) in the lumbar spine with a "limbus" lesion at L4; this is not a true Scheuermann's lesion by definition.*

spaces have to be affected for the diagnosis to be made. The outcome is chronic grumbling backache and often, in the long run, a round back or kyphotic deformity (Fig. 22.7).

The cause is thought to be microfractures falling on weakened endplates. The endplates may be weakened through alterations in the blood supply as growth speeds up. The condition is very common, and the symptoms disappear when the skeleton matures. Most patients end up with little deformity, but occasionally a patient will present with significant deformity that requires surgical correction. During the symptomatic phase, NSAIDs and activity restriction are the mainstays of treatment. If it appears that a kyphotic deformity is developing, bracing will be required until growth is completed.

Scoliosis

Idiopathic, congenital, neuropathic, or myopathic scoliotic patients usually do not have back pain. Anything other than a painless right thoracic or left lumbar curve should alert the clinician to the possibility of an underlying tumor or infection. Other red flags in the scoliotic patient include short segment curves, rapid acceleration of the deformity, and/or neurological symptoms/signs.

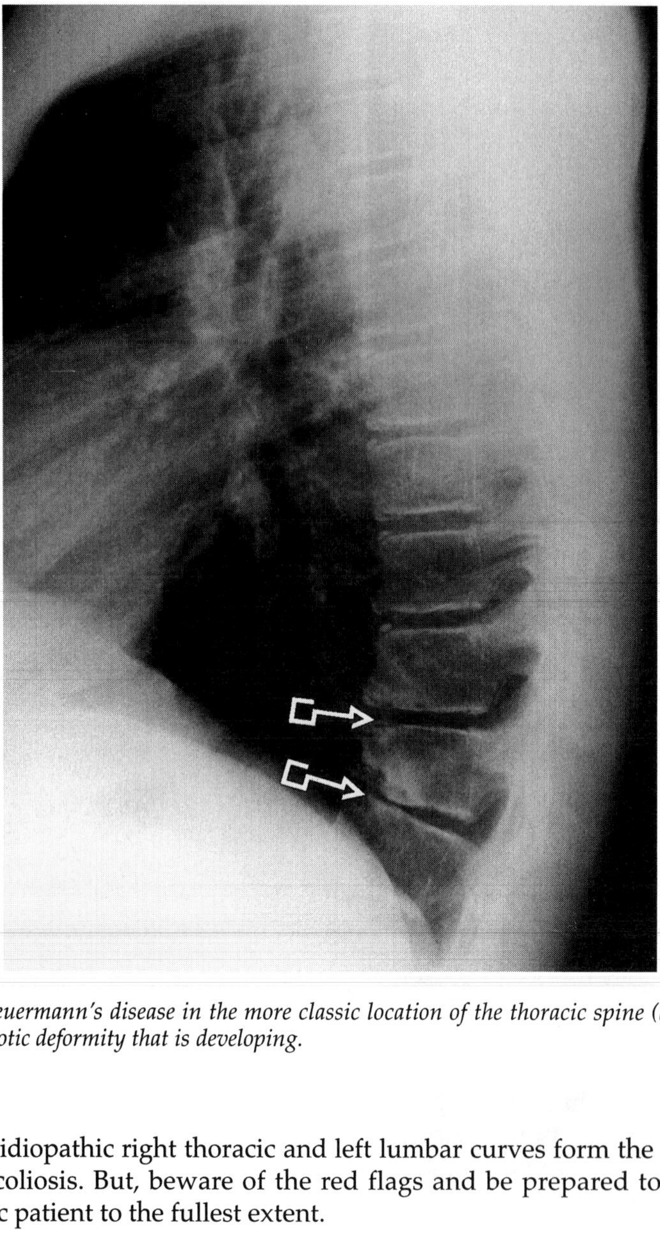

Figure 22.7 *Scheuermann's disease in the more classic location of the thoracic spine (arrows). Notice the round back or kyphotic deformity that is developing.*

The painless idiopathic right thoracic and left lumbar curves form the vast majority of patients with scoliosis. But, beware of the red flags and be prepared to investigate the atypical scoliotic patient to the fullest extent.

Infectious/Inflammatory

Discitis

This may be one of the most elusive diagnoses to pin down in the pediatric population. It is most common in the 2- to 6-year-old patient because the disc space is still vascularized by an arterial/venous system that perforates the endplates.(27, 38) After 6 years, these vessels regress and the disc becomes an avascular structure. Before 6 years of age, these vessels may deposit bacteria in the disc cavity 2 to 4 weeks after a remote infection such as pharyngitis.

The young child presents with a sudden change in function , that is, withdrawal from activities and lack of desire to walk, both rather nonspecific symptoms. The older the child, the more apparent it will be that the change in function is due to back pain. Some patients will present with abdominal pain, which is apt to deflect the clinician away from consideration of discitis.

Fever may or may not be present and the pulse will be rapid. Physical examination will reveal a back in spasm, that is, no ROM allowed, and a scoliosis and/or palpable muscle spasm. Leg symptoms and signs (neurological changes) are routinely absent. Straight leg raising is often reduced because anything that moves tissue in the area of the discitis will produce back pain.

Investigation Plain radiographs are initially negative, but within 2 to 4 weeks they will show disc space narrowing and endplate "fuzziness" (Fig. 22.8) at the levels most often affected (T12–L1, L4–L5, L5–S1). The bone scan will be positive immediately and weeks before the plain radiographic changes (Fig. 22.9) (38).

The only consistently abnormal laboratory test is an elevated erythrocyte sedimenatation rate (ESR). The white blood cell count (WBCC) is often equivocal. Attempts to culture an organism (source/throat swab, site/biopsy, and serum/blood culture) are fruitless in more than 50% of cases.

The standard for diagnosis is quickly becoming the MRI (Fig. 22.10).(34)

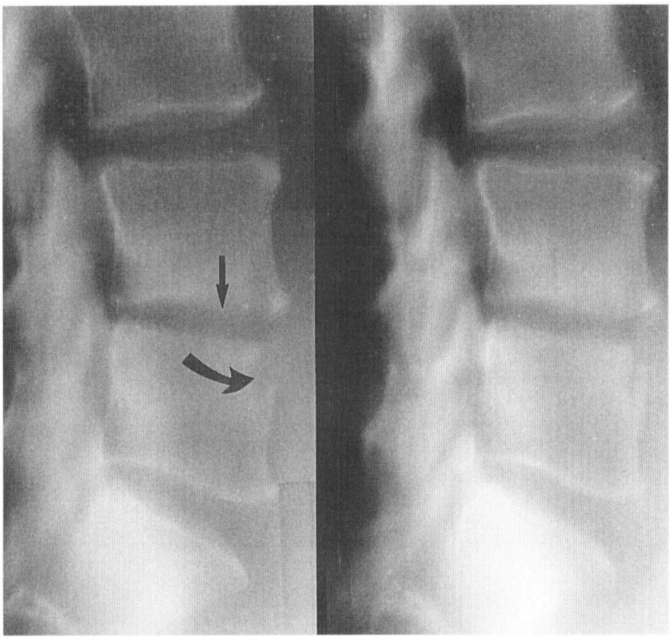

Figure 22.8 *Adjacent tomographic cuts showing disc space narrowing at L4–L5, fuzziness of the endplates (straight arrow), and "kissing" defects at the anterior aspect of the vertebral bodies (curved arrow); obviously, this condition is more than a benign discitis.*

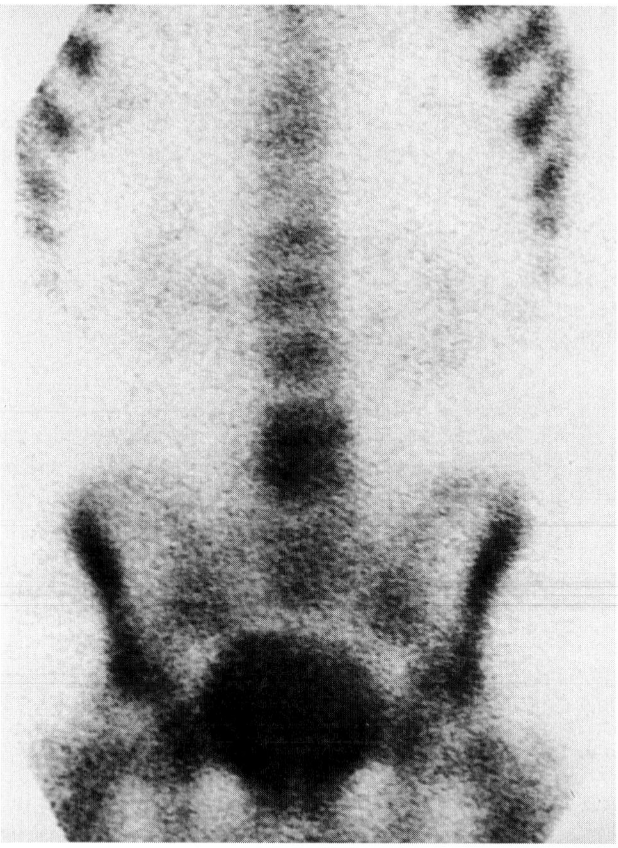

Figure 22.9 *A bone scan in an L4–L5 discitis.*

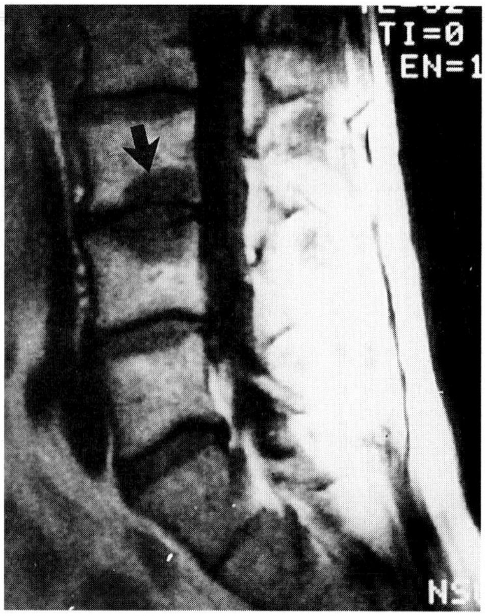

Figure 22.10 *An MRI (T1 sagittal) in an early discitis in a young patient. The decreased signal intensity (blackness—arrow) on either side of the disc space represents edema (remember, water is darker than fat on T1).*

Treatment Discitis is, by and large, a benign condition that has led many authors to recommend (5, 38): (1) avoiding a biopsy of the disc space, (2) bed rest for a number of weeks, and (3) the avoidance of antibiotics. This is a difficult treatment position for you, as the attending physician, to take. In the face of a negative blood culture and a normal WBCC in a pediatric patient with back pain and an elevated ESR and a positive bone scan or MRI, it is hard to accept that your patient will arrive at a successful outcome without the use of antibiotics.

Osteomyelitis

Vertebral osteomyelitis is a completely different story from discitis in the pediatric population. The topic was well covered in Chapter 4. It presents a serious risk of abscess formation, neurological compression and spinal deformity in the undiagnosed or untreated patient.(38)

This patient is older, sometimes immunocompromised, but is always very sick with fever, elevated ESR and WBCC and a positive culture of the infected vertebrae.

The appearance of the bone scan will not be too much different from that of discitis, but MRI or CT scan will show bony erosions (Fig. 22.11).

If the diagnosis is made early, both before abscess formation and neurological compression has occurred and without the threat of pending spinal deformity, conservative treatment (bed rest and antibiotics) may save the day. Abscess formation, neurological compression, pending or actual deformity, and failed antibiotic therapy constitute the indications for surgical intervention. It is routine that in this patient population the anterior approach be used.

Inflammatory/Spondyloarthropathies

These are very rare causes of back pain in the child. Juvenile ankylosing spondylitis is the most common condition, with a prevalence of approximately 30/100,000. Back

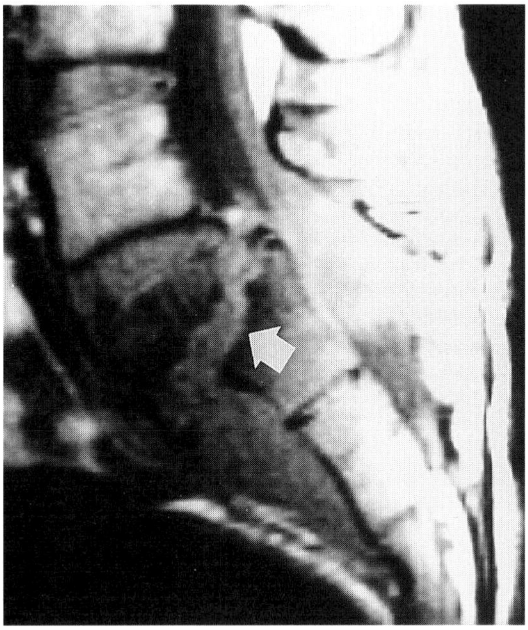

Figure 22.11 *An MRI (T1 sagittal) in a young diabetic with a severe erosive lesion (osteomyelitis) at L5–S1 (arrow).*

pain is usually well down the list of concerns in these patients but does occur. Its management is passively attached to the treatment of the other manifestations of the arthropathy.

Intervertebral Disc Calcification

This is predominantly a condition of the cervical rather than the lumbar spine (Fig. 22.12). It does occur in the lumbar spine and can cause pain and stiffness.(32) It is a perfectly benign condition and should not lead you to overreact. Most lesions will spontaneously disappear, but a few will persist into adulthood as benign observations on lumbar spine radiograph.(26)

Neoplasms

Bone and neurogenic tumors in the pediatric population are fortunately rare. The patients present with back pain, most often complain of pain at night and will all have positive CT scans or MR imaging. Their diagnosis and management was covered in Chapter 4.

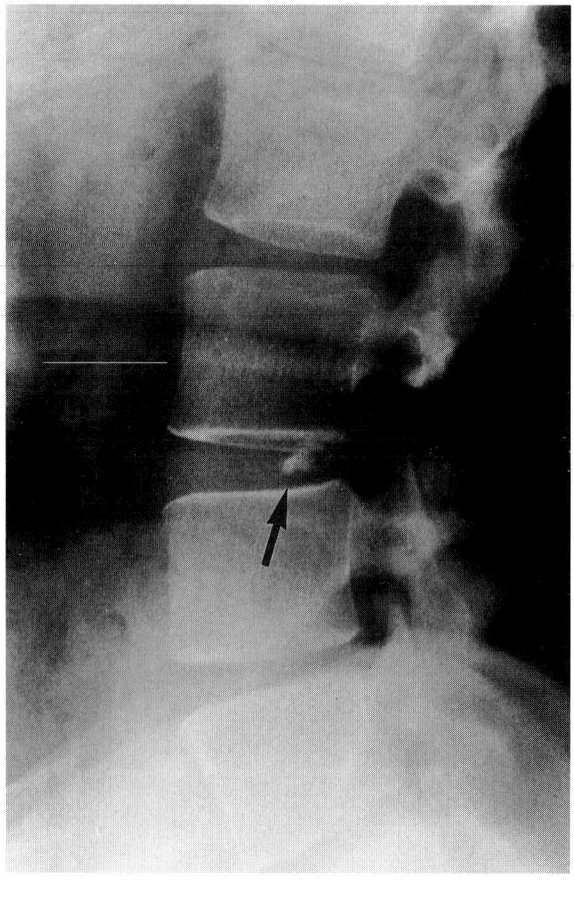

Figure 22.12 *A small amount of intervertebral disc calcification at L3–L4 (arrow).*

The Tethered Cord

Tethering (anchoring) of the end of the spinal cord to the sacrum will result in failure of ascent of the cord to its natural position at L1–L2. The tethering prevents ascent of the cord as the spine grows and may cause back pain.

The cause may be simply a thick, nonpliable filum terminale but diastematomyelia, lipomas and dermoid need to be ruled out. All patients will have a spina bifida on radiograph (Fig. 22.13).(31)

The majority of the patients who are symptomatic have back pain and a mild scoliosis. Most often, neurological signs (weakness/sensory loss) may be present but are often missed early in the deformity. With growth and stretching of the cord cavus feet, equinus deformities and shortening of one leg may appear.

The diagnosis is made on MRI (Fig. 22.14).(1, 31, 35) Mild cases of tethered cord with few or no symptoms require no treatment intervention. Patients with progression of the sciatica, masses in the spinal canal, or progressive neurological deficit require surgery to untether the cord and remove any abnormal mass. The surgery is best done as early in life as possible; waiting will only complicate things.

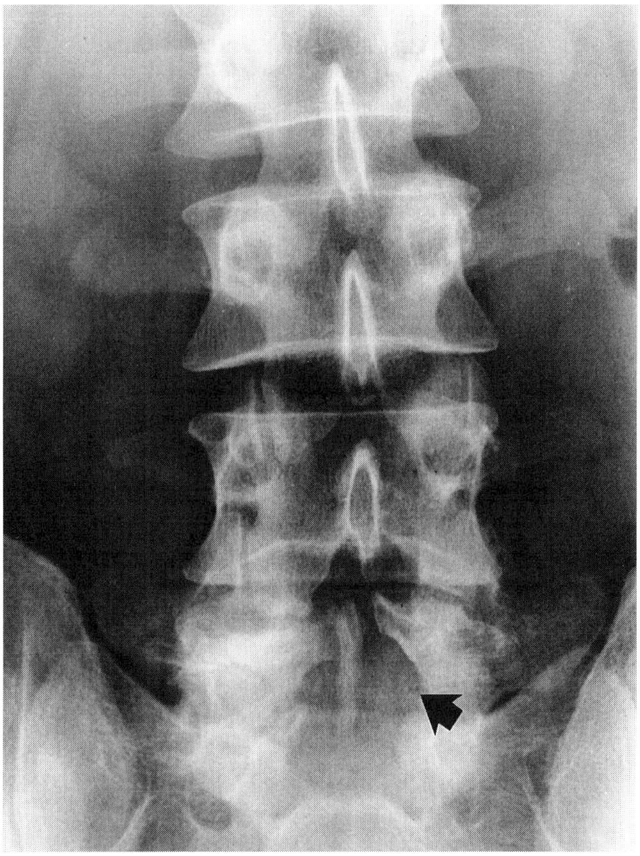

Figure 22.13 *A rather large spina bifida (arrow) of L5 and S1 that may signify some unusual pathology in the thecal sac.*

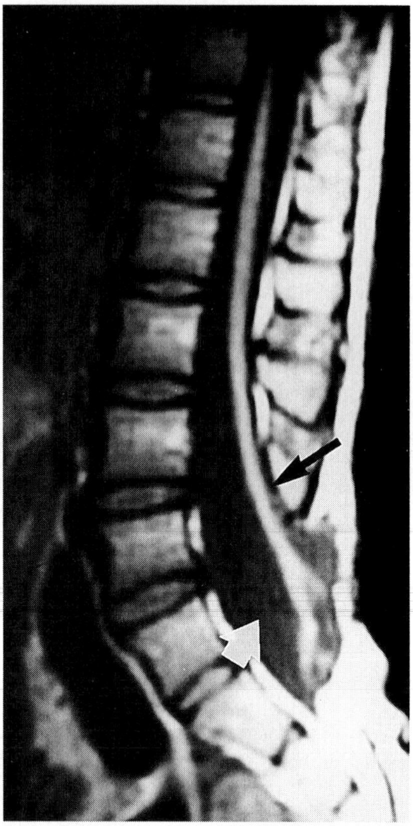

Figure 22.14 *A tethered cord (black arrow) and a large common dural sac (white arrow) bulging into a spina bifida defect at L5 and S1.*

Psychogenic Back Pain

This is a rare entity in the children. Before labeling a back pain "psychogenic" be sure you have pulled out all stops to rule out underlying infections, inflammations, and tumors.

Conditions of No Clinical Significance

Inconsequential conditions that almost do not merit description but that do appear on radiographic reports are:

Spina bifida occulta (Fig. 22.15).
Schmorl's node (Fig. 22.16).
Limbus vertebra (Fig. 22.17).
Single vertebral body epiphysitis (Fig. 22.6).

LOW BACK PAIN IN SPORTS MEDICINE

Introduction

Sport has achieved new meaning in society in the past two decades. High-performance and weekend athletes of all ages are pushing their bodies to new heights of performance,

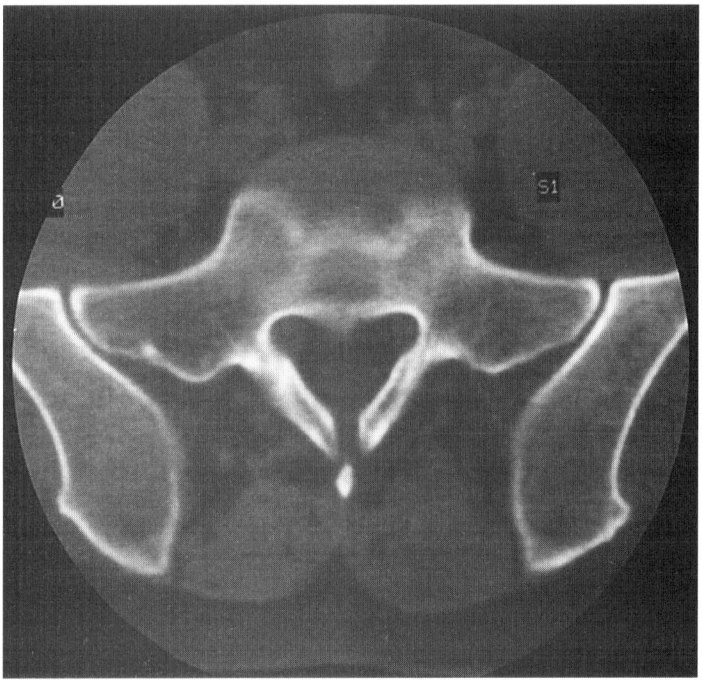

Figure 22.15 *A benign spina bifida of S1 on axial CT.*

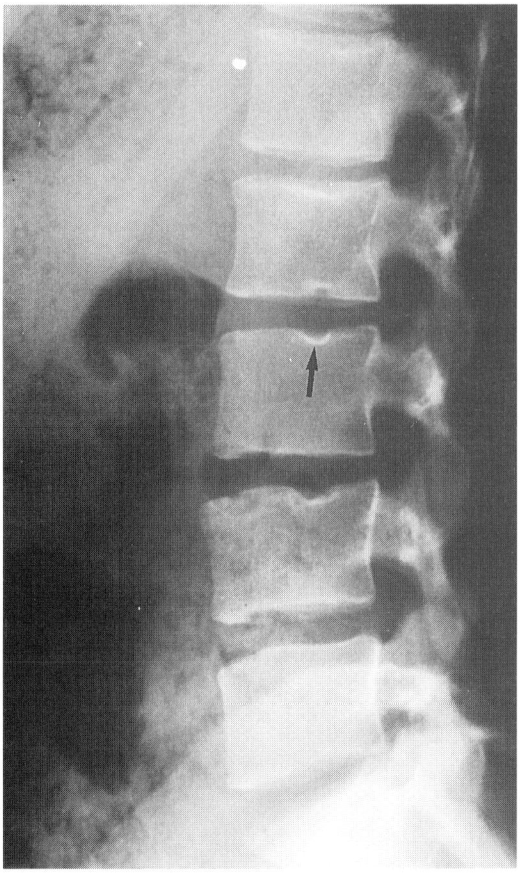

Figure 22.16 *There are multiple Schmorl's nodes (arrow) and almost an appearance of Scheuermann's epiphysitis, which are still insignificant findings in a young patient with minor low back pain.*

which results in a dramatic increase in injuries.(12) The low back has not been spared from the onslaught.

Fortunately, most sport-related injuries to the low back are soft tissue in nature and self-limiting with regard to duration of symptoms. More severe injuries such as fractures can occur to the spinal column and its neurological contents, an event much more common in the cervical spine.

Sport-specific injuries can be more structural (bone and nerve tissue) in their effect and are summarized in Table 22.4. All these structural lesions are no different in presentation, evaluation, and treatment from that described in previous chapters, and readers are referred to these sections for a complete description.

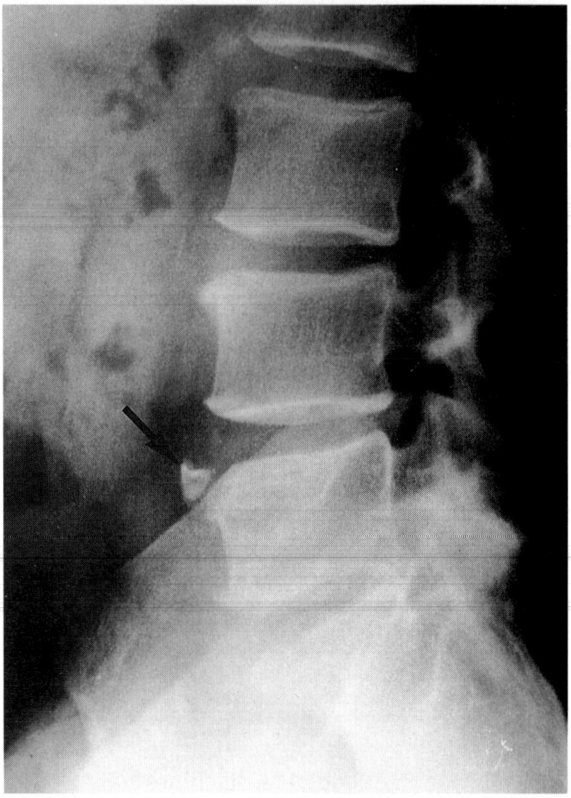

Figure 22.17 *A limbus vertebrae, not a fracture (arrow).*

Table 22.4. Sport-Specific Structural Lesions

Sport	Structural Lesion
Gymnastics (15, 18), football (linemen), ballet, weight lifting, polevaulting, hurdling	Spondylolysis
Golf	Facet joint
Water skiing (17)	DDD at TL junction
Basketball, Football, Wrestling	DDD lumbar

Key: DDD = Degenerative disk disease; TL = thoracolumbar.

Principles of Treatment

The treatment of the sport-injured patient requires alot of patience on the part of the physician or therapist. Often, multiple parties need to be treated (Table 22.5).

Above all, be conservative. Aggressive surgical treatment applied to an athlete often ends a career. Be conservative in the prescription of pain and mood-altering drugs. Athletes, by definition, are deeply committed to exercise, and that should become the foundation of all treatment programs. For the more acutely debilitating injuries, one or two days of bed rest may be needed at the onset of symptoms, but very quickly the patient should progress to an exercise program. Whether or not modalities (especially ice) are used as an introduction to the exercise effort is left up to the discretion of the therapist. Manipulation is useful to reduce axial pain early in treatment but should give way early to the exercise effort.(16) Obviously, in the early days of treatment, the inciting sport needs to be avoided unless the injury is a minor soft-tissue lesion that will respond to aggressive exercise. Avoid the use of braces and exotics such as acupuncture and transcutaneous electrical nerve stimulation units.

The high-performance athlete quickly becomes deconditioned and needs to start on aerobic fitness within days of injury. This is best accomplished with walking exercises, especially in a swimming pool. Graduated aerobics are biking and cross-country ski machines. The impact of running may set the athlete back if started too soon in the rehabilitation program.

The early goal is to maintain flexibility and strength, and these exercises should be introduced as soon as feasible. If they can be accomplished without increasing pain, then dynamic resistive sport-specific flexibility and strengthening exercises are started. The final stage of rehabilitation is the pursuit of endurance exercises.

Along the way, spend time with the parent, trainers, and coaches to educate them on the nature of the injury, the anticipated rehabilitation time, and a program for the return to sport.

Prevention of Sport Injury to the Spine

Tremendous progress in prevention of serious injury to the cervical spine has been made in sports such as football by redesigning equipment and banning head tackling. Fortunately, these injuries are rare in the lumbar spine.

Fancy isokinetic testing machines have been used to assess the athlete and spot weaknesses in low back function. To date, these machines have not worked out.(2)

Table 22.5. An Overview of the Sport-Injured Back

Age of Athletes	Nature of Injury	Parties to be Treated
Young	Soft tissue	Patient
Middle-aged	Skeletal	Parents
Older	Neurological	Coach
		Owner
		Colleagues

Conclusion

The sport-injured back is a challenge, usually managed by nonsurgical methods. The early intervention with surgery often has an adverse effect on the high-performance athlete. If there is a clear-cut lesion, such as a disc herniation, a prescribed treatment program should not exceed 6 weeks before failure is decided and surgery performed. All other structural lesions are treated conservatively, especially those requiring fusion, for example, spondylolisthesis. It is the rare high-performance athlete that returns to acceptable performance standards after a lumbar fusion.

REFERENCES

1. Altman NR, Altman DH. MR imaging of spinal dysraphism. Am J Neuroradiol 1987;8:655–658.
2. Beimborn DS, Morrissey MC. A review of the literature related to trunk muscle performance. Spine 1988;13:655–660.
3. Briggs GG, Freeman RK, Yaffee SJ. Drugs in Pregnancy and Lactation: A Reference Guide to Fetal and Neonatal Risk. Ed. 3. Baltimore: Williams and Wilkins; 1990.
4. Bunnell WP. Back pain in children. Orthop Clin North Am 1982;13:587–604.
5. Curd JG, Thorne RP. Diagnosis and management of lumbar disc disease. Hosp Pract 1989; 15:135–148.
6. DeOrion JK, Bianco JA. Lumbar disc excision in children and adolescents. J Bone Joint Surg 1982;64(7):991–996.
7. Dietemann J, Runge M, Badoz A, et al. Radiology of posterior lumbar apophyseal ring fractures: report of 13 cases. Neuroradiology 1988;30:337–344.
8. Ebersold MJ, Quast LM, Bianco AJ Jr. Results of lumbar discectomy in the pediatric patient. J Neurosurg 1987;67:643–647.
9. Ehni G, Scheider J. Posterior lumbar vertebral rim fracture and associated disc protrusion in adolescence. J Neurosurg 1988;68:912–916.
10. Epstein JA, Epstein N, Marc J. Lumbar intervertebral disk herniation in teenage children: recognition and management of associated anomalies. Spine 1984;9:427–431.
11. Epstein JA, Benton J, Browder J, Lavine LS, Rosenthal AH, Warren R. Treatment of low back pain and sciatic syndromes during pregnancy. New York State J Med 1959;59:1757–1768.
12. Farfan HF. The effects of torsion on the intervertebral joints. Can J Surg 1969;12:336.
13. Fast A, Shapiro D, Ducommun EJ, et al. Low back pain in pregnancy. Spine 1987;12:368–371.
14. Garrido E, Humphreys RP, Hendrick EB, Hoffman HJ. Lumbar disc disease in children. Neurosurgery 1978;2:22–26.
15. Goldstein JD, Berger PE, Windler GE, et al. Spine injuries in gymnasts and swimmers: an epidemiologic investigation. Am J Sports Med 1991;19:463–468.
16. Haldeman S. Spinal manipulative therapy in sports medicine. Clin Sports Med 1988;7:277–287.
17. Horne J, Cockshott WP, Shannon HS. Spinal column damage from water ski jumping. Skeletal Radiology 1987;16:612–614.
18. Jackson DW, Wiltse LL, Cirincione RJ. Spondylolysis in the female gymnast. Clin Orthop 1976;117:68–73.
19. Kurihara A, Kataoka O. Lumbar disc herniation in children and adolescents. Spine 1989;5: 443–451.
20. LaBan MM, Perrin JC, Latimer FR. Pregnancy and the herniated lumbar disc. Arch Phys Med and Rehab 1983;64:319–321.

21. Lorenz M, McCulloch J. Chemonucleolysis for herniated nucleus pulposus in adolescents. J Bone Joint Surg 1988;67(A):1402–1404.
22. MacLennan AH, Nicolson R, Green RC, Bath M. Serum relaxin and pelvic pain of pregnancy. Lancet 1986;2:243–245.
23. Mantle MJ, Greenwood RM, Currey HL. Backache in pregnancy. Rheumatol and Rehab 1977; 16:95–101.
24. Mattison DR, Angtuaco T, Miller FC, Quirk JG. Magnetic resonance imaging in maternal and fetal medicine. J Perinatol 1989;9:411–419.
25. Maxwell C, Spiegal A. The rehabilitaion of athletes following spinal injuries. The Spine in Sports. Philadelphia: Hanley and Belfus; 1990, pp 281–292.
26. McGregor JC, Butler P. Disc calcification in childhood: computed tomographic and magnetic resonance imaging appearances. Br J Radiol 1986;59:180–182.
27. Menelaus MB. Discitis: An inflammation affecting the intervertebral discs in children. J Bone Joint Surg 1964;46(B):16–23.
28. Ostgaard HC, Andersson GB. Previous back pain and risk of developing back pain in a future pregnancy. Spine 1991;16:432–436.
29. Ostgaard HC, Andersson GBJ. Postpartum low-back pain. Spine 1991;17:53–55.
30. Ostgaard HC, Zetherstrom G, Roos-Hansson E, Svanberg B. Reduction of back and posterior pelvic pain in pregnancy. Spine 1994;19:894–900.
31. Raghaven N, Barkovich AJ, Edwards M, et al. MR imaging in the tethered spinal cord syndrome: am J Roentgenol 1989;152:843–852.
32. Sonnabend DH, Taylor TKF, Chapman GK. Intervertebral disc calcification syndromes in children. J Bone Joint Surg 1982;64B:25–31.
33. Svenson H, Andersson GBJ, Hagstad A, Jansson P. The relationship of low-back pain to pregnancy and gynecologic factors. Spine 1990;15:371–375.
34. Szalay EA, Green NE, Heller RM. Magnetic resonance imaging in the diagnosis of childhood discitis. J Pediatr Orthop 1987;7:164–167.
35. Szalay EA, Roach JW, Smith H, et al. Magnetic resonance imaging of the spinal cord in spinal dysraphisms. J Pediatr Orthop 1987;7:164–167.
36. Turner PG, Green JH, Galasko CSB. Back pain in childhood. Spine 1989;14:812–814.
37. Weinreb JC, Wolbarsht LB, Cohen JM, Brown CE, Maravilla KR. Prevalence of lumbosacral intervertebral disk abnormalities on MR images in pregnant and asymptomatic nonpregnant women. Radiology 1989;170:125–128.
38. Wenger DR, Bobechko WP, Gilday DJ. The spectrum of intervertebral disc space infection in children. J Bone Joint Surg 1978;60(A):100–108.

Index

page numbers in *italics* denote figures; those followed by *t* denote tables